Lovell and Winter's
Pediatric Orthopaedics

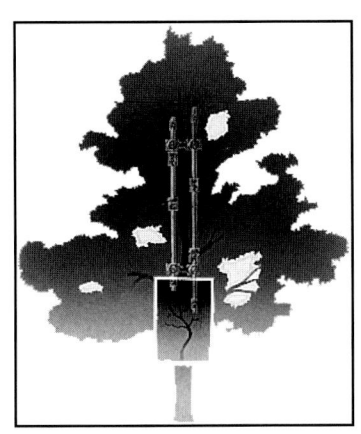

Lovell and Winter's Pediatric Orthopaedics

EDITED BY

Raymond T. Morrissy, MD
Medical Director and Chief of Orthopaedics
Scottish Rite Children's Medical Center
Clinical Professor of Orthopaedics
Emory University School of Medicine
Atlanta, Georgia

Stuart L. Weinstein, MD
Ignacio V. Ponseti Professor of Orthopaedic Surgery
University of Iowa College of Medicine
Iowa City, Iowa

With 31 Contributors

Volume I

Fourth Edition

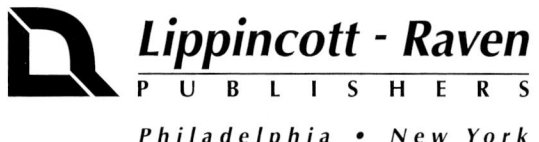

Philadelphia • New York

Acquisitions Editor: James D. Ryan
Developmental Editor: Delois Patterson
Project Editor: Molly E. Dickmeyer
Production Manager: Caren Erlichman
Production Coordinator: David Yurkovich
Designer: Doug Smock
Compositor: Bi-Comp
Printer: Quebecor/Kingsport

Copyright © 1996 by Lippincott–Raven Publishers.

Copyright © 1990, 1986, 1978, 1975 by J.B. Lippincott Company. All rights reserved. This book is protected by copyright. No part of it may be reproduced, stored in a retrieval system, or transmitted, in any form or by any means—electronic, mechanical, photocopy, recording, or otherwise—without the prior written permission of the publisher, except for brief quotations embodied in critical articles and reviews. Printed in The United States of America. For information write Lippincott–Raven Publishers, 227 East Washington Square, Philadelphia, PA 19106.

Library of Congress Cataloging-in-Publication Data

Pediatric orthopaedics.
    Lovell and Winter's pediatric orthopaedics / edited by Raymond T.
Morrissy and Stuart L. Weinstein. — 4th ed.
      p.   cm.
    Includes bibliographical references and index.
    ISBN 0-397-51397-6 (set : alk. paper). — ISBN 0-397-51598-7 (vol.
1 : alk. paper). — ISBN 0-397-51599-5 (vol. 2 : alk. paper)
    1. Pediatric orthopedics. I. Lovell, Wood. W. 1915– .
II. Winter, Robert B. 1932– . III. Morrissy, Raymond T.
IV. Weinstein, Stuart L.V.
    [DNLM: 1. Orthopedics—in infancy & childhood. WS 270 L911 1996]
RD732.3.C48P43 1996
617.3'0083—dc20
DNLM/DLC
for Library of Congress   95-31125
                                                                             CIP

    The material contained in this volume was submitted as previously unpublished material, except in the instances in which credit has been given to the source from which some of the illustrative material was derived.
    Great care has been taken to maintain the accuracy of the information contained in the volume. However, neither Lippincott–Raven Publishers nor the editors can be held responsible for errors or for any consequences arising from the use of information herein.
    The authors and publisher have exerted every effort to ensure that drug selection and dosage set forth in this text are in accord with current recommendations and practice at the time of publication. However, in view of ongoing research, changes in government regulation, and the constant flow of information relating to drug therapy and drug reactions, the reader is urged to check the package insert for each drug for any change in indications and dosage and for added warnings and precautions. This is particularly important when the recommended agent is a new or infrequently employed drug.
    Materials appearing in this book prepared by individuals as part of their official duties as U.S. Government employees are not covered by the above-mentioned copyright.

9 8 7 6 5 4 3 2 1

To Orthopaedic Residents and Fellows
that through continued inquiry and learning
they may find medicine to be fun for a lifetime

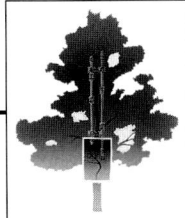

Contributors

Behrooz A. Akbarnia, M.D.
Associate Clinical Professor
Department of Orthopaedic
  Surgery
University of California, San Diego,
  School of Medicine
San Diego, California;
Adjunct Professor of Orthopaedic
  Surgery
St. Louis University School of
  Medicine
St. Louis, Missouri

George S. Bassett, M.D.
Associate Professor of
  Orthopaedics
University of Southern California
  School of Medicine;
Children's Hospital of Los Angeles
Los Angeles, California

Loui G. Bayne, M.D.
Director of Hand Clinic
Scottish Rite Children's Medical
  Center;
Clinical Professor of Orthopaedics
Emory University School of
  Medicine
Atlanta, Georgia

Michael T. Busch, M.D.
Scottish Rite Children's Medical
  Center
Atlanta, Georgia

William G. Cole, M.B.B.S., M.Sc., Ph.D.
Head, Division of Orthopaedic
  Surgery
The Hospital for Sick Children;
Professor of Genetics and
  Molecular Medicine
University of Toronto
Toronto, Ontario
Canada

Bronier L. Costas, M.D.
Assistant Director of Hand Clinic
Scottish Rite Children's Medical
  Center;
Clinical Assistant Professor of
  Orthopaedics
Emory University School of
  Medicine
Atlanta, Georgia

Donald R. Cummings, C.P.
Director, Prosthetics
Scottish Rite Hospital for Children;
Adjunct Faculty
Prosthetic/Orthotics Program
University of Texas Southwestern
  Medical School at Dallas
Dallas, Texas

Jon R. Davids, M.D.
Director, Motion Analysis
  Laboratory
Shriners Hospital
Greenville, South Carolina

Dennis P. Devito, M.D.
Scottish Rite Children's Medical
  Center
Atlanta, Georgia

James G. Gamble, M.D., Ph.D.
Professor of Orthopaedic Surgery
Stanford University School of
  Medicine;
Lucile-Salter Packard Children's
  Hospital at Stanford
Stanford, California

Michael J. Goldberg, M.D.
Professor and Chairman
Department of Orthopaedics
Tufts University School of
  Medicine and New England
  Medical Center
Boston, Massachusetts

Walter B. Greene, M.D.
Professor of Orthopaedic Surgery
  and Pediatrics
University of North Carolina
  School of Medicine
Chapel Hill, North Carolina

Richard H. Gross, M.D.
Professor of Orthopaedic Surgery
  and Pediatrics
Medical University of South
  Carolina
Charleston, South Carolina

H. Theodore Harcke, M.D.
Professor of Radiology and
  Pediatrics
Jefferson Medical College
Philadelphia, Pennsylvania;
Chairman, Department of Medical
  Imaging
Alfred I. duPont Institute
Wilmington, Delaware

John A. Herring, M.D.
Chief of Staff
Scottish Rite Hospital for Children;
Professor of Orthopaedic Surgery
University of Texas Southwestern
  Medical Center
Dallas, Texas

Douglas K. Kehl, M.D.
Department of Orthopaedic
  Surgery
Scottish Rite Children's Medical
  Center;
Associate Clinical Professor of
  Orthopaedic Surgery
Emory University School of
  Medicine
Atlanta, Georgia

Richard E. Lindseth, M.D.
Professor of Orthopaedic Surgery
Indiana University School of
  Medicine
Indianapolis, Indiana

Randall T. Loder, M.D.
Assistant Professor of Surgery
Section of Orthopaedics
University of Michigan School of
 Medicine
Ann Arbor, Michigan

John E. Lonstein, M.D.
Clinical Associate Professor
Department of Orthopaedic
 Surgery
University of Minnesota Medical
 School;
Staff, Minnesota Spine Center
Gillette Children's Hospital
St. Paul, Minnesota

Gary M. Lourie, M.D.
Assistant Director of Hand Clinic
Scottish Rite Children's Medical
 Center;
Clinical Assistant Professor of
 Orthopaedics
Emory University School of
 Medicine
Atlanta, Georgia

Raymond T. Morrissy, M.D.
Medical Director and Chief of
 Orthopaedics
Scottish Rite Children's Medical
 Center;
Clinical Professor of Orthopaedics
Emory University School of
 Medicine
Atlanta, Georgia

Vincent S. Mosca, M.D.
Associate Professor of
 Orthopaedics
Chief, Pediatric Orthopaedics
University of Washington School of
 Medicine;
Director, Department of
 Orthopaedics
Children's Hospital and Medical
 Center
Seattle, Washington

Colin F. Moseley, M.D.
Clinical Professor of Orthopaedics
University of California, Los
 Angeles, UCLA School of
 Medicine;
Chief of Staff
Shriners Hospital for Crippled
 Children
Los Angeles, California

Thomas S. Renshaw, M.D.
Professor of Orthopaedic Surgery
 and Pediatrics
Yale University School of Medicine
New Haven, Connecticut

David D. Sherry, M.D.
Assistant Professor of Pediatrics
University of Washington School of
 Medicine
Director of Clinical Pediatric
 Rheumatology
Children's Hospital and Medical
 Center
Seattle, Washington

Paul D. Sponseller, M.D.
Associate Professor and Head
Division of Pediatric Orthopaedics
Johns Hopkins University School
 of Medicine
Baltimore, Maryland

Dempsey S. Springfield, M.D.
Visiting Orthopaedic Surgeon
Massachusetts General Hospital;
Associate Professor of
 Orthopaedics
Harvard Medical School
Boston, Massachusetts

J. Andy Sullivan, M.D.
Chairman
Department of Orthopaedic
 Surgery and Rehabilitation,
University of Oklahoma Health
 Sciences Center College of
 Medicine
Oklahoma City, Oklahoma

George H. Thompson, M.D.
Professor of Orthopaedic Surgery
 and Pediatrics
Case Western Reserve University
 School of Medicine;
Director, Pediatric Orthopaedics
Rainbow Babies and Children's
 Hospital
Cleveland, Ohio

Vernon T. Tolo, M.D.
John C. Wilson, Jr, Professor of
 Orthopaedics
University of Southern California
 School of Medicine;
Head, Division of Orthopaedics
Children's Hospital
Los Angeles, California

William C. Warner Jr, M.D.
Assistant Professor of Orthopaedics
University of Tennessee, Memphis,
 College of Medicine
Staff
The Campbell Clinic
Memphis, Tennessee

Stuart L. Weinstein, M.D.
Ignacio V. Ponseti Professor of
 Orthopaedic Surgery
University of Iowa College of
 Medicine
Iowa City, Iowa

David J. Zaleske, M.D.
Associate Professor of
 Orthopaedics
Harvard Medical School;
Chief, Pediatric Orthopaedic Unit
Massachusetts General Hospital
Boston, Massachusetts

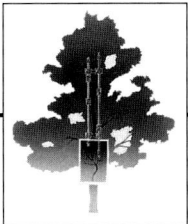

Preface

As we go about our daily practice of pediatric orthopaedics, we might be tempted to answer the question from our colleagues in other fields "What's new?" with the usual response, "Not much." However, when organizing the fourth edition of *Pediatric Orthopaedics*, a different answer became apparent; there is much that is new, and there is much that is better understood and supported by solid clinical or basic scientific data. Since the publication of the third edition, significant advances have taken place in molecular genetics, imaging techniques, diagnostic and therapeutic modalities, and surgical and medical technology. Additional information has also been accumulated on the natural history and long-term sequelae of various pediatric orthopaedic conditions.

To address this rapidly expanding knowledge base of pediatric orthopaedics, the fourth edition has been completely reorganized for a new, fresh approach. A second editor has been added, and 16 new authors bring their expertise to the text. In addition, several past contributors have written different chapters in which their expertise could be better utilized. Some subjects have been appropriately deemphasized, such as polio, whereas there are new chapters dealing with orthopaedic genetics, history taking and examination of the pediatric patient, syndromes and localized disorders affecting bone, neuromuscular disorders, and fracture treatment, a major portion of pediatric orthopaedic practice.

Each author has been asked to synthesize and evaluate both the old and new knowledge on their subjects, answer the important questions regarding each condition, and critically evaluate existing information about the disease and its treatment. They have persevered with two active editors who questioned, suggested, commented, and cajoled during the entire process.

As with the previous edition, the text focuses on the decision-making process that precedes and governs the selection of treatment. Additional goals for the fourth edition of *Pediatric Orthopaedics* are to emphasize basic scientific knowledge as it relates to the diagnosis and treatment of a particular disease or condition and to increase the amount of clinically relevant material regarding each entity. Each author provides the reader with the basic science that relates to the condition under discussion and the scientific basis for treatment decisions. Also, when current recommended treatment decisions are based on empiric (or even less) information, this is clearly pointed out.

The task of editing 32 chapters consisting of hundreds of pages of text while trying to make all of it as current as possible is a challenge. But the role of the editor should be more: to ensure that the content of each chapter is as current, accurate, well reasoned, and concisely presented as possible. This is a time-consuming, difficult, and often trying interaction between the editors and the authors, but one that is well worthwhile. It is much like a discussion with a colleague in which views and opinions are challenged. It can be simultaneously stimulating and trying, but usually you are intellectually better for it at the conclusion.

The editors trust that the work of these authors will inform and stimulate you in your orthopaedic care of infants, children, and adolescents, as would a good colleague.

Raymond T. Morrissy, M.D.
Stuart L. Weinstein, M.D.

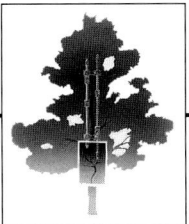

Preface to the First Edition

The field of pediatric orthopaedics has changed significantly in recent years. In the main, textbooks have kept abreast of change, to the extent that there is now a broad and useful literature addressed to the techniques of treatment of the orthopaedic disorders of children. The editors believe, however, that their fellow surgeons will have increasingly shared the desire for a work focused especially upon the decision-making process that precedes and governs the selection of surgical technique. Basic research and clinical specialization have had a dual effect upon clinical decision making: They have broadened the field of choice, and at the same time have made judicious choice more difficult.

Chapters that will aid the reader at the critical junctures at which decisions must be made have been contributed by authorities of eminence, persons who have long and successful experience dealing with the conditions about which they have written. The reader will notice that each topic is covered in depth, and that the emphasis on decision making will facilitate his assessment of the indications and contraindications for a particular treatment approach.

Although we have attempted to match depth with breadth, children's fractures have not been included because the subject is well covered in other textbooks that have recently appeared.

We would like to state that our task has been made not only worthwhile but pleasurable by the continued thoughtful and kind cooperation of the contributors whose names appear in the pages of this book. They have our deepest thanks.

Wood W. Lovell, M.D.
Robert B. Winter, M.D.

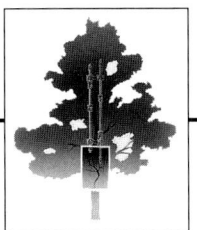

Acknowledgments

The editors would like to acknowledge the great fortune that we have had to practice our profession in the finest medical system in the world during a period of unprecedented advances in research and innovation combined with extraordinary cross-fertilization provided by our scientific societies and publishers. This text stands as testimony to these advances and provides an information base for our colleagues that physicians of past generations would certainly envy.

We would like to give special thanks to those who have contributed to this book. These individuals were selected because they have worked hard to attain their knowledge and expertise and have the special talent of being able to relate the knowledge and expertise to others. In addition, we readily acknowledge the work of all of our colleagues in orthopaedics and other fields of medicine who have contributed to our knowledge.

Finally, we acknowledge the opportunity to be involved in teaching residents and fellows. Their stimulating inquiries have been a large part of what has made orthopaedic surgery fun and exciting for us over the past two decades.

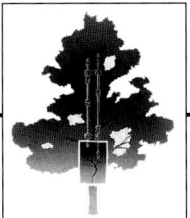

Contents

VOLUME I

1 **Development and Maturation of the Neuromusculoskeletal System** 1
James G. Gamble

Molecular Embryology 2
  Human Genome 2
  HOX, Homeotic Genes, and Basic Body Design 3
  Extracellular Matrix Formation 4
Embryogenesis 5
  Fertilization and Cell Cleavage 5
  Gastrulation, the Trilaminar Disc, and the Three Germ Layers 7
  Neurulation and Neurogenesis 8
  Differentiation of Somites and Organogenesis 8
  Fetal Period 9
Skeletogenesis and Neuromuscular Integration 9
  Spine Development 9
  Limb Precursors 13
  Apical Ectodermal Ridge and Limb Formation 14
  Neuromuscular Development 15
  Limb Rotation 15
  Synovial Joint Development 16
Bone Formation 18
  Intramembranous Bone Formation 18
  Endochondral Ossification 18
  Mechanical Loading and Bone Development 19
  Growth Plate Development 20

2 **Imaging Techniques and Applications** 25
H. Theodore Harcke

General Considerations 25
  Clinical Effectiveness 26
  Availability and Time 26
  Biologic Effect 26
  Cost 27
  Other Risks 27
Radiography Without Contrast 28
  Plain Films and Fluoroscopy 28
  Directional Tomography 30
  Digital Radiography 30
  Bone Densitometry 30
Radiography With Contrast 31
  Angiography 31
  Arthrography 31
  Myelography 32
Computed Tomography 32
Scintigraphy 34
Ultrasonography 39
Magnetic Resonance Imaging 43
Summary 46

3 **The Pediatric Orthopaedic Examination** 51
Richard H. Gross

Focused Examination 51
  Gathering Information 52
  Recording Information 53
Normal Development 54
  Normal Development of the Newborn 55
  Normal Development in Early Childhood 57
Examining and Recording Joint Motion and Function 61
Limb Lengths 63
Examinations of Specific Anatomic Areas 65
  Skin 65
  Spine 65
  Shoulder and Upper Limb 68
  Elbow, Forearm, and Wrist 72
  Hand 73
  Hip 74

Knee and Leg 79
Foot and Ankle 84
Conclusion 89

4 Normal Gait and Assessment of Gait Disorders 93
Jon R. Davids

Normal Gait 95
The Gait Cycle 97
　Ankle 101
　Knee 103
　Hip 103
The Running Cycle 106
Maturation of Gait 107
Common Gait Deviations 107
　Ankle 108
　Knee 108
　Hip 109
Gait Analysis 110
　Observational Gait Analysis 110
　Instrumented Gait Analysis 110

5 Genetic Aspects of Orthopaedic Conditions 117
William G. Cole

Molecular Basis of Inheritance 117
　Chromosomes 117
　Gene Structure 118
　Transcription and RNA Processing 118
　Translation 118
　Posttranslational Modification and Protein Assembly 119
Molecular Basis of Mutations 119
　Point Mutations 119
　Deletions and Insertions 120
　Detection of Mutations 120
Chromosome Disorders 121
　Abnormalities of Autosomal Chromosome Number 121
　Abnormalities of Autosomal Chromsome Structure 121
　Abnormalities of Sex Chromosomes 122
Single-Gene Disorders 122
　Autosomal Dominant Disorders 123
　Autosomal Recessive Disorders 126
　X-Linked Disorders 127
　Other Patterns of Single-Gene Inheritance 129
Multifactorial Disorders 131
Teratologic Disorders 131
　Principles of Teratology 131
　Teratogenic Agents 131

Genetic Counseling and Prenatal Diagnosis 132
　Indications for Genetic Counseling 132
　Diagnostic Precision 133
　Estimation of Recurrence Risk 133
　Burden of Genetic Diseases 133
　Neonatal and Prenatal Diagnosis 133
Treatment of Genetic Diseases 134

6 Metabolic and Endocrine Abnormalities 137
David J. Zaleske

Factors Influencing Skeletal Development 137
Mineral Phase 141
　Calcium and Phosphorus Homeostasis 141
　Rickets and Osteomalacia 146
Organic Phase 163
　Bone Physiology 163
　Osteogenesis Imperfecta 164
　Idiopathic Juvenile Osteoporosis 170
　Osteopetrosis 172
　Periosteal Reaction and Soft Tissue Calcification and Ossification 174
　Connective Tissue Syndromes 179
Endocrinopathies and Conditions With Indefinite Pathophysiology 182
　Normal Variant Short Stature 184
　Growth Hormone Deficiency and Hypopituitarism 185
　Hypothyroidism 186
　Gonadal Abnormalities and Sex Steroids 187
　Glucocorticoid-Related Abnormalities 188
　Fibrous Dysplasia 189

7 The Osteochondrodysplasias 203
George S. Bassett

Achondroplasia 205
　Clinical Features 205
　Growth and Development 206
　Radiographic Features 206
　Medical Considerations 207
　Orthopaedic Implications 209
Hypochondroplasia 213
　Clinical Features 213
　Radiographic Features 213
　Orthopaedic Implications 214
Metatropic Dysplasia 214
　Clinical Features 214
　Radiographic Features 214
　Medical Considerations 215
　Orthopaedic Implications 215
Chondroectodermal Dysplasia 216
　Clinical Features 216

Radiographic Features 216
Orthopaedic Implications 217
Diastrophic Dysplasia 218
Clinical Features 218
Radiographic Features 219
Medical Considerations 220
Orthopaedic Implications 220
Kniest Dysplasia 222
Clinical Features 222
Radiographic Features 222
Medical Considerations 223
Orthopaedic Implications 223
Spondyloepiphyseal Dysplasia Congenita 224
Clinical Features 224
Radiographic Features 225
Medical Considerations 226
Orthopaedic Implications 227
Spondyloepiphyseal Dysplasia Tarda 227
Clinical Features 228
Radiographic Features 228
Orthopaedic Implications 228
Pseudoachondroplastic Dysplasia 229
Clinical Features 229
Radiographic Features 230
Orthopaedic Implications 231
Multiple Epiphyseal Dysplasia 232
Clinical Features 232
Radiographic Features 232
Orthopaedic Implications 234
Chondrodysplasia Punctata 235
Clinical Features 235
Radiographic Features 236
Medical Considerations 236
Orthopaedic Implications 236
Metaphyseal Chondrodysplasia 237
Clinical Features 237
Radiographic Features 238
Medical Considerations 239
Orthopaedic Implications 239
Dyschondrosteosis 239
Clinical Features 239
Radiographic Features 240
Orthopaedic Implications 240
Cleidocranial Dysplasia 240
Clinical Features 241
Radiographic Features 241
Orthopaedic Implications 242
Larsen Syndrome 242
Clinical Features 242
Radiographic Features 243
Orthopaedic Implications 243

8 Syndromes of Orthopaedic Importance 255
Michael J. Goldberg

Neurofibromatosis 256
　Nonorthopaedic Manifestations 256
　Orthopaedic Manifestations 257
Proteus Syndrome 260
Arthrogryposis 262
　Arthrogryposis Multiplex Congenita 262
　Other Forms of Arthrogryposis 265
Down Syndrome 271
Fetal Alcohol Syndrome 274
Nail-Patella Syndrome 277
De Lange Syndrome 279
Familial Dysautonomia 280
Rubinstein-Taybi Syndrome 281
Progeria 283
Russell-Silver Dwarfism 284
Turner Syndrome 284
Noonan Syndrome 285
Prader-Willi Syndrome 285
Beckwith-Wiedemann Syndrome 286
Stickler Syndrome 287
VACTERLS and VATER Association 288
Goldenhar Syndrome 288
Trichorhinophalangeal Syndrome 290
Mucopolysaccharidoses 291
　Morquio Syndrome 292

9 Localized Disorders of Bone and Soft Tissue 305
Paul D. Sponseller

Congenital and Developmental Disorders 305
　Soft Tissue or Generalized Disorders 305
　Disorders Involving Bone or Joint 317
Acquired Disorders 334
　Myositis Ossificans 334
　The Osteochondroses 337
　Congenital Quadriceps Fibrosis 338
　Reflex Sympathetic Dystrophy 339

10 Diseases Related to the Hematopoietic System 345
Walter B. Greene

Disorders of Erythrocytes 345
　Iron Deficiency Anemia 345
　Diamond-Blackfan Anemia 346
　Fanconi Anemia 347
　Sickle Cell Disorders 347
　Thalassemia 353

Disorders of Granulocytes 354
  Schwachman-Diamond Syndrome 355
  Chronic Granulomatous Disease 355
Disorders of Lymphocytes and the Immune System 356
  X-Linked Agammaglobulinemia 356
  Cartilage-Hair Hypoplasia 357
  Acquired Immunodeficiency Syndrome 357
Disorders of the Monocyte-Macrophage System 358
  Gaucher Disease 359
  Neimann-Pick Disease 363
  Langerhans Cell Histiocytosis 363
Disorders of Hemostasis 369
  Thrombocytopenia With Absent Radius Syndrome 370
  Hemophilia 371
Leukemia 380

11 Juvenile Rheumatoid Arthritis and Seronegative Spondyloarthropathies 393
David D. Sherry and Vincent S. Mosca

Juvenile Rheumatoid Arthritis 394
  Pauciarticular Onset 394
  Polyarticular Onset 396
  Systemic Onset 396
Seronegative Spondyloarthropathies 397
  Ankylosing Spondylitis 397
  Other Seronegative Spondyloarthropathies 398
Etiology 398
Pathology and Radiology 399
Differential Diagnosis of Childhood Arthritis and Arthralgia 401
  Septic Arthritis 402
  Leukemia 402
  Systemic Lupus Erythematosus 402
  Acute Rheumatic Fever 402
  Henoch-Schönlein Purpura 402
  Toxic Synovitis of the Hip 403
  Reflex Neurovascular Dystrophy 403
  Pigmented Villonodular Synovitis 403
  Sarcoidosis 403
  Lyme Disease 403
  Foreign Body Synovitis 403
  Hypermobility Syndrome 403
  Miscellaneous Conditions 404
Approach to the Child With Joint Swelling, Limited Motion, and Pain 404
  History 404
  Physical Examination 405
  Laboratory Tests 406
  Radiography 406
  Arthrocentesis and Synovial Biopsy 406

Management of Arthritis Syndromes in Children 407
  Medical Therapy 407
  Intraarticular Steroid Injections 409
  Physical and Occupational Therapy 409
  Other Issues 409
Orthopaedic Surgical Treatment 410
  Special Considerations 410
  Synovectomy 410
  Soft Tissue Release 411
  Osteotomy 412
  Arthrodesis 412
  Total Joint Arthroplasty 413
  Epiphyseodesis 413
Joint-Specific Orthopaedic Treatment 414
  Hip 414
  Knee 414
  Foot and Ankle 417
  Cervical Spine 417
  Hand and Wrist 418
  Elbow 419
  Shoulder 419
Orthopaedic Surgery in Seronegative Spondyloarthropathies 419

12 Bone and Soft Tissue Tumors 423
Dempsey S. Springfield

Origins 423
Classification 424
Evaluation 424
  Chief Complaint 425
  Medical History 425
  Review of Systems 425
  Physical Examination 426
  Plain Radiograph Examination 426
  Additional Diagnostic Studies 427
  Staging 430
  Biopsy 431
Specific Bone Tumors 433
  Bone-Forming Tumors 433
  Cartilaginous Tumors 439
  Lesions of Fibrous Origin 444
  Miscellaneous Lesions 448
  Soft Tissue Tumors 454
Chemotherapy for Musculoskeletal Tumors 462

13 Cerebral Palsy 469
Thomas S. Renshaw

Basic Brain Development 469
Etiology 470
Prevalence 470

Classification 470
    Neuropathic Types 470
    Anatomic Patterns 471
Associated Problems in Other Systems 472
    Central Nervous System 472
    Gastrointestinal System 472
    Genitourinary System 472
Diagnosis 472
    History 472
    Physical Examination 472
    Other Tests 473
Common Types of Cerebral Palsy and Their Management 473
    Spastic Quadriplegia 473
    Spastic Diplegia 482
    Spastic Hemiplegia 493
    Athetoid Cerebral Palsy 494
Upper Extremity Involvement 494
    Nonsurgical Treatment 495
    Surgical Treatment 495

14 Myelomeningocele 503
Richard E. Lindseth

Classification and Pathology 503
Neurologic Abnormality 505
Genetics, Etiology, and Prenatal Diagnosis 506
Natural History 507
    Hydrocephaly 507
    Arnold-Chiari Deformity 508
    Tethered Cord Syndrome 508
    Latex Hypersensitivity 509
Effect of Myelomeningocele on Developmental Sequence 509
Treatment 510
    Spine 511
    Hip 521
    Thoracic Paraplegia 522
    Upper Lumbar Paraplegia 523
    Middle and Lower Lumbar Paraplegia 523
    Knee 525
    Foot 527
    Orthotic Devices 532

15 Neuromuscular Disorders 537
George H. Thompson

History 537
Physical Examination 538
Diagnostic Studies 538
    Hematologic Studies 538
    Electromyography 539
    Nerve Conduction Studies 539
    Muscle Biopsy 539
    Nerve Biopsy 539
    Other Studies 539
    Genetic and Molecular Biology Studies 540
Muscular Dystrophies 540
    Sex-Linked Muscular Dystrophies 540
    Autosomal Recessive Muscular Dystrophies 549
    Autosomal Dominant Muscular Dystrophies 550
    Myotonia 551
    Congenital Myopathies 552
    Congenital Muscular Dystrophy 555
Spinal Muscular Atrophy 555
    Clinical Classification 555
    Functional Classification 556
    Genetic Research 556
    Clinical Features 556
    Diagnostic Studies 556
    Radiographic Evaluation 556
    Treatment 557
Friedreich Ataxia 558
    Clinical Features 558
    Genetic Research 560
    Treatment 560
Hereditary Motor Sensory Neuropathies 561
    Classification 561
    Diagnostic Studies 561
    Genetic Research 562
    Treatment 562
Poliomyelitis 565
    Pathology 565
    Management 565
    Treatment Guidelines 567
    Postpoliomyelitis Syndrome 570

16 Bone and Joint Sepsis 579
Raymond T. Morrissy

Bone and Joint Infection 579
    Definition 579
    Epidemiology 580
    Etiology 580
    Pathophysiology of Osteomyelitis 581
    Pathophysiology of Septic Arthritis 585
Diagnosis 586
    History 586
    Examination 587
    Laboratory 587
    Organisms 589
    Imaging 590
    Aspiration 593
Differential Diagnosis 594
    Osteomyelitis 594
    Septic Arthritis 595

Treatment **596**
    Organism Identification **596**
    Antibiotic Selection **596**
    Antibiotic Delivery **597**
    Surgery **599**
Results **601**
Special Conditions **601**
    Spine **601**
    Pelvis and Sacroiliac Joint **603**

The Neonate **605**
Sickle Cell Disease **607**
Chronic Recurrent Multifocal Osteomyelitis **609**
Subacute Osteomyelitis **611**
Puncture Wounds of the Foot **612**
Lyme Arthritis **615**
Gonococcal Arthritis **615**
Tuberculosis **616**

VOLUME 2

17 Scoliosis 625
John E. Lonstein

Patient Evaluation **625**
    History **625**
    Physical Examination **626**
    Radiologic Evaluation **627**
    Pulmonary Function Testing **632**
Adult Sequelae of Untreated Spinal Deformity **633**
Nonstructural Scoliosis **635**
    Postural Scoliosis **635**
    Leg Length Discrepancy **635**
    Hysterical Scoliosis **636**
Structural Scoliosis **636**
    Idiopathic Scoliosis **636**
    Congenital Scoliosis **667**

18 Kyphosis 687
William C. Warner Jr.

Postural Kyphosis **689**
Congenital Kyphosis **690**
    Patient Presentation **691**
    Treatment **692**
    Complications of Treatment **694**
Scheuermann Disease **694**
    Natural History **697**
    Radiographic Examination **697**
    Treatment **698**
Postlaminectomy Kyphosis **699**
Radiation Kyphosis **704**
    Treatment **705**
Miscellaneous Causes of Kyphotic Deformities **705**
    Achondroplasia **705**
    Pseudoachondroplasia **705**
    Spondyloepiphyseal Dysplasia Congenita **708**
    Diastrophic Dwarfism **708**
    Mucopolysaccharidosis **708**
    Marfan Syndrome **708**

Posttraumatic Deformities **709**
Tuberculosis **709**
Neurofibromatosis **709**
Juvenile Osteoporosis **709**

19 Spondylolysis and Spondylolisthesis 717
John E. Lonstein

Definitions **717**
Classification **717**
Natural History **719**
    Progression **719**
    Pain **719**
Etiology **719**
    Hereditary Factors **719**
    Trauma and Biomechanical Factors **720**
    Posture **720**
    Growth **720**
Patient Evaluation **720**
    History **720**
    Physical Examination **720**
    Radiologic Evaluation **721**
Treatment **723**
    Spondylolysis **723**
    Sponylolisthesis **725**

20 The Cervical Spine 739
Randall T. Loder

Normal Embryology, Growth, and Development **739**
    Embryology **739**
    Growth and Development **740**
    Normal Radiographic Parameters **741**
Congenital and Developmental Problems **744**
    Torticollis **744**
    Klippel-Feil Syndrome **755**
    Os Odontoideum **755**
    Developmental and Acquired Stenoses and Instabilities **756**
    Other Syndromes **760**

Trauma 763
  Fractures and Ligamentous Injuries of the Occipital Complex to the C1–C2 Complex 764
  Fractures and Ligamentous Injuries of C3–C7 765
  Spinal Cord Injury Without Radiographic Abnormality 767
  Transient Quadriparesis 767
  Special Injury Mechanisms 769
Inflammatory and Septic Conditions 770
  Juvenile Rheumatoid Arthritis 770
  Intervertebral Disc Calcification 771
  Pyogenic Osteomyelitis and Discitis 772
  Tuberculosis 772
Hematologic and Oncologic Conditions 773
  Benign Tumors 773
  Malignant Tumors 774

21 The Upper Limb 781
Loui G. Bayne, Bronier L. Costas, and Gary M. Lourie

General Principles 782
Incidence 782
Genetics and Inheritance 783
Classification of Upper Limb Malformations 783
Failure of Formation of Parts 783
  Transverse Arrest 784
  Longitudinal Deficiencies 796
  Failure of Differentiation or Separation of Parts 801
  Synostosis 801
  Radial Head Dislocation 804
  Syndactyly 805
  Arthrogryposis 808
  Trigger Digits 810
  Camptodactyly 811
  Clinodactyly 813
  Delta Phalanx 814
  Duplication 815
  Preaxial Polydactyly, or Duplicate Thumbs 815
  Triphalangeal Thumb 817
  Central Polydactyly, or Polysyndactyly 819
  Postaxial Polydactyly, or Little-Finger Polydactyly 819
Macrodactyly 821
Congenital Constriction Band Syndrome 822
General Skeletal Abnormalities 825
  Madelung Deformity 825
  Obstetric Brachial Plexus Injury, or Birth Palsy 826
Trauma to the Pediatric Hand 828
  Skeletal Injuries 828
  Mallet Finger 829
  Distal Phalanx Fracture and Nail Bed Injury 830
  Flexor Digitorum Profundus Avulsion and the Reverse Mallet Finger Fracture 830
  Phalangeal Neck Fractures, or Supracondylar Fractures 831
  Middle Phalanx Fractures 832
  Intraarticular Fracture of the Proximal Interphalangeal Joint 834
  Fractures of the Shaft of the Proximal Phalanx 834
  Metacarpal Fractures 836
  Injury of the Metaphalangeal and Proximal Interphalangeal Joints 837
  Carpal Injuries 840

22 Leg Length Discrepancy and Angular Deformity of the Lower Limbs 849
Colin F. Moseley

Effects 850
  Mechanisms of Compensation 850
  Gait 850
  Hip 851
  Knee 851
  Spine 851
Growth 853
Etiology 856
  Interference With Length 856
  Inhibition of Growth 858
  Stimulation of Growth 861
  Patterns of Growth 862
Patient Assessment 862
  History of Discrepancy 862
  Clinical Assessment 863
  Radiologic Assessment 864
Data Analysis 868
  Arithmetic Method 871
  Growth Remaining Method 872
  Straight-Line Graph Method 872
  Patterns of Inhibition 874
  Inadequate Data 874
Determination of Treatment Goals 875
  Equal Leg Lengths 875
  Unequal Leg Lengths 875
  Level Pelvis 875
  Vertical Lumbar Spine 875
  Equalization by Prosthetic Fitting 875
  Correction of Coexisting Problems 875
Treatment 876
  General Principles 876
  Shoe Lift 876
  Prosthetic Fitting 876
  Epiphyseodesis 877
  Femoral Shortening 879
  Growth Stimulation 880
  Leg Lengthening 880

Angular Deformity **891**
　Etiology and Pathogenesis **891**
　Radiologic Evaluation **892**
　Indications and Goals **892**
　Patient Assessment **893**
　Preoperative Planning **893**
　Operative Strategy **894**
　Gradual and Acute Correction **895**
Summary **896**

23　Developmental Hip Dysplasia and Dislocation **903**
Stuart L. Weinstein

Normal Growth and Development of the Hip Joint **904**
　Acetabular Growth and Development **904**
　Growth of the Proximal Femur **905**
　Determinants of Acetabulum Shape and Depth **906**
Pathoanatomy **907**
　Dislocations in Newborns **907**
　Acetabular Development in Developmental Hip Dysplasia **908**
Etiology, Epidemiology, and Diagnosis **908**
　Causes of Developmental Dysplasia of the Hip **908**
　Risk Factors and Incidence **910**
　Diagnosis **911**
Natural History **916**
　Course in Newborns **916**
　Course in Adults **916**
　Course of Dysplasia and Subluxation **917**
Treatment **922**
　Treatment of Hip Dislocation **922**
　Treatment of Acetabular Dysplasia in Children 6 Months to 2 Years of Age **931**
Sequelae and Complications **931**
　Residual Femoral and Acetabular Dysplasia **931**
　Growth Disturbance of the Proximal Femur **937**

24　Legg-Calvé-Perthes Disease **951**
Stuart L. Weinstein

History **951**
Epidemiology and Etiology **952**
Pathogenesis **954**
　Radiographic Stages **956**
　Pathogenesis of Deformity **958**
　Patterns of Deformity **961**
Natural History **963**
　Long-Term Follow-Up Results **965**
　Prognostic Factors **968**
Clinical Presentation **973**
Physical Examination **973**

Imaging **974**
Differential Diagnosis **974**
Treatment **977**
　Patient Management **978**
　Nonoperative Treatment **979**
　Surgical Treatment **980**
　Treatment Options in the Noncontainable Hip and the Late-Presenting Case **982**
Future Developments **983**

25　Slipped Capital Femoral Epiphysis **993**
Douglas K. Kehl

Epidemiology **993**
Pathoanatomy **994**
Etiology **994**
Clinical Presentation **996**
Radiographic Features **998**
Natural History **1000**
Treatment **1002**
　Treatment to Prevent Further Slippage **1002**
　Treatment to Reduce the Degree of Slippage **1009**
　Salvage Procedures **1015**
Prophylactic Pinning of the Contralateral Hip **1017**
Complications **1017**

26　Developmental Coxa Vara; Transient Synovitis; and Idiopathic Chondriolysis of the Hip **1023**
Douglas K. Kehl

Developmental Coxa Vara **1023**
　Historical Review **1025**
　Incidence **1026**
　Etiology **1026**
　Clinical Presentation **1027**
　Radiographic Findings **1027**
　Natural History **1027**
　Treatment **1028**
　Results **1030**
Transient Synovitis of the Hip **1033**
　Historical Review **1033**
　Etiology **1033**
　Incidence **1034**
　Clinical Presentation **1034**
　Radiographic Findings **1034**
　Natural History **1035**
　Treatment **1036**
Idiopathic Chondrolysis of the Hip **1037**
　Historical Review **1037**
　Etiology **1037**
　Incidence **1038**
　Clinical Presentation **1038**
　Radiographic Findings **1038**

Pathology 1040
Natural History 1041
Treatment 1042

27 The Lower Extremity 1047
Vernon T. Tolo

In-Toeing and Out-Toeing 1047
Etiology 1048
Clinical Features 1048
Imaging Studies 1049
Natural History 1050
Treatment 1051
Complications 1052
Bowlegs and Knock-Knees 1054
Normal Development 1054
Clinical Features 1054
Imaging Studies 1055
Causes and Treatment of Bowlegs 1055
Causes and Treatment of Knock-Knees 1060
Knee Disorders 1061
Recurvatum Deformity 1061
Osgood-Schlatter Disease 1063
Larsen-Johansson Disease 1064
Bipartite Patella 1065
Popliteal Cyst 1065
Osteochondritis Dissecans 1065
Discoid Lateral Meniscus 1067
Tibial Disorders 1069
Toddler's Fracture of the Tibia 1069
Stress Fracture of the Proximal and Middle Tibia 1069
Posteromedial Bowing of the Tibia 1070
Idiopathic Toe Walking 1071

28 The Child's Foot 1077
J. Andy Sullivan

Terminology 1078
Standard Radiography 1078
Normal Alignment 1078
Metatarsus Adductus 1078
Incidence 1078
Etiology 1079
Clinical Features 1079
Radiographic Evaluation 1080
Natural History 1080
Treatment 1081
Skewfoot 1081
Incidence 1083
Clinical Features 1083
Radiographic Evaluation 1083
Treatment 1083
Congenital Calcaneovalgus Foot 1083

Flexible Flatfoot 1085
Incidence 1085
Etiology 1085
Pathoanatomy 1085
Natural History 1085
Clinical Features 1085
Radiography 1086
Treatment 1086
Congenital Vertical Talus 1089
Etiology and Genetics 1089
Clinical Features 1090
Natural History 1090
Radiographic Evaluation 1090
Pathoanatomy 1091
Treatment 1092
Tarsal Coalition 1093
Etiology and Incidence 1094
Natural History 1094
Clinical Features 1094
Radiographic Evaluation 1095
Pathophysiology 1096
Treatment 1098
Accessory Navicular Bone 1099
Clinical Features 1100
Radiographic Evaluation 1100
Pathoanatomy 1100
Natural History 1100
Treatment 1101
Osteochondroses 1101
Koehler Disease 1101
Freiberg Infarction 1101
Congenital Clubfoot 1103
Incidence 1103
Etiology 1103
Clinical Features 1104
Radiographic Evaluation 1104
Pathoanatomy 1104
Natural History 1106
Treatment 1106
Adolescent Bunion 1116
Incidence 1116
Etiology 1116
Clinical Features 1116
Radiographic Evaluation 1116
Pathophysiology 1117
Treatment 1117
Tailor Bunionette 1119
Heel Pain in Children 1119
Clinical Features 1119
Sever Disease 1120
Pump Bump 1120
Cavus 1120
Etiology 1120

Clinical Features 1121
Radiographic Evaluation 1121
Natural History 1122
Pathoanatomy 1122
Treatment 1122
Calcaneocavus 1123
Miscellaneous Foot Problems 1124
Congenital Hallux Varus 1124
Curly Toes 1125
Overriding of the Fifth Toe 1126
Idiopathic Toe Walking 1127
Cleft Feet 1127
Macrodactyly 1128
Polydactyly 1128
Ingrown Toenails 1129
Subungual Exostosis 1131

29 The Limb-Deficient Child 1137
John A. Herring and Donald R. Cummings

Classification of Limb Deficiencies 1137
Congenital Abnormalities 1137
What to Tell Parents 1138
Guide to Decision Making 1141
Specific Lower Extremity Deficiencies 1142
Proximal Focal Femoral Deficiency 1142
Fibular Deficiency 1149
Tibial Deficiency 1154
Foot Deficiencies 1157
Acquired Amputation 1158
Etiology 1158
Complications 1161
Above-Knee Amputation 1162
Knee Disarticulation 1162
Below-Knee Amputation 1162
Upper Extremity Amputations 1164
Multiple Congenital Amputations 1164
Prosthetics 1166
Lower Extremity Prosthetics 1167
Gait Evaluation 1173
Upper Extremity Prosthetics 1174
Indications for Replacement 1177

30 Sports Medicine 1181
Michael T. Busch

Care of the Young Athlete 1181
Nutrition 1182
Heat Illness and Fluids 1182
Strength Training 1184
Drug Abuse 1184
Antiinflammatory Drugs 1184
Overuse Syndromes 1185
Classic Stress Fractures 1185

Repetitive Physeal Injuries 1187
Apophyseal Conditions 1188
Tendinoses 1191
Shin Pain 1192
Iliotibial Band Friction Syndrome 1194
Breaststroker's Knee 1195
Valgus Overload Injuries of the Elbow 1195
Sports Trauma 1197
Epidemiology 1197
Prevention 1198
Athletic Trainers 1199
Types of Injuries and Treatment 1199
Patellofemoral Disorders 1208
Anatomy and Biomechanics 1208
Anterior Knee Pain 1209
Chondromalacia 1215
Saphenous Nerve Entrapment 1215
Dorsal Defects of the Patella 1215
Fat Pad Impingement 1216
Plica Syndrome 1216
Acute Patellar Dislocation 1217
Recurrent Patellar Dislocations 1218

31 Management of Fractures and Their Complications 1229
Dennis P. Devito

General Features of Fractures in Children 1230
Anatomic Differences 1230
Biomechanical Differences 1230
Physiologic Differences 1230
Injury to the Physis 1231
Physeal Anatomy 1231
Physeal Fractures 1231
Physeal Arrest 1233
Fractures of the Shoulder Region 1236
Clavicle Fractures 1236
Acromioclavicular Separation 1237
Scapular Fracture 1238
Shoulder Dislocation 1238
Humeral Fractures 1238
Fractures and Dislocations About the Elbow 1241
Supracondylar Fracture 1242
T-Condylar Fracture 1247
Lateral Condyle and Epicondyle Fracture 1247
Medial Epicondyle and Condyle Fracture 1251
Fracture-Separation of the Distal Humeral Physis 1252
Fractures of the Proximal Radius and Ulna 1253
Forearm and Wrist Fractures 1257
Midshaft Fracture 1259
Distal-Third Fracture 1262

Distal Physis Fracture 1264
Forearm Fracture-Dislocations 1264
Pelvic Fractures 1268
Classification 1269
Management 1270
Acetabular Fractures 1270
Fractures and Dislocations of the Hip 1271
Proximal Femur Fractures 1271
Hip Dislocation 1277
Femoral Shaft Fractures 1277
Management 1278
Fractures and Dislocations About the Knee 1285
Distal Femoral Physeal Fractures 1285
Knee Dislocation 1287
Intraarticular Avulsions 1289
Patellar Disorders 1290
Tibial Fractures 1293
Regions of Tibial Fracture 1293
Management 1295
Ankle Fractures 1300
Common Patterns of Ankle Fractures 1300
Transitional Fractures 1302
Foot Fractures 1303
Talus Fractures 1303
Calcaneus Fractures 1307
Metatarsal Fractures 1307

32 The Role of the Orthopaedic Surgeon in Child Abuse 1315

Behrooz A. Akbarnia

Definition 1316
Prevalence 1316
Diagnosis 1316
The Parents 1317
The Child 1317
Clinical Manifestations 1317
Skin Lesions 1317
Head Injuries 1318
Internal Injuries 1319
Orthopaedic Manifestations 1319
Physeal Fractures 1319
Metaphyseal Fractures 1319
Diaphyseal Fractures 1321
Miscellaneous Fractures 1322
Spinal Injuries 1322
Decision Making 1323
Dating Fractures 1325
Management 1328
Medical Neglect 1331
The Orthopaedic Surgeon, Child Abuse, and the Law 1331
Preparation for Court Testimony in Child Abuse Cases 1331

Lovell and Winter's Pediatric Orthopaedics

Volume **I**

Chapter 1

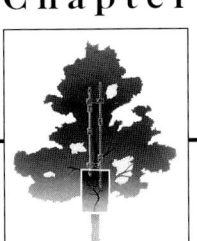

Development and Maturation of the Neuromusculoskeletal System

James G. Gamble

Molecular Embryology
   Human Genome
   HOX, Homeotic Genes, and Basic Body
      Design
   Extracellular Matrix Formation
Embryogenesis
   Fertilization and Cell Cleavage
   Gastrulation, the Trilaminar Disc, and
      the Three Germ Layers
   Neurulation and Neurogenesis
   Differentiation of Somites and
      Organogenesis
   Fetal Period

**Skeletogenesis and Neuromuscular
   Integration**
   Spine Development
   Limb Precursors
   Apical Ectodermal Ridge and Limb
      Formation
   Neuromuscular Development
   Limb Rotation
   Synovial Joint Development
Bone Formation
   Intramembranous Bone Formation
   Endochondral Ossification
   Mechanical Loading and Bone
      Development
   Growth Plate Development

Advances in our understanding of human embryology, developmental anatomy, and molecular genetics stand as one of the greatest intellectual achievements of the 20th century. Using a variety of experimental techniques, scientists have uncovered the morphologic events and discovered many of the biochemical reactions that cause two gametes to fuse and to grow into a fully developed neonate 266 days later. The process of development from a zygote to a neonate requires the activation and the precise expression of many complex genetic programs that are encoded in chromosomal DNA. Development depends on more than just DNA, however; it depends on the coordinated interaction of genetic and microenvironmental factors (e.g., biochemical gradients, morphogen concentrations, mechanical forces, cellular migrations, cellular adhesions).

Each system of the body has a unique embryologic origin and developmental pattern. Development of any embryologic system involves physical growth plus the production and organization of cellular diversity. A single fertilized cell, the zygote, is the ultimate source for all adult cell types, including bone cells, muscle cells, neurons, and lymphocytes. The process by which cells acquire special features and unique functions is called differentiation. The organization of differentiated cells into tissues and organs to create anatomic form and structure is called morphogenesis. These and other general embryologic concepts provide the basis of our understanding of many congenital anomalies and musculoskeletal variations.

Using the powerful methods of biochemistry and molecular genetics, scientists have determined the chromosomal locus and the precise molecular defect causing several diseases, such as Duchenne muscular dystrophy, familial hypercholesterolemia, Huntington disease, and Ehlers-Danlos syndrome.[1,12] Rapid advances in the field of molecular biology promise to revolutionize the way we think about and treat many congenital diseases and other pediatric orthopaedic problems. Genes causing congenital anomalies and many other diseases are being identified and cataloged regularly. Human genes can be manipulated in the laboratory and inserted into microorganisms or into other eukaryotic cells. Transgenic animals containing functional human genes have been produced from mice, sheep, and cows, showing promise for easy and economical production of pure antibodies, hormones, and other medicinally important proteins.[6,12] We stand on the brink of possessing the ability to influence and even to change human genetic destiny.

The purpose of this chapter is to present some of the important concepts in this exciting field and to review some of the major principles of embryology and developmental anatomy, particularly as they relate to pediatric orthopaedic conditions.

CONCEPT: Morphogenesis is the production of anatomic form and structure. Development is an increase in molecular and cellular complexity coupled with tissue organization and physical growth. Differentiation is the increase in cellular specialization.

MOLECULAR EMBRYOLOGY

Soon after fertilization of the haploid egg by a haploid sperm, the resulting diploid zygote undergoes an explosion of genetic activity and cellular proliferation, producing an embryo that initially resembles the embryos of many other vertebrates, such as salamanders, rabbits, and chickens. The cells of an early embryo are said to be pleuripotential, which means that any particular cell can follow more than one developmental pathway. Actually, soon after fertilization, it is possible to physically separate and clone the individual cells of an early embryo. Each subsequent developmental phase incrementally adds positional information and biochemical specificity to cells, resulting in the eventual appearance of embryonic organ structures in their appropriate places.

Although morphogenesis is incredibly complex, it involves a limited repertoire of cellular processes, such as cell divisions, cell shape changes, cell migrations, cell growth, changes in cell composition, and changes in extracellular matrix composition. Cells become progressively more restricted during differentiation as they acquire the structural and functional features required for specialization. Gradually, the human embryo accumulates all the special morphologic features that become the human neonate. The molecular events that initiate these embryologic changes are choreographed by a series of perfectly timed and properly executed gene expressions.

CONCEPT: Cells lose their pleuripotential ability as they become structurally and functionally more specialized.

Biochemical interactions between different groups of tissues commonly occur during the early phases of embryologic development. These interactions are termed inductive events when one tissue induces or directs another tissue to follow a particular developmental course. Both intracellular and extracellular inductive cues appear to be necessary for certain cells to assume a precise and predetermined position at a particular time. Cells in slightly different locations within the embryo begin to activate different sets of genes, changing the mix of intracellular and extracellular proteins that open up specific pathways of tissue development. For instance, cells that are induced to occupy a position in the central core of the limb bud express genes for type II collagen; these cells eventually become the cartilage precursors of the appendicular skeleton.

CONCEPT: Precise control of the timing and the order of gene-directed protein synthesis is the molecular basis of cellular differentiation and morphogenesis.

Human Genome

The complete set of nucleic acid instructions for making a human—the blueprint for all cellular structures and biochemical reactions—is called the human genome. The information in the genome is in the form of nucleotides present in tightly coiled threads of DNA, which are packed and organized into structures called chromosomes. Each DNA molecule contains many genes, which are the basic functional units of heredity. A gene is actually a certain group of nucleotide bases—adenine, thymine, guanine, cytosine—whose sequence within the DNA molecule provides the information necessary for cells to synthesize a particular structural protein or an enzyme, which is also a protein. Generally, one gene encodes the information necessary to make one protein.

The haploid human genome is estimated to contain at least 100,000 genes scattered along 3 billion base pairs within the 23 chromosomes.[1,6] All nucleated cells contain the same complement of genomic DNA that was present in the zygote. During embryogenesis, however, only certain genes are activated while other genes are permanently repressed, thus producing different populations of proteins that make up the different histologic cell types. mRNA transcribed from activated genes transmits the protein coding instructions from the nucleus to the cytoplasm, where mRNA

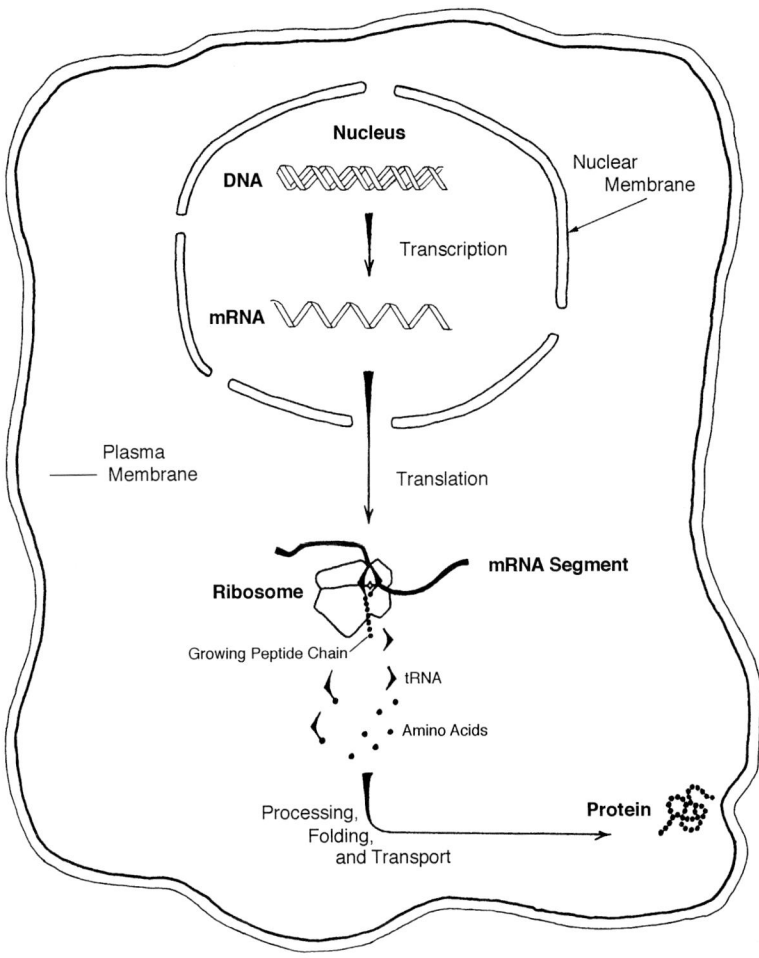

FIGURE 1-1. Triplets of DNA nucleotides encode the sequence information for amino acids comprising the polypeptide chains of proteins. RNA polymerase transcribes the DNA sequence information into mRNA, which enters the cytoplasm to function as a blueprint for protein biosynthesis. Ribosomes bind to the end of the mRNA and move along the messenger, sequentially presenting mRNA triplets to the appropriate tRNA molecule carrying a specific amino acid. Other enzymes and translation factors catalyze peptide bond formation to synthesize the protein, which is subsequently used by the cell or exported for use elsewhere.

serves as a template for protein synthesis. The protein-synthesizing machinery of the cell (i.e., ribosomes, transfer RNA) then translates the codons of the mRNA into a string of amino acids that comprise a protein molecule (Fig. 1-1).

CONCEPT: A gene is the DNA sequence from which mRNA is transcribed to direct the synthesis of a specific protein.

Synthesis of the right proteins at the right time and in the right place results in the appropriate biochemical reactions required for morphogenesis and development. Specificity is crucial, and control of specific gene expression is one of the central features of developmental biology.

CONCEPT: Two copies of the total genome (roughly 6 billion base pairs) are present in all nucleated cells, but different cells selectively activate only certain genes while repressing all others.

HOX, Homeotic Genes, and Basic Body Design

One of the fundamental questions concerning the events of morphogenesis is the following: how does it happen that organ structures emerge from an initially homogenous field of cells and come to reside in particular places, as exemplified by the formation of vertebral bodies or the development of the foot? How is it that a finger forms on the end of a hand? Answers to these and other questions are becoming clear as a result of research on the role of the homeotic genes in morphogenesis.[13,27] Homeotic genes, so named because of the ability of these genes when mutated to transform one body segment into the likeness of another body segment,[13] are involved in establishing a molecular coordinate system throughout the embryo—coordinates that define the basic body plan. Homeotic genes may be thought of as providing the information necessary to tell cells where to go, which should go, and exactly how many should report for duty.

An interrelated group of homeotic genes called *HOX* genes govern the basic body design in many different types of embryos. Homeotic mutations can cause bizarre changes; for example, the homeotic mutation in *Drosophila* causes antennae on the head to be transformed into an extra pair of thoracic legs. Homeotic genes assign distinct positional identities to cells along the anteroposterior axis, telling one group of undifferentiated cells that they are to be part of the head, another group that they are to be part of the thorax, and another the abdomen. Most homeotic mutations result in severe insults that cause deformities affecting body design, usually resulting in embryonic death.

CONCEPT: Homeotic genes are responsible for the basic body design.

As the embryo accumulates more and more cells, the diversity of cell populations increases and the variety of biochemical reactions taking place within the embryonic cells increases. The cells are no longer similar in appearance. For example, billions of differentiated cells called neuroblasts form a mass of tissue recognizable as a rudimentary brain, whereas another mass of entirely different cells form embryonic muscle groups. From a reductionist point of view, it is convenient to think of embryonic cells as eventually producing 11 distinct organ systems composed of characteristic tissues that arise from the process of differentiation. These 11 organ systems are the circulatory, digestive, endocrine, urinary, immune, integumentary, muscular, nervous, reproductive, respiratory, and skeletal systems. Although we often think and speak and even medically treat the systems as separate entities, in vivo, all 11 systems function as one integrated human body.

Having said that, three organ systems are recognized that are of particular interest to pediatric orthopaedic surgeons: namely, the nervous system, the muscular system, and the skeletal system. The brain and spinal cord, the sensory and motor nerves, and the sense organs comprise the nervous system. The function of the nervous system is to receive stimuli, to integrate information, and to initiate and direct action. The muscular system is characterized by three muscle tissue types: skeletal, cardiac, and smooth. A distinguishing feature of these tissues is the presence of two proteins, actin and myosin, that polymerize into the contractile elements. The function of the muscular system is to produce body movement. The skeletal system is composed of bones, cartilage, and ligaments; it provides protection and support for the body, acts as a reservoir for mineral metabolism, and it forms the levers for movement of the body segments and for locomotion.

Extracellular Matrix Formation

The correct migration of cells from one area of the embryo to a new area depends on the composition of the extracellular matrix. During organogenesis individual cells change their relative positions and become associated with other cell types. Migrating cells have the ability to selectively recognize other types of cellular environments and to adhere to certain cells while migrating over others. Several cell adhesion molecules have been identified, including cadherins, whose cell adhesive properties depend on calcium ions; and immunoglobulin adhesion molecules, whose cell binding domains resemble those of antibody molecules. In addition to cell-surface recognition, migrating cells use two major methods of communication to reach their destinations: detection of diffusible substances such as morphogens, growth factors, and hormones, and cues in the extracellular matrix composition. The extracellular matrix does more than just offer an inert scaffolding; it can critically influence cell development, migration, proliferation, and metabolic functions. Three major components comprise the extracellular matrix: collagens, proteoglycans, and glycoproteins, also called substrate adhesion molecules.

Collagen is the major structural protein of the body, making up nearly half of the total body protein. Collagens provide strength, stability, and molecular binding capacity to the tissues. Collagens are long, thin molecules that self-assemble to form fibrils, usually 60 to 70 nm in diameter. Type I collagen, found in the extracellular matrices of bone, tendon, and skin, comprises about 90% of the body's total collagen (Table 1-1). In addition, several other types of collagen have special functions. Type II collagen is present in cartilage and also in the notochord. Type III collagen is mostly found in blood vessels. Type IV collagen is nec-

TABLE 1-1 **Major Collagen Types**

TYPE	CHARACTERISTICS	PRIMARY LOCATIONS
I	90% of all collagen; thick, tightly packed 67-nm banded fibrils give a high tensile strength	Bone, ligament, tendon, skin
II	Small, 67-nm banded fibrils; high in carbohydrate; forms thin compressible fibrils	Cartilage, vitreous body, nucleus pulposus
III	Small, banded reticulin fibrils; interchain disulfide bonds	Skin, blood vessels, internal organs other than bone
IV	Appearance of "chicken-wire;" cell-attachment sites; binds to laminin	Basement membranes

TABLE 1-2 *Repeating Disaccharide Units of the Most Common Glycosaminoglycans of Extracellular Matrix Proteoglycans*

GLYCOSAMINOGLYCAN	MAJOR REPEATING DISACCHARIDE UNIT	PRIMARY LOCATIONS
Hyaluronic acid	Glucuronic acid–N-acetylglucosamine	Bone, connective tissues
Chondroitin sulfate	Glucuronic acid–N-acetylgalactosamine sulfate	Cartilage, cornea, arteries
Dermatan sulfate	Glucuronic or iduronic acid–N-acetylgalactosamine sulfate	Skin, heart, vessels
Keratin sulfate	Galactose–N-acetylglucosamine sulfate	Cartilage, cornea
Heparan sulfate	Glucuronic or iduronic acid–N-acetylgalactosamine sulfate	Lung, arteries, cell surfaces

essary for the formation of the basal lamina, in which the fibrils are like fine chicken wire and assemble into a felt-like surface. Tissues contain many other minor collagen types that are important for regional specificity and cellular function.

Proteoglycans are enormous aggregates of protein and polysaccharide, in which the polysaccharide portion makes up most of the molecular mass, often 95% or more. Usually, one of the sugar residues of the repeating disaccharides has an amino group, so that the polysaccharide is called a glycosaminoglycan (Table 1-2). The glycosaminoglycans are bound covalently to a core protein to form the proteoglycan subunits. Because the glycosaminoglycan chains are strongly hydrophilic, when they are bound to the core protein, they electrostatically repel each other and come to occupy a large volume in the extracellular space, taking the form of giant hydrated gels. The proteoglycan subunits bind noncovalently to long hyaluronate chains, forming proteoglycan aggregates that often exceed a molecular weight of hundreds of millions (Fig. 1-2). Proteoglycans stimulate as well as modulate cell movement. For example, heparan sulfate proteoglycans are essential for the proliferation of Schwann cells around axons of the dorsal root ganglia.

Glycoproteins are responsible for arranging the extracellular collagen and the proteoglycans into an ordered mesh. Integrin, a class of surface receptor glycoproteins embedded in the plasma membrane of cells, binds the cells to many of the extracellular matrix proteins, such as fibronectin. Fibronectin is another glycoprotein that is synthesized by many cells, including chondrocytes, fibroblasts, and epithelial cells. Fibronectin is a general adhesive molecule, linking cell integrin receptors to molecules of collagen and proteoglycans. Fibronectin is an important molecule in embryogenesis. When the neural crest cells migrate from the dorsal edge of the neural tube to other regions of the embryo, extracellular matrices containing fibronectin provide the "tracks" over which the migrating cells travel. All mesodermal cell migrations during gastrulation appear to depend on fibronectin pathways. Laminin is a major glycoprotein of basal laminae, and like fibronectin, it binds cells to collagen and to glycosaminoglycans. The cell binding region of laminin mostly recognizes neurons and epithelial cells.

The ratio of collagen to proteoglycan in the extracellular matrix varies from one embryonic region to another and from one connective tissue type to another. For example, cartilage has a high percentage of proteoglycans relative to the collagen content and is soft and pliable yet resistant to compression. Ligaments are predominantly collagen with a little proteoglycan and are relatively weak in compression but strong in tension.

CONCEPT: The extracellular matrix is a highly structured collection of collagen, proteoglycans, and other macromolecules that are essential for cellular recognition, migration, and adhesion.

EMBRYOGENESIS

Traditionally, gestation has been divided into the embryonic period and the fetal period. The embryonic period is considered to be the time from fertilization to the end of the eighth week of gestation; the remainder of gestation is called the fetal period. The five major stages of embryonic development are fertilization, cleavage, gastrulation, neurulation, and organogenesis (Table 1-3). By the end of the embryonic period, all of the major organ systems have been established, and the basic body plan is complete.

Fertilization and Cell Cleavage

At the moment of fertilization, the pronucleus of the sperm passes through the cell membrane of the oocyte and the two gamete pronuclei subsequently undergo a process of fusion to restore the diploid state (Fig. 1-3). Fertilization can be subdivided into three distinct phases:

1. Enzymatic penetration of the oocyte by the sperm and entry of the sperm pronucleus into the cytoplasm

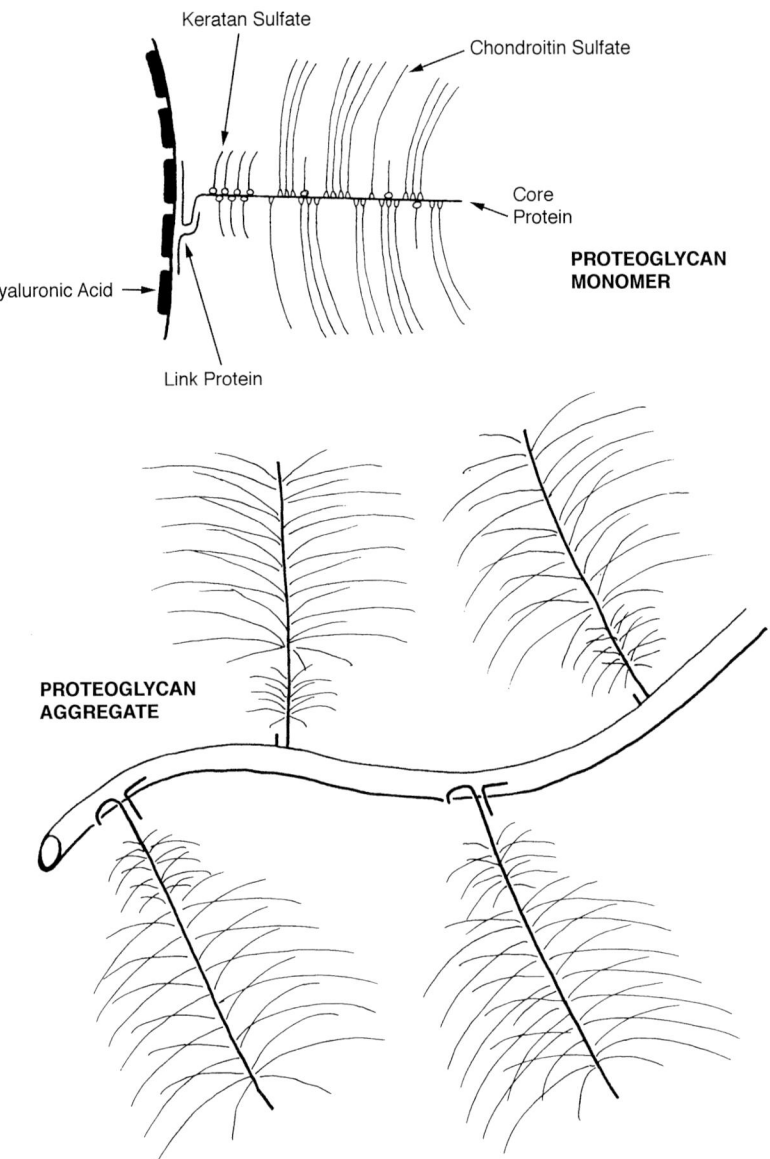

FIGURE 1-2. Glycosaminoglycans (keratan sulfate and chondroitin sulfate) attach to core proteins, forming proteoglycan monomers, which bind at regular intervals to a central strand of hyaluronic acid. The repulsion of multiple negative charges on the glycosaminoglycan chains causes maximum volume expansion of the aggregate. (Adapted from Lehninger AL, Nelson DI, Cox MM. Principles of biochemistry, 2nd ed. New York: Worth, 1993:314.

2. Immediate activation of the second meiotic division and extrusion of the second polar body from the oocyte
3. Fusion of the haploid sperm pronucleus with the haploid oocyte pronucleus to form a zygote containing 46 chromosomes—one set of 23 chromosomes from the father's gamete and the other set of 23 from the mother's gamete.

The sperm pronucleus is physically larger than the oocyte pronucleus but the oocyte contributes virtually

TABLE 1-3	Stages of Embryonic Development
Fertilization	Female and male gametes combine to form a zygote
Cleavage	The zygote divides into a ball of smaller cells, each receiving different parts of the maternal cytoplasm
Gastrulation	Migration and proliferation of cells to form the three primary germ layers, the ectoderm, the mesoderm, and the endoderm
Neurulation	Formation of the notochord, the neural crest, and the precursors of the central and peripheral nervous system
Organogenesis	Differentiation of the primary cell types to generate the organs

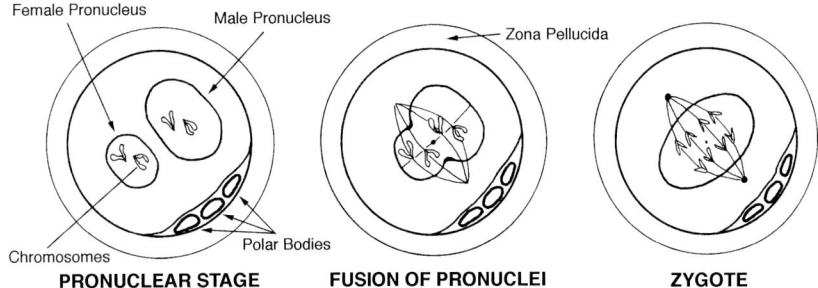

FIGURE 1-3. Fertilization occurs when sperm enzymes dissolve a hole in the zona pellucida, through which the sperm is able to contact and penetrate the oocyte plasma membrane. Entry of the sperm nucleus induces the second meiotic division. Subsequently, the female pronucleus, containing 23 chromosomes, and the larger male pronucleus, also containing 23 chromosomes, fuse to form the diploid zygote nucleus, containing 46 chromosomes. Note that virtually all the zygote cytoplasm, including all the subcellular organelles, comes from the oocyte. (Adapted from Larsen WJ. Human embryology. New York: Churchill Livingstone, 1993:18).

all the cytoplasm to the zygote, including subcellular organelles such as mitochondria, Golgi apparatus, and lysosomes.

Within 24 hours after fertilization, the zygote undergoes a succession of rapid cell divisions not accompanied by cellular growth. This means that the large single-celled zygote gets divided into a smaller group of cells called blastomeres. By 4 days, there are about 32 blastomeres, collectively still the same overall size as the zygote but packed into a tight ball that has the appearance of a small mulberry, hence the name morula, from the Latin term "morum," meaning "mulberry." The cells of the morula divide and grow in size until they form a hollow ball of about 1000 cells called a blastocyst. Although all the roughly 1000 cells of the blastocyst morphologically resemble each other, they are quite different biochemically because each cell contains a slightly different portion of the original maternal cytoplasm present in the oocyte. Each cell of the blastocyst is in contact with a different set of neighbors and experiences a somewhat different biochemical environment. Cell location and orientation in the blastocyst is not a purely random event but is genetically influenced. Each cell has a positional address from the molecular standpoint. The centrally located cells of the blastocyst, the inner cell mass, are induced to form a bilaminar disc composed of the epiblast (primary ectoderm) and the hypoblast (primary endoderm). It is the inner cell mass that subsequently becomes the embryo proper. The outer cell mass, also called the trophoblast, is the source of cells for the placenta.

Gastrulation, the Trilaminar Disc, and the Three Germ Layers

At the beginning of the third week of gestation, some cells of the inner mass begin to divide and migrate from the surface of the bilaminar disc, causing a faint midline primitive groove to appear on the surface (Fig. 1-4), signaling the initiation of gastrulation. As a result of this cell migration, the inner cell mass of the blastocyst becomes a trilaminar embryonic disc during gastrulation, establishing the three primary tissue layers: the ectoderm, the mesoderm, and the endoderm. The three primary tissues of the inner cell mass eventually become all of the organ systems. The ectoderm produces the central and peripheral nervous system, the sensory organs, the epidermis and its appendages. The mesoderm becomes bone, cartilage, muscle, heart, vessels, kidneys, gonads, and the spleen. The endoderm is the origin of the liver and pancreas; the linings, such as those of the respiratory and gastrointestinal tracts; the bladder and most of the urethra; plus the thyroid, parathyroid, and thymus glands.

Soon after the appearance of the primitive groove, the notochord begins to form, first in the cranial region and then rapidly extending in the caudal direction. Both the primitive streak and the notochord are strong inductive tissues that are responsible for initiating and orchestrating the formation of future organ systems. A group of genes encoding a zinc finger protein have been identified as being necessary for proper mesenchymal cell emigration from the primitive streak. Abnormalities in this gene prevent normal cell migration and interfere with the progress of gastrulation.[11,15] The cellular events of gastrulation firmly define the craniocaudal axis and set the stage for bilateral symmetry, coupled with craniocaudal asymmetry.

CONCEPT: The process of gastrulation defines the embryonic axes and results in the appearance of three primary germ layers: the ectoderm, the mesoderm, and the endoderm.

Anything that produces even a minor perturbation in the proper sequence of gastrulation can cause skeletal and visceral malformations, such as imperforate anus, sacral agenesis, or sirenomelia. Although it can

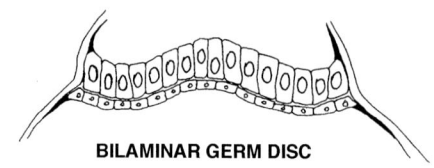
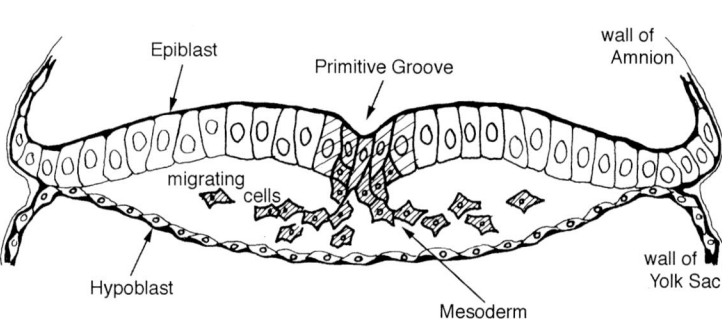

FIGURE 1-4. Transverse view of the cranial half of the inner cell mass of the bilaminar disc, and the cell migrations from the region of the primitive groove toward the hypoblast, resulting in the appearance of the mesoderm and the formation of the trilaminar disc. The epiblast becomes the ectoderm, and the hypoblast becomes the endoderm. (Adapted from Moore KL. The developing human, 4th ed. Philadelphia: WB Saunders, 1988:52.)

be said that all the events of embryogenesis are important, the extraordinary importance of gastrulation was underscored by the pioneering embryologist, Wolpert,[25,27] who noted that it is not birth, marriage, or death but gastrulation that is truly the most important event in your life.

Neurulation and Neurogenesis

The process of neurulation begins during the third week, with the formation of the neural plate on the surface of the embryonic ectoderm.[14] The underlying notochordal cells induce the differentiation of the neural plate cells. During the fourth week, the central cells of the neural plate divide in such a way as to produce an invagination, whereas cells along the lateral edges become elevated to form the neural folds. The elevated neural fold cells approach the midline and eventually join over the top of the invagination to close the neural tube (Fig. 1-5). The closure of the neural tube proceeds bidirectionally, ending with closure of the cranial and caudal neuropores. By the end of the fourth week, the embryonic nervous system consists of a closed tubular structure detached from the overlying ectoderm (Fig. 1-6).

Neuroepithelial cells lining the walls of the neural tube proliferate and differentiate to form the neuroblasts, which ultimately become the gray matter of the brain and spinal cord. The lumen of the neural tube becomes the ventricular system of the brain and the central canal of the cord. Neural crest cells detach from the neural plate and migrate to form the sympathetic ganglia and a variety of nonneuronal structures, such as the adrenal medulla and the melanocytes.

Genes control the initial shape and structure of the embryonic and fetal brain. The individual's experience in the world, however, subsequently fine-tunes the pattern of neural connections underlying cerebral function.[24] Throughout life, experience continues to change and modulate the quality of cortical connections, allowing adults to acquire new skills and new knowledge, such as the knowledge of interesting embryologic concepts.

If the neural tube fails to properly close, neural tissue remains exposed to the surface, producing rachischisis. If the caudal neuropore fails to properly close at the end of the fourth week, the clinical consequences can range from the mild condition of spina bifida occulta to the severe condition of a myelomeningocele (Fig. 1-7).

Differentiation of Somites and Organogenesis

As the notochord and the neural tube evolve from the ectoderm, cells of the paraxial mesoderm on each side of the notochord organize from a cranial to caudal direction, forming the 42 to 44 pairs of somites. Each somite is a tight collection of undifferentiated mesenchymal cells that becomes, in a segmental fashion, the axial skeleton, the head and trunk musculature, and the associated dermis. Shortly after they appear, each somite separates into three subdivisions known as the sclerotome, the myotome, and the dermatome (Fig. 1-8). Under the influence of morphogens produced by the notochord and the neural tube, the cells derived from the sclerotome form the rudimentary vertebral bodies and the vertebral arches (Fig. 1-9). Cells from

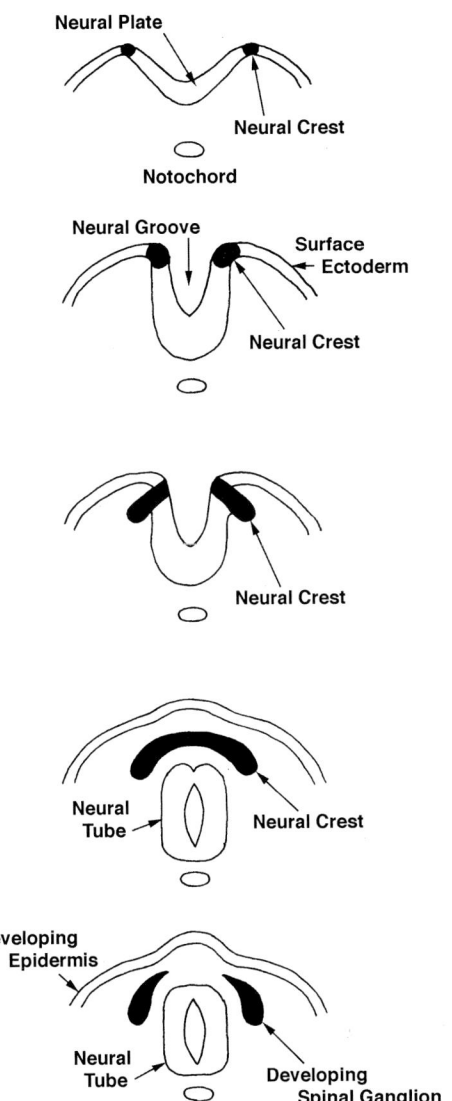

FIGURE 1-5. Transverse sections through progressively older embryos up to the end of the fourth week of gestation showing formation of the neural groove and neural crest that closes into the neural tube. (From Moore KL. The developing human, 4th ed. Philadelphia: WB Saunders, 1988:58).

the myotome differentiate into myoblasts, and cells from the dermatome contribute to the skin.

CONCEPT: Somites give rise to the sclerotome, the myotome, and the dermatome, which generate skeletal, muscular, and dermal tissues.

Organogenesis kicks into high gear during the fourth week, when the eyes appear and a four chamber heart starts to beat. At about the same time, the limb buds sprout from the lateral embryonic wall and begin to elongate. During the time from the fourth to the eighth week of gestation, all the major external and internal structures develop, and by the end of the eighth week, the embryo clearly has a human appearance.

CONCEPT: The second month of gestation is the period of organogenesis during which the basic structure of all organ systems is established.

Contracting rubella (German measles) during the period of organogenesis can severely affect fetal development, particularly the development of the central nervous system. Exposure to drugs such as thalidomide can disrupt the limb formation sequence, causing phocomelia.

Fetal Period

Early in the fetal period, the arms, legs and mouth begin to move. Reflexes such as the startle and the sucking reflex appear. The fetus assumes a position such that the hips are flexed and externally rotated, the knees are flexed, the legs are internally rotated and the feet are supinated. The skeleton undergoes considerable growth and ossification, and the head becomes covered with hair as all the epidermal appendages appear. The mother starts to feel the baby kick by the end of the fourth month. The third trimester is a period of rapid physical growth, refinement of organ structure, and a time of continued neurologic development, with formation of most major nerve tracts in the brain and spinal cord.

SKELETOGENESIS AND NEUROMUSCULAR INTEGRATION

At the cellular and the biochemical level, all the individual bones have a remarkably similar composition (i.e., osteocytes, osteoclasts, marrow cells, proteoglycans, collagen, and mineral). One of the facts about the skeleton, however, is that the individual bones have different lengths, widths, and characteristic shapes. It is by the process of pattern formation, the ordered spatial arrangement of cells to produce anatomic structure, that individual bones acquire their characteristic shapes.[26] Pattern formation produces a unique temporospatial orientation of precursor cells, such as that which occurs when a group of chondrocytes in the shoulder region assemble and synthesize a cartilaginous matrix in the rough shape of a scapula and those in the arm bud synthesize a precursor of a humerus. In this section are other examples of pattern formation and the developmental details of spine and limb formation are reviewed.

Spine Development

The spine has its embryologic origins in the cells that are induced to migrate out of the somite and toward the notochord and the neural tube (see Fig. 1-9). As a mass of sclerotomal cells collects segmentally at the

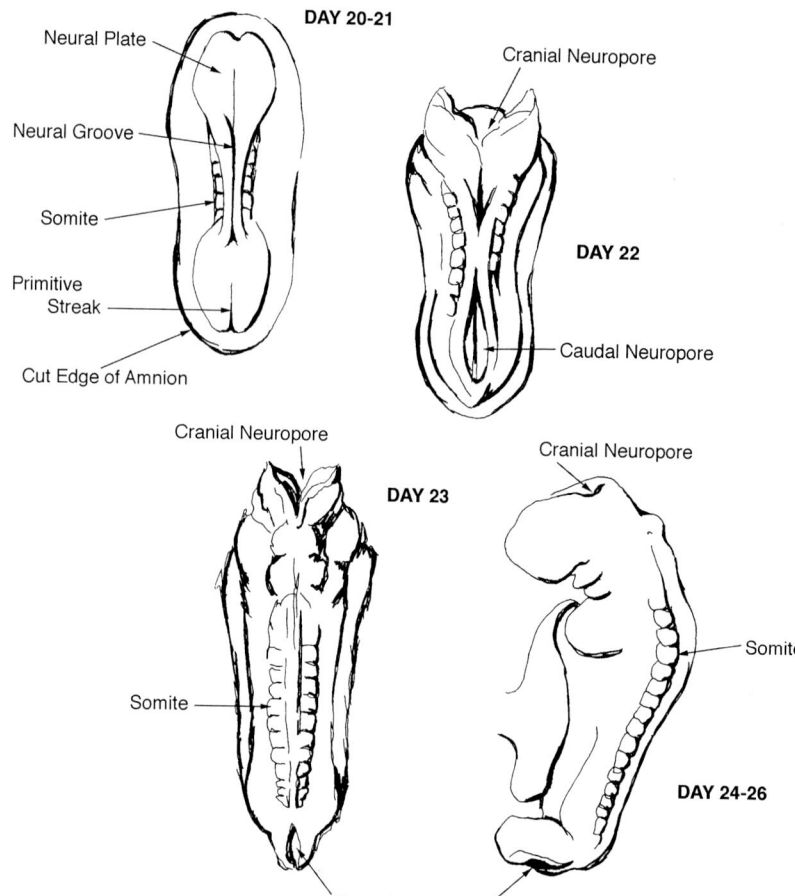

FIGURE 1-6. Progressively older embryos with the amniotic membrane cut away, showing the neural tube increasing in length as it "zippers-up" from both the cranial and the caudal ends. The neuropores become progressively smaller, and the cranial neuropore closes around day 24 of gestation. The caudal neuropore closes a few days later. Somites appear in the wake of neural tube closure. (Adapted from Larsen WJ. Human embryology. New York: Churchill Livingstone, 1993:75.)

embryonic midline, surrounding the neural tube and the notochord, the sclerotomal cells begin to separate into a cranial portion and a caudal portion. The cranial portion of each sclerotome recombines with the caudal portion of the directly superior sclerotome in a resegmentation process known as a metameric shift. After the metameric shift, spinal nerves, which originally left the neural tube to go to the center of the sclerotome, are able to pass between the precartilaginous vertebral bodies to innervate the segmental myo-

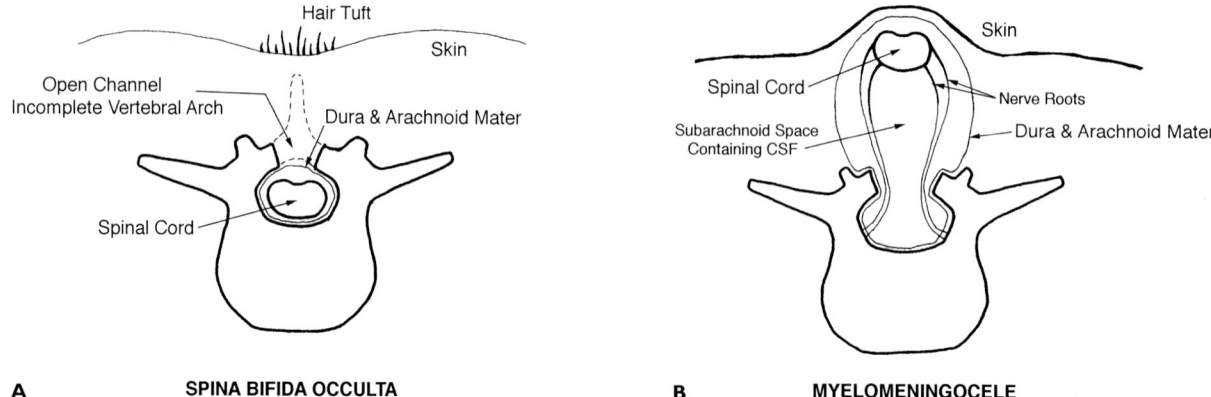

FIGURE 1-7. (A) Spina bifida occulta is an open bony channel that results from incomplete vertebral arch formation but has adequate dermal and epidermal coverage. It may be revealed by a small dimple, a tuft of hair, or a nevus overlying the incomplete arch. (B) Defective neural arch and dermal development can result in a myelomeningocele, in which a cyst, or a cele, protrudes and contains meninges in addition to portions of the spinal cord and spinal nerves. (Adapted from Larsen WJ. Human embryology. New York: Churchill Livingstone, 1993:86.)

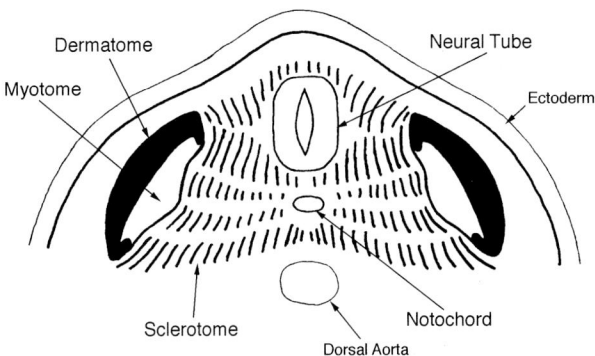

FIGURE 1-8. A transverse section through an embryo illustrates the relative locations of the dermatome, the myotome, and the sclerotome. (Adapted from Moore KL. The developing human, 4th ed. Philadelphia: WB Saunders, 1988:334.)

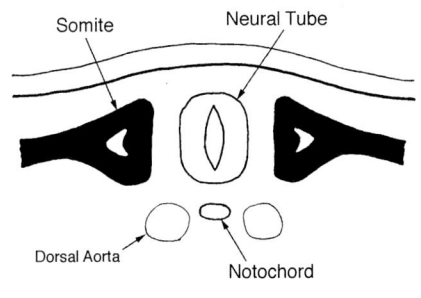

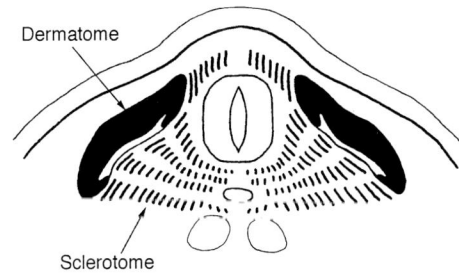

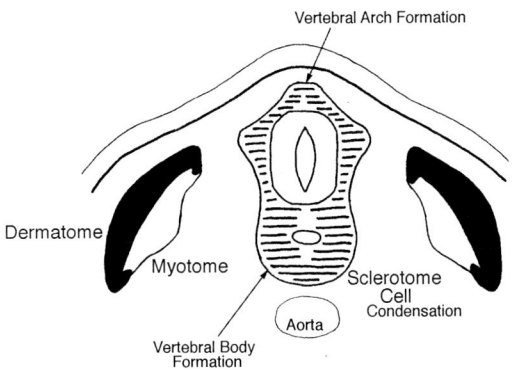

FIGURE 1-9. Ventromedial cells of the sclerotome migrate toward the midline of the embryo to surround the neural tube and the notocord, where these cells collect and divide before the metameric shift, forming the precursors of the vertebral arch and vertebral body. (Adapted from Larsen WJ. Human embryology. New York: Churchill Livingstone, 1993:67.)

tomes (Fig. 1-10). Because the segmental arteries initially grew into the area between the original sclerotomes, the arteries come to lie near the center of each precartilaginous vertebral body after the resegmentation.

The atlas and axis form by a mechanism that is different from that of the other vertebral bodies. Parts of the first cervical sclerotome plus the cranial portion of the second cervical sclerotome contribute cells, forming both the odontoid process and the arch of the atlas. Separation of the cranial portion of the second cervical sclerotome is incomplete because some of the cells fail to undergo the craniocaudal resegmentation. As a result, the residual cells form the odontoid, which remains connected to the body of the axis.[11,16]

In the cervical region, the eight cervical somites generate seven cervical vertebrae because the cranial portion of the first cervical sclerotome contributes to the formation of the occiput and the caudal portion of the eighth cervical sclerotome contributes to T1. The caudal portion of the C1 sclerotome then fuses with the cranial portion of the C2 sclerotome to form the atlas (Fig. 1-11). In this way, the eight cervical spinal nerves become associated with seven cervical vertebra. The first cervical spinal nerve passes between the base of the skull and the first cervical vertebra; the eighth cervical nerve exits below the seventh cervical vertebra and above the first thoracic vertebra (see Fig. 1-11). The remainder of the nerve roots exit below their corresponding vertebral bodies.

CONCEPT: The relation of the spinal nerves and arteries to the vertebrae is the result of the craniocaudal rearrangement of the sclerotomes.

The intervertebral discs form in the area between the resegmented vertebral bodies after the split of the sclerotomes. The nucleus pulposus originates from cells of the notochord, whereas the annulus fibrosis originates from the sclerotomal cells left behind after the resegmentation (Fig. 1-12). Occasionally persistent notochordal remnants remain in the region of the clivus at the base of the skull or in the sacrococcygeal region, creating a special class of neoplasms called chordomas.

The position of the spinal cord relative to the vertebral bodies changes with growth. At the end of the first trimester, the cord extends the entire length of the embryo. The embryonic trunk, the vertebral column, and the dura, which remains attached to the coccyx, grow at a faster rate than the cord, so that the terminal end of the cord gradually rises to a higher level. At birth, the end of the cord is at the level of the third lumbar vertebra, and the spinal nerves run obliquely downward to exit at a lower level of the vertebral column. At skeletal maturity, the cord terminates at the L1–L2 level (Fig. 1-13).

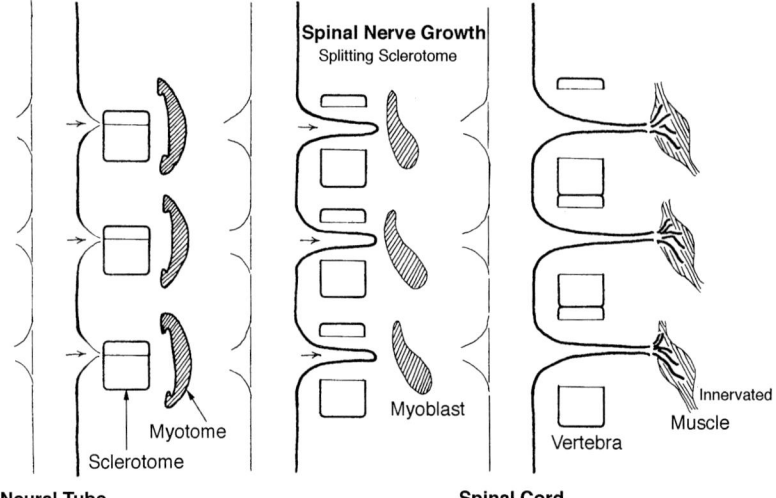

FIGURE 1-10. Morphogenesis of the vertebra. Each vertebral sclerotome splits into a cranial and a caudal portion. The cranial portion recombines with the caudal portion of the next superior sclerotome, permitting the segmental spinal nerves to grow out and innervate the myotome derivatives. (Adapted from Larsen WJ. Human embryology. New York: Churchill Livingstone, 1993:68).

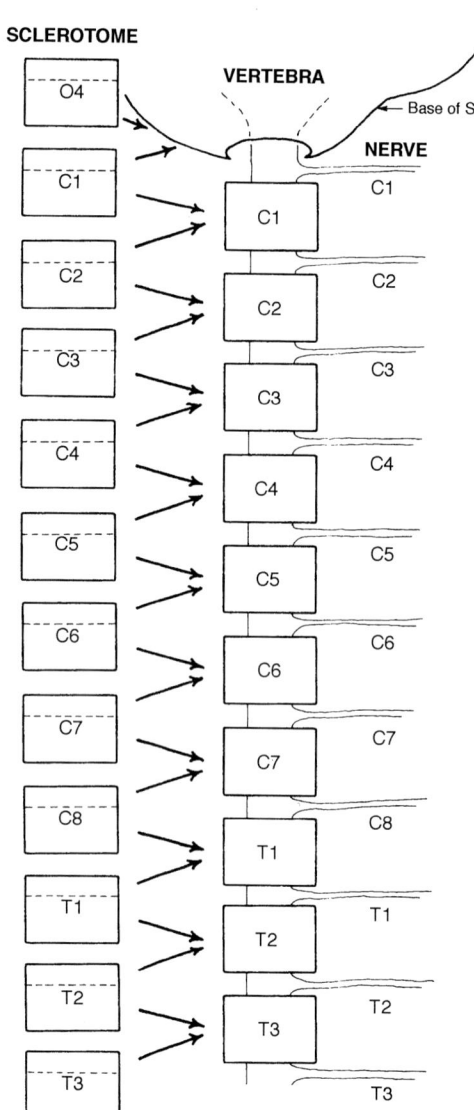

FIGURE 1-11. The cervical spine has eight nerves but seven cervical vertebrae as a result of the resegmentation of the sclerotomes. The cranial portion of the first cervical sclerotome combines with the fourth occipital sclerotome to contribute to the base of the skull, whereas the eighth cranial somite contributes to C7 and to T1. This resegmentation explains the superior relation of the cervical nerve roots to their corresponding vertebral bodies and the inferior relation of the remaining nerve roots to their corresponding vertebral bodies. (From Larsen WJ. Human embryology. New York: Churchill Livingstone, 1993:69.)

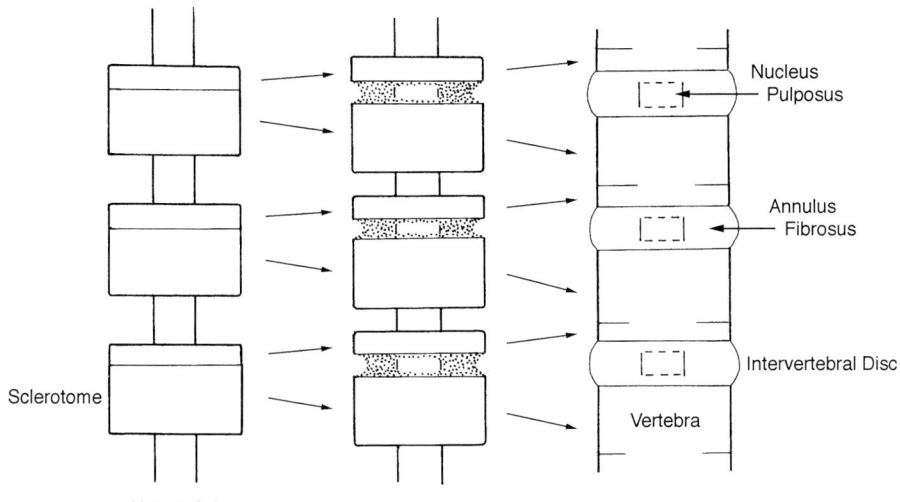

FIGURE 1-12. After cranial–caudal resegmentation, the residual sclerotomal cells coalese to form the annulus fibrosis of the disc, while the enclosed notochordal cells differentiate into the nucleus pulposus. Notochordal cells that are trapped within the vertebral bodies usually degenerate and disappear as the vertebral body undergoes further maturation. (Adapted from Larsen WJ. Human embryology. New York: Churchill Livingstone, 1993:70.)

Defects of formation or of segmentation can produce congenital spinal abnormalities. Defects of formation are recognized as wedged vertebrae, hemivertebrae, or butterfly vertebrae. Defects of segmentation result in unsegmented bars, laminar synostosis, or block vertebra. Because the cells of the sclerotome become the ribs and the vertebrae, rib anomalies such as fused or absent elements often accompany severe vertebral defects. Furthermore, during the same time that the sclerotomes are undergoing their metameric shift to form the vertebral bodies, the heart, kidneys, trachea, and esophagus are differentiating, so that a noxious influence during this time can produce the VACTER (vertebral, anal atresia, cardiac, tracheoesophageal, renal) association. The close temporospatial relation of vertebral body formation and nephrogenesis means that an insult during this time has an effect on both systems, which explains the clinical association of congenital vertebral anomalies with renal anomalies.

Limb Precursors

A morphogenetic field is a collection of cells that are committed as a group to become a particular organ, such as the heart, an eye, or a limb. One of the first morphogenetic fields to be identified was the limb field. Positional cues in the early limb bud facilitate skeletal pattern formation.[10,21] It is the expression of appropriate developmental genes that gives cells a mo-

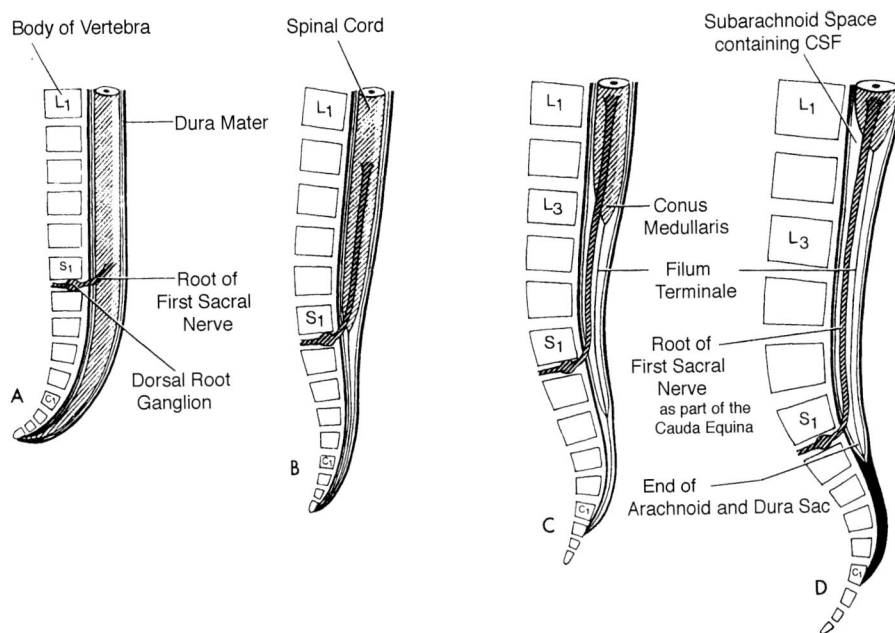

FIGURE 1-13. The position of the caudal end of the spinal cord changes in relation to the vertebral bodies during the various stages of development. (**A**) At 8 weeks of gestation, the cord extends all the way to the end of the coccygeal segments. (**B**) At 24 weeks, the cord ends at S1. (**C**) In the newborn, the cord ends at L3. (**D**) In the adult, the cord ends at the level of L1. (From Moore KL. The developing human, 4th ed. Philadelphia: WB Saunders, 1988:373.)

lecular positional address. Interpretation of this molecular positional information, coupled with local biochemical and biophysical signals, leads to the proliferation of the appropriate cells and to a refinement of skeletal precursor shape. Both epithelial-mesenchymal and mesenchymal-mesenchymal cell interactions are necessary for this process to proceed normally. Some of the signaling agents that have been discovered thus far include the retinoids, transforming growth factor-β, fibroblast growth factors, and a family of proteins named "hedgehog" after the appearance of certain Drosophila mutants. Fibroblast growth factors provide the signal that makes the limb bud elongate and allows the sequential placement of bony precursors along the length of the limb. Retinoids appear to mediate large-scale pattern changes, such as the division of the upper limb bud into the brachium and the forearm. Transforming growth factor-β directs differentiation of skeletal precursor cells, whereas the hedgehog proteins—and one protein in particular, named "sonic"—appear to be involved in determining individual bone identity, such as deciding which metacarpal will be part of the thumb and which will go on to become an index finger.

Apical Ectodermal Ridge and Limb Formation

Appendicular bones trace their origin to the mesenchymal cells of the limb field that arise from the somatic layer of the lateral plate mesoderm. These cells migrate laterally to cause a bulge under the embryonic epidermis. This bulge is called the limb bud. The upper limb buds appear first as small bulges along the lateral walls opposite somites C5 to T1. Within the limb bud, skeletal precursors initially appear as mesenchymal condensations, which are focal areas of densely packed, undifferentiated cells.[17,18] Mesenchymal condensations bear only a minimal resemblance to the future bone at that site. Under the influence of morphogens such as transforming growth factor-β, these mesenchymal cells synthesize and secrete large amounts of type II collagen. As the cartilaginous extracellular matrix accumulates, the founding cells enlarge (hypertrophy), whereas the cells at the periphery flatten into an investing sheath called the perichondrium. In this way, the basic shape of an individual bone is first formed in cartilage.[20]

The upper limb buds appear at the beginning of the fourth week, and the lower limb buds appear a few days later opposite the third to the fifth lumbar and the first three sacral somites. The proximal parts of the limb buds appear and differentiate earlier than the distal parts. At each stage of development, the lower limb lags slightly behind that of the upper limb.

CONCEPT: There is a cranial-to-caudal and a proximal-to-distal sequence in limb development.

Each limb bud consists of an inner mesodermal core and an outer ectodermal cap of pseudostratified columnar epithelium called the apical ectodermal ridge (AER).[18] The AER is essential for the formation of the limb and exerts a permissive effect on limb growth and elongation. Growth and differentiation of the limb bud depend absolutely on biochemical interactions between mesoderm and the overlying ectodermal AER. If the AER is removed surgically, no further distal limb development occurs, and only those parts of the limb already laid down behind the AER continue to develop.

The limb bud elongates as a result of mesenchymal cell proliferation in a region directly under the AER, a special region called the progress zone. Evidence indicates that one of the AER-signaling molecules is fibroblast growth factor 2.[2] The AER directs the flipper-like limb buds to elongate and to eventually flatten at the ends into the paddle-like hand and foot plates.[5]

Initially, an uninterrupted stretch of primitive mesenchymal cells occupies the core of the limb bud but within 2 weeks, the mesenchyme differentiates into cartilage, and shallow surface constrictions appear at the sites of future joints. Cartilage replaces mesenchyme in a proximodistal sequence (Fig. 1-14).

The proximodistal axes of human limbs are highly polarized. Limbs originate at the shoulder/pelvis with a single bone (humerus/femur); after the appearance of a joint (elbow/knee), two additional bones, the radius/tibia and the ulna/fibula, extend outward to the multiple bones of the wrist/ankle and the fingers/toes.[6] Mathematical models are known that describe such a sequence. Polynomial equations called Bessel functions can explain limb polarization based on competing morphogen concentrations. The anteroposterior (thumb/little finger) axis of the limb seems to be determined by a special region of cells called the zone of polarizing activity, which secretes both retinoic acid and the hedgehog protein. By day 33, the shoulders, arms, forearms, and paddle-like hand plates have formed, whereas the feet appear as tapering distal tips of the lower limb buds. By the early part of the sixth week, chondrification has started in the humerus, radius, and ulna; a few days later, chondrocytes appear in the femur and tibia.

By the end of the sixth week, the limb buds clearly have an external resemblance to mature limbs.[16,22] Early in the seventh week, all the skeletal elements of the upper limb, except the distal phalanges, are undergoing chondrification. Finger rays are visible in the hands as radial thickenings of the digital plates.[28]

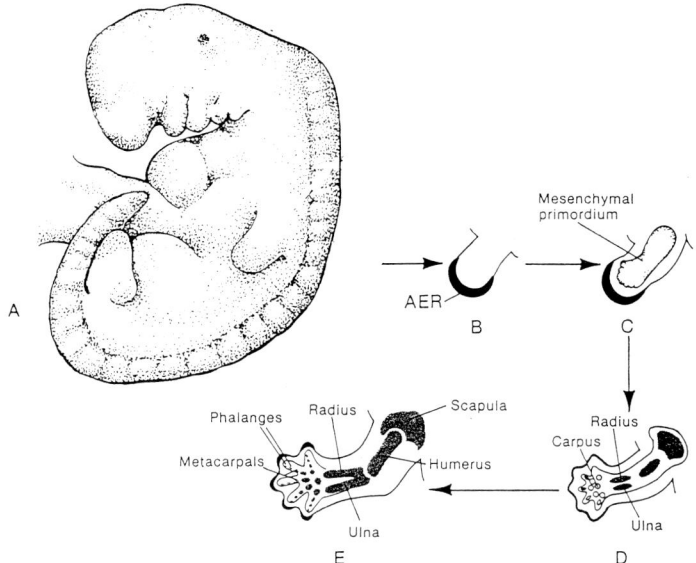

FIGURE 1-14. Developmental sequence of the limbs. (**A**) The limb buds sprout from the lateral somatic mesoderm and grow laterally and caudally. (**B**) Magnified view of the limb bud shows the ectodermal covering and the apical ectodermal ridge. (**C**) Continuous tube of mesenchyme occupies the center of the limb bud. (**D**) Centers of the chondrification appear in a proximodistal gradient. (**E**) By the end of 6 weeks, cartilaginous miniatures of the bones-to-be are present. The hand plate is still in the shape of a mitten, and the apical ectodermal ridge remains only at the tips of each digit. (From Moore KL. The developing human, 4th ed. Philadelphia: WB Saunders, 1988:346).

By a process of programmed cellular death called apoptosis, the cells in the interdigital necrotic zones begin to die. Death of these cells occurs in the absence of any obvious external insult and is thought to be a form of cellular suicide, in which a genetic death program is activated that causes the release of lysosomal enzymes that kill the cells. A gene named *REAPER* has been shown to encode a small peptide that controls apoptosis in *Drosophila*, and presumably in other organisms also.[23] Failure of apoptosis in the human foot or hand plate results in the condition of syndactyly.

CONCEPT: Programmed cell death, apoptosis, is a part of normal development.

The foot passes through a developmental stage when it is in a position of equinus, supination, and forefoot adduction, externally resembling that of a clubfoot. During the eleventh week, as ankle movement increases, the foot gradually returns to a more neutral position.[5,8] Another interesting observation is that the incidence of cartilaginous talocalcaneal bridges in the region of the sustentaculum tali is high during the ninth and tenth weeks but most of the bridges disappear by the time of birth.[9]

Neuromuscular Development

Ganglia invade and innervate the somites as they are taking shape, establishing a "one nerve, one somite" relation that remains, no matter how far the derivatives of the somite migrate during their subsequent development. For example, the shoulder girdle and the upper limb buds initially appear at the embryonic neck because they form opposite the lower cervical and first thoracic somites and are innervated by cervical ganglia. The shoulder and limb anlagen subsequently migrate caudally and rotate but they retain their original somite-ganglion relations (Fig. 1-15). If caudal migration of the shoulder anlagen is somehow prevented, as may occur because of the presence of an omovertebral bone or a cartilaginous bar, the result is a high-riding scapula of Sprengel deformity.

CONCEPT: Upper and lower extremity innervation retains the original pattern of somite innervation.

During the fifth week, cells migrate out of the myotome and invade the limb buds, forming dorsal and ventral condensations of myoblasts that are the precursors of the limb musculature. The individual myoblasts undergo cell fusion to form large conglomerate syncytia called myotubes. Newly synthesized contractile proteins, actin and myosin, polymerize within the myotubes to form the sarcomeres. Movement of muscle begins as innervation takes place in the eighth week. At about sixteen weeks, the multiple cellular nuclei migrate to their final subsarcolemma position. Generally, the dorsal muscle mass produces the extensor/supinator group of the upper limb and the extensor/abductor group of the lower limb. The ventral muscle mass of the limb buds produces the flexor/pronator group of the upper and the flexor/adductor group of the lower limb.

Limb Rotation

The limb buds protrude outward at about right angles to the embryonic torso, with the longitudinal axes of the upper and lower limb buds being relatively parallel. As the result of differential growth rates between

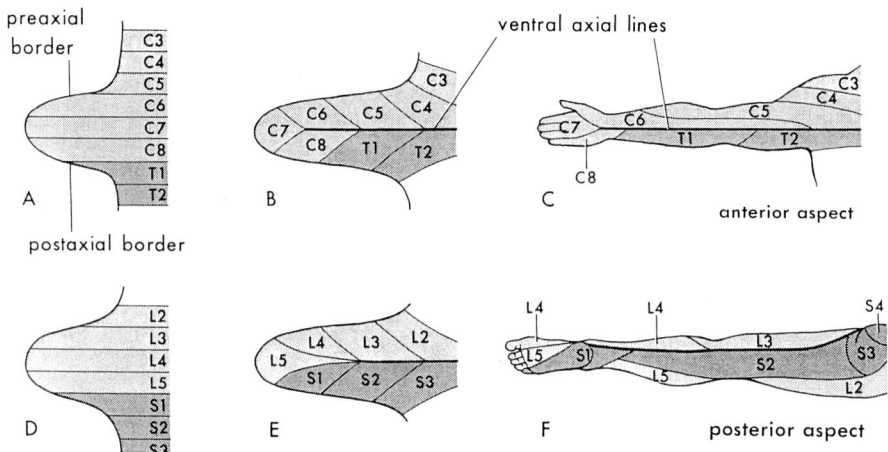

FIGURE 1-15. (**A** and **D**) The ventral aspect of the limb buds early in the fifth week of gestation show the primitive segmental arrangement of the dermatomal patterns. (**B** and **E**) Similar views after growth of the buds. (**C** and **F**) The adult pattern. Most of the original ventral surface of the lower limb lies on the back of the adult limb because of the medial rotation of the lower limb with further development. In the upper limb, the ventral line extends along the anterior surface of the arm and forearm; in the lower limb, the ventral axial line extends along the medial side of the thigh and knee, toward the posteromedial aspect of the leg and the heel. (From Moore KL. The developing human, 4th ed. Philadelphia: WB Saunders, 1988:357.)

the ectoderm and the mesenchyme, the limbs gradually begin to rotate and then to slightly flex at the sites of the future elbows/knees. The upper limbs rotate externally to put the forearm flexors in a medial position, the extensors lateral, the thumbs ventral, and the elbows dorsal.[7] The lower limbs rotate internally to place the extensors in a ventral position and the flexors dorsal. The anatomic consequences of lower limb rotation can be observed in the well-known spiral twisting of the hip capsule. Figure 1-16 summarizes the timeline of upper and lower limb development.

Intrauterine molding of the fetal lower limbs during the third trimester causes the hips to assume a posture of flexion and external rotation, with the thighs held in lateral rotation. The knees are flexed and the legs are usually crossed and held in medial rotation, whereas the feet are somewhat supinated.[19]

CONCEPT: Final limb position is due to external rotation of the upper limb buds, internal rotation of the lower limb buds, plus intrauterine molding of the fetus.

Synovial Joint Development

As mentioned earlier in this chapter, the skeletal precursors of the limb appear initially as a continuous central core of scleroblastema (primitive skeletal mesenchyme) induced by the AER. It is during the sixth week that joints begin to form at the appropriate locations within the scleroblastema. The rudimentary joints initially appear as areas of densely packed homogenous cells called the interzone.

Cells within the interzone differentiate into three distinct groups: chondrogenic cells lying next to the scleroblastema; synovial precursor cells; and central interzonal cells that become the intraarticular elements of the joints (Fig. 1-17). The chondrogenic cells become the articular cartilage. The outer layers of the synovial precursor cells assume a more fibrous phenotype and produce the joint capsule, whereas the inner layers produce the highly vascular synovial membranes. Some of the cells of the central interzone produce the intraarticular structures (e.g., menisci, cruciate ligaments), whereas the remainder of the cells undergo apoptosis, forming small spaces that coalesce into a joint cavity containing synovial fluid.[17] Homeotic genes appear to be responsible for determining the exact location of the joints, and local cellular signals appear to activate the process of cavitation because a basic joint cleft appears before muscular innervation and before any movement occurs in the limb. Soon after cavitation, however, the newly innervated muscles result in limb movement that is essential for proper joint development. In certain pathologic conditions, such as arthrogryposis multiplex congenita, decreased or absent muscular activity appears to be the proximate cause of stiff, abnormally shaped joints that are clinically apparent at the time of birth.

CONCEPT: Normal joint development requires muscular activity and limb movement.

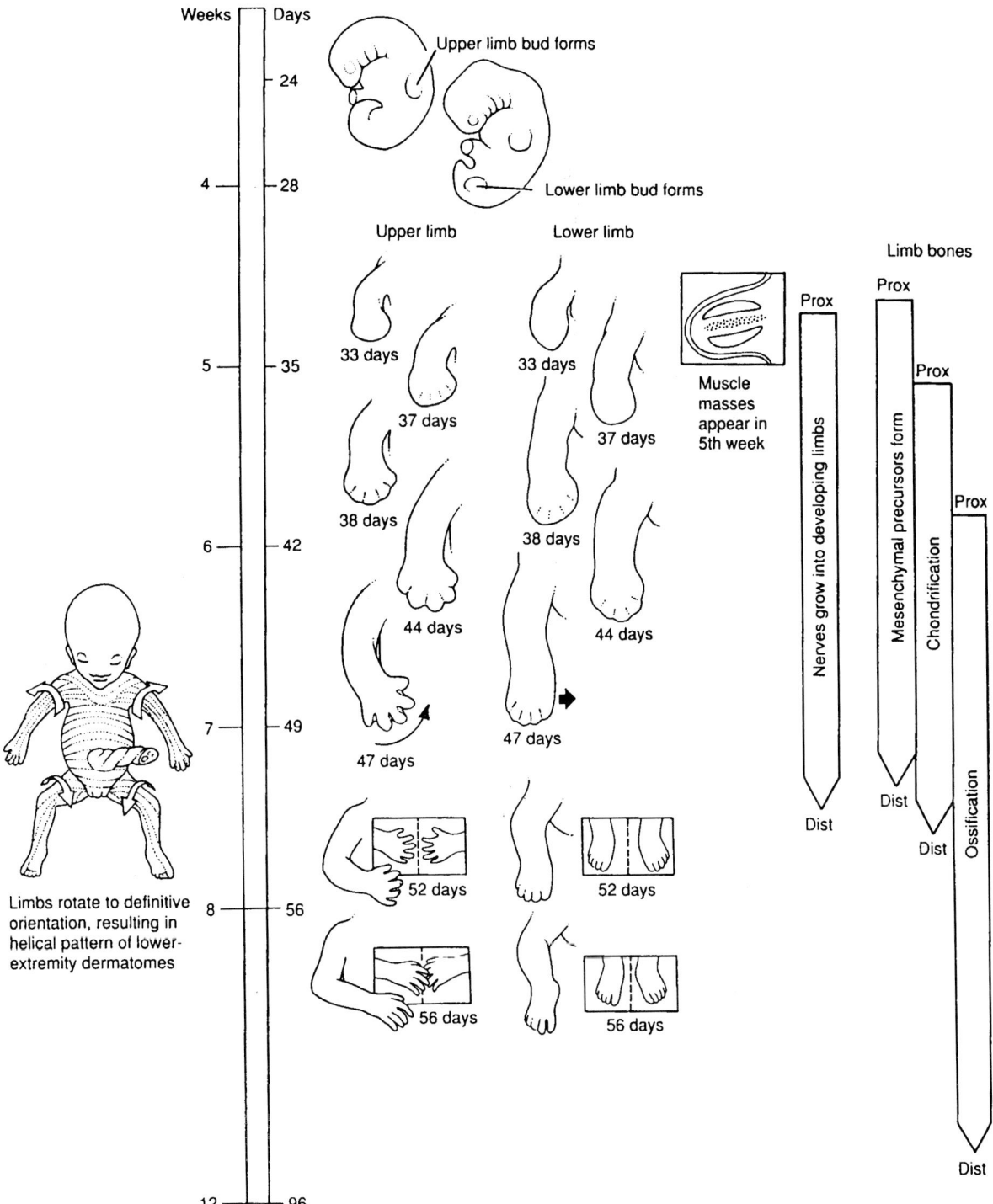

FIGURE 1-16. Timeline of upper and lower limb development. (From Larsen WJ. Human embryology. New York: Churchill Livingstone, 1993:282.)

The knee goes through an intermediate cavitation stage, in which it is divided into three large chambers. If the cells comprising the walls of these chambers fail to undergo apoptosis, the result is the clinically familiar synovial plica. The most common wall remnant is the infrapatellar plica (ligamentum mucosum). This is followed by the less frequent suprapatellar plica and finally by the least common but probably most symptomatic wall remnant, the mediopatellar plica.

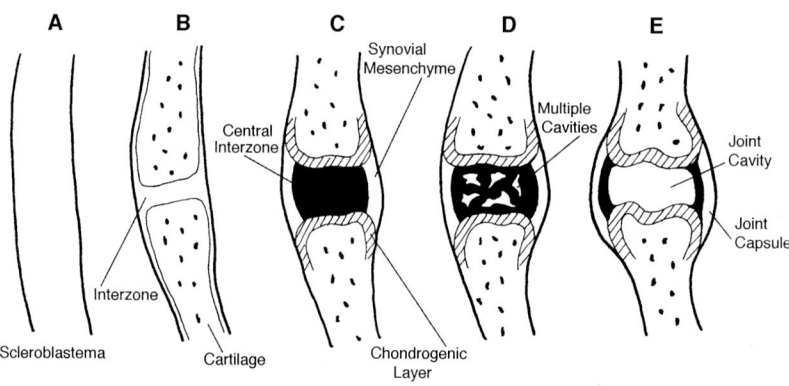

FIGURE 1-17. (A) The early limb bud, with a continuous central core of scleroblastema. (B) Appearance of the interzone, which is the site of the future joint. (C) The three-part interzone consists of the central interzone, the synovial mesenchyme, and the chondrogenic layer. (D) Multiple cavities appear within the central interzone, the area of the future joint space. (E) The multiple cavities coalesce into one joint cavity, characteristic of a mature joint.

BONE FORMATION

The general process of bone formation is known as osteogenesis. There are two distinct mechanisms of osteogenesis: intramembranous and endochondral bone formation. In both mechanisms, bone does not form de novo; it is made either in an area occupied by fibrous mesenchyme or in an area of cartilaginous tissue. The clavicle and the mandible, which are the first bones to begin ossification early in the seventh week, are intramembranous bones that form by direct transformation of the fibrous mesenchyme; they do not have cartilaginous precursors. The next fetal bones to undergo osteogenesis are the scapula and humerus, followed by the radius and the ulna. These skeletal elements form by bony replacement of a cartilaginous precursor through the process of endochondral ossification. Except the clavicle, all the bones of the appendicular and the axial skeleton form by endochondral ossification. Continuous modeling and remodeling of the skeletal elements to define and further refine their shape requires both endochondral and intramembranous mechanisms.

Intramembranous Bone Formation

Intramembranous bone formation occurs when osteoblasts are induced to differentiate directly from a layer of loose fibrous mesenchyme. After receiving the appropriate induction signal, the mesenchymal cells become more rounded and basophilic, indicating the presence of ample endoplasmic reticulum, ribosomes, and Golgi, the cellular machinery necessary for the synthesis and secretion of proteins. These plump, rounded cells are called osteoblasts, and the proteins that they secrete make up the extracellular substance called osteoid, the organic matrix of bone. High levels of the enzyme alkaline phosphatase and the appearance of matrix vesicles in the osteoid mark the commencement of ossification. Cells that become completely surrounded by the mineralized osteoid are called osteocytes.

The first bit of new bone has the shape of an irregular spicule, which gradually lengthens and joins with other spicules, anastomosing into a structure called a trabeculae. Spicules and trabeculae grow into a three-dimensional lattice-like network known as the primary spongiosa. Osteoblasts cover the surface of the spongiosa and deposit new layers of bone matrix on the preexisting bony scaffold. This process repeats numerous times as the bone tissue builds up layer on layer. While new bone is being deposited on some surfaces, excess bone is being removed from other surfaces by a special group of multinucleated phagocytic cells called osteoclasts. Remodeling is the net result of bone formation at some sites and of bone resorption at others. Continued appositional growth coupled with trabecular remodeling increases the size and refines the shape of a bone.

Endochondral Ossification

The process of endochondral ossification begins as the condensed scleroblastema divides and differentiates into chondroblasts in the central portion of the limb bud. The chondroblasts mature into chondrocytes as they synthesize the extracellular matrix of the cartilaginous anlagen. Interstitial and appositional chondrocyte growth plus the continued synthesis of a hyaline matrix causes the cartilaginous anlagen to increase in size. Eventually, bone tissue completely replaces the cartilage anlagen as the chondrocytes go through a sequence of cellular changes—proliferation, maturation, hypertrophy and apparent degeneration—before ossification. As the cartilage model continues to grow, the central chondrocytes hypertrophy and massively increase their cellular volume. Calcium salts begin to precipitate in the matrix partitions separating the hypertrophic cells, and capillary buds penetrate the perichondrium and begin to invade the hypertrophic cells. Osteoblasts appear in the wake of the capillary invasion and begin to lay down a thin collar of osteoid around the midsection of the cartilage model. The perichondrium is called a periosteum.

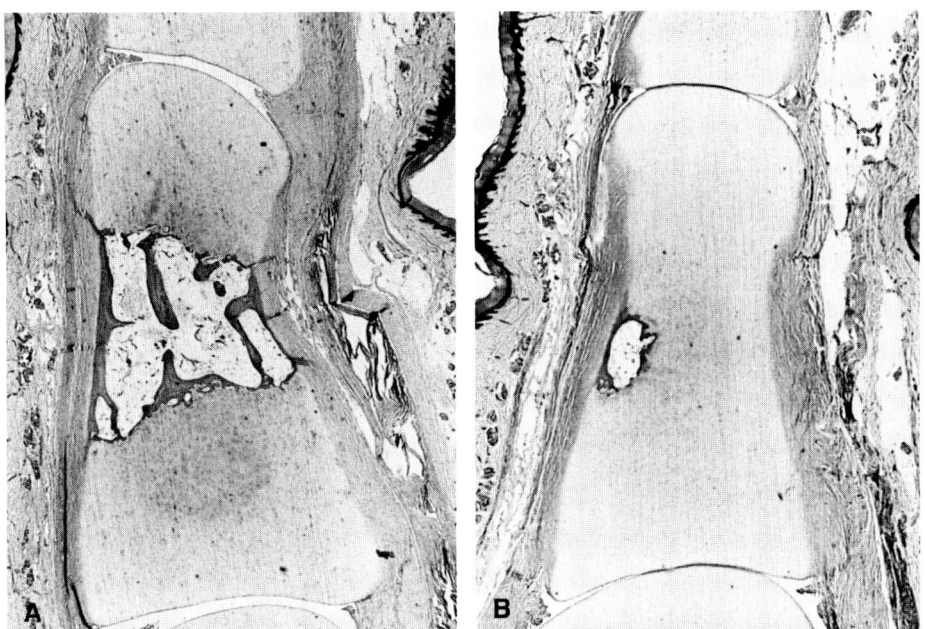

FIGURE 1-18. (A) The primary ossification center in the central portion of a fetal phalynx. Note the central symmetric location of the center and how the synovial mesenchyme conforms to the shape of the joint space. (B) Delayed formation of the primary ossification center in a case of digital duplication. The lack of vascular invasion delays ossification and is responsible for the peripheral, eccentric, gradually expanding center. (From Ogden JA. Pediatric Orthopaedics, 3rd ed. Philadelphia: JB Lippincott, 1990:2.)

The bone collar surrounds the midsection of the cartilage model as more capillaries, accompanied by more osteoblasts, invade the middle of the calcified cartilage and establish the primary ossification center (Fig. 1-18). In this vascularized environment, osteoblasts deposit layers of osteoid on the residual calcified cartilage, and bone tissue gradually replaces the formerly solid mass of cartilage (Fig. 1-19). Eventually, osteoclasts begin the remodeling process in the center of the primary ossification center, leaving a central medullary cavity as the ossification front proceeds toward the ends of the cartilage anlagen.

Mechanical Loading and Bone Development

Experimental observations confirm that cartilaginous anlagen of long bones grows in organ culture and even develops the rough outline of diaphyseal and epiphyseal regions, presumably under the sole influence of the genetic programs.[20] Subsequent skeletal morphogenesis fails in organ culture, however, due at least partly to the absence of mechanical-biochemical interactions. Clinical observations have confirmed that abnormal limb movement can alter the pattern of bone growth and ossification. For example, a decrease or an absence of normal joint forces can delay the appearance of secondary ossification centers,[22] such as that which occurs in patients with myelomeningocele, infantile poliomyelitis, and arthrogryposis.

Carter and associates[3] have used a biomechanical model to study skeletogenesis. They have proposed that mechanical stresses, created by an increasingly active embryonic neuromuscular system, play a major role in the developmental biology of bones. Carter predicted that endochondral ossification is accelerated by intermittently applied shear stress and is inhibited by high compressive-dilatational stress. Theoretic calculations based on this model have successfully

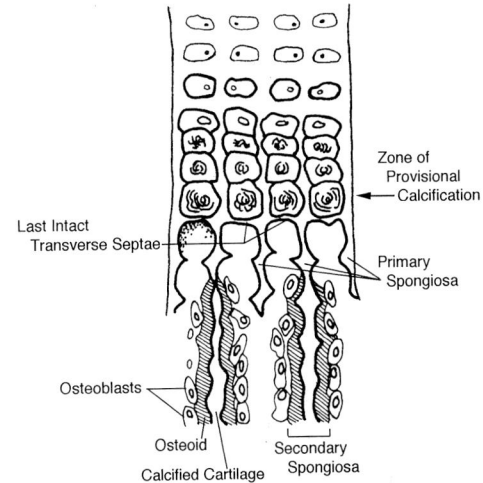

FIGURE 1-19. Within the growth plate, the primary spongiosa are the calcified bars that extend into the metaphysis and are the remnants of the longitudinal septa of the hypertrophic zone. Secondary spongiosa form by the addition of layers of woven bone on top of the primary spongiosa.

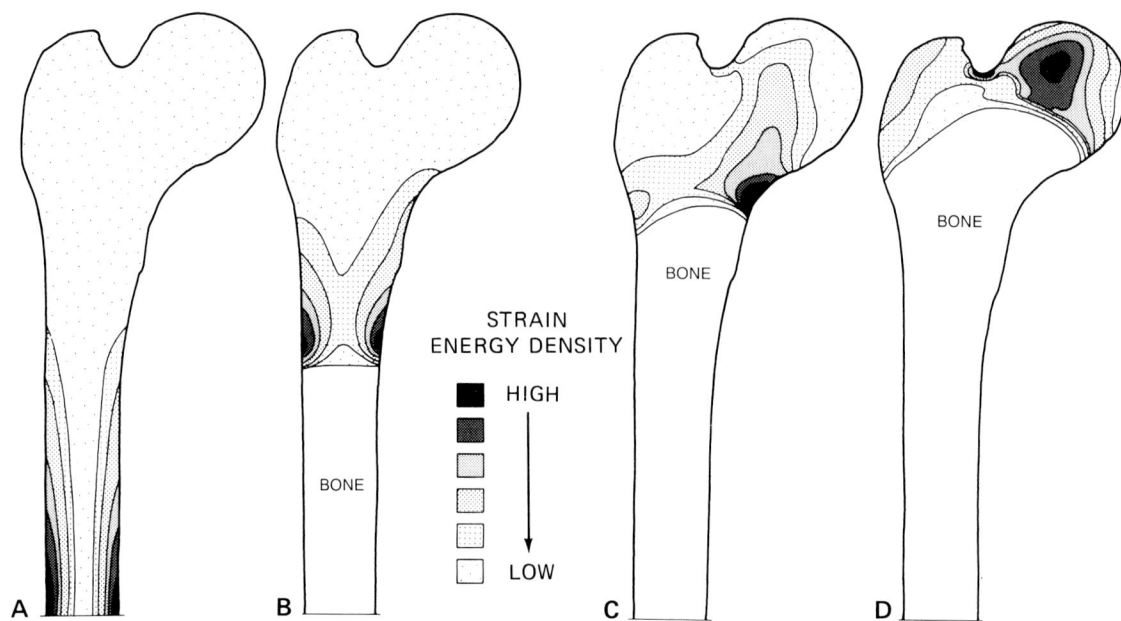

FIGURE 1-20. Distributions of cartilage strain energy imposed by mechanical loading at various stages of ossification. (**A**) At 8 weeks of gestation. (**B**) At 11 weeks of gestation. (**C**) At 30 weeks. (**D**) At 4 months of age. The pattern of changing high-strain energy calculations presages the pattern of progressive ossification in the cartilaginous femur. (From Carter DR, Orr TE, Fyhrie DP, Schurman DJ. Influence of mechanical stress on prenatal and postnatal skeletal development. Clin Orthop 1987;219:237.)

simulated the morphologic features of a variety of embryonic bones, such as the femoral anlagen (Fig. 1-20), the radiohumeral joint, and the sternum.[4] This model was able to predict the key features of bone formation, including:

- development of the primary ossification site
- appearance of a tubular diaphysis and marrow cavity
- location and geometry of the growth plate
- appearance and location of the secondary ossification center.[3]

The high correlation between the known ossification pattern of the cartilaginous anlagen and the mechanical stress history implies an important causal role for mechanical forces in skeletal morphogenesis.

Growth Plate Development

It is convenient to think about the growth plate, or physis, as being composed of three parts. The first part is the growth cartilage, which is divided into recognizable cellular zones. The second part is the metaphysis, which is the region where bone replaces the remnants of calcified cartilage. The third part of the physis is the circumferential fibrous structures, consisting of the perichondrial ring of LaCroix and the groove of Ranvier.

The perichondrial ring of LaCroix and the ossification groove of Ranvier surround the growth plate. Although both the ring and the groove are part of the same anatomic structure, they have different biologic functions. The perichondrial ring contains a thin extension of the metaphyseal cortex that has been referred to as the "bone bark." The ring contains circumferential collagen fibers that provide a peripheral supporting girdle around the physis and is continuous with the fibrous layer of the metaphyseal periosteum. The ossification groove is a wedge-shaped collection of cells jutting out into the growth cartilage in the region of the reserve and proliferative zones. The groove is an area of intense cellular division, a germinal zone that replenishes the supply of reserve chondrocytes by providing cells for the growth in diameter of the physis (Fig. 1-21). Together, the perichondrial ring of LaCroix and the ossification groove of Ranvier support and expand the width of the growth plate.

Within the growth cartilage, chondrocytes undergo a series of biochemical and morphologic changes that result in the production of longitudinal bone growth. These cellular changes are responsible for the recognizable histologic zones of the growth cartilage: the reserve zone, the proliferating zone, and the hypertrophic zone. The hypertrophic zone is subdivided further into three additional zones: the zone of maturation, the zone of degeneration, and the zone of provisional calcification. Growth cartilages from different bones have a different overall thickness due

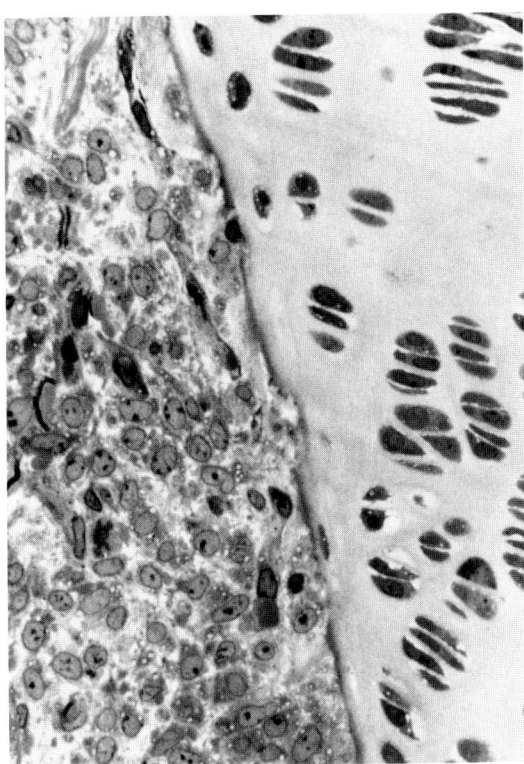

FIGURE 1-21. Photomicrograph of the zone of Ranvier shows the demarcation of the hypertrophic cells from the highly cellular germinal zone that contributes cells toward widening of the physis. (From Ogden JA. Pediatric orthopaedics, 3rd ed. Philadelphia: JB Lippincott 1990:19.)

to the relative numbers and the orientation of the chondrocytes in the various zones (Fig. 1-22). Generally, the greater the number of chondrocytes, the taller the plate and the faster the growth rate of the bone.

To a large extent, the cellular physiology within each of the zones depends on the quality of the blood supply and hence on the oxygen tension and the substrate concentrations. Three major arterial systems supply the growth plate: the epiphyseal arteries, the nutrient artery, and the perichondrial arteries (Fig. 1-23). The epiphyseal arteries send branches through the cartilaginous epiphysis within cartilage canals to supply the growth plate cells. The capillaries from this arterial system penetrate only to the level of the proliferating zone; the hypertrophic zone remains avascular. Thus, embryonic growth cartilage, unlike adult articular cartilage, has a vascular supply (Fig. 1-24).

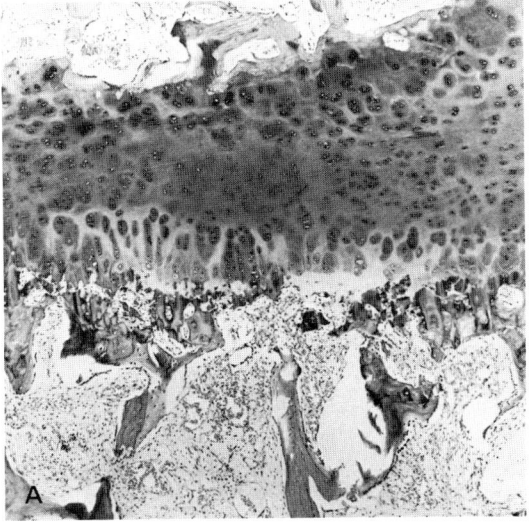
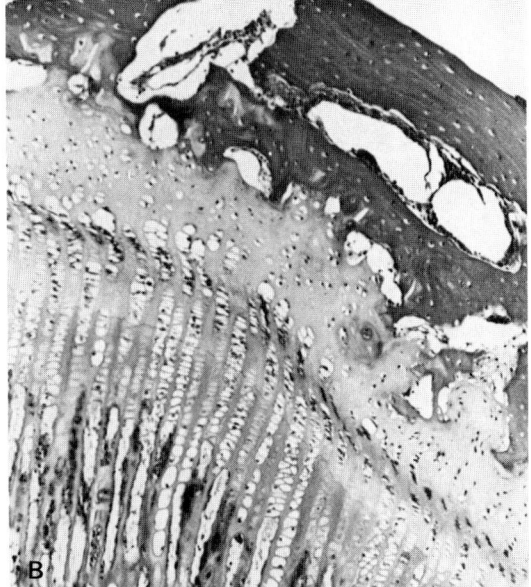
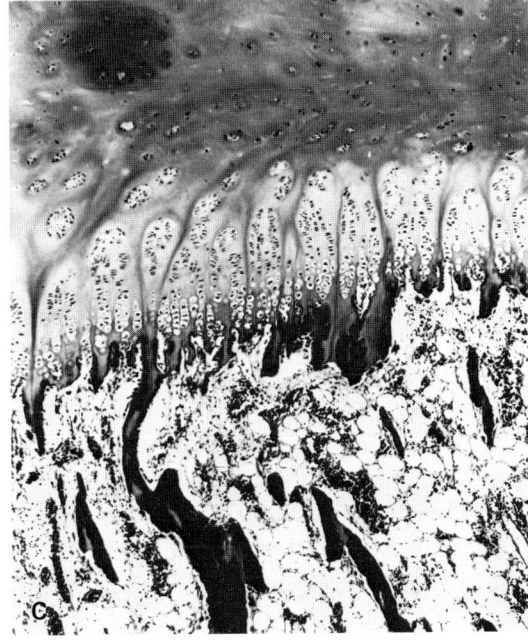

FIGURE 1-22. Variations in physeal morphology. (**A**) Slow-growing phalangeal physis with limited cell column formation. (**B**) Rapidly growing distal femoral physis with elongated cell columns. (**C**) Some rapidly growing physes form clone-like groupings of hypertrophic cell columns divided by longitudinal cartilaginous columns. (From Ogden JA. Pediatric orthopaedics, 3rd ed. Philadelphia: JB Lippincott, 1990:17.)

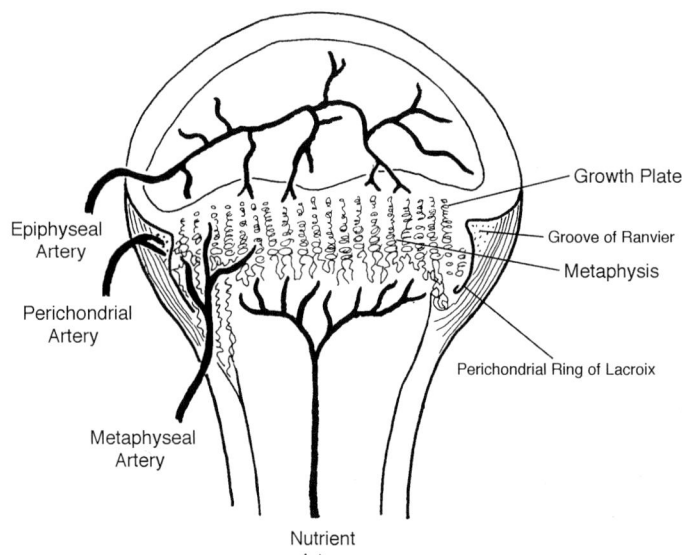

FIGURE 1-23. Schematic of the blood supply to a typical long bone. The epiphyseal artery supplies the secondary ossification center and provides circulation to the growth cartilage. The perichondrial artery supplies the groove of Ranvier and LaCroix ring. Vascular buds from the metaphyseal and nutrient arteries grow into the degenerating, hypertrophic lacunae. (From Gamble JG. The musculoskeletal system. Physiological basics. New York: Raven Press, 1988:49.)

The nutrient artery enters the diaphysis and terminates in an extensive capillary network at the junction of the metaphysis and the growth cartilage. This arterial system is responsible for importing the osteoblasts. Closed capillary loops from the nutrient arterioles grow into the residual hypertrophic lacunae after dissolution of the transverse cartilaginous septa.

The perichondrial arteries supply the ring of Lacroix and the groove of Ranvier. Capillaries from this system communicate with the epiphyseal and metaphyseal capillaries in addition to the vessels of the joint capsule. This anastomosis is a potential conduit for extension of metaphyseal osteomyelitis into the epiphysis or into the joint space, producing a septic arthritis.

The reserve zone of the growth cartilage contains chondrocytes that are widely separated by a hyalin extracellular matrix. The reserve chondrocytes synthesize and secrete the macromolecules of the hyaline extracellular matrix. Arterioles and venules traverse this zone on their way to the proliferative zone but minimal oxygen is unloaded within the cartilage canals of the reserve zone. The local oxygen tension is low (~20 mm Hg) and the calcium content is also low. Functionally, the reserve zone is the source for a continuous supply of chondrocytes to the proliferative zone.

A major cellular feature of the proliferative zone is mitosis of the chondrocytes. As the cells divide, they align in longitudinal columns parallel to the long axis of the bone. Oxygen tension is high in this zone (57 mm Hg), and the chondrocytes use aerobic metabolism to synthesize and store glycogen, presumably as a future energy source for calcium pumping. It is important to realize that the cells of the proliferative zone do not actually move down the zone but the epiphysis essentially moves away from the cells as a result of cellular division. In this sense, mitosis in the proliferative zone is thought to be the "jack" responsible for long bone growth.

Cells in the hypertrophic zone enlarge to five or six times their original size and ultimately perish at the bottom of the zone. In the top zone of maturation, the chondrocytes begin to enlarge and to consume their glycogen stores. Mitochondria of the hypertrophic chondrocyte, which have the capacity to pump and to store ions, become loaded with calcium. In the middle zone of degeneration, the chondrocytes begin to show signs of intracellular disorganization and deterioration. Oxygen tension is low (24 mm Hg), and the cells shift to a catabolic metabolism, depleting the remainder of their glycogen and releasing the calcium previously stored within the mitochondria. In the bottom zone of provisional calcification, calcium salts diffuse from the chondrocytes and deposit in the extracellular matrix of the longitudinal septa. The proteoglycans disaggregate, and crystals appear in matrix vesicles. The growth cartilage terminates, and the metaphysis begins at the last intact transverse septa.

The major physiologic events occurring within the metaphysis are bone formation and bone remodeling. Bone formation begins with dissolution of the last intact transverse septa of the hypertrophic zone, followed by invasion of the hypertrophic lacunae by vascular sprouts from the nutrient arterioles. The vascular sprouts enter lacunae previously occupied by hypertrophic chondrocytes, bringing with them perivascular osteoblasts that adhere to the primary spongiosa and begin to synthesize osteoid. The combination of primary spongiosa covered by mineralized osteoid is called secondary spongiosa. Remodeling begins immediately. Osteoclasts resorb the secondary

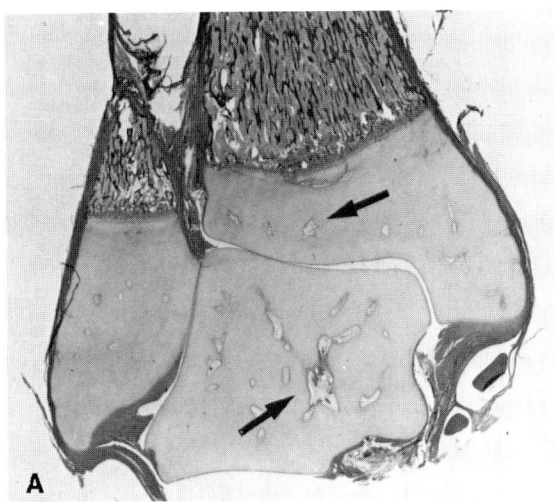

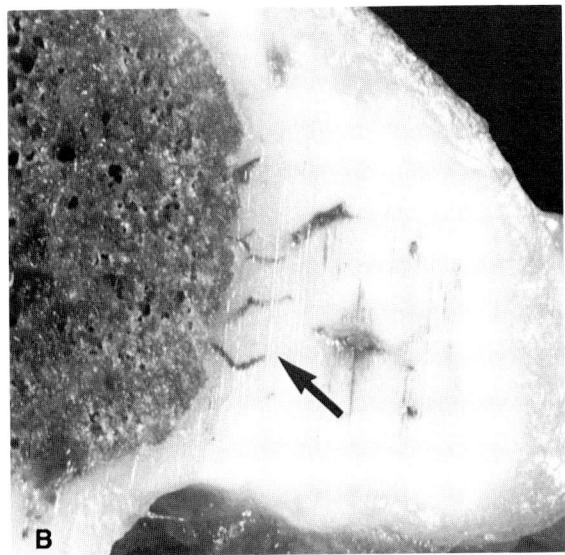

FIGURE 1-24. Blood vessels are present within an infant's epiphyseal cartilage. (**A**) The vessels in cartilage canals course throughout the epiphyseal cartilage of the distal tibia, fibula, and talus before ossification. (**B**) The metaphyseal and epiphyseal osseous vasculature incorporates the cartilaginous vessels as ossification progresses. (From Ogden JA. Pediatric orthopaedics. Philadelphia: JB Lippincott, 1990:27.)

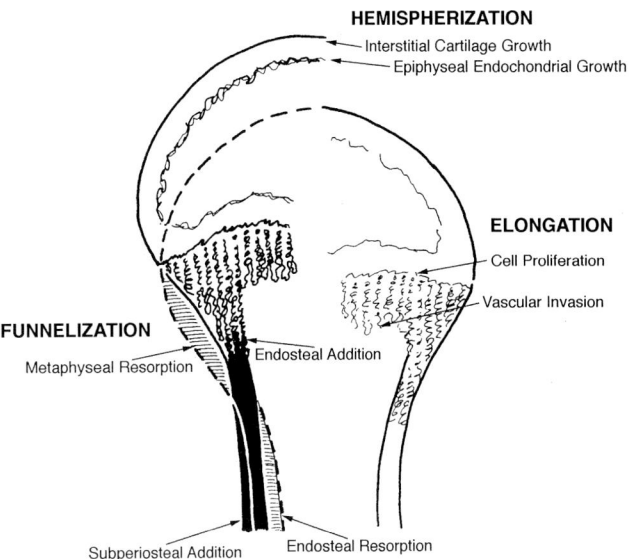

FIGURE 1-25. The growing-remodeling process of a typical long bone. Selective bone resorption coupled with new bone deposition in the epiphyseal, metaphyseal, and diaphyseal regions results in growth and shape changes. (Adapted from Ham AW. Some histophysiologic problems peculiar to calcified tissue. J Bone Joint Surg [Am] 34:1952;701.)

spongiosa, and osteoblasts follow closely, making lamellar bone in the wake of osteoclastic resorption.

Growth plates tend to be relatively flat in the fetus but with increasing age and with increasing mechanical loads, the physis develops undulations to help neutralize shear stresses.

Bones grow in width and thickness in addition to length. Because the metaphysis is larger than the diaphysis, the metaphysis must be cut back to the width of the diaphysis during the remodeling process. This metaphyseal process is termed funnelization. In an area called the cut-back zone, osteoclasts resorb, or cut back, the bulbous peripheral bone of the metaphysis and osteoblasts make new bone at a decreased radius of curvature. In this way, the wide metaphysis gradually narrows to the width of the diaphysis as the epiphysis grows away from the shaft of the bone. The region of the metaphyseal cut-back zone contains thin, fenestrated bone and this area is a common site for the collection of subperiosteal pus in cases of osteomyelitis.

The width of the diaphysis increases with growth as a result of intramembranous appositional bone formation by cells derived from the periosteum. As osteoblasts lay down new subperiosteal layers, osteoclasts resorb older bone on the endosteal surface, increasing the diameter of the medullary canal. The rate of bone formation on the outside is slightly greater than the rate of resorption on the inside, so that the cortex grows in thickness and in diameter. This modeling process is called cylinderization.

The size of the epiphysis increases by endochondral ossification. Growth at the bulbous ends of a bone is called hemispherization, and it is best understood by noting that the epiphysis is covered by two types of cartilage: a thin layer of growth cartilage directly below a thicker layer of articular cartilage. Endochondral ossification takes place in the thin growth cartilage, enlarging the hemisphere of the epiphysis, but the growth cartilage is much thinner and the cells divide at a slower rate than their compatriots in the physis. Thus, the bone acquires its final shape by the combined action of endochondral and intramembranous bone formation during the processes of funnelization, cylinderization, and hemispherization (Fig.

1-25). Bone formation and resorption continue through life, constantly adjusting and remodeling the structure of the skeleton under the influence of hormones and various cytokines in an attempt to match the biomechanical properties of the bone to the functional demands placed on the body.

References

1. Bishop JE, Waldholz M. Genome. New York: Simon & Schuster, 1990:1.
2. Bryant SV, Muneoka K. Views of limb development and regeneration. Trends Genet 1986;2:153.
3. Carter DR, Orr TE, Fyhrie DP, Schurman DJ. Influence of mechanical stress on prenatal and postnatal skeletal development. Clin Orthop 1987;219:237.
4. Carter DR. Mechanical loading history and skeletal biology. J Biomech 1987;20:1095.
5. Gardner E, Gray DJ, O'Rahilly. The prenatal development of the skeleton and joints of the human foot. J Bone Joint Surg 1959;41:847.
6. Gilbert SF. Developmental biology. 4th ed. Sunderland, MA: Sinauer Associates, 1994.
7. Guidera KJ, Ganey TM, Keneally, Ogden JA. The embryology of lower-extremity torsion. Clin Orthop 1994;302:17.
8. Kawashima T, Uhthoff HK. Development of the foot in prenatal life in relation to idiopathic club foot. J Pediatr Orthop 1990;10:232.
9. Kawashima T, Uhthoff HK. Prenatal development around the sustentaculum tali and its relation to talocalcaneal coalitions. J Pediatr Orthop 1990;10:238.
10. Kelley RO. Early development of the vertebrate limb: an introduction to morphogenetic tissue interactions using scanning electron microscopy. Scanning Microsc 1985;11:827.
11. Larsen WJ. Human embryology. New York: Churchill Livingstone, 1993.
12. Levine J, Suzuki D. The secret of life. Redesigning the living world. Boston: WGBH Education Foundation, 1993:1.
13. McGinnis W, Kuziora M. The molecular architects of body design. Sci Am 1994;270(2):58.
14. Moore KL. The developing human, clinically oriented embryology, 4th ed. Philadelphia: WB Saunders, 1988.
15. Nieto MA, Sargent MG, Wilkinson DG, Cooke J. Control of cell behavior during vertebrate development by Slug, a zinc finger gene. Science 1994;264:835.
16. Ogden JA, Grogan DP. Prenatal development and growth of the musculoskeletal system. In: Albright JA, Brand RA, eds. The scientific basis of orthopaedics. New York: Appleton and Lange, 1987:47.
17. O'Rahilly R, Gardner E. The embryology of bone and joints. Bone and joints. IAP monograph No. 17. Baltimore, Williams & Wilkins, 1976:1.
18. Saunders JW. The proximo-distal sequence of origin of the parts of the chick wing and the role of the ectoderm. J Exp Zool 1948;108:363.
19. Staheli LT, Corbett M, Wyss C, King H. Lower extremity rotation problems in children. J Bone Joint Surg [Am] 1985;67:39.
20. Thorogood P. Morphogenesis of cartilage. In: Hall BK, ed. Cartilage. 2nd vol. Development, differentiation and growth. New York: Academic Press, 1983:223.
21. Tickle C. On making a skeleton. Nature 1994;368:587.
22. Trueta J. Studies of the development and decay of the human frame. Philadelphia: WB Saunders, 1968:37.
23. White K, Grether ME, Abrams JM, et al. Genetic control of programmed cell death in *Drosophila*. Science 1994;264:677.
24. Wiesel TN. Genetics and behavior. Science 1994;264:1647.
25. Wolpert L. Cellular basis of skeletal growth during development. Br Med Bull 1981;37:215.
26. Wolpert L. Pattern formation in biological development. Sci Am 1978;239:154.
27. Wolpert L. Positional information and pattern formation. Curr Top Dev Biol 1971;6:183.
28. Zaleske DJ. Development of the upper limb. Hand Clin 1985;1:383.

Chapter 2

Imaging Techniques and Applications

H. Theodore Harcke

General Considerations
  Clinical Effectiveness
  Availability and Time
  Biologic Effect
  Cost
  Other Risks
Radiography Without Contrast
  Plain Films and Fluoroscopy
  Directional Tomography
  Digital Radiography
  Bone Densitometry
Radiography With Contrast
  Angiography
  Arthrography
  Myelography
Computed Tomography
Scintigraphy
Ultrasonography
Magnetic Resonance Imaging
Summary

Revolutionary advances in medical imaging have occurred in the past 25 years. Largely because of computer technology, this field continues to develop and foster new and improved capabilities for evaluating the musculoskeletal system. Through constant exposure during training and practice, orthopaedic surgeons become comfortable with conventional radiographs and quite skilled in the recognition of osseous pathology. For the other imaging modalities of nuclear medicine (scintigraphy), computed tomography (CT), ultrasonography, digital radiography, and magnetic resonance imaging (MRI), it is impractical for most orthopaedic surgeons to maintain the same familiarity that exists with plain films. Still, the orthopaedic surgeon should have sufficient knowledge of these techniques to ensure that they are used appropriately in practice.

A key responsibility of the radiologist is to serve as consultant and assist in the selection of an imaging strategy—the sequence of studies that answers the clinical question in the most effective manner. To control health care costs, it is important for the orthopaedic surgeon to bring to the consultant information obtained from the history and physical examination and to pose the questions that he or she desires to be answered.

The purpose of this chapter is to provide an overview of musculoskeletal imaging for the orthopaedic surgeon. With the knowledge of the principles of each imaging technique and an understanding of its strengths and weaknesses, more effective communication with the radiologist will be possible. Certain strategies exist for the evaluation of common clinical problems. These strategies develop through experience and through controlled clinical research studies. Accepted strategies are noted but it must be recognized that as technology changes and experience grows, the accepted strategy may be discarded for a new one.

GENERAL CONSIDERATIONS

As a preliminary step to the consideration of each imaging technique, it is important to establish common criteria for comparison. Although clinical effectiveness is the primary consideration, several practical issues influence the choice of technique.

Clinical Effectiveness

Concepts that are frequently employed for evaluating technique are sensitivity and specificity. Sensitivity refers to the ability of a test to detect abnormality when it is present. Specificity relates to the correctness of a positive test for a particular abnormality when abnormality is detected. No medical test is perfect, and this is true of the various imaging modalities. The sensitivity and specificity of each imaging modality vary with the disease process. Plain radiographs, for example, are quite sensitive and specific in the detection of long bone fractures. The sensitivity decreases, however, if the detection of fractures in the ribs or spine is considered. In clinical practice, it is common to use a combination of studies that increases the overall sensitivity and specificity over those of individual techniques. Accuracy is the measure that incorporates both sensitivity and specificity.

Availability and Time

Not all types of studies are readily available. When a study is easy to obtain and the results become known in a short time, that study becomes popular, even when it is not the most sensitive or specific. Conversely, new and technically sophisticated studies frequently are not readily available or require scheduling; this limits their use. In emergency situations, it becomes impractical to select an imaging technique by criteria other than availability and timely results.

Biologic Effect

The public concern over the effects of irradiation is recognized. Some new techniques produce images without ionizing irradiation, and this may be a compelling reason to consider one study over another. These techniques, however, may pose other risks. The practicing pediatric orthopaedic surgeon finds the degree of anxiety varies among families and is often an openly stated problem for parents. In discussing the risks of radiation exposure from the use of diagnostic radiographs and radioisotope tracers, it is important to understand that public perception of these risks is often distorted because of lack of familiarity with the actual level of risk. Diagnostic imaging techniques that employ an x-ray beam or radioisotope tracer are considered to give low-level exposure. These exposure levels must be differentiated from radiation levels used in cancer treatment.

The health risks of low-level radiation exposure have been studied carefully. The chief issues are the carcinogenic and genetic effects. Although irradiation-induced cancer is known to occur at sufficiently high exposures, a variety of studies of low-level exposure from medical, occupational, and military sources have led to a spectrum of positive, negative, and equivocal results.[79] The genetic risk from irradiation to human gonadal tissue is based on animal experiments and carries even more uncertainty than data on carcinogenesis. Effects in humans have not been observable, presumably because of low frequency of occurence. For the purpose of irradiation protection, it is necessary to make certain assumptions between radiation dose and effect. The internationally accepted basic assumption for diagnostic radiography is a linear relation, without threshold between dose and the probability of an effect. This "no-threshold" hypothesis is a deliberately cautious assumption and because of it, an attempt is made to reduce exposure through every reasonable means (e.g., technologic improvements, gonadal shielding). Because level at which a direct link between carcinogenesis and irradiation occurs has not been established, a small cancer risk must be postulated from even the lowest irradiation levels. Consequently, it is impossible to tell a parent or patient whether a study is "safe" or how many studies a patient may undergo without concern. Scientific studies customarily express irradiation risk in relation to a large population, not to an individual (e.g., the increased risk of cancer cases per million per unit of radiation dose). Webster has summarized our knowledge in his statement that "there is no proven body of fact that establishes an increase in human cancer after low doses of X or γ irradiation, such as those received environmentally, occupationally, or from medical diagnostic procedures; that is irradiation levels below about 10 rad (0.1 Gy)."[117]

A most helpful way of presenting the concept of risk to parents is by relating the assumed risk of irradiation to a comparative risk encountered in daily living. Such comparisons show, for example, that the risk of developing cancer and dying as a result of irradiation received from a chest radiograph is equivalent to the risk of death by cancer from flying 1000 miles by jet or living 2 months in Denver.[107] Information such as this is intended to place irradiation risk in the proper perspective for the patient and family. Another practical approach is to consider each study as a risk-versus-benefit relation. The information obtained from an x-ray study should benefit the patient to a degree that offsets the irradiation risk. Stated another way, a patient who refuses a necessary x-ray study faces a greater risk that some harmful effect could result from failure to obtain the needed information.

Ultrasonography, which involves no ionizing irradiation, has been reported to show some in vitro cellular effects. Its safety in clinical practice is based on finding no independently confirmed significant biologic effects in mammalian tissues exposed in vivo to unfocused ultrasound with intensity levels below 100 mW/cm^2.[6] Diagnostic equipment operates in the safe range and widespread usage to date has produced no adverse effects.

Magnetic resonance imaging exposes patients to both high magnetic fields and radiofrequency (RF) pulses. Because of the uncertainty of the response of surgical clips and other hardware, MRI studies are contraindicated in patients having vascular clips in the central nervous system or those who have pacemakers. Although metallic fixation that is used in orthopaedic procedures is not a contraindication to MRI, the devices can alter the magnetic field homogeneity, creating signal voids and artifacts.[69]

The use of contrast material in a study adds the risk of adverse side effects. Most of these are mild or moderate non–life-threatening events that require only observation and support. The principle concern is the possibility of a severe anaphylactoid or idiosyncratic type of reaction that is life-threatening. There are two categories of agents; the older ionic (high-osmolar) varieties and the newer nonionic (low-osmolar) types. The ionic agents are reported to have a 5% to 12% incidence of side effects, compared with 1% to 3% for nonionic agents. The reason that nonionic agents have not replaced ionic agents is that they have a significantly higher cost. Whereas some institutions have switched completely to nonionic agents, others use both and choose the agent based on clinical and risk factors for the individual patient. As a result of these usage patterns, the rate of fatal outcomes for contrast media studies is about 0.9 per 100,000.[5] It should be noted that the radiopharmaceutic agents used in nuclear medicine studies of the skeleton do not cause allergic reaction. Invasive studies using catheters and needles carry the possibility of specific additional complications.

Cost

The high costs of medical care have been discussed both in the popular press and in the professional literature. If managed care is implemented, some imaging studies will be capitated and the contract will dictate where and under what conditions (e.g., prior approval) they can be obtained. Children may be sent to adult centers, where technologists have little pediatric experience and quality may be a problem. It is worth intervening in the system to have studies performed where quality pediatric imaging is provided. Studies performed using the new imaging techniques are generally more expensive than conventional radiographic studies, so their use is more likely to be constrained. When ordering tests, however, it is also important to consider the positive aspects of more costly imaging studies. If a series of imaging studies leads to a quick and accurate diagnosis, the savings in hospital days can more than offset the expense of the studies. In a similar manner, if a series of studies accurately defines a problem in a manner that permits more effective surgery, the patient benefits by a decrease in morbidity, which also translates into cost savings. Using multiple tests to make an early diagnosis of infection allows prompt initiation of effective treatment, with a reduction of short-term complications and prevention of costly long-term sequelae. Negative results are defensible. The negative result may prevent an unnecessary surgical procedure or treatment that would have been more costly.

Other Risks

In pediatrics, sedation or anesthesia may be required to obtain an adequate imaging study. This entails added risk, particularly when the patient's general medical condition is compromised. General radiography and ultrasonography seldom require sedation. Typically, children younger than 4 to 5 years of age require sedation for MRI; this is usually true for CT also. Nuclear medicine studies using tomography may require some sedation. The invasive studies, arthrography and myelography, are also performed under sedation or general anesthesia, depending on age and clinical circumstances. Most facilities are prepared to perform studies that require sedation on an outpatient basis. Experience with pediatric sedation is sometimes lacking in adult centers, and inadequate sedation can result in a poor quality or unsuccessful examination. Choice of agent depends on many factors, especially the length of the procedure. Magnetic resonance imaging studies in particular have an extended duration (e.g., 1 hour) and are quite susceptible to motion artifact. Oral sedation with chloral hydrate is a popular technique because of the relative safety of the drug; a common error is too small a dose. Doses in the 80 to 100 mg/kg range (maximum, 2.5 g) have given a 96% success rate in pediatric MRI.[42] Intravenous sedation is often selected by pediatric centers because it is reliable, rapid-acting, and can be controlled. Pentobarbital at a dose of 2 to 6 mg/kg (maximum, 200 mg) is a standard regimen. Proper precautions must be taken when administering either an oral or intravenous medication, and the child should be monitored during and after the procedure in accordance with the American Academy of Pediatrics guidelines.[4]

RADIOGRAPHY WITHOUT CONTRAST

Plain Films and Fluoroscopy

The conventional radiographic image is produced by differential attenuation of an x-ray beam. Selective attenuation by body parts permits identification of four primary densities: bone, water, fat, and air. Correct radiographic exposure has a great deal to do with the information obtained. With overexposure of a body part, the film is dark and the soft tissues are poorly seen. The obliteration of fat-muscle planes that accompany edema and inflammation cannot be detected, and the potential to recognize the presence of fluid in a joint space is lost. Tiny calcifications in the soft tissues are obscured. Likewise, underexposure results in a light film that prevents discrimination of differences in osseous structures. Subtle changes in mineralization and the trabecular pattern of bone are not evident and significant skeletal lesions may be missed on underpenetrated films.

The plain film is almost always the initial imaging technique used in orthopaedics. It is the most widely available, is obtained more easily and quickly than other imaging studies, and is least expensive. A negative aspect of the plain film is the associated radiation exposure. Several measures are taken to reduce this risk, so that the benefit to the patient outweighs the prospective hazard. Dose reduction is achieved by placing the radiographic film between two intensifying screens in the light-proof holder or cassette. External lead shielding is used to protect gonadal tissue.

The use of an x-ray image intensifier is a variation of conventional radiographic technique that substitutes a phosphoreceptor for film. The advantage of this process is that motion is displayed. The resolution of the image produced on an image intensifier is less than that obtained with film, and use results in increased x-ray exposure because of the amount of time the patient is exposed. Effective use of the image intensifier entails brief intermittent exposure instead of prolonged viewing, coning the radiographic beam to the area of interest, and limiting the total exposure time to the absolute minimum. This affords the best protection for the patient and can be supplemented in some cases by lead shielding to block scattered irradiation. The orthopaedic surgeon, who should always wear a lead apron, also benefits by short exposure times. He or she can supplement the apron with a thyroid shield and leaded eye glass if desired. Leaded rubber surgical gloves are designed to reduce scattered irradiation only; they are not intended to allow the hand to be in the field of view. Positioning with props and localizing with long-handled instruments insure that the surgeon's hand is never in the primary beam. This is helpful in obtaining special projections such as tangential views of a curved surface of bone or in establishing the exact relation of superimposed structures. The orthopaedic surgeon finds fluoroscopy useful in fracture reduction and pin placements. Small field of view portable image intensifiers are available but are limited to use with small body parts. They should be used with the same care as their full-sized counterparts.

The radiograph compresses three dimensions into two. This limitation is overcome by the standard practice of obtaining 90-degree orthogonal views of the area of interest. Difficulties in interpretation of radiographs arise because bones have irregular surfaces and groups of bones project onto others. Some of these difficulties are overcome by the use of special views and multiple projections.

The orthopaedic surgeon must always be cognizant of the pitfalls of position. Much of the information from radiographs is obtained with the assumption that structures have been projected onto the film in a standard manner. Basic aspects of position relate to such simple things as whether the radiograph was obtained with the patient supine or erect. In scoliosis radiographs, for example, films are assumed to be taken with the patient erect, and variation from this routine should be noted on the film to avoid confusion. Obliquity of the pelvis can result in a false interpretation of hip malposition when an infant is being evaluated for congenital dislocation or dysplasia.[10]

Closely related to the question of position is the concept of projection. This becomes important when judging spatial relations, such as the location of a pin tip with respect to a joint space or growth plate. An important concept is that an object outside a bone may be projected to lie within it; however, it is never possible to project an object outside a bone when it truly lies within, regardless of the position from which the object is viewed. A corollary to this rule is that two objects may be projected to appear closer together than they are but they can never be projected to appear further apart. Applying these principles to common orthopaedic practice means that the orthopaedic surgeon may obtain a projection in which the tip of a pin appears to lie within bone when it really does not. It is not possible, however, to project the tip of a pin outside the bone when it truly is contained within it. Likewise, the separation at a fracture or osteotomy may not be apparent in one projection when the margins of a bone appear superimposed but if separation is seen between the margins of a bone, it is real; it is not possible that this is an artifact of projection.

The immature skeleton is a dynamic structure that is constantly undergoing change and is subject to some developmental variation. Fortunately, development of paired parts is usually symmetric. If the radiographic appearance of a symptomatic area of the skeleton is confusing (e.g., whether the radiograph shows a lesion or developmental process), the contralateral part can be radiographed for comparison. Other sources of help are reference texts devoted to normal development and the variations in development that simulate disease (Fig. 2-1).[63,65,102]

In the pediatric skeleton, the appearance of ossification centers and the subsequent maturation and closure of growth centers are predictable within certain levels of confidence. Most tables indicate the normal range of variation. The usual method of assessing skeletal maturation, commonly called bone age, is depicted in Greulich and Pyle's *Radiographic Atlas of Skeletal Development of the Hand and Wrist*.[43] This pictorial method allows a left hand radiograph to be compared with those of a studied group. Contained in the volume but rarely consulted are charts that show the standard deviation for the population studies. When these tables are consulted, it becomes apparent that at certain ages, the standard deviation can be as much as 11 months. Conservatively assuming that plus or minus two standard deviations is a reflection of normality, it means that bone age assessment may normally range over 3½ years. Another common

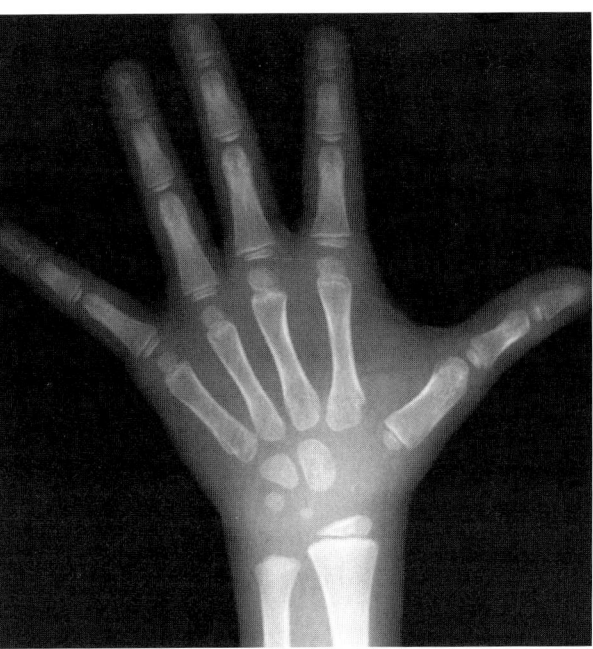

FIGURE 2-2. Discordant bone age in a 7-year-old boy. The carpal bones and radial epiphysis match the 4-year to 4-year, 6-month standards. The phalangeal epiphyses are more mature and correspond to the 6-year standard. Distal phalangeal centers are considered to be more reliable than carpal centers.

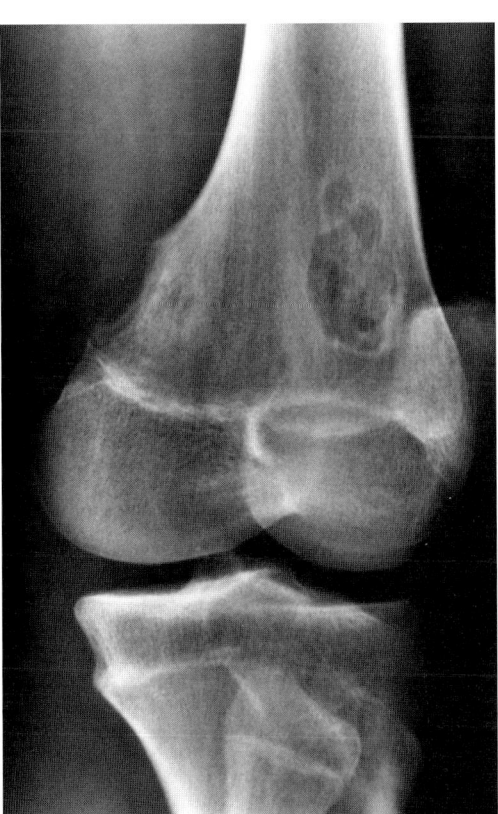

FIGURE 2-1. The lesion in the distal femoral metaphysis shows cortical disruption, periosteal reaction, and at first impression could be mistaken for tumor. This location and appearance is classic for the cortical desmoid, a normal developmental variation. A nonossifying fibroma (benign cortical defect) is also present.

pitfall when viewing the atlas superficially is concentrating mainly on the appearance of carpal bones (Fig. 2-2). Discrepancy between carpal development and that of the epiphyses of the phalanges often is found. When this occurs, it is recommended practice to use the more advanced development depicted by the distal epiphyses as the most reliable indicator of maturation.[41]

Measurement has become an integral part of the orthopaedic use of plain films. It is a useful technique for comparing serial studies and for establishing normal and abnormal criteria to assist in patient diagnosis and management. Compilations of tables of measurement have been published and are referred to daily by practicing orthopaedists and radiologists.[64] Although these tables are useful, it must be recognized that they are not absolute and certainly are not infallible. Many studies have documented the potential for variability in measurement. This is recognized in the evaluation of scoliosis,[24] congenital hip dysplasia,[76] and femoral anteversion.[58] The important lesson to learn from such studies is that all measurements are subject to variation as a result of magnification factors introduced by variation in distances between the x-ray tube, the patient, and the film; selection of landmarks; position of the patient; projection; and even the device used to perform the measurement. Protractors and goniometers have a variation in calibration, with some being calibrated to no finer than 5-degree increments. Even when measurements are made electronically, as is possible with computer techniques, the potential for the same types of variation exists.

Serial radiographs best document both physiologic and pathologic changes in the skeleton over time. In studying a radiographic examination, the orthopaedic surgeon should not overlook information contained on previous studies of the same part or of other parts of the skeleton. Often, these hold the key to accurately assessing and interpreting the findings.

Directional Tomography

Conventional radiographic tomography employs tube and film movement to blur the detail of structure above and below a focal plane. This has the effect of clearly showing the structures in a plane of interest. Linear and multidirectional (i.e., cycloidal) movement is possible, with the latter technique theoretically yielding better detail. In orthopaedic applications, either is suitable. Serial tomographic sections are obtained by moving the focal plane. The advantage of conventional tomography over CT is the ability to examine long segments of the body in planes that are sagittal and coronal. At times, osseous changes can be appreciated better in these planes than in the axial (i.e., cross-sectional) and reconstructed planes produced by CT. For example, spine tomograms performed in both anterior and lateral projections have been quite valuable in the assessment of congenital anomalies. In cases wherein metal instrumentation limits use of CT and MRI, tomography can provide details of bone morphology and location of bone fragments. Conventional tomography of the foot for anomalies and of the elbow joint after injury continues to be helpful. I have found conventional tomography of the hip to be less helpful than CT. Although I previously used tomograms to map physeal arrest, I prefer MRI when metal is not present.

Digital Radiography

Replacement of the conventional radiographic film as the medium for data storage and transmission is proceeding slowly. The electronic acquisition, processing, and transmitting of radiographic images will ultimately make radiography filmless. Digital images displayed on monitors can be manipulated electronically to enhance contrast and define edges, can be rapidly transmitted over long distances for consultation, and can be easily stored. Digital imaging systems contain software that permits direct measurement of distances and angles on the display.[3] The transition from current methods to filmless systems will not occur rapidly because of the cost.

The development of a digital counterpart of the conventional or analog radiograph is accomplished by different systems. In some, the x-ray beam passes through the patient and interacts with a detector rather than x-ray film. Another popular system uses a sensitive plate in the same manner as a standard film cassette. The exposed plate is scanned by a laser beam, and a digital image is constructed. Digital systems already in use have another advantage: they significantly reduce radiation exposure, compared with that from plain films.[68] Digital images possess the fine detail that permits complete substitution of a digital system for a conventional one.

Bone Densitometry

Assessment of bone mineral density can be useful in patients having metabolic bone disease and skeletal dysplasia. Although several types of equipment are used to determine bone density, they all measure the attenuation of a beam of energy as it passes through bone. Patients are scanned by the tightly collimated beam, and a study takes 5 to 20 minutes, during which time no movement can occur. This is a factor to consider in studying children. Equipment varies according to the nature of the energy beam; it can be a radioisotope emission or an x-ray photon. Methods also vary in the area surveyed (e.g., a local region such as the wrist, hip, or lumbar spine versus the whole body scan).

Single-photon absorptiometry and dual-photon absorptiometry measure photons from a radioisotope source. Single-photon absorptiometry instrumentation can survey limited areas such as the forearm and os calcis, which primarily contain cortical bone. With dual-photon absorptiometry equipment, the proximal femur and lumbar spine are studied and a better assessment is obtained because more trabecular bone is included. Turnover of bone occurs more rapidly in trabecular than in cortical bone, so this is theoretically a more sensitive measure.

Quantitative CT[13] and dual-energy x-ray absorptiometry (DEXA) use x-ray beams. Both systems initially focused on assessing the lumbar spine but DEXA units can scan either a region or the whole body. Radiation exposure is lowest for single-photon absorptiometry and DEXA and is highest for quantitative CT and dual-photon absorptiometry. Precision of measurement varies from 2% to 5%, depending on the technique and population studied.[56] As use in children increases, more disease-specific knowledge is being acquired. Although a patient can serve as his or her own control through serial studies, there is a need for age-, gender-, and race-specific normal values in pediatrics. Such data are slowly being acquired.[38,39,99] There are several potential applications of bone densitometry to patient management (e.g., serial measurement may be used postoperatively to judge new bone formation at a surgical site).[27]

RADIOGRAPHY WITH CONTRAST

Angiography

Delineation of vascular anatomy is accomplished by taking rapid-sequence radiographs in conjunction with the injection of contrast material into a vessel supplying the area of interest. The major use of angiography is in trauma. It is here the orthopaedic surgeon becomes involved in decisions related to emergency angiography and the need for treatment of vascular injury to take precedence over skeletal injury.

There are numerous alternatives to conventional angiography that can be used in nonemergency situations to assess vessels. Digital subtraction angiography (DSA) is a computer-based technique that permits delineation of arterial anatomy after a less hazardous intravenous injection of contrast material. Sequential images from an image intensifier are converted to digital data and subtracted from a precontrast image to remove bone and enhance contrast-filled vessels. The resolution obtained from DSA is less than that achieved using conventional angiographic technique, and DSA is effective only in studying vessels larger than 3 to 4 mm in diameter. In some instances, two-dimensional and Doppler ultrasonography may substitute for angiography. It is accurate in identifying small aneurysms, ectasia, and thrombus in larger vessels.[119]

The role of angiography in the evaluation of bone tumors has decreased with the advent of MRI.[97] There are also MRI techniques that depict vascular anatomy. Magnetic resonance angiography is being used as a noninvasive method for seeing vessels. Angiography has not proved to be specific in different tumor types or in simply differentiating benign from malignant lesions. It is used in planning for resection and when preoperative embolization or chemotherapy is employed.[84,90]

Arthrography

Arthrography combines conventional radiographic techniques with the use of contrast material to see joint components. Air and iodinated contrast medium may be used alone or in combination. The ionic iodinated contrast materials are still the most popular of the positive contrast agents; however, use is increasing of the significantly more expensive nonionic contrast agents (e.g., iohexol, ioxaglate sodium meglumine) of low osmolarity. These agents have been found to reduce postprocedural pain and improve image quality by prolonging intraarticular localization.[94]

Arthrography is most effective when the concentration of contrast material is dense enough to be seen on the image intensifier but not so dense as to obscure cartilage. In the knee, 2 to 3 mL of undiluted contrast material with 10 to 20 mL of air is recommended. For the shoulder, 10 mL of air and 5 mL of undiluted contrast material is effective. For the hip, elbow, and ankle, it is helpful to dilute the contrast agent to some degree. I prefer a 50% dilution of 5 mL of contrast agent and 5 mL of saline solution. Volume varies with age. In the infant hip, 2 to 4 mL are adequate. Because contrast material is absorbed quite rapidly by the synovium, some arthrographers have added epinephrine to the injection to decrease resorption. I have not found this to be of value and believe that it contributes to poststudy pain and persistence of joint fluid. Nonionic agents give better quality images without this effect.

The quality and accuracy of an arthrogram depend on the skill of the arthrographer. In most practices, the number of arthrograms has decreased because of the use of arthroscopy and MRI.[45] Conversely, the combined use of arthrography and CT, arthrotomography, has proved to be a new dimension for this procedure. Cross-sectional anatomy is best demonstrated when the CT images are obtained about 30 minutes from the time the contrast material was introduced.

There are instances when conventional arthrography and arthrotomography have an advantage over MRI. In the detection of nonopaque loose bodies and evaluation of bone irregularity at articular surfaces, arthrography provides detail that is not appreciated on MRI because cortical bone produces no signal (Fig. 2-3). Arthrography can define communication between a cyst and the joint space. It is also a dynamic study, which has the advantage of showing what occurs when joints move, although motion MRI studies are being developed.

Hip arthrography remains important in the preoperative or intraoperative assessment of hip dislocation and dysplasia.[51,59] An excellent tool in the operating room, it gives the orthopaedic surgeon an opportunity to see key relations as femoral head position is varied. This is valuable in the performance of closed reduction and in the evaluation of focal femoral deficiency. In assessing the femoral head and acetabulum in Perthes disease or after trauma or infection, arthrography is the most effective method for detecting incongruity.

Shoulder arthrography is used to evaluate the rotator cuff and the glenoid labrum and when loose

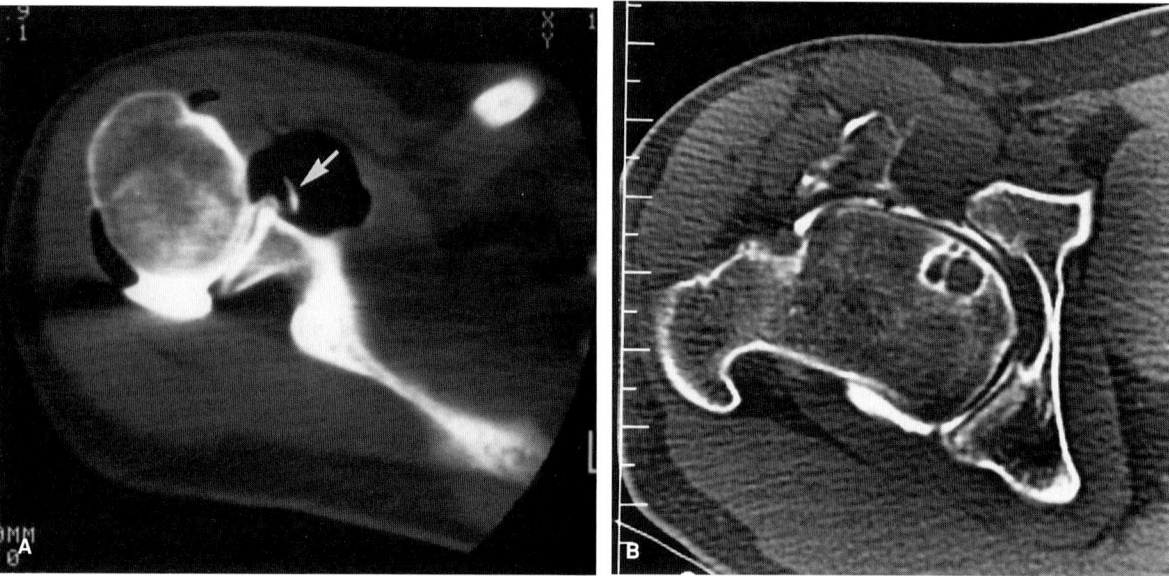

FIGURE 2-3. Arthrotomography (computed tomography [CT] after arthrography) improves the sensitivity of the arthrogram. (A) The anterior detachment of the capsule (*arrow*) in this 15-year-old girl was seen only on the CT images. (B) The cartilage is thinned but intact over the cyst in the deformed femoral head of this 18-year-old man with Perthes disease.

bodies, recurrent dislocation, or a frozen joint is suspected.[21] The role of wrist arthrography is controversial. Because the wrist is subdivided into multiple compartments, multiple injections may be required. The radiocarpal joint is the primary site examined but clinical information and physical examination may direct attention to other compartments.

Myelography

Although myelography has proved to be an excellent study having a high degree of accuracy, the invasive nature of the technique and its potential complications have fostered its replacement first by CT and then MRI. Generally, the MRI study has become the preferred first step for evaluation of the spinal canal and its contents. Myelography is used as a follow-up study in situations in which MRI fails to provide answers. Improved water-soluble contrast agents do not ionize in aqueous solutions and therefore possess lower osmolarity. They are less toxic to the nervous system and are absorbed into the bloodstream and excreted through the kidneys. The postmyelogram headache is still encountered with the new agents but with reduced frequency.

The major advantage of myelography is that it permits examination of the entire cord at one time and establishes the dynamics of cerebrospinal fluid flow in the presence of lesions that could create a block. I have experienced a few other situations in which myelography was helpful. For posttraumatic assessment of the cord in the presence of metallic fixation, MRI is limited by hardware that disturbs the homogenicity of the magnetic field and creates signal-void artifacts. Myelography in conjunction with CT may be effective in such instances. Patients with severe scoliosis can be evaluated by MRI but the planar format of the images makes interpretation difficult. Myelography with multiple projections has given clarification to confusing MRI studies in these patients.

COMPUTED TOMOGRAPHY

The CT image is made by a computer, using a complex algorithm that converts beam attenuation data into a detailed map of the attenuation at points within the plane examined. Translation of attenuation measurements into shades on the gray scale produces an image that depicts the various body densities. Attenuation values are expressed as Hounsfield units (HU). The CT image presents a thin section of body anatomy. By moving the patient slightly and repeating the process, a volume of anatomy is studied with serial CT slices. Slice thickness is selected and prelocation of the planes of section is made by using a scout image, which is a two-dimensional digital image of the body similar to a standard radiograph.

The major advantage offered by CT is the cross-sectional anatomic display, showing structures in a plane not obtainable with conventional radiography. An additional benefit of CT is the ability to manipulate the gray scale used for display and to reconstruct new images in other planes.

Accurate reconstruction of sagittal or coronal images requires contiguous thin axial slices and is best suited to regions of high contrast, such as the spine. Software technology has advanced such that CT data can be reconstructed into three-dimensional images (Fig. 2-4). Most work to date has dealt with the hip joint and the acetabular characteristics specifically.[8,74] It must be emphasized that a routine three-dimensional reconstruction of the hip in the immature child shows bone but not cartilage. The information obtained from Figure 2-4 is therefore an incomplete representation of the acetabulum. With CT comes the ability to measure the attenuation in a given area and relate it to standards for soft tissue, fat, and bone and to perform measurements between points within the slice. Such measurements should be used with caution because they are not absolute, and significant differences can exist between scanners.

To enhance the ability of CT to distinguish between objects of similar density, contrast material is injected intravenously or into a body cavity such as a joint or the thecal sac. Computed tomography images are not perfect; a structure or lesion that only partially occupies the thickness of a slice is subject to partial volume-averaging, which can misrepresent the true density of the lesion or allow it to be undetected. Artifacts are produced when metal is present within the slice, this poses limitations on some postsurgical evaluations. I would emphasize that the high quality of three-dimensional reconstruction relies on having thin contiguous or overlapping slices. This raises the dose above that of a routine study and both two-dimensional and three-dimensional CT studies should be obtained only in complex cases having clear indications. Young children usually require sedation for CT examination. The radiation dose received by a child during a CT examination is within the range of other diagnostic radiographic procedures, particularly those involving fluoroscopy and multiple films. Although the dose for a single slice seems high in comparison with that for other procedures, the beam is well collimated and scatter is limited. The irradiation issue for CT is the number of slices and the sensitivity of tissue included in the field of study. Computed tomography is most effective when radiography or bone scintigraphy has documented an area of abnormality that needs further clarification (Fig. 2-5). An exception to this rule is the use of CT to evaluate the spine when clinical symptoms provide the information that directs the evaluation to a specific location.

Computed tomography and MRI have become competitive modalities to some extent; however, each has strengths and weaknesses. In spinal stenosis, CT and MRI are roughly equivalent in providing diagnostic information. In neoplastic disease, CT is best for defining calcific deposits, pathologic fractures, and the nature and extent of the osseous component of a lesion (Fig. 2-6). Magnetic resonance imaging is superior in delineating the extent of marrow and soft tissue involvement. Use of CT in acute trauma is preferred because it more rapidly and clearly defines anatomic relations in all dimensions. It provides a clear picture of the extent of fractures and characterizes the position of bony fragments in the spine, hip, acetabulum, or shoulder.[80] Special orthopaedic applications of CT have been advocated to define important anatomic relations that are not easily determined from plain radiographs. In the hip, the position of the femoral head after reduction and casting is established easily by a minimum number of slices.[108] Computed tomog-

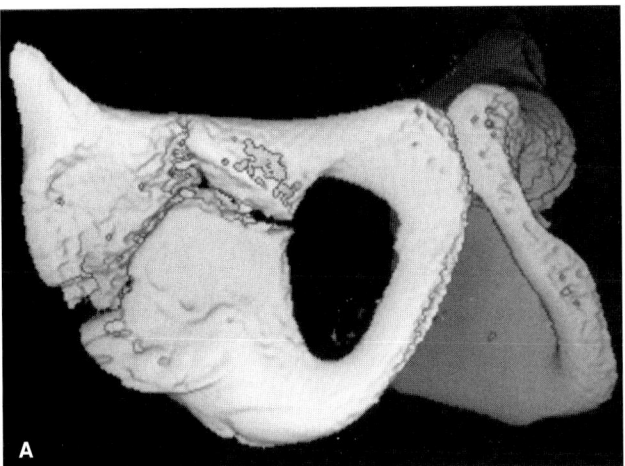
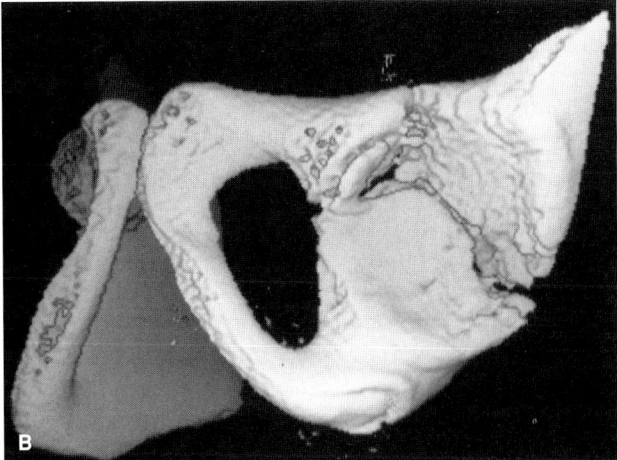

FIGURE 2-4. Three-dimensional reconstruction of the pelvis made from axial computed tomography sections. (**A**) The right acetabulum in this child with developmental dysplasia of the hip shows deficiency of the posterosuperior bony margin. (**B**) Normal left acetabulum is shown for comparison.

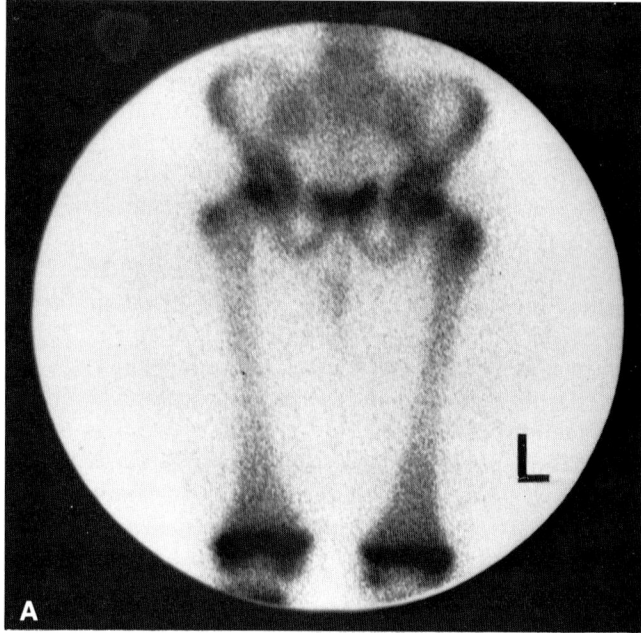

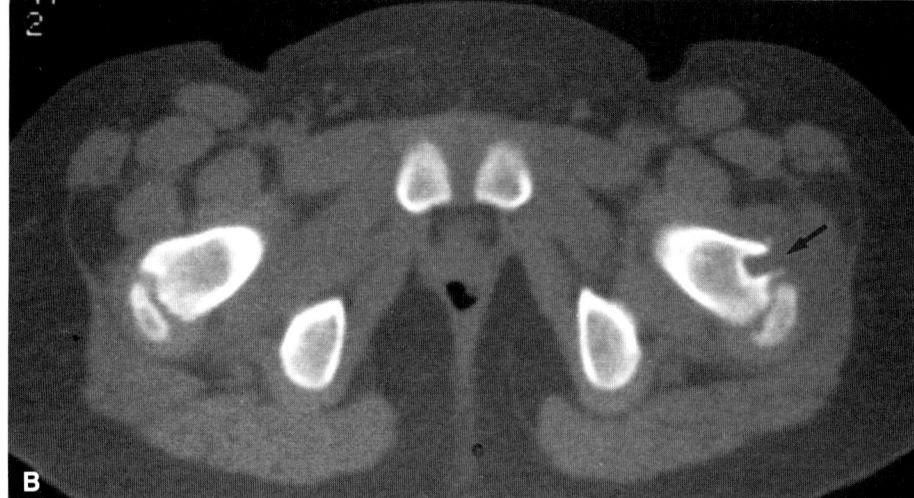

FIGURE 2-5. This 2-year-old child with subacute osteomyelitis presented with left hip pain. Radiographs revealed no pathology. (A) Bone scintigraphy showed increased uptake in the greater trochanter. (B) Knowing the general area of the abnormality allowed its exact nature and location (*arrow*) to be determined using computed tomography. Pus was found at surgery.

raphy is an alternative method for determining torsional relations of the femur.[58] I recommend CT when plain films fail to show suspected tarsal coalition.[75,103]

SCINTIGRAPHY

In skeletal imaging, the most commonly used radiopharmaceutic agent is a technetium 99m (^{99m}Tc)–labeled phosphate compound. The phosphate portion of the compound determines its behavior in the body; it is circulated in the bloodstream and as it diffuses within the tissues, it is absorbed to hydroxyapatite crystals. Binding occurs in direct relation to the amount of blood flow and the metabolic activity of the bone. The ^{99m}Tc radiolabel (half-life, 6 hours) provides the means for determining the location of the phosphate molecule. Gallium 67 (^{67}Ga), indium 111 (^{111}In), and Technetium-labeled hexamethyl propylene amine oxine (^{99m}Tc-HMPAO) are used on a limited basis in skeletal imaging, specifically for the diagnosis of infection. When ^{111}In and ^{99m}Tc-HMPAO are used, it is to label or tag a sample of leukocytes in vitro. The labeled leukocytes are then injected. The radiotracer thallium 201 (^{201}Tl), best known for its use in cardiac studies, is also used to monitor bone tumors.

The bone-seeking tracers gain their advantage over other imaging techniques because of high sensitivity to pathologic change. In conventional radiography, 30% to 50% of the calcium within bone must be lost before change becomes evident. It also requires 7 to 10 days before periosteal new bone formation becomes apparent on a radiograph. In bone scintigraphy, pathologic alterations of the skeleton caused by

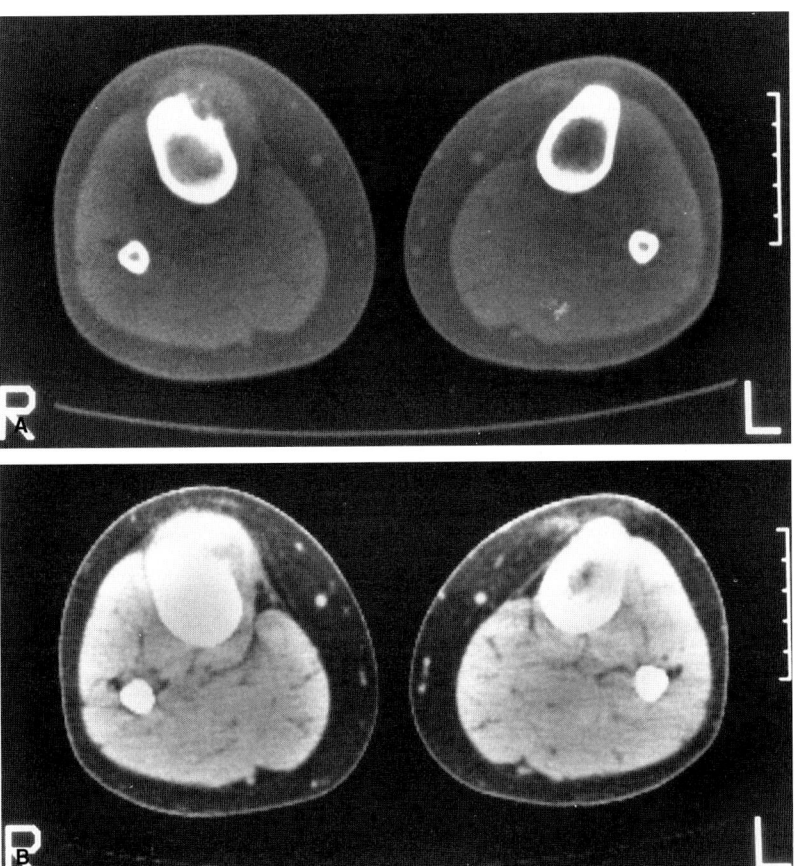

FIGURE 2-6. Computed tomographic images of a 12-year-old girl with osteosarcoma of the proximal right tibia. (**A**) The bone window best defines calcifications and marrow changes. (**B**) The soft tissue window shows the extraosseous extent of the changes. (This patient's magnetic resonance imaging study is seen in Fig. 2-15.)

trauma and infection become evident as early as 24 to 48 hours after the triggering event. This sensitivity in detecting bone pathology is the major advantage of bone scintigraphy. A disadvantage of bone scintigraphy, with technetium phosphates in particular, is the lack of specificity. The bone image of a patient who has sustained trauma may look no different from that of a patient having a bone tumor. Similarly, tumor and infection can give similar patterns of abnormal uptake. The bone scan cannot distinguish between a benign and malignant process.

In pediatric patients, prompt diagnosis and treatment of acute bone and joint infection are mandatory, and the need for emergency bone scans must be recognized. Commercial radiopharmacies supply 24-hour delivery of agents on a unit-dose basis for hospitals that do not wish to maintain materials for emergency cases. It takes about 4 hours to complete a bone scan on a child. There are three phases in which imaging can be performed. Phase one is the flow phase, which shows immediate vascular perfusion at the time of injection. The soft tissue phase occurs in the 5 to 15 minutes after injection; this second phase reflects regional tissue perfusion. The two early phases indicate the presence of soft tissue hyperemia. From the distribution, I get a sense of whether inflammation is superficial or deep and whether it involves a joint. For example, the pattern in cellulitis is different from that of arthritis. The orthopaedic surgeon must wait at least 2 hours before the third or bone phase, when the injected tracer has optimally localized in bone and the soft tissues have cleared. This phase shows the pattern of tracer uptake in bone. It may take from 5 to 15 minutes to obtain each individual scintigraphic image and because every study requires multiple images, patients may be under the camera for 1 to 2 hours. Rushing a study results in a poor quality scan and inadequate information.

To obtain adequate detail of the small bones in infants and children, it is necessary to supplement the usual high-resolution images with magnification views. These can be obtained by use of a pinhole collimator or electronically when the nuclear medicine camera is linked to a computer. Pinhole views make the difference between detecting or missing lesions in and about the joints, where growth plate uptake is normally prominent. The orthopaedic surgeon should identify the joint or joints suspected of involvement and request a magnification view of both the symptomatic site and the asymptomatic contralateral side, when applicable. Some camera-computer systems are designed to produce tomographic images. This process, called single-photon emission computed tomography (SPECT), is performed by rotating the camera detector around the patient. Use of SPECT imaging has increased the sensitivity of the bone scan in detecting spinal lesions, such as spondylolysis[18] (Fig. 2-7) and vertebral infection (i.e., discitis).[110] All patients with back pain who are studied by bone scintigraphy require SPECT imaging, otherwise some lesions are missed.

The radiation exposure in bone scintigraphy depends on the dose administered. The pediatric patient receives a portion of an adult dose, calculated based on relative weight. The total body exposure from a bone scan is comparable with that received from a radiographic skeletal survey. Target organs such as the bladder and growth plates, wherein the isotope accumulates in higher concentration, receive increased exposure. The less commonly used tracers, gallium, indium, and thallium, give higher levels of exposure than ^{99m}Tc.[30] For this reason, they are reserved for problem cases of infection, as noted later in this section.

Bone scintigraphy is rarely the first imaging modality used when patients present with musculoskeletal problems. Plain films are customarily obtained first, with the bone scan used to screen the skeleton when the radiographs show no abnormality and the clinical history or physical examination makes a skeletal etiology high on the list of differential diagnoses. In virtually every category of bone disease, scintigraphy has been used successfully to identify skeletal abnormalities that are not seen radiographically. The normal bone scan is also of value because it makes a significant skeletal abnormality highly unlikely.

Bone scintigraphy is used to detect occult infection and to localize the site of infection in instances in which an inflammatory process is present clinically. By the use of multiphase imaging, cellulitis, septic arthritis, and osteomyelitis can be differentiated. Studies have established that prior diagnostic aspiration of a

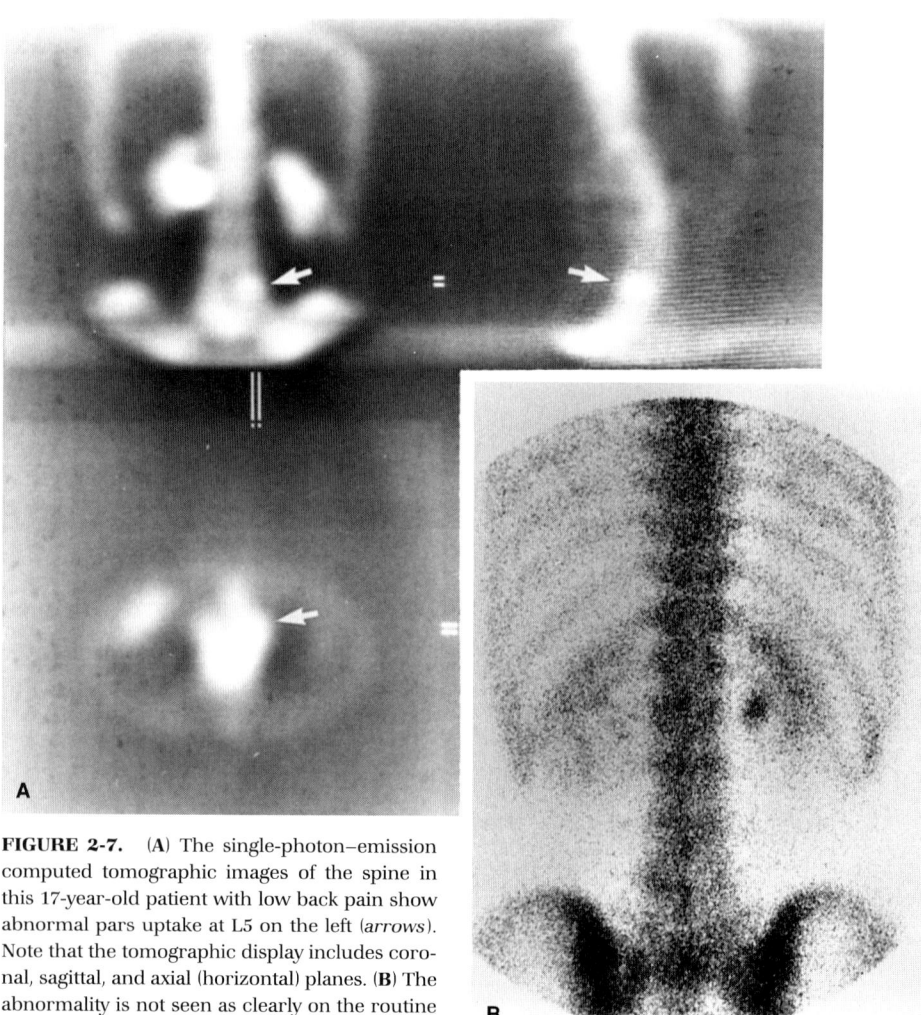

FIGURE 2-7. (A) The single-photon–emission computed tomographic images of the spine in this 17-year-old patient with low back pain show abnormal pars uptake at L5 on the left (*arrows*). Note that the tomographic display includes coronal, sagittal, and axial (horizontal) planes. (B) The abnormality is not seen as clearly on the routine (planar) image, which is a posterior view.

bone or joint does not cause a scintigraphic study to be abnormal.[12,83] Joint inflammation characteristically shows symmetric involvement on both sides of the joint. The two early phases show more increased activity than the third (bone) phase. Osteomyelitis typically shows focally increased activity in all three phases (Fig. 2-8). When bone infection is adjacent to a joint, there is asymmetric localization, with the most intense increase at the site of involvement. Variable success rates are reported with bone scintigraphy, ranging from 65% to 90%.[37,81,111] Results improve when multiphase imaging and magnification views have been employed. In neonatal osteomyelitis, the frequent occurrence of false-negative images has been reported.[7] Accuracy of bone scanning increases when atypical patterns, such as "cold" osteomyelitis, are recognized. Early in the course of infection, edema can reduce blood flow to the affected area of bone, and images show normal or decreased tracer activity.[91]

Problems with the use of scintigraphy to diagnose infection occur in the presence of some other insult to the bone, such as infarction, trauma, or surgery. In these instances and other situations in which the increased tracer uptake that accompanies a healing process cannot be distinguished from the increased uptake that relates to infection, combined ^{99m}Tc phosphate and gallium imaging increases accuracy.[77] The pattern of ^{99m}Tc and gallium uptake is compared; focal gallium accumulation that does not correspond to ^{99m}Tc uptake indicates an inflammatory focus.

The use of labeled leukocytes in pediatrics has included few bone cases. There are theoretic advantages to the use of labeled leukocytes instead of gallium as a study to follow primary screening by routine bone scintigraphy. Accumulation in noninfected skeletal lesions is less frequent and of lower intensity than with gallium. A blood sample is taken, the leukocyte fraction isolated and incubated with the radiotracer (e.g., ^{111}In, ^{99m}Tc-HMPAO). After in vitro labeling, the patient's cells are reinjected. In adults, accuracy with ^{111}In-labeled leukocytes has depended on whether the process is acute or chronic,[23] and false-positive cases can occur.[100] One small series of patients found HMPAO-labeled leukocytes superior to conventional bone scintigraphy.[73] In the case of a negative equivocal bone scan and a strong suspicion of infection, I use ^{99m}Tc HMPAO-labeled leukocytes in older children, when a sufficient volume of blood for labeling can be obtained. Infants and young children still have a gallium scan as the sequel. The higher irradiation burden war-

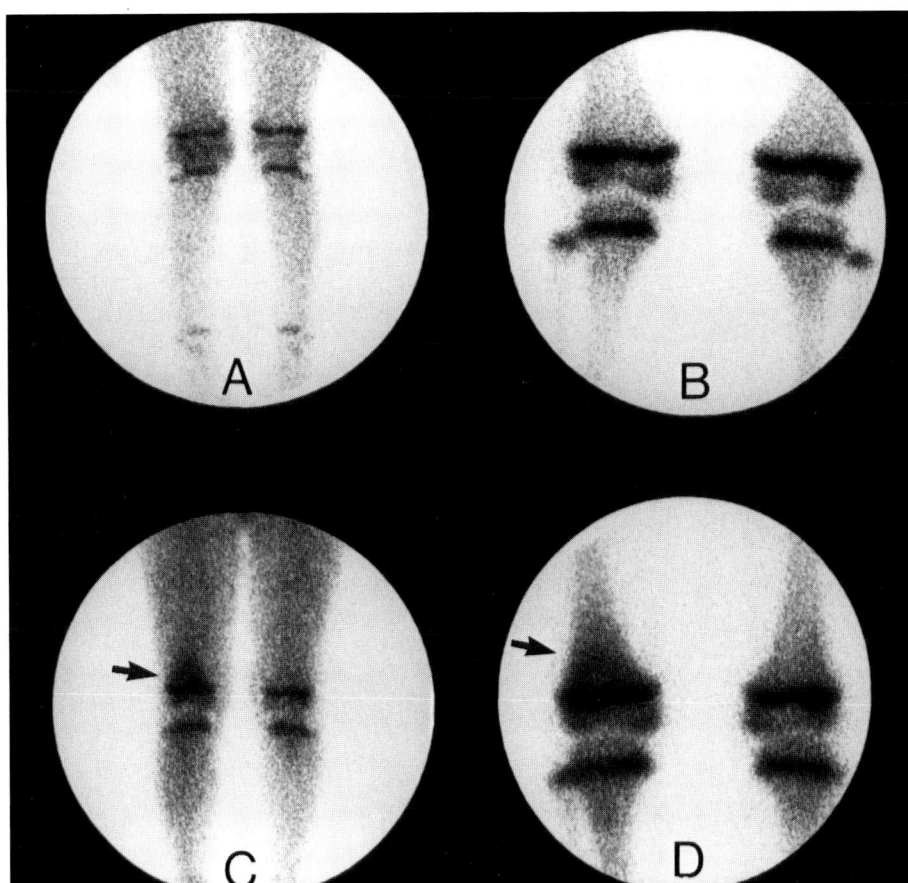

FIGURE 2-8. Multiphase bone scintigraphy in two patients with inflammatory disease. (**A**) In septic arthritis, blood pool imaging shows increased uptake in the right knee joint and (**B**) no focal increase in bone uptake on the delayed image. (**C**) In osteomyelitis, increased metaphyseal uptake (*arrow*) is noted on both the blood pool image and (**D**) the delayed bone image (*arrow*).

rants use of these studies only in complex clinical situations;[34] labeling with technetium is preferable to indium from the standpoint of patient exposure.

Bone imaging shows decreased isotope activity at areas of avascular necrosis, whereas radiographs are normal.[28] Magnification (i.e., pinhole) images are required. These permit the differentiation of Perthes disease from other causes of hip pain, especially transient synovitis. Although both scintigraphy and MRI can be used, I find it most convenient to follow plain films with a bone scan. Scintigraphy surveys a greater region and can identify areas in the spine, pelvis, or distal femur that refer pain to the hip. It should be noted that transient photopenia in the femoral head can occur with joint effusion.[66] Patients having Perthes disease are usually followed-up radiographically after diagnosis; however, if the orthopaedic surgeon desires to know the progress of revascularization of the femoral head at a point in time,[19,29] it is mandatory to match tracer uptake on magnification scintigraphs with areas of ossification on radiographs.

The differentiation of bone infarction and infection in patients with hemoglobinopathies has pitfalls. Both conditions show a range of uptake, depending on the age of the process, and a clear distinction is not possible. The purpose of scintigraphy is to establish the presence of an osseous lesion; this then may be evaluated by aspiration, biopsy, or additional imaging with gallium or labeled leukocytes.

In neoplastic disease, the purpose of the bone scan is to detect osseous metastases. It cannot distinguish between benign and malignant tumors or between tumor and infection. Computed tomography and MRI seem to be more effective in mapping tumor extent because they can define soft tissue and marrow involvement.[16] For osteosarcoma, scintigraphy is more sensitive than radiography in detecting bone metastasis but it is not as sensitive as chest radiography and CT in detecting pulmonary metastasis. Ewing tumors cause increased bone uptake but soft tissue and lung metastases are not detected. Thallium uptake in osteosarcoma and Ewing sarcoma has been recognized. Imaging of tumors with thallium before and after chemotherapy has confirmed an association between tracer uptake and histologic response to treatment.[92] Response to chemotherapy is considered in planning definitive follow-up surgery.

Occult benign tumors, such as osteoid osteoma and osteoblastoma, typically have markedly increased uptake, which makes them easy to detect in the spine or hip, where they are difficult to see radiographically. The nidus is the most active part of the lesion and usually a good quality scan with magnification (i.e., pinhole) images shows the nidus to be more intense than the adjacent sclerotic bone, which also exhibits increased tracer accumulation. A CT scan of the lesion is helpful for preoperative planning, and one method for localizing the nidus is to place a marking pin under CT guidance. An alternative technique for localizing the nidus during resection is the use of a surgical radiation probe or portable gamma camera. The tracer is injected a few hours before surgery. In the operating room, the surgical site and resected fragments are monitored. This ensures accurate removal and minimizes the volume of resected bone.[48,67] Special localization techniques are not always required but are helpful when a lesion cannot be readily identified by image intensifier at surgery or is in an area where resection of a minimal volume of bone is desired.

In suspected child abuse, some investigators advocate scintigraphy instead of a skeletal survey because of its increased sensitivity;[109] others have found radiography to be more convenient and highly successful.[86] A practical scheme that I employ is to obtain a skeletal

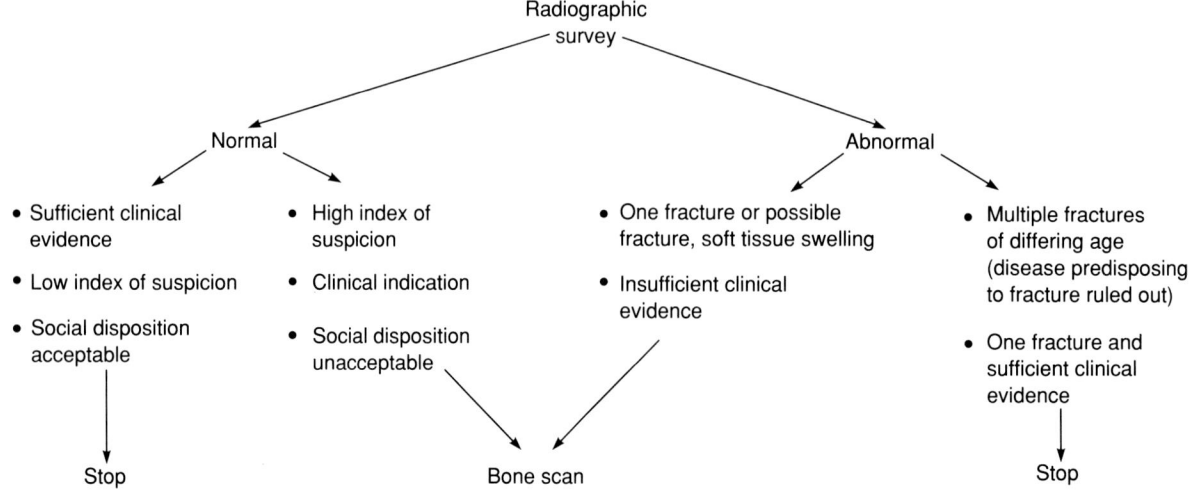

FIGURE 2-9. Skeletal imaging strategy in cases of suspected child abuse.

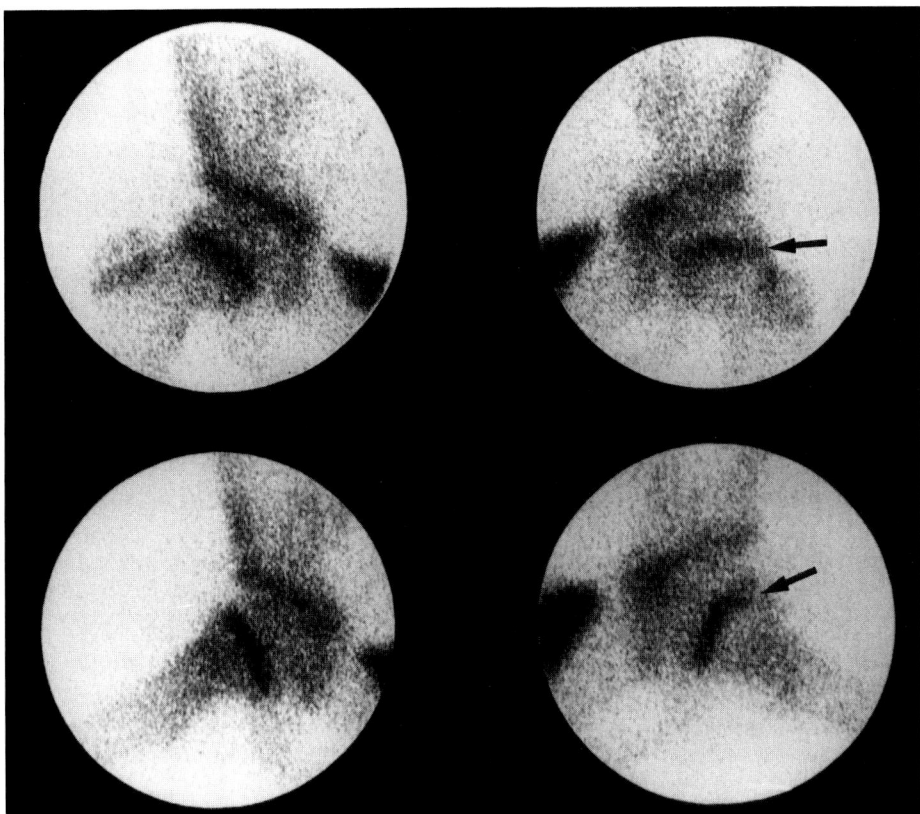

FIGURE 2-10. Bone tracers provide physiologic information about growth plates. This 9-year-old girl with coxa valga had been treated for left congenital dislocation of the hip as an infant. Radiographically, the proximal femoral growth plates appeared to be open. Magnification bone scintigraphy showed closure (absent plate activity) of the anterolateral portion of the plate in the left hip (*right, arrows*). Views of the normal right hip are provided for comparison (*left*).

survey first; it reveals the trauma that needs clinical attention. When additional information is desired for social or legal reasons, it can be supplemented by scintigraphy (Fig. 2-9).

Use of scintigraphy in evaluation of growth plates after trauma (Fig. 2-10) is advocated because the physiologic status is reflected by isotopic activity.[53] Stimulation by adjacent trauma causes increase; plate activity decreases in the process of closing. The isotope study is used in conjunction with correlative anatomic imaging.

Scintigraphy has been used to evaluate specific orthopaedic surgical procedures when the sensitivity of radiographic studies has been low. It has been accurate in confirming intact vascular perfusion after surgery and in assessing the viability of vascularized grafts.[78] Assessment of spinal fusion for pseudarthrosis has shown low sensitivity and specificity, with both false-positive and false-negative results.[85] Joint prostheses are used infrequently in children. In adults, labeled-leukocyte imaging has improved the accuracy of distinguishing between infected and noninfected loosening of hardware.[95]

It is important to correlate the results of a bone scan with those of all other available imaging modalities. In this way, the orthopaedic surgeon can overcome the lack of specificity inherent in this imaging modality. In instances in which the bone scan reveals a lesion that was not visible on an initial study (e.g., plain radiographs), it directs attention to the precise area of the skeleton to be studied by a high-resolution anatomic technique, such as CT.

ULTRASONOGRAPHY

Ultrasonography is a high-frequency mechanical vibration that is totally different in nature from ionizing irradiation. Its safety is established.[6] As a sound wave crosses the boundary between two tissues having different acoustic properties, some of the energy fails to cross and is reflected, creating an echo. By receiving the echo and knowing the direction and time of travel, the position of the interface can be plotted. This same principle is used in sonar and radar, and the technology had its genesis in these applications. The acoustic properties of body tissues determine whether ultrasonography is practical for imaging. When the sound beam encounters rigid inelastic tissue, such as bone, complete reflection occurs, and there is no image of deeper tissues. Gas in the body also prevents imaging because its elasticity is too different from that of adjacent soft tissue. Practical applications of sonography are limited to viewing soft tissues in the direct path of the beam. The same type of equipment used in hospitals for obstetric and abdominal sonographic examinations is suitable for musculoskeletal applications. Ultrasonographic examinations are dependent, however, on the skill and experience of the operator. Outside of North America, sonographic examinations often are performed by orthopaedic surgeons, although this is not usually the case in the United States and Canada. North American surgeons have believed that the time to learn and perform examinations, equipment expense, and liability considerations preclude their direct involvement. With the exception of developmental dislocation of the hip (DDH), use of ultrasonography does not eliminate the requirement for plain films. Sonography has the potential to replace some CT and MRI examinations when the personnel performing the study have acquired the requisite skill.

The ability of ultrasonography to differentiate solid and cystic lesions and to identify subtle changes in tissue texture has led to its use in evaluating and characterizing soft tissue masses and localizing tumors, abscesses, hematomas, and simple cysts.[50] For example, in a child with swelling behind the knee, ultrasonography is an ideal way to confirm it is a popliteal cyst. Similarly, with an inflammatory swelling or draining sinus, sonography can rapidly determine whether there is a discrete fluid collection. Recognition of the ability of ultrasonography to document muscle tears[71] and tendon ruptures[70] has led to its use in evaluating sports injuries. Some foreign bodies (e.g., wood and fiber, which are not visible on plain radiographs) can be detected with ultrasonography.[33] When abnormalities are sonographically visible within the soft tissues, the equipment can be used to guide needle aspirations or to place drainage tubes.

The use of ultrasonography to evaluate the infant hip has gained wide acceptance. Ultrasonography can distinguish cartilage and related soft tissue structures of the hip that are not visible radiographically. Work in Europe and in the United States has found sonography to be more sensitive than the clinical and radiographic assessment of the hip in infancy.[15,40,49,72,120] In addition to the assessment of hip position, it is also possible to assess acetabular configuration. In 1993, the two primary developers of hip sonography, Graf and Harcke, merged their methods and proposed a "dynamic minimum standard exam." The standard examination uses a coronal view to assess acetabular landmarks and a transverse (i.e., axial) view to assess stability with stress (Fig. 2-11). A proper examination must consider the morphologic characteristics of the bony acetabulum and labrum, together with femoral head position at rest and during Barlow- and Ortolani-type maneuvers.

High-frequency linear transducers (5 and 7.5 MHz) are required for infant hip examinations. Cartilage produces fewer echoes than other soft tissue structures, and the femoral head can be identified easily, regardless of the plane of examination. A lateral approach to the hip has been the most popular and is the position recommended in the standard examination. Some advocate sonographic examination from an anterior approach.[20,112] In addition to dislocation, which is easily identified, sonography shows improved sensitivity for identifying laxity and subluxation. This has led to reassessment of criteria for treatment in the first 4 weeks of life. Most minor instability that sonography recognizes in the newborn period tightens up without treatment.[14,35]

Use of sonography in evaluating infants suspected of having DDH can be divided into two categories: initial assessment and management. Universal hip screening with ultrasonography is performed in some areas of Europe. In these areas, this has led to overtreatment, with several infants being placed in abduction devices and called for reexamination.[113,115] I believe that universal sonographic screening programs such as those undertaken in Europe are not economically practical in the United States because of the resources required. I recommend using ultrasonography to supplement universal clinical screening.[47] Referral for ultrasonographic assessment is based on a questionable or abnormal physical examination or an increased risk factor. My risk factors include family history of DDH, oligohydramnios, breech delivery, torticollis, and foot deformity (Fig. 2-12). I generally discourage ultrasonography in the immediate newborn period because instability and minor developmental immaturity can self-correct. Clinically unstable hips (i.e., those that are Barlow-Ortolani–positive, or those that do not feel normal) should be checked by ultrasonography before committing to Pavlik or other treatment. Again, this can be done within the first 2 weeks of life on a nonemergency basis. The first sonogram establishes the baseline position at rest and in flexion-abduction; it also defines the status of the acetabulum. The follow-up studies then document improvement or failure to respond. The orthopaedic surgeon should wait to check the hip that feels stable but clicks until age 2 to 4 weeks. I believe that these need to be checked to verify the accuracy of the assessment. Sonography of infants having a normal clinical examination and a risk factor is recommended at 4 to 6 weeks of life to detect dysplasia and clinically unrecognized instability. This scheme using sonography to augment the clinical examination does not identify every DDH case[9] but it is proposed as a rational way to improve clinical screening within current health care restraints.

In infants being followed up for congenital dislocation of the hip, sonography can be used to monitor hip position and development. Dynamic splints, such as the Pavlik harness, permit evaluation while the hip is held in flexion and abduction.[44] Hip position can be tested within the limits of the harness and with stress maneuvers. Sonography has been tried with rigid casting; this requires a modified approach to the examination or cutting a window in the cast. We have abandoned this in favor of a limited CT examination (i.e., 1–2 sections) through the cast.[51] In assessments of acetabular development, the coronal sonogram shows one midplane section of the acetabulum, whereas the radiograph is the projection of the complete, three-dimensional acetabulum onto the two-dimensional film. Some discrepancy between sonography and radiography may occur. For this reason, I recommend that an anteroposterior radiograph of the pelvis be obtained in patients finishing treatment to document bony acetabular configuration.[44] Because orthopaedic

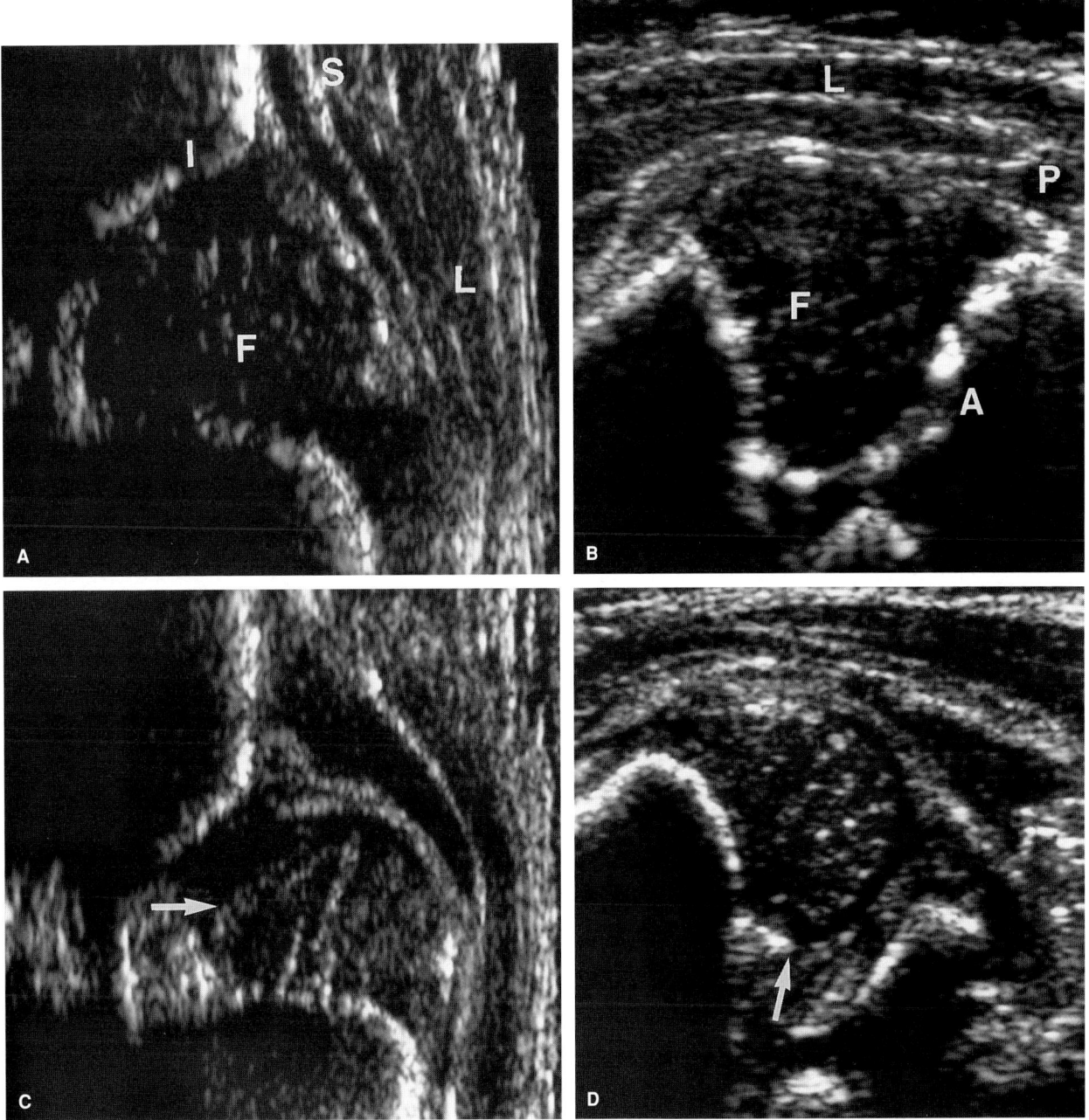

FIGURE 2-11. The standard hip examination includes coronal and transverse views. (**A**) Normal coronal neutral view. (**B**) Normal transverse flexion view. In subluxation, femoral head displacement is evident (*arrow*) in both views: (**C**) coronal neutral and (**D**) transverse flexion. (A, acetabulum [ischium]; F, femur; I, iliac bone; L, lateral; P, posterior; S, superior.)

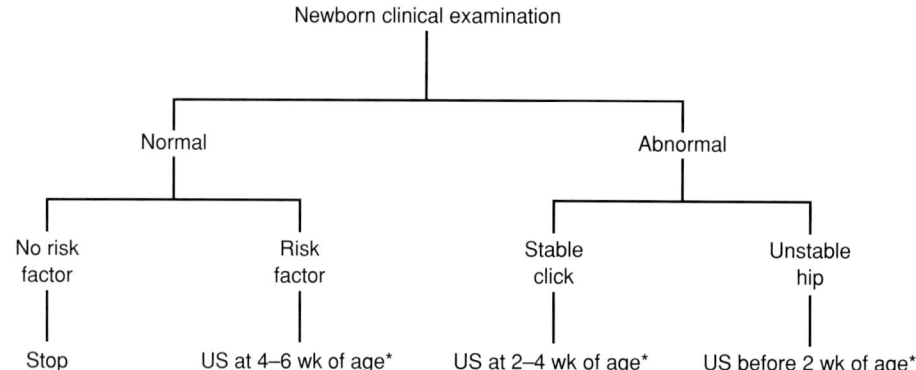

FIGURE 2-12. Protocol for sonographic ultrasound (US) support of infant hip screening. (*, observe or treat, depending on results and clinical findings.)

surgeons have experience using radiographs to monitor DDH, this becomes the baseline with which later radiographs are compared as the infant grows.

After the age of 1 year, the ossification of the femoral head has progressed to the point at which sonography is no longer reliable in establishing the relation between the femoral head and acetabulum.[52] After this age, hip sonography is performed to establish the presence or absence of fluid in the hip joint. In this role, it has not replaced another imaging study[2] but serves as a rapid and accurate means of documenting an effusion.[62,82] An anterior approach in the axis of the femoral neck is used (Fig. 2-13). When fluid is detected in the hip joint, aspiration can be performed, with

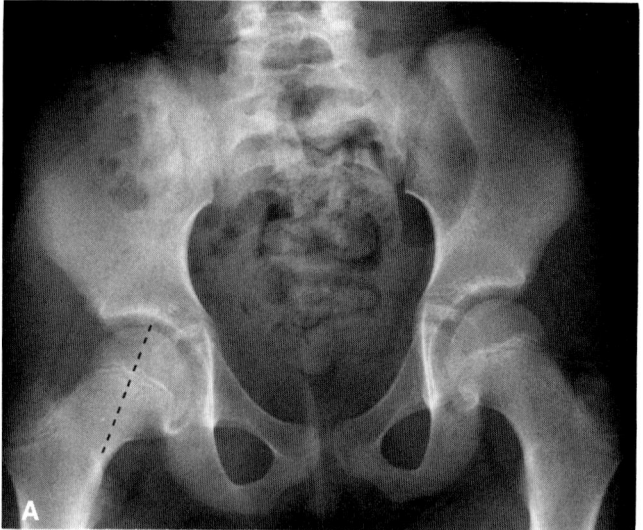

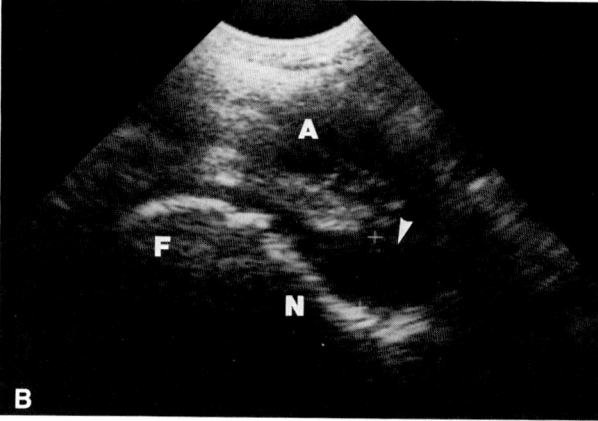

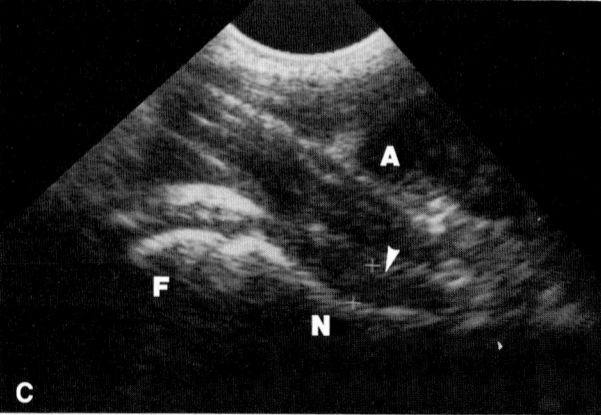

FIGURE 2-13. Sonographic evaluation of the hip for joint effusion is performed anteriorly. (**A**) Normal radiograph of a child with transient synovitis. The beam is directed in the axis of the femoral neck (N) (*dashed line*). (**B**) Sonogram of the right hip shows accumulation of fluid in the inferior recess of the capsule. The margin is convex in configuration (*arrowhead*) and measures 0.9 cm between the cursors. Aspiration yielded 6 mL of sterile fluid. (**C**) Sonogram of the normal left hip for comparison. The capsule margin is concave (*arrowhead*) and measures 0.5 cm between the cursors. (A, anterior; F, femoral head.)

sonographic guidance, if desired. Sonography does not differentiate between types of effusion (i.e., septic versus aseptic).[87] Although sonograms show changes in the proximal femur with late Perthes disease and slipped capital femoral epiphysis, there is no compelling reason to abandon the use of radiographs.

Tendons give distinct echo patterns in comparison with adjacent fat and muscle. Evaluation of the patellar and Achilles tendons is not difficult because these structures are readily identified. Applications center on diagnosis of traumatic and inflammatory changes.[31,32,70] The thickness and echo pattern within a tendon change with edema. Disruption of the tendon can be identified after acute injury. Where experienced sonographers are available, the initial plain film could be followed by ultrasonography instead of MRI. For chronic injuries, areas within the tendon where scar formation has occurred show increased echoes. Evaluation of the shoulder has centered on the detection of rotator cuff abnormalities. Although some reports show results that compare sonography favorably with shoulder arthroscopy[118] and arthrography,[106] other studies have been unable to reproduce their success.[116] Sonography of the shoulder must also be judged against MRI.

The major difficulty in establishing the credibility of musculoskeletal applications of ultrasonography has revolved around its being operator-dependent. When care has been taken to obtain suitable experience and skill, this technique has been found to be effective and quite popular for pediatric applications. An important factor to the orthopaedic surgeon is availability of ultrasonography at the time the patient is seen. Accommodations must be made in scheduling so that this service is provided in a timely manner.

MAGNETIC RESONANCE IMAGING

The newest of the imaging techniques, MRI, produces images without the use of ionizing irradiation. Clinical units are available in many regions for routine inpatient and outpatient evaluations.

The property of magnetic resonance is found in anatomic nuclei, which have an odd number of protons or neutrons and therefore show a net charge. These nuclei behave as magnetic dipoles and, when present in sufficient quantity, produce a signal that can be measured. Clinical imaging uses the magnetic resonance properties of the hydrogen nucleus, the most abundant in the human body. In a strong magnetic field, the nuclei align themselves with the field axis. They absorb and emit a specific RF energy, depending on the type of nucleus and its chemical environment. Because the nuclei are spinning, they act like tiny gyroscopes, and the pulse of RF energy causes them to tilt and come out of alignment with the field, a movement known as precession. After the disturbance that is induced in the aligned nuclei is removed, the excited nuclei return to their original alignment. The process of excitation and realignment is measured as relaxation time. Reference is most often made to T1 and T2 relaxation times. Variations in the relaxation time of hydrogen nuclei in different body tissue are the basis for the contrast between tissue types and the production of a usable image. In bone marrow, for example, the red and yellow marrow show different signal intensity on the same image because of differing amounts of fat and water. Intensities also change when the pulse sequence is shifted from T1- to T2-weighting. Because marrow distribution varies with age, the normal MRI images vary also.[89]

The process of creating the image is complex and involves variation in the timing sequences of the RF pulses and changes in the magnetic field to establish spatial relation. From a practical standpoint, the orthopaedic surgeon recognizes a similarity between MRI and CT images. Both represent a thin, planar, cross-sectional image of the body. Axial, coronal, and sagittal planar sections can be obtained with MRI, depending on the information desired. Magnetic resonance images are capable of differentiating soft tissue structures that cannot be differentiated by CT. By varying pulse sequences, the contrast between different tissues can be manipulated to highlight both normal differences and pathologic changes. When performing MRI studies, it is therefore essential that appropriate parameters be selected because this may determine the results of the study. Much of the clinical research in musculoskeletal MRI has been devoted to the determination of effective techniques.[96] It is the radiologist's responsibility to stay current with changes in the discipline and tailor each study to best provide the information required.

The orthopaedist should think of MRI as a technique for imaging soft tissue, cartilage, and bone marrow. To understand bone images, the magnetic resonance characteristics of fatty and hematopoietic marrow must be appreciated, and the orthopaedist must have knowledge of the variation in marrow distribution with age. Pathologic processes are detected because they alter the signal characteristics of normal tissue. Magnetic resonance imaging reflects the presence of edema in marrow and muscle when it occurs in response to injury or infection because it is sensitive to the increase in extracellular water. The hydrogen nuclei in bone, however, are bound tightly and do not produce signal intensities of the magnitude produced by the nuclei in soft tissues. Magnetic resonance images therefore show a signal void from bone. In the standard MRI—in which high signal is white and low signal is black, with intermediate shades of gray— calcified bone is black and therefore is not visible. Thus, a practical distinction between MRI and CT is that CT shows calcium well and MRI does not.

Despite the high cost of studies, the use of MRI has increased dramatically. A complete MRI examination takes 30 to 60 minutes. For most of that time, the patient is inside the cylindrical bore of the magnet. As the image is being acquired, there must be no motion; for infants and young children, this requires sedation. The restricted field of view and requirement for region-specific techniques with an MRI scanner mean that a request to study "head, cervical and thoracic spine" is actually a request for three studies. In such cases, the duration of the procedure may excede the period of effective sedation, necessitating general anesthesia. Physicians requesting MRI studies need to be as specific as possible in designating the critical location. The improving quality of MRI images is partly related to development of specialized RF coils tailored to a particular anatomic site (e.g., knee and shoulder) and to selection of pulse sequences. There is a growing body of knowledge about pediatric musculoskeletal applications, and this is being incorporated to the diagnosis and management of pediatric problems. The literature is also filled with adult studies but caution should be exercised because findings may not hold true in infants and children.

Magnetic resonance imaging is the preferred approach in evaluating children for lesions of the spinal canal and spinal cord. It is equal or superior to myelography for congenital lesions such as syringomyelia, diastematomyelia, tethering of the cord (Fig. 2-14), and lipomeningoceles.[11,46,61] Acquired lesions, such as intraspinal tumors and demyelinating diseases, also are identified more effectively. For diagnosis of disc disease, the National Institutes of Health consensus report judged MRI to be equivalent to CT myelography in the evaluation of herniated cervical and thoracic discs.[93] At the lumbar level, MRI was considered equal to or better than CT and more accurate than myelography. An important observation with this highly sensitive imaging technique is that disc abnormalities must be correlated with clinical findings. Not all discs that are abnormal on MRI cause symptoms.[36] Magnetic resonance imaging is a sensitive method for demonstrating spinal infections, such as discitis.[25] In cases of suspected spinal infection in which plain films are normal, MRI is considered to be an alternative to scintigraphy[110] from the standpoint of sensitivity and to be comparable or better than CT for showing extent of disease. Typically, I go from plain film to scintigraphy to gain the advantage of the broad bone survey; however, in the case of focal clinical findings and appropriate laboratory values, it is not inappropriate to go from plain film to an MRI of the spine.

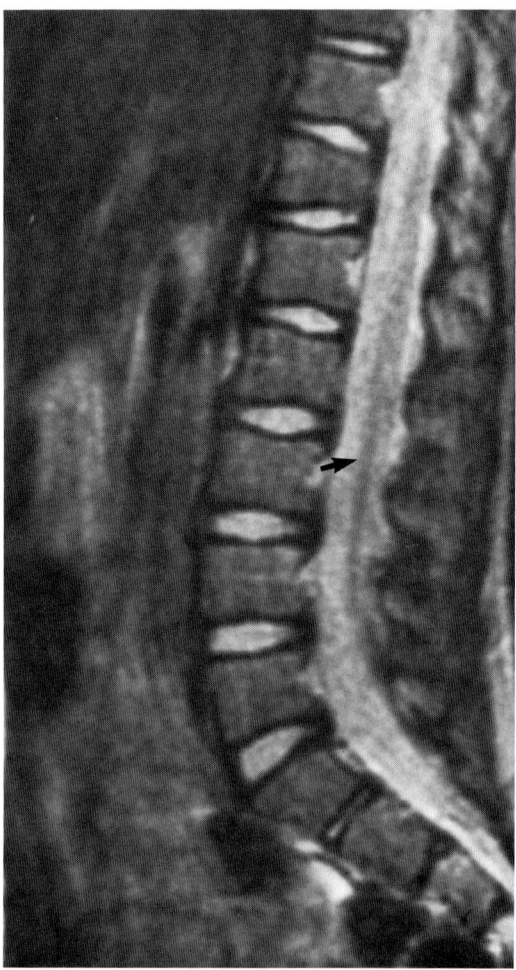

FIGURE 2-14. Sagittal magnetic resonance imaging study made with T1-weighted pulse sequence of a 6-year-old boy with tethered cord. The cord terminates at the L3 level (*arrow*), and the filum is thickened distally.

Magnetic resonance imaging evaluation of tumors arising in the paraskeletal soft tissue and in bone is being promoted enthusiastically. Thus far, the characteristics of benign and malignant tumors show considerable overlap, and the technique is not reliable in predicting tumor histology. The success, however, of MRI over CT in detecting and defining the soft tissue involvement, marrow extent, and epiphyseal and joint space invasion of musculoskeletal tumors is reported in children, just as in adults (Fig. 2-15).[17,88] Magnetic resonance imaging is well suited for delineating the involvement of tumor with ligaments, tendons, and neurovascular tissue. Skip areas within a bone can be recognized but the use of MRI in detecting distant metastatic disease has not been advocated because total body imaging is not technically feasible at this time.

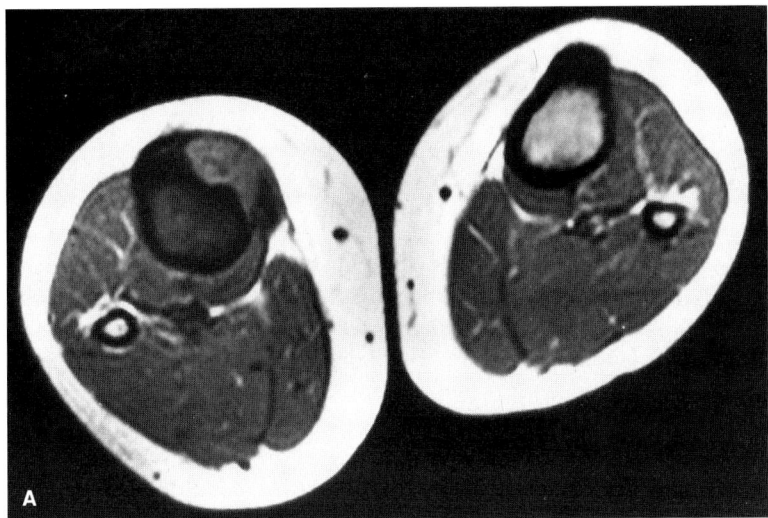

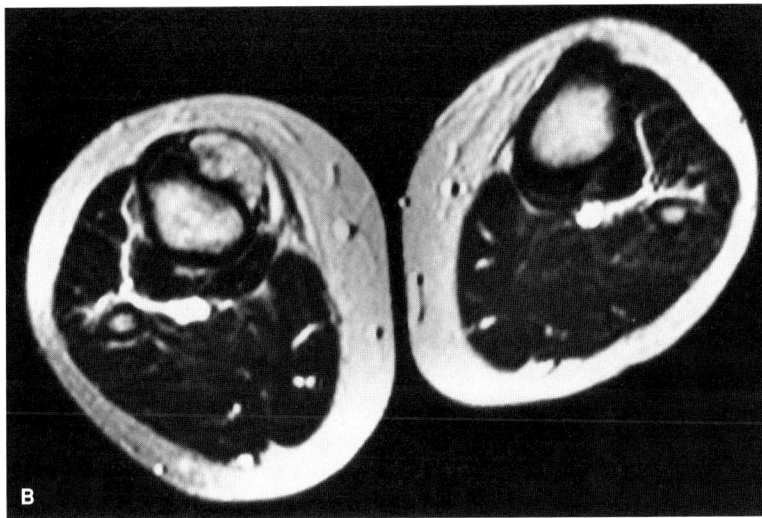

FIGURE 2-15. Axial magnetic resonance imaging scans of a 12-year-old girl with osteosarcoma of the proximal right tibia. (**A**) T1-weighted image shows that the marrow and soft tissue component have low signal intensity. (**B**) T2-weighted image shows reversal of signal, which is consistent with tumor.

Infectious processes are detectable by MRI and use of the modality is growing in this area. By demonstrating marrow and soft tissue changes, MRI has a high sensitivity for detecting osteomyelitis but has not shown equally high specificity.[101] Uncomplicated septic effusions, for example, have caused marrow changes that were mistaken for osteomyelitis.[26] A limitation of MRI is that the specific location or locations to be studied must be selected. It does not provide the broad survey that is obtained with bone scintigraphy or show the osseous changes as well as does CT. In some areas of the skeleton, such as the sacroiliac joints, MRI has been found to have an advantage over scintigraphy.[17] The major value for magnetic resonance imaging may be in cases of subacute and chronic osteomyelitis, in which it can separate active inflammation from chronic fibrosis and guide surgical debridement.[22]

In cases of ischemic bone disease, MRI shows marrow changes both acutely and during healing. There are other disorders that can similarly affect marrow. Controversy still exists regarding the use of MRI and scintigraphy to identify avascular necrosis because case reports document cases wherein one method has been positive and the other negative and vice versa. In cases in which a child with normal radiographs is suspected of having Perthes disease, I still use scintigraphy. In management of patients, it has been shown that compared with less expensive plain films, the information gained from MRI did not justify its expense.[57]

Use of MRI in acute trauma has been hampered by difficulty in monitoring patients while they are in the magnet. For subacute nonosseous trauma, MRI is competing with arthrography and arthroscopy.[98,104] Magnetic resonance imaging has been helpful in assessing osteochondritis dissecans and osteochondral fractures to identify loose fragments.[91] Discoid meniscus is readily identified.[105] Rotator cuff abnormality in the shoulder is also successfully identified by MRI.

Accuracy is related to whether tears are full or partial thickness.[114]

A role for MRI in the assessment of physeal closure has been established, and I prefer this technique over radiographic tomography because of the ability to show detailed cartilage and marrow anatomy. The physiologic process of maturation and closure is shown by optimal pulse sequences that depict physeal cartilage.[54] These gradient or field-echo sequences show physeal and articular cartilage with bright signal intensity. Injury to the growth plate with subsequent bar formation can be documented in detail.[60] The ability to obtain sagittal and coronal sections makes it feasible to map the extent of a physeal bar (Fig. 2-16).[55] Although these studies show the presence and distribution of cartilage in the physis, they provide no information about cartilage growth potential; I use scintigraphy to assess plate physiology.

Although MRI can show anatomic detail that permits diagnosis of congenital hip dislocation, prudent use of resources dictates that MRI be reserved for special cases, such as posttreatment avascular necrosis or assessment of acetabular cartilage in residual dysplasia.[30] In classification of congenital anomalies, proximal femoral focal deficiency, MRI can distinguish cartilage elements and their morphology.[88]

It is clear that MRI has a growing role in evaluating the musculoskeletal system in children. Studies of the spinal cord and related structures and tumor imaging can already be considered as accepted indications. The use of MRI as a first or second step in the diagnosis of ischemic disease, infection, and joint abnormalities has yet to be justified based on clinical effectiveness and cost-effectiveness.

SUMMARY

To provide guidance in selecting an appropriate sequence of imaging techniques for a given diagnostic problem, the algorithm concept is being used. This is a step-by-step sequence in which the results from one step determine the course of action to be taken as the succeeding step. In clinical practice, the orthopaedist must consider physical examination, laboratory data, and results from diagnostic procedures such as aspiration in addition to imaging information to determine the need for an additional imaging study.

As the orthopaedic surgeon and radiologist struggle with their selection of imaging techniques, they also must keep in mind two important practical points. First is availability. Regardless of the reports in the literature attesting to the superiority of one method over another, a modality cannot be used when it is not available, and an appropriate substitute technique must be selected. Second, some institutions and individuals perform some procedures better than others. If the orthopaedic surgeon has a particularly skilled sonographer or arthrographer with whom to work, he or she may favor that technique over another that is not performed with the same degree of accuracy. All of the discussions regarding choice of technique are a tribute to the technologic advances in imaging. When the orthopaedic surgeon and radiologist communicate effectively in both investigation and clinical work, patients benefit from these advances.

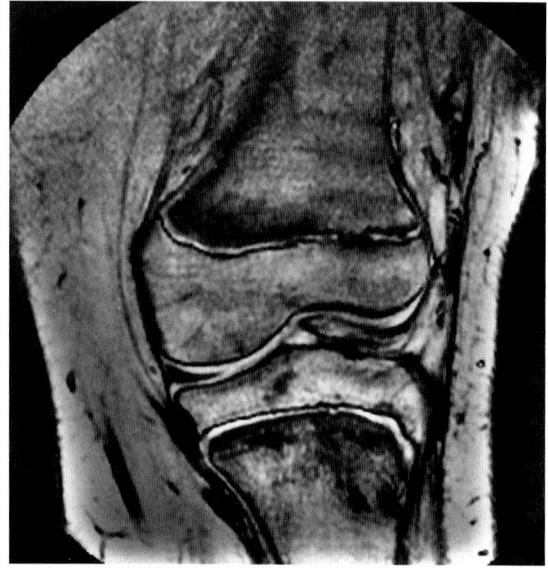

FIGURE 2-16. Coronal magnetic resonance imaging study of the knee in an 11-year-old girl after trauma shows growth plate damage in both the distal femur and proximal tibia. Note the low signal in the tibial metaphysis, where there has been a fracture. This study was conducted with field echo pulse sequence.

References

1. Adelstein SJ. Uncertainty and relative risks of radiation exposure. JAMA 1987;258:655.
2. Alexander JE, Seibert JJ, Glasier CM, et al. High-resolution hip ultrasound in the limping child. J Clin Ultrasound 1989;17:19.
3. Altongy JF, Harcke HT, Bowen JR. Measurement of leg length inequalities by micro-dose digital radiographs. J Pediatr Orthop 1987;7:311.
4. American Academy of Pediatrics Committee on Drugs. Guidelines for monitoring and management of pediatric patients during and after sedation for diagnostic and therapeutic procedures. Pediatrics 1992;89:1110.
5. American College of Radiology. Manual on iodinated contrast media. Reston, VA: American College of Radiology, 1991.
6. American Institute of Ultrasound in Medicine. Bioeffects considerations for safety of diagnostic ultrasound. J Ultrasound Med 1988;7(Suppl 9):S1.
7. Ash J, Gilday DL. The futility of bone scanning in neonatal osteomyelitis: concise communication. J Nucl Med 1980;21:417.
8. Azuma H, Taneda H, Igarashi H. Evaluation of acetabular coverage: three-dimensional CT imaging and modified pelvic inlet view. J Pediatr Orthop 1991;11:765.

9. Boree NR, Clarke NMP. Ultrasound imaging and secondary screening for congenital dislocation of the hip. J Bone Joint Surg [Br] 1994;76:525.
10. Blank E. Some effects of position on the roentgenographic diagnosis of dislocation at the infant hip. Skeletal Radiol 1981;7:59.
11. Bradford DS, Heithoff KB, Cohen M. Intraspinal abnormalities and congenital spine deformities: a radiographic and MRI study. J Pediatr Orthop 1991;11:36.
12. Canale ST, Harkness RM, Thomas PA, et al. Does aspiration of bones and joints affect results of later bone scanning? J Pediatr Orthop 1985;5:23.
13. Cann CE. Quantitative CT for determination of bone mineral density. Radiology 1988;166:509.
14. Clarke NMP. Sonographic clarification of the problems of neonatal hip instability. J Pediatr Orthop 1986;6:527.
15. Clarke NMP, Harcke HT, McHugh P, et al. Real-time ultrasound in the diagnosis of congenital dislocation and dysplasia of the hip. J Bone Joint Surg [Br] 1985;67:406.
16. Cohen MD. Clinical utility of magnetic resonance imaging in pediatrics. Am J Dis Child 1986;140:947.
17. Cohen MD. Magnetic resonance imaging of the pediatric musculoskeletal system. Semin Ultrasound CT MR 1991;12:506.
18. Collier BD, Hellman RS, Krasnow AZ. Bone SPECT. Semin Nucl Med 1987;17:247.
19. Conway JJ. A scintigraphic classification of Legg-Calve-Perthes disease. Semin Nucl Med 1993;23:274.
20. Dahlstrom H, Oberg L, Friberg S. Sonography in congenital dislocation of the hip. Acta Orthop Scan 1986;57:402.
21. Dalinka MK, Osterman AL, Albert AS, et al. Arthrography of the wrist and shoulder. Orthop Clin North Am 1983;14:193.
22. Dangman BC, Hoffer FA, Rand FF, et al. Osteomyelitis in children: gadolinium-enhanced MR imaging. Radiology 1992;182:743.
23. Datz FL, Thorne DA. Effect of chronicity of infection on the sensitivity of the In-111-labeled leukocyte scan. AJR 1986;147:809.
24. DeSmet AA. Radiology of spinal curvature. St. Louis: CV Mosby, 1985:40.
25. duLac P, Panuel M, Devced P, et al. MRI of disc space infection in infants and children. Pediatr Radiol 1990;20:175.
26. Erdman WA, Tamburro F, Jayson HT, et al. Osteomyelitis: characteristics and pitfalls of diagnosis with MR imaging. Radiology 1991;180:533.
27. Eyres KS, Bell MJ, Kanis JA. New bone formation during leg lengthening. J Bone Joint Surg [Br] 1993;75:96.
28. Fasting OJ, Langeland N, Bjerkreim I, et al. Bone scintigraphy in early diagnosis of Perthes' disease. Radiology 1975;115:407.
29. Fisher RL, Roderique JW, Brown DC, et al. The relationship of isotopic bone imaging findings to prognosis in Legg-Perthes disease. Clin Orthop 1980;150:23.
30. Fisher R, O'Brien TS, Davis KM. Magnetic resonance imaging in congenital dysplasia of the hip. J Pediatr Orthop 1991;11:617.
31. Fornage BD. Achilles Tendon: US examination. Radiology 1986;159:759.
32. Fornage BD, Rifkin MD, Touche DH, et al. Sonography of the patellar tendon: preliminary observations. AJR 1984;143:179.
33. Fornage BD, Schernberg FL. Sonographic diagnosis of foreign bodies of the distal extremities. AJR 1986;147:567.
34. Gainey MA, Siegel JA, Smergel EM, et al. Indium-111-labeled white Blood Cells: cosimetry in children. J Nucl Med 1988;29:689.
35. Gardiner HM, Dunn PM. Controlled trial of immediate splinting versus ultrasonographic surveillance in congenitally dislocatable hips. Lancet 1990;336:1553.
36. Gibson MJ, Szypryt EP, Buckley JH, et al. Magnetic resonance imaging of adolescent disc herniation. J Bone Joint Surg [Br] 1987;69:699.
37. Gilday DL, Paul DJ, Patterson J. Diagnosis of osteomyelitis in children by combined blood pool and bone imaging. Radiology 1975;117:331.
38. Gilsanz V, Gibbens DT, Roe TF, et al. Vertebral bone density in children: effect of puberty. Radiology 1988;166:847.
39. Glastre C, Braillon P, David L, et al. Measurement of bone mineral content of the lumbar spine by dual energy x-ray absorptiometry in normal children: correlations with growth parameters. J Clin Endocrinol Metab 1990;70:1330.
40. Graf R. Ultrasonography of the infantile hip. In: Sanders RC, Hill MC, eds. Ultrasound annual 1985. New York: Raven Press, 1985.
41. Graham CB. Assessment of bone maturation—methods and pitfalls. Radiol Clin North Am 1972;10:185.
42. Greenberg SB, Faerber EN, Aspinall CL, et al. High dose chloral hydrate sedation for children undergoing MR imaging: safety and efficacy in relation to age. AJR 1993;161:639.
43. Greulich WW, Pyle SI. Radiographic atlas of skeletal development of the hand and wrist. 2nd ed. Stanford, CA: Stanford University Press, 1959:50.
44. Grissom LE, Harcke HT, Kumar SJ, et al. Ultrasound evaluation of hip position in the Pavlik harness. J Ultrasound Med 1988;7:1.
45. Hall FM. Arthrography: past, present, and future. AJR 1987;149:561.
46. Han JS, Benson JE, Kaufman B, et al. Demonstration of diastematomyelia and associated abnormalities with MR imaging. AJNR 1985;6:215.
47. Harcke HT. Screening newborns for developmental dysplasia of the hip: the role of sonography. AJR 1994;162:395.
48. Harcke HT, Conway JJ, Tachdjian MO, et al. Precise scintigraphic localization of bone lesions during operative intervention. J Nucl Med 1982;23:50.
49. Harcke HT, Grissom LE. Sonographic evaluation of the infant hip. Semin Ultrasound CT MR 1986;7:331.
50. Harcke HT, Grissom LE, Finkelstein MS. Evaluation of the musculoskeletal system with sonography. AJR 1988;150:1253.
51. Harcke HT, Kumar SJ. The role of ultrasound in the diagnosis and management of congenital dislocation and dysplasia of the hip. J Bone Joint Surg [Am] 1991;73:622.
52. Harcke HT, Lee MS, Sinning L. Ossification center of the infant hip: sonographic and radiographic correlation. AJR 1986;147:317.
53. Harcke HT, Mandell GA. Scintigraphic evaluation of the growth plate. Semin Nucl Med 1993;23:266.
54. Harcke HT, Synder M, Caro PA, Bowen JR. Growth plate of the normal knee: evaluation with MR imaging. Radiology 1992;183:119.
55. Havranek P, Lizler J. Magnetic resonance imaging in the evaluation of partial growth plate arrest after physeal injuries in children. J Bone Joint Surg [Am] 1991;73:1234.
56. Henderson RC. Assessment of bone mineral content in children. J Pediatr Orthop 1991;11:314.
57. Henderson RC, Renner JB, Sturdivant MC, et al. Evaluation of magnetic resonance imaging in Legg-Perthes disease: a prospective, blinded study. J Pediatr Orthop 1990;10:289.
58. Hernandez RJ, Tachdjian MO, Poznanski AK, et al. CT determination of femoral torsion. AJR 1981;137:97.
59. Heinrich SD, MacEwen GD, Zembo MM. Hip dysplasia, subluxation, and dislocation in cerebral palsy: an arthrographic analysis. J Pediatr Orthop 1991;11:488.
60. Jaramillo D, Hoffer FA. Cartilaginous epiphysis and growth plate: normal and abnormal MR imaging findings. AJR 1992;158:1105.
61. Jospan T, Worthington BS, Holland IM. A comparative study

62. Kallio P, Ryoppy S, Jappinen S, et al. Ultrasonography in hip disease in children. Acta Orthop Scand 1985;56:367.
63. Keats TE. An atlas of normal roentgen variants that may simulate disease. 3rd ed. Chicago: Year Book Medical Publishers, 1984.
64. Keats TE, Lusted LB. Atlas of roentgenographic measurement. 5th ed. Chicago: Year Book Medical Publishers, 1985.
65. Keats TE, Smith TH. An atlas of normal developmental roentgen anatomy. Chicago: Year Book Medical Publishers, 1977.
66. Kloiber R, Pavlovsky W, Portner O, et al. Bone scintigraphy of hip joint effusions in children. AJR 1983;140:995.
67. Kumar SJ, Harcke HT, MacEwen GD, et al. Osteoid osteoma of the proximal femur: new techniques in diagnosis and treatment. J Pediatr Orthop 1984;4:669.
68. Kushner DC, Cleveland RH, Herman TE, et al. Radiation dose reduction in the evaluation of scoliosis: an application of digital radiography. Radiology 1986;161:175.
69. Lackman RW, Kaufman B, Han JS, et al. MR imaging in patients with metallic implants. Radiology 1985;157:711.
70. Laine HR, Harjula A, Peltokallio P. Ultrasound in the evaluation of the knee and patellar regions. J Ultrasound Med 1987;6:33.
71. Laine HR, Harjula A, Peltokallio P. Experience with real-time sonography in muscle injuries. Scand J Sports Sci 1985;7(2):45.
72. Langer R. Ultrasonic investigation of the hip in newborns in the diagnosis of congenital hip dislocation: classification and results of a screening program. Skeletal Radiol 1987;16:275.
73. Lantto T, Kaukonen JP, Kokkola A, et al. Tc-99m HMPAO labelled leukocytes superior to bone scan in the detection of osteomyelitis in children. Clin Nucl Med 1992;17:7.
74. Lee DY, Choi IH, Lee CK, et al. Assessment of complex hip deformity using three-dimensional CT image. J Pediatr Orthop 1991;11:13.
75. Lee MS, Harcke HT, Kumar SJ, et al. Subtalar joint coalition in children: new observations. Radiology 1989;172:635.
76. Lemperg R, Liliequist B, Mattsson S. Asymmetry of the epiphyseal nucleus in the femoral head in stable and unstable hip joints. Pediatr Radiol 1973;1:191.
77. Lewin JS, Rosenfield NS, Hoffer PB, et al. Acute osteomyelitis in children: combined Tc-99m and Ga-67 imaging. Radiology 1986;158:795.
78. Lisbona R, Rennie WJF, David RK. Radionuclide evaluation of free vascularized bone graft viability. AJR 1980;134:387.
79. Lyon JL. Radiation exposure and cancer. Hosp Pract 1984;19:159.
80. Magid D, Fishman EK, Ney DR, et al. Acetabular and pelvic fractures in the pediatric patient: value of two- and three-dimensional imaging. J Pediatr Orthop 1992;12:621.
81. Majd M, Frankel RS. Radionuclide imaging in skeletal inflammatory and ischemic disease in children. AJR 1976;126:832.
82. Marchal GJ, Val Holsbeeeck MT, Raes M. Transient synovitis of the hip in children: role of ultrasound. Radiology 1987;162:825.
83. McCoy JR, Morrissy RT, Seibert J. Clinical experience with the technetium-99m scan in children. Clin Orthop 1981;154:175.
84. McLean O, Freiman DB. Angiography of skeletal disease. Orthop Clin North Am 1983;14:257.
85. McMaster MJ, Merrick MV. The scintigraphic assessment of the scoliotic spine after fusion. J Bone Joint Surg [Br] 1980;62:65.
86. Merten DF, Radkowski MA, Leonidas JC. The abused child: a radiological reappraisal. Radiology 1983;146:377.
87. Miralles M, Gonzalez G, Pulpeiro JR, et al. Sonography of the painful hip in children: 500 consecutive cases. AJR 1989;152:579.
88. Moore SG, Bisset GS, Siegel MJ, et al. Pediatric musculoskeletal MR imaging. Radiology 1991;179:345.
89. Moore SG, Dawson KL. Magnetic resonance appearance of red and yellow marrow in the femur: spectrum with age. Radiology 1990;175:219.
90. Moser PP, Madewell JE. An approach to primary bone tumors. Radiol Clin North Am 1987;25:1049.
91. Murray IPC. Photopenia in skeletal scintigraphy of suspected bone and joint infection. Clin Nucl Med 1982;7:13.
92. Nadel HR. Thallium-201 for oncological imaging in children. Semin Nucl Med 1993;23:243.
93. National Institutes of Health Consensus Development Conference statement—magnetic resonance imaging. Oncology 1988;2:53.
94. Obermann WR, Kieft GJ. Knee arthrography: a comparison of iohexol, ioxaglate sodium meglumine, and metrizoate. Radiology 1987;162:729.
95. Palestro CJ, Kim CK, Swyer AJ, et al. Total hip arthroplasty: periprosthetic indium-111-labeled leukocyte activity and complimentary technetium-99m-sulfur colloid imaging in suspected infection. J Nucl Med 1990;31:1950.
96. Peterfy CG, Linares R, Steinbach LS. Recent advances in magnetic resonance imaging of the musculoskeletal system. Radiol Clin North Am 1994;32:291.
97. Pettersson H, Springfield DS, Enneking WF. Radiologic management of musculoskeletal tumors. New York: Springer-Verlag, 1987:9.
98. Polly DW Jr, Callaghan JJ, Sikes RA, et al. The accuracy of selective magnetic resonance imaging compared with the findings of arthroscopy of the knee. J Bone Joint Surg [Am] 1988;70:192.
99. Rubin K. Schirduan V, Gendreau P, et al. Predictors of axial and peripheral bone mineral density in healthy children and adolescents, with special attention to the role of puberty. J Pediatr 1993;123:863.
100. Salzman L, Lee VW, Grant P. Gallium uptake in myositis ossificans—potential pitfalls in diagnosis. Clin Nucl Med 1987;12:308.
101. Schauwecker DS. The scintigraphic diagnosis of osteomyelitis. AJR 1992;158:9.
102. Schmidt H, Freyschmidt J. Borderlands of normal and early pathologic findings in skeletal radiography. 4th ed. New York: Thieme Medical Publishers, 1993.
103. Seltzer SE, Weissman BN, Braunstein EM, et al. Computed tomography of the hindfoot. J Comput Assist Tomogr 1984;8:488.
104. Silver I, Silver DM. Tears of the meniscus as revealed by magnetic resonance imaging. J Bone Joint Surg [Am] 1988;70:199.
105. Silverman JM, Mink JH, Deutsch AL. Discoid meniscus of the knee: MR imaging appearance. Radiology 1989;173:351.
106. Soble MG, Kaye AD, Guay RC. Rotator cuff tear: clinical experience with sonographic detection. Radiology 1989;173:319.
107. Sorenson JA. Perception of radiation hazards. Semin Nucl Med 1986;16:158.
108. Stanton RP, Capecci R. Computed tomography for early evaluation of developmental dysplasia of the hip. J Pediatr Orthop 1992;12:727.
109. Sty JR, Starshak RJ. The role of bone scintigraphy in the evaluation of the suspected abused child. Radiology 1983;146:369.
110. Sty JR, Wells RG, Conway JJ. Spine pain in children. Semin Nucl Med 1993;23:296.
111. Sullivan DC, Rosenfield NS, Ogden J, et al. Problems in the scintigraphic detection of osteomyelitis in children. Radiology 1980;135:731.

112. Suzuki S, Kasahara Y, Futami T, et al. Ultrasonography in congenital dislocation of the hip. J Bone Joint Surg [Br] 1991;73:879.
113. Szoke N, Kuhl L, Heinrichs J. Ultrasound examination in the diagnosis of congenital hip dysplasia of newborns. J Pediatr Orthop 1988;8:12.
114. Traughber PD, Goodwin TE. Shoulder MRI: Arthroscopic correlation with emphasis on partial tears. J Comput Assist Tomogr 1992;16:129.
115. Tonnis D, Storch K, Ulbrich HJ. Results of newborn screening for CDH with and without sonography and correlation of risk factors. J Pediatr Orthop 1990;10:145.
116. Vick CW, Bell SA. Rotator cuff tears: diagnosis with sonography. AJR 1990;154:121.
117. Webster EW. On the question of cancer induction by small x-ray doses. AJR 1981;137:647.
118. Wiener SN, Seitz WH. Sonography of the shoulder in patients with tears of the rotator cuff: accuracy and value for selecting surgical options. AJR 1993;160:103.
119. Yeh HS. Ultrasonography of orthopedics and soft tissues of extremities. In: Sanders RC, Hill MC, eds. Ultrasound annual 1985. New York: Raven Press, 1985.
120. Zieger M. Ultrasound of the infant hip. Part II. Validity of the method. Pediatr Radiol 1986;16:488.

Chapter 3

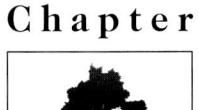

The Pediatric Orthopaedic Examination

Richard H. Gross

Focused Examination
  Gathering Information
  Recording Information
Normal Development
  Normal Development of the Newborn
  Normal Development in Early Childhood
Examining and Recording Joint Motion and Function
Limb Lengths
Examinations of Specific Anatomic Areas
  Skin
  Spine
  Shoulder and Upper Limb
  Elbow, Forearm, and Wrist
  Hand
  Hip
  Knee and Leg
  Foot and Ankle
Conclusion

The examination is the cornerstone of the practice of pediatric orthopaedics. The history directs the examination, the examination points to the diagnosis, and the diagnosis influences the treatment. Outcome often depends on an accurate history and physical examination. Performing a good physical examination is a learned motor skill, requiring practice to become proficient and a knowledge of the pertinent anatomy and structural effects of the suspected condition. Practice, a fortuitous word that describes what doctors do, also implies that physicians continue to improve their capabilities. Every patient affords an opportunity to practice diagnostic skills. Although repeatedly practicing careful examinations enhances skills, a pattern of performing hasty assessments results in atrophy of diagnostic acumen. In this sense, practice is a lifelong art.

Because it is impossible to describe the pertinent anatomy and the detailed manner in which that anatomy is altered for every condition encountered in the pediatric orthopaedic examination, the material in this chapter must be complemented by studying the various pathologic entities described in these volumes.

The situations encountered in the operating room, clinic, and office can enhance the surgeon's skill in physical assessment and in conceptualizing alterations in structure and function. Imaging studies, including radiography, computed tomography scans, and magnetic resonance images, offer other opportunities to correlate clinical findings with the underlying pathology. Alterations in motion and function may be obvious or so subtle that only skillful assessment can detect them. The patient's history may be unambiguous and readily available from parents or grandparents, or it may be confusing or totally lacking, as in the case of a fractured long bone in an abused infant.

FOCUSED EXAMINATION

Examining the child requires ingenuity on the part of the physician, because the directed examination of an adult is often impossible in the case of a frightened child. An exhaustive examination of the child's musculoskeletal system cannot be performed during every patient visit. The mature physician makes many rapid and often barely conscious decisions about the focus of the history taking and the emphasis of the examination within moments after the initial encounter. Information triage is essential in selecting the pertinent examination maneuvers to detect the conditions responsible for the presenting complaint. The examiner's approach is tailored to the age of the patient and to the suspected pathology.

The concept of the focused examination does not exclude a systematic approach. It acknowledges, for example, that a detailed assessment of hand function is not done for a toddler presenting because of parental concern about a toeing-in pattern. In this case, a systematic examination of torsional and angular alignment of the lower limb is performed. Necessary historical and physical assessment factors are integral parts of the focused examination.

The first component of this technique is knowledge of the disease process. Without understanding the anatomic direction of the movement of the femoral head relative to the neck in a patient with slipped capital femoral epiphysis and the effect of that femoral head movement on hip range of motion, the examination maneuvers necessary to detect this condition would not be performed or performed without understanding the findings. Without the knowledge that hip pathology in the child often masquerades as knee pain, an examination of the hip may not be performed at all. Being aware that soft tissue swelling is the cardinal clinical sign of an underlying osteomyelitis directs a careful assessment of these structures. The invariable presence of rotation in structural idiopathic scoliosis has emphasized accurately evaluating and recording this finding using ancillary aids such as the scoliometer. The complaint that a 9-month-old child is not using a hand well directs attention to an evaluation of the tone of the upper and lower limbs. Knowledge of the disease process focuses the examination.

The second component is knowledge of the functional anatomy. This understanding is as basic as knowing the arrangement of the keys when trying to play the piano. For example, an unstable hip in a newborn may be discovered with a gentle examination performed in a manner designed to displace the femoral head posteriorly, but the condition may not be discovered with a more vigorous but less directed examination, with the hip in a position that does not allow displacement of the femoral head.

The final component is the experience gained from previous examinations. Accumulating experience does not necessarily require a lengthy period; using each examination as an opportunity to build on previous competence can be rewarding in a relatively short time. For example, a newborn examination requested for possible hip instability may reveal absence of the normal flexion contracture of the hip at this age. Using this situation as a stimulus to learn the range of hip motion in the newborn quickly adds to the examiner's skill. However, a perfunctory examination for instability could be performed in which the absence of the hip flexion contracture was not noticed, cheating the patient of good care and the examiner of valuable experience.

Gathering Information

Gathering essential information in a timely fashion is an integral part of the physician-patient encounter. Many practices use a written form that is completed before the initial interview and examination (see Appendix 3-1). Pertinent developmental history is also included, as are the names and addresses of physicians who should receive a copy of the examination. Height and weight are recorded, and when available, an initial nursing interview can document helpful information such as medications, allergy profile, and general medical and surgical history.

The information obtained from the questionnaire and the nursing encounter should be verified during the interview and examination. The interviewing style of the physician is important; patient and parental satisfaction with the encounter depends more on the physician's manner and communication style than on the length of time spent with the patient.[54] Patients and their parents expect physicians to be friendly, concerned, and sympathetic and to take the time to answer questions and provide explanation. Open-ended questions are often more yielding than factual inquiries. For example Baird and Gordon suggest it is better to ask "When did you feel something was wrong?" than "How long has your child had this problem?"[5] Taking a history in a relaxed manner while demonstrating a real interest in the problem increases the confidence of the patient and family and results in a more complete and meaningful clinical story. The word "story" is used purposefully instead of history, because story implies a unique and personal component. The history would be appropriate for charting or presentation in a conference setting, but listening to the story gives the physician insight into the patient's background and expectations. It allows the physician to know the patient and family better, which increases their confidence in the physician.

Evaluating complaints of pain can be taxing. Popoff developed a method of analyzing the patient's description to guide the physician in separating organic and psychogenic pain.[71] In general, organic pain is intermittent, can be described clearly, is produced and relieved by specific activity, is well localized, and can awaken the patient from a sound sleep. Psychogenic pain is often vague or bizarre, and it tends to be described as continuous and poorly localized.

It is not produced or relieved by specific activity, and it does not awaken the patient from a sound sleep.

The examination is performed in a manner dictated by the age of the patient and the presenting problem. Experienced physicians process a great deal of information rapidly in deciding what examination maneuvers to perform and in what order. In general, observation is the initial component of the examination. Spontaneous active range of motion, use of the limbs in dressing or moving about the room, swelling, and splinting or guarding are noteworthy findings. The child's interactions with the environment, parents, and physician are of particular interest before the physical examination is started. Palpation and measurement of the passive range of motion constitute the hands-on examination, with the order determined by the presenting problem. In general, the most threatening or potentially painful portion of the examination is reserved for the final part.

The contralateral limb often serves as a valuable baseline in unilateral conditions such as pain and is better usually first. A toddler's fracture may be suspected by observing guarding of the affected limb. Gently performing a passive range of motion can eliminate the ankle as a site of pathology, and systematic palpation of the tibia can reveal the site of tenderness, directing the radiographic attention to that site. For a complaint of knee pain, an older patient can be asked to localize the site of pain; absence of tenderness in that area can direct attention to the hips, and an assessment of hip motion is added to that of the knee motion. The American Academy of Orthopaedic Surgeons has published a handbook for the clinical measurement of joint motion.[34]

Observation of gait is best done with minimal clothing, and the physician should maintain a supply of paper shorts, which are useful for children who come only with bulky clothing. Sutherland's classic paper on the development of mature gait is helpful in interpreting the observations of young children.[86] Observation of gait usually should be done serially. When observing the gait of an in-toeing child, the examiner should use the first pass to observe the direction of the feet in relation to the line of progression, the second pass to determine the relation of the patella to the line of progression, and a third pass to observe motion of the entire limb.

After the examination is completed, the physician must organize her or his findings and synthesize the information gathered. The family is then informed of the physician's findings and recommendations for treatment. Patients or parents expect to learn the cause and nature of the condition for which they went to the doctor, and they tend to be dissatisfied if excessive medical jargon is used to explain the condition. A study of young British physicians found that feedback training could improve interviewing skills, but it did not increase their skill in delivering information.[59] Skill in information giving can be developed and assessed by asking the patient or parents if they understood the explanation offered them and if they have any further questions.[58] The presence of siblings in the examination room has been found to decrease the parents' capability for retention of information given by the physician.[46] The use of a skeletal model can help in explaining anatomic findings. Videotapes and pamphlets can also be helpful, but these should be substituted for conversation.

Recording Information

The examination is useless unless it is accurately documented. There are several compelling reasons for good documentation. Documenting the patient's current status provides a baseline for ongoing observation and more effective care. Reports are sent to referring physicians, who appreciate accurate and informative accounts. The record may be used by insurance carriers to justify or deny payment for a particular treatment plan or to determine the level of payment for the services. The medical records may become legal documents in the event of litigation involving the patient, even if the lawsuit does not involve the physician.

The record of an initial encounter should include an explanation of the reason for the visit, pertinent history and physical findings, interpretation of imaging studies, an impression, and recommendations or disposition. For follow-up visits, the record is generally abbreviated, but interim history should be recorded, with any change in physical findings, imaging studies, or disposition. A follow-up record may be as complete as an initial record or as brief as a notation that postoperative cast change was performed, including a concise description of the status of the affected area.

For an extensive or complex history, dictating the history in the family's presence ensures that it is complete and accurate. The examination can also be dictated at the time it is performed, eliminating the need for notes that must be reinterpreted later.

Language can be critical when relating findings to others or for comparison during subsequent examinations. For example, what is a hip click? Is it a normal or abnormal finding? Are other terms more descriptive of the physical findings? We communicate by means of language, and if the language is ambiguous, the communication is ineffective. For recording an examination of a hip of a child with Legg-Perthes disease, "20 degrees of abduction in extension" is much more meaningful than describing "moderate loss of abduction," especially if another examiner may see the child for the next visit. Phrases such as "nearly

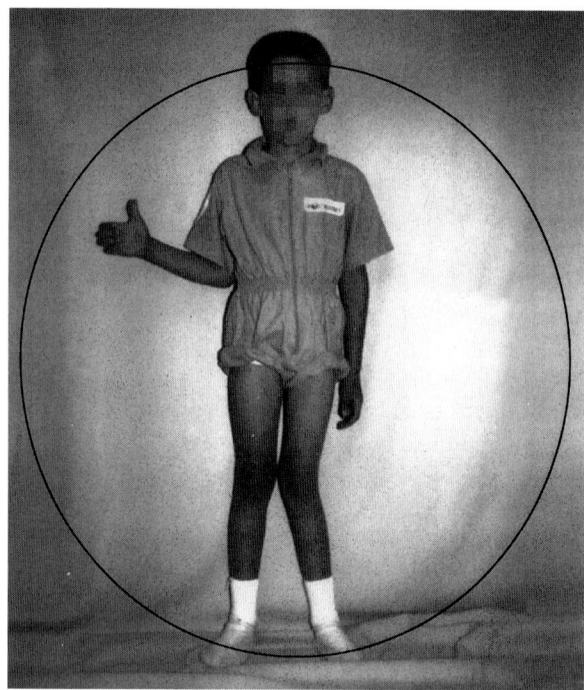

FIGURE 3-1. Salter's concept of placing the patient in an imaginary circle. The left leg distal to the deformity is pointing toward the center of the circle, demonstrating a valgus deformity. The right arm is normal.

full range of motion" or "mild atrophy" are of less value than "lacking 5 degrees of full extension" or "2 cm of calf atrophy." The physician should record information as if someone else will be performing the next examination and depending on the record to determine if there has been any interval change.

A hinged goniometer should be used for angular measurement. With practice, the examiner can achieve accuracy in estimating angular measurements, but even for experienced examiners, goniometric measurements are more accurate.[15,76,91] If a goniometer is not available, angles can be estimated by mentally dividing a 90-degree arc of motion into two 45-degree segments or three 30-degree segments and then superimposing the observed angle into these mental arcs.

Photographs can be an invaluable method of documentation. They are cheaper and more quickly obtained than radiographs, and they have no potentially harmful side effects. If documentation of the patient's status is helpful for conditions such as physiologic bowing, photographs are excellent for later comparison.

The terminology used in orthopaedic assessment is often confusing for those without experience. This chapter does not address the sources of confusion, which are largely centered on the terms "varus" and "valgus." The tricky part is determining which body part is being described, and there is no science in the way the terms are used; the current usage of the terms is the opposite of their original Latin meanings. Salter described a simple and understandable method for picking the term judged correct by modern usage.[78] The patient is conceptually placed inside an imaginary circle (Fig. 3-1). If the direction of the part distal to the angular deformity conforms with the circle, a varus deformity is present. If the part distal to the deformity points outside the circle, a valgus deformity is present. An angular deformity of the proximal tibia in which the distal fragment points toward the midline (conforming with the shape of the circle) would be designated as tibia vara, and a deformity of the elbow in which the forearm is directed toward the body would be cubitus varus. The site of the deformity is designated by the anatomic term (e.g., cubitus, coxa, pes). Generally, these terms are well understood because of continuous use by orthopaedic surgeons, but they may be confusing to pediatricians or family practitioners. Houston and Swischuk have suggested using the terms bowlegs and knock-knees instead, and there is probably some merit to this when discussing these entities with primary care physicians.[45]

NORMAL DEVELOPMENT

Childhood is so familiar that it it is easy to overlook the almost unbelievable transformation from the tiny newborn to the fully grown teenager. Such a transformation involves an incredibly ordered but dynamic growth process. Many of the orthopaedic conditions of childhood are related to disorders of the growth process or to conditions that alter growth in some way. Growth may be absent in some congenital limb deficiencies, retarded in the presence of extrinsic pressure on the growth plate, or even accelerated in the presence of conditions such as juvenile arthritis. Communication requires a standardized terminology for describing the conditions affecting growth. An international working group published the following recommendations for terminology in 1982, and familiarity and usage of this system by the orthopaedist is highly recommended.[25,82] A schema depicting the different effects of errors of development is illustrated (Fig. 3-2).

Malformations result from an interruption of normal organogenesis and are usually genetic in origin. The fetal malformation is present from the time of organogenesis (weeks 4–8). Examples of malformations are polydactyly, Poland syndrome, and proximal focal femoral deficiency.

Disruptions are morphologic defects of an organ or body part resulting from the extrinsic breakdown of or interference with an originally normal developmental process. For example, abnormalities of struc-

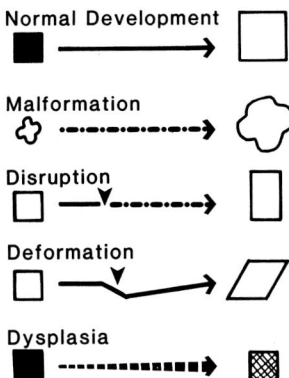

FIGURE 3-2. Dunne and Clarren's modification of Spranger's schema illustrating the types of errors in morphogenesis. A *solid line* indicates development is structurally normal, but the shape can still be influenced by deformation. *Broken lines* depict disruption in developmental potential. (From Dunne KB, Clarren SK. The origin of prenatal and postnatal deformities. Pediatr Clin North Am 1986;33:1277.)

ture may be associated with congenital constricting bands in limbs that were normal at the time of organogenesis. Drugs or toxic substances may cause disruptions.

Dysplasias result from abnormal organization of cells into tissues, leading to abnormal tissue differentiation, such as the connective tissue defect responsible for the defective bone in osteogenesis imperfecta.

Deformations are abnormalities in form, shape, or position of body parts caused by mechanical molding. Deforming forces may be intrinsic, such as central nervous system disorders resulting in hypomobility; extrinsic, such as uterine constraint; or both. Deforming forces mold or bend tissues. The fetus is more susceptible to deformations because it grows seven times as fast as the infant, although infants with habitual sleeping positions may also demonstrate deformations.

Differentiating malformations, which cannot be directly treated, from deformations, which may respond well to removal of the deforming force in the neonate, is important. Many severe deformations may appear to be malformations unless carefully assessed.[19] An example is the condition of congenital hyperextension of the knee, in which the leg may appear grotesquely misshapen at first glance, but it is actually a normally formed leg perhaps constrained by a breech presentation or in a bicornuate uterus. Treatment is simple, unlike that for dislocation of the knee secondary to tibial hemimelia, a structural malformation.

Normal Development of the Newborn

Illingworth stated that a thorough knowledge of the normal should be just as much the basis of the study of children as is physiology and anatomy for medicine in general; it is essential for the study of the abnormal and of disease.[49]

Professor Illingworth's statement remains valid. Orthopaedic surgeons are often the first to be consulted when there is concern about a child's delay in walking or in the acquisition of some other motor skill or for reassurance when the parents are worried about the child's motor capabilities. For the 12-month-old child who is favoring one hand over the other, the time when handedness becomes evident in normal development becomes very important. Although there are volumes of information on the normal development of children, the space restrictions of this chapter dictate selection. The neurologic status of the normal newborn is presented, followed by the normal developmental sequence in early childhood. There are excellent resources for the interested reader to study this fascinating subject in greater depth.[12,48,49,68] What follows are the basic tools necessary to evaluate a significant neurodevelopmental delay.

The newborn is largely reflexive but does have some social characteristics. Within minutes of birth, the infant follows a face-like pattern more than other patterns of similar brightness. A black and white pattern evokes more interest than a plain gray one. The newborn infant turns his eyes toward sound. Within a week, the baby can differentiate the mother from strangers.[49]

The normal newborn has a predominance of flexor tone (Fig. 3-3). The concept of tone is important in many aspects of pediatric orthopaedic examination, but it is an essential component of the newborn examination. Tone is the quality in muscle that resists movement or stretch. When a normal muscle is slowly stretched, there is a gentle but appreciable resistance, and when it is stretched past a comfortable resting position, it springs back when the stretch is released. This increased flexor tone is responsible for the lack of complete hip and knee flexion in newborns. Flexor tone is first evident at about 32 weeks of gestation, initially in the lower extremities. By term, all limbs are

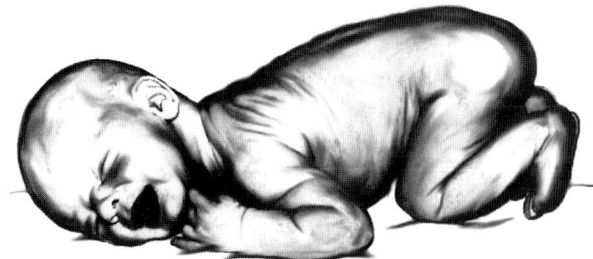

FIGURE 3-3. Physiologic flexion contractures are normal findings in the newborn. (Adapted from Illingworth RS. The development of the infant and young child—normal and abnormal. 9th ed. New York: Churchill Livingstone, 1987.)

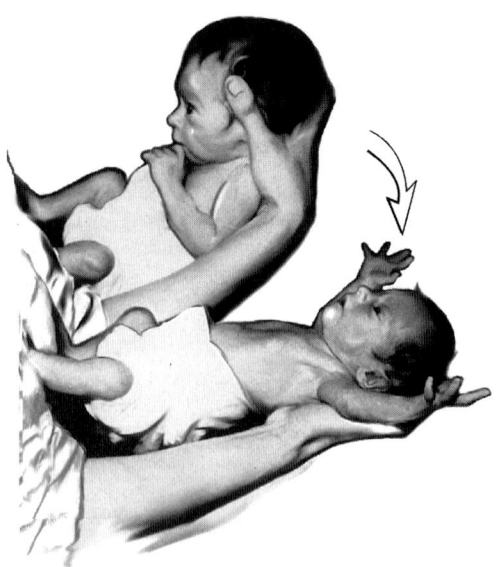

FIGURE 3-4. Method of Dubowitz and Illingworth for testing the Moro reflex. The child is supported at angle of 45 degrees with the examiner's hand under the infant's head, then the head is dropped a short distance. The infant's arms spread, and the hands open. This phase of the Moro reflex is followed by adduction of the arms, as in an embrace. (Adapted from Illingworth RS. The development of the infant and young child—normal and abnormal. 9th ed. New York: Churchill Livingstone, 1987.)

maintained in flexion posture, and passive manipulation reveals strong flexor tone in all extremities and the neck. The normal newborn moves limbs in an alternating manner when stimulated.

Myriad reflexes in the newborn can be evaluated. These include primitive reflexes, which should disappear, and others, such as the knee jerk, that persist throughout life. Postural reflexes, such as neck and body righting and the parachute posture, appear later and are not present at birth. The reflexes for the newborn discussed in this chapter are those considered of value by Illingworth, who has devoted his career to the study of early development of the child.

Of the facial reflexes, only the oral reflexes are selected by Illingworth. The "rooting" reflex is a feeding reflex, allowing the baby to find the mother's nipple. When the corner of the mouth is lightly stimulated, the tongue moves toward that point, and the lower lip is opened. If the finger is moved laterally, the head turns to follow it.

The Moro response, a vestibular reflex, is present in the normal newborn and in many premature babies. Any maneuver producing sudden extension of the neck provokes a Moro reflex. Baird and Gordon think the best way to test the Moro reflex is to lift the child from the supine position with one of the examiner's hands under the thoracic spine and the other hand under the head (Fig. 3-4).[5] The hand under the head is then suddenly withdrawn, allowing neck extension. A positive response is sudden abduction and extension of the upper limbs, with spreading of the fingers followed by an embrace. In normal infants, this reflex disappears by about 4 months of age. The startle response, a mass myoclonic reflex, is normal in infants and young children. The elbow remains flexed in the startle reflex. Although sometimes confused, the startle response is not equivalent to the Moro reflex.

The grasp reflex consists of two parts: grasp and arm contraction. The head should be in the midline; if the head is rotated, the reflex is more easily obtained on the side toward which the occiput is directed. The grasp is elicited by introducing an examiner's finger into the infant's palm from the ulnar side. The palm is stimulated, and the fingers flex and grasp. The examiner then places traction on the infant's arm by pulling the finger gently upward. The muscles of the arm and shoulder girdle contract, and the baby can be suspended for a moment by his grasped fingers on the examiner's finger. The grasp reflex disappears by 2 or 3 months of age (Fig. 3-5).

The tonic neck reflexes are symmetrical and asymmetrical. The asymmetrical form is more often performed. When the baby is resting in the supine position, the limb toward which the face lies is extended at the elbow, and the limb on the side of the occiput is flexed. When the head is rotated, there is some tendency for the baby to assume the position just described, but the classically described fencing position is never obligatory in the neurologically normal baby. The tonic neck reflex disappears in 2 to 3 months. In

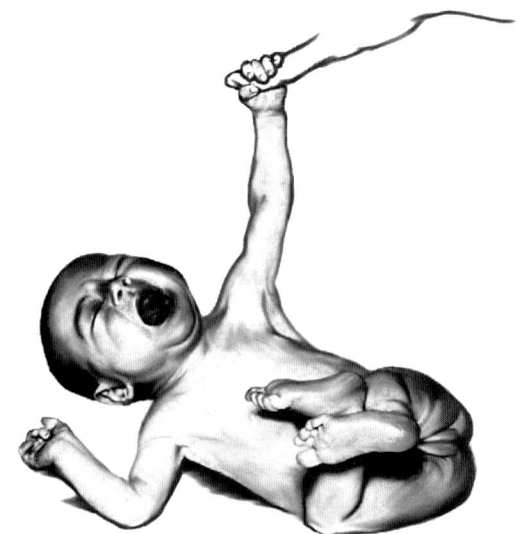

FIGURE 3-5. Grasp reflex. The examiner's finger is placed in the baby's hand. The baby grasps the hand and can momentarily be suspended by pulling the grasping hand upward. (Adapted from Illingworth RS. The development of the infant and young child—normal and abnormal. 9th ed. New York: Churchill Livingstone, 1987.)

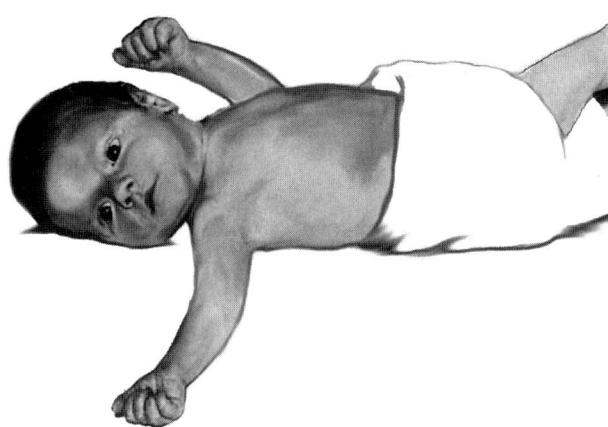

FIGURE 3-6. Asymmetrical tonic neck reflex. When the baby's head is turned to the side, the elbow on the side of the occiput flexes, and the elbow on the side of the face extends. (Adapted from Illingworth RS. The development of the infant and young child—normal and abnormal. 9th ed. New York: Churchill Livingstone, 1987.)

the infant with cerebral palsy, the reflex persists, and the fencer's position may be obligatory when the head is rotated (Fig. 3-6).

The biceps, knee, and ankle reflexes are tested by tapping the tendons. In the newborn, the fingertip suffices admirably to tap the patellar and Achilles tendons; the effects of the reflex contraction of the quadriceps and gastrosoleus can be directly observed. The biceps is more difficult to observe directly. Placing the tip of the index finger of the examiner's nondominant hand on the tendon and then tapping with a fingertip of the dominant hand affords the examiner a tactile impression of the quality of the reflex contraction.

Before attempting to elicit ankle clonus, the hip is flexed and abducted, and the knee is flexed. The ankle is then rapidly but gently dorsiflexed. Clonus is an indicator of increased tone but by itself does not indicate a neuromuscular deficit.

Johnson described methods of examining the newborn and infant for neuromuscular weakness.[50] The shoulder stabilizers can be assessed by lifting the baby with the examiner's fingers on the lateral chest walls under the armpits. The baby tends to slip through the hands if there is shoulder girdle weakness. Grasping the baby's hands and pulling the baby to a sitting position gives an indication of muscle tone. Tone may be assessed by rapidly alternating flexion and extension of the limbs; a weakened extremity resists with less force or muscle tone. Placing a corner of a sheet over the infant's face results in a reflex or voluntary attempt by the baby to remove the sheet. Placing the baby prone on the examiner's hand and allowing the baby's hips to flex while stimulating the posterior thighs or feet with the other examiner's hand can afford easier assessment of the activity of hip ex-

tensors and hamstrings. Stimulating the sole of the foot results in dorsiflexion of the ankle in the normal newborn.

Normal Development in Early Childhood

Neurologic Maturation

The general sequence of development is the same in all children, but the timing of developmental milestones varies from child to child. The rate depends on maturation of the central nervous system, and this cannot be rushed. A 5-month-old infant cannot be taught how to walk. Primitive reflexes must disappear before a child can walk. Development proceeds in a cephalocaudad direction; head control and hand control precede the ability to control the lower limbs.[49]

The examination of the infant uses these principles. In the first few months, emphasis is on the acquisition of head control. The easiest way to assess head control is to suspend the prone baby in the examiner's hand. The newborn has no head control, but by 2 months of age, the baby should be able to hold his or her head in the same plane as the rest of the body and, by 3 months of age, above the plane of the rest of the body (Fig. 3-7). Similarly, by 3 to 4 months of age, the head should not lag when the baby is pulled from a supine to a sitting position. By 6 months of age, the infant should be able to grasp objects, including a bottle, and should be able to sit with hand support or minimal external support. As development continues to proceed in a cephalocaudal direction, better motor control of the legs becomes evident with each passing month. By the ninth month, pulling up to furniture is possible, as is sitting on the floor without

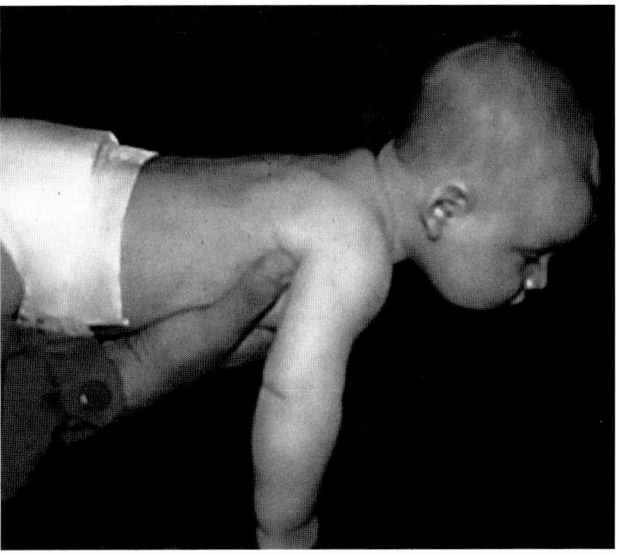

FIGURE 3-7. Head control in 3-month-old child. When supported, the head is held above the plane of the body.

TABLE 3-1 Average Developmental Achievement by Age

AGE	ACHIEVEMENT
1 mo	Little change from newborn; may hold head up momentarily when held in prone position
2 mo	Maintains head in plane of body when held in prone position; partial head control when pulled from supine to sitting
3 mo	Head held up above plane of body when supported in prone position; only slight head lag when pulled up to sitting position; disappearance of tonic neck and grasp reflex
4 mo	When prone, can lift head and chest off bed, with weight on forearms
6 mo	When prone, lifts head and chest off bed, with weight on hands; when held in standing position, almost full weight on legs; sits with support
8 mo	Sits without support; reaches for toys
10 mo	Crawls; can pull to sitting position; can stand holding on to furniture
12 mo	Walks independently or with hand support
18 mo	Handedness becoming established
2 y	Jumps, knows full name, helps put things away
3 y	Goes upstairs alternating feet; stands momentarily on one foot; knows age and gender
4 y	Hops on one foot; climbs well; throws ball overhand
5 y	Skips; dresses and undresses

support. Independent ambulation occurs around 1 year of age, with a wide variation of normal. The 1-year-old child can also throw objects on the floor and speak two or three words. Handedness is not established until about 18 months of age; if there is a definite preference for one hand in the first year of life, a careful assessment of the other hand and upper limb is warranted. Table 3-1 lists developmental milestones of particular interest to the orthopaedic surgeon.

Evaluating an infant's development consists initially of learning from the parents what developmental milestones have been achieved and comparing these with the norms for that age. One method of inquiry that works well is to ask what the child is doing now that he or she was not able to do 3 months earlier; the interval asked about depends on the circumstances. The next step is to watch the infant for a few moments, noticing spontaneous motion and head control. The older infant can be observed reaching and grasping for a toy or interesting object. If the toy is placed nearby on the table or floor, the crawling ability can be evaluated. Only after a period of observation should formal reflex testing be done, and if a careful history and period of observation have been performed, there will be few surprises. If a further check on development would be helpful in the clinic setting, the revised Denver Developmental Screening Test can be administered by a nurse familiar with the test. If the screening results indicate delay, referral to a pediatrician familiar with developmental testing is warranted.

Establishing developmental delay often is not a clear-cut issue. There are considerable variations in the attainment of developmental milestones and myriad causes for delay. A few children are advanced. About 3% learn to walk independently by 9 months of age. The relation between advanced physical development and intelligence is not clear, although early acquisition of language skills may be predictive.

If a child is delayed in one sphere of development but "on time" for the rest, there is little reason for concern. Some children, for no apparent reason, may eliminate the stage of creeping. Illingworth described a girl who could walk before she could sit. Familial factors seem to have some influence, as does race; infants of African descent mature more rapidly than Caucasian infants.[49] The major concern is whether a neuromuscular condition is responsible for delayed developmental milestones. When is a neurologic consultation indicated? Available information seems to indicate that walking should have occurred by 18 months in virtually any neuromuscularly normal child. Boys with Duchenne muscular dystrophy have been reported to walk at an average age of 17 months. In general, delayed walking is accompanied by other historical or physical findings that clarify the need for further investigation or consultation.

The neurologic evaluation need not be exhaustive. The quality and symmetry of deep tendon reflexes can be easily assessed, regardless of age. Retention of primitive reflexes is an important finding, because these reflexes interfere with the motor control necessary to walk. If there is a question of delayed development, the primitive infant reflexes (usually the asymmetric tonic neck, Moro response, or extensor thrust) are repeated. Bleck described seven primitive reflexes that he assesses in the following sequence.[14]

1. Asymmetrical tonic neck reflex (see Fig. 3-5)
2. Neck-righting reflex. The head of the supine child is turned to the side, and if the shoulders and trunk turn with the head, the reflex is positive. This reflex normally disappears by 10 months of age (Fig. 3-8).
3. Moro reflex (see Fig. 3-4)
4. Symmetrical tonic neck reflex. The child is placed in the crawling position on hands and knees. When the neck is flexed, the upper limbs flex, and the lower limbs extend. When the neck is extended, the upper limbs extend, and the lower limbs flex (Fig. 3-9).

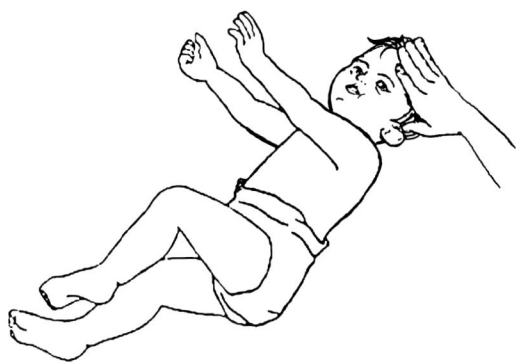

FIGURE 3-8. Neck righting reflex. When the head is turned, the trunk and limbs turn to same side. (Adapted from Bleck EE. Orthopaedic management in cerebral palsy. Philadelphia: JB Lippincott, 1987.)

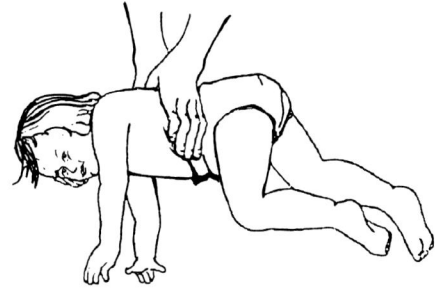

FIGURE 3-10. Parachute reflex. The child is held above a table and dropped slightly, simulating a fall. The normal response is extension of the limbs and placement of the hands as if to break the fall. (Adapted from Bleck EE. Orthopaedic management in cerebral palsy. Philadelphia: JB Lippincott, 1987.)

5. Parachute reflex. The child is lifted while in the prone position and quickly lowered to the table top, simulating a fall. The normal response, found after about 1 year of age, is extension of the arms and placement of the hands as if to break the fall. The parachute reaction has been especially helpful in predicting ambulatory potential when performed at about 1 year of age. The infant is held above the table in a prone position and suddenly lowered toward the table, simulating a fall. The normal 1-year-old child can extend the arms and legs (like a parachute unfolding) to cushion the expected fall. In a child with spastic hemiplegia, this response may be one sided; in a child with quadriplegia, it may not exist. This response is responsible for the frequency of distal radius fractures in children with normal development as they protect themselves from falls (Fig. 3-10).
6. Foot placement reaction. The child is held by the chest wall and axilla and then lifted so the dorsum of each foot is brought up against the underside of the table top or chair. The normal response, even in infants, is placement of the foot on the table top or chair. This reflex persists in some fashion until 3 or 4 years of age (Fig. 3-11).
7. Extensor thrust. The child is held in the same manner as for the foot placement reaction, but the feet are lowered toward the top of the table or chair. Normal infants flex their legs with this maneuver, and extension of the lower limbs indicates neurologic impairment (Fig. 3-12).

There has been little further refinement of this widely used sequence of reflex testing over the past two decades, and the reflexes selected by Bleck had already been well described. They comprise a mixture of physiologic obligatory reflexes in the newborn (Moro) that persist in the presence of profound cerebral palsy, reflexes that are never normal (extensor thrust and asymmetric tonic neck), and acquired normal reflexes (parachute position) that may be delayed. Bleck emphasizes that his reflex profile is not meaningful before the child is 12 months of age.

Physical Development

Although there are published standards available for various physical measurements throughout childhood, acceptance of these published normal values does not apply to all populations. The measurements vary on the basis of geography, socioeconomic status, genetic influences, and even altitude.[1,28] The standards still used in the United States were calculated from

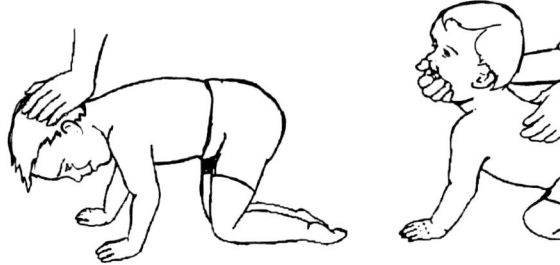

FIGURE 3-9. Symmetrical tonic neck reflex. Flexion of the head causes flexion of the arms and a tendency toward hip extension. Extension of the head causes extension of arms and flexion of the hips and legs. (Adapted from Bleck EE. Orthopaedic management in cerebral palsy. Philadelphia: JB Lippincott, 1987.)

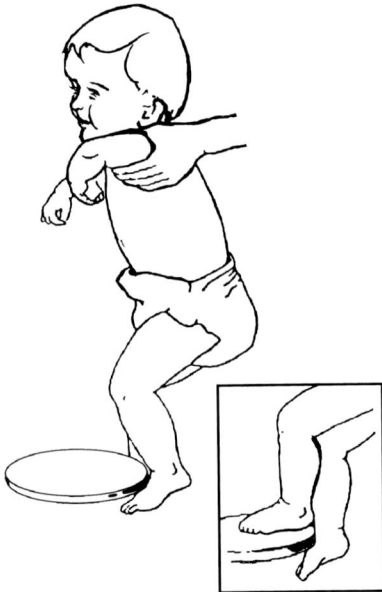

FIGURE 3-11. Foot placement reaction. The child is lifted so the dorsal sides of the feet are against the underside of the table. Symmetrical or asymmetrical placement of the feet on a table constitute a normal response. (Adapted from Bleck EE. Orthopaedic management in cerebral palsy. Philadelphia: JB Lippincott, 1987.)

work done in the 1940s, and these standards probably reflect the status of shorter children than those growing up in the 1990s. The mean height of schoolchildren in Oslo, Norway, has increased about 5 cm during this time, with a general upward slope of the height of the schoolchildren from 1920 to the present, except one dip during the war years of the 1940s.[16] The role of socioeconomic status is reflected in a study from Poland, which found the height of 18-year-old sons of college-educated men to be more than 6 cm greater than that of conscripts for military service from the families of peasant farmers.[13] Standards of measurements can be helpful, especially if the examiner knows the population from which the standards were developed and demurs from overzealous application of these standards to other populations.[42,90] Age influences the range of motion, with the degree of flexibility differing by gender and diminishing at a variable rate throughout life.[64,73,75,85,87]

Standards formulated from the study of normal children do afford the examiner guidelines by which to gauge whether growth is occurring within the normal range. In early childhood, dramatic changes occur in lower limb alignment, passing from physiologic bowlegs to physiologic knock-knees.[77] Rotation of the lower limbs changes considerably during early childhood and less rapidly afterward.[85] After 9 years of age, there can be immense differences in height velocity between early- and late-maturing children. Skeletal age gives better information in this regard than chronologic age, and radiography is required. A clinical method of comparing physical maturation to chronologic age has been described by Tanner; standards are available to compare breast development in girls and genital development in both sexes (see Appendix 3-2).[17,89] It is not necessary for the orthopaedist to have thorough knowledge of Tanner's standards, but an overall familiarity is valuable. Determining the age of menarche while evaluating a young female with scoliosis is one way of discerning the status of physical maturity. Most girls approaching skeletal maturity are uncomfortable with the idea of having a Tanner standard evaluation performed by a male physician. In this situation, a trained nurse may perform the Tanner assessment. Many helpful standards are available in the volume compiled by Hensinger, but the *Handbook of Normal Physical Measurements* by Hall and coauthors is also easily consulted in a clinical setting for basic information.[37]

Smith's *Recognizable Patterns of Human Malformations* contains an appendix that lists anomalies by region.[80] For instance, if an infant has brachydactyly, clinodactyly, and hypertelorism, consulting the appendix under each of those headings would reveal Aarskog syndrome to be common to all. Although the orthopaedist usually is not a competent dysmorphologist, clinical acumen grows with more awareness of the possible patterns and combinations of malformations.

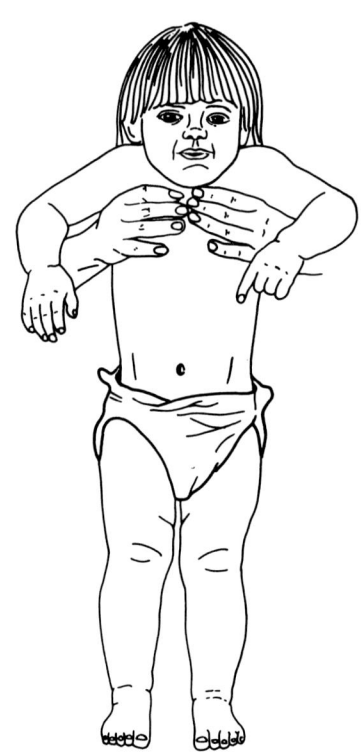

FIGURE 3-12. Extensor thrust. When the soles of the feet are pressed to a table, there is progressive extension of the legs from the feet proximally. (Adapted from Bleck EE. Orthopaedic management in cerebral palsy. Philadelphia: JB Lippincott, 1987.)

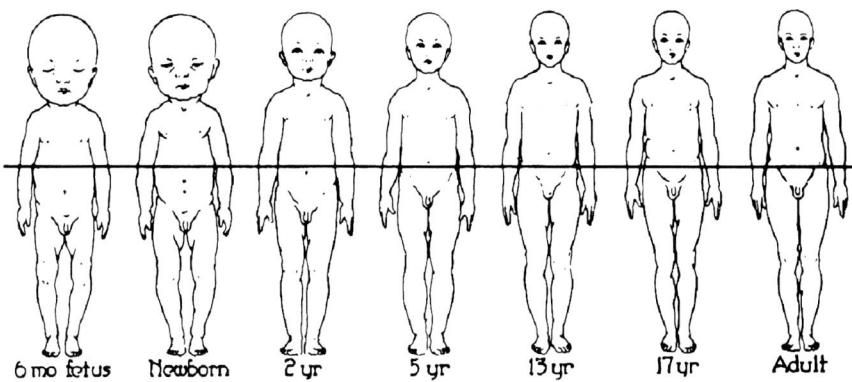

FIGURE 3-13. Relation of the center of gravity to body segments. At birth, the head and body are about 1.7 times as long as the legs; by maturity, the segments are nearly equal. (From Hensinger RN. Standards in pediatric orthopedics. New York: Raven Press, 1986.)

Body proportions change markedly throughout growth. In fetal life, the head is disproportionately large, and even at birth, it accounts for about one quarter of the length of the entire body. Subcutaneous fat is not deposited until the last month of a normal intrauterine pregnancy, and the difference in appearance of a premature from a term newborn is largely secondary to the presence or absence of subcutaneous fat. The head also grows rapidly in infancy, and the head circumference is normally greater than chest circumference for the first year. The upper to lower segment ratio reflects differences in body proportions; it is the ratio of the distance from the top of the head to the symphysis pubis divided by the distance from the symphysis pubis to the soles of the feet. At birth, the ratio is about 1.7; it becomes 1 at about 10 years of age; and it is normally less than 1 after 10 years of age (Fig. 3-13). Rapidly growing body structures are subject to many influences, including the general health and nutritional status; for example, leg length growth has prematurely ceased in adolescent female gymnasts undergoing heavy physical training.

Psychosocial Development

The orthopaedic surgeon does not have expertise in the field of psychosocial development but is qualified to be an interested observer. Psychosocial factors influence the coping skills of patients with chronic conditions and their families and can affect orthopaedic treatment strategies. For example, it is not worthwhile to prescribe brace treatment unless the brace will be worn. Arduous treatment programs, such as leg lengthening procedures, may be extremely taxing on the emotional resources of the family. Children with chronic disabilities often require so much of the family's energy that siblings may feel neglected or resentful.

To determine the situation, the orthopaedic surgeon can ask open-ended questions, such as "How are things going?" or "How are you all getting along?" Inquiries about friends and progress in school are often rewarding. Physical disability can sometimes be sought by a child eager to avoid an uncomfortable social or school situation. If the family perceives a genuine interest on the part of their physician, they are glad to share their concerns, and psychologic support can be obtained when indicated.

EXAMINING AND RECORDING JOINT MOTION AND FUNCTION

The pediatric orthopaedic examination must assess possible contracture and spasticity. Although these are extremely useful words, their definitions are not precise.

Contracture indicates loss of the normal excursion of a joint or muscle-tendon unit. The fact that the anatomic basis of contractures can be located in different anatomic structures is often confusing. Babies have physiologic contractures of upper and lower limbs.[22,30,70,73,92] A hip flexion contracture may be caused by a bony deformity, such as that accompanying a slipped capital femoral epiphysis, or muscular defect, such as a tight iliopsoas muscle in a child with cerebral palsy. A capsular contracture is often found in the posterior knee capsule of children with spina bifida. A displaced torn meniscus blocks knee extension, producing a flexion contracture of cartilaginous origin. Synovial fluid accumulation, such as that found in children with juvenile arthritis, impedes normal joint motion, and the resultant loss of motion may be called a contracture. Immobilization may be responsible for the development of contracture, such as in the presence of a gastrocnemius contracture found after a cast has been applied with the foot in equinus.

For two-joint muscles, such as the hamstrings or gastrocnemius, examination for contracture must control the movement of one joint before ranging the second joint. The initial maneuver in assessing the popliteal angle is stabilization of the flexed femur on the pelvis, and then the knee is extended.

The ability to assess contractures is key for the pediatric orthopaedic examination. For many years, children have been regarded as "loose," and contracture was considered to be a problem of older children or adults. However, work indicates contracture may cause conditions such as growing pains.[10] Contracture assessment most often is performed on the lower limbs in early childhood. In later childhood, especially with participation in throwing sports, contracture assessment is also valuable in the evaluation of the elbow and shoulder.

Spasticity is another condition impeding joint motion. Spasticity refers to an increase in tone of a muscle. Normally, humans have a slight tension in their muscles, enough to keep them from being floppy but not enough to impair contracting a given muscle to move a joint through a normal range of motion. Conditions with decreased tone, such as neuropathies, are characterized by a flabby feel of the muscle, with decreased muscle strength and excursion. There is little resistance to passive joint motion in the presence of hypotonia. Spastic muscles have increased tone, and it is more difficult to put a joint spanned by spastic muscles through a normal range of motion. For example, spastic hamstrings may impede knee extension. Spastic muscles are more difficult to control, because they are under more obligatory reflex control, and relaxation is impaired to some degree. Spasticity is characteristic of upper motor neuron impairment, and cerebral palsy is the most common cause. The degree of actual spasticity can vacillate tremendously in any given muscle, depending on apprehension, room temperature, time of day, and a host of other variables.

When evaluating the range of motion in a patient with a spastic condition, the endpoint is often less certain. With gentle persistence, a spastic muscle relaxes, and greater excursion can be achieved. As a result, different quantitative values may be obtained for the same examination. A review by Perry documented the imprecision of quantitative evaluations of muscles with spasticity.[69] Measurements varied significantly from day to day or even hour to hour. With sitting and standing, ankle dorsiflexion was less than when supine. Knee flexion allowed greater ankle dorsiflexion in 95% of children with cerebral palsy. To cope with this variability, the examiner can make a record for the popliteal angle, such as "initial resistance at 55 degrees, with persistence 40 degrees." Some observers think that reliability within 15 degrees of joint motion can be achieved with goniometric measurements of patients with spasticity,[39] but others think goniometric evaluations are of such limited value that they should not be used for decision making.[2] A description of the quality of resistance, such as fixed, initial resistance with subsequent relaxation, or constant resistance; the effect of sustained resistance by the examiner; and the overall tone of the patient at the time of examination is useful. The position of adjacent joints is also pertinent. For example, the physician should notice whether dorsiflexion of the ankle was examined with hip and knee flexion or extension. Because foot position also affects ankle dorsiflexion, ankle motion is recorded in a manner such as "lacks 5 degrees of dorsiflexion to neutral, with knee extended and foot supinated."

Spastic muscles often function in patterns of movement. The flexor pattern of the lower limb is ankle dorsiflexion with hip and knee flexion, as occurs during the swing phase of gait. A patient with moderate spasticity of the lower limb often has difficulty dorsiflexing the ankle with the knee extended. Sometimes the phrase "out of phase" is used to describe muscles that are not patterned to contract simultaneously. A patient unable to dorsiflex the ankle with the knee extended may automatically dorsiflex the ankle when asked to further flex the thigh when the patient is sitting with the knee dangling over the end of the table. This maneuver is most commonly called the confusion test (Fig. 3-14). Many normal children also have a positive confusion test result, because flexor pattern is a normal component of gait. The confusion test is considered important for decision making by some physicians but not by others.[7,24]

The ability of orthopaedic surgeons in developed countries to evaluate and record muscle strength has atrophied since the conquest of poliomyelitis. However, evaluation of muscle strength remains an inte-

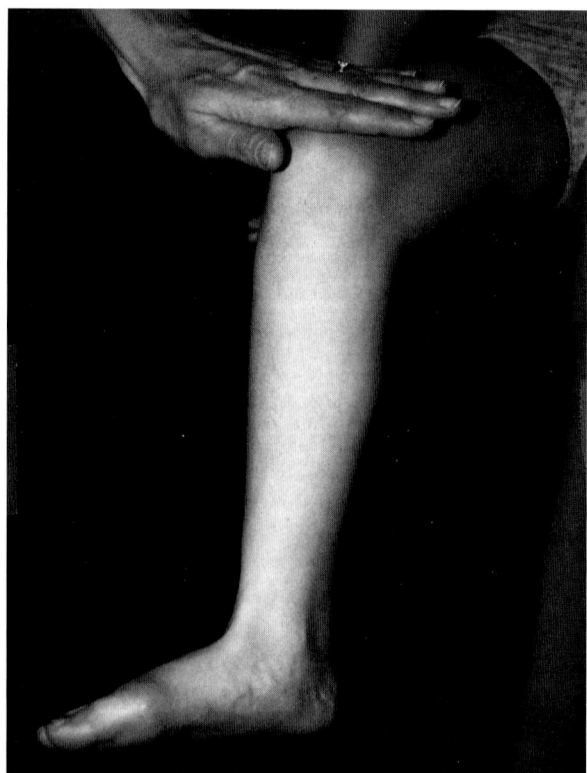

FIGURE 3-14. Confusion test. Asking the patient to touch the examiner's hand with the knee induces a flexion pattern. If the anterior tibial muscle is activated by this maneuver, as shown, the test result is positive.

gral part of the orthopaedic examination, and some competence with strength evaluation and recording is essential. For purposes of the office orthopaedic examination, muscles can be sorted into functional groups. For example, when determining the functional level of the lower limbs in a patient with spina bifida, it is unnecessarily cumbersome to test the semitendinosus, gracilis, and semimembranosus separately; the examiner is interested in the activity of the medial hamstrings as a group. In general, proximal muscles, such as hip abductors, are tested as a group; more distal muscles, such as the flexor pollicis longus or extensor digitorum communis are easier to isolate and evaluate separately. Detailed descriptions of individual muscle testing are available.[44]

The time-honored grading of muscle strength, initially described Lovett[56] in 1917, is still useful in the evaluation of neuromuscular conditions:

0. No evidence of contraction
1. Trace: slight contraction, no joint motion with gravity eliminated
2. Poor: complete range of motion with gravity eliminated
3. Fair: complete range of motion against gravity
4. Good: complete range of motion against gravity with some resistance
5. Normal: complete range of motion against gravity with full resistance.

Additional categories have been proposed to further describe muscle function in neuromuscular conditions.[62]

6. Indeterminant (transferred): muscle has been transferred or released, and strength cannot be measured
7. Indeterminant (spastic, contracture): cannot estimate true strength
8. Indeterminant (abnormal movement, such as athetosis)
9. Unknown: limb in cast or uncooperative patient.

However, this classification cannot quantitate differences in strength between, for example, a very strong quadriceps in a trained athlete's uninjured leg and a weakened but still strong quadriceps in an injured leg. Entities such as anterior knee pain are characterized by pain in part of the arc of motion, and more refined isometric techniques are sometimes necessary to evaluate strength. Repetitive testing may be important in revealing lack of endurance, a more subtle form of weakness.

LIMB LENGTHS

Leg length discrepancy or the possibility of leg length discrepancy is a relatively common presenting symptom in the field of children's orthopaedics. Because leg length discrepancy is discussed in detail in another chapter, the importance of this feature is briefly mentioned here. It is worthwhile to discern when the discrepancy was first suspected, because different causes of leg length discrepancy are accompanied by different patterns of physical findings. Congenital shortening mandates a careful evaluation of deficiency of the postaxial side of the leg. Congenital shortening is often accompanied by contracture of the iliotibial band, genu valgum secondary to hypoplasia of the lateral femoral condyle, and various degrees of fibular hypoplasia (Fig. 3-15). Shortening secondary to injury or sepsis can be accompanied by a variety of bony and soft tissue problems. It is important not to focus so much on the leg length discrepancy that other significant findings go unnoticed.

There are several methods of measuring leg length discrepancy.[18] The classic method, called the true leg length discrepancy, is to measure the distance from the anterior superior iliac spine to the medial malleolus with the patient supine (Fig. 3-16). This is regarded as more accurate than measuring the distance from the umbilicus, which has been called the apparent leg length, but both measurements can be affected by abduction or adduction at the hips, angular deformity of the legs, and flexion posturing of the hip or knee. The legs should be perpendicular to an imaginary

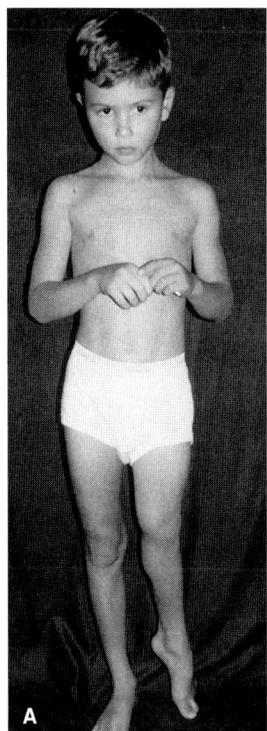
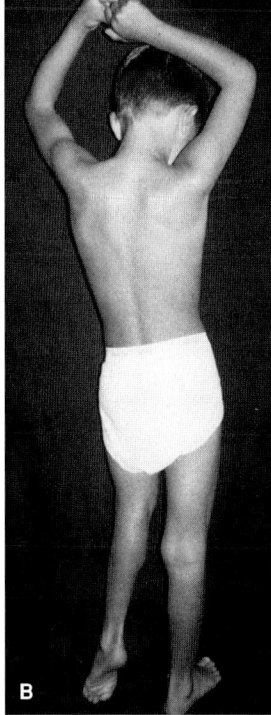

FIGURE 3-15. (A) Appearance of a lower limb with a congenital short femur. The angulation and rotation of the knee result from hypoplasia of the postaxial limb bud. (B) Knee valgus is evident when the limb is internally rotated; it is not apparent with external rotation of the limb.

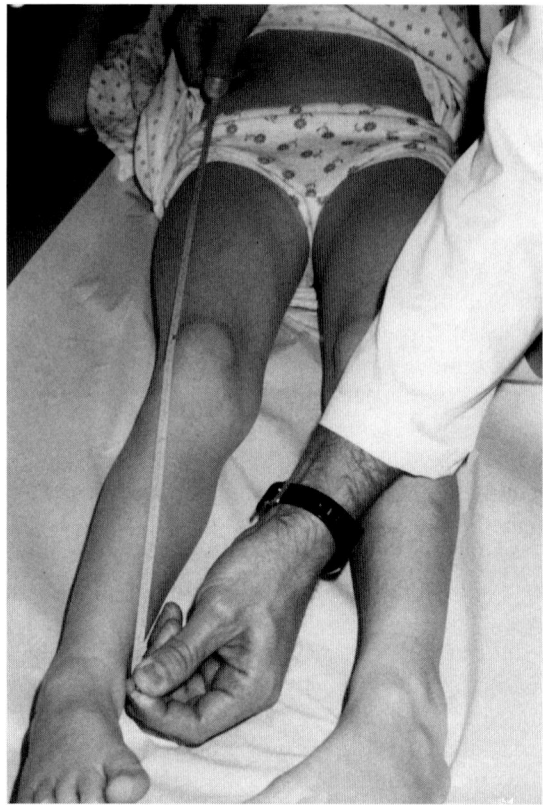

FIGURE 3-16. Classically, leg length discrepancy is measured from the anterior superior iliac spine to the medial malleolus. These measurements are not reliable unless a line between the iliac spines is perpendicular to the legs and the hips and knees are extended completely. Positioning of the tape relative to the patella can also affect the measurement.

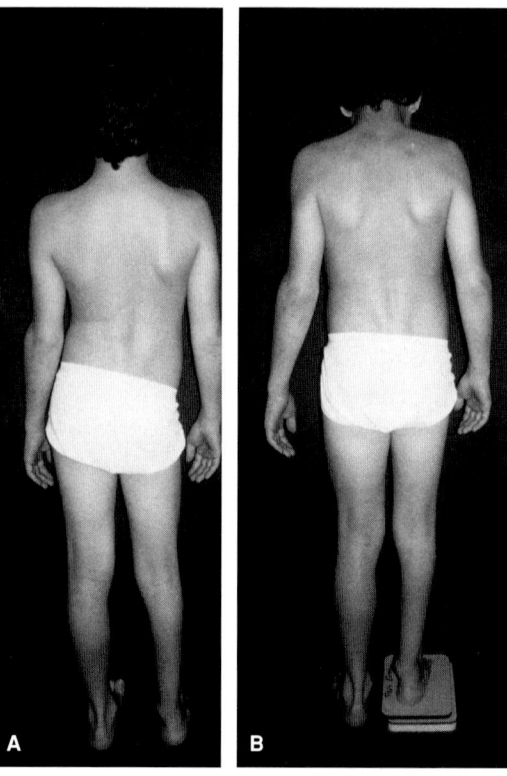

FIGURE 3-17. (A) In a patient with a leg length discrepancy, the elastic top of the patient's underwear is not parallel to the floor. (B) The pelvis is leveled by placing blocks under the short leg.

line between the anterior superior iliac spines; any deviation from this perpendicular relation produces factitious lengthening of the abducted leg and shortening of the adducted leg. If there is a fixed flexion contracture of the knee or hip, the femoral segments can be measured from greater trochanter or, less optimally, from the anterior superior iliac spine to the lateral or medial joint line of the knee. The tibia can be measured from the joint line to the medial malleolus.

Leg length discrepancy can also be evaluated with the patient in a standing position. Underwear conforms to the tilt of the pelvis, and tilted underwear indicates the presence of leg length discrepancy (Fig. 3-17). The dimples over the posterior superior iliac spines, when evident, also give a direct indication of pelvic height. The examiner should be seated on a small stool behind the patient with the examiner's head at about the patient's waist level. The extended index fingers detect the site of the iliac crests, and with the eyes at the height of the crests, the examiner can detect approximately 5 mm of difference in height (Fig. 3-18). The patient can bend forward to accentuate the position of the iliac crests. Blocks can be placed

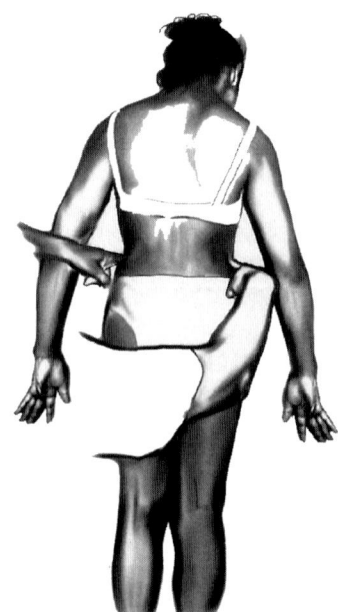

FIGURE 3-18. With the examiner's eyes at the level of the iliac crests while palpating the crest with an extended index finger, differences of 5 mm of pelvic height can be visualized.

under the feet to equalize the height of the iliac crests; the height of the block necessary to square the pelvis is equal to the leg length difference. When leg length discrepancy is measured carefully by the same observer, reproducibility in the range of 5 mm of error should be attainable. Interobserver errors are greater, often because of a failure to use the same bony landmarks for measurement.[18]

EXAMINATIONS OF SPECIFIC ANATOMIC AREAS

Skin

The skin often is the site of valuable information, such as the hue of lupus or the woody subcutaneous tissue of scleroderma. A search for café-au-lait spots is warranted when the physician examines a patient for scoliosis or an anteromedial bow of the tibia. The orthopaedist is often the first physician to make the diagnosis of neurofibromatosis and observing the skin of the parents may reveal the characteristic cutaneous nodules of the adult with neurofibromatosis. Multiple contusions may signify an active child, abuse, or hemophilia. Vascular malformations may or may not have associated purplish patches in addition to hypertrophy of the affected body part. Hairy patches or skin dimples over the spinal midline usually herald an underlying spinal dysraphism. Localized elevation in skin temperature indicates the presence of an inflammatory process; localized reduction in skin temperature accompanying a purplish hue to the limb suggests reflex sympathetic dystrophy. The most sensitive portion of the examiner to temperature is the dorsal skin overlying the middle phalanges of the fingers; this surface of the examiner's hand is placed against the skin being tested for temperature, with the examiner's hand in a loose fist.

Spine

Examination of the spine may be performed for the conditions resulting from trauma, congenital or acquired deformities, infections, or neoplasms. The problem may be obvious, as in cases of severe spinal deformity, or subtle, as in the case of voluntary guarding secondary to an osteoid osteoma. History is key, especially in problems secondary to infection or neoplasia.

Problems involving the child's cervical spine are unusual. Balancing their infrequency, however, are the potential serious consequences of many such problems. The cervical region is the most mobile portion of the spinal column. When examining for traumatic injury, there is no other anatomic area that requires the same care as that for the younger child's cervical spine.[43] Because the young child has a relatively larger head and the plane of the facet joints is more horizontal than in the adult, relatively more catastrophic spinal cord injuries in the young child occur in the cervical region. If instability is suspected, especially in the young child who is not able—because of pain or disposition—to cooperate by actively moving the neck, the physician should splint the neck and obtain appropriate imaging studies to ensure no harm would result from an examination. Stability is best assessed by radiographs of the spine obtained while the child actively flexes and extends the neck; the spine does not lend itself to clinical stability testing as the knee does. If no instability is discovered by imaging studies, active and passive motion may be assessed. Flexion and extension, lateral rotation, and lateral bending are evaluated.

Although special goniometers have been used for quantifying cervical spine motion, a standard goniometer is equally as reliable.[96] The examiner should record the presenting position of the head, such as head rotated to which side, tilted (bent) to which side, and flexion or extension. The motions of flexion, extension, left and right side bending, and left and right rotation are evaluated. Normally, the child's neck mobility allows enough lateral bending that the ear (bending) or chin (rotation) touches the adjacent shoulder. Nontraumatic conditions such as torticollis or rotary subluxation cause child to splint the head and neck in an unusual position. Conceptualizing the course of the sternocleidomastoid muscle from the medial clavicle to the mastoid process helps in understanding the clinical presentation of torticollis; shortening the distance from origin to insertion tilts the head toward the affected side but rotates the face toward the side opposite the contracture (Fig. 3-19). Palpation of the sternocleidomastoid while the neck is being rotated can be helpful in differentiation of torticollis from rotatory subluxation, although visual estimates are less accurate than goniometric measurements in the evaluation of cervical spine motion.[96]

The neck may be shortened in patients with congenital anomalies such as Klippel-Feil syndrome, with variable amounts of loss of motion. Congenital elevation of the scapula may be confused with a short neck, but palpation of the scapula with the clavicle as a reference point indicates whether the scapula is elevated. Because skeletal dysplasias are associated with an increased incidence of cervical spine problems, special attention to the cervical spine is indicated in patients with short stature, especially if limb shortening is concentrated in the proximal segment (i.e., rhizomelic shortening).

The thoracolumbar spine is the site of several significant problems seen in pediatric orthopaedic practice. Examination of the spine may sometimes be

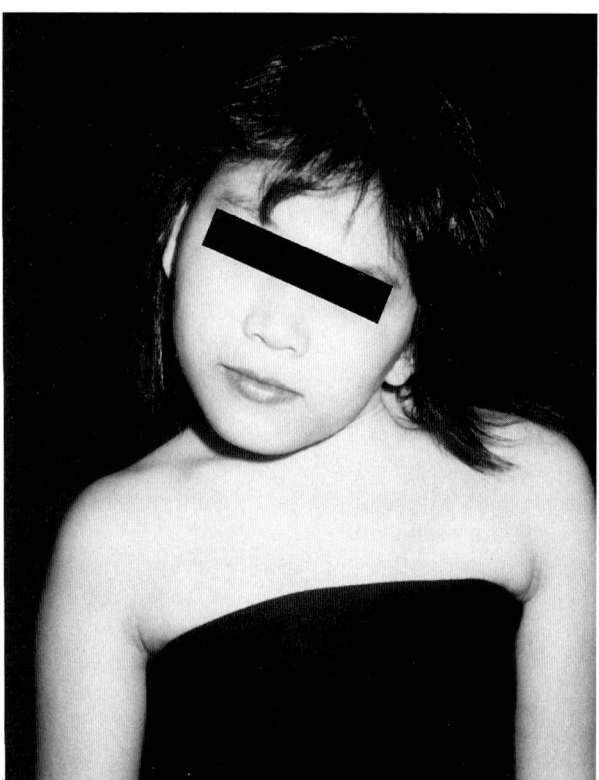

FIGURE 3-19. Presenting position of a child with torticollis. The head is rotated 30 degrees to the right and tilted 15 degrees to the left. The left shoulder is elevated 1 cm. The left sternocleidomastoid muscle is contracted.

impaired by modesty, and a two-piece bathing suit is ideal garb for girls. A systematic approach is best. The patient is initially observed in the standing position. The skin is observed for unusual pigmentation or dimpling. Any shoulder asymmetry is evaluated. The height of the iliac crests is determined with weight equally borne on both legs. The trunk is viewed from the front, back, and side of the patient. Compensation of the spine is evaluated by comparing the relation of the occiput with the gluteal cleft, measuring any lateral displacement of the occiput in centimeters. The patient is asked to bend forward, and any trunk rotation recorded. While in the forward-bending position, the spine is observed from three perspectives: from the cephalad and caudal ends of the spine to detect rotation and from the side to evaluate sagittal plane alignment. These maneuvers complete the basic assessment of the spine.

If shoulder asymmetry is documented, spine deformity must be differentiated from scapular displacement, such as seen in a patient with Sprengel deformity. The scapula may also appear elevated secondary to a thoracic curve, but rotation of the spine accompanies any curve of sufficient magnitude to elevate the scapula. Shoulder asymmetry secondary to posture is rarely an isolated finding.

Occasionally, differentiating a lumbar curve from a primary leg length discrepancy can be difficult. Lumbar curves can give the appearance of a leg length discrepancy. Palpation of the iliac crests with the examiner seated so the patient's crests are at the examiner's eye level is helpful; if a discrepancy is found, the short leg may be elevated with blocks, and the effect on the curve is assessed (Fig. 3-20). A lumbar curve secondary to leg length discrepancy does not demonstrate a rotational component.

Spine rotation accompanies any significant idiopathic curve, and curves secondary to such conditions as prior irradiation or congenital scoliosis may or may not have an apparent rotational component. The scoliometer described by Bunnell is a valuable adjunct to rotational assessment (Fig. 3-21). The patient is in the forward-bending position, and the scoliometer is applied to the portion of the spine with the greatest degree of rotation. It is important that the patient's arms are hanging freely and are not supported on a knee. Bunnell's original work with the scoliometer as a screening technique concluded that less than 5 degrees of trunk rotation is unlikely to be associated with structural changes. Ashworth and colleagues concluded that a baseline of 7 degrees would eliminate many false-negative results.[3] When two curves are evident, comparison of the angle of trunk rotation can often indicate which curve is more structural. A fleshy body habitus can mask truncal rotation and falsely reduce the measured angle of trunk rotation. With the prominence of the right rib cage accompanying idiopathic scoliosis, the reduced thoracic kyphosis may not be appreciated unless viewed from the patient's left side (Fig. 3-22).

It is best to observe the patient in a forward-bending position from three perspectives: from the cephalad and caudal ends of the spine and from the side.[61] If forward bending is limited because of tight hamstrings, viewing from the head end can be more rewarding, especially in the lumbar region. Viewing from the side reveals the sagittal contour of the spine. The head should be centered over the pelvis, with a gentle cervical lordosis, thoracic kyphosis, and lumbar lordosis. Particular attention should be given to the presence of any angular localized kyphotic deformities, which are clearly different from the normal gentle kyphotic posture of the entire thoracic spine. Postural kyphosis is characterized by flexibility of the kyphosis with forward bending; structural kyphosis is characterized by a persistent sharp kyphotic posture of the spine during forward bending (Fig. 3-23).[55] Any kyphotic position of the thoracolumbar junction of the lumbar spine is abnormal. Thoracolumbar kyphosis

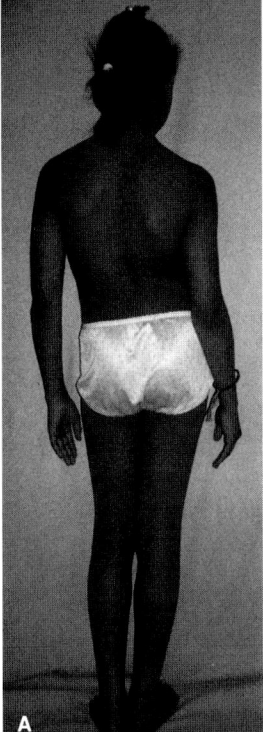
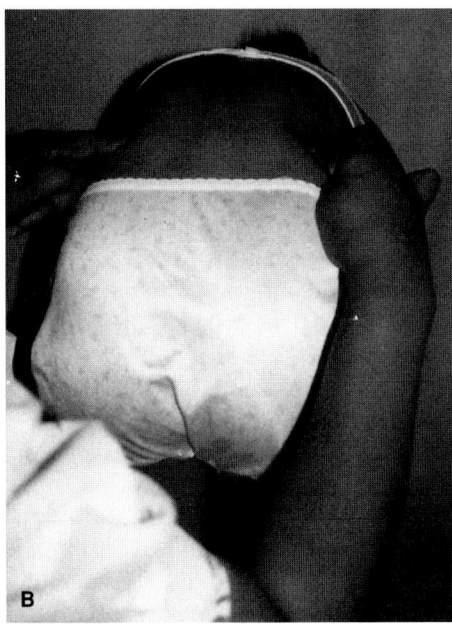

FIGURE 3-20. (A) Apparent leg length discrepancy accompanying lumbar scoliosis. (B) A level pelvis can be confirmed by palpating the iliac crests while the patient bends forward.

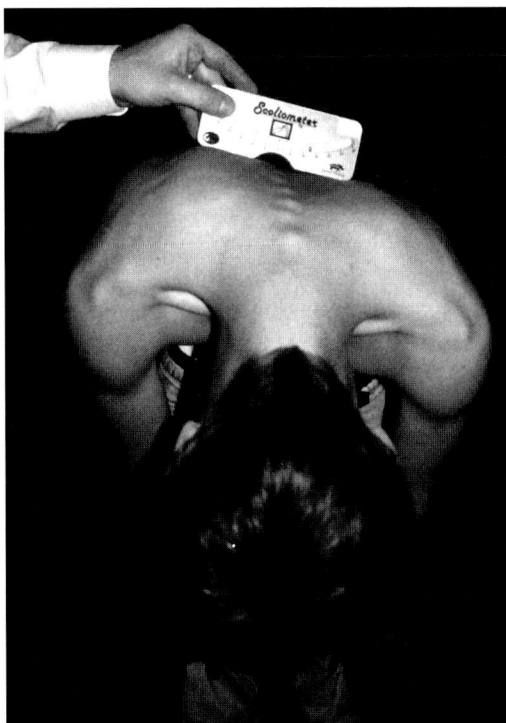

FIGURE 3-21. The scoliometer, which is similar to the inclinometer found on a sailboat, is an easily used tool for reproducibly documenting truncal rotation. The arms should be hanging freely.

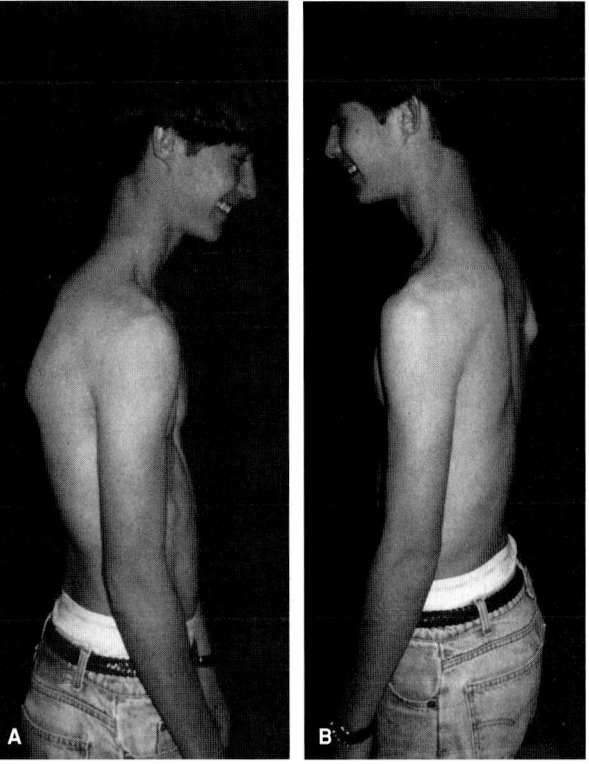

FIGURE 3-22. With the characteristic right rib hump of idiopathic scoliosis, thoracic lordosis may not be appreciated unless evaluated from the patient's left side. (A) The patient's right side. (B) The patient's left side.

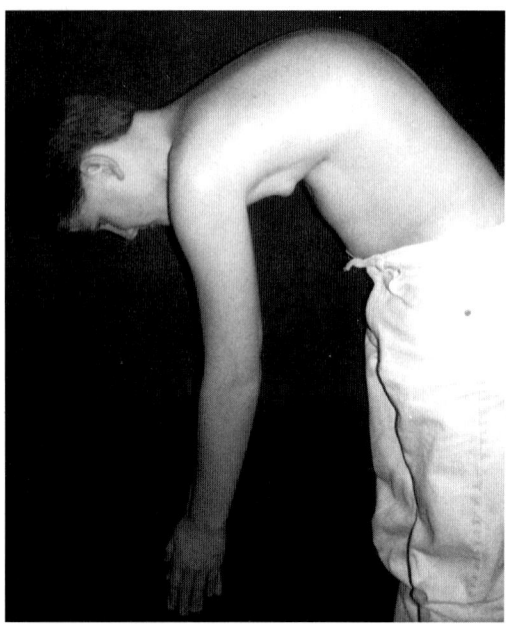

FIGURE 3-23. Characteristic sharp, V-shaped thoracic hump of structural kyphosis.

may result in subcostal skin folds as a result of shortening of the anterior abdominal wall. The normal lumbar lordosis should flatten but not reverse during forward bending.

With more severe grades of spondylolisthesis, a forward displacement of the trunk on the pelvis can be seen, often with knee flexion secondary to hamstring contracture (Fig. 3-24). Painful conditions result in the patient's splinting the particular segment of the spine affected, usually the lumbar spine in conditions such as spondylosis or disc space infection. In such cases, the lumbar spine is flattened in the standing and forward-bending positions. Asking the child with a painful back condition to pick up an object off the floor underscores the severity of the voluntary guarding.

The relation of hamstring tightness to sagittal spine posture has long been recognized, but it is still not explained. Tight hamstrings accompany spondylolisthesis and many painful conditions of the spine, limiting forward bending at the waist. Evaluating the degree of hamstring contracture must complement assessment of kyphotic or painful conditions. Measuring the popliteal angle has become a popular and reliable method of evaluating hamstring contracture. This is performed with the patient supine, with the hip flexed to 90 degrees and the knee flexed (Fig. 3-25). The knee is then extended, and the number of degrees by which the knee fails to reach full extension is recorded as the popliteal angle. The sit-reach test is widely used to test flexibility in the field of sports medicine. The patient is in a seated position with the knees extended and asked to touch the toes while keeping the knees extended. The number of inches between the toes and fingers is recorded. The lumbosacral spine and pelvis share the movement required to perform the sit reach test, and this can sometimes be noticed by the kyphotic appearance of the lumbar spine of patients with tight hamstrings while sitting with the knees extended (Fig. 3-26). Some children with very tight hamstrings have difficulty sitting at all with the knees extended.

Shoulder and Upper Limb

Although all joints have individual characteristics, the shoulder has several features that are unique. Shoulder motion is a combination of glenohumeral motion and scapulothoracic motion. The glenohumeral joint is a true diarthrodial joint, but there is no joint between the scapula and thorax. A flat bone, the scapula, is powered by surrounding muscles, allowing it to glide over the posterolateral thorax, coupled with the clavicle anteriorly to rotate through the sternoclavicular joint. Although physicians often refer to the glenohumeral joint as the shoulder joint, shoulder motion also depends on other components. A standard ratio for the contribution of glenohumeral to scapulothoracic motion is 3 : 2, but considerable variations have

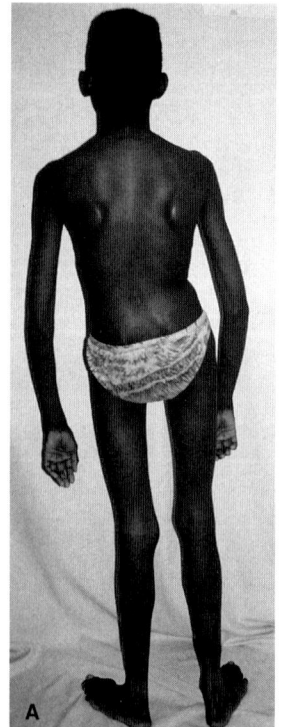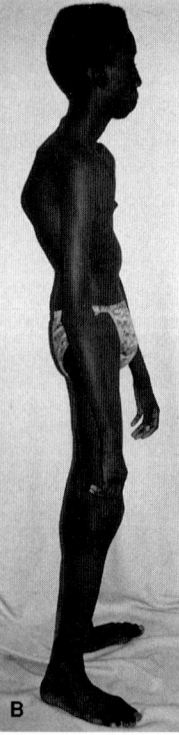

FIGURE 3-24. (A) The back and (B) side views of this patient show the anterior displacement of the lumbar spine secondary to severe spondylolisthesis. Notice the shortening of the trunk and head height relative to the legs; at the age of this patient, the ratio of trunk plus head height to leg plus pelvis height normally is 1 : 1.

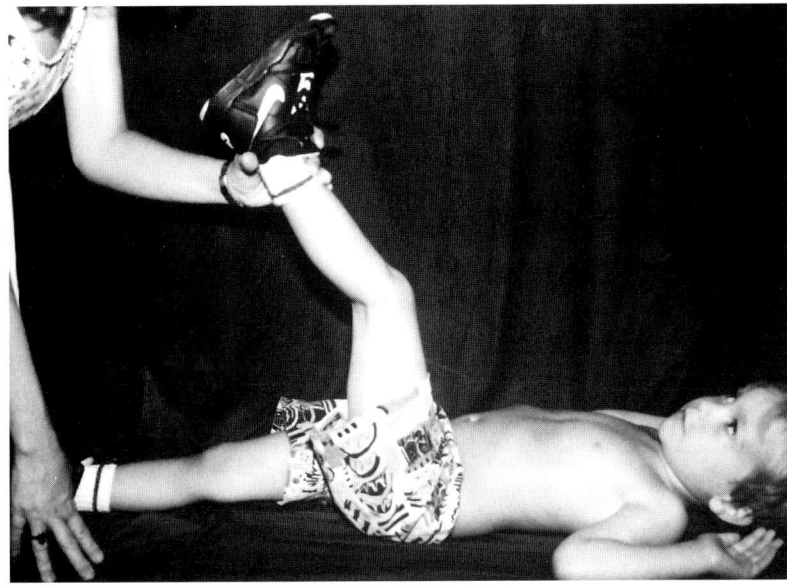

FIGURE 3-25. Popliteal angle. The thigh is flexed to 90 degrees, then the knee is maximally extended. The contralateral thigh is stabilized against the table. The angle recorded is that between complete knee extension and actual knee extension.

been reported. The glenohumeral joint is inherently unstable without muscular support. Examination of the shoulder therefore includes the entire complex that enables the remarkable ability to place the upper limb and hand in space and to provide a stable connection for the limb to the body when heavy lifting is done. When the shoulder is considered in this way, the scapula, clavicle, proximal humerus, and all intervening ligaments and muscles acting on the bony components are included in an evaluation of the shoulder.

Most shoulder problems presenting to orthopaedic surgeons involve pain or instability. However, painless deformity or impaired motion is a more common indication for pediatric shoulder evaluation. Proper shoulder assessment requires inspection, palpation, evaluation of stability, quantitating joint motion, and neurologic examination. The strategies to accomplish this necessarily vary with the patient's age and presenting complaint.

Orthopaedic consultation for an infant is most often required for paralysis or deformity of the shoulder. With birth palsies or fractures, impairment of spontaneous motion is obvious to parents and primary care physicians. Hawkins and Bokor use the term "attitude" to denote the general contour and symmetry of the shoulder.[40] The attitude of the shoulder in an infant with birth palsy is described as adducted and internally rotated, with a further description of any spontaneous motion observed. Asymmetry of grasp and Moro reflexes can easily be observed. A similar attitude, however, may be seen in a newborn with a birth fracture

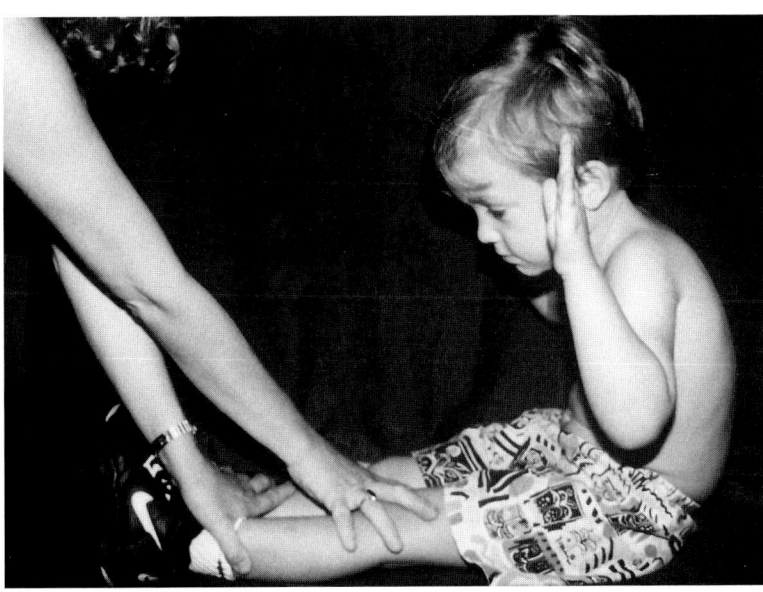

FIGURE 3-26. The kyphotic posture of the lumbar spine of the patient shown in Figure 3-25 produces "sacral sitting," which compensates for tight hamstrings.

of the clavicle. Palpation in this instance reveals swelling and tenderness of the easily accessible subcutaneous clavicle, and differentiation is not difficult. Rarely, congenital posterior dislocation of the shoulder may mimic birth palsy. Palpation of the proximal humerus alerts the examiner to this possibility. In the infant, active range of motion is elicited by the Moro reflex, and passive range is tested as for a child of any age.

Shoulder motion in the toddler is no longer reflexive, although active cooperation is not yet possible. The toddler naturally reaches for items of interest (e.g., toys, penlights, keys), and reaching for any item offers the examiner an opportunity to observe active shoulder motion. At this age, observation as the initial phase of the examination optimally includes observation of the active range of motion before any physical examination is performed, especially if tenderness is suspected.

The Society of American Shoulder and Elbow Surgeons has developed a protocol for the active shoulder examination, somewhat simplifying the more traditional parameters.[40] They have introduced the concept of elevation instead of abduction and flexion. Elevation is the degree of upward mobility of the shoulder in the same sagittal plane as flexion, but the patient is allowed to use whatever additional abduction desired to get the greatest amount of mobility over the head. Internal and external rotation should be measured with the arm at the side and in 90 degrees of abduction. Generally, there is slightly more external rotation with the arm at the side and slightly more internal rotation with the shoulder abducted 90 degrees. In the adult or older child, internal rotation is recorded according to the body part touched by the thumb of the arm being internally rotated. Usually, some part of the spine can be touched—the high thoracic spine with mobile shoulders and the lower lumbar spine or greater trochanter for restricted shoulders.

Tachdjian illustrated a method for rapid qualitative assessment of shoulder motion (Fig. 3-27).[88] Active

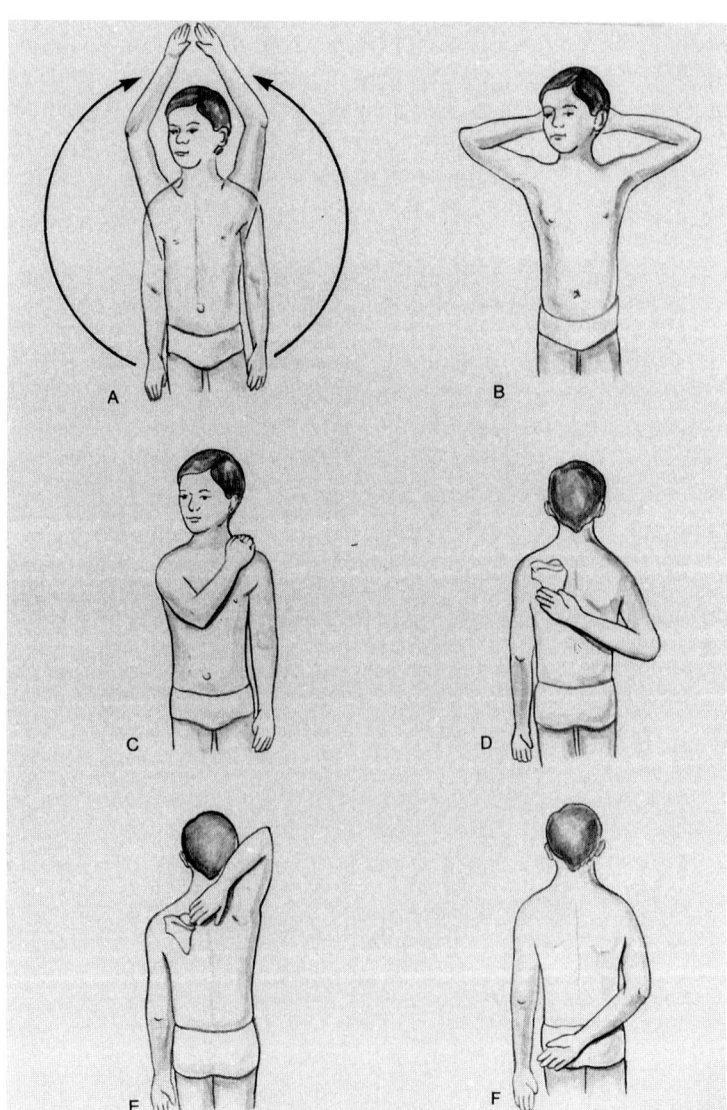

FIGURE 3-27. Tachdjian's rapid assessment of shoulder motion. (**A**) Elevation. (**B**) Abduction and external rotation. (**C**) Internal rotation and adduction. (**D**) Extension, internal rotation, and adduction. (**E**) Elevation, internal rotation, and adduction. (**F**) Extension, adduction, and internal rotation. (From Tachdjian MO. Pediatric orthopedics. vol. 1. Philadelphia: WB Saunders, 1990.)

external rotation by patients of all ages is evaluated with the arm at the side and recorded in degrees. Useful information for a child too young to cooperate with this type of instructed examination can still be acquired by observing the child's reach for interesting objects placed in space, and the examiner can quantitate the motions observed.

The hands-on portion of the examination is performed last. Depending on the presenting complaint, the examination may focus on suspected tenderness, swelling, instability, or contracture. Conditions commonly seen in athletes such as acromioclavicular sprains, clavicle fractures, and anterior shoulder instability require palpation for tenderness or maneuvers designed to stress the glenohumeral capsule.

In adolescence, shoulder instability is relatively common. It also can be present in younger children with habitual laxity. Translation of the humerus on the glenoid is tested by placing one hand on the scapula and the other on the humerus, and applying anterior, posterior, and inferior stress to the humerus. This is performed in the seated and supine positions. The apprehension test is performed in the sitting position. The examiner is behind the shoulder being examined. The shoulder is abducted to 90 degrees and then slowly externally rotated. Additional stress may be applied by the other hand, with the thumb applying anterior stress to the posterior humeral head while the fingers remain on the anterior humeral head in case there is more instability than anticipated. If there is anterior instability of the shoulder, the patient demonstrates obvious concern or guarding during this maneuver.

Shoulder girdle problems may be congenital, such as Sprengel deformity, or acquired, such as scapular winging after trauma or accompanying some of the muscular dystrophies or syringomyelia.[93] An understanding of the primary muscular forces about the scapula is essential. The scapula may be rotated, retracted toward the midline, protracted away from the midline, elevated, or depressed, depending on the pattern of muscle weakness. Scapular elevators include the upper trapezius and levator scapulae. The middle trapezius and rhomboids retract, and the serratus anterior protracts. Depression is accomplished by the serratus anterior and lower trapezius, aided by the stabilizing effect of the large thoracohumeral muscles (i.e., pectoralis major, latissimus dorsi) on the proximal humerus. Evaluating these muscles by functional groups is more sensible than individual muscle testing. Shrugging the shoulders against resistance tests the elevators. Retraction of the scapulas toward each other is easily evaluated, but protraction is better evaluated by reaching for an object in front of the body or leaning against a wall or the floor as in a pushup position (Fig. 3-28). Depression is tested by having the seated patient attempt to push off the surface of the table and elevate the body. Without stabilization of the shoulder girdle by the scapular depressors, this maneuver is not possible.

Glenohumeral control is a result of the synergistic relation between the deltoid and the muscles of the rotator cuff; the exact pattern depends on the plane of motion. For example, flexion requires the anterior deltoid, and abduction in the coronal plane requires the posterior deltoid. Studies of shoulder motion with nerves to the rotator cuff or deltoid blocked reveal that a strong person can attain full arm elevation with one component of this force couple blocked, but a weaker person cannot. Without scapulothoracic stabi-

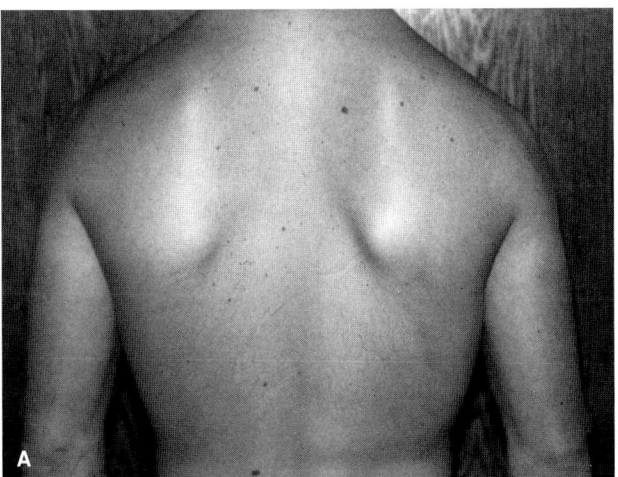
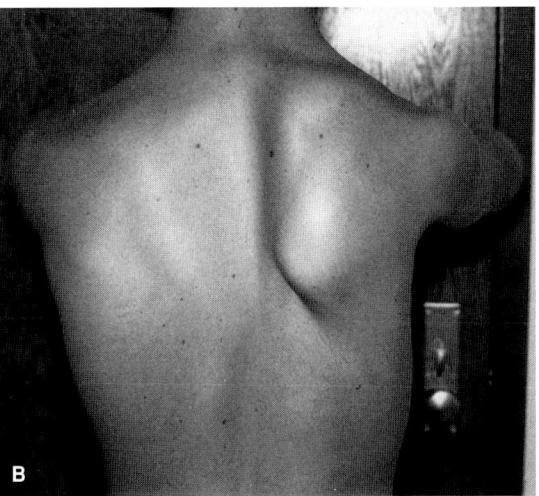

FIGURE 3-28. Scapular winging. (**A**) The right scapula is protracted, with an increased prominence of the inferomedial border. (**B**) When the patient leans forward on his arms, the absence of scapulothoracic stability is obvious.

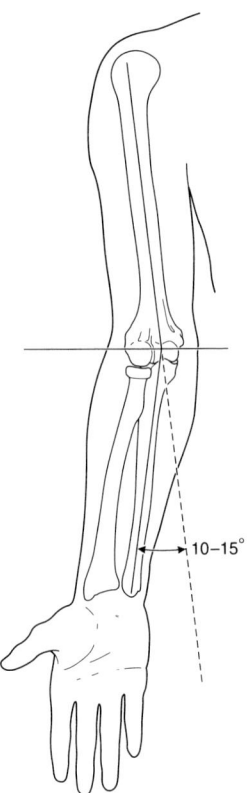

FIGURE 3-29. The angle between the humerus and forearm is called the carrying angle of the elbow. A normal carrying angle is about 10 to 15 degrees of valgus. (From Clark CR, Bonfiglio M. Orthopaedics. Essentials of diagnosis and treatment. New York: Churchill Livingstone, 1994.)

lization, however, glenohumeral motion is impaired, as in facioscapulohumeral dystrophy, in which the deltoid is spared relative to the scapular stabilizers. In this instance, stabilizing the scapula manually against the thorax allows the patient to demonstrate the actual capability of the glenohumeral motors. The total muscle picture must be considered when evaluating strength about the shoulder.

Elbow, Forearm, and Wrist

The elbow is more superficial than the shoulder and more accessible to examination. Alignment of the elbow is easily ascertained by observation with the limb in the anatomic position, with the elbow extended and the forearm supinated (Fig. 3-29). The angle between the humerus and forearm is called the carrying angle and is usually between 10 and 15 degrees of valgus, with slightly higher measurements recorded for most girls. Beals found a slight increase in carrying angle with age but could not differentiate any gender difference.[11] Flexion and extension of the elbow are easily measured; normally, the elbow may be completely extended (a few degrees of hyperextension is not unusual, especially in younger children), and flexion is limited only by soft tissue impingement of the forearm against the arm. Rotation is more complex and may be affected by disorders of the elbow, forearm, or wrist. Pronation and supination are usually tested with the humerus against the torso (Fig. 3-30). This is acceptable if care is taken to ascertain and prevent any motion of the humerus, because patients with limitation of rotation quickly learn to compensate with shoulder motion. Generally, there is about 80 to 90 degrees of pronation and supination, with some individual variation. Pencils may be placed in the palms and held with the flexed fingers to more easily discern pronation and supination. The major active pronators are the pronator teres and pronator quadratus; the major supinators are the biceps and supinator. More daily activities require pronation than supination, and

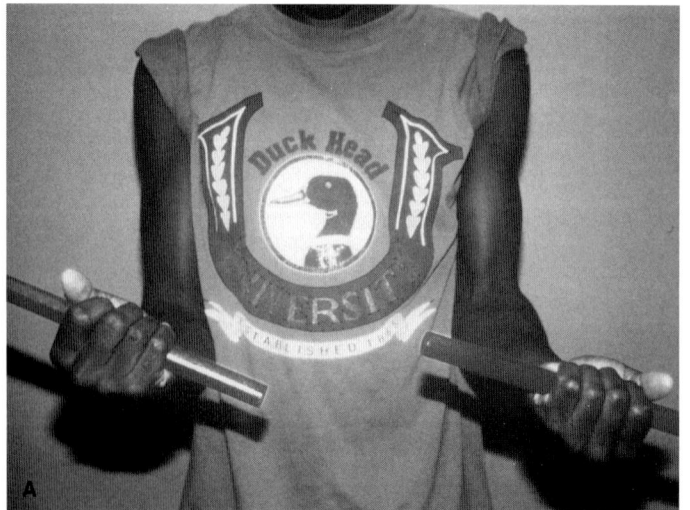
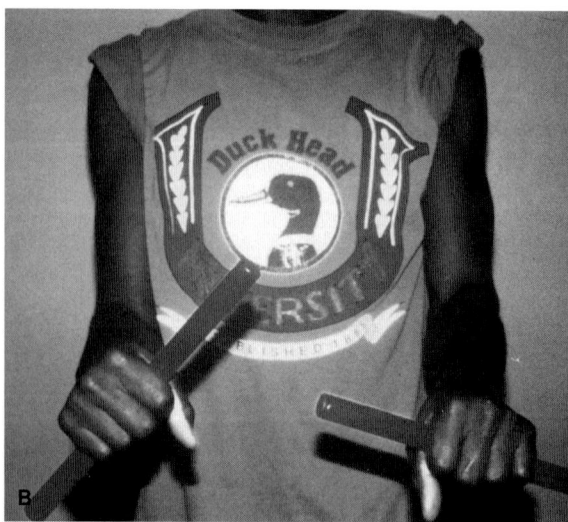

FIGURE 3-30. Evaluation of pronation and supination. The arm must be held at the side to obtain accurate measurements. (**A**) Supination. (**B**) Pronation. (Courtesy of John Todd, M.D., Pensacola, FL.)

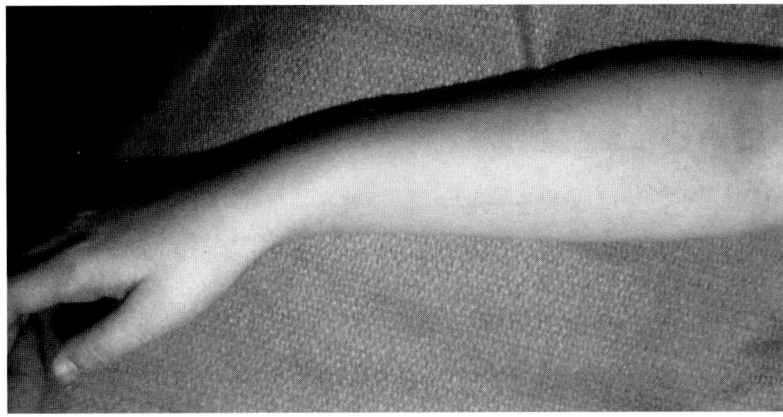

FIGURE 3-31. Appearance of the forearm after a greenstick fracture. The distal fragment is pronated relative to the proximal fragment.

about 50 degrees of each provides sufficient motion for activities of daily living.

The medial and lateral epicondyles are palpable unless there is massive soft tissue swelling. Normally, the medial and lateral epicondyles form an equilateral triangle with the olecranon. The ulnar nerve usually is palpable in the notch between the medial epicondyle and the olecranon. The radiohumeral joint is palpable just distal to the lateral epicondyle. Normally, there is a sulcus in the area bordered by the radial head, the lateral epicondyle, and the lateral olecranon, in which the radiohumeral joint may be palpated. In the presence of an elbow effusion, this site allows palpation of the joint where it is subcutaneous. Displacement of the radial head can be detected. Palpation of the radial head while rotating the forearm may be rewarding in conditions such as multiple hereditary exostosis, in which the radial head may be displaced during portions of the arc of motion. Palpation is valuable in detecting minimally displaced fractures about the elbow, especially those involving the radial head.

Examination of the forearm has received little attention. The radius and ulna constitute the link from elbow to wrist. The forearms are compared for length and contour. Normally, the radial styloid is longer than the ulnar, and a line drawn between the two styloids forms an angle of about 10 degrees with the long axis of the forearm. The ulnar border is subcutaneous, and deformity is readily observed. The radius is deeper, especially in its proximal half, and bony deformities are better concealed from inspection. With the common greenstick fracture of the forearm, different rotational attitudes can be found in the forearm proximal and distal to the fracture (Fig. 3-31). Apex dorsal angulation results in a pronated posture distal to the fracture; apex volar angulation results in a supinated posture distally. With shortening of the ulna, ulnar deviation of the hand on the wrist is evident. Similarly, radial shortening results in radial deviation.

Wrist motion is evaluated in flexion, extension, and radial and ulnar deviation. Wrist extension is usually possible to 80 degrees, flexion to 70 degrees, radial deviation to 20 degrees, and ulnar deviation to 30 degrees.

Nerve impairment in the forearm is evaluated by examining the hand and is discussed in the next section. Sensation to the forearm is from designated terminal sensory nerves; the exception is the musculocutaneous nerve that supplies the biceps and brachialis along with sensation of the radial volar forearm.

Hand

The hand is one of the most complex structures in the body, incorporating the anatomic features necessary for complex fine and gross activities into a compact, mobile package. Examination of the child's hand is performed for congenital anomalies, fracture, or effects of neuromuscular disorders. The attitude of the hand is first observed. Generally, the fingers are in a position of comfortable flexion. Watching the hand while the child is playing or undressing is rewarding, because these activities involve placement of the hand in space, grasp, release, and finger and thumb posture and function. Because hands with impaired sensation are shunned for everyday tasks, adequate sensation is implied by normal usage of the hand. Probably more information is gained from observing the functional use of the hand than by the static examination. If the patient has a definite preference for one hand, it is isolated by the examiner to better evaluate the capabilities of the hand in question.

Static examination documents proportions of the hand and fingers. The color and temperature of the skin and the quality of nail beds are briefly assessed. Sensory testing of the hand is often important in the detection of nerve impairment accompanying fracture of the elbow or forearm. The pattern of peripheral

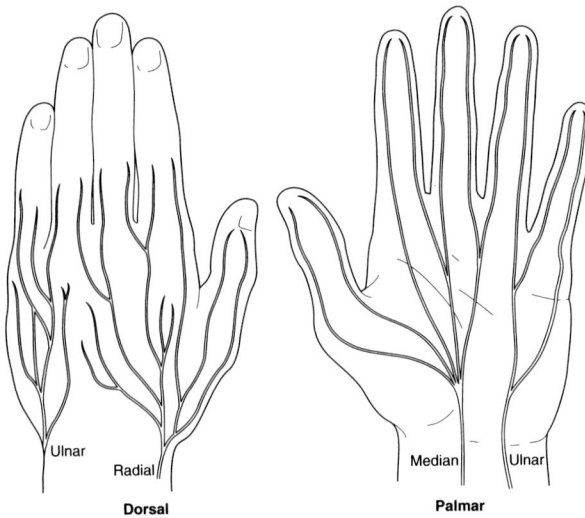

FIGURE 3-32. Sensory distribution of the hand. (From Clark CR, Bonfiglio M. Orthopaedics. Essentials of diagnosis and treatment. New York: Churchill Livingstone, 1994.)

nerve sensory distribution to the hand is basic knowledge for orthopaedic practice (Fig. 3-32).

Evaluation of motor function to the hand is often critically important in cases of a displaced elbow or proximal forearm injuries. All extensor muscles are supplied by the radial nerve, and all finger and thumb extensors are supplied by the deep branch (i.e., posterior interosseous nerve) after it enters the supinator muscle. Extension of all fingers and abduction of the thumb are impaired by radial nerve injury. The deep branch of the radial nerve has no sensory distribution. The median nerve supplies flexor muscles on the radial side of the forearm. Like the radial nerve, the median nerve has a deep branch, known as the anterior interosseous, which has no sensory distribution. The anterior interosseous supplies the radial part of the flexor digitorum profundus, the flexor pollicis longus, and the pronator quadratus. The anterior interosseous nerve is frequently impaired after supracondylar fracture of the humerus. The best way to test for function of this nerve is active flexion of the interphalangeal joint of the thumb. The ulnar nerve supplies the flexor digitorum profundus to the ulnar side of the hand, the ulnar lumbical muscles, the adductor of the thumb, and all the interossei. The best test of ulnar function is the ability to adduct and abduct the fingers. This is most easily seen or palpated by asking the child to touch an object requiring abduction of the index finger.

Congenital deletions occur in myriad forms about the hand and are often associated with deficiencies of other organ systems. The deficiency is described anatomically, but functional and sensory assessments are critically important in decision making. Stereognosis can be easily tested in an older child be asking the child to close the eyes and differentiate a quarter (i.e., serrated edge) from a nickel (i.e., smooth edge). For congenital deficiencies and neuromuscular conditions, the most important observation that can be made is how the child uses the affected hand. If the hand is isolated because of sensory impairment, no reconstruction can restore functional use.

Hip

The hip is the site of several important pediatric orthopaedic problems. Because the hip has a deep location compared with joints such as the knee or elbow, direct observation must be supplanted by other techniques to ensure accurate technique. For example, when examining rotation of the elbow, motion of humerus indicating substitution of shoulder motion for elbow rotation may be easily observed. When hip motion is restricted, the patient often compensates with increased lumbar spine motion to tilt the pelvis and move the thigh. Monitoring pelvic motion is a necessary component of evaluating hip motion.[8] Similarly, capsular distention of the hip joint cannot be observed as it is in the knee; indirect methods must be used for detection. Although strategies used for the actual examination depend on the patient's age, the basics of detecting soft tissue swelling and impairment of normal motion and function are constant.

Examination of the hip begins with observation of the attitude of the hip. Guarding of the hip in a position of flexion, abduction, and external rotation is characteristic of inflammatory or other painful conditions. The spastic neuromuscular hip is often held in an adducted position. If the patient is ambulatory, observation of the standing position and gait is helpful. It is important to observe the position of the spine, because many hip conditions are accompanied by hip flexion deformity for which the patient may compensate with increased lumbar lordosis.

The infant's hip usually is examined to detect instability or suspected sepsis. The normal neonate has a hip flexion contracture of approximately 30 degrees, although various studies have reported contractures from 20 to 60 degrees.[11,36,79,92] The contracture is thought to be a result of the relatively greater tone in flexor muscles in the neonate, but it probably is also related to the flexed in utero position of the hip. Dislocation of the hip eliminates the flexion contracture. There is a tendency toward greater external than internal hip rotation during the first year of life, presumably secondary to contracture of the posterior hip capsule, which diminishes after walking commences. Paradoxically, this external rotation contracture occurs at the time of life when femoral anteversion is greatest, and the external rotation contracture is sufficient to mask physical findings related to femoral anteversion at this age.

When examining the patient for sepsis, the attitude of the hip at rest is noteworthy. Soft tissue swelling of the proximal thigh heralds the presence of inflammation or fracture. Range of motion is assessed in flexion, extension, abduction, adduction, and rotation. A hip with intracapsular swelling is most comfortable in abduction, flexion, and external rotation, and it is least comfortable in adduction, extension, and internal rotation. The neonate with hip sepsis may not demonstrate these characteristic findings; soft tissue swelling and pseudoparalysis of the affected limb are more likely in the infant with hip joint sepsis.[53]

To detect neonatal hip instability, the baby is examined in the supine position. The goal of the examination is to detect laxity of the capsule, which allows the femoral head to slip over the posterior acetabulum. Instability similar to that of the dysplastic newborn hip can sometimes be detected in the older child with a neuromuscular condition. The best way to detect such motion is to have one hand control pelvic motion and use the other hand to mobilize the femur and displace the femoral head if laxity is present (Fig. 3-33).[35] The webbed space of the hand controlling the femur is placed over the flexed knee, the thumb rests medially in the region of the lesser trochanter, and the long finger rests laterally in the region of the greater

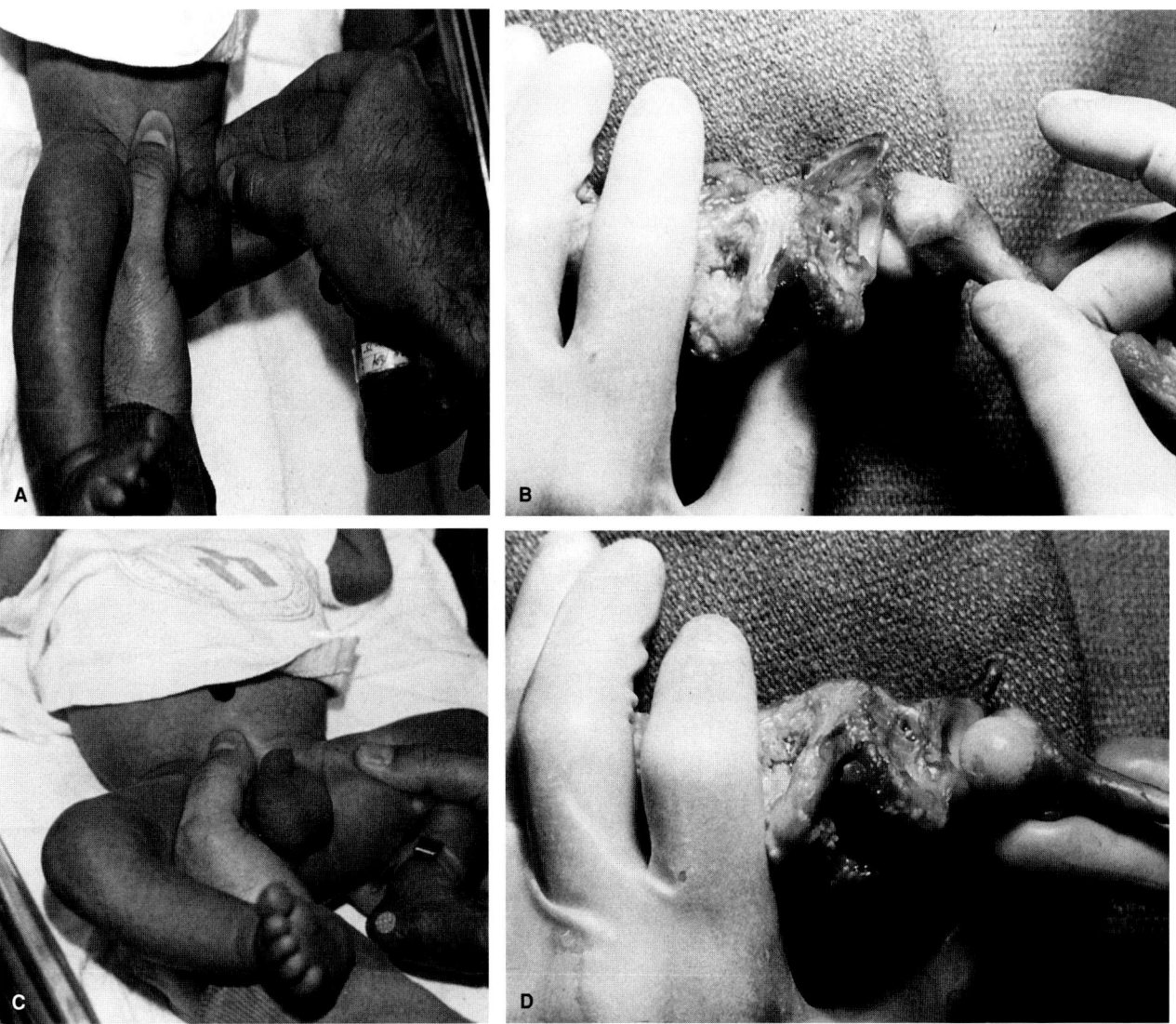

FIGURE 3-33. (A) To displace an unstable hip, the femur is adducted. Mild posteriorly directed pressure is applied with the web space of the examiner's hand, and lateral pressure is applied with the thumb on or near the patient's lesser trochanter. (B) Anatomy of the dislocated infant hip. (C) To reduce the displaced hip, the femur is abducted, and gentle upward pressure is applied on the greater trochanter. (D) Anatomy of reducing the unstable hip. (From Gross RH, Wisnefske M, Howard TC, Hitch M. Infant hip screening. In: Nelson JP, ed. The hip. Proceedings of the tenth open scientific meeting of The Hip Society, 1982. St Louis: CV Mosby, 1982:50.)

trochanter. The other hand is placed under the sacrum, with the thumb on the symphysis pubis. The hips are flexed 90 degrees and in neutral adduction-abduction. By a gentle rocking motion, applying lateral pressure on the lesser trochanter while posteriorly directed pressure is applied to the femur, the unstable femoral head slides over the posterior lip of the acetabulum and out of the joint. The femoral head dislocated can be reduced by releasing the posterior pressure on the femur and applying upward pressure on the greater trochanter with the long finger as the femur is abducted. An alternate method is to place one hand on each femur, moving one femur at a time.

Little force is required to displace an unstable hip if the baby is relaxed. Crying can produce muscular guarding, which Barlow believed could mask the findings of a dislocatable hip. The amount of pressure required to displace the hip is no more than that used to firmly palpate an abdomen. The portion of the examination that displaces the femoral head has become known as the Barlow maneuver, honoring the orthopaedist who provided the classic description of this examination and the natural history of hip instability in the newborn.[6] The portion of the maneuver reducing the hip has become known as the Ortolani maneuver, honoring the Italian pediatrician credited with the earliest description of the examination for neonatal hip instability.[66] The critical finding when testing for instability is the sensation of the femoral head displacing over the acetabulum to a dislocated position.

The terminology used to describe findings of the examination for neonatal hip instability is important for communicating with and conceptualizing the findings described by another examiner. There is no single word other than "dislocatable" that describes the sensation of the femoral head being displaced from the acetabulum. The term click is often used, but it is a subjective description. Most of the physical events described as clicks are probably extracapsular in origin. At least 10% of all newborns have evidence of clicks on hip examination, but it is hard to know exactly what constitutes a click.[29] The clicks seem unrelated to prognosis or decision making. In a study of newborn hip examinations, my colleagues and I found that insistence on describing the actual mobility of the femoral head as dislocatable, subluxatable, or stable and eliminating the use of click greatly reduced the number of false-positive examinations.[35]

Other findings associated with examination for developmental dysplasia of the hip are only found in the presence of an established dislocation with secondary muscle and capsular contracture that prevents reduction with the Ortolani maneuver. These secondary changes of restriction of abduction with the hips flexed 90 degrees, asymmetric skin folds, and femoral

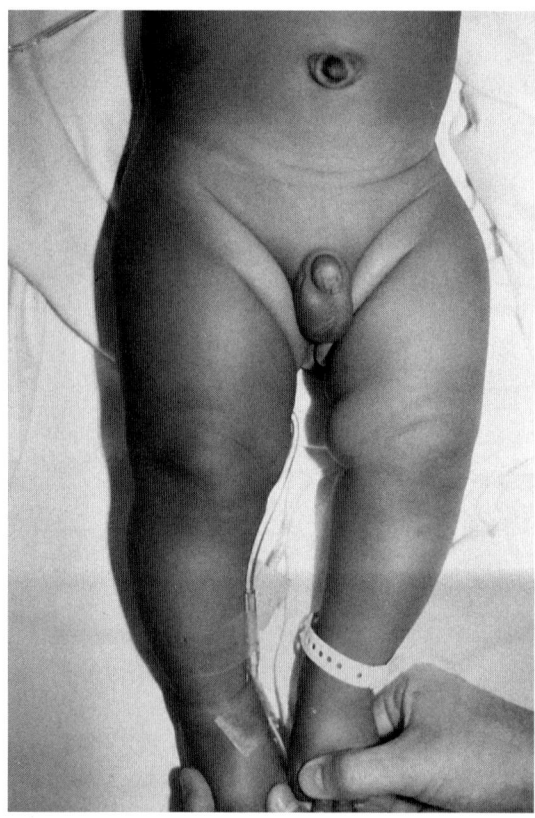

FIGURE 3-34. The femur on the side of a displaced hip, in this case on the patient's left side, is laterally displaced relative to a line between the anterior superior iliac spine and the patella. Assessing the position of the femur in this manner aids in detection of bilateral dislocation when the findings are subtle.

shortening due to the proximal migration of the femoral head are usually not evident for at least 2 to 3 months. The shortening of the femoral segment when the hips are adducted and flexed 90 degrees is known as the Galeazzi sign. It is important to ensure that the pelvis is flat on the table when quantitating hip abduction, because the act of abducting both hips simultaneously can tilt the pelvis to compensate for an adduction contracture and give the appearance of equal abduction. Removing the diaper when assessing hip abduction makes this error less likely. An additional finding in an established dislocation of the hip that is not often observed is lateral displacement of the femur relative to the midline (Fig. 3-34). Bilateral dislocated hips give the appearance of a widened perineum. Lateral displacement of the femoral shaft can be suspected by observation and verified by palpation of the femurs.

Examination for hip flexion contracture is performed in the same way for all ages. Two techniques are described, and both are reliable if performed carefully. The Thomas test requires that both hips be flexed as the initial part of the test, and while one hip is held in flexion, the other hip is extended (Fig. 3-35). The

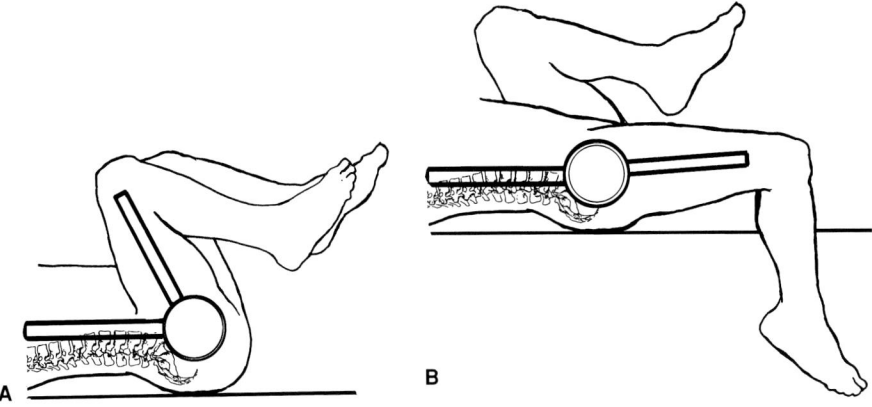

FIGURE 3-35. The Thomas test. (**A**) By flexing both hips, the lumbar spine and pelvis are stabilized against the examination table. (**B**) The spine and pelvis are stabilized by holding the leg not being examined in flexion while the leg being examined is extended. The angle between the plane of the table and the femur on the side being examined is measured with a goniometer.

purpose of maintaining contralateral hip flexion is to stabilize the lumbar spine and pelvis. If a hip flexion contracture is present, the patient must compensate with pelvic extension and a secondary lumbar lordosis to maintain an erect position. By flexing the knees with the patient supine on the examination table, extension of the pelvis and lumbar lordosis are prevented. A flexion contracture of the hip becomes evident on attempts to extend the hip. The angle between the thigh in maximum extension and the table represents the degree of contracture. Extension of the contralateral hip can allow pelvic extension and mask a hip flexion contracture.

The other method of quantitating hip flexion contracture is that of Staheli.[83] The patient is prone, with the legs flexed over the edge of the examination table. With one hand guiding the femur, the hip is extended while the other hand stabilizes the pelvis; the degree of contracture is that measured when the pelvis starts to extend.

Green and Griffin have emphasized the role of abduction contracture of the contralateral hip in the pathophysiology of developmental dysplasia of the hip.[33] With abduction contracture of a hip, the contralateral hip is swept into adduction, and the femoral head of an adducted hip is not centered in the acetabulum. Testing for an abduction contracture may be done with the patient prone or supine. One hand is on the pelvis to detect motion, and the other hand adducts the femur of the hip being tested from an initial position of abduction and extension until pelvic motion is detected. The abduction contracture is measured with a goniometer at this point (Fig. 3-36).

Hip rotation usually is evaluated in flexion and extension. The anterior capsule and iliopsoas are relaxed in flexion and taut in extension, allowing more external rotation in flexion. Rotation in extension has a greater effect on stance and gait. Rotation in flexion is assessed with the patient supine and with the hips and knees flexed 90 degrees. The position of the tibias serve as markers for quantitative measurement. Rotation in extension may be assessed in the supine or prone position. In the prone position, the knees are flexed 90 degrees, the tibias can serve as markers for measuring degrees with a goniometer. Hip rotation in extension is part of the torsional profile described by Staheli[84] (Fig. 3-37), which is a convenient method of examining the in-toeing child. Other examiners, however, have documented considerable intraobserver and interobserver variation in quantitating torsional profile measurements, with measurements varying as much as 15 to 25 degrees.[57]

For a patient with a hip flexion contracture, the prone examination for rotation is difficult. In the supine position, the maximally extended legs are rolled internally and externally, the patellas serve as markers for quantification. Alternately, in the supine position, the knees may be dangled over the end of the table, and the tibias may then serve as markers for goniometric measurement of hip rotation. Because younger children are often examined for torsional problems in a

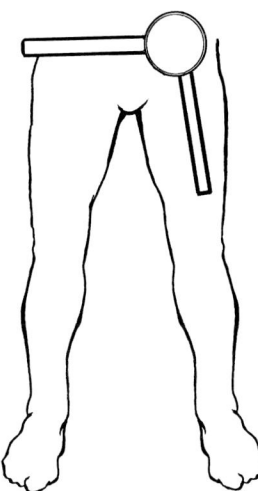

FIGURE 3-36. Assessment of abduction contracture. The starting position is prone or supine, with the hip extended, abducted, and neutrally rotated. A line between the iliac crests serves as a reference for measuring the lack of abduction to the neutral position.

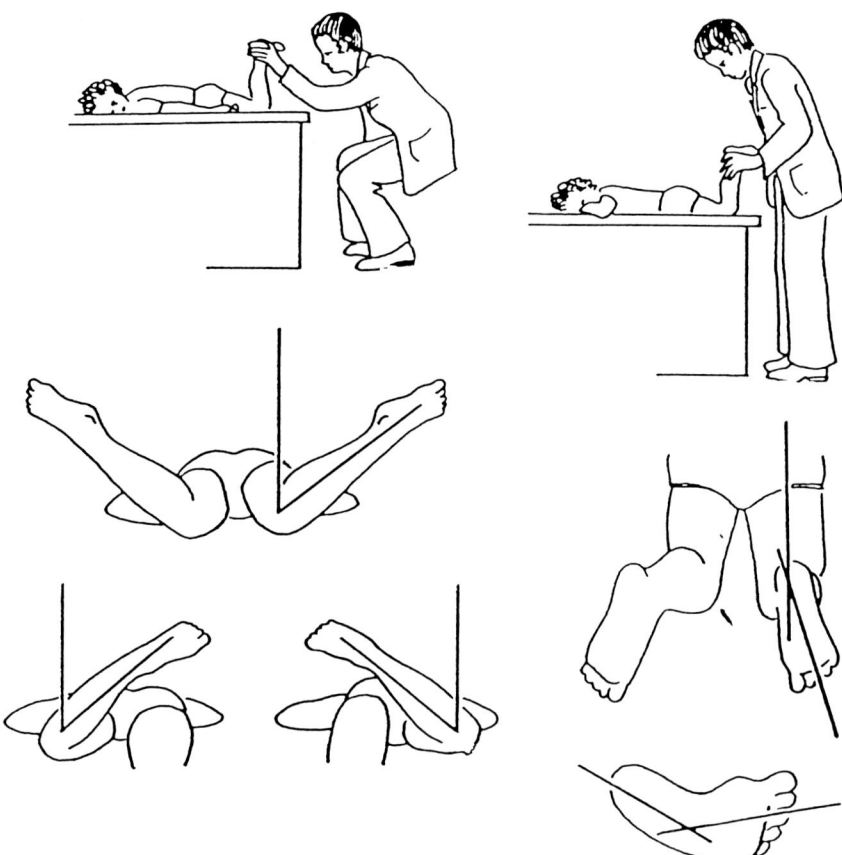

FIGURE 3-37. Torsional profile. With the patient in the prone position, the hip internal and external rotation, the thigh-foot angle, and the foot angle are quantitated. (From Staheli LT. Torsional deformity. Pediatr Clin North Am 1977;24:799.)

prone position and older children for conditions such as slipped capital femoral epiphysis in the supine position, both methods are useful.

Adduction varies in flexion and extension, and the position of the knee can be an additional variable in those with spasticity or contracture of the hamstrings. With the patient supine, the hips and knees are flexed 90 degrees, and the hips are abducted. The femurs serve as markers for quantification. The knee may then be extended and any effect on abduction as a result of increased tension on the medial hamstrings, especially the gracilis and semitendinosus, observed. Position of the pelvis must be monitored by a hand on the anterior superior iliac spines, the most accessible portion of the pelvis to palpation. A common pitfall is underestimation of the amount of contracture when compensatory motion of the pelvis is undetected. The pelvis may be stabilized by hanging the leg not being examined over the edge of the examination table.

The Ober test detects contracture of the iliotibial band.[65] To perform the Ober test, the patient is placed in the side-lying position. The hip not being examined is flexed and held against the chest. One hand must ensure that the pelvis remains stable. With the other hand, the hip on the side being examined is abducted in a slightly flexed position with the knee flexed 90 degrees. With the knee held at 90 degrees of flexion, the hip is then extended completely while still held in an abducted position. The hip is then adducted. In the presence of an iliotibial band contracture, the hip cannot be adducted to a neutral position (Fig. 3-38). The amount of adduction is recorded. A supple iliotibial band should allow about 20 degrees of adduction, often allowing the knee to touch the examining table.

Muscle strength about the hip can be measured in the conventional pattern with the method used for manual muscle testing. Flexion and adduction are as-

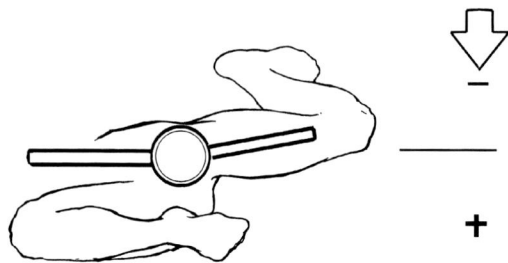

FIGURE 3-38. The Ober test. In the starting position, the contralateral hip is in flexion, the ipsilateral hip is abducted and extended, and the knee is flexed to 90 degrees. The leg is allowed to adduct; the number of degrees (x) lacking adduction from the anatomic position is recorded as −x degrees.

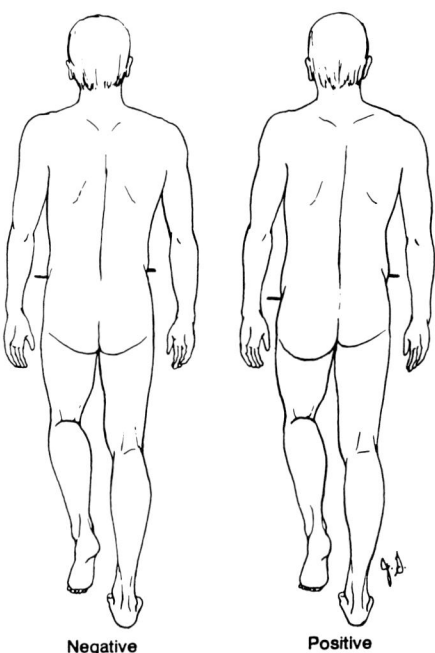

FIGURE 3-39. The Trendelenburg test. With the patient standing, the contralateral knee is flexed while the hip remains extended. A drop of the contralateral pelvis signifies a positive test result. A trunk shift toward the weight-bearing limb also indicates abductor weakness. (From Clark CR, Bonfiglio M. Orthopaedics. Essentials of diagnosis and treatment. New York: Churchill Livingstone, 1994.)

sessed in the supine position, but abduction requires the patient to lie on the side not being tested and abduction of the hip. The examiner must ensure that flexion of the hip is not allowed, because this permits substitution of the tensor fascia and other hip flexors for the abductor muscle. The patient usually tries to roll back into a more supine position. Extensors are evaluated with the patient prone.

Functional tests augment static testing. The time-honored Trendelenburg test is performed by having the patient stand and lift the contralateral leg by flexing the knee, leaving the hip extended (Fig. 3-39). A drop of the pelvis on the unsupported side denotes a positive test. Because patients with abductor weakness attempt to shift the body's center of gravity toward the supporting leg, any trunk shift must be carefully monitored. The delayed Trendelenburg test requires the patient maintaining the single-leg stance position for 15 to 30 seconds to fatigue the abductor muscles. This can detect lesser degrees of hip abductor weakness. Hopping on one leg can give an overall assessment of strength and endurance of the entire lower limb of the patient.

The sacroiliac joint is occasionally the site of sepsis or other inflammatory processes, but recognition of disorders in this joint is often delayed. Localized tenderness is routine but cannot be discovered if the entire examination is performed with the patient in the supine position. Pain is also elicited by compression of the iliac wings, with ipsilateral straight leg raising, the Gaenslen maneuver (i.e., hyperextension of the hip over the end of the table while the other hip is flexed), or the Patrick maneuver.[44] The Patrick maneuver is also known as the fabere test, consisting of flexion, abduction, and external rotation of the hip on the affected side. This maneuver, by "taking up" all the available hip motion, transfers the stress to the sacroiliac joint, producing pain in the presence of inflammation.

Knee and Leg

Complaints referable to the knee are among the most common musculoskeletal problems in children. The knee, unlike the hip, is relatively subcutaneous and is much more easily examined. The knee may be visualized as an ingeniously designed hinge-rotary joint with a huge sesamoid (i.e., patella) and controlling guy wires in three corners (i.e., medial and lateral hamstrings and the quadriceps). Menisci cushion the joint and fill in the empty spaces imposed by the basic architecture of a rounded articular femoral surface sitting on a slightly concave tibial surface. The knee is no different than other joints in the sense that problems may arise from any of these structures, but it is different in that so many aspects can be directly examined.

Although patient complaints can steer the examination, it is hard to overemphasize the frequency with which hip problems in children present as knee pain. Always consider the possibility of hip problems when assessing complaints related to children's knees. The hip capsule is innervated by branches of the femoral and obturator nerves.[32] The femoral nerve supplies sensation to the anterior thigh, and the obturator supplies the medial thigh and knee. Neither nerve supplies sensation below the knee, and pain referred from the hip usually is described as being in the thigh.

Inspection of the knee and thigh reveals atrophy of the thigh, swelling, ecchymosis or other skin changes, and the alignment of the knee. The angle of genu varum or valgum is measured with a goniometer,[41] and the anatomic site of angulation is documented (Fig. 3-40). When observing the patient from behind, the knee flexion crease gives valuable information about whether angular deformities are above or below the knee. Popliteal cysts are evident on inspection of the posterior knee.

Palpation is performed next. Differentiation between intraarticular and extraarticular swelling can be difficult, as can determining whether there is an actual effusion. Extraarticular swelling, such as a subcutaneous hematoma, is diffuse and not restricted by synovial reflections. Localized extraarticular fluid

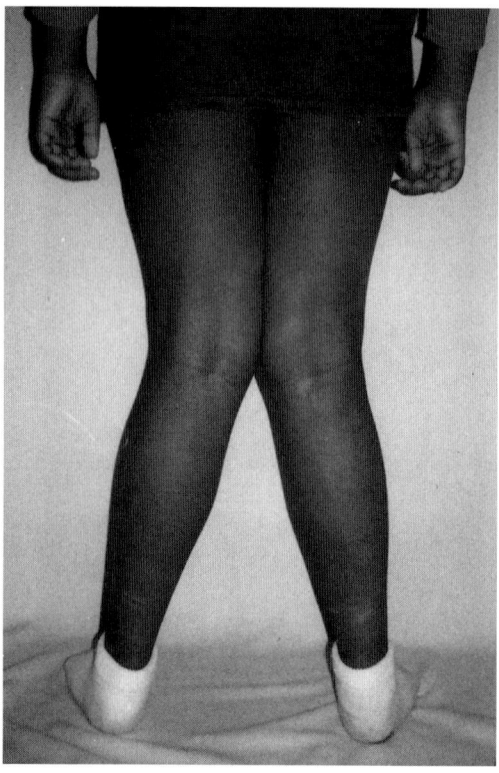

FIGURE 3-40. Assessment of the angular configuration of the legs from behind. In this instance, the angle of the flexion crease denotes deformity of the distal femur.

accumulations can occur in conditions such as prepatellar bursitis or pes anserinus bursitis. An intraarticular effusion is bounded by the suprapatellar pouch and the synovial reflections about the joint space. A helpful maneuver to determine whether there is a small intraarticular effusion is to "milk" the fluid in the suprapatellar pouch medially toward the sulcus between the vastus medialis and the medial femoral condyle. Normally, this area is concave, and a convex fluid bulge can be detected if intraaarticular fluid is displaced to this region. Differentiating swelling of the synovium from effusion in patients with conditions such as juvenile arthritis or hemophilia can be very difficult.

Palpation is more helpful around the knee than the hip for delineating the site of tenderness. The joint line can be palpated medially and laterally unless there is a large effusion; joint line tenderness suggests meniscal pathology. A helpful maneuver to ensure that elicited tenderness is localized to the joint line is serial palpation of the femoral condyle, joint line, and tibial plateau, numbering the sites as 1, 2, and 3. The patient is then asked to identify the site of tenderness by number. The medial and lateral sides of the joint are palpated. The patellofemoral joint, distal pole of the patella, ligamentous origins and insertions, pes anserinus, and tibial tubercle are other sites of potential tenderness.

The examination includes assessment of the range of motion and specific diagnostic maneuvers for detection of meniscal pathology, ligamentous instability, and muscular weakness. Normally, the knee completely extends, but young children and a few patients with conditions such as ligamentous laxity may normally demonstrate a few degrees of hyperextension. Passive extension to 0 degrees should be unencumbered, and flexion should be limited only by posterior soft tissue impingement. The loss of only a few degrees of extension is important. With the patient in a supine position with both ankles held off the table at the same level, the examiner can see if one knee is elevated and can detect small knee flexion contractures. Flexing the hips and the knees to 90 degrees gives the starting position for measuring the popliteal angle, which quantitates hamstring contracture (see Fig. 3-25). Complete extension of the knee with the hip flexed is recorded as a popliteal angle of 0 degrees; the number of degrees lacking from full knee extension is the popliteal angle. The popliteal angle in children 1 to 3 years of age is less than 15 degrees, and the mean angle increases abruptly at 4 years of age to an average of 24 degrees and remains at that level throughout childhood.[51] With the patient in the prone position, knee flexion contracture can be identified by allowing the feet to dangle over the end of the table so the knee can extend as completely as possible. Flexing the patient's knee while he or she is prone produces hip flexion in the presence of quadriceps contracture or spasm, a diagnostic maneuver called the Ely test (Fig. 3-41).

Maneuvers to test meniscal integrity involve rota-

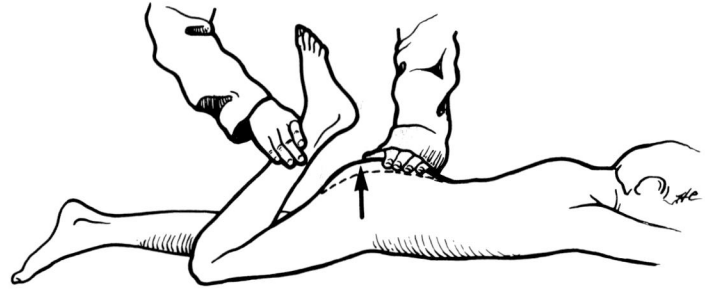

FIGURE 3-41. The Ely test. The patient is prone, with the hips and knees extended. Flexing one knee stretches the quadriceps; the hip flexes with the knee flexion in the presence of quadriceps contracture. (From Bleck EE. Orthopaedic management in cerebral palsy. Philadelphia: JB Lippincott, 1987.)

tion coupled with flexion and extension of the knee; the object is to impinge or displace the unstable fragment, reproducing symptoms. The McMurray sign is elicited with the patient supine, the knee fully flexed, and the tibia internally rotated. The sign is positive if a painful joint-line click is palpated as the knee is extended to 90 degrees. In the younger child with a discoid meniscus, there may be a clunking sensation, although this is unusual, because many discoid menisci remain asymptomatic well into adult life. The Apley grind test is performed with the patient prone and the knees flexed 90 degrees. The examiner leans on the foot to apply compressive force to the knee and rotates the leg; pain implies a torn meniscus. Pain may also occur with forced flexion or extension of the knee.

The evaluation of ligamentous instability has undergone several refinements. Instability was formerly classified by the direction in which the tibia was displaced, such as medial or lateral. As orthopaedic surgeons recognized that pure one-plane instabilities were unusual, a more complex and more descriptive terminology evolved. Although evaluation of instability is more often associated with sports medicine than pediatric orthopaedics, a working knowledge of knee instability is helpful for pediatric orthopaedic assessment. The increased laxity of the knee in younger children was documented by Baxter.[9] Trauma, especially accompanying a femoral fracture in childhood and adolescence, requires assessment of ligamentous stability. Preoperative evaluation of knee instability in the presence of congenital shortening may be pivotal to planning strategy for lengthening procedures. For a working classification of ligamentous instabilities, the following proposal by Kennedy[52] for categorizing ligamentous injuries has stood the test of time.

A. **One-plane instabilities**
 1. Medial
 2. Lateral
 3. Posterior
 4. Anterior

B. **Rotatory instabilities**
 1. Anteromedial
 2. Anterolateral
  a. In flexion
  b. Approaching extension
 3. Posterolateral
 4. Posteromedial

C. **Combined instabilities**
 1. Anterolateral-posterolateral rotatory
 2. Anterolateral-anteromedial rotatory
 3. Anteromedial-posteromedial rotatory

An exhaustive description of the underlying pathology of the various instabilities is not presented here; such descriptions are complex and available elsewhere for the interested reader. Maneuvers employed to detect instability are described, because they are an essential part of the examination.

One-plane medial instability is the simplest form of instability. The medial collateral ligament can be isolated with the knee flexed 30 degrees and applying a valgus stress. Laxity of the medial collateral ligament at 30 degrees of flexion combined with a stable examination with the knee completely extended denotes a one-plane instability of the medial collateral ligament. Similarly, minor lateral instability may only be recognizable with the knee flexed 30 degrees, but instability in extension implies a major instability. With the proximity of the peroneal nerve to the lateral structures, careful testing of dorsiflexion and sensation at the base of the first and second toes is necessary.

Posterior one-plane instability is diagnosed as a characteristic "sag" of the proximal tibia when the patient is supine with the hip flexed 45 degrees, the knee flexed 90 degrees, and the foot supported. When viewed from the side, the tibia is displaced posteriorly. The tibia may be displaced anteriorly to its normal position, but the direction of the instability is clearly posterior. In the presence of posterior instability, contraction of the quadriceps results in anterior displacement of the tibia.[23] From the same starting position, anterior instability is characterized by the ability to displace the proximal tibia anteriorly by pulling the tibia toward the examiner. A false-negative maneuver may occur if the hamstrings are contracted during the attempt to pull the tibia anteriorly. Anterior instability rarely occurs as an isolated finding.

Rotatory instabilities are described according to the motion of the tibia relative to the femur. If the medial plateau of the tibia rotates anteriorly with anterior displacement of the proximal tibia, the patient has an anteromedial instability. This can be ascertained from the starting position previously described or with the patient sitting with the knee flexed over the edge of the examination table. Anteromedial instability indicates disruption of the medial capsular ligaments and the anterior cruciate ligament.

Anterolateral instability is evaluated in 90 degrees of flexion and as the knee is approaching extension. This instability results from injury or insufficiency of the anterior cruciate and lateral capsular ligaments. The major feature is an anterior gliding of the lateral tibial plateau on the lateral femoral condyle as the knee approaches extension from a starting position of flexion. The relative tightening of the iliotibial band in flexion provides some stability in this position, but that protection is lost as the knee extends. The subluxation of the lateral tibial plateau is sometimes dramatic, and this maneuver is known as the jerk test. This may be performed with the patient supine on the examination table or standing. An internal rotation stress is applied to the tibia as the knee is brought from a flexed to an extended position. At about 30 degrees, the lateral tibial plateau is felt to subluxate anteriorly, producing the jerk.

Posterolateral and posteromedial instabilities result from major injuries to the knee. These conditions imply that the medial or lateral tibial plateau displaces posteriorly secondary to the lack of stability of the capsular structures and the popliteus tendon for posterolateral instability. The external rotation recurvatum test is helpful for the diagnosis of posterolateral instability. The patient is supine, and the affected leg is held by the big toe. If there is posterolateral instability, the tibia rotates externally and slides posteriorly. The knee appears to be in varus, recurvatum, and excessive external tibial rotation. Testing for posteromedial instability, which generally accompanies other instabilities, is less well defined.

A most useful test of knee instability is the Lachman test, although the same maneuver was previously described by Ritchey.[67] The Lachman test is performed with the patient supine and the knee flexed about 20 degrees. A support under the thigh is helpful to obtain relaxation. An anteriorly directed force is applied to the proximal tibia without enhancing or restricting axial rotation. The amount of tibial displacement is estimated in millimeters, and the firmness of the endpoint is subjectively evaluated. Anterior displacement indicates laxity of the posterolateral position of the anterior cruciate ligament; anteromedial position is more directly tested with the knee flexed 90 degrees. The Lachman test is more comfortable for the patient with an acutely injured knee than other types of testing for instability and should always be performed for injuries such as fractures of the tibial spine, which are associated with stretch injuries of the anterior cruciate.

Another maneuver, the Wilson test, may appear to be testing ligamentous integrity but is designed to detect existence of osteochondral defects in their common location on the lateral aspect of the medial femoral condyle. The knee is flexed to 90 degrees, internally rotating the tibia on the femur and extending the knee slowly with the tibia maintained in internal rotation.[94] In the presence of an osteochondritic lesion of the medial femoral condyle, the patient experiences pain as the knee approaches 30 degrees short of full extension. If the pain is relieved by externally rotating the tibia, which removes the spine from the lesion, a diagnosis of osteochondritis of the medial femoral condyle is strongly suspected.

The extensor mechanism is a common site of pediatric orthopaedic symptomatology.[47] The Q angle has become a standard method of describing extensor mechanism mechanics (Fig. 3-42). The Q angle is formed by the angle between the quadriceps muscle

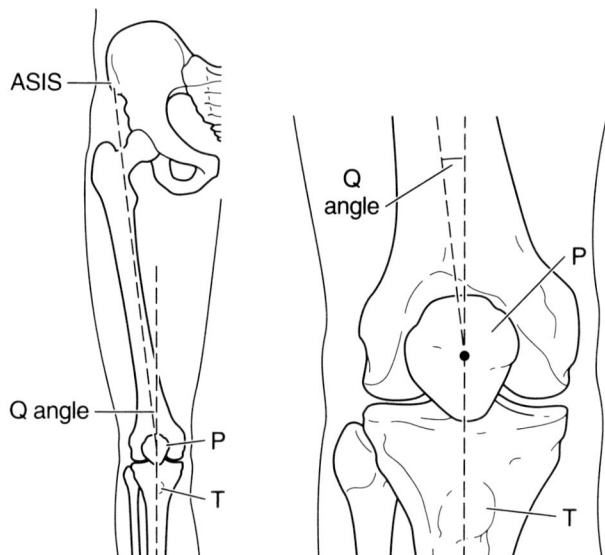

FIGURE 3-42. The Q angle is formed by a line from the anterior superior iliac spine to the center of the patella (P) and a line from the center of the patella to the tibial tubercle (T). (From Clark CR, Bonfiglio M. Orthopaedics. Essentials of diagnosis and treatment. New York: Churchill Livingstone, 1994.)

and the patellar tendon; the apex of the angle is located in the middle of the patella. The patient is in the supine position. The first line is drawn from the anterior superior iliac spine to the middle of the patella, and the second line is from the middle of the patella to the tibial tubercle. The larger the Q angle, the greater is the tendency toward lateral displacement of the patella with contraction of the quadriceps. The Q angle increases with genu valgum or external rotation of the tibia on the femur.

Patellar mobility is tested with the patient in the supine position, with the knee flexed 30 degrees and in full extension. In full extension, the patella can be displaced laterally up to one half of its width, but at 30 degrees of flexion, the femoral condyles should securely hold the patella. If the patient feels or anticipates discomfort while laterally directed pressure is placed on the patella, this finding is described as a positive apprehension test result. An extremely unstable patella may be dislocated laterally. Compressing the patella against the femur longitudinally and transversely against the femur produces pain with many patellofemoral disorders, but this test is nonspecific. An alternate maneuver is to place a hand just proximal to the superior patella, blocking proximal mobility of the patella during contraction of the quadriceps and producing pain as the patellar and femoral surfaces are compressed against each other.

Eilert compares medial and lateral force vectors on the patella by applying medial and lateral pressure to the patella with the finger while the patient contracts the quadriceps muscle. The medial force vector is

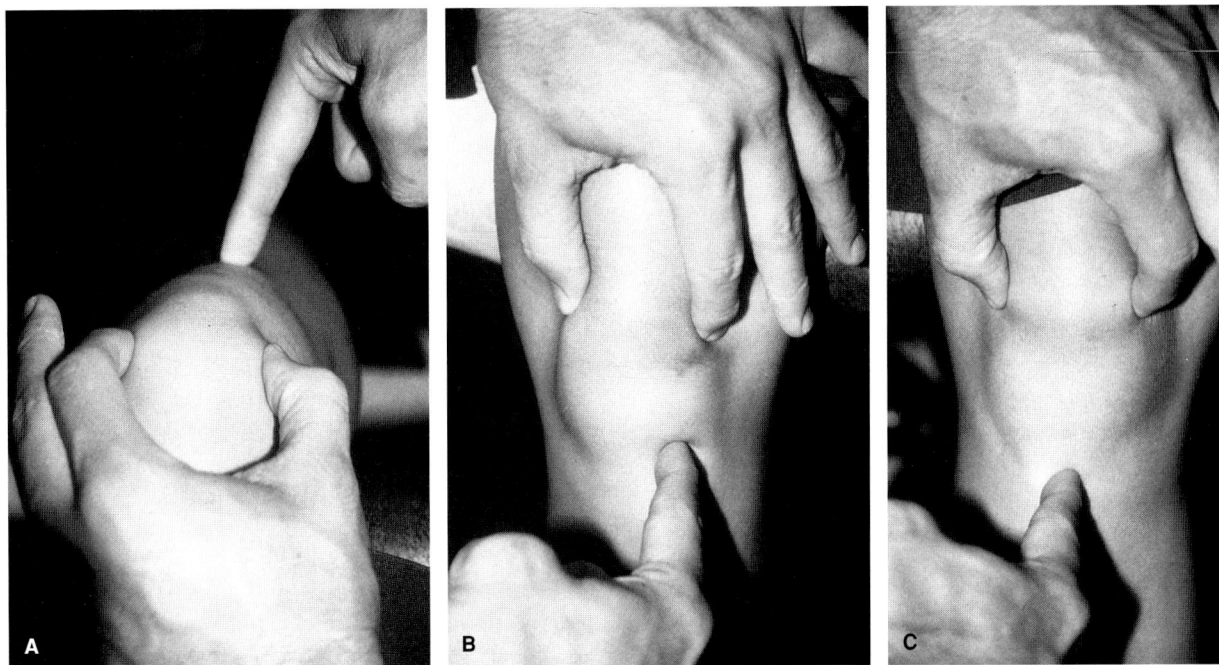

FIGURE 3-43. The Helfet test. (**A**) When the knee is flexed, the tibial tubercle is aligned with the midpatella. (**B**) Normally, in extension, the femur and patella internally rotate so the tubercle is aligned with the lateral patella. (**C**) With disruption of the "screw home" mechanism, the tubercle remains aligned with the midpatella.

often weaker in the presence of anterior knee pain.[26] The medial and lateral patellofemoral articulations are palpated for tenderness. The lateral retinaculum is often contracted in a patient with patellofemoral instability and restricts medial mobility of the patella. Contracture of the iliotibial band may contribute to lateral retinacular contracture.[74] This may be confirmed by the Ober maneuver.

The patellofemoral joint is viewed with the knees flexed 90 degrees over the edge of the table. In this position, each patella should be centered in the outline made by the soft tissues of the thighs. With lateral displacement, the "grasshopper eyes" appearance may be noticed as the patellas are tilted superolaterally. Patellar tracking is observed during active flexion and extension of the knee. This is done from the starting position of the knees flexed 90 degrees over the end of the examination table, allowing the relation of the tibial tubercle and the patella to be observed. Ordinarily, with the "screw home" mechanism accompanying the last few degrees of knee extension, the femur and patella internally rotate or the tibia externally rotates.[31] In complete extension, the tibial tubercle is ordinarily aligned with the middle of the patella. As the knee flexes, the tibia internally rotates, and the tibial tubercle assumes a position aligned with the lateral aspect of the patella (Fig. 3-43). The lack of this rotational component of patellofemoral motion indicates a pathologic process interfering with normal joint dynamics. This was originally identified by Helfet and is sometimes known as the modified Helfet test.

In the sagittal plane, patella alta can be assessed with the patient sitting and the knees flexed 90 degrees. In this position, the patella should be in the sulcus between the femoral condyles; normally, the proximal pole of the patella should be in a line extended along the anterior surface of the femoral shaft. In a patient with patella alta, the patella is prominent and tilted toward the ceiling, with a sulcus distal to the inferior pole. Patella baja, also called inferior patella, results in the patella sitting inferior to the femoral condyles.

The patient is asked to extend the knee, and the character and strength of the vastus medialis obliquus is assessed. Hypoplasia of the vastus medialis accompanies disorders of the extensor mechanism, and this component of the quadriceps is easiest to observe. Strength of the quadriceps may be roughly quantitated by asking the patient to extend the knee against resistance or hold the knee extended against manual resistance directed at the floor. An older child should be able to generate sufficient quadriceps strength to maintain knee extension against a force exerted by the examiner on the distal tibia great enough to lift the buttock off the table via the lever of the extended knee. An alternate method is to have the supine patient lift the extended knee about 10 cm (4 in) off the table, hold for a count of three, return to the starting position, and repeat. Patients with functional quadriceps weakness

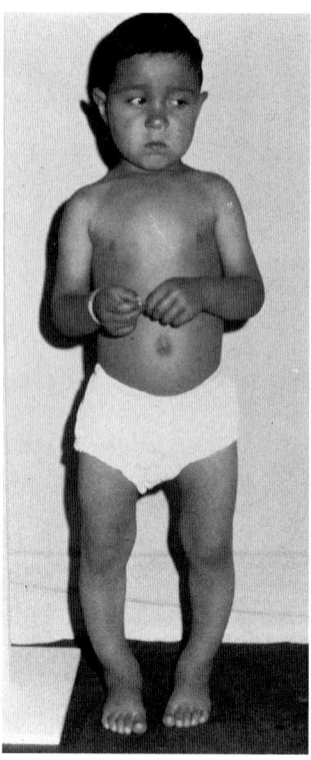

FIGURE 3-44. Instead of the gentle continuous bow associated with physiologic bowing, a localized sharper bend, seen here in the distal tibia, indicates a bony deformity.

have difficulty repeating this lift 10 times. Testing in this manner also provides a convenient baseline with which to compare at later visits. Hopping on one leg 20 times can give information about the functional capability of the quadriceps. Quadriceps circumference should be measured in the bulk of the muscle, using a bony landmark such as the tibial tuberosity as a reference point.[20]

The plica, which is a normal fold of synovium, achieved a certain degree of notoriety as a cause of anterior knee pain after arthroscopic evaluation of painful knees became widespread. Although it has probably been a convenient but innocent culprit as the cause of pain in many arthroscopic examinations, it can rarely be a cause of anterior knee pain. Mital and Hayden described a method of clinical testing based on the location of the medial plica sliding over the medial femoral condyle.[63] The knee is held in a position of 30 degrees of passive flexion; the opposite examiner's forearm from the hand being used to examine the patella can support the knee. The patella is displaced medially, producing local pain if the plica is inflamed. They were not able to palpate the plica in most of their patients.

The leg is relatively accessible to physical examination, because the tibia is subcutaneous along its entire anteromedial border. The most common alignment problem in young children requiring special attention to the leg is bowlegs, with tibia vara a possible etiologic entity. A visual clue to differentiating physiologic bowlegs from anatomic tibia vara is to notice whether the bowing is gently distributed throughout the legs or concentrated in the region of the proximal tibia (Fig. 3-44). Localized bowing of the shaft of the bone suggests a metabolic or growth disorder. Anterolateral bowing of the shaft strongly suggests congenital pseudoarthrosis and is easily differentiated from the more benign posteromedial bowing.

With the patient undressed, a visual estimate of the alignment of the limb can be made. As orthopaedic surgeons have recognized the importance of the mechanical axis of the limb in planning for reconstructive procedures, this concept has assumed greater clinical relevance. The mechanical axis is defined by the relation of the center of the hip, knee, and ankle joints and is a radiographic measurement. As experience is gained in comparing radiographic measurements with clinical appearance, a visual estimate can be made with more confidence. The act of recording the examiner's visual impression of the lower limbs of a child with an angular deformity results in a more critical assessment of limb alignment.

Localized swelling can be recognized by inspection or palpation. In the young child unable to walk, detection of swelling is more difficult because of the more generous layer of subcutaneous fat at this age. However, by gentle systematic palpation, the swelling and tenderness associated with an occult fracture can be identified by starting at the foot and working up the leg.

Foot and Ankle

The foot is a common site of pediatric orthopaedic problems, but it is also a difficult area to examine and describe. The relatively large number of joints in the foot can make accurate assessment of motion in a particular joint complex. For example, the actual motion of the ankle joint measured radiographically is less than that measured clinically because of the additive motion from other joints.[4] Nonetheless, with standardized measurement techniques, clinically useful assessment of foot motion is not difficult. The particular physical findings discovered with examination of the foot are often the expression of a systemic pathologic condition or disorder of the central or peripheral nervous system. Awareness of the association of cavus foot deformities with neuromuscular conditions directs the examiner to neurologic and muscle examinations.[72]

Because there are various ways in which foot joint motion may be characterized, the terminology used in the American Academy of Orthopaedic Surgeons

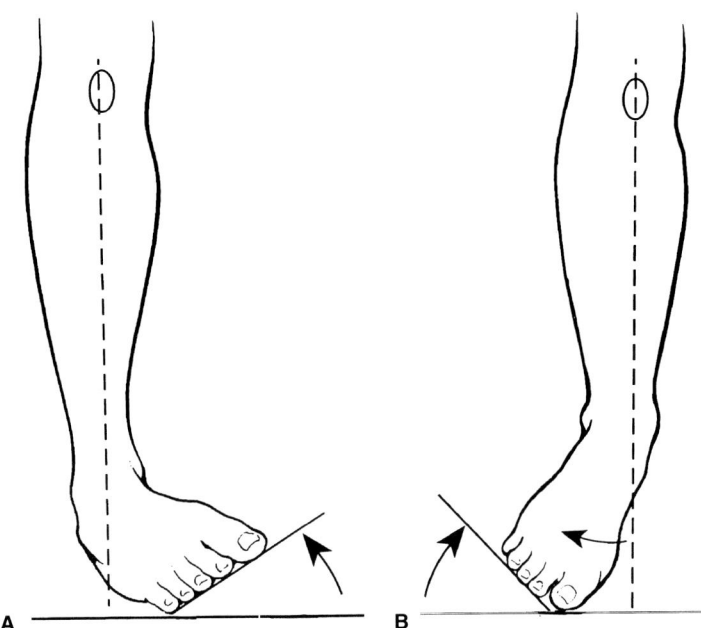

FIGURE 3-45. (A) Supination and (B) pronation of the foot. (From Greene WB, Heckman JD. The clinical measurement of joint motion. Rosemont, IL: American Academy of Orthopaedic Surgeons, 1994.)

handbook on joint motion is used here.[34] Ankle motion is measured only in dorsiflexion and plantar flexion. The starting point is with the foot at a right angle to the tibia. The goniometer is placed along the lateral border of the foot, and degrees of dorsiflexion and plantar flexion of the lateral border are measured.[27] Some foot motion is inevitably included in the angle measured, but this is of little functional significance.

Inversion (i.e., turning the heel inward) and eversion (i.e., turning the heel outward) denote motion at the subtalar joint. Many clinical writings interchange valgus for eversion and varus for inversion and sometimes use valgus for pronation (i.e., pes planovalgus). Pronation and supination refer to more complex motions (Fig. 3-45). Supination includes inversion and adduction and plantar flexion of the midfoot. Pronation includes eversion, abduction, and dorsiflexion of the midfoot. Adduction and abduction of the foot occur in the plane of the metatarsals; sometimes varus and valgus are used interchangeably (i.e., metatarsus adductus or varus). In-toeing and out-toeing are terms used interchangeably with internal and external rotation to describe foot position during gait.

In-toeing or out-toeing positions are frequent presenting complaints for infants and young children. Examination consists of a dynamic phase, observing gait, and the static examination. During gait observation, the degree of in-toeing or out-toeing to the line of progression is ascertained. The patellar positions during gait can identify whether the rotational deformity is above (i.e., femoral anteversion) or below (i.e., tibial torsion) the knee. Optimally, several passes of the child's gait are observed. On the first pass, the positions of the feet are observed; on the second pass, the positions of the patellas are evaluated; and on the third pass, an overall assessment is made.

The torsional profile described by Staheli is a rapid and effective static method of examination for rotational problems in children. The child is prone with the knees flexed 90 degrees (see Fig. 3-37). The tibias serve as reference markers to measure internal and external rotation of the hips. The bimalleolar axis is identified; normally, the fibular malleolus is about 10 to 30 degrees posterior to the medial malleolus. The thigh–foot angle documents the resting position of the feet. The lateral border of the foot is examined for adduction or abduction posture. Similar maneuvers may be performed anteriorly in the supine or sitting positions, but reproducibility may be impaired because of the more subjective parameters for measurement. With the patient in a sitting position and each patella positioned straight ahead, the malleoli are palpated and the degree of torsion estimated.

For foot problems other than in-toeing or out-toeing, examination is more complex. Mann stresses the need for a routine procedure for examination of inspection, palpation, and manipulation.[60] In addition to skin and posture, inspection includes observation of gait, with attention to rotation, heel strike and heel rise, limp, and amount of pronation during stance phase. Whether the ankle is dorsiflexed by the tibialis anterior or the toe extensors and whether there is excessive weight bearing on the medial or lateral borders of the foot are important observations. The patient is asked to stand on the toes. This necessitates muscular strength and normal subtalar mechanics.

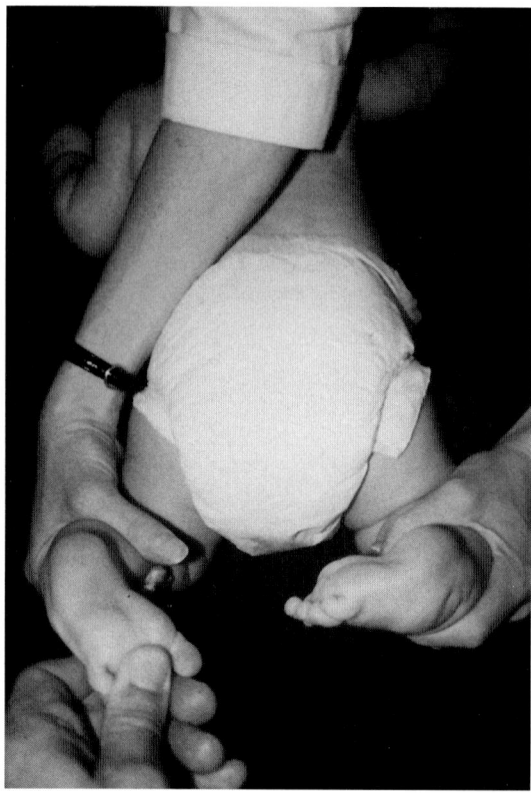

FIGURE 3-46. Prone position for evaluation of adduction, supination, and internal rotation of the infant clubfoot. Passive mobility can be documented photographically in this manner.

lation is applicable to the infant's foot when clubfoot or congenital vertical talus is suspected. The rotational relation of the resting foot to the knee is assessed and described in anatomic terms. Skin folds or creases are identified. The head of the talus is palpated. The resiliency of the heel cord is determined. With manipulation, the rigidity of the deformity can be ascertained. A postural deformation may be easily corrected; a structural malformation is unyielding. Ankle motion is quantitated. The infant is placed in the prone position for evaluation of subtalar motion and foot adduction or abduction (Fig. 3-46).

Although an estimate of subtalar motion can be made with the patient in the sitting position by holding the calcaneus in one hand and the forefoot with the other, subtalar motion is best evaluated with the patient prone and the knees flexed.[34,60] Because the axis of the subtalar joint is about 40 to 45 degrees off the horizontal, flexing the knees to 130 degrees puts the axis of the subtalar joint parallel with the table top (Fig. 3-47). The calcaneus is then inverted and everted, and the degrees of motion are recorded. The position of the subtalar joint also affects the amount of foot joint motion at the talonavicular and calcaneocuboid joints, where much of pronation and supination occur. When the subtalar joint is inverted, the axes of the calcaneocuboid and talonavicular joints are divergent, and motion at these joints is inhibited. When the subtalar joint is everted, the axes of the calcaneocuboid and talonavicular joints are parallel, and motion is facilitated.

Many foot deformities are characterized by alterations in the relation of the forefoot to the hindfoot. The forefoot may be in equinus (i.e., cavus foot), supination (i.e., clubfoot), pronation (i.e., pes cavus), or abduction (i.e., congenital vertical talus). To evaluate this relation, one hand is placed on the calcaneus, and the other manipulates the forefoot. If a disruption in the normal relation is found, the rigidity of the deformity is documented.

Subtalar mechanics are also tested by rotating the body on the weight-bearing limb. Supination of the foot occurs as the leg is externally rotated, and pronation occurs as the foot is internally rotated. The great toe is dorsiflexed, increasing tension on the plantar aponeurosis. Normally, this causes the longitudinal arch to rise. In a patient with an elongated plantar aponeurosis accompanying pes planovalgus, dorsiflexion of the great toe has no effect on the arch.

The routine of inspection, palpation, and manipu-

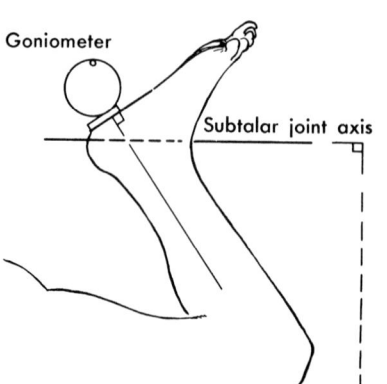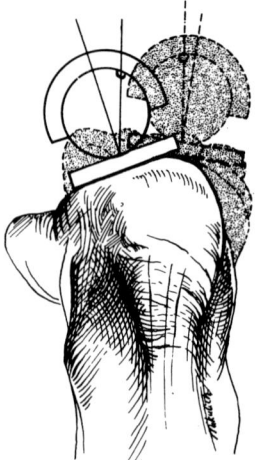

FIGURE 3-47. Method of Mann for evaluation of subtalar motion. With the knees flexed 135 degrees, the axis of subtalar motion is parallel with the table top. The hindfoot is inverted and everted, and the motion is recorded with a goniometer. (From Mann RA. Principles of examination of the foot and ankle. In: Mann RA, Coughlin MJ, eds. Surgery of the foot and ankle. St Louis: CV Mosby, 1992:45.)

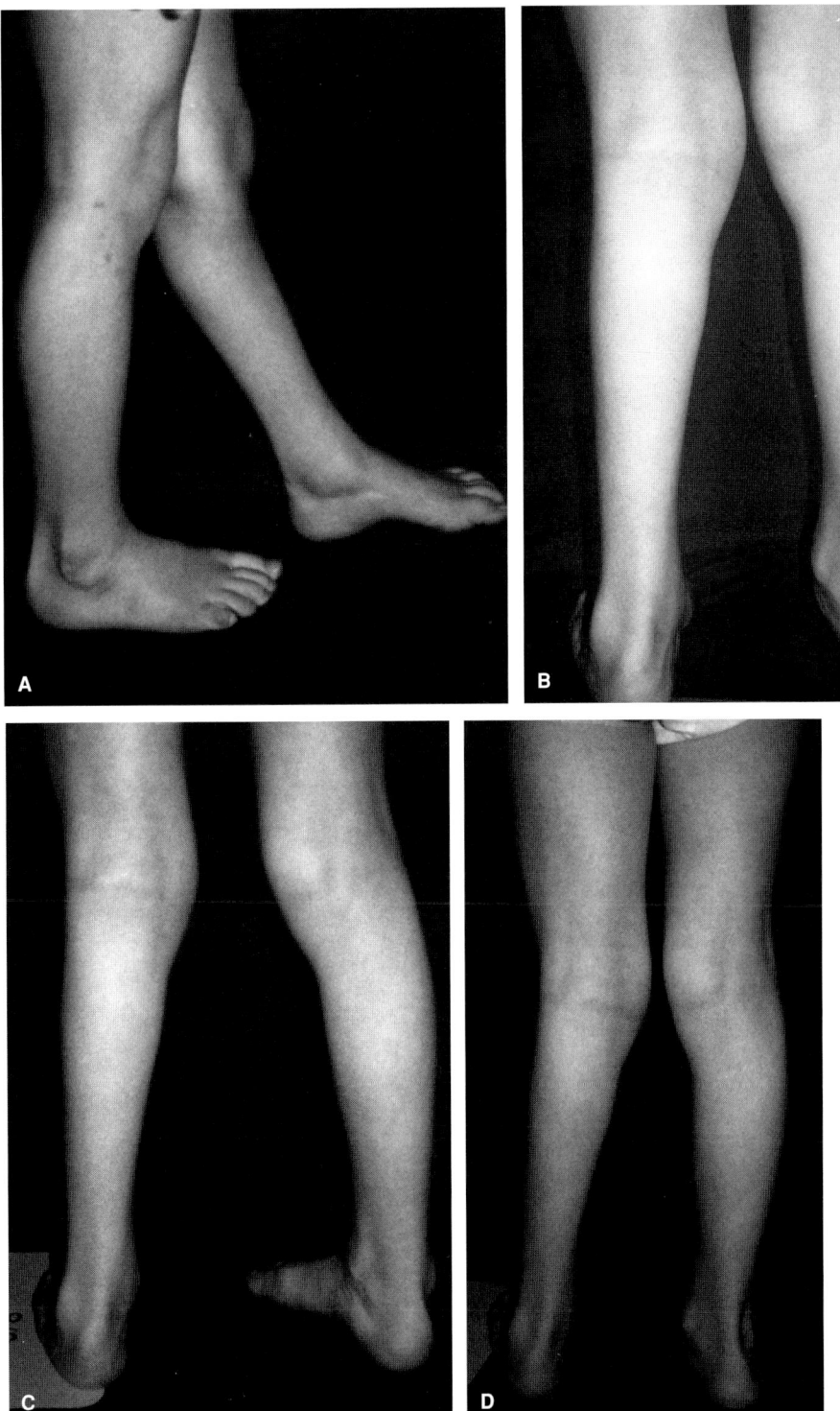

FIGURE 3-48. Block test. (A) Cavus foot, viewed from the medial side. The first metatarsal is plantarflexed, and the first metatarsophalangeal joint is hyperextended. (B) The left hindfoot is inverted 5 degrees relative to the long axis of the leg. The unaffected right hindfoot is everted. (C) In the method described by Coleman, a block is placed under the hindfoot and lateral forefoot and the first metatarsal head is allowed to plantar flex. The hindfoot is neutral relative to the long axis of the leg. (D) In an alternate method, the block is placed under the fifth metatarsal head. The hindfoot is everted.

The cavus foot, characterized by a high arch, plantar flexion of the first metatarsal, and usually inversion of the hindfoot, requires an extra maneuver, the block test, for adequate assessment of the relation of the forefoot to the hindfoot. The forefoot of a cavus foot is fixed in pronation because of the plantar-flexed first metatarsal. The hindfoot may be supple or fixed. However, on weight bearing, the hindfoot is in an inverted position, regardless of whether it is supple or fixed, because the depressed first metatarsal head tilts the entire foot toward an inverted position. The block test can differentiate whether or not there is fixed hindfoot deformity (Fig. 3-48). A block (the same blocks used to evaluate leg length discrepancy are suitable), de-

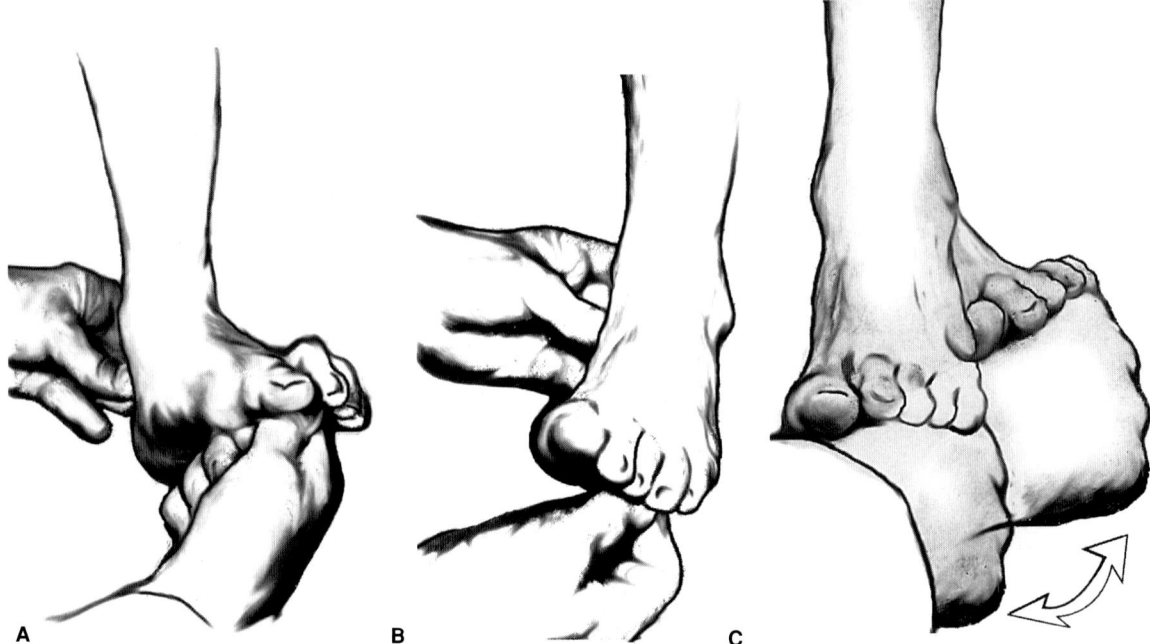

FIGURE 3-49. Effect of pronation and supination of the foot on measured ankle motion. (**A**) Pronation allows eversion of the hindfoot to occur, factitiously increasing apparent dorsiflexion. (**B**) Supination blocks eversion of hindfoot, providing more accurate assessment of ankle motion in the presence of tight heel cord. (**C**) The difference in achievable dorsiflexion with the foot pronated and supinated. (Adapted from Harris RI, Beath T. Hypermobile flat-foot with short tendo-Achilles. (J Bone Joint Surg [Am] 1948;48:116.)

scribed by Coleman as usually 1 to 1.5 in (2.5–3.75 cm) high, is placed under the lateral aspect of the foot.[21] The purpose of the block is to allow the pronated and plantar-flexed first metatarsal to hang free and negate any tilting effect this rigidly plantar-flexed metatarsal may have had on the heel. If the heel assumes a neutral position when the block is under the lateral foot, the hindfoot is not rigid but is accommodating the forefoot deformity. This differentiation is important in planning treatment.

Pes planovalgus is a frequent complaint prompting pediatric orthopaedic examination. Harris and Beath discovered the effects of tight heel cords and subtalar motion on measured ankle joint motion.[38] To evaluate the effect of heel cord contracture on ankle joint motion, the knee is extended, and the foot is supinated before dorsiflexion of the ankle is attempted, measuring the lateral border of the foot with the long axis of the tibia. If the foot is allowed to pronate, further apparent ankle dorsiflexion is achieved, but the additional motion achieved actually occurs at the subtalar joint (Fig. 3-49). Allowing knee flexion during ankle dorsiflexion during gastrocnemius contracture allows additional apparent ankle dorsiflexion, because the gastrocnemius origin is from the distal femur. Because standing necessitates knee extension, gastrocnemius contracture is associated with an everted posture of the hindfoot.

Bunions or hallux valgus deformities can occur in older children. The severity of deformity is described by the angle between the first metatarsal and the proximal phalanx. The toe may pronate on the first metatarsal (Fig. 3-50). Pronation of the foot describes rotation about an axis from the toes to the heel, and

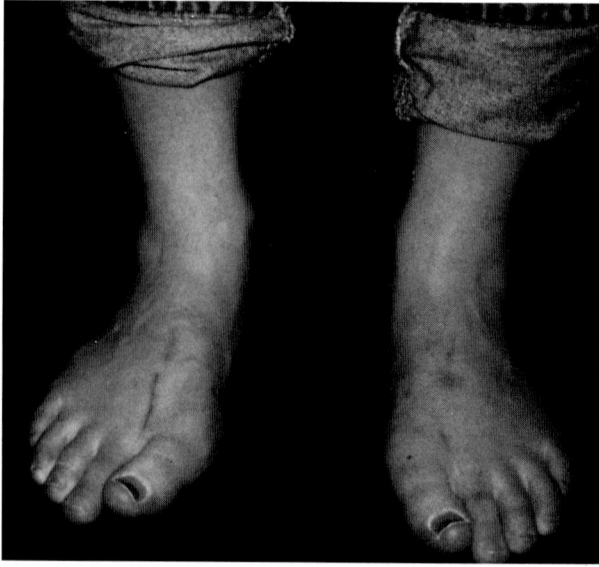

FIGURE 3-50. Recurrent bunion deformity with pronation of the great toes.

pronation of the toe describes lateral rotation of the dorsal surface of the toe along the long axis of the toe.

The examination is completed with an assessment of strength of muscles about the foot and ankle. If normal gait and function have already been documented during the observation portion of the examination, detailed muscle testing is unnecessary. If any deviation has been found, the strength of the major muscle groups should be assessed. Older children can cooperate by actively resisting the examiner's hand in dorsiflexion, plantar flexion, supination (includes inversion), and pronation (includes eversion). The feet of younger children may be tickled. In a few moments, a normal foot demonstrates active motion in all spheres.

The positions of the toes are assessed. Clawing is a term used to describe a condition similar to clawing of the fingers with hyperextension of the metatarsal-phalangeal joints and flexion deformity of the interphalangeal joints. Relatively mild clawtoes have a normal posture at rest, but they deform with contraction of the dorsiflexors. Long-standing clawtoes become fixed. Pushing the metatarsal heads dorsally corrects flexible clawtoes.

Radiographs and photographs usually are obtained for documentation of gait. Another way to record the weight-bearing pattern of the foot during gait is the Shutrack carbon paper system used by Yngve in his report on results of clubfoot surgery.[95] The child walks on a strip of pressure-sensitive paper, which can be incorporated in the permanent record for later comparison. Smith and colleagues recommended having the child who weighs less than 10 kg stand on a copying machine and using the photocopy obtained for documentation of foot posture.[81]

CONCLUSION

The examination methods described in this chapter are limited. Although the variety of pediatric orthopaedic conditions precludes adequate description of all of the examination maneuvers, the principles of understanding the underlying anatomy and recognizing the alterations in anatomy and expected function are timeless. Many orthopaedists develop their own methods of examination, which may work better for them than the maneuvers described here. Tailoring the examination method is acceptable as long as the necessary information is gleaned. A consistently competent pediatric orthopaedic examination is produced by practice.

References

1. Ahlberg A, Moussa M, Al-Nahdi M. On geographical variations in the normal range of joint motion. Clin Orthop 1988;234:229.
2. Ashton BB, Pickles B, Roll JW. Reliability of goniometric measurements of hip motion in cerebral palsy. Dev Med Child Neurol 1978;20:87.
3. Ashworth M, Hancock J, Ashworth L, Tessier K. Scoliosis screening: an approach to cost-benefit analysis. Spine 1988;13:1187.
4. Backer M, Kofoed H. Passive ankle mobility. Clinical measurement compared with radiography. J Bone Joint Surg [Br] 1989;71:696.
5. Baird HW, Gordon EC. Neurological evaluation of infants and children. Clin Dev Med 1983;84:85.
6. Barlow TG. Early diagnosis and treatment of congenital dislocation of the hip. J Bone Joint Surg [Br] 1962;44:292.
7. Barnes MJ, Herring JA. Combined split anterior tibial tendon transfer and intramuscular lengthening of the posterior tibial tendon. J Bone Joint Surg [Am] 1991;73:734.
8. Bartlett MD, Wolf LS, Shurtleff DB, Staheli LT. Hip flexion contractures: a comparison of measurement methods. Arch Phys Med Rehabil 1985;66:620.
9. Baxter MP. Assessment of normal pediatric knee laxity using the Genucom. J Pediatr Orthop 1988;8:546.
10. Baxter MP. "Growing pains" in childhood—a proposal for treatment. J Pediatr Orthop 1988;8:402.
11. Beals RK. The normal carrying angle of the elbow. A radiographic study of 422 patients. Clin Orthop 1976;119:194.
12. Bernbeck R, Sinios A. Neuro-orthopedic screening in infancy. Munich: Urban & Schwarzenberg, 1978.
13. Bielicki T. Growth and economic well-being: 20th century. In: Falkner F, Tanner JM, eds. Human growth, 2nd ed. New York: Plenum Press, 1986:283.
14. Bleck EE. Orthopaedic management in cerebral palsy. Philadelphia: JB Lippincott, 1987.
15. Boone DC, Azen SP, Lin CM. Reliability of goniometric measurements. Phys Ther 1978;58:1355.
16. Brundtland GH, Liestrol K, Walloe L. Height, weight, and menarchal age of Oslo schoolchildren during the last 60 years. Ann Hum Biol 1980;7:307.
17. Buckler JMH. A reference manual of growth and development. Melbourne: Blackwell, 1979.
18. Carey RPL. Clinical examination and measurement of limb length inequality. In: Menelaus MB, ed. The management of limb inequality. Edinburgh: Churchill Livingstone, 1991:49.
19. Chapple CC, Davidson DT. A study of the relationship between fetal position and certain congenital deformities. J Pediatr 1941;18:483.
20. Clark CR, Bonfiglio M. Orthopaedics. Essentials of diagnosis and treatment. New York: Churchill Livingstone, 1994.
21. Coleman SS. Complex foot deformities in children. Philadelphia: Lea & Febiger, 1983.
22. Coon V, Donato G, Houser C, Bleck EE. Normal ranges of motion of the hip joint in infants, six weeks, three months, and six months of age. Clin Orthop 1975;110:256.
23. Daniel DM, Stone ML, Barnett PEA. Use of the quadriceps active test to diagnose posterior cruciate ligamentous disruption and measure posterior laxity of the knee. J Bone Joint Surg [Am] 1988;70:386.
24. Davids JR, Holland WC, Sutherland DH. Significance of the confusion test in cerebral palsy. J Pediatr Orthop 1993;13:717.
25. Dunne KB, Clarren SK. The origin of prenatal and postnatal deformities. Pediatr Clin North Am 1986;33:1277.
26. Eilert RE. Adolescent anterior knee pain. In: Heckman JD, ed. Instr Course Lect 1993;42:497.
27. Elveru RA, Rothstein JM, Lamb RL. Goniometric reliability in a clinical setting. Subtalar and ankle joint measurements. Phys Ther 1988;68:672.
28. Eveleth PB. Population differences in growth. In: Falkner F, Tanner JM, eds. Human growth, 2nd ed. New York: Plenum Press, 1986:221.

29. Finlay HVL, Maudsley RH, Busfield PI. Dislocatable and dislocated hip in the newborn infant. Br Med J 1967;4:377.
30. Forero N, Okamura LA, Larson MA. Normal ranges of hip motion in neonates. J Pediatr Orthop 1989;9:391.
31. Frankel VH, Burstein AH, Brooks DB. Biomechanics of internal derangement of the knee. J Bone Joint Surg [Am] 1971;53:945.
32. Gardner K. The innervation of the hip joint. Anat Rec 1948;101:353.
33. Green NE, Griffin PP. Hip dysplasia associated with abduction contracture of the contralateral hip. J Bone Joint Surg [Am] 1982;64:1723.
34. Greene WB, Heckman JD. The clinical measurement of joint motion. Rosemont, IL: American Academy of Orthopaedic Surgeons, 1994.
35. Gross RH, Wisnefske M, Howard TC, Hitch M. Infant hip screening. In: Nelson JP, ed. The hip. Proceedings of the tenth open scientific meeting of The Hip Society, 1982. St Louis: CV Mosby, 1982:50.
36. Haas SS, Epps CH Jr, Adams JP. Normal ranges of hip motion in the newborn. Clin Orthop 1973;91:114.
37. Hall JG, Forster-Iskenius UG, Allanson JE. Handbook of normal physical measurements. Oxford: Oxford University Press, 1989.
38. Harris RI, Beath T. Hypermobile flat-foot with short tendo-Achilles. J Bone Joint Surg [Am] 1948;48:116.
39. Harris SR, Smith LH, Krukowski L. Goniometric reliability for a child with cerebral palsy. J Pediatr Orthop 1985;5:348.
40. Hawkins RJ, Bokor DJ. Clinical evaluation of shoulder problems. In: Rockwood CA, Matsen FA, eds. The shoulder. Philadelphia: WB Saunders, 1990:149.
41. Heath CH, Staheli LT. Normal limits of knee angle in white children—genu varum and genu valgum. J Pediatr Orthop 1993;13:259.
42. Hensinger RN. Standards in pediatric orthopedics. New York: Raven Press, 1986.
43. Herzenberg JE, Hensinger RN, Dedrick DK, Phillips WA. Emergency transport and positioning of young children who have an injury of the cervical spine. J Bone Joint Surg [Am] 1989;71:15.
44. Hoppenfeld S. Physical examination of the spine and extremities. New York: Appleton-Century-Crofts, 1976.
45. Houston CS, Swischuk LE. Varus and valgus. No wonder they are confused. N Engl J Med 1980;302:471.
46. Huckabay LM. Effect of having siblings in the exam room on parents' retention of clinicians' instructions. Nurse Pract 1992;17:56.
47. Hughston JC, Walsh WM, Puddu G. Patellar subluxation and dislocation. Philadelphia: WB Saunders, 1984.
48. Illingworth RS. Basic developmental screening, 2nd ed. Oxford: Blackwell, 1977.
49. Illingworth RS. The development of the infant and young child—normal and abnormal, 9th ed. New York: Churchill Livingstone, 1987.
50. Johnson EW. Examination for muscle weakness in infants and small children. JAMA 1958;168:1306.
51. Katz K, Rosenthal A, Yosiplvitch Z. Normal range of popliteal angles in children. J Pediatr Orthop 1992;12:229.
52. Kennedy JC. The injured adolescent knee. Baltimore: Williams & Wilkins, 1979.
53. Knudsen CJM, Hoffman EB. Neonatal osteomyelitis. J Bone Joint Surg [Br] 1990;72:846.
54. Korsch BM, Gozzi EK, Francis V. Gaps in doctor-patient communication. 1. Doctor-patient interaction and patient satisfaction. Pediatrics 1968;42:855.
55. Lambrinudi C. Adolescent and senile kyphosis. Br Med J 1934;2:800.
56. Lovett RW. Fatigue and exercise in treatment of infantile paralysis: study of one thousand eight hundred and thirty-six cases. JAMA 1917;69:168.
57. Luchini M, Stevens DB. Validity of torsional profile examination. J Pediatr Orthop 1983;3:41.
58. Maguire P, Fairbairn S, Fletcher C. Consultation skills of young doctors: I. benefits of feedback training in interviewing as students persist. Br Med J 1986;292:1773.
59. Maguire P, Fairbairn S, Fletcher C. Consultation skills of young doctors: II. most young doctors are bad at giving information. Br Med J 1986;292:1576.
60. Mann RA. Principles of examination of the foot and ankle. In: Mann RA, Coughlin MJ, eds. Surgery of the foot and ankle. St Louis: CV Mosby, 1992:45.
61. McCarthy R. Evaluation of the patient with deformity. In: Weinstein S, ed. The pediatric spine: principles and practice. New York: Raven Press, 1994:185.
62. McDonald CM, Jaffe KM, Shurtleff DB. Assessment of muscle strength in children with myelomeningocele: accuracy and stability of measurements over time. Arch Phys Med Rehabil 1986;67:855.
63. Mital MA, Hayden J. Pain in the knee in children: the medial plica syndrome. Orthop Clin North Am 1979;10:713.
64. Nigg BM, Fisher V, Allinger TL, et al. Range of motion of the foot as a function of age. Foot Ankle 1992;3:336.
65. Ober FR. The role of the iliotibial band and fascia: a factor in the causation of low back disorders and sciatica. J Bone Joint Surg 1936;18:105.
66. Ortolani M. The classic, congenital hip dysplasia in the light of early and very early diagnosis. Clin Orthop 1976;119:6.
67. Paessler HH, Michel D. How new is the Lachman test? Am J Sports Med 1992;20:95.
68. Paine RS, Oppé TE. Neurological examination of children. Clin Dev Med 1966;20/21.
69. Perry J. Determinants of muscle function in the spastic lower limb. Clin Orthop 1993;288:10.
70. Phelps E, Smith LJ, Hallum A. Normal ranges of hip motion of infants between nine and 24 months of age. Dev Med Child Neurol 1985;27:785.
71. Popoff L. Pain indexes: an aid in differential diagnosis of organic and psychogenic illness. Med Digest 1970;(Oct):43.
72. Rasool MN, Govender S, Naidoo KS, Moodley M. Foot deformities and occult spinal abnormalities in children: a review of 16 cases. J Pediatr Orthop 1992;12:94.
73. Reade E, Hom L, Hallum A, Lopopolo R. Changes in popliteal angle measurement in infants up to one year of age. Dev Med Child Neurol 1984;26:774.
74. Reid DC, Burnham RS, Saboe LA. Lower extremity flexibility patterns in classical ballet dancers and their correlation to lateral hip and knee injuries. Am J Sports Med 1987;15:347.
75. Roach KE, Miles TP. Normal hip and knee active range of motion: the relationship to age. Phys Ther 1991;71:656.
76. Rothstein JM, Miller PT, Roeltger RF. Goniometric reliability in a clinical setting. Elbow and knee measurements. Phys Ther 1983;63:1611.
77. Salenius P, Vankka E. The development of the tibiofemoral angle in children. J Bone Joint Surg [Am] 1975;57:259.
78. Salter RB. Textbook of disorders and injuries of the musculoskeletal system. 2nd ed. Baltimore: Waverly Press, 1983.
79. Schwarze DJ, Denton JR. Normal values of neonatal lower limbs: an evaluation of 1,000 neonates. J Pediatr Orthop 1994;13:758.
80. Smith DW. Recognizable patterns of human deformation. In: Markowitz M, ed. Major problems in clinical pediatrics. 3rd ed. Philadelphia: WB Saunders, 1982.
81. Smith JT, Bleck EE, Gamble JG, et al. Simple method of documenting metatarsus adductus. J Pediatr Orthop 1991;11:679.
82. Spranger J, Bernischke K, Hall JG. Errors of morphogenesis. Concepts and terms. J Pediatr 1982;100:160.

83. Staheli L. The prone hip extension test. Clin Orthop 1977;123:12.
84. Staheli LT. Torsional deformity. Pediatr Clin North Am 1977;24:799.
85. Staheli LT, Corbett M, Wyss C, King H. Lower-extremity rotational problems in children. Normal values to guide management. J Bone Joint Surg [Am] 1985;67:39.
86. Sutherland DH, Olshen R, Cooper L, Woo S. The development of mature gait. J Bone Joint Surg [Am] 1980;62:336.
87. Svenningsen S, Terjesen T, Auflem M, et al. Hip motion related to age and sex. Acta Orthop Scand 1989;60:205.
88. Tachdjian MO. Pediatric orthopedics, vol 1. Philadelphia: WB Saunders, 1990.
89. Tanner J. Growth and endocrinology of the adolescent. In: Gardner L, ed. Endocrine and genetic diseases of childhood. Philadelphia: WB Saunders, 1975.
90. Tanner JM. Use and abuse of growth standards. In: Falkner F, Tanner JM, eds. Human growth, vol 3. New York: Plenum Press, 1986.
91. Watkins MA, Riddle DL, Lamb RL, et al. Reliability of goniometric measurements and visual estimates of knee range of motion obtained in a clinical setting. Phys Ther 1991;71:90.
92. Waugh KG, Minkel JL, Parker R, et al. Measurement of selected hip, knee, and ankle joint motions in newborns. Phys Ther 1983;63:1616.
93. Williams B. Orthopaedic features in the presentation of syringomyelia. J Bone Joint Surg [Br] 1979;61:314.
94. Wilson JN. A new diagnostic sign in osteochondritis dissecans of the knee. J Bone Joint Surg [Am] 1967;49:477.
95. Yngve D. Foot-progression angle in children. J Pediatr Orthop 1990;10:467.
96. Youdas JW, Carey JR, Garrett TR. Reliability of measurements of cervical spine motion—comparison of three methods. Phys Ther 1991;71:98.

APPENDIX 3-1.   *Chart for a patient profile.*

PATIENT PROFILE

DATE:_____ PATIENT'S NAME:_____

BIRTHDATE:_____ M__F__ AGE: YEARS____MONTHS_____

What is the reason for today's visit?_____

When did this problem first start?_____

Is the problem better since you first noticed it? Yes___No___
Is the problem worse since you first noticed it? Yes___No___
Is the problem the same? Yes___No___

Is there a family history of this problem? Yes___No___
Has this problem been treated previously? Yes___No___
Please list all treating physician(s). _____

Past medical history:
Major illnesses?   Yes___No___
Operations?   Yes___No___
Medications?   Yes___No___
Allergies?   Yes___No___
List any medications allergic to:_____

Your child's birth history:
Premature?   Yes___No___Reason?_____
Problems?   Yes___No___Reason?_____
Breech?   Yes___No___Reason?_____
Caesarean?   Yes___No___Reason?_____

Birthweight:_____ lb, _____ oz; number of pregnancies: _____ ;

number of children: _____ ; your child sat up at age _____ months;

your child walked at age _____ months; your child spoke at age _____ months.

Do you have a family doctor or pediatrician who should get a copy of your child's

medical report? Doctor's name:_____ Address:_____

_____ Telephone:_____

SIGNATURE OF PARENT OR GUARDIAN: _____

APPENDIX 3-2. *Tanner's stages of development.*

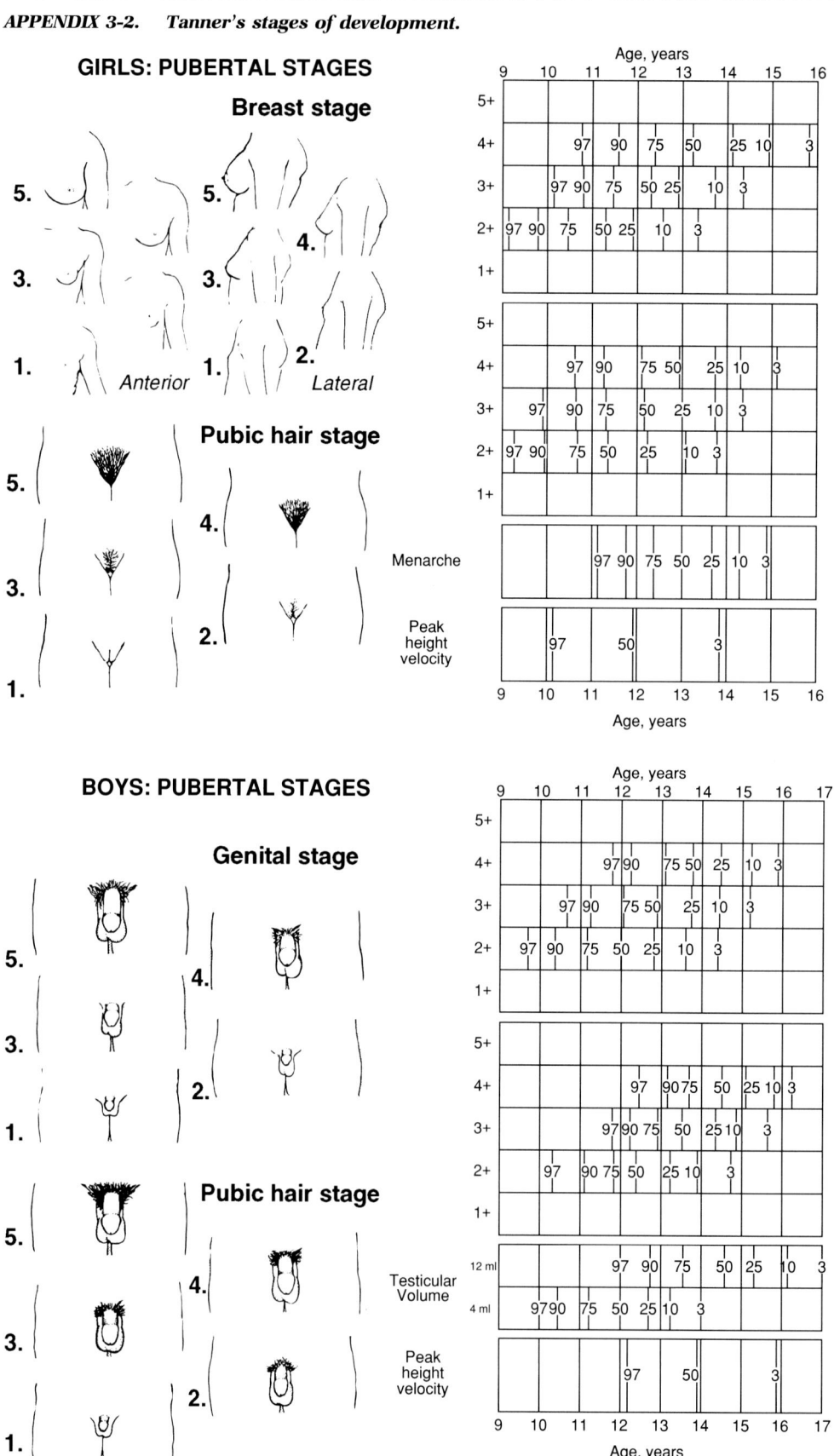

(Adapted from Buckler JMH. A reference manual of growth and development. Melbourne: Blackwell, 1979.)

Chapter 4

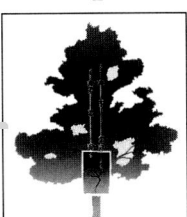

Normal Gait and Assessment of Gait Disorders

Jon R. Davids

Normal Gait
The Gait Cycle
  Ankle
  Knee
  Hip
The Running Cycle
Maturation of Gait

Common Gait Deviations
  Ankle
  Knee
  Hip
Gait Analysis
  Observational Gait Analysis
  Instrumented Gait Analysis

The evolutionary forces that engendered life's emergence from the primordial slime and subsequent domination of the local environment greatly favored organisms with the ability to move from one spot to another. Locomotion evolved from reptilian slithering to advanced quadrupedal and bipedal gait. Quadrupedal locomotion is greatly favored in the animal kingdom because it promotes stability and speed.[21] A quadruped's center of mass is located between the front and hindlimbs, which form a stable base of support. Speed is enhanced by the use of the trunk musculature to augment stride length and power. Ventral flexion of the trunk allows the animal to bring the flexed hindlimbs forward beyond the planted forelimbs. After weight has been transferred to the hindlimbs, the hips, shoulders, and trunk extend in synchrony to advance the forelimbs forward to complete a single cycle.[21]

Bipedal gait sacrifices stability and speed to free the upper extremities for prehensile functions, imparting a tremendous evolutionary advantage. An upright position requires the center of mass to be balanced above the base of support, an inherently less stable and energy-efficient alignment.[27,30,42,53,70] The diminished ability to use the trunk musculature to advance the swing limb limits stride length and power, compromising the speed of ambulation.

The early human fascination with normal gait and its deviations is revealed in the primitive cave paintings that illustrate hunters pursuing their prey. The modern era of motion analysis began with artists and mathematicians who were primarily interested in anatomy, aesthetics, and body segment motion.[27,81,91] Eadward Muybridge, a British photographer working in California, was the first to photograph fast motion.[45] In 1872, his technique, which was the forerunner of modern motion pictures, was initially financed by Leland Stanford, who sought to win a wager by proving that a trotting horse, at some point in its stride, had all four feet off the ground at the same time. Muybridge's work was later supported by the University of Pennsylvania, where he created elegant studies of animal and human locomotion (Fig. 4-1). This extensive body of work has been collected into three volumes and can still be found in the art section of large bookstores.[45]

Etienne-Jules Marey was the first to develop a method of graphic notation derived from recording devices attached to the animal or person being studied.[11,27,45,81] His "experimental shoe," described in 1873, is the direct forerunner of the electrical foot switch developed in the 1950s. In 1894, Braune and Fischer performed the first systematic study of human gait.[11] Their subjects were Prussian soldiers who were

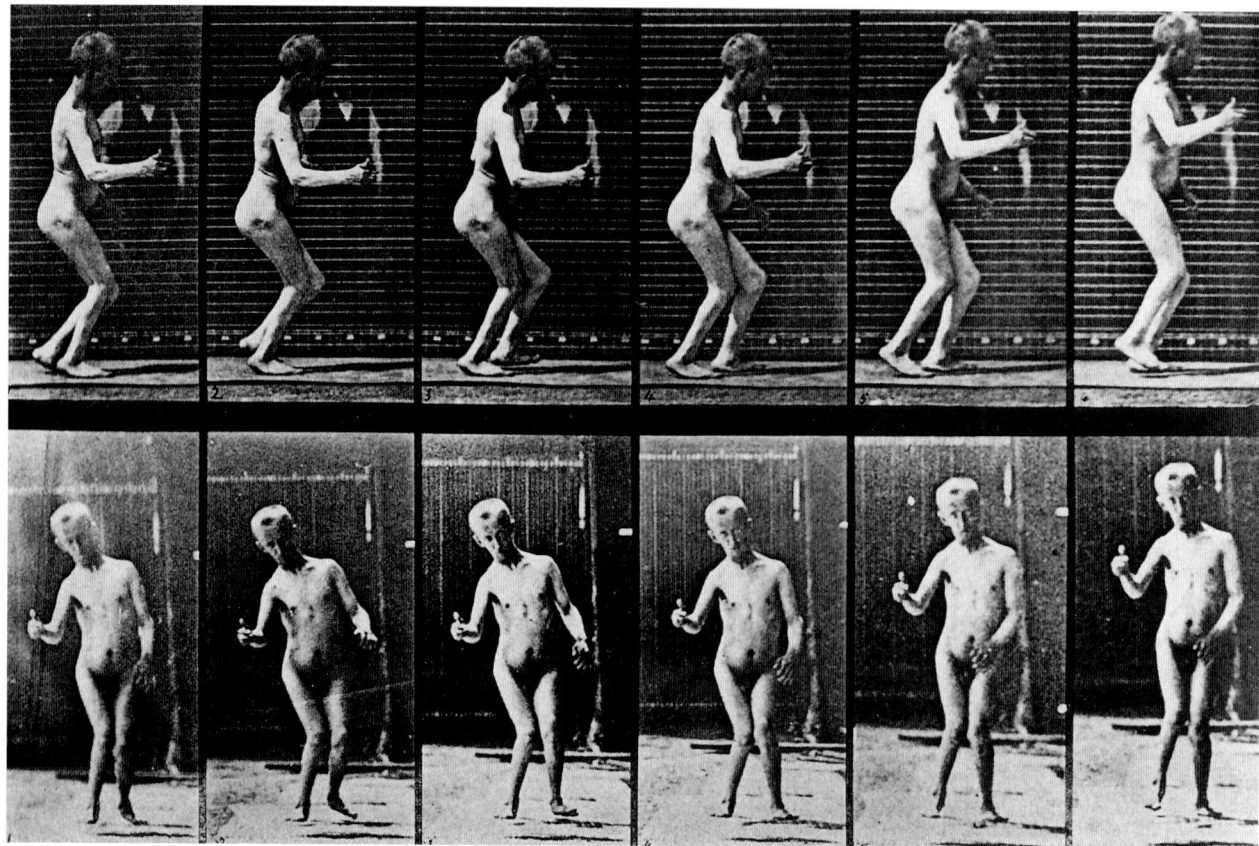

FIGURE 4-1. Muybridge's study of a young man with Little disease, published in 1887. The subject exhibits many of the common gait deviations seen in children with cerebral palsy. (From Muybridge E. Complete human and animal locomotion. New York: Dover Publications, 1980.)

placed into rubberized suits with electrical tubes attached to define the body segments (Fig. 4-2). It took 8 hours to dress each volunteer, primarily because of concerns about potential electrocution. The mathematical analysis of the data was performed by hand and took several months to reduce. Their analysis, however, was as mechanically sophisticated as that performed by computer-driven instrumented motion analysis systems.[11] Shortly after World War II, Dr. Verne T. Inman, an orthopaedist and functional anatomist, and defense industry–based colleagues in engineering and physiology became involved in lower limb prosthetics research.[30,70] This collaboration led to the development of the first modern motion analysis laboratory. Inman's work was advanced and the value of motion analysis was disseminated by two of his students and orthopaedic residents, Jacqueline Perry and David H. Sutherland. There are approximately 65 clinical motion analysis laboratories in North America.

Instrumented motion analysis has had a significant impact on virtually all fields within orthopaedics, primarily by facilitating the quantitative analysis of an individual's functional deficits of movement. Instrumented motion analysis before and after intervention allows assessment of the outcome in an objective manner previously not possible in orthopaedics. Although some investigators may be discouraged by the cost and labor intensity of performing instrumented motion analysis, the central role of outcome studies in the health care reform packages being debated in the United States suggests that the application of this technique will play a crucial part in the redefinition of the clinical practice of orthopaedics in the future.

In pediatric orthopaedics, instrumented motion analysis has advanced treatment concepts in cerebral palsy, myelodysplasia, muscle disease, and limb deficiency. The study of patients with cerebral palsy revealed several principles: the separation of primary gait abnormalities due to the underlying neurologic lesion from secondary or compensatory gait deviations; the value of reducing the energy expenditure associated with pathologic gait by interventions aimed at reestablishing normal mechanical parameters; and recognition of the significance of muscles that cross two joints.[20,21,22] Instrumented motion analysis has identified common gait deviations at the hip, knee, and ankle.[5,16,21,22,25,32,46,54,55,64,77,83,87,92,97,108,113] The efficacy of orthoses, tendon releases, tendon transfers, and dor-

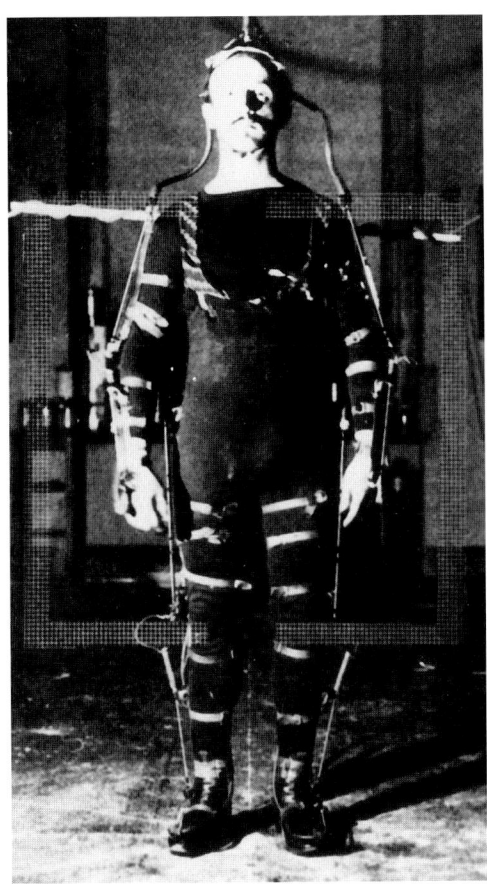

FIGURE 4-2. Rubberized suit with electrical tubes attached to various body segments used by Braune and Fisher to study human gait in 1894. (From Braune W, Fisher D. The human gait. Berlin: Spinger-Verlag, 1987.)

sal rhizotomy have been studied with motion analysis.[10,12,14,19,26,49,50,56,57,72,89,94]

In cases of myclodysplasia, instrumented motion analysis has been used to evaluate the impact of orthotic design on gait and assess the surgical treatment of calcaneus gait by anterior tibial tendon transfer to the os calcis and Achilles tenodesis.[4,29] For children with Duchenne muscular dystrophy, the pathomechanics of the deterioration of their gait have been elucidated, with implications for the timing and nature of surgical intervention.[28,86] Children with congenital and acquired limb deficiencies have been studied to evaluate various reconstructive procedures, such as Van Nes rotationplasty, and assess prosthesis design.[18,37,80]

Adult orthopaedics has also proven to be fertile ground for the application of instrumented motion analysis. The issues of adult joint disease examined include the energy costs of various arthrodeses, prediction of the efficacy of high tibial osteotomy, and functional recovery after knee and hip arthroplasty.[2,9,36,40,68,75,105] In sports medicine, the various adaptations and their significance in gait of anterior cruciate ligament deficiency and the biomechanics of throwing, swimming, running, and cycling have been assessed by motion analysis.[3,8,23,39,65,66,95] Instrumented motion analysis has also been applied to adults with stroke, closed head injury, acquired limb deficiency, and spinal cord injury.[35,58,64,67,98,99,100,102,104]

Using the results of instrumented motion analysis, this chapter defines and describes normal gait, running gait, and the maturation of gait. The most common gait deviations seen in the practice of pediatric orthopaedics are delineated. A technique of observational gait analysis is described, and the technology and technique of instrumented motion analysis are considered, primarily to facilitate a critical review of studies that employ instrumented motion analysis.

NORMAL GAIT

The primary goal of gait is to provide a smooth, energy-efficient transfer of the body through space.[20,27,30,53,63,91,101] Normal gait is an extremely complex process that is built on the manipulation of selective synergistic motor patterns (i.e., "hard wired" spinal cord reflexes) and incorporation of learned sequential motor patterns.[21,24,31] The remarkable similarity of gait between individuals is thought to be a consequence of the underlying demand for energy-efficient locomotion.[30,70] Mechanically, this phenomenon is observed by considering the excursion of the body's center of gravity, located anterior to the second sacral vertebra, during gait. Although the body grossly appears to be walking a straight path, the center of gravity actually follows a sinusoidal course in the coronal and sagittal planes (Fig. 4-3). The maximum vertical displacement of the body's center of gravity occurs at the point of minimal horizontal displacement, which is a relatively energy-efficient pattern.[21,30] In the sagittal plane, the body's center of gravity is at its highest point (i.e., minimum velocity, maximum potential energy) in midstance and at its lowest point (i.e., maximum velocity, maximum kinetic energy) in terminal stance, when the two limbs are farthest apart.[109,112] The transformation of potential to kinetic energy and the use of the kinetic energy to accelerate the body and create potential energy is a cyclic process occurring throughout gait. This form of energy transfer is effective but costly, with only 30% to 50% of the potential energy recovered as kinetic energy.[21,63] Gait is therefore most efficient when the magnitude of the energy transferred is minimized. This is accomplished by minimizing the excursion of the center of gravity, one of three significant mechanisms of energy conservation, and is best appreciated by applying basic mechanical principles to the analysis of normal gait.

Dynamic mechanical modeling of gait considers the motions that occur at joints and body segments

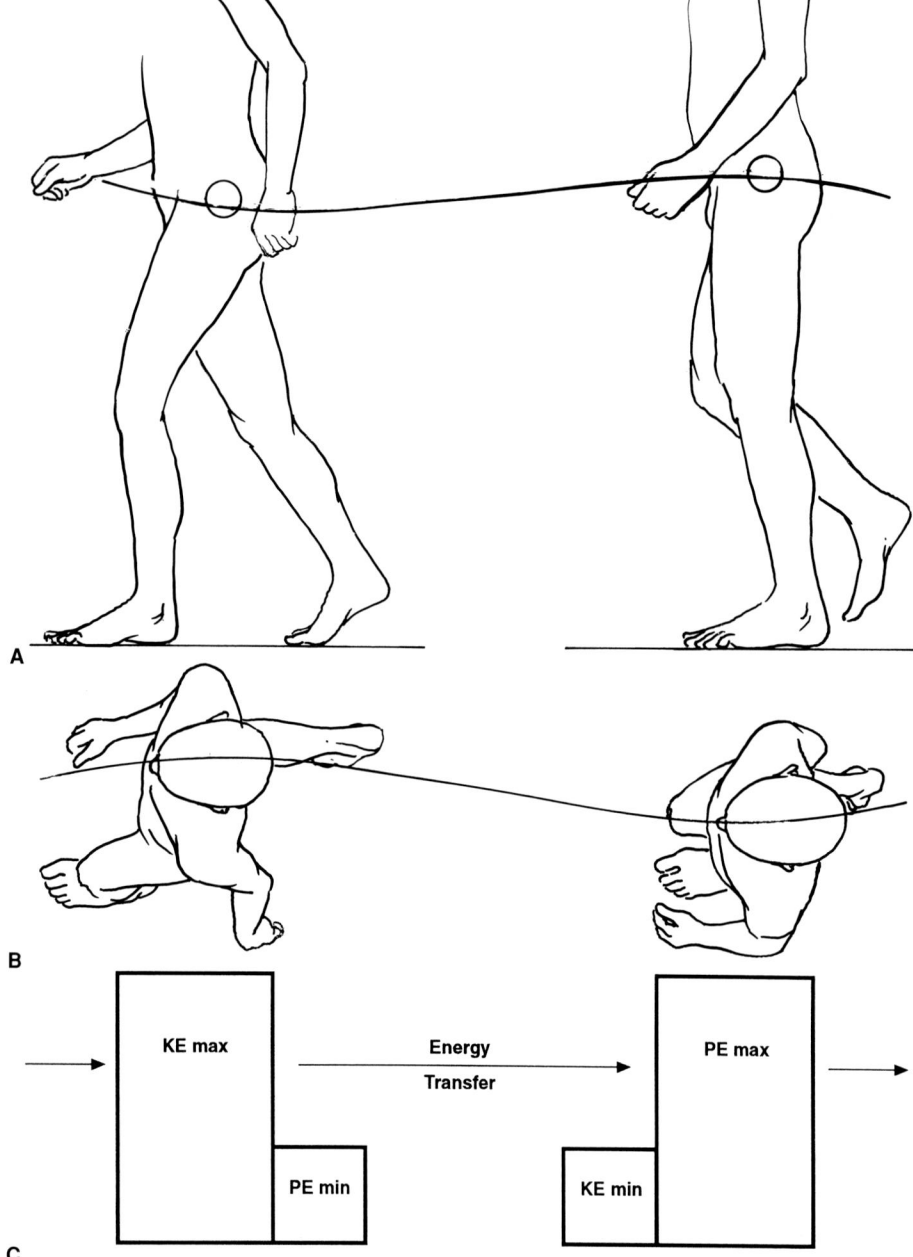

FIGURE 4-3. The excursion of the body's center of gravity follows a sinusoidal path in the (**A**) sagittal and (**B**) coronal planes. Notice that the maximal excursion in one plane occurs in synchrony with minimal excursion in the other plane. (**C**) Kinetic energy is maximal in double support periods (left-side figures), and potential energy is maximal in single-limb support periods (right). (Adapted from Gage JR. Gait analysis in cerebral palsy. In: Clinics in developmental medicine. Oxford: MacKeith Press, 1991; and Inman VT, Ralston H, Todd F. Human walking. Baltimore: Williams & Wilkins, 1981.)

(i.e., kinematics) and the forces that produce the motion (i.e., kinetics). Kinematic data describe gait and its deviations, including sagittal, coronal, and axial joint angles, velocities, and accelerations.[48,111] Kinetic data address the causes of motion and movement abnormalities, including the ground reaction forces, joint moments, and joint powers.[48,111] A joint moment is the product of the force generated by a muscle and the distance of the muscle from the joint's estimated center of rotation.[20,47,90,112] The ground reaction forces produce an external moment about the joints, and the moments generated by the muscles that cross the joint are called internal moments. Joint power is the product of a joint moment and the joint's angular velocity.[20,47,90,112] Power generation occurs when a muscle contracts concentrically (i.e., shortens) to produce a joint motion in the same direction that the muscle pulls.[48] Power absorption occurs when the joint motion is opposite to the direction of the muscle pull and the muscle exhibits an eccentric (i.e., lengthening) contraction.[48]

This mechanical model recognizes three major mechanisms by which the body conserves energy during gait.[21,22] The first mechanism involves minimizing the excursion of the center of gravity.[27,30,53,63,70,87] This is accomplished by synchronized pelvic, hip, knee, and ankle motions. The efficacy of this mechanism is illustrated by the analysis of above-knee amputee gait, in which the energy cost is approximately double that for nonamputee gait.[99,103] The second mechanism uses external moments (instead of internal moments) to stabilize joints during the gait cycle.[20–22,48,74,76,82,85,91,109,112] Because of proper positioning of the ankle in midstance, which is controlled by eccentric contraction of the soleus, the ground reaction force vector falls in front of the knee, generating an extension moment in which stability at the knee is provided by ligaments instead of muscle action. Incompetence of the ankle plantar flexors after overlengthening of the heel cord in children with cerebral palsy leads to poor control of ankle position in midstance, posterior displacement of the ground reaction force vector at the knee, and creation of an external flexion moment. With time, this overwhelms the internal knee extension moment generated by the quadriceps, resulting in a progressive crouch gait, which is extremely energy inefficient.[83,87] A similar coupling occurs at the hip, where the ground reaction force vector falls behind the joint center to generate an extension moment, which is stabilized by the anterior hip ligaments.[63] The final mechanism involves the efficient transfer of energy between body segments.[21,22] Early work suggests that two-joint muscles—such as the rectus femoris, which can generate power when serving as a hip flexor while simultaneously absorbing power in its role as a knee extensor during rapid walking—serve a central role in the efficient transfer of energy between nonadjacent segments.[110–112] The physiologic confirmation of this mechanical model is under investigation.[38]

THE GAIT CYCLE

A single gait cycle, also called stride, functionally defines the events occurring between two sequential floor contacts by the same limb. The gait cycle is logically divided into two phases, stance and swing, respectively defined by the presence or absence of floor contact for the limb being considered. Normal walking allows each limb to accomplish three tasks during each gait cycle: weight acceptance, single-limb support, and limb advancement (Fig. 4-4).[63] Pathologic deviations of gait compromise the achievement of these tasks and increase the energy cost of ambulation. The events of gait are temporally described as occurring at specific percentages of the gait cycle. Stance phase constitutes the first 60% of the gait cycle and contains two periods of "double support," when both limbs are in contact with the floor. The first period occurs immediately after the initiation of stance phase and the second just before the end of stance. Clinically, stance phase is further divided into five subphases, each of which has a functional objective: initial con-

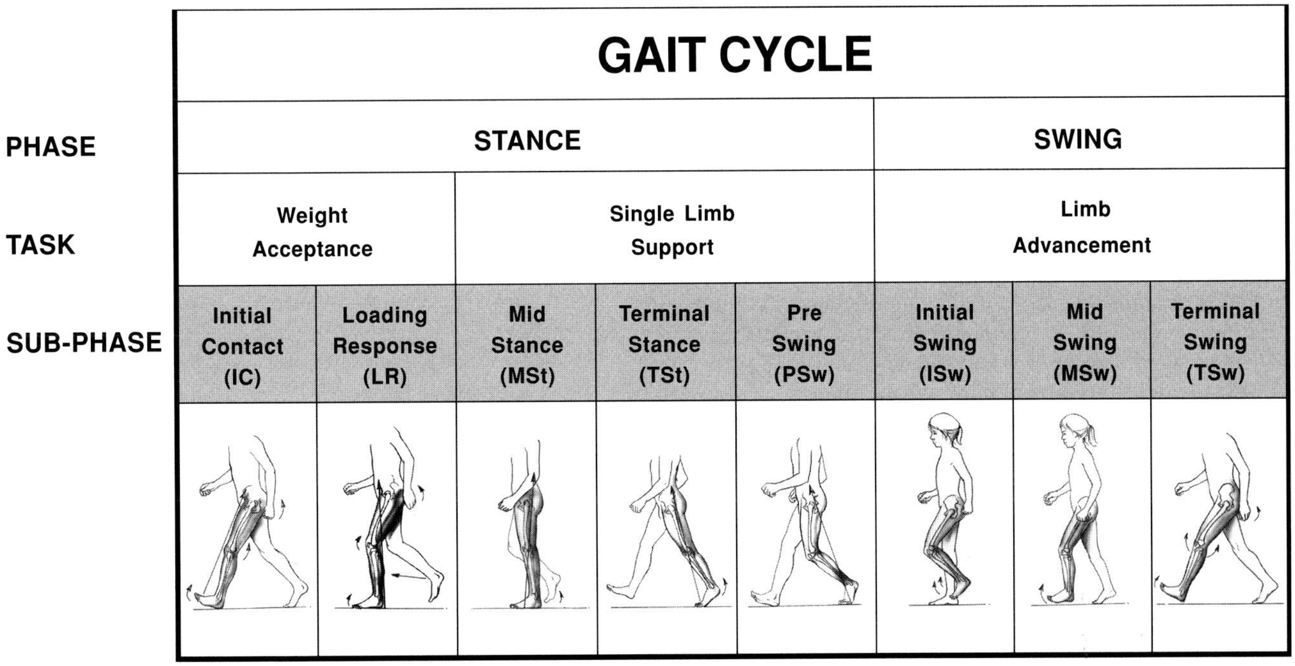

FIGURE 4-4. The division of the gait cycle into phases, tasks, and subphases facilitates the analysis of normal and pathologic gaits.

TABLE 4-1 Stance Phase of the Gait Cycle

Initial Contact (see Fig. 4-5)
 Interval: 0% of the gait cycle
 Task: weight acceptance
 Critical events: the ankle is positioned so the heel strikes first as the foot comes in contact with the floor
 Kinematics
  Ankle: 0 degrees
  Knee: 0 degrees
  Hip: 25 degrees flexion
 Kinetics
  Ankle: external plantar flexion moment, which is balanced by internal dorsiflexion moment by tibialis anterior
  Knee: external extension moment; hamstring activity decelerates the advancing limb
  Hip: external flexion moment, controlled by hamstring extension moment, which also contributes to deceleration

Loading Response (see Fig. 4-6)
 Interval: 0%–10% of the gait cycle
 Task: weight acceptance; shock is adsorbed, primarily by the quadriceps, as forward moment is preserved
 Critical events: controlled ankle plantar flexion and knee flexion; hip stability
 Kinematics
  Ankle: 10 degrees plantar flexion
  Knee: 15 degrees flexion
  Hip: 25 degrees flexion
 Kinetics
  Ankle: external plantar flexion moment; internal dorsiflexion moment by tibialis anterior decelerates and stabilizes the foot and advances the tibia anterior to the ground reaction force vector
  Knee: external flexion moment; internal extension moment by quadriceps stabilizes the knee in flexion and absorbs the shock of floor contact
  Hip: diminishing external flexion moment as the body advances; activity of the hip extensors and abductors stabilize the hip and pelvis

Midstance (see Fig. 4-7)
 Interval: 10%–30% of the gait cycle
 Task: single-limb support; the body progresses over the foot in a controlled manner; forward momentum is generated by the contralateral swing limb
 Critical events: controlled tibial advancement
 Kinematics
  Ankle: 5 degrees dorsiflexion
  Knee: 0 degrees
  Hip: 0 degrees
 Kinetics
  Ankle: external dorsiflexion moment; internal plantar flexion moment by the soleus decelerates ankle dorsiflexion, stabilizes the tibia, and controls the position of the ground reaction force vector at the knee and hip
  Knee: external moment changes from flexion to extension as the ground reaction force vector moves anteriorly; internal muscle moments are no longer necessary for joint stability after the vector passes in front of the knee
  Hip: external moment changes from flexion to extension as the ground reaction force vector moves posteriorly; internal extension moment generated by the gluteus maximus is no longer required; the pelvis is stabilized in the coronal plane by action of the gluteus medius (i.e., internal abduction moment).

Terminal Stance (see Fig. 4-8)
 Interval: 30%–50% of the gait cycle
 Task: single-limb support; the body passes in front of the foot, and forward progression is accelerated by kinetic energy generated primarily by the ankle plantar flexors
 Critical events: heel rise
 Kinematics
  Ankle: 10 degrees dorsiflexion
  Knee: 0 degrees
  Hip: 20 degrees extension
 Kinetics
  Ankle: maximum external dorsiflexion moment is opposed by internal plantar flexion moment from the gastrocnemius, leading to heel rise as the body advances forward; this muscle is the principal source of power, accelerating the limb as it enters the swing phase
  Knee: external extension moment is diminishing, but no internal muscle moments are required to maintain stability
  Hip: maximal external extension moment is attained as the body advances

Preswing (see Fig. 4-9)
 Interval: 50%–60% of the gait cycle.
 Task: swing limb advancement; the principal objective is preparation and positioning of the limb for swing.
 Critical events: passive knee flexion
 Kinematics
  Ankle: 20 degrees plantar flexion
  Knee: 40 degrees flexion
  Hip: 0 degrees
 Kinetics
  Ankle: passive plantar flexion as the limb is unloaded
  Knee: passive flexion as the limb is unloaded; the rectus femoris, a biarticular muscle, may assist in energy transfer between the knee and hip in this subphase
  Hip: passive flexion as the limb is unloaded

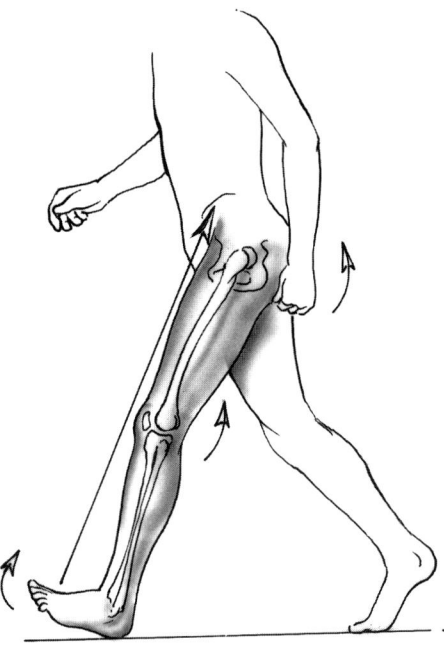

FIGURE 4-5. Initial contact. The long arrow represents the ground reaction force vector. Its position relative to each joint determines the external moment. The smaller arrows represent the net internal moments that are generated by the muscles crossing each joint.

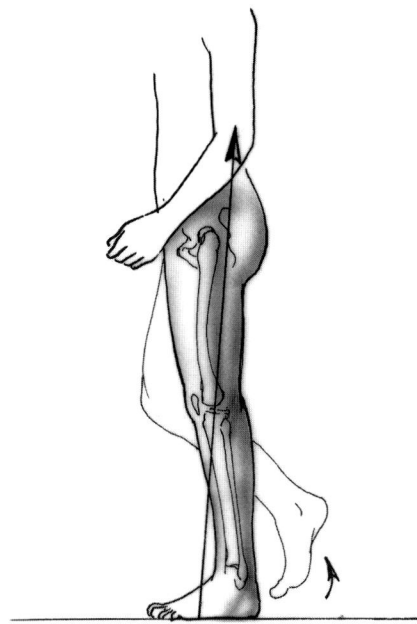

FIGURE 4-7. Midstance. After the ground reaction force vector (long arrow) falls in front of the knee, generating an external extension moment, and behind the hip, generating an external extension moment, internal muscle-generated moments are no longer necessary for joint stability. This is one of the energy-efficient mechanisms often lost in pathologic gait deviations. Tibial advancement over the foot constitutes the second or ankle rocker and is controlled by an internal ankle plantar flexion moment (*small arrow*).

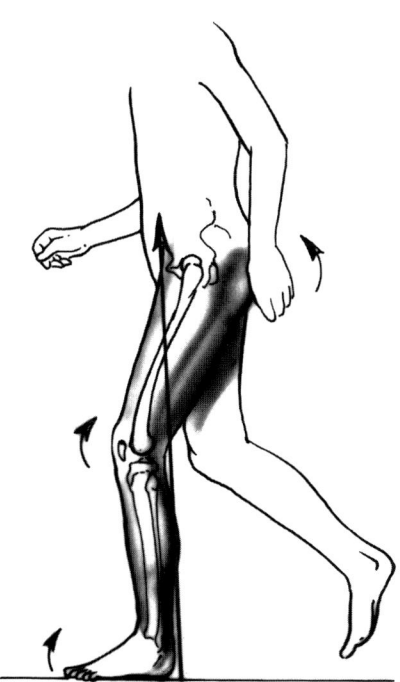

FIGURE 4-6. Loading response. Shock absorption by the quadriceps and controlled ankle plantar flexion are the central events. The ankle plantar flexion sets up the first or heel rocker. (*Long arrow*, ground reaction force vector; *curved arrows*, net interval moments generated by muscles crossing each joint.)

tact, loading response, midstance, terminal stance, and preswing (Figs. 4-5 through 4-9; Table 4-1).

The swing phase constitutes the remaining 40% of the gait cycle and begins at the point where the limb is unloaded and the foot comes off the ground. The limb is advanced from behind the body to in front of the body, reaching out to take the next step. Foot clearance and correct positioning for the initiation of the subsequent stance phase are critical components of swing-limb advancement.[63] The velocity of gait can be altered by changing the stride length (i.e., distance covered by a single gait cycle) or changing the cadence (i.e., number of gait cycles per unit time).[43,47,110] Changes in cadence are primarily accomplished by altering the duration of swing phase.[21] A period of variable acceleration (i.e., initial swing), a transitional period (i.e., midswing), and a final period of deceleration and limb positioning (i.e., terminal swing) are the recognized subphases of swing. Kinetic analysis of the joints in swing phase is much simpler because there is no external moment generated by the ground reaction force vector. External moments may be generated by gravitational and inertial forces and are usually dominated by the internal muscle-generated moments (Figs. 4-10 through 4-12; Table 4-2).[48]

In addition to analysis by phase, task, and sub-

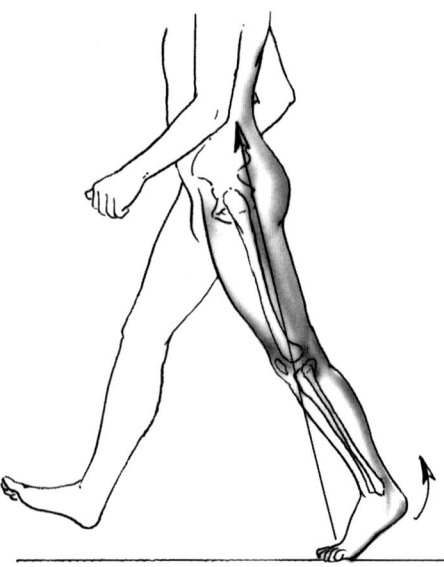

FIGURE 4-8. Terminal stance. Heel rise occurs as the body advances and the ankle plantar flexors resist the large external dorsiflexor moment. (This constitutes the third or forefoot rocker). (*Long arrow*, ground reaction force vector; *curved arrow*, internal plantar flexion moment.)

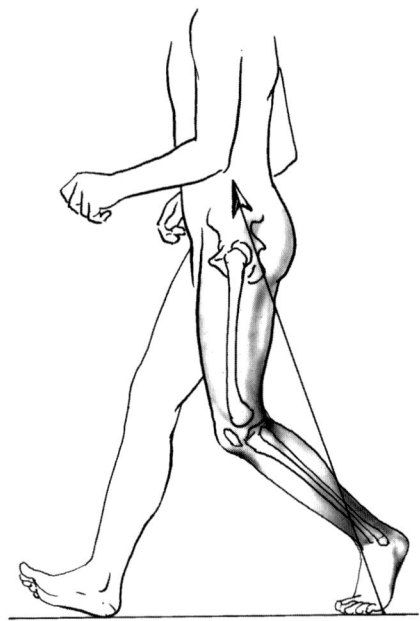

FIGURE 4-9. Preswing. "Passive" ankle plantar flexion, knee flexion, and hip flexion (i.e., no internal muscle moments) occur as the limb is unloaded. (*Long arrow*, ground reaction force vector.)

TABLE 4-2 *Swing Phase of the Gait Cycle*

Initial Swing (see Fig. 4-10)

Interval: 60%–75% of the gait cycle
Task: swing limb advancement; variable acceleration is possible
Critical events: foot clearance
Kinematics
    Ankle: 10 degrees plantar flexion
    Knee: 60 degrees flexion
    Hip: 15 degrees flexion
Kinetics
    Ankle: the pretibial musculature generates a dorsiflexion moment; diminished plantar flexion alignment contributes to foot clearance
    Knee: at a normal cadence, increased knee flexion is determined by external flexion moments generated by inertial and gravitational forces; at a slower cadence, an internal flexion moment generated by the lateral hamstrings may be present[63,100]; at a faster cadence, the rectus femoris contributes to limb acceleration by generating an extension moment at the knee[21,110]
    Hip: the flexors and adductors generate an internal flexion moment, which contributes to limb advancement and acceleration

Midswing (see Fig. 4-11)

Interval: 75%–90% of the gait cycle
Task: swing limb advancement
Critical events: vertical alignment of the tibia; foot clearance
Kinematics
    Ankle: 0 degrees
    Knee: 25 degrees flexion
    Hip: 25 degrees flexion
Kinetics
    Ankle: internal dorsiflexion moment from the tibialis anterior supports the ankle and prevents footdrop
    Knee: external moment from inertial forces begin to extend the knee
    Hip: external moment from inertial forces cause further hip flexion

Terminal Swing (see Fig. 4-12)

Interval: 90%–100% of the gait cycle
Task: swing limb advancement, achievement of maximal step length, position the foot for initial contact, and deceleration of swing limb
Critical events: knee extension to neutral
Kinematics
    Ankle: 0 degrees
    Knee: 0 degrees
    Hip: 25 degrees flexion
Kinetics
    Ankle: internal dorsiflexion moment maintains the foot in the proper position for initial contact
    Knee: internal extension moment by the quadriceps extends the knee for stance; internal flexion moment by the hamstrings decelerates and stabilizes the advancing swing limb
    Hip: internal extension moment by the hamstrings contributes to deceleration

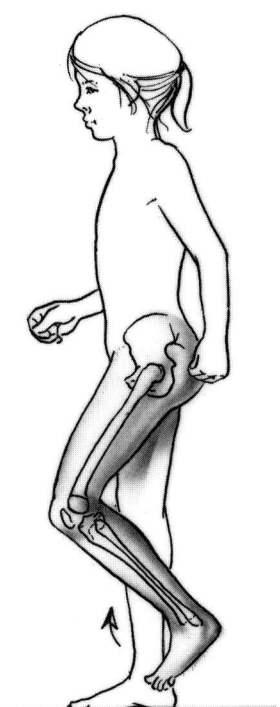

FIGURE 4-10. Initial swing. Hip flexion, knee flexion, and ankle dorsiflexion contribute to limb clearance. (*Curved arrow*, internal ankle dorsiflexion moment.)

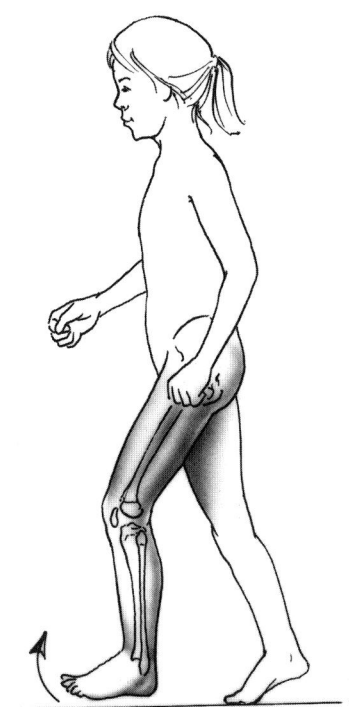

FIGURE 4-11. Midswing. Gravitational and inertial external moments dominate at the hip and knee. The ankle position for clearance is determined by an internal dorsiflexion moment (*curved arrow*).

phase, the functional assessment of gait is facilitated by considering the kinematics and kinetics of anatomic areas, such as joints and body segments, throughout the gait cycle.

Ankle

Stance Phase

Ankle function during stance phase is best considered in terms of three rockers (Fig. 4-13).[34,60] The first or heel rocker begins at initial contact and extends through the loading response. Correct ankle position at initial contact ensures that the heel strikes the floor first, creating an external plantar flexion moment. The 10 degrees of plantar flexion seen in the loading response is resisted by the internal moment generated by the ankle dorsiflexor muscles. This deceleration of ankle plantar flexion contributes to tibial advancement and shock absorption. The second or ankle rocker occurs during midstance, and the external moment favors dorsiflexion. The 5 degrees of dorsiflexion is resisted by the internal moment generated by the ankle plantar flexor muscles. This deceleration of ankle dorsiflexion controls tibial advancement and contributes to stance stability by ensuring that the ground reaction force vector is anterior to the knee and posterior to the hip, creating an external extension moment at each joint. This promotes joint stability through ligaments and without muscle action, which

is energy efficient. The third or forefoot rocker occurs during terminal stance as the body advances over the stance limb. The greatest external moment of the gait cycle, favoring ankle dorsiflexion, occurs at this

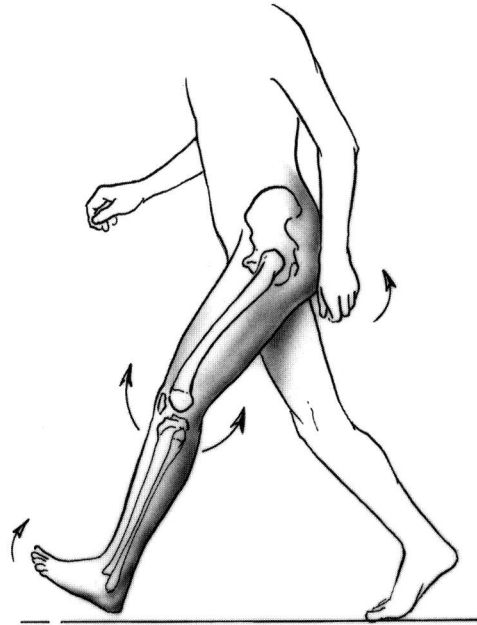

FIGURE 4-12. Terminal swing. Internal muscle moments at the hip, knee (i.e., simultaneous flexion and extension moments), and ankle decelerate the limb and position it correctly for the initiation of the subsequent stance phase. (*Curved arrows*, internal moments generated by the muscles crossing each joint.)

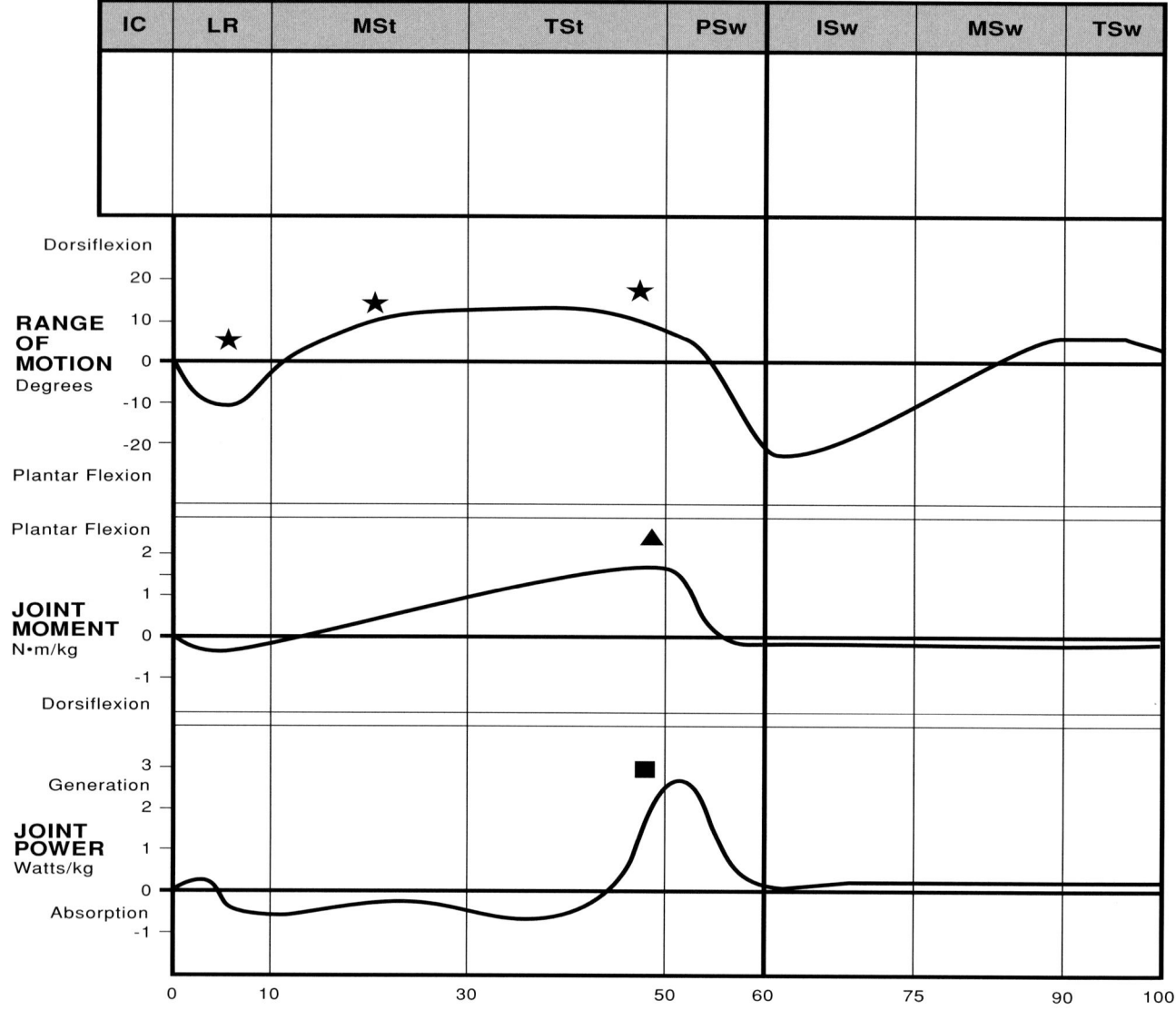

FIGURE 4-13. Normal motion, moments, and powers of the ankle. Motion is in the sagittal plane. Notice the three rockers (★) that occur during stance phase. The joint moment curve describes the net internal muscle moment, generated in response to the external moments from the ground reaction force, gravity, and inertia. The internal plantar flexion moment generated at the end of the terminal stance (TSt) subphase (▲) is the greatest muscle moment occurring at any joint at any time in the gait cycle. The TSt power generation (■) reflects the crucial role of the ankle plantar flexors in accelerating the limb as it enters the swing phase (i.e., energy transfer). (IC, initial contact; LR, loading response; MSt, midstance; PSw, Preswing; ISw, initial swing; MSw, midswing; TSw, terminal swing; adapted from Ounpuu MS, Gage JR, Davis RB. Three-dimensional lower extremity joint kinetics in normal pediatric gait. J Pediatr Orthop 1991;11:341; Pathokinesiology Department, Physical Therapy Department. Observational gait analysis handbook. Downey: The Professional Staff Association of Rancho Los Amigos Medical Center, 1989; Perry J. Gait analysis: normal and pathologic function. Thorofare: Slack, 1992; and Sutherland DH, Valencia FG. Pediatric gait. In: Drennan JC, ed. The child's foot and ankle. New York: Raven Press, 1992:19.)

point.[48,52,63,74,85] The ankle plantar flexors meet the challenge, generating the greatest internal muscle moment occurring at any joint at any time in the gait cycle. The net joint moment favors ankle plantar flexion and accelerates the advancing limb. Minimal ankle movement at this point (during the forefoot rocker) causes the heel to rise, maintaining momentum and efficiently transferring energy between body segments.[20,63,85]

Before instrumented analysis and mechanical

modeling, heel rise was erroneously perceived as active ankle plantar flexion and referred to as "push off," which implies propulsion and is misleading. Although the ankle plantar flexors are active, they are resisting the external dorsiflexion moment, effectively stabilizing the ankle joint and promoting controlled tibial advancement over the forefoot. A child with a calcaneal gait pattern (e.g., L5-level myelodysplasia) loses heel rise, has uncontrolled tibial advancement over the foot, has instability, and has poor energy transfer proximally during terminal stance. Twenty degrees of ankle plantar flexion does occur during preswing as the body weight is transferred to the other limb. This plantar flexion takes place during a period of unloading in response to external moments generated by inertia and gravity forces, not as a result of active internal muscle moments.

Swing Phase

Active ankle dorsiflexion begins during the initial swing to assist in early swing-limb clearance. The internal dorsiflexion moment in midswing resists inertia and gravity forces to promote clearance. In terminal swing, the internal muscle moments position the ankle for initial contact so the heel strikes the floor first, generating the first or heel rocker.

Knee

Stance Phase

The knee exhibits a single flexion wave during stance phase (Fig. 4-14). Full extension at initial contact provides stability for weight acceptance and contributes to optimal foot position. Flexion at the knee in the loading response is the principal means of shock absorption and is a consequence of the external flexion moment generated by the ground reaction force.[15] The alignment of this vector behind the knee is controlled by the heel rocker. Although knee flexion promotes shock absorption, it must not compromise knee stability. Competent quadriceps function to generate an internal knee extension moment to prevent excessive knee flexion and instability.[55] The knee extends in midstance to promote stability and advancement. The ankle rocker correctly aligns the ground reaction force vector such that an external knee extension moment is generated, promoting energy-efficient knee stability. Maximum knee extension is attained in terminal stance, maintaining stability during forward progression. As the stance limb is unloaded in preswing, the knee flexes, driven primarily by the external flexion moment from the ground reaction force vector, which falls behind the knee as the body advances forward.[20] Approximately two thirds of the knee flexion necessary for swing-limb clearance occurs in the preswing subphase.

Swing Phase

A second flexion wave of greater magnitude occurs during swing phase. The principal function of this flexion wave is limb clearance.[63] Further knee flexion occurs during initial swing, which is crucial for foot clearance because the ankle is in equinus at this point.[44] Variable acceleration of the swing limb during initial and midswing subphases, generated by internal muscle flexion moments, is a central mechanism for decreasing the duration of swing phase.[21] A shorter swing phase allows more strides per unit of time (i.e., greater cadence), which increases the velocity of gait. After the tibia has attained a vertical alignment, clearance has been achieved, and the primary function at the knee becomes limb advancement and stride length.[63] The knee therefore extends, primarily because of an external moment derived from the forces of inertia and gravity. Optimal stride length is achieved by further knee extension in terminal stance. Internal (i.e., muscle) and external (i.e., gravitational and inertial) moments contribute to knee extension and limb positioning for the initial contact subphase. An internal flexion moment by the hamstrings decelerates the advancing limb before beginning the stance phase.

Hip

Stance Phase

The hip exhibits a single extension wave during stance phase (Fig. 4-15). At initial contact, the hip is flexed to promote limb position. During the loading response subphase, the ground reaction force vector falls in front of the hip joint, generating the second highest external moment of the entire gait cycle.[48,63] The internal muscle extension moment generated by the hamstrings stabilizes the hip. In the coronal plane, the weight of the contralateral swing limb causes the ground reaction force vector to fall medial to the stance-limb hip, creating an adduction moment that is resisted by the internal muscle moment of the gluteus medius.[41,51] In the transverse plane, the pelvis is rotated forward over the stance limb. In midstance, the hip is extending as the body advances. After the ground reaction force vector falls at or behind the hip joint, an external extension moment is generated, and hip stability is provided by the anterior ligaments, an energy-efficient mechanism. In the coronal plane, the hip adduction moment persists. In the transverse plane, the pelvis rotates back to neutral, and by terminal stance, it is rotated backward over the trailing stance limb. Pelvic rotation contributes to apparent hip hyperextension at the end of the stance phase. As the limb is unloaded in the preswing subphase, the hip begins to flex, primarily because of inertial and gravitational external moments. In the coronal plane,

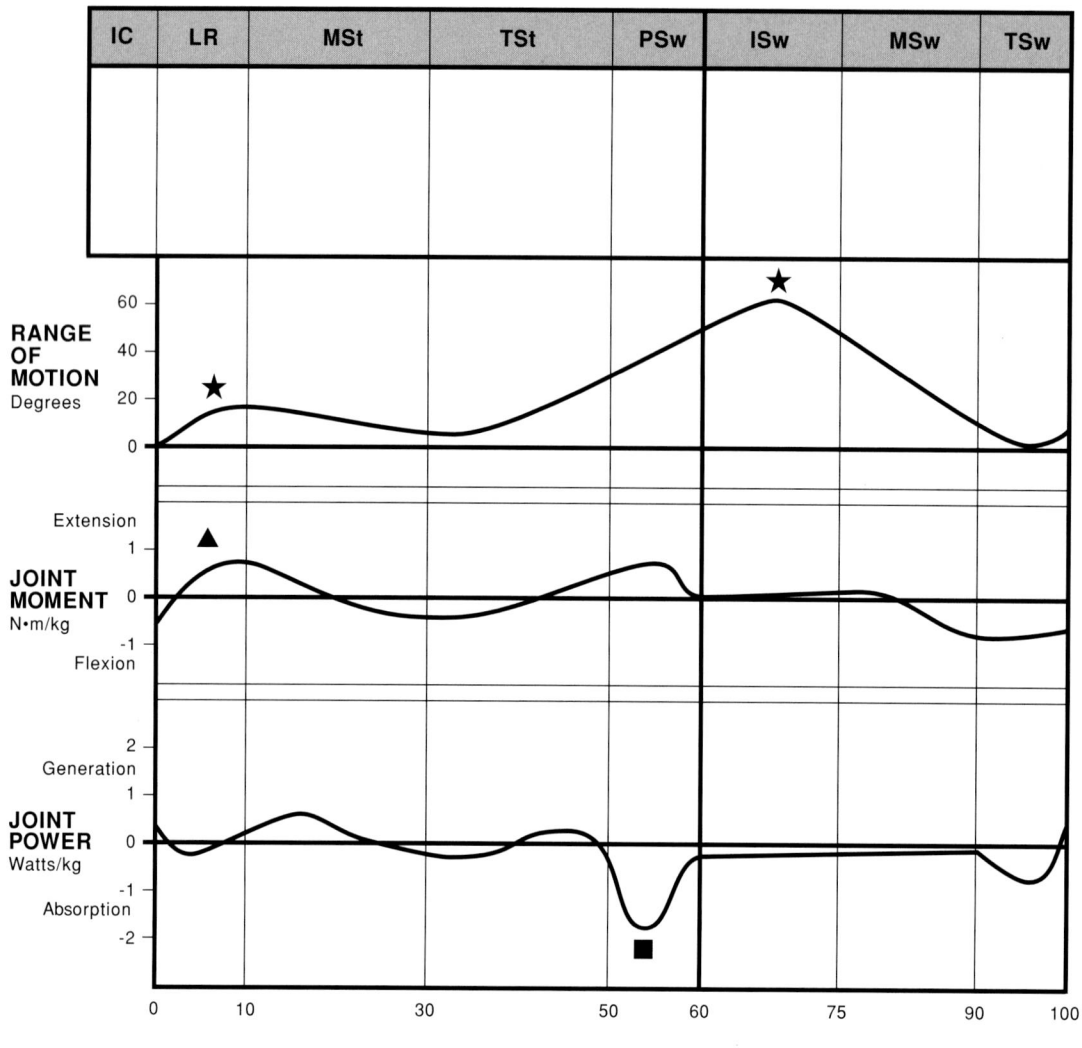

FIGURE 4-14. Normal motion, moments, and powers of the knee. Sagittal plane motion of the knee is characterized by two flexion waves (★). Stance-phase knee flexion (during loading response [LR] subphase) reflects shock absorption, and the swing-phase flexion wave promotes limb clearance. The quadriceps are the primary shock absorbers at the knee, generating the internal muscle extension moment seen during the LR subphase (▲). Power absorption occurs during LR and terminal stance (■). The relatively low level of power generation and absorption reflects the transfer of energy across the knee (between body segments above and below) by two joint muscles, such as the rectus femoris, biceps femoris, and gastrocnemius. (IC, initial contact; MSt, midstance; Tst, terminal stance; PSw, Preswing; ISw, initial swing; MSw, midswing; TSw, terminal swing; adapted from Ounpuu MS, Gage JR, Davis RB. Three-dimensional lower extremity joint kinetics in normal pediatric gait. J. Pediatr Orthop 1991;11:341; Pathokinesiology Department, Physical Therapy Department. Observational gait analysis handbook. Downey: The Professional Staff Association of Rancho Los Amigos Medical Center, 1989; Perry J. Gait analysis: normal and pathologic function. Thorofare: Slack, 1992; and Sutherland DH, Valencia FG. Pediatric gait. In: Drennan JC, ed. The child's foot and ankle. New York: Raven Press, 1992:19.)

the adduction moment diminishes as the contralateral limb begins weight acceptance.

Swing Phase

The hip exhibits a single flexion wave in swing phase. During the initial swing subphase, internal muscle flexion moments may contribute to hip flexion. The remaining flexion in swing phase is a consequence of inertial and gravitational external moments.[48,112] The hip flexion contributes to limb clearance early in swing and limb positioning for weight acceptance after the terminal swing subphase. In the transverse plane, the pelvis rotates forward with the swing limb to promote stride length and to position the swing limb correctly for weight acceptance.

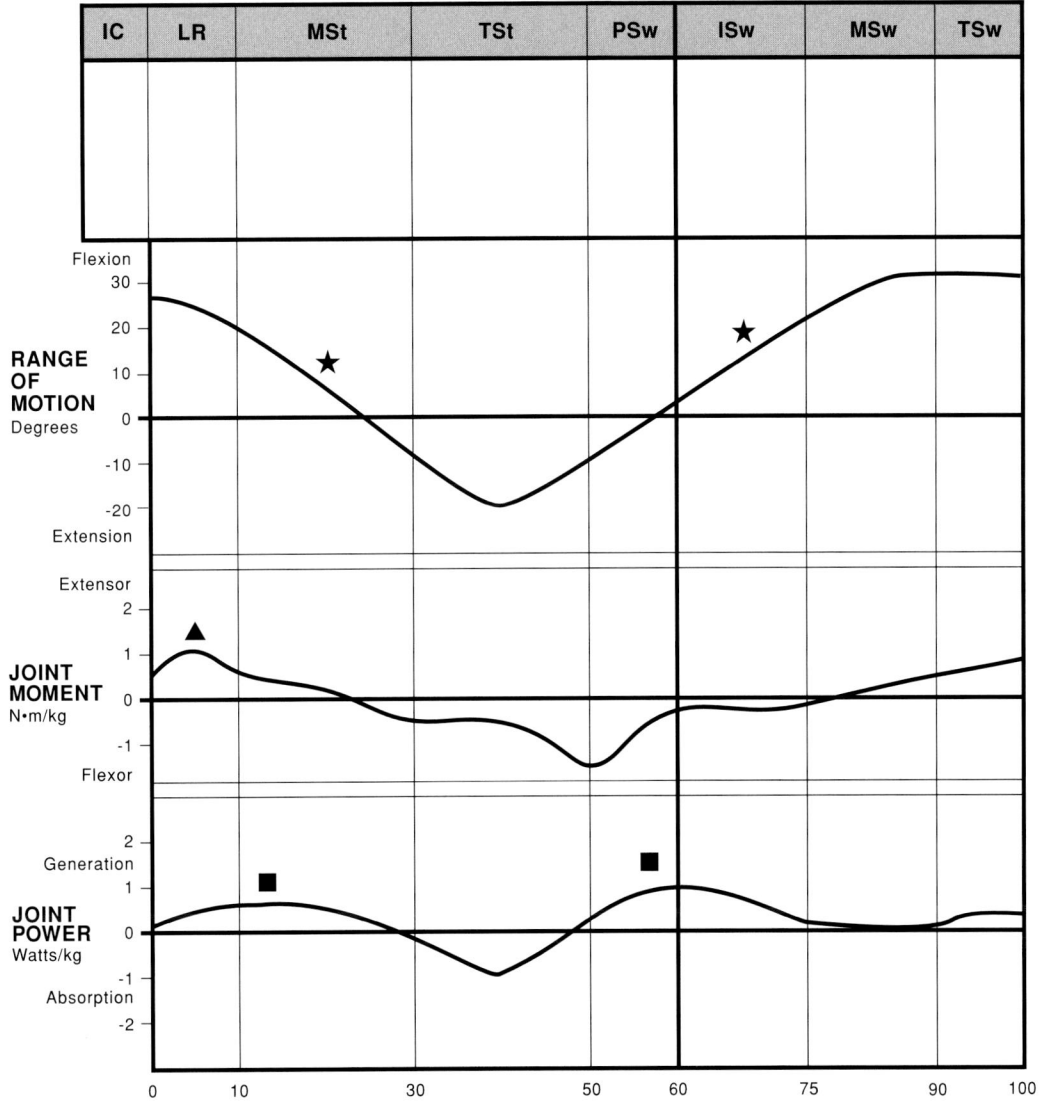

FIGURE 4-15. Normal motion, moments, and powers of the hip. Sagittal plane motion of the hip is characterized by an extension wave in stance phase and a flexion wave in swing phase (★). The extensor moment generated by the hamstrings in the loading response subphase (▲) is the second greatest internal muscle moment in the gait cycle. The two periods of power generation (■) serve to accelerate the limb in the stance and swing phases. (IC, initial contact; LR, loading response; MSt, midstance; Tst, terminal stance; PSw, Preswing; ISw, initial swing; MSw, midswing; TSw, terminal swing; adapted from Ounpuu MS, Gage JR, Davis RB. Three-dimensional lower extremity joint kinetics in normal pediatric gait. J. Pediatr Orthop 1991;11:341; Pathokinesiology Department, Physical Therapy Department. Observational gait analysis handbook. Downey: The Professional Staff Association of Rancho Los Amigos Medical Center, 1989; Perry J. Gait analysis: normal and pathologic function. Thorofare: Slack, 1992; and Sutherland DH, Valencia FG. Pediatric gait. In: Drennan JC, ed. The child's foot and ankle. New York: Raven Press, 1992:19.)

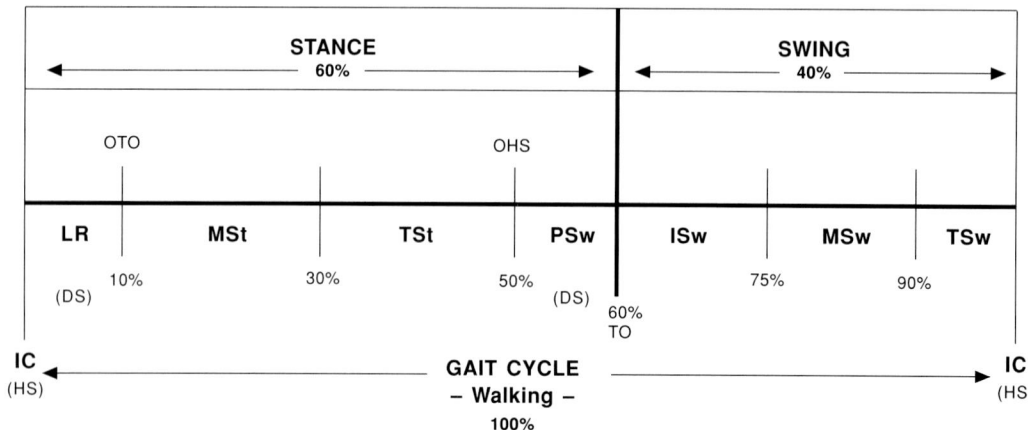

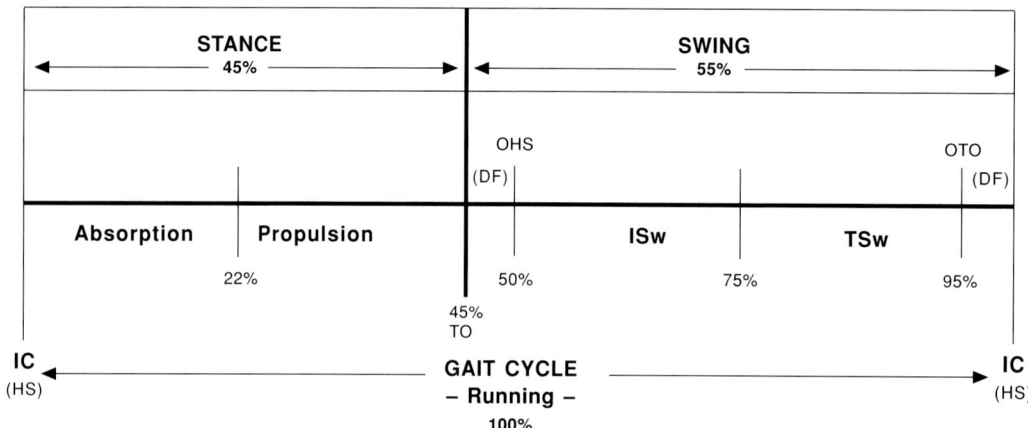

FIGURE 4-16. Comparison of the walking and running gait cycles. In walking, the stance phase constitutes more of the gait cycle than the swing phase. In running, this relation is reversed. In walking, heel strike (HS) and opposite heel strike (OHS) occur before opposite toe-off (OTO) and toe-off (TO), respectively, creating two periods of double support (DS), when both feet are touching the ground. In running, HS and OHS occur after OTO and TO, respectively; both periods of DS are lost, and two additional periods of double float (DF) are created. (IC, initial contact; LR, loading response; MSt, midstance; Tst, terminal stance; PSw, Preswing; ISw, initial swing; MSw, midswing; TSw, terminal swing; adapted from Gage JR. Gait analysis in cerebral palsy. In: Clinics in developmental medicine. Oxford: MacKeith Press, 1991; Mann RA, Hagy J. Biomechanics of walking, running, and sprinting. Am J Sports Med 1980; 8:345; and Ounpuu S. The biomechanics of running: a kinematic and kinetic analysis. Instr Course Lect 1990:305.)

THE RUNNING CYCLE

As the velocity of gait increases, bipedal ambulators progress from walking to running to sprinting. The transitional velocity at which an individual switches from one form of ambulation to the other is not constant; it is a function of leg length.[47] For this reason, children begin to run at lower velocities than adults. Walking is differentiated from running and sprinting by the pattern of ground contact.[43,47,71] In walking, there is always ground contact with one or both feet, but running and sprinting are characterized by "double float" periods when neither foot is on the ground (Fig. 4-16).

In terms of the gait cycle, walking can be differentiated from running by the duration of the stance phase. In walking, the two periods of double support (i.e., both feet in contact with the floor) ensure that the duration of the stance phase is greater than 50% of the gait cycle.[21,43,47] In running, both periods of double support are lost. The toe-off motion occurs before the opposite heel strike, creating two periods of double float (i.e., neither foot in contact with the floor), which constitute portions of the swing phase. In running, the duration of the stance phase constitutes less than 50% of the gait cycle.[21,43,47]

Running and sprinting are most easily differentiated by the position of the foot at initial contact.[43,47] In running, the initial contact is made with the heel, as in walking. In sprinting, the initial contact is made with the toe, which is advantageous at higher velocities.

Biomechanical analysis of running divides the

stance phase into two subphases. During absorption, the hip and knee flex, and the ankle dorsiflexes. Kinetic studies of children running suggest that the knee and ankle are primary and secondary energy absorbers, respectively, during this subphase.[47] The propulsion subphase is characterized by active hip and knee extension and ankle plantar flexion. Kinetic analysis reveals that the ankle is the primary power generator, contributing two and three times the power generated by the hip and knee, respectively.[47] This period of active ankle plantar flexion that occurs during the propulsion subphase of running can correctly be called the push-off period.

MATURATION OF GAIT

The widely recognized developmental milestones of infants, such as rolling over, sitting, crawling, and standing, are thought to primarily reflect the physiologic maturation of the neuromuscular system.[17] Animal models of spinal cord injury and the presence of mass flexion and extension reflexes in neonates suggests the existence of "hard-wired" motor synergies emanating from the spinal cord.[24,31] With maturation, these spinal cord reflexes are manipulated to produce and control a reciprocating gait pattern. With further development, complex learned motor activities can be incorporated into the neuronal circuitry.[21] With appropriate training, such learned activities can be performed with increasing ease. In all likelihood, the development of a mature gait pattern represents a combination of physiologic maturation of the neuromuscular system and incorporation of complex, learned motor activities.[7,79,84,88,96]

Landmark studies by Sutherland, employing instrumented gait analysis, characterized the different stages in the maturation of gait.[84,87,88,91] In toddler gait, the upper extremities are held in abduction with elbow extension. Reciprocal arm movement does not occur. The foot and ankle exhibit a toe-strike pattern at initial contact, increased stance-phase dorsiflexion, and increased swing-phase plantar flexion. The knee shows diminished flexion throughout the gait cycle. The hip is externally rotated during the stance and swing phases. The stance phase is characterized by diminished single-limb stance time and a widened base of support in double stance. In the swing phase, circumduction (i.e., hip abduction) is used to clear the externally rotated, extended, and plantar-flexed extremity.

By 2 years of age, significant maturation is exhibited. Reciprocal arm swing is achieved by most children. Heel strike occurs at initial contact, and ankle dorsiflexion facilitates limb clearance during the swing phase. The knee flexion wave also occurs during the stance phase. Rotation at the hip has normalized. The stance phase is characterized by increased single-limb stance time, and the movement during swing phase shows normalized clearance mechanisms.

By 3 years of age, most adult kinematic patterns are developed. Subsequent changes in time-distance parameters, such as cadence, velocity, and step length, continue to occur until 7 years of age, when an adult gait pattern is achieved.

Sutherland's analysis of more than 300 children identified five statistically significant parameters of gait maturity[88]:

1. Single-limb stance duration increases with age and maturation.
2. Walking velocity increases with age and limb length.
3. Cadence decreases with age and limb length.
4. Step length increases with age and limb length.
5. The ratio of the interankle distance to the pelvic width decreases with age and maturation.

COMMON GAIT DEVIATIONS

Mechanical modeling of gait assumes mobile body segments powered by internal muscle activity and external, applied forces. The pathologic processes that affect gait usually compromise joint mobility and muscle activity by three general mechanisms: deformity, muscle dysfunction, and pain.[2,62,63]

In deformity, soft tissue contractures limit joint motion. Fixed contractures create rigid deformity, and elastic contractures lead to dynamic deformity. Ligament laxity causes instability that can contribute to joint deformity. Osseous tissues may be altered by trauma, infection, vascular compromise, and abnormally applied mechanical forces to create a bony deformity that limits joint mobility.

Disorders of the neuromuscular system can cause dynamic muscle weakness that alters gait. Children with lower motor neuron lesions or primary muscle diseases can often compensate for the function deficit. This capacity to substitute depends on the preservation of proprioception and selective control.[62,63] Primary compensatory mechanisms include changing the timing of other muscle actions during gait and use of postural adjustments to substitute for deficient muscle forces. Children with upper motor neuron lesions have the most challenging functional deficits. Their gait deviations are a consequence of spasticity, persistent primitive locomotor patterns (i.e., mass flexion or extension reflexes), poor selective control, and impaired proprioception.[21,63]

Pain can contribute to joint deformity and muscle dysfunction. After an injury, the body assumes a natural resting joint position that minimizes intraarticular pressure.[63] This mechanism contributes to soft tissue and osseous tissue changes over time. Neurologic control mechanisms exist that protect joint structures from destructive pressures.[63] These protective reflexes limit the ability to activate certain muscles after an injury, which over time causes disuse atrophy and contributes to a vicious cycle of progressive functional deficits. An antalgic gait reflects the body's efforts to compensate for pain or instability in the stance-phase limb by minimizing the duration and magnitude of loading and is a gait pattern characterized by diminished single-limb stance time.

Within this framework, gait abnormalities may be seen as primary, if they are the direct result of a mechanical change related to the injury or disease process; secondary, when a primary deviation at another joint causes a pathologic deviation at the reference joint; or compensatory, reflecting an adaptation to an applied pathologic condition. It is an error to intervene when a compensatory gait deviation successfully substitutes for a functional deficit. Treatment is appropriate when the compensations are inadequate or when they require excessive energy cost, joint strain, or muscle overuse.[2,22,62]

Ankle

Excessive Ankle Plantar Flexion

The primary causes of excessive ankle plantar flexion in the stance phase include plantar flexor muscle spasticity, contracture, and impaired proprioception. Compensatory ankle plantar flexion is seen as a substitution pattern for weak quadriceps or for ankle or forefoot pain. Increased ankle plantar flexion in midstance and terminal stance, called vaulting, may occur as a compensatory mechanism to facilitate swing clearance of a relatively long contralateral limb. The consequences include diminished shock absorption by limiting knee flexion in the loading response subphase and decreased forward progression of the tibia over the foot and ankle that interferes with the heel and ankle rockers. The primary causes of excessive ankle plantar flexion in the swing phase include weakness or impaired selective control of the ankle dorsiflexors and plantar flexor spasticity or contracture. Excessive ankle plantar flexion during the swing phase interferes with foot clearance and foot positioning for initial contact.

Excessive ankle plantar flexion is clinically described as an equinus gait and is commonly seen in patients with cerebral palsy, muscle diseases such as Duchenne muscular dystrophy, and posttraumatic conditions such as anterior compartment nerve injury or compartment syndrome.

Excessive Ankle Dorsiflexion

The most common primary cause of excessive ankle dorsiflexion during the stance phase is weakness of the ankle plantar flexors. This is seen in conditions such as L5-level myelodysplasia and after overlengthening of the heel cord in children with cerebral palsy. This circumstance is clinically described as a calcaneous gait. Fixed ankle-foot orthoses and the solid-ankle, cushioned-heel prosthetic foot also limit ankle plantar flexion in the loading response subphase. A common secondary cause of excessive ankle dorsiflexion in the stance phase is excessive knee flexion due to hamstring contracture or spasticity, as seen in cerebral palsy. Excessive ankle dorsiflexion may serve as a compensation for forefoot pain and as a mechanism to shorten the step length of the opposite limb.[52,63]

The consequences of excessive ankle dorsiflexion are significant in all of the subphases of stance. In the loading response and midstance subphases, exaggeration of the heel and ankle rockers increases the demand on the quadriceps (i.e., knee extensors) and diminishes limb stability. The crouch gait in cerebral palsy is a consequence of this deviation. In the terminal stance and preswing subphases, heel rise is compromised, which diminishes the step length of the opposite limb. This decreases the subsequent shock absorption demands of the loading response. Excessive ankle dorsiflexion during the swing phase is unusual and interferes with the foot position for initial contact.

Knee

Inadequate Flexion and Excessive Extension

Primary inadequate flexion and excessive extension of the knee in the stance phase are usually caused by quadriceps spasticity or contracture. The stiff knee gait in cerebral palsy is an example of this deviation. Hyperextension of the knee in stance phase, called recurvatum gait, may be a primary consequence of overly aggressive medial and lateral distal hamstring lengthening in children with cerebral palsy. The most common secondary cause of these deviations is increased stance-phase ankle plantar flexion, which in the extreme also causes knee hyperextension or recurvatum deformity. Inadequate flexion or excessive extension of the knee in the stance phase may also reflect a compensatory deviation for knee or patellofemoral pain or indicate a weakness of the quadriceps, classically seen in children with polio. The consequences of the deviation in the stance phase are decreased shock absorption ability or demand, decreased forward progression of the tibia, and potential injury to the posterior knee joint structures.

A common primary cause of inadequate flexion

and excessive extension of the knee in the swing phase is quadriceps spasticity or contracture, as seen in cerebral palsy. Hip flexor weakness is a secondary cause of this deviation in swing phase. During the terminal swing subphase, inadequate flexion or excessive extension of the knee may occur as a compensatory mechanism for knee pain or quadriceps weakness. The principal consequence of this deviation in initial and midswing subphases is impaired foot clearance. Suboptimal positioning of the limb for initial contact and loading response is the principal consequence of this deviation in terminal swing.

Excessive Flexion and Inadequate Extension

The primary causes of excessive flexion and inadequate extension of the knee in the stance phase include hamstring spasticity or contracture, as seen in cerebral palsy patients, and quadriceps weakness, as seen in patients with polio. The jump gait and crouch gait deviations seen in children with cerebral palsy are characterized by increased knee flexion in stance phase.[92] Secondary causes are related to increased ankle dorsiflexion in the stance phase, usually a consequence of ankle plantar flexor weakness, as seen in L5-level myelodysplasia or after excessive lengthening of the heel cord in cerebral palsy patients. This deviation is rarely used as a compensatory mechanism, because it is energy inefficient. The consequences of excessive flexion and inadequate extension of the knee in the stance phase are increased demands on the quadriceps, increased joint reaction forces at the knee and patellofemoral joint, diminished limb stability, and decreased step length of the contralateral limb.

The primary causes of excessive flexion and inadequate extension of the knee in the swing phase are hamstring spasticity or contracture and persistence of primitive locomotor reflex patterns (i.e., inability to extend the knee while flexing the hip), as seen in patient with cerebral palsy.[63] Increased knee flexion in the initial and midswing subphases may be a compensatory mechanism to facilitate limb clearance in the face of ankle plantar flexion or diminished hip flexion. Similarly, this deviation during the terminal swing allows forefoot strike at initial contact, which would be a compensatory mechanism for a child with heel pain. The consequences of excessive flexion and inadequate extension of the knee the in swing phase are diminished step length and impaired positioning of the foot for heel strike at initial contact.

Hip

Inadequate Extension and Excessive Flexion

The primary causes of inadequate extension and excessive flexion of the hip in the stance phase include hip flexor spasticity or contracture, as seen in cerebral palsy patients; hamstring or hip extensor weakness, as seen in those with myelodysplasia; iliotibial band contracture, as seen in children with Duchenne muscular dystrophy; and hip joint pain. The most common secondary cause of this deviation in the stance phase is excessive ankle dorsiflexion, as seen in L5-level myelodysplasia patients and in the crouch gait pattern of patients with cerebral palsy.

The consequences of inadequate extension and excessive flexion of the hip in stance phase are the result of forward trunk lean. Children have the flexibility to compensate for this deformity by increasing their lumbar lordosis.[52,63] This places increased strain across the lumbar spine over time. Incomplete compensation for forward trunk lean moves the ground reaction force vector anteriorly, increasing the external extension moment at the knee and dorsiflexion moment at the ankle.

The most common primary cause of this deviation in the swing phase is hip flexor spasticity or contracture. Compensatory increased hip flexion during the swing phase in used to facilitate limb clearance in the face of inappropriate ankle plantar flexion or knee extension. The main consequence of this deviation in swing phase is increased energy cost.

Excessive Adduction

The primary causes of excessive adduction of the hip during the stance phase are adductor muscle spasticity or contracture and ipsilateral abductor muscle weakness. Secondary causes include contralateral hip abductor muscle contracture and scoliosis with pelvic obliquity. The consequences of this deviation in the stance phase are a decreased base of support in the coronal plan and diminished limb stability.

Excessive adduction of the hip is seen as a primary deviation in the swing phase caused by adductor muscle spasticity or contracture. A common secondary cause is limb length inequality. A significantly short contralateral limb causes pelvic obliquity in the stance phase, effectively adducting the reference limb in swing phase. Compensatory hip adduction in the swing phase occurs when the hip adductors substitute for weak hip flexors to assist with limb clearance.[52,63] The principal consequence of excessive hip adduction in swing phase is a relative increase in the limb length, which can cause problems with clearance. In cerebral palsy patients, the scissor gait deformity is a combination of excessive hip adduction and flexion combined with increased femoral anteversion in the swing phase.

A child who exhibits contralateral pelvic drop when asked to stand on one leg, a sign of ipsilateral hip abductor muscle weakness, is said to have a positive

Trendelenburg sign. Contralateral pelvic drop during the stance phase of the reference limb is called a Trendelenburg gait. A common compensation for this inefficient gait deviation is lateral trunk lean over the stance limb, which effectively moves the body's center of mass closer to the stance-phase hip joint and diminishes the demand on the gluteus medius muscle, the principal hip abductor; this movement is called the gluteus medius lurch.

Excessive Abduction

The primary cause of excessive abduction of the hip during the stance phase is abductor muscle contracture. Secondary causes are limb length inequality, in which the ipsilateral limb is significantly short, and scoliosis with pelvic obliquity. Excessive abduction of the hip in the stance phase may also be a compensatory mechanism for a relatively long limb. The consequences in the stance phase are to increase the base of support in the coronal plane and decrease the relative length of the stance limb.

The primary cause of excessive abduction of the hip in the swing phase is ipsilateral abductor muscle contracture. Compensatory excessive hip abduction in swing is seen as a substitution pattern for weak hip flexors.[52,63] This deviation is also used, in combination with pelvic rotation and hiking, as a means to clear a relatively long limb (i.e., absolute length or due to inadequate knee flexion or ankle dorsiflexion). This complex deviation is called circumduction. The principal consequence of excessive hip abduction in the swing phase is to decrease the functional length of the ipsilateral limb.

GAIT ANALYSIS

Observational Gait Analysis

A systematic method of observational gait analysis promotes a comprehensive assessment of gait deviations and functional deficits and avoids the common pitfall of focusing exclusively on the most striking component of a complex multilevel problem. The technique described has three phases: preparation, observation, and interpretation.

The preparation begins with determination or confirmation of the underlying diagnosis by taking a clinical history. It is essential to determine the principal gait problems as perceived by the child, the parents, and the referring physician or therapist. A physical examination should assess the active and passive range of motion of the hips, knees, ankles, and subtalar joints. A thorough neurologic evaluation should include muscle strength, selective control, tone, spasticity (i.e., response to fast stretch), contracture (i.e., response to slow stretch), presence or persistence of primitive mass reflexes, sensation, and proprioception.

The observation phase begins with a gross analysis of the child's gait, focusing on velocity, cadence, step length, stability, and antalgia. This is followed by serial horizontal analyses, beginning at the ankle and proceeding to the hip, of each anatomic area relative to the eight subphases of the gait cycle: initial contact, loading response, midstance, terminal stance, preswing, initial swing, midswing, and terminal swing. Analysis of one limb is completed at each joint before analysis of the opposite limb. Sagittal-plane analysis is performed from the right and left sides. Coronal-plane analysis is performed with the child walking toward and away from the observer. The observations are entered as they are made on a standardized form (Fig. 4-17).

Interpretation begins with horizontal summation, by anatomic area, of the data collected. This approach can identify the gait deviations at each joint. Vertical summation of the data can identify the functional deficits with respect to gait tasks and the subphases of the gait cycle. A review of the gait deviations and functional deficits helps to determine the primary deviations, secondary deviations, and compensatory deviations. Appropriate interventions can be determined and implemented at this point.

Instrumented Gait Analysis

There are five modalities, used in various combinations, that constitute instrumented gait analysis. Movement measurements evaluate the magnitude and timing of limb-segment motion and generate kinematic data, such as linear position and angular orientation. Dynamic electromyography (EMG) assesses the timing and magnitude of skeletal muscle function. Force platforms determine the magnitude and direction of the stance phase ground reaction force. Force data, when combined with the kinematic data, allow the calculation of kinetic parameters, such as moments and powers. Stride analysis can be performed by direct or indirect methods and determines parameters such as velocity, cadence, step length, and stride length. Energetics evaluates the energy expenditure and efficiency of gait.

Movement Measurements

Biomechanical analysis of limb movement in gait reduces the skeletal segments to rigid bodies moving through space, which are interconnected by frictionless joints. There are two main types of automated video systems used to generate kinematic data.[63,90] The

	GAIT CYCLE							
PHASE	STANCE					SWING		
TASK	Weight Acceptance		Single Limb Support			Limb Advancement		
SUB-PHASE	Initial Contact (IC)	Loading Response (LR)	Mid Stance (MSt)	Terminal Stance (TSt)	Pre Swing (PSw)	Initial Swing (ISw)	Mid Swing (MSw)	Terminal Swing (TSw)

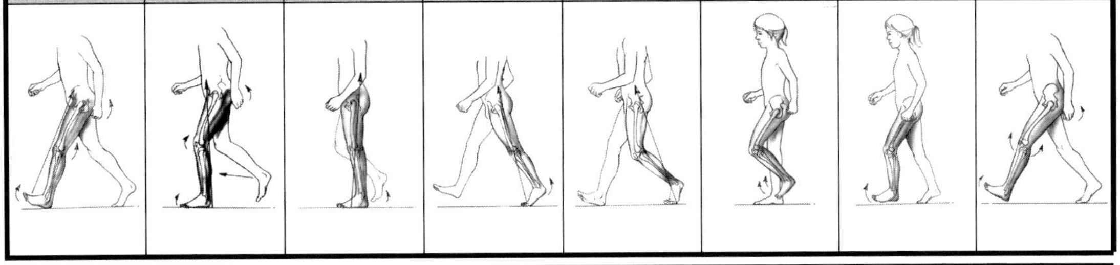

A

NAME ____________ Side: Right / Left		Weight Acceptance		Single Limb Support			Swing Limb Advancement			Gait Deviations
Anatomic Area	Deviation	IC	LR	MSt	TSt	PSw	ISw	MSw	TSw	(By Anatomic Area)
ANKLE	↑ Dorsiflexion									
	Neutral									
	↑ Plantar Flexion									
	Varus									
	Valgus									
KNEE	↑ Flexion									
	Neutral									
	↑ Extension									
	Varus									
	Valgus									
HIP	↑ Flexion									
	Neutral									
	↑ Extension									
	Adduction									
	Abduction									
FUNCTIONAL DEFICITS (By Gait Tasks)										

B

FIGURE 4-17. Standardized form used when performing observational gait analysis. (IC, initial contact; LR, loading response; MSt, midstance; Tst, terminal stance; PSw, Preswing; ISw, initial swing; MSw, midswing; TSw, terminal swing; adapted from Pathokinesiology Department, Physical Therapy Department. Observational gait analysis handbook. Downey: The Professional Staff Association of Rancho Los Amigos Medical Center, 1989).

first and most widely used technique consists of video cameras that generate digital data by tracking passive, retroreflective markers fixed to body landmarks based on surface anatomy. A central computer analyzes this data to determine the three-dimensional coordinates of each marker throughout the gait cycle. To generate accurate, reproducible data, all cameras must record data simultaneously, and the image space must be calibrated frequently. Each marker must be traced throughout the duration of the gait cycle by at least two cameras to enable three-dimensional calculations. When attempting to study both limbs simultaneously, five or six cameras are required.

This first technique has several limitations. First, it assumes that surface anatomy, which determines marker placement, is consistently related to the underlying osseous anatomy. It also considers the marker position to be stable throughout the gait cycle. The margin of error is acceptable when calculating limb-segment movement. However, more sophisticated kinetic analysis requires determination of the joint centers from the surface anatomy, which remains a controversial and less widely accepted practice. Research is directed at validation and improvement of this technique. Second, the cameras require a minimum distance of 5 to 7 cm between markers for recognition.[63,90] This can make it difficult to analyze small anatomic areas, such as the foot and ankle of a child. Third, any event that blocks the marker from the camera, such as a swinging hand, an assistive device, or the overlap of two markers in the camera field, causes the computer to lose track of the marker. This is called "marker dropout" and can only be corrected by manual sorting of the marker trajectories, which can be labor intensive. Sampling rates are limited to 50 to 60 images per second.[27,91] Technologic advances should improve the sampling rate in the near future.

The second type of automated video system uses active markers to designate anatomic sites. Each marker is a light-emitting diode that is activated sequentially by a central computer. A computer-controlled optical detector tracks the markers in a similar sequence. This technique facilitates data differentiation and has fewer problems with marker spacing and dropout.[63,90] Problems with this system include background reflections of the markers from the floor and walls and electronic interference when simultaneously recording EMG during the gait cycle. As a result, this second technique is less widely used in clinical motion analysis laboratories.

Dynamic Electromyography

EMG documents the electrical activity associated with skeletal muscle contraction on a visual record.[6,63,73,87,114] Dynamic EMG uses surface or internal electrodes to record these myoelectric potentials. Surface electrodes are pairs of metal pads that are placed directly on the skin overlying the muscle to be studied. They are easy to apply and cause no pain or discomfort. Unfortunately, they pick up signals from other muscles in the same area, which can interfere with the signal from the muscle being studied. This phenomena is called "muscle cross talk" and limits the use of surface electrodes to superficial muscles such as the gluteus maximus or muscle groups such as the medial or lateral hamstrings.[59,90] Internal electrodes are 50-μm diameter wires that are introduced through the skin with a 27-gauge needle and embedded in the muscle belly. The principal advantage of the internal electrode is its ability to record the activity of a specific muscle without interference from surrounding muscles.[33] It is ideal for studying deeper or smaller muscles such as the iliacus or posterior tibialis.[63,90] The disadvantages associated with the use of fine wire electrodes include pain on insertion, difficulty of accurate placement, and wire movement with muscle contraction.[61,90,114] Moreover, the temporal parameters of gait in children with cerebral palsy can change after insertion of fine wire electrodes.[115]

Controversies encumber the interpretation of EMG data, particularly with respect to the determination of muscle force. The raw EMG signal is quantified by computer-based digital sampling, rectification (i.e., transposition of the negative signals to the positive side of the graphic display to avoid the positive and negative signals cancelling each other out in subsequent data processing), and integration (i.e., summing of the digitized, rectified EMG signals over time).[63,90] The signal is then normalized to a selected reference value, usually that generated by a maximal effort manual muscle test.[61,112] Other investigators notice improved reproducibility when the selected reference value is the peak EMG activity generated by the muscle during a representative gait cycle.[63,112] The former technique is difficult to apply in children with cerebral palsy who have poor selective control. The latter technique fails to differentiate between weak and strong muscular activity.[63]

The use of dynamic EMG to determine the timing of muscle activity is widely accepted, even though the determination of actual on and off is subjective, with the minimum significant signal arbitrarily defined as being $\geq$5% of the maximal manual muscle test.[33,59,73,114] There is poor consensus concerning the relation of muscle force to the EMG signal, with linear and nonlinear correlations having been reported.[63,90,112] Potentially significant confounders include the type of muscle contraction (i.e., concentric versus eccentric versus isometric), the speed of the contraction, the joint position (i.e., affecting the resting muscle length and the muscle's moment arm), and electromechanical delay.[63]

Force Platform

As the body advances forward over the stance-phase limb, a three-dimensional ground reaction force, which is equal in magnitude and opposite in direction to the force being experienced by the stance-phase limb, is generated. The magnitude of the vertical, horizontal, and axial components of the ground reaction force can be determined by a force platform.[15,48,63,78,90,93] This device is a rigid plate mounted on four piezoelectric triaxial transducers. With each corner having a transducer sensitive to applied loads in three dimensions, the vertical force and horizontal shear forces (i.e., mediolateral and progressional) can be measured directly. Summation of this data allows the examiner to calculate the center of pressure, which is the point on the foot about which the ground reaction force has zero moment, and calculate its progression.[63,90,93]

By combining the position of the ground reaction force vector with the position of the joint centers, which are derived from the kinematic data, the external joint moments can be calculated.[48] These moments reflect the demands applied to the joints by body-segment position, gravity, and inertia. The external moments determine the requirements for the internal moments generated by the muscles. Further kinetic analysis combines the position of the ground reaction force vector with the joint angular velocity, which is derived from the kinematic data, to determine joint powers.[48]

To obtain accurate data, the child must walk across the force platform in a spontaneous, natural fashion. Deliberately stepping onto the platform, an action called targeting, compromises the data collected and is avoided by mounting the platform flush with the floor and camouflaging it with a thin "skin" that matches the rest of the floor. The foot of the reference limb must strike the platform completely while the opposite foot remains clear. Children who use assistive devices such as walkers or crutches cannot be studied with a standard force platform, because only a portion of their body weight is supported by the stance-phase limb.

Stride Analysis

Gait can be characterized by temporal and distance parameters. Velocity is the distance per unit time; cadence is the steps per unit time; stride length is the distance between two sequential initial contacts by the same limb; step length is the distance between the initial contact by each foot; and single-limb stance time is the period during which the opposite limb is in the swing phase with no floor contact. Compensations for diminished velocity include increased cadence and, when possible, increased stride length.[1,111] In children, changes in temporal and distance parameters with age are primarily a function of increasing limb length.[63,84,88,96] Adults have a wide range of safe and comfortable walking velocities, influenced primarily by voluntary variability.[106] Age has no significant effect until the person is older than 60 years of age.[63]

Stride analysis can be performed by several techniques. The indirect method uses kinematic data. A single foot or ankle marker is tracked with respect to time and distance over a predetermined gait cycle sequence.

Direct techniques measure the foot contact with the floor. This is accomplished with a foot switch system, which consists of individual pressure sensors that are placed beneath the heel and the metatarsal heads.[33,63,87,90,108] Time and distance parameters can be determined directly from the activation patterns of the different sensors. Insertable insole pressure sensors enable analysis of more complex patterns of foot pressure distribution.

Energetics

Measurement of the energy required for walking provides a comprehensive parameter of gait performance and a means of quantifying the physiologic cost of various gait deviations.[13,21,69,90,103,107] Total body calorimetry, which is a measurement of the body's heat and work production, is the most accurate technique of energy use assessment but is not clinically practical.

Indirect calorimetry assumes that anaerobic metabolism contributes little to energy production during steady-state ambulation at a self-determined walking velocity.[103,106,107] In this model, the energy needs of gait are completely met by the aerobic metabolism of inspired oxygen (O_2). The magnitude of O_2 consumed reflects the energy requirements for walking. Indirect calorimetry uses open spirometry to measure O_2 consumption.[107] While ambulating, the child inspires ambient air and expires air into a closed capture system. Analysis and comparison of the O_2 content of the ambient and expired air determines the child's O_2 consumption over time. The O_2 consumption is reported as the O_2 rate, expressed in milliliters per kilogram minute, and is a reflection of the intensity of the effort required to ambulate.[103,107]

When comparing gait patterns, the most valuable parameter is the O_2 cost, which is a measure of gait efficiency. In general, children are studied at their self-determined walking speed, which represents the most energy-efficient compromise between progression and stability. The O_2 cost is defined as the O_2 rate divided by the walking velocity, which is expressed as milliliters per kilogram meter, and it describes the amount of energy needed to walk a standard distance.[103,107] Children with cerebral palsy tend to have O_2 rates similar to healthy normal children, indicating a common range of energy used for walking.[13,69,101] However, the self-selected walking velocity is significantly less for the children with cerebral palsy. Their relatively energy-inefficient gait is best described by the O_2 cost, which is greater than the controls.[13,69]

Investigators have found a linear relation between the O_2 rate and the heart rate through a wide range of walking velocities in children with cerebral palsy and in normal children, validating the use of this more easily measured parameter as an index of energy expenditure.[69]

ACKNOWLEDGMENTS

I wish to recognize the contributions of David H. Sutherland, M.D., Jacqueline Perry, M.D., and James R. Gage, M.D., to the field of motion analysis, and to refer interested readers to references 21, 63, 87, and 88.

References

1. Andriacchi TP, Ogle JA, Galante JO. Walking speed as a basis for normal and abnormal gait measurements. J Biomech 1977;10:261.
2. Andriacchi TP. Evaluation of surgical procedures and/or joint implants with gait analysis. Instr Course Lect 1990;39:343.
3. Andriacchi TP, Birac D. Functional testing in the anterior cruciate ligament-deficient knee. Clin Orthop 1993;288:40.
4. Banta HV, Sutherland DH, Wyatt MP. Anterior tibial transfer to the os calcis with Achilles tenodesis for the calcaneal deformity in myelomeningocele. J Pediatr Orthop 1981;1:125.
5. Barto PS, Supinski RS, Skinner SR. Dynamic EMG findings in varus hindfoot deformity and spastic cerebral palsy. Dev Med Child Neurol 1984;26:88.
6. Basmajian JV, DeLuca CJ. Muscles alive: their functions revealed by electromyography. 5th ed. Baltimore: Williams & Wilkins, 1985.
7. Beck RJ, Andriacchi TP, Kuo KN, et al. Changes in the gait patterns of growing children. J Bone Joint Surg 1981;63:1452.
8. Berchuck M, Andriacchi TP, Bach BR, Reider B. Gait adaptations by patients who have a deficient anterior cruciate ligament. J Bone Joint Surg [A] 1990;72:871.
9. Berman AT, Zarro VJ, Bosacco SJ, Israelite C. Quantitative gait analysis after unilateral or bilateral total knee replacement. J Bone Joint Surg [A] 1987;69:1340.
10. Boscarino LF, Ounpuu S, Davis RB, et al. Effects of selective dorsal rhizotomy on gait in children with cerebral palsy. J Pediatr Orthop 1993;13:174.
11. Braune W, Fischer D. The human gait. Berlin: Springer-Verlag, 1987.
12. Brodke DS, Skinner SR, Lamoreux LW, et al. Effects of ankle-foot orthoses on the gait of children. J Pediatr Orthop 1989;9:702.
13. Butler P, Engelbrecht M, Major RE, et al. Physiological cost index of walking for normal children and its use as an indicator of physical handicap. Dev Med Child Neurol 1984;26:607.
14. Cahan LD, Adams JM, Perry J, Beeler LM. Instrumented gait analysis after selective dorsal rhizotomy. Dev Med Child Neurol 1990;32:1037.
15. Chao EVS, Laughman RK, Schneider E, Stauffer RN. Normative data of knee joint motion and ground reaction forces in adult level walking. J Biomech 1983;16:219.
16. DeLuca PA. Gait analysis in the treatment of the ambulatory child with cerebral palsy. Clin Orthop 1991;264:65.
17. Devivo DC. Developmental milestones in pediatrics. In: Rudolph A, ed. Pediatrics. 18th ed. Norwalk: Appleton & Lange, 1987.
18. Engsberg JR, Lee AG, Tedford KG, Harder JA. Normative ground reaction force data for able-bodied and below-knee-amputee children during walking. J Pediatr Orthop 1993;13:169.
19. Etryre B, Chambers CS, Scarborough NH, Cain TE. Preoperative and postoperative assessment of surgical intervention for equinus gait in children with cerebral palsy. J Pediatr Orthop 1993;13:24.
20. Gage JR. An overview of normal walking. Instr Course Lect 1990;39:291.
21. Gage JR. Gait analysis in cerebral palsy. In: Clinics in developmental medicine. Oxford: MacKeith Press, 1991.
22. Gage JR. Gait analysis: an essential tool in the treatment of cerebral palsy. Clin Orthop 1993;288:126.
23. Glousman R. Electromyographic analysis and its role in the athletic shoulder. Clin Orthop 1993;288:27.
24. Grillner S. Neurobiological bases of rhythmic motor acts in vertebrates. Science 1985;228:143.
25. Hicks R, Durinick N, Gage JR. Differentiation of idiopathic toe-walking and cerebral palsy. J Pediatr Orthop 1988;8:160.
26. Hoffer MM. Ten year follow-up of split anterior tibial tendon transfer in cerebral palsied patients with spastic equinovarus deformity. J Pediatr Orthop 1985;5:432.
27. Hoffinger SA. Gait analysis in pediatric rehabilitation. Phys Med Rehab Clin North Am 1991;2:817.
28. Hsu JD, Furumasu J. Gait and posture changes in the Duchenne muscular dystrophy child. Clin Orthop 1993;288:122.
29. Hullin MG, Robb JE, Loudon IR. Ankle-foot orthosis function in low-level myelomeningocele. J Pediatr Orthop 1992;12:518.
30. Inman VT, Ralston H, Todd F. Human walking. Baltimore: Williams & Wilkins, 1981.
31. Joseph J. Neurological control of locomotion. Dev Med Child Neurol 1985;27:822.
32. Kalen V, Adler N, Bleck EE. Electromyography of idiopathic toe walking. J Pediatr Orthop 1986;6:31.
33. Kadaba MP, Wooten ME, Gainey J, Cochran GVB. Repeatability of phasic muscle activity: performance of surface and intramuscular wire electrodes in gait analysis. J Orthop Res 1985;3:350.
34. Katoh Y, Chao EYS, Laughman RK, et al. Biomechanical analysis of foot function during gait and clinical applications. Clin Orthop 1983;177:23.
35. Kozin SH, Keenan MAE. Using dynamic electromyography to guide surgical treatment of the spastic upper extremity in the brain-injured patient. Clin Orthop 1993;288:109.
36. Kroll MA, Otis JC, Sculco TP, et al. The relationship of stride characteristics to pain before and after total knee arthroplasty. Clin Orthop 1989;239:191.
37. Lewallen R, Kyck G, Quanbury A, et al. Gait kinematics in below-knee child amputees: a force plate analysis. J Pediatr Orthop 1986;6:291.
38. Lieber RL. Skeletal muscle structure and function. Baltimore: Williams & Wilkins, 1992.
39. Limbird TJ, Shiavi R, Frazer M, Borra H. EMG profiles of knee joint musculature during walking: changes induced by anterior cruciate ligament deficiency. J Orthop Res 1988;6:630.

40. Long WT, Dorr LD, Healy B, Perry J. Functional recovery of noncemented total hip arthroplasty. Clin Orthop 1993;288:73.
41. Lyons K, Perry J, Gronley JK, et al. Timing and relative intensity of hip extensor and abductor muscle action during level and stair ambulation: am EMG study. Phys Ther 1983;63:1597.
42. Mann RA, Hagy JL, White V, Liddell D. The initiation of gait. J Bone Joint Surg [A] 1979;61:232.
43. Mann RA, Hagy J. Biomechanics of walking, running, and sprinting. Am J Sports Med 1980;8:345.
44. Mansour JM, Audu ML. Passive elastic moment at the knee and its influence on human gait. J Biomech 1986;19:369.
45. Muybridge E. Complete human and animal locomotion. New York: Dover Publications, 1980.
46. Norlin R, Odenrick P. Development of gait in spastic children with cerebral palsy. J Pediatr Orthop 1986;6:674.
47. Ounpuu S. The biomechanics of running: a kinematic and kinetic analysis. Instr Course Lect 1990;39:305.
48. Ounpuu MS, Gage JR, Davis RB. Three-dimensional lower extremity joint kinetics in normal pediatric gait. J Pediatr Orthop 1991;11:341.
49. Ounpuu S, Muik E, Davis RB, et al. Rectus femoris surgery in children with cerebral palsy. Part I: the effect of rectus femoris transfer location on knee motion. J Pediatr Orthop 1993;13:325.
50. Ounpuu S, Muik E, Davis RB, et al. Rectus femoris surgery in children with cerebral palsy. Part II: a comparison between the effect of transfer and release of the distal rectus femoris on knee motion. J Pediatr Orthop 1993;13:331.
51. Pare EB, Stern JT, Schwartz JM. Functional differentiation within the tensor fasciae latae. J Bone Joint Surg [A] 1981;63:1457.
52. Pathokinesiology Department, Physical Therapy Department. Observational gait analysis handbook. Downey: The Professional Staff Association of Rancho Los Amigos Medical Center, 1989.
53. Perry J. Mechanics of walking. Phys Ther 1967;47:778.
54. Perry J, Hoffer MM, Giovan P, Antonelli D, Greenberg R. Gait analysis of the triceps surae in cerebral palsy. J Bone Joint Surg [A] 1974;56:511.
55. Perry J, Antonelli D, Ford W. Analysis of knee-joint forces during flexed-knee stance. J Bone Joint Surg [A] 1975;57:961.
56. Perry J, Hoffer MM, Antonelli D, et al. Electromyography before and after surgery for hip deformity in children with cerebral palsy. J Bone Joint Surg [A] 1976;58:201.
57. Perry J, Hoffer MM. Preoperative and postoperative dynamic electromyography as an aid in planning tendon transfers in children with cerebral palsy. J Bone Joint Surg [A] 1977;59:531.
58. Perry J, Waters RL, Perrin T. Electromyographic analysis of equinovarus following stroke. Clin Orthop 1978;131:47.
59. Perry J, Easterdays CS, Antonelli D. Surface versus intramuscular electrodes for electromyography of superficial and deep muscles. Phys Ther 1981;61:7.
60. Perry J. Anatomy and biomechanics of the hindfoot. Clin Orthop 1983;177:9.
61. Perry J, Ireland ML, Gronley J, Hoffer MM. Predictive value of manual muscle testing and gait analysis in normal ankles by dynamic electromyography. Foot Ankle 1986;6:254.
62. Perry J. Pathologic gait. Instr Course Lect 1990;39:325.
63. Perry J. Gait analysis: normal and pathologic function. Thorofare, NJ: Slack, 1992.
64. Perry J. Determinants of muscle function in the spastic lower extremity. Clin Orthop 1993;288:10.
65. Pink M, Jobe FW, Perry J, et al. The normal shoulder during the butterfly swim stroke: an electromyographic and cinematographic analysis of twelve muscles. Clin Orthop 1993;288:48.
66. Pink M, Jobe FW, Perry J, et al. The painful shoulder during the butterfly stroke: an electromyographic and cinematographic analysis of twelve muscles. Clin Orthop 1993;288:60.
67. Pinzur MS. Dynamic electromyography in functional surgery for upper limb spasticity. Clin Orthop 1993;288:118.
68. Prodromos C, Andriacchi T, Galante J. A relationship between gait and clinical changes following high tibial osteotomy. J Bone Joint Surg [A] 1985;67:1188.
69. Rose J, Gamble JG, Medeiros J, et al. Energy cost of walking in normal children and in those with cerebral palsy: comparison of heart rate and oxygen uptake. J Pediatr Orthop 1989;9:276.
70. Saunders JBdeCM, Inman VT, Eberhart HD. The major determinants in normal and pathologic gait. J Bone Joint Surg [A] 1953;35:543.
71. Schwab GH, Moynes DR, Jobe FW, Perry J. Lower extremity electromyographic analysis of running gait. Clin Orthop 1983;176:166.
72. Segal LS, Sienko Thomas SE, Mazur JM, Mauterer M. Calcaneal gait in spastic diplegia after heelcord lengthening: a study with gait analysis. J Pediatr Orthop 1989;9:697.
73. Shiavi R, Green N, McFadyen B, et al. Normative childhood EMG gait patterns. J Orthop Res 1987;5:283.
74. Simon JR, Mann R, Hagy JL, Larsen LJ. Role of the posterior of calf muscles in normal gait. J Bone Joint Surg [A] 1978;60:465.
75. Skinner HB. Pathokinesiology and total joint arthroplasty. Clin Orthop 1993;288:78.
76. Skinner SR, Antonelli D, Perry J, Lester DK. Functional demands on the stance limb in walking. Orthopaedics 1985;8:355.
77. Skinner SR, Lester DK. Gait electromyographic evaluation of the long-toe flexors in children with spastic cerebral palsy. Clin Orthop 1986;207:70.
78. Soames RW. Foot pressure patterns during gait. J Biomed Eng 1985;7:120.
79. Statham L, Murray MP. Early walking patterns of normal children. Clin Orthop 1971;79:3.
80. Steenhoff JRM, Daanen HAM, Taminiav AHM. Functional analysis of patients who have had a modified Van Nes rotationplasty. J Bone Joint Surg [A] 1993;75:1451.
81. Steindler A. A historical review of the studies and investigations made in relation to human gait. J Bone Joint Surg [A] 1953;35:540.
82. Sutherland DH. An electromyographic study of the plantar flexors of the ankle in normal walking on the level. J Bone Joint Surg [A] 1966;48:66.
83. Sutherland DH, Cooper L. The pathomechanics of progressive crouch gait in spastic diplegia. Orthop Clin North Am 1978;9:143.
84. Sutherland DH, Olsen R, Cooper L, Woo S. The development of mature gait. J Bone Joint Surg [A] 1980;62:336.
85. Sutherland DH, Cooper L, Daniel D. The role of ankle plantar flexors in normal walking. J Bone Joint Surg [A] 1980;62:354.
86. Sutherland DH, Olsen R, Cooper LB, et al. The pathomechanics of gait in Duchenne muscular dystrophy. Dev Med Child Neurol 1981;23:3.
87. Sutherland DH. Gait disorders in childhood and adolescence. Baltimore: Williams & Wilkins, 1984.
88. Sutherland DH, Olsen RA, Biden EN, Wyatt MP. The development of mature walking. London: MacKeith Press, 1988.
89. Sutherland DH, Santi M, Abel MF. Treatment of stiff-knee gait in cerebral palsy: a comparison by gait analysis of distal rectus femoris transfer versus proximal rectus release. J Pediatr Orthop 1990;10:433.
90. Sutherland DH, Kaufman KR. Motion analysis: lower extremity. In: Nickel VL, Botte MJ, eds. Orthopaedic rehabilitation. 2nd ed. New York: Churchill Livingstone, 1992:223.

91. Sutherland DH, Valencia FG. Pediatric gait. In: Drennan JC, ed. The child's foot and ankle. New York: Raven Press, 1992:19.
92. Sutherland DH, Davids JR. Common gait abnormalities of the knee in cerebral palsy. Clin Orthop 1993;288:139.
93. Takegami Y. Wave pattern of ground reaction force of growing children. J Pediatr Orthop 1992;12:522.
94. Thometz J, Simons S, Rosenthal R. The effect on gait of lengthening of the medial hamstrings in cerebral palsy. J Bone Joint Surg [A] 1989;71:345.
95. Tibone JE, Antich TJ. Electromyographic analysis of the anterior cruciate ligament-deficient knee. Clin Orthop 1993; 288:35.
96. Todd FN, Lamoreux LW, Skinner SR, et al. Variations in the gait of normal children. J Bone Joint Surg [A] 1989;71:196.
97. Tylkowski CM, Simon SR, Mansour JM. Internal rotation gait in spastic cerebral palsy. In: Nelson JP, ed. The hip. St. Louis: CV Mosby, 1982:89.
98. Water RL, Yakura JS, Adkins RH. Gait performance after spinal cord injury. Clin Orthop 1993;288:87.
99. Waters RL, Perry J, Antonelli D, Hislop H. The energy cost of walking of amputees—influence of level of amputation. J Bone Joint Surg [A] 1976;58:42.
100. Waters RL, Garland DE, Perry J, et al. Stiff-legged gain in hemiplegia: surgical correction. J Bone Joint Surg [A] 1979;61:927.
101. Waters RL, Hislop HJ, Thomas L, Campbell J. Energy cost of walking in normal children and teenagers. Dev Med Child Neurol 1983;25:184.
102. Waters RL, Lunsford BR. Energy cost of paraplegic ambulation. J Bone Joint Surg [A] 1985;67:1245.
103. Waters RL, Lunsford BR. Energy expenditure of normal and pathologic gait: application to orthotic prescription. In: Bunch WH, ed. Atlas of orthotics. St. Louis: CV Mosby, 1985.
104. Waters RL, Campbell J, Perry J. Energy cost of three-point crutch ambulation in fracture patients. J Orthop Trauma 1987;1:170.
105. Waters RL, Barnes G, Husserl T, et al. Comparable energy expenditure following arthrodesis of the hip and ankle. J Bone Joint Surg [A] 1988;70:1032.
106. Waters RL, Lunsford BR, Perry J, Byrd R. Energy-speed relation of walking: standard tables. J Orthop Res 1988;6:215.
107. Waters RL. Energy expenditure. In: Perry J. Gait analysis: normal and pathologic function. Thorofare, NJ: Slack, 1992:443.
108. Wills CA, Hoffer MM, Perry J. A comparison of foot-switch and EMG analysis of varus deformities of the feet of children with cerebral palsy. Dev Med Child Neurol 1988;30: 227.
109. Winter DA. Biomechanical motor patterns in normal walking. J Motor Behav 1983;15:302.
110. Winter DA. Energy generation and absorption at the ankle and knee during fast, natural, and slow cadence. Clin Orthop 1983;175:147.
111. Winter DA. Kinematic and kinetic patterns in human gait: variability and compensating effects. Hum Movement Sci 1984;3:51.
112. Winter DA. The biomechanics and control of human gait. Waterloo: University of Waterloo Press, 1987.
113. Winters TF, Gage JR, Hicks R. Gait patterns in spastic hemiplegia. J Bone Joint Surg [A] 1987;69:437.
114. Wootten ME, Kadaba MP, Cochran GV. Dynamic electromyography. II. Normal patterns during gait. J Orthop Res 1990;8:259.
115. Young CC, Rose SE, Biden EN, et al. The effect of surface and internal electrodes on the gait of children with cerebral palsy, spastic diplegic type. J Orthop Res 1989;7:732.

Chapter 5

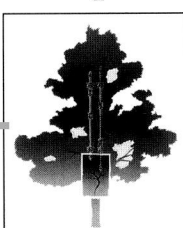

Genetic Aspects of Orthopaedic Conditions

William G. Cole

Molecular Basis of Inheritance
   Chromosomes
   Gene Structure
   Transcription and RNA Processing
   Translation
   Posttranslational Modification and
     Protein Assembly
Molecular Basis of Mutations
   Point Mutations
   Deletions and Insertions
   Detection of Mutations
Chromosome Disorders
   Abnormalities of Autosomal
     Chromosome Number
   Abnormalities of Autosomal
     Chromosome Structure
   Abnormalities of Sex Chromosomes

Single-Gene Disorders
   Autosomal Dominant Disorders
   Autosomal Recessive Disorders
   X-Linked Disorders
   Other Patterns of Single-Gene
     Inheritance
Multifactorial Disorders
Teratologic Disorders
   Principles of Teratology
   Teratogenic Agents
Genetic Counseling and Prenatal Diagnosis
   Indications for Genetic Counseling
   Diagnostic Precision
   Estimation of Recurrence Risk
   Burden of Genetic Diseases
   Neonatal and Prenatal Diagnosis
Treatment of Genetic Diseases

Many orthopaedic conditions are associated with genetic anomalies that produce congenital, developmental, metabolic, immunologic, and neoplastic disorders. Identification of the genes responsible for many of these conditions has resulted in more precise diagnoses and yielded insights into the pathogenesis, classification, prognosis, and treatment of the disorders. Further advances are likely to influence the orthopaedic care of families with genetic disorders of the musculoskeletal system. This chapter summarizes the principles of genetics as they apply to orthopaedic conditions and highlights the advances in knowledge in this field.

MOLECULAR BASIS OF INHERITANCE

Chromosomes

Chromosomes are rod-shaped organelles in the nucleus. The chromosomes contain genes, which are the DNA units of genetic information. They are linearly arranged along the chromosomes, and each gene occupies a particular position or locus.

The karyotype of a cell refers to its complement of chromosomes.[39] Human somatic cells contain 23 pairs of chromosomes, referred to as euploidy. Twenty-two of them are autosomes that occur in males and females. The remaining pair, the sex chromosomes, are designated XX in females and XY in males. The members of a pair of autosomes and a pair of X chromosomes contain matching genetic information.

During the metaphase of mitosis, the chromosomes consist of two chromatids joined at the centromere, which is the primary constriction of the chromosome. The centromere divides the chromosome into the short p arm and into the long q arm. Cytogenetic techniques divide the arms into banded regions that are used to indicate the sites of chromosomal rearrangements and the loci of genes. For example, the COL1A1 gene for one of the type I collagen protein chains is located on chromosome 17 at locus q21.3–22. The latter notation indicates that the gene is located on the q arm of chromosome 17 at the band 21.3–22.

Somatic cells divide during growth, development and repair by the process of mitosis. The daughter cells contain the identical genetic profile to their parent cell. Germline cells undergo meiosis during gametogenesis. In this process, the diploid number of 46 chromosomes is reduced to the haploid number of 23, including one of each of the autosomes and either an X or a Y chromosome. The random assortment of each of the chromosome pairs during meiosis is central to the mendelian inheritance pattern of single-gene disorders and some forms of chromosomal rearrangements.

Gene Structure

About 100,000 genes are present in the human genome of about 7 billion base pairs of DNA. Genes are made up of linearly aligned nucleotides. Each unit or nucleotide of DNA consists of a deoxyribose sugar, a purine or pyrimidine base, and a phosphate group. There are two purine bases, adenine (A) and guanine (G), and two pyrimidines, thymine (T) and cytosine (C). The nucleotides form long polynucleotide chains.

DNA forms a double-stranded structure, called the double helix, in which the component polynucleotide chains run in opposite directions and contain complementary sequences. Central to the Watson and Crick model of the DNA double helix is the complementary sequences of the chains, which are held together by hydrogen bonding between complementary pairs of nucleotide bases. An A of one chain pairs with a T of the other, and a G of one chain pairs with a C of the other.

A typical gene is illustrated in Figure 5-1. The coding sequence is divided into exons that are separated by noncoding introns or intervening sequences. The exons contain codons that encode specific amino acids. Each codon contains three nucleotides. Exons often delimit functional domains within the protein. The 5' or upstream end of the gene contains promotor sequences that regulate the expression of the gene. The promotor immediately precedes the start site of transcription of messenger RNA (mRNA).

Transcription and RNA Processing

During transcription, an exact RNA copy of the gene, called pre-mRNA, is synthesized from the start site of transcription to the 3' untranslated region. The pre-mRNA undergoes several modifications to form mRNA, which is transported from the nucleus to the cytoplasm and ribosomes. After the introns are spliced out, the remaining exons form a continuous coding sequence. The coding region is flanked by a 5' untranslated region that contains sequences essential for ribosomal binding and translation. The 3' untranslated region contains sequences that are important for mRNA stability. The polyadenylation signal contains sequences that result in the addition of a poly-A nucleotide tail, a polyadenosine sequence that characterizes most mRNAs.

Translation

Translation of the DNA code copied by the mRNA to the amino acid code of the corresponding protein is achieved on the ribosomes. The key to the genetic code is the codon, which is a group of three bases. Because each codon contains three of the four nucleotide bases, there are 64 possible triplet combinations. In humans, there are only 20 relevant amino acids, and most of them are encoded by more than one codon. Three of the codons are called stop or nonsense codons because they designate the site of termination of translation.

The first codon of the coding sequence of mRNA encodes the amino acid methionine. This codon establishes the translational reading frame, ensuring that the correct amino acids are added sequentially to the growing polypeptide chain. Addition of the appropriate amino acids is achieved by specific transfer RNAs (tRNAs) for each amino acid. They contain the anticodon sequences that recognize the complementary codon sequences of the mRNA. As an amino acid is added to the carboxyl end of the polypeptide chain, the mRNA slides exactly one codon length along the ribosome and brings the next codon into line for interaction with its specific tRNA. The proteins are synthesized from the amino to the carboxyl terminus, which corresponds to translation of the mRNA from 5' to 3'.

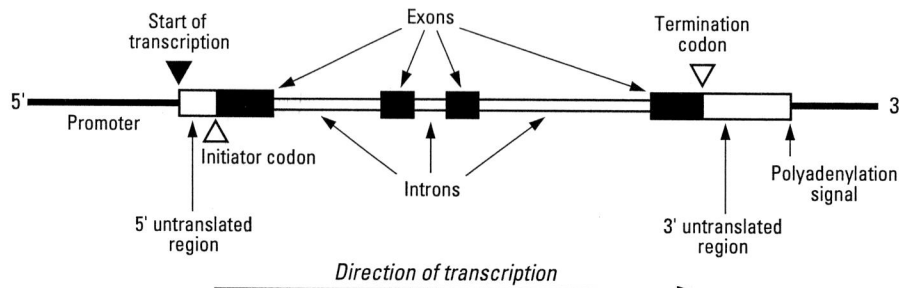

FIGURE 5-1. General structure of a typical human gene, showing the main functional domains. (From Thompson MW, McInnes RR, Willard HF. Genetics in medicine. 5th ed. Toronto: WB Saunders, 1991.)

Translation ceases at the first stop codon. The completed polypeptide is released from the ribosome.

Posttranslational Modification and Protein Assembly

Many proteins undergo numerous posttranslational modifications in the rough endoplasmic reticulum, Golgi apparatus, and outside the cell. For example, the core proteins of collagen and glycosaminoglycans undergo extensive enzymatic modification. Many proteins are produced with terminal extensions that are removed to convert the pre-pro-proteins into functional proteins. The functional proteins are assembled into complex polymers.

MOLECULAR BASIS OF MUTATIONS

A mutation is any permanent change in the sequence or arrangement of DNA. It can occur in somatic cells, as observed in many cancers, but when it occurs in germline cells, the mutation can be transmitted to subsequent generations. Permanent changes in DNA sequence are rarely deleterious but add to genetic diversity among individuals. Loci that have many alternative forms, called alleles, are polymorphic.

Mutations occur on various scales, from genome mutations that involve misaggregation of chromosomes to chromosome mutations that involve chromosome rearrangements and specific gene mutations.

Point Mutations

Point mutations are the commonest mutations. These nucleotide substitutions can result in several molecular outcomes:[39]

> Missense mutations that alter the amino acid sequence
> Nonsense mutations that introduce a premature termination codon
> Alteration of promotor sequences
> mRNA splicing mutations that result in exon loss

Although point mutations are often considered to occur randomly, there are mutational hot spots in the genome, commonly at CG dinucleotides, and mutations tend to recur at such sites. Transitions, which exchange one pyrimidine for the other or one purine for the other, are more common than transversions that exchange a purine for a pyrimidine or vice versa. Transitions and transversions are responsible for most of the mutations of the type I collagen genes in osteogenesis imperfecta and of the type II collagen gene in the spondyloepiphyseal dysplasias.

Advanced paternal age is a frequent factor in cases of sporadic point mutations and is referred to as the paternal age effect on new mutations.[26,37] It is common in achondroplasia. Germline mosaicism for the new mutation also occurs in achondroplasia and other skeletal dysplasias. It accounts for the birth of affected siblings from clinically normal parents.[4] The paternal age effect and germline mosaicism are explained by differences in gametogenesis in males and females. Spermatogonia go through a few mitotic divisions before embarking on the meiotic divisions that lead to mature sperm.[7] Some of the products of the mitotic divisions are returned to the "cell bank" to replenish the supply of spermatogonia. Mutations occurring during DNA replication can accumulate, providing a basis for paternal age effect and for germline mosaicism.

Missense Mutations

A missense mutation occurs when a single nucleotide substitution alters the sense of a codon and a different amino acid is added to the elongating polypeptide. Mutations of this kind are common in many structural proteins, such as the collagens in osteogenesis imperfecta and in some of the chondrodysplasias.

Nonsense Mutations

Nonsense mutations occur when a single nucleotide substitution converts a codon for an amino acid to a termination codon. The introduction of a termination codon into the sequence results in the premature termination of translation and a truncated protein. Such proteins are rarely functional because they lack the carboxyl terminal domains that are usually required for formation of the secondary and higher orders of protein structure. The mRNAs containing a premature translational termination codon are often retained within the nucleus. Because the mutant allele is essentially functionless, it produces a state of haploid insufficiency. This type of mutation produces the common mild form of osteogenesis imperfecta.

Promotor Mutations

Point mutations within the promotor may alter the transcription of the gene. They have been identified in the β-globin gene and in the factor IX gene in hemophilia B. Few other mutations of this type have been identified in humans.

Mutations of the 3′ untranslated region may result in altered transcription or instability of mRNA, reducing the production of the relevant protein. Such mutations have been identified in the β-globin gene but not in the genes producing musculoskeletal diseases.

mRNA Splicing Mutations

Mutations of mRNA splicing are common in large genes that contain numerous exons and introns. Commonly, the point mutations occur in the consensus sequences at the exon-intron boundaries. The adjoining exon is usually spliced out, resulting in a shortened protein chain. If the exon normally starts and finishes with complete codons, the normal translational reading frame is retained, and the amino acid sequence is normal beyond the spliced-out exon. The resulting protein functions abnormally, because it is shorter than normal and because it lacks the functional domain encoded by the lost exon. If the exon contains split codons at its ends, the translational reading frame beyond the spliced-out exon is abnormal, and the amino acid sequence is incorrect. An often-encountered premature translational termination codon results in the synthesis of a truncated protein.

Abnormal splicing can also occur because of point mutations that create a new or cryptic splice site. The consequences of such mutations are often complex, because splicing may remove part of an exon and include intron sequences. Lethal forms of osteogenesis imperfecta and spondyloepiphyseal dysplasia frequently result from such mutations of the type I and II collagen genes, respectively.

Deletions and Insertions

Small and large deletions and insertions produce major changes in gene structure and in the transcript. These genetic variations result from several types of molecular alterations:

- Frameshift mutations due to incomplete codon gain or loss
- Complete codon deletions or insertions
- Gene deletions and duplications
- Insertion of duplicated elements

A protein of abnormal length and sequence may be produced. The protein may be partially functional, as observed with the shortened forms of dystrophin produced by deletions in the *DMD* gene in patients with the Becker form of muscular dystrophy.[17]

Detection of Mutations

Genetic mutations are identified by specifying the locus that is the cause of the disease and defining the range of mutations in the disease.

Identification of the disease locus involves several approaches. In some diseases, candidate genes are selected and tested for their association with the disease. For example, the type I collagen genes were the candidate genes in osteogenesis imperfecta because the protein is found in all of the major tissues affected by the disease and because protein anomalies were directly identified in these tissues. The candidate gene can be directly studied for mutations in affected individuals. Alternatively, linkage analysis is used to determine whether genetic markers or polymorphisms in or flanking the candidate gene are coinherited with the disease phenotype in families.

Knowledge concerning the disease locus is often lacking, and a list of candidate genes cannot be prepared. The chromosome and region of the chromosome containing the disease gene may be revealed by cytogenetic analysis. Translocations may disrupt a gene, producing the disease, and a microdeletion may indicate loss of contiguous genes. Linkage and gene mapping studies can then focus on these regions. Similar conditions in the mouse or other species in which the disease locus has been determined can be used as a guide for analysis of the corresponding part of the human genome. However, no leads may be forthcoming, necessitating a general genome search to identify the disease gene.

The general genome studies rely on access to families, preferably of at least three generations, in whom the members have been carefully evaluated for the disease. Blood is collected from each member. DNA is extracted for analysis of polymorphic DNA markers, which are distributed throughout the genome, particularly in regions containing the highest concentrations of genes. Linkage of a DNA marker to a disease locus is a statistical exercise. After a linked gene marker has been identified, additional studies are required to identify the disease locus. Candidate genes are sought in the region. Such an approach was successfully used in identifying the Marfan locus, which was at the same site as the fibrillin gene.[12] A similar approach successfully identified the fibroblast growth factor receptor 3 (*FGFR3*) gene as the achondroplasia locus.[31]

Mutations can be identified in the disease gene or in its products. Protein analysis may be used to verify that an individual is affected, but it is infrequently used to define the abnormal amino acid sequence, because it is more easily deduced from the abnormal DNA sequence. A popular method of identifying mutations is to prepare mRNA from cells that express the gene. The mRNA, with its compact protein coding sequence, is converted to complementary DNA (cDNA). The cDNA is amplified millions of times by the polymerase chain reaction (PCR), which is one of the most widely used techniques in molecular biology. The amplified PCR products are screened for mutations such that only a portion of the cDNA need be sequenced.

If mRNA and cDNA are not available, genomic DNA is used for mutational analysis. It is much more difficult to localize the mutation, because genes contain more noncoding than coding sequences. However, PCR is used to amplify all exons and exon-intron boundaries for mutational screening and for DNA sequencing of abnormal fragments.

CHROMOSOME DISORDERS

Chromosome disorders are more frequent than all of the single-gene disorders together.[3] They occur in about 0.7% of live births, 2% of all pregnancies of women older than 35 years of age, and in 50% of all spontaneous first-trimester abortions. They are being recognized with increasing frequency because of improvements in cytogenetic techniques. Chromosome abnormalities of number or structure can involve autosomes or sex chromosomes.

Abnormalities of Autosomal Chromosome Number

Incidence

An abnormal chromosome number, called aneuploidy, occurs in about 4% of pregnancies. Most aneuploid patients are trisomic; they have three instead of the normal pair of a particular chromosome. Monosomy, which is the loss of one member of a pair, occurs less commonly. The most common trisomies of an entire autosome compatible with postnatal survival are trisomy 21 (i.e., Down syndrome), trisomy 18, and trisomy 13. They all produce growth retardation, mental retardation, and multiple congenital anomalies. It is likely that the additional dosage of the specific genes on the extra chromosome are responsible for the abnormal phenotype.[14]

Down Syndrome

About one child in 800 is born with Down syndrome, and the frequency is higher among pregnancies of mothers older than 35 years. At birth, the babies are dysmorphic and hypotonic. They have short stature, brachycephaly, up-slanted eyes with epicanthal folds, Brushfield spots on the margin of the iris, depressed nasal bridge, low-set ears with overfolded helices, and short and broad hands with a single, transverse, simian palmar crease and clinodactyly. Cardiac malformations, duodenal atresia, tracheoesophageal fistula, and leukemia are more common than in normal babies. Congenital dislocation of the hip, patellofemoral instability, and atlantoaxial instability are common orthopaedic anomalies.

The specific karyotype has little effect on the phenotype but is important for counseling. In 95% of patients, trisomy 21 results from meiotic nondisjunction of the chromosome 21 pair. The recurrence risk increases with maternal age, particularly in women older than 30 years of age. Nondisjunction usually occurs during maternal meiosis I and occasionally during paternal meiosis I. The cause of nondisjunction is uncertain.

About 4% of patients have 46 chromosomes, one of which is a robertsonian translocation between chromosome 21q and the long arm of chromosome 14 or 22. The resulting karyotype for a robertsonian translocation between chromosome 14 and 21 is 46,XX or XY,−14,+t(14q21q), with a loss of chromosome 14, designated as −14, and a new hybrid 14q21q chromosome, designated as +t(14q21q). This karyotype produces a trisomy 21 state. The translocation forms of Down syndrome are not related to maternal age, but there is a high recurrence risk, particularly when the mother is a carrier of the translocation. A carrier involving chromosomes 14 and 21 has only 45 chromosomes because one of each of these chromosomes is missing and is replaced by the translocation chromosome t(14q21q). Down syndrome is produced when the fetus inherits a normal chromosome 21 from one parent and an unbalanced complement of chromosomes, including a normal chromosome 21 and the translocation chromosome, from the other parent. The unbalanced chromosome complement appears in 15% of the progeny of carrier mothers, which is less than the expected proportion, and it rarely appears in the progeny of carrier fathers.

Rarely, Down syndrome is produced by the inheritance of a translocation chromosome t(21q21q), made up of two chromosome 21 long arms from one parent and a normal chromosome 21 from the other parent. Carriers usually only have children with Down syndrome.

About 1% of cases of Down syndrome are mosaic for the trisomy state. There is wide variability in the severity of the phenotype, probably because of the variable proportion of trisomic and euploid cells. Germline mosaicism may account for the higher than expected recurrence risk in young mothers.

Abnormalities of Autosomal Chromosome Structure

Structural anomalies occur less frequently than anomalies of chromosome number. They are balanced if the chromosome set has the normal complement of DNA or unbalanced if there is additional or missing DNA.

Unbalanced rearrangements alter the amount of genetic information and commonly produce abnormal phenotypes. Duplication of part of a chromosome produces a partial trisomy, and deletion leads to a partial monosomy. Increasingly, small deletions and insertions are detected by cytogenetic techniques. The phenotypes of some of the deletion syndromes can be readily explained by the loss of contiguous genes. For example, in the Langer-Giedion syndrome, deletion of chromosome 8q24.11–q24.13 produces mental retardation, dysmorphism, and osteochondromas. The osteochondromas occur because the deletion includes the *EXT* locus, which is abnormal in some patients with autosomal dominant multiple exostoses.

Balanced rearrangements do not usually have a phenotypic effect, because all of the genetic information is present, although it is arranged differently. Occasionally, such rearrangements do disrupt a gene at the site of chromosome break. Balanced rearrangements increase the risk of unbalanced rearrangements in progeny.

Abnormalities of Sex Chromosomes

Sex chromosome aneuploidy produces syndromes that are associated with abnormally tall and short statures. The 47,XXY chromosome constitution, called the Klinefelter syndrome, and the 47,XYY constitution produce abnormally tall stature in males. Trisomy X (47,XXX) is the female counterpart of Klinefelter syndrome with tall stature, and 45,X and its variants (e.g., Turner syndrome) are associated with short stature. The Turner syndrome also includes gonadal dysgenesis, abnormal facies, webbing of the neck, and an increased frequency of renal and cardiovascular anomalies.

SINGLE-GENE DISORDERS

In contrast to the chromosomal disorders, single-gene defects are not detectable by current cytogenetic methods. Single-gene defects alter one or both copies of a gene. Alternate forms of a gene are called alleles. Many genes have only one allele, and others have many alleles that contain nonpathologic changes of DNA sequence. These loci are polymorphic. Mutant alleles contain changes in DNA sequence that can produce single-gene disorders.

The genetic constitution at one or more loci is the genotype. The detectable expression of the genotype is called the phenotype. Single-gene disorders are produced by a specific allele at a single locus of one or both members of a chromosome pair. If the alleles are identical, the individual is homozygous for that trait; if they are dissimilar, the individual is heterozygous; and if they have have two different mutant alleles, the individual is a compound heterozygote. Males are hemizygous for X-linked genes because they only have one X chromosome.

Patterns of transmission of single-gene defects are determined by pedigree analysis. They may involve genes on autosomes (i.e., autosomal inheritance) or genes on the X chromosome (i.e., X-linked inheritance).[23] The phenotypes are dominant if the disease is expressed when only one chromosome carries a mutant allele and recessive if both chromosomes need to carry the mutant allele.

For many genetic diseases, there is little detailed knowledge of the critical factors that link the genotype and phenotype. Many other genetic and environmental factors modify the expression of the genotype; some affected individuals show minimal or no clinical anomalies, but others show severe changes.

Penetrance is the probability that a gene defect will have any phenotypic expression at all. In pedigrees, particularly autosomal dominant pedigrees, some affected individuals fail to express the genotype. The penetrance of a gene can be defined as the proportion of individuals with the appropriate genotype who express it.

Variable expressivity refers to different severities of the phenotype among individuals who have the same genotype. Many autosomal dominant disorders show variable expressivity. For example, patients with Marfan syndrome may have few or all of the classic features of the condition.

Another form of variable expressivity is called anticipation, which refers to the apparent worsening of the disease in successive generations. This is a feature of pedigrees of myotonic dystrophy, Huntington disease, and fragile X mental retardation, and it is caused by variable and unstable expansions of DNA. Myotonic dystrophy, for example, is caused by the unstable expansion of a CTG trinucleotide repeat located in the 3′ untranslated region of a gene on chromosome 19 that encodes a protein kinase.[29]

Variable expressivity can also be a function of the age of onset of the phenotype. Some single-gene disorders, such as achondroplasia, are evident at birth and are therefore congenital. Others, such as pseudoachondroplasia, are not apparent at birth but become so after the patient is 2 to 3 years of age, when growth retardation and dysmorphism appear.

Many single-gene defects give rise to the diverse phenotypic effects referred to as pleiotropy. For many diseases, there is no obvious causative link between their diverse manifestations. It is likely, however, that links will be established as more knowledge is obtained about the molecular pathology of the single-gene disorders. For example, the pleiotropic musculoskeletal, ocular, and cardiovascular manifestations of Marfan syndrome are causally linked by fibrillin, the microfibrillar protein at fault in this syndrome, that is distributed throughout all of the affected tissues.[12]

In contrast to the considerable heterogeneity that exists in the phenotypic expression within and between the single-gene disorders, the underlying molecular changes in their mutant loci are similar, reflecting the limited number of ways in which a single gene can be altered.

Autosomal Dominant Disorders

About one half of the known single-gene defects are autosomal dominant traits. Affected individuals are heterozygous for the mutation; they have one normal and one mutant allele of the gene. However, the product of the normal allele is unable to compensate for the abnormality produced by the mutant allele. Matings of two heterozygous individuals can produce homozygous autosomal dominant traits. The homozygotes are usually much more severely affected, often with perinatal death, than heterozygotes.

Many autosomal dominant disorders have major musculoskeletal anomalies. They include many of the chondrodysplasias, osteogenesis imperfecta, Marfan syndrome, Ehlers-Danlos syndrome, acrocephalosyndactyly syndromes, absent tibial syndromes, Charcot-Marie-Tooth disease types IA and IB, and neurofibromatosis 1.

In typical families, the autosomal dominant trait is transmitted from generation to generation by affected individuals who transmit the mutant gene to about one half of their offspring (Fig. 5-2). Males and females are equally affected, and unaffected individuals do not carry or transmit the mutant gene. Typical multigeneration autosomal dominant pedigrees (see Fig. 5-2) are common in families with neurofibromatosis, osteogenesis imperfecta type I, and Marfan syndrome. However, there is wide variability of penetrance and expression of the genotype in such families. For example, in families with the common type I form of osteogenesis imperfecta, some members have grey-blue scleras and severe osteoporosis with multiple fractures but others have grey-blue scleras, a characteristic feature of the disease, without clinical evidence of bone fragility. Similar variability is observed in families with neurofibromatosis 1 and Marfan syndrome when the clinical manifestations are correlated with the inheritance of the mutant allele. Many of the individuals shown to carry the mutant allele lack the major clinical features required for a firm clinical diagnosis and are unaware that they have the disease. The latter observation applies particularly to young people who are likely to develop more obvious features with age.

Atypical autosomal dominant pedigrees occur with new dominant mutations. About one half of the individuals with osteogenesis imperfecta or Marfan syndrome and most of those with achondroplasia have new autosomal dominant mutations. The mutation occurs in the ovum or sperm involved in the formation of the fertilized ovum for the first affected individual in the family. New dominant mutations are often associated with increased paternal age, presumably due to an increased level of mutagenesis during spermatogenesis in older men. The affected individuals transmit the trait to one half of their offspring, typical of an autosomal dominant inheritance pattern.

Some families with osteogenesis imperfecta and Marfan syndrome show an apparently autosomal recessive form of inheritance, with clinically normal parents and multiple affected offspring. In most instances, genetic testing has shown that one parent is mosaic for the dominant mutation and transmits the trait to multiple children. Presumably, a spontaneous mutation has occurred early in embryogenesis of the mosaic parent, and some of the somatic cells and gametes carry the mutation. Mosaic parents may show some minor clinical features of the disease. Genetic testing of dermal fibroblasts, hair follicles, and leukocytes reveals the proportion of cells carrying the mutant allele. The sperm can be similarly tested.

Rapid progress is being made in identifying mutant genes in autosomal dominant disorders that produce musculoskeletal anomalies. Several disorders illustrate important principles and are discussed in the following sections.

Osteogenesis Imperfecta

Many of the principal features of autosomal dominant diseases are illustrated by recent findings in osteogenesis imperfecta. The majority of cases are inherited as autosomal dominant traits or occur from new autosomal dominant mutations. The mutations usu-

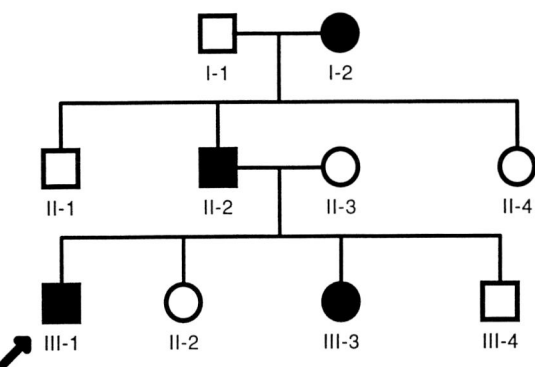

FIGURE 5-2. Typical autosomal dominant pedigree. Each individual is identified by a generation number and the position in each generation. Males are indicated by squares and females by circles. Filled symbols indicate clinically affected individuals. The proband (*arrow*) is the family member through whom the family history was ascertained.

ally involve one or other of the two genes that encode the chains of type I collagen, the principal collagen of the tissues affected by the disease. The COL1A1 gene on chromosome 17 encodes the pro-α1(I) chain, and the COL1A2 gene on chromosome 7 encodes the pro-α2(I) chain. Each type I collagen molecule contains two α1(I) chains and one α2(I) chain.

Although osteogenesis imperfecta is clinically and genetically heterogeneous, the genetic patterns are relatively simple.[5,9] The common type IA form with grey-blue scleras, osteoporosis, mild bone fragility, normal teeth, ligament laxity, and premature deafness is caused by mutations of the COL1A1 gene in which the mutant allele is functionless. The mutant allele usually produces an mRNA containing a premature stop codon that would be expected to produce a truncated and functionless α1(I) collagen chain. However, the nucleus retains most of the mutant mRNA, and the cytoplasm contains predominantly normal α1(I) mRNA, although in one half of the normal amounts. The type I collagen produced by the osteogenesis imperfecta type IA cells is normal, but the amount produced is about one half of normal. Each family has been shown to have its own private mutation leading to premature stop codons at different sites of the mRNA. Despite this genetic heterogeneity, there is a final common pathway of type I collagen deficiency that accounts for this type of osteogenesis imperfecta. Nonetheless, because the severity of the disease varies between and within families, it is likely that modifying genes and epigenetic factors also play a role in the pathogenesis of the disease.

All other forms of osteogenesis imperfecta, which include the moderate and severe forms, are caused by autosomal dominant mutations of the COL1A1 or COL1A2 genes that result in the production of a mixture of normal and mutant collagen chains and type I collagen molecules. The most common mutation involves the substitution of a glycine residue in one of the 338 glycine-X-Y triplets, the mandatory repetitive triplet sequence required for triple helix formation (Fig. 5-3). Proline is often in the X position and hydroxyproline in the Y position of the triplets. Abnormal helix formation occurs after substitution of glycine, the smallest amino acid, with the larger amino acids alanine, valine, arginine, aspartic acid, and glutamic acid. Collagen α chains carrying these substitutions are able to combine with normal chains to produce type I collagen molecules. In cases of COL1A1 mutations, one half of the α1(I) chains are expected to be mutant and one half should be normal. Because type I collagen molecules contain two α1(I) chains, it is expected that about 25% of the molecules will be normal and 75% will contain one or two mutant α1(I) chains. The particular α1(I) chain composition of the type I collagen molecules enhances the impact of the heterozygous COL1A1 mutation.

Similarly, with COL1A2 mutations, about one half of the α2(I) chains will be normal and one half will be mutant. Because type I collagen molecules only contain one α2(I) chain, about one half of the molecules will be normal and one half will contain the mutant α2(I) chain. The mutant molecules, whether containing mutant α1(I) or α2(I) chains, are more sus-

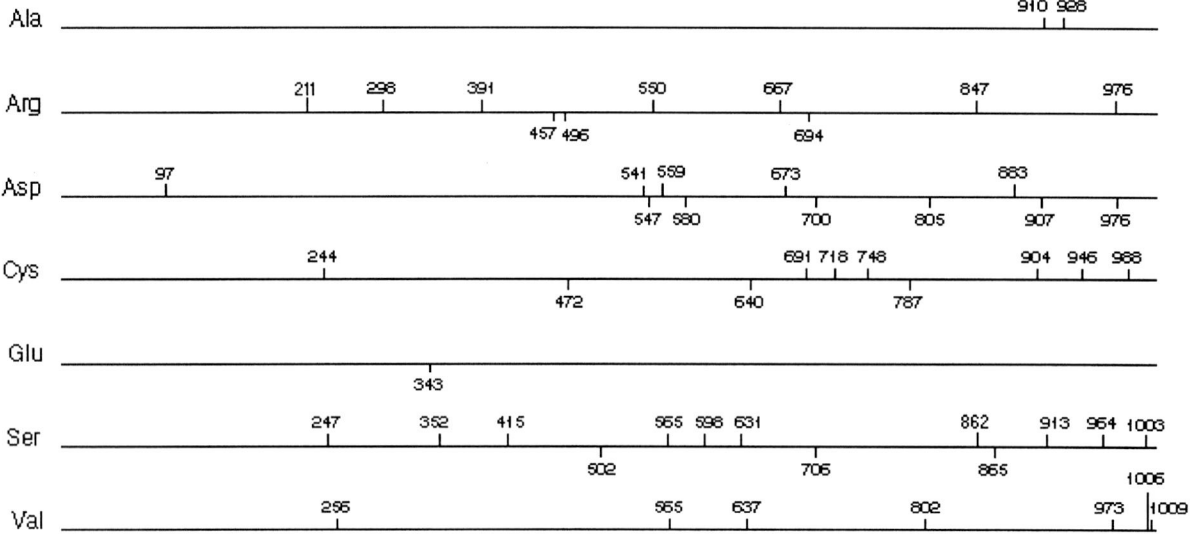

FIGURE 5-3. The diagram indicates the position of glycine substitutions in the type I collagen chains in perinatal lethal osteogenesis imperfecta. The substitutions by alanine, arginine, aspartate, cysteine, glutamine, serine, and valine are shown separately. The numbers above the line indicate the glycine residues substituted in the α1(I) chain, and substitutions in the α2(I) chain are shown below the line.

ceptible to degradation and are poorly secreted. Once secreted, they interfere with formation of the extracellular matrix of bone and other type I collagen–containing tissues. These mutations act in a dominant-negative fashion because the mutant collagen chains impair the function of the normal α chains.

Most of these families also have their own private mutations, as shown for the perinatal lethal forms of osteogenesis in Figure 5-3. There are a few examples of unrelated families with the same mutation. Variability in the severity of the disease has also been observed in such families, indicating that modifying genes and epigenetic factors contribute to the pathogenesis of the dominant-negative forms of osteogenesis imperfecta.

Little is known about the factors that are important in determining the clinical severity of the disease resulting from dominant-negative mutations of the type I collagen genes. However, most of the perinatal lethal cases result from mutations that involve the carboxyl-terminal half of the collagen chains (see Fig. 5-3). Substitutions of glycine by cysteine yield a gradient of severity, with lethal cases at the carboxyl terminus, moderately severe cases in the middle, and milder cases in the amino terminus of the α chains.

Mosaic cases giving rise to an apparently autosomal recessive form of inheritance are common. As a result, the empiric risk of recurrence in a family with a sporadic form of osteogenesis imperfecta is about 6%. The risk can be better assessed by genetic testing of the parents, but it is still only a rough estimate because the proportion of affected gametes is usually unknown. Intrauterine DNA testing for osteogenesis imperfecta is available in specialized centers.

Spondyloepiphyseal Dysplasia

The chondrodysplasias are a diverse group of genetically determined diseases affecting the structure and function of cartilage. Spranger grouped the disorders with similar features into families.[35] One family consists of a heterogeneous group of spondyloepiphyseal dysplasias. The severity of these disorders varies markedly among the lethal forms of achondrogenesis type II and hypochondrogenesis, the severely dwarfing forms of spondyloepiphyseal dysplasia congenita and Kniest syndrome, the marfanoid form of Stickler syndrome or hereditary arthro-ophthalmopathy, and mild forms with premature osteoarthritis. Heterozygous mutations of type II collagen, the principal collagen of cartilage, are found in this family of spondyloepiphyseal dysplasias. The general categories of mutations found in osteogenesis imperfecta are also found in this family of dysplasias.

The Stickler syndrome is caused by null mutations of the COL2A1 gene on chromosome 12 that encode the pro-α1(II) chains of type II procollagen.[36] The type of mutations observed in patients with Stickler syndrome are similar to those found in the COL1A1 gene in patients with osteogenesis imperfecta type IA. In both of these diseases, the mutant allele of the respective genes is functionless and leads to the production of normal collagen, although in about one half of the normal amounts.

The other members of this family of type II collagenopathies are caused by heterozygous mutations that alter the structure of the triple helical domain of type II collagen.[9,36] Unlike the marfanoid habitus of individuals with Stickler syndrome, these individuals are often severely dwarfed. The dominant-negative effects of the mutations are severe because type II collagen molecules contain three α1(II) chains. About 12.5% of the molecules contain three normal chains, and 87.5% of them contain one, two, or three mutant chains. As in osteogenesis imperfecta, the mutant molecules are poorly secreted, more susceptible to degradation, and impair normal formation of the extracellular matrix.

Achondroplasia

Achondroplasia is the most common form of short-limb dwarfism. It is inherited as an autosomal dominant trait with complete penetrance. About 87% of cases are caused by new mutations. There is a considerable reduction in the effective reproductive fitness of patients with achondroplasia.

Patients with achondroplasia have less phenotypic heterogeneity than occurs in other skeletal dysplasias such as osteogenesis imperfecta and the type II collagen family of spondyloepiphyseal dysplasias. The clinical and radiographic features are remarkably constant, and the growth plates are histologically normal despite the severe retardation of longitudinal growth. The similarity of phenotype between unrelated patients can be explained by the molecular defects in achondroplasia.

The gene for achondroplasia was assigned to chromosome 4 at locus p16.3 by linkage analysis, and mutations were identified in the gene for fibroblast growth factor receptor 3 (FGFR3).[15,22,31,41] Transcripts of this gene are most abundant in the nervous system and may account for the megaloencephaly of some patients. Outside the nervous system, the highest levels are found in the cartilage anlage of all bones and in the resting chondrocytes of the growth plate.[27] All patients have missense mutations that change glycine residue 380 to arginine or, less often, change a nearby amino acid residue.[15,38] The codon for amino residue 380 includes a CG dinucleotide, which is a "hot spot" for mutations. These mutations are expected to alter the structure of the transmembrane domain of the receptor and to produce similar functional abnormalities, accounting for the relatively invariant phenotype of achondroplasia.

Hypochondroplasia is a milder form of achondroplasia that has also been linked to chromosome 4 at locus p16.3. The milder phenotype is likely to be due to mutations in other domains of the FGFR3 protein. Thanatophoric dwarfism, a lethal chondrodysplasia, shares some phenotypic features with achondroplasia and may be caused by a particularly severe mutation at the achondroplasia locus.[1]

Homozygous achondroplasia, arising from achondroplasia matings, is extremely severe and often lethal. The same mutations as those observed in heterozygous cases of achondroplasia have been detected in homozygous achondroplasia.

Neurofibromatosis 1

Also known as von Recklinghausen's disease, neurofibromatosis 1 produces anomalies of the nervous system, café-au-lait spots, fibromatous skin lesions, pseudarthroses, scoliosis, and an increased risk of malignancies. It shows complete penetrance in that all individuals carrying the mutation express the mutation. However, expression is highly variable, and some individuals within affected families have extremely severe disease although others may have café-au-lait spots as their only manifestation of neurofibromatosis 1.

The gene responsible for this disease, *NF1*, is located on chromosome 17 at locus q11.2.[19] It is a very large gene that encodes a protein called neurofibromin. It is a GTPase-activating protein that acts as a tumor-suppressor gene.[21,25] The protein is most abundant in the nervous system.

The mutations of *NF1* include deletions, insertions, missense mutations, and nonsense mutations.[42] About 80% of these mutations potentially encode a truncated protein because of premature termination of translation. The disease expression is probably the result of haploid insufficiency, because the truncated proteins are likely to be functionless. The normal allele produces a reduced amount of normal neurofibromin that is insufficient for normal development and function of the tissues that express the *NF1* gene.

Patients with affected mothers often have a more severe disease than patients with affected fathers.[24] This phenomenon probably reflects genomic imprinting, which is a poorly understood process that alters the relative expression of the paternally and maternally derived genes.

In a few cases, the mutation is transmitted from a clinically unaffected father in whom some of the sperm contain a mutant *NF1* allele. This process is an example of gonadal or germline mosaicism.

In about 50% of patients, the disease arises from a new mutation that is not inherited from either parent. The spontaneous mutation rate is about 1 in 10,000 gametes, which is one of the highest levels in humans. This high rate presumably reflects the large size of the gene and its resulting susceptibility to deletions, insertions, point mutation, and major rearrangements. In most cases, the new mutation occurs in the paternally derived gene. This finding suggests that the mutation may occur during mitotic division that takes place in male gametogenesis but not in female gametogenesis. Because there is little or no evidence of accumulation of mutations, reflected by the absence of a paternal age effect, the mutations may be accumulating in cells that are not involved in the process of replenishment of the germ cell bank.

In neurofibromatosis 1, malignant tumors are homozygous for *NF1* gene anomalies, and benign tumors are still heterozygous for *NF1* anomalies. The malignant process arises by somatic mutation of the normal *NF1* allele and results in homozygous loss of tumor-suppressor activity of the gene.[21,32]

Autosomal Recessive Disorders

Autosomal recessive disorders account for about one third of the single-gene defects.[39] Affected individuals are homozygous, having inherited a mutant allele from each parent (Fig. 5-4). The clinically normal parents are heterozygotes, also called carriers. Carrier frequency varies considerably, but for common autosomal recessive disorders such as cystic fibrosis, it affects about 1 in 45 individuals. The mutant alleles in a population occur much more frequently in carriers than in affected individuals. For example, about 98% of the cystic fibrosis alleles are present in asymptomatic carriers and only 2% in homozygous patients.

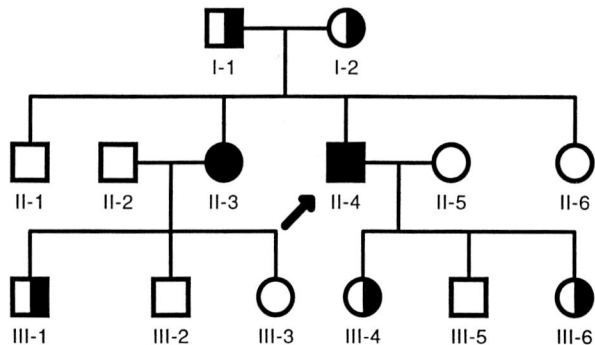

FIGURE 5-4. Typical autosomal recessive pedigree. Homozygous affected individuals are indicated by *filled symbols*. Asymptomatic carriers, who are heterozygotes, are indicated by *half-filled symbols*. The proband is indicated by the *arrow*.

Males and female are equally likely to be affected. Autosomal recessive traits are more frequent in consanguineous marriages, particularly if the mutant gene is rare.

Many autosomal recessive diseases produce inborn errors of metabolism, a term introduced by Garrod.[20] They result from deficiencies of specific enzymes, which leads to a block in a normal metabolic pathway, with accumulation of the substrate and a deficiency of the product. Because most enzymes are normally present in vast excess, a major reduction in their activity is required before a metabolic pathway is blocked. As a result, carriers rarely express inborn errors of metabolism because the activity of the enzyme produced by the normal allele is sufficient to ensure normal metabolic activity. In the homozygous state, the activity of the specific enzyme is often reduced to about 5% or less of normal values. Reductions of this magnitude are usually required before a metabolic pathway is blocked.

The consequences of an enzyme deficiency result from the accumulation of its substrate, the deficiency of its product, or both. Substrates may be readily diffusible and are found in excessive amounts in all body fluids and in all tissues. An example is phenylalanine, which accumulates in phenylketonuria, the classic example of an autosomal recessive disease. In diseases of this kind, the widespread accumulation of the substrate may result in pathologic changes in tissues that are not normally involved in the particular metabolic pathway. Damage to the developing nervous system in phenylketonuria results from this mechanism. Most of the inborn errors of amino acid metabolism produce types of changes similar to those observed in phenylketonuria. Homocystinuria is one of the few inborn errors of amino acid metabolism that produces musculoskeletal anomalies. Affected individuals have a marfanoid appearance.

Nondiffusible substrates accumulate within the cells that are normally involved in the metabolic process. Cell function deteriorates, eventually producing cell death, as the substrate progressively accumulates intracellularly. The diseases are often referred to as storage diseases, because the affected tissues progressively enlarge. Typical examples include lysosomal storage diseases such as Gaucher disease and the mucopolysaccharidoses. The lysosomal enzymes are responsible for the degradation of macromolecules such as the mucopolysaccharides of the extracellular matrix. Deficiencies of the lysosomal enzymes involved in the degradative cascade of the mucopolysaccharides produce a heterogeneous group of diseases, some of which manifest severe skeletal anomalies. This group includes Hurler, Scheie, Sanfilippo A to D, Morquio A and B, Maroteaux-Lamy, and Sly syndromes.

Similar clinical phenotypes, such as Sanfilippo A to D syndromes, can occur with different enzyme deficiencies, a phenomenon referred to as locus heterogeneity. Partial and complete deficiencies of the enzymes can also alter the severity of the phenotype, referred to as clinical heterogeneity. These syndromes may also show wide variation in clinical severity due to allelic heterogeneity, in which different defects occur in the one gene.

The clinical manifestations of some enzyme deficiencies are caused by a deficiency of the normal product rather than to an accumulation of the substrate. For example, some forms of congenital hypothyroidism result from enzyme defects in the synthesis of thyroxine.

Autosomal recessive diseases are also produced by other mechanisms, including defects in receptor proteins, membrane transport, and cell organelles. Cystic fibrosis is caused by mutations of a protein called cystic fibrosis transmembrane conductance regulator. Disorder of peroxisomes, which are subcellular organelles, produce a variety of diseases, including rhizomelic chondrodysplasia punctata.

X-Linked Disorders

X-linked disorders are readily identified by their characteristic patterns of inheritance (Fig. 5-5). Males are unaffected or affected, because they have only one X chromosome and are therefore hemizygous for X-linked genes. Females are homozygous unaffected, homozygous affected, or heterozygous, because they have a pair of X chromosomes.

Heterozygous females show variable expression of X-linked disorders because of the normal random inactivation of one or other of the X chromosomes in their somatic cells. The random inactivation of the X chromosome is called the Lyon hypothesis, which accounts for the similar levels of expression of one

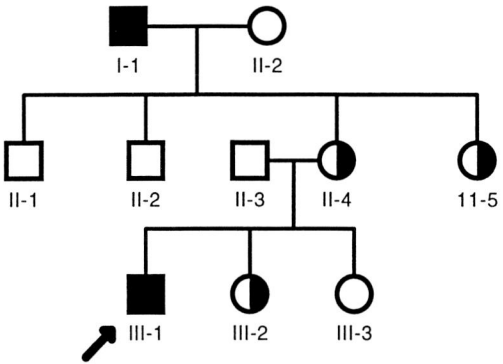

FIGURE 5-5. Typical X-linked recessive pedigree. Affected hemizygous males are indicated by the *filled squares*. Asymptomatic carrier females are indicated by the *half-filled circles*.

allele in males and a pair of alleles in females. This process is also referred to as dosage compensation; the level of expression of one dose of an X-linked gene in a male is equivalent to that of two doses of an X-linked gene in a female.

At the 16- to 64-cell stage of embryogenesis, random inactivation of the paternal or maternal X chromosome occurs in each somatic cell. The descendants of each cell have the same inactive X chromosome. As a result, the somatic cells of females are mosaic, with some cells expressing one X chromosome and the remainder expressing the other. The inactive X chromosome is condensed, and with the exception of the pseudoautosomal region, its genes are not expressed. Because heterozygous females have various proportions of cells expressing either X-linked allele, there is marked variability in the expression and clinical phenotypes. Some females appear normal, but others, referred to as manifesting heterozygotes, have the typical phenotype displayed by hemizygous males.

X-linked disorders are classified as dominant, recessive, and atypical forms of inheritance.

X-Linked Dominant Disorders

CLASSIFICATION AND INCIDENCE. An X-linked phenotype is classified as dominant if it is expressed in heterozygous females. A characteristic feature of such pedigrees is that all the daughters and none of the sons of affected males are affected. The affected females transmit the mutation in a manner similar to an autosomal dominant trait because they have a pair of X chromosomes. As a result, affected females transmit the mutation to one half of their children, regardless of the offspring's gender. Affected females are usually less severely affected than affected males because of random inactivation of one of the X chromosomes. The expression depends on the proportion of cells that express the normal or mutant allele.

Typical X-linked dominant disorders with musculoskeletal manifestations include X-linked hypophosphatemic rickets and Rett syndrome. Rett syndrome is lethal in males at birth, but heterozygous affected females are severely mentally retarded.

HYPOPHOSPHATEMIC RICKETS. This disorder is also called vitamin D–resistant rickets. It resembles metaphyseal chondrodysplasia-type Schmid, which results from mutations of type X collagen. This collagen is specific to the hypertrophic zone of the growth plate. These disorders are differentiated by the low serum inorganic phosphorus levels in the children with hypophosphatemic rickets.

The males always express the disease, because they are hemizygous, with only one X chromosome.

Variable expression occurs in heterozygous females because of random inactivation of the paternal and maternal X chromosomes.[18]

X-Linked Recessive Disorders

CLASSIFICATION AND INCIDENCE. An X-linked phenotype is classified as recessive if it is expressed in all males but expressed only in homozygous females. The latter situation is rare, because expression in females is usually limited to the manifesting heterozygotes in whom the normal X chromosome has by chance been inactivated in most somatic cells.

The X-linked gene causing the disorder is transmitted from an affected male through all his daughters. Consequently, a daughter's sons have a 50% chance of inheriting the gene. Males do not directly transmit the gene to their sons.

Typical X-linked recessive disorders include hemophilia A, which produces a deficiency of factor VIII, and Duchenne muscular dystrophy, which produces a deficiency of dystrophin.

DUCHENNE MUSCULAR DYSTROPHY. In males, this X-linked recessive disorder is lethal in the late teenage years. It is caused by mutations of the large *DMD* gene that encodes the protein dystrophin, a normal component of the muscle membrane. About one third of cases are new mutations, and the remainder are inherited from carrier females. Most of the mutations are deletions.[17] Affected males infrequently reproduce, and the disease it is transmitted by carrier females who are usually clinically unaffected. Some mutations produce Becker muscular dystrophy, which has a milder phenotype.

Atypical X-Linked Disorders

CLASSIFICATION. The inheritance pattern of an X-linked disorder may not fall into the typical dominant or recessive patterns. The fragile X syndrome is an example of a disorder with an atypical X-linked inheritance pattern.

FRAGILE X SYNDROME. After Down syndrome, fragile X syndrome is the most common cause of mental retardation in males. Females can be affected, although the phenotype is usually milder and is characterized by learning disabilities or mild mental retardation. Postpubertal males have a marfanoid appearance, macroorchidism, and mental retardation. They also have lax joints, resembling milder forms of Ehlers-Danlos syndrome.

The name for fragile X syndrome came from a characteristic cytogenetic anomaly. The chromatin in the fragile site at position Xq27.3 fails to condense during mitosis. The molecular defect is attributable to an amplification of a region containing a variable CGG trinucleotide repeat in the 5' untranslated region of the *FMR1* gene.[16] Expression of the *FMR1* gene is deficient in affected males, although normal individuals, carrier females, and males with the premutation all show normal expression.[28] Normal allele sizes vary from 6 to 54 repeats, premutations from 52 to 200 repeats, and affected individuals from 200 to more than 1000 repeats.[16] Expansion of premutations to full mutations occurs only after passage through the female germline. Males can pass on the premutation for this condition to their daughters, but it is only after female gametogenesis that sufficient trinucleotide expansion occurs to silence the *FMR1* gene and give rise to the clinical manifestations found in grandsons of the premutation males.[13]

Huntington disease and myotonic dystrophy are caused by unstable expansion of trinucleotide repeats in other genes. They, like fragile X syndrome, also have a parental sex bias in the transmission of the mutation with respect to the age of onset or clinical expression.[2]

Other Patterns of Single-Gene Inheritance

Most single-gene disorders are inherited in accordance with mendelian principles. However, alternative modes of inheritance have been identified in humans. For example, some neuromuscular and ocular diseases are caused by mutations of mitochondrial rather than nuclear DNA. They are inherited from the mother, because mitochondria are transmitted in the ovum but not in sperm. As a result, women transmit their mitochondrial DNA to all their children, but men do not transmit their mitochondrial DNA to any of their children.

Other patterns include mosaicism, genomic imprinting, and uniparental disomy.

Mosaicism

All somatic cells are usually considered to contain identical nuclear DNA derived from a single zygote. However, mutations can produce cell clones that are genetically different from the original zygote.[2] Such individuals are said to be mosaic. Mosaicism can be somatic, gonadal, or both.

SOMATIC MOSAICISM. Mutations that occur early in embryogenesis may produce somatic and gonadal mosaicism; later in embryogenesis or in postnatal life, they are limited to producing somatic mosaicism. Some unusual clinical manifestations and inheritance patterns have been observed. Asymmetrical Marfan syndrome affects one side of the body, and segmental neurofibromatosis type 1 affects a segment of the body. These mutations appear to arise early in embryogenesis and produce somatic and gonadal mosaicism, with transmission of the typical disease to offspring. Many mutations, however, occur later in embryogenesis and are limited to somatic cells.

McCUNE-ALBRIGHT SYNDROME. This syndrome is a sporadic disease that produces polyostotic fibrous dysplasia, café-au-lait spots, sexual precocity, and other dysfunctional endocrinopathies. Activating missense mutations in the gene for the α-subunit of G_s, the G protein that stimulates cyclic adenosine monophosphate formation, have been identified in these patients.[33] The mutations are found in variable abundance in different affected endocrine and nonendocrine cells, including osteoblast precursors, consistent with the mosaic distribution of abnormal cells generated by somatic cell mutation early in embryogenesis. However, because the mutations are not transmitted to offspring, the mutations presumably occur after cells are committed to form gametes.

Other examples of sporadic segmental and symmetrical disorders that probably arise by a similar mechanism of somatic mosaicism include Proteus syndrome and other hemihypertrophy and local gigantism syndromes.

MALIGNANT TUMORS. Somatic mosaicism also plays a major role in the cascade of genetic events leading to the development of malignant neoplasms.[8,11] Using retinoblastoma, which can be associated with osteosarcomas, as a model, the inherited types can be explained by a germline mutation of the *RB1* gene, followed by a somatic mutation of the remaining normal allele in a given cell. In the sporadic form, the two mutations are somatic in origin, affecting both copies of the normal allele of the *RB1* gene in the same cells. A similar mechanism applies to the development of malignant tumors in individuals with neurofibromatosis type 1. However, more complex arrangements occur, with combinations of somatic mutations and chromosomal rearrangements. The chromosomal rearrangements in tumors, such as the t(11:12)(q24;q12) translocation in Ewing sarcoma, alter the structure or regulation of cellular oncogenes or tumor-suppressor genes.[11] Mutations involving the tumor-suppressor gene *P53* are common in many malignant tumors.

GERMLINE MOSAICISM. Germline mosaicism has been observed in autosomal dominant diseases such as osteogenesis imperfecta and Marfan syndrome and in X-linked disorders. In affected families, multiple affected children can be shown by genetic testing to be heterozygous for the mutation, although the parents are clinically normal. Such pedigrees were previously considered to show autosomal recessive inheritance of the trait, with the resulting prediction that 25% of offspring would be homozygous for the mutation and clinically affected. The predicted recurrence risk may be greater, depending on the proportion of germline cells containing the mutant gene. If there is only one affected child, the prediction of recurrence risk is difficult. If neither of the parents are mosaic for the mutation, the recurrence risk is equal to the spontaneous occurrence rate of the disease in that ethnic group, which is usually low. However, the recurrence rate is significantly higher if either parent has germline mosaicism. In the absence of genetic testing of germline cells, the empiric recurrence risk of autosomal dominant or X-linked disorders for phenotypically normal parents is about 6%. The affected heterozygous children will transmit the mutation to one half of their offspring.

Genomic Imprinting

Genomic imprinting refers to the concept that certain genes are marked, or imprinted, in some way such they are expressed differently when they are inherited from the mother than when they are inherited from the father.[2] The process of imprinting often involves differences in DNA methylation that alter the transcriptional regulation of the paternally derived and the maternally derived genes.

Genomic imprinting is an important process in many human diseases, including familial cancers, chromosomal deletion syndromes, and single-gene disorders such as retinoblastoma, neurofibromatosis 1, Beckwith-Wiedemann syndrome, Huntington disease, and myotonic dystrophy. More severe forms of myotonic dystrophy and neurofibromatosis 1 occur when the mutant gene is inherited from the mother. More severe forms of Huntington disease and autosomal dominant spinocerebellar ataxia occur when the mutant gene is inherited from the father.

The Beckwith-Wiedemann syndrome is a generalized overgrowth syndrome. Hemihypertrophy, Wilms tumors, and other tumors are common in affected persons. Cytogenetic duplication of a band p15 of chromosome 11 occurs in these patients, and it is paternal in origin.[43] There is increased expression of the insulin-like growth factor type 2 gene (*IGF2*) that maps to this band. The maternal *IGF2* allele is normally repressed but is activated in some maternally inherited forms of the syndrome. These women carry chromosomal rearrangements involving chromosome 11 at locus p15 that appear to activate the *IGF2* gene. The syndrome results from increased expression of *IGF2* by a paternal duplication or maternal activation of the gene.

The chromosome deletion disorders, Prader-Willi and Angelman syndromes, highlight further the importance of genomic imprinting and parental origin of genetic material.[2,8] The Prader-Willi syndrome produces hypotonia, obesity with hyperphagia, hypogonadism, mental retardation, short stature, and small hands and feet. The Angelman syndrome is clinically distinct. Affected individuals have a happy disposition, mental retardation, repetitive ataxic movements, abnormal facies with a large mouth and protruding tongue, and an unusual type of seizure. Despite their clinical dissimilarity, these syndromes share the same cytogenetic deletion of chromosome 15 (15q11q13). In Prader-Willi syndrome, the deletion is inherited from the father, and in Angelman syndrome, it is inherited from the mother.

Uniparental Disomy

Individuals with uniparental disomy have cells that contain two chromosomes of a particular type that have been inherited from only one parent.[2,8] Isodisomy exists when one chromosome is duplicated, and heterodisomy exists when both homologs have been inherited from one parent. Examples include patients with Prader-Willi syndrome lacking cytogenetic anomalies in whom both copies of chromosome 15 had been inherited from the mother. Conversely, some cases of Angelman syndrome lacking cytogenetic anomalies result from the inheritance of both copies of chromosome 15 from the father. Some of these individuals carry two identical copies of the same chromosome 15 and have uniparental isodisomy, and others carry two different copies of chromosome 15 from one parent and have uniparental heterodisomy. These findings suggest that it is the lack of the q11–13 region of the paternal chromosome 15 that leads to the Prader-Willi syndrome and the lack of the equivalent region of the maternal chromosome 15 that produces the Angelman syndrome. These observations also indicate that both parental chromosome contributions serve necessary and complementary functions in normal growth and development.

Uniparental disomy has been observed in a few patients with cystic fibrosis who had unexplained short stature at birth. It is unclear whether there is a higher frequency of uniparental disomy in patients with intrauterine growth retardation syndromes such as the Russell-Silver syndrome, which is also associated with limb length discrepancy.

Uniparental disomy can involve the X and Y chromosomes. For example, a boy with hemophilia A inherited both sex chromosomes from his father with no contribution of sex chromosomes from his mother. Although such events occur rarely, they add to the difficulties of predicting recurrence risks.

MULTIFACTORIAL DISORDERS

Many diseases of orthopaedic importance show multifactorial inheritance.[6] Neural tube defects, congenital talipes equinovarus, and developmental dislocation of the hip are examples of multifactorial disorders that involve a combination of multiple genetic and environmental factors. Little is known about the genetic or environmental factors involved in the pathogenesis of clubfeet or developmental dislocation of the hip. However, folic acid intake during pregnancy appears to be an important nutritional factor in the pathogenesis of neural tube defects.

Many of the mutifactorial disorders behave as multifactorial threshold traits.[6] There appears to be an underlying continuous variation in liability to each multifactorial disease that has to exceed a threshold before the abnormal phenotype appears.

Several additional principles have emerged from studies of multifactorial inheritance of diseases.[39] The disorders are familial but do not show the inheritance patterns typical of single-gene defect disorders. The risk to first-degree relatives is about the square root of the population risk, but the risk is much lower for second-degree relatives. For example, the risk of congenital talipes equinovarus in the general population is about 0.001, but it is 25 times higher in first-degree relatives, only five times higher in second-degree relatives, and only twice as common in third-degree relatives. If the disorder is more common in one sex, the recurrence risk is higher for relatives of the less susceptible sex. The recurrence risk is higher when there is more than one affected family member and when the malformation is more severe. The recurrence risk is also increased when the parents are consanguineous.

Genetic counseling about multifactorial disorders involves the provision of empiric risk, which is the recurrence risk observed in similar families. It may not be accurate for a given family. Progress in defining the genes at fault can be expected to improve the risk estimates. Preventative measures, such as taking folic acid in the periconception time, may diminish the risk of neural tube defects. The pregnancy can also be monitored using α-fetoprotein levels in maternal serum and amniotic fluid and monitored by ultrasonography of the fetus.

TERATOLOGIC DISORDERS

Principles of Teratology

The effects of known teratogens on the fetus are determined by the timing of exposure and dosage.[10,34] During blastocyst formation, teratogens usually result in fetal death and spontaneous abortion. During the period of organogenesis, 18 to 60 days postconception, the fetus is most vulnerable to the effects of teratogens. Easily recognizable structural defects are the usual result. Later in pregnancy, teratogens may produce no anomaly or subtle changes.

Most teratogens act by interfering with metabolic processes. They may act on cell membranes or the metabolic machinery of cells. The final common pathway of these various levels of action is cell death or a failure of replication, migration, or fusion of cells. These changes often involve specific organs but can produce more general changes in the fetus.

Exposure of the father to teratogens does not appear to play a significant role in the development of birth defects. Most agents that interfere with the DNA of sperm produce sterility rather than teratogenic effects in the fetus.

Current methods for detecting potential teratogens are inadequate. Interspecies differences in sensitivity are common. For example, thalidomide is teratogenic in rabbits but not in rats and mice. Many agents known to be teratogenic in animals, such as glucocorticoids in rats, do not produce any detectable anomalies in humans.

Most known teratogenic agents in humans have been identified from clinical observations of unexpected outbreaks of malformations. In most instances, however, unexpected clusters of cases result from natural fluctuations in the frequency of specific birth defects, as shown by birth defect registers. Epidemiologists associated with birth defects registers play an important role in assessing whether apparent outbreaks are potentially important.

Teratogenic Agents

The selected items in the following list are teratogenic agents in humans.[34]

- Drugs and environmental chemicals
- Androgens
- Aminopterin
- Chlorobiphenyls
- Coumadin
- Cyclophosphamide
- Diethylstilbestrol
- D-penicillamine
- Goitrogens and antithyroid drugs
- Isoretinoin
- Methyl mercury
- Phenytoin
- Tetracyclines
- Thalidomide
- Valproic acid
- Infections

Cytomegalovirus
Rubella
Syphilis
Toxoplasmosis
Maternal metabolic imbalance
Alcoholism
Diabetes mellitus
Phenylketonuria
Virilizing tumors
Ionizing radiation

There is continuing concern about the possible adverse effects of drugs and other environmental factors on the developing fetus. However, relatively few agents have proven to be teratogenic.

Thalidomide

Lenz in Germany and McBride in Australia reported an increased frequency of limb-deficient babies born to mothers who used thalidomide as a sedative during the pregnancy. The agent was shown from clinical studies to produce its major effects during the period of limb formation.

Warfarin

Teratogenic effects occur from exposure of the fetus to warfarin from the sixth to the ninth week of gestation. Stippling of the epiphyses is one of the characteristic changes. Exposure during the second and third trimesters produces severe neural anomalies.

Retinoic Acid

Retinoic acid has been used in the treatment of severe cystic acne. Recipient females are often of childbearing age and are at risk from the potent teratogenic effects of this agent. It produces craniofacial, cardiac, thymic, and central nervous system defects. Megadoses of vitamin A are also teratogenic. Vitamin A, retinoic acid, and its analogs should be avoided during pregnancy. If women of childbearing age use these agents, unplanned pregnancies should be avoided by contraception.

Alcohol

Alcohol is the most common teratogen to which a pregnancy is likely to be exposed.[10,34] Regular intake of two alcoholic drinks each day during pregnancy results in a slightly reduced birthweight. Chronic intake of 8–10 drinks each day, is likely to produce babies with low birthweights, craniofacial anomalies, mental retardation, incoordination, short stature, and increased frequency of congenital heart disease. A gradient of severity of these effects are seen with intermediate levels of alcohol intake. Alcohol should be avoided during pregnancy.

Radiation

Pregnant women should avoid unnecessary exposure to radiographs and isotopes. Doses in excess of 1 Gy should be avoided, and doses in excess of 10 Gy produce microcephaly, growth retardation, and mental retardation. Women of childbearing age should not be exposed to unnecessary radiation if they may be or are known to be pregnant.

Infections

Syphilis was the first known infectious teratogen. Its deleterious effects on the fetus can be prevented by routine testing of pregnant women and treatment when necessary. The virus that causes acquired immunodeficiency syndrome (AIDS) has emerged as a major teratogen. Rubella embryopathy is preventable by vaccination of young girls. When the fetus is exposed to the virus in the first trimester, blindness, deafness, cataracts, microphthalmos, congenital heart disease, limb deficiencies, and mental retardation occur. Cytomegalovirus infection and toxoplasmosis also produce birth defects.

Diabetes Mellitus

Abnormal embryogenesis occurs more often in babies of diabetic mothers, particularly if their diabetes is poorly controlled in the first trimester of the pregnancy. For example, cardiac malformations occur three to four times more often in babies of diabetic than normal mothers, and anencephaly and myelomeningocele occur in 1% to 10% of babies born to diabetic mothers. Caudal regression syndrome with sacral hypoplasia and fusion of the legs is a rare disorder, but it is more common in the babies of diabetic mothers.

GENETIC COUNSELING AND PRENATAL DIAGNOSIS

Genetic counseling aims to provide sufficient information for an individual or couple to make an informed decision about future pregnancies and to assist them in coming to terms with the issues they face.[30]

Indications for Genetic Counseling

Anybody who suspects that there may be an increased risk of producing a child with a birth defect should receive formal genetic counseling. Appropriate genetic counseling requires diagnostic precision and knowledge of the recurrence risk, burden of the disorder, and reproductive options. There are several indications for genetic counseling:[20,30]

Couples who have a stillbirth or multiple miscarriages
A child with a birth defect
Mental retardation
Family history of any of the above problems
Relatives with known genetic diseases, such as muscular dystrophy
Exposure to radiation, drugs, or infections during pregnancy
Advanced maternal age
Consanguinity
Chromosomal translocations

Diagnostic Precision

The most important element in counseling is establishing the correct diagnosis. A precise diagnosis cannot be made for about one half of the children presenting with mental retardation or dysmorphic features. However, there is a large amount of empiric data that can be used for counseling in this group.

Estimation of Recurrence Risk

After diagnostic evaluation, an estimate of the recurrence risk is made. It is a numeric estimate of the likelihood of a particular disorder occurring in subsequent children, such as a 1 in 4 risk of an autosomal recessive disorder and a 1 in 2 risk of an autosomal dominant disorder. The recurrence risk for multifactorial disorders after a single affected child is about 3% to 5%.

Many families do not have a grasp of probabilities and need a careful discussion to give meaning to any risk estimate. For example, a 1 in 4 risk applies to each pregnancy, but many families believe that they can have three more children without worry if they already have one abnormal child.

Another aspect of risk is the background level of risk for major birth defects. About 1 in 25 children are born with a major defect. In this setting, risks of 1 in 2 and 1 in 4 are high, and risks of 1 in 100 are low.

Burden of Genetic Diseases

The burden of genetic diseases is important in genetic counseling. Clinodactyly is a common autosomal dominant condition with a high recurrence risk of 1 in 2, although it has minimal or no burden to those who have it. Clubfeet and congenital dislocation of the hip are multifactorial diseases with lower risks of recurrence. The potential burden of these conditions is minimized by early diagnosis and treatment. In contrast, the burden of additional children with Duchenne muscular dystrophy, severe osteogenesis imperfecta, or severe chondrodysplasias is considerable, because there are no curative treatments available.

There may be disparities between the doctor's concept of burden and the family's concept. Some families are prepared to accept a 1 in 4 risk of a perinatally lethal disorder, knowing that the child will die at or soon after birth or be normal. Other families may not be willing to accept the burden of recurrent deformities such as clubfeet, despite the lower risk and the availability of treatment.

Neonatal and Prenatal Diagnosis

General neonatal screening programs for inborn errors of metabolism such as phenylketonuria and hypothyroidism have been highly successful. The severe consequences of these diseases have been prevented by early diagnosis and treatment.

Prenatal diagnosis is used more selectively but is being offered to an increasing number of families as the number of diseases that can be detected in early pregnancy increases. The most common indication is a maternal age of 35 years or older. The indications for prenatal diagnosis are shown in the following list:

Advanced maternal age (≥35 years)
Known chromosomal anomaly in one parent or in a previous pregnancy
Previous neural tube defect, high serum level of α-fetoprotein, or neural tube defect suspected from ultrasound results
Family history of disorders detectable by biochemical or DNA technology, including Duchenne and Becker muscular dystrophy, myotonic dystrophy, hemoglobinopathies, hemophilia A or B, Huntington disease, cystic fibrosis, and other rare detectable genetic diseases

In most instances, prenatal diagnosis does not reveal an abnormality, providing reassurance to the parents. The availability of prenatal diagnosis increases the number of families willing to have children instead of refrain from having them because of a fear of birth defects.

Serum α-Fetoprotein Screening

α-Fetoprotein is a fetal protein produced by the yolk sac and liver. It reaches a peak in fetal serum at about 13 weeks of gestation and decreases thereafter. Amniotic levels are high in the fetus with a lesion that is not covered by skin, such as open spina bifida, anencephaly, and exomphalos. The protein leaks into the amniotic fluid and into the maternal circulation. An elevated maternal serum level of α-fetoprotein is not diagnostic of open spina bifida but is an indication for further investigation. Abnormally high levels also occur in cases of fetal death, cystic hygroma, polycystic kidneys, and Turner syndrome.

Ultrasound Screening

Real-time ultrasonography is used to visualize the fetus and fetal movements. Ultrasonography is commonly undertaken to check gestational age. However, more extensive studies by experienced ultrasonographers are required when examining for fetal abnormalities in at-risk pregnancies. Such examinations are increasingly undertaken as screening investigations in all pregnancies.

Amniocentesis and Chorionic Villus Sampling

Ultrasound-guided amniocentesis is a relatively safe procedure when undertaken at 16 weeks of gestation. The risk of fetal loss is about 0.5% to 1%. The amniotic fluid is most often used for determination of α-fetoprotein levels. The amniotic cells are used for karyotype analysis, determining enzyme levels in inborn errors of metabolism, and DNA diagnosis using direct detection of a previously defined mutation or indirect detection using polymorphisms. Chorionic villus sampling can be undertaken between 9 and 11 weeks of the pregnancy and allows earlier diagnosis of many genetic diseases and first-trimester termination. The risk of fetal loss is about 4%.

Prenatal Counseling

Families at risk for genetic diseases and birth defects should seek counseling before the mother becomes pregnant. This approach ensures that there is sufficient time available to establish the diagnosis, recurrence risk, burden of the disorder, reproductive alternatives, and suitability for prenatal diagnosis. These options may be limited when counseling is sought during the pregnancy. Parents must be fully informed about the risks of investigational procedures and anticipated delays in receiving test results. They must be given all test results and appropriate explanations of their significance. Parents require much support at this difficult time and are responsible for the decision to terminate the pregnancy.

TREATMENT OF GENETIC DISEASES

Early treatment of phenylketonuria and hypothyroidism has effectively prevented mental retardation and other consequences of these diseases. However, they are the exceptions, because treatment is not available for most genetic diseases, and when available, it is relatively ineffective. Table 5-1 lists the various levels at which intervention is possible.

Most methods of treatment, such as metabolic manipulations and protein replacement, occur beyond the level of the gene. However, bone marrow transplants have been successfully used to cure diseases such as congenital immune deficiencies, infantile malignant osteopetrosis, thalassemia, lysosomal storage diseases, infantile agranulocytosis, and chronic granulomatous disease. The normal genes of the transplanted cells produce the protein, usually an enzyme, which corrects the metabolic defect. The donor marrow cells continue to replicate, providing a continuing source of the normal protein.

TABLE 5-1. Levels of Treatment of Genetic Diseases

LEVEL OF INTERVENTION	TREATMENT STRATEGY
Mutant gene	Modification of somatic genotype
	Modulation of gene expression
Mutant mRNA	Modulation of mutant mRNA expression
Mutant protein	Protein replacement or stimulation of residual function
Metabolic or biochemical dysfunction	Specific metabolic manipulation
Clinical phenotype	Nonspecific medical or surgical intervention
The family	Genetic counseling; carrier detection and pre-symptomatic diagnosis

From Valle D. Genetic disease: an overview of current therapy. Hosp Pract 1987;22:167.

Somatic gene therapy is in its infancy but is likely to become available for many genetic diseases. Gene transfer is used to replace a gene that is nonfunctional, such as the *DMD* gene in boys with Duchenne muscular dystrophy. For other diseases, the adverse effects of the mutant allele are blocked by specific gene therapy directed to the mutant sequence. Therapy of the latter kind is most applicable to diseases in which many affected individuals share the same mutation. Designing gene therapy is more difficult for diseases in which most individuals have their own mutations, as occurs in osteogenesis imperfecta.

There are many challenges to achieving safe and effective somatic gene therapy. One of the challenges is to target the therapy to specific cells. Transplantations of modified autologous bone marrow cells are likely to be suitable for hematologic diseases and for some bone diseases. Specific cell surface receptor–mediated gene transfer is likely to be more suitable for other diseases, as in transferring a replacement gene into the skeletal and cardiac muscles cells of young children with Duchenne muscular dystrophy.

Less dramatic solutions are likely to be applicable in patients with autosomal dominant disorders that give rise to haploid insufficiency. In such patients, the protein produced is qualitatively normal but is reduced in amount because only the normal allele is functional. In this situation, the amount of normal protein produced from the normal allele is increased by specific pharmacologic modulation of gene expression. Therapy of this kind is potentially curative for one half of the cases of osteogenesis imperfecta and Marfan syndrome.

References

1. Aterman K, Welch JP, Taylor PG. Presumed homozygous achondroplasia: a review and report of a further case. Pathol Res Pract 1983;178:27.
2. Austin KD, Hall JG. Nontraditional inheritance. Pediatr Clin North Am 1992;39:335.
3. Borgaonkar DS. Chromosomal variation in man: a catalog of chromosomal variants and anomalies. 5th ed. New York: Alan R Liss, 1989.
4. Bowen P. Achondroplasia in two sisters with normal parents. Birth Defects 1974;10:31.
5. Byers PH, Wallis GA, Willing MC. Osteogenesis imperfecta: translation of mutation to phenotype. J Med Genet 1991;28:433.
6. Carter CO. Genetics of common single malformations. Br Med Bull 1976;32:21.
7. Clermont Y. Renewal of spermatogonia in man. Am J Anat 1966;118:509.
8. Cohen MM, Rosenblum-Vos LS, Prabhakar G. Human cytogenetics: a current overview. Am J Dis Child 1003;147:1159.
9. Cole WG. Collagen genes: mutations affecting collagen structure and expression. Prog Nucleic Acid Res Mol Biol 1994;47:29.
10. Danks DM, Rogers JG. Birth defects. In: Robinson MJ, ed. Practical paediatrics. 2nd ed. London: Churchill Livingstone, 1990:19.
11. Delattre O, Zucman J, Melot T, et al. The Ewing family of tumors—a subgroup of small round-cell tumors defined by specific chimeric transcripts. N Engl J Med 1994;331:294.
12. Dietz HC, Cutting GR, Pyeritz RE, et al. Marfan syndrome caused by a recurrent de novo missense mutation in the fibrillin gene. Nature 1991;352:337.
13. Driscoll DJ. Genomic imprinting in humans. Mol Genet Med 1994;4:37.
14. Epstein CJ. The consequences of chromosome imbalance: principles, mechanisms and models. New York: Cambridge University Press, 1986.
15. Francomano CA, Ortiz de Luna RI, et al. Localization of the achondroplasia gene to the distal 2.5 Mb of human chromosome 4p. Hum Mol Genet 1994;3:787.
16. Fu Y, Kuhl DP, Pizzuti A, et al. Variation of the CGG repeat at the fragile X site results in genetic instability: resolution of the Sherman paradox. Cell 1991;67:1047.
17. Gillard EF, Chamberlain JS, Murphy EG, et al. Molecular and phenotypic analysis of patients with deletions within the deletion-rich region of the Duchenne muscular dystrophy (DMD) gene. Am J Hum Genet 1989;45:507.
18. Glorieux F, Scriver CR. Loss of a PTH sensitive component of phosphate transport in X-linked hypophosphatemia. Science 1972;175:997.
19. Goldgar DE, Green P, Parry DM, Mulvihill JJ. Multipoint linkage analysis in neurofibromatosis type 1: an international collaboration. Am J Hum Genet 1989;44:6.
20. Harper PS. Practical genetic counselling. 2nd ed. Bristol: Wright, 1984.
21. Legius E, Marchuk D A, Collins FS, Glover TW. Somatic deletion of the neurofibromatosis type 1 gene in a neurofibrosarcoma supports a tumour suppressor gene hypothesis. Nature Genet 1993;3:122.
22. Le Merrer M, Rousseau F, Legeai-Mallet L, et al. A gene for achondroplasia—hypochondroplasia maps to chromosome 4p. Nature Genet 1994;6:314.
23. McKusick VA. Mendelian inheritance in man. Catalogs of autosomal dominant, autosomal recessive, and X-linked phenotypes. 9th ed. Baltimore: The Johns Hopkins University Press, 1990.
24. Miller M, Hall JG. Possible maternal effect of severity of neurofibromatosis. Lancet 1978;11:1071.
25. Nakafuku M, Nagamine M, Ohtoshi A, et al. Suppression of oncogenic Ras by mutant neurofibromatosis type 1 genes with single amino acid substitutions. Proc Natl Acad Sci USA 1993;90:6706.
26. Penrose LS. Parental age in achondroplasia and mongolism. Am J Hum Genet 1957;9:167.
27. Peters K, Ornitz D, Werner SM, Williams L. Unique expression pattern of the FGF receptor 3 gene during mouse organogenesis. Dev Biol 1993;155:423.
28. Pieretti M, Zhang F, Fu Y, et al. Absence of expression of the FMR-1 gene in fragile X syndrome. Cell 1991;66:817.
29. Redman JB, Fenwick SK, Fu TH, et al. Relationship between parental trinucleotide GCT repeat length and severity of myotonic dystrophy in offspring. JAMA 1993;269:1960.
30. Rogers JG. Genetic counselling. In: Robinson MJ, ed. Practical paediatrics. 2nd ed. London: Churchill Livingstone, 1990:55.
31. Shiang R, Thompson LM, Zhu Y-Z, et al. Mutations in the transmembrane domain of FGFR3 cause the most common genetic form of dwarfism, achondroplasia. Cell 1994;78:335.
32. Shannon K M, O'Connell P, Martin GA, et al. Loss of the normal NF1 allele from the bone marrow of children with type 1 neurofibromatosis and malignant myeloid disorders. N Engl J Med 1994;330:597.

33. Shenker A, Weinstein LS, Sweet DE, Spiegel AM. An activating G_s α mutation is present in fibrous dysplasia of bone in the McCune-Albright syndrome. J Clin Endocrinol Metab 1994:79:750.
34. Shepard TH. Catalog of teratologic agents. 6th ed. Baltimore: Johns Hopkins University Press, 1989.
35. Spranger J. Bone dysplasia "families." Pathol Immunopathol Res 1988;7:76.
36. Spranger J, Winterpacht A, Zabel B. The type II collagenopathies: a spectrum of chondrodysplasias. Eur J Pediatr 1994;153:56.
37. Stoll C, Roth M-P, Bigel P. A reexamination of parental age effect on the occurrence of new mutations for achondroplasia. In: Papadatos CJ, Bartsocas CS, eds. Skeletal dysplasias. New York: Alan R Liss, 1982:419.
38. Superti-Furga A, Eich G, Bucher HU, et al. A glycine 375-to-cysteine substitution in the transmembrane domain of the fibroblast growth factor receptor-3 in a newborn with achondroplasia. Eur J Pediatr 1995 (in press).
39. Thompson MW, McInnes RR, Willard HF. Genetics in medicine. 5th ed. Toronto: WB Saunders, 1991.
40. Valle D. Genetic disease: an overview of current therapy. Hosp Pract 1987;22:167.
41. Velinov M, Slaugenhaupt SA, Stoilov I, et al. The gene for achondroplasia maps to the telomeric region of chromosome 4p. Nature Genet 1994;6:318.
42. Weiming X, Yu Q, Lizhi L, et al. Molecular analysis of neurofibromatosis type 1 mutations. Hum Mutat 1992;1:474.
43. Weksberg R, Shen DR, Fei YL, et al. Disruption of insulin-like growth factor 2 imprinting in Beckwith-Wiedemann syndrome. Nature Genet 1993;5:143.

Chapter 6

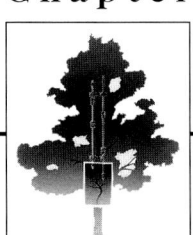

Metabolic and Endocrine Abnormalities

David J. Zaleske

Factors Influencing Skeletal Development
Mineral Phase
  Calcium and Phosphorus Homeostasis
  Rickets and Osteomalacia
Organic Phase
  Bone Physiology
  Osteogenesis Imperfecta
  Idiopathic Juvenile Osteoporosis
  Osteopetrosis
  Periosteal Reaction and Soft Tissue
    Calcification and Ossification
  Connective Tissue Syndromes

Endocrinopathies and Conditions With
  Indefinite Pathophysiology
  Normal Variant Short Stature
  Growth Hormone Deficiency and
    Hypopituitarism
  Hypothyroidism
  Gonadal Abnormalities and Sex Steroids
  Glucocorticoid-Related Abnormalities
  Fibrous Dysplasia

Metabolic bone disease includes systemic disorders of calcium and phosphorus that affect osseous tissue. The immature skeleton forms bone through turnover, which is affected by all the disorders considered to be metabolic bone disease, and bone is formed at the interface between vascular tissue and proliferating cartilage, which can be affected by genetic and endocrine disturbances that interfere with growth.[73,385,403]

The advances in molecular biology tend to blur traditional disciplines and definitions.[330,426] Pediatric patients with metabolic and endocrine abnormalities are usually under the care of pediatric endocrinologists, nephrologists, or gastroenterologists in addition to a primary pediatrician. The pediatric orthopaedic surgeon is presented with children with alterations in morphology. He or she may have to participate in the diagnosis and needs to understand the basic science for an intelligent approach to treatment. This chapter describes the physiology and pathophysiology of the formation of bone and cartilage in the immature skeleton as the basis for pediatric orthopaedic care.

FACTORS INFLUENCING SKELETAL DEVELOPMENT

Genetic, metabolic, endocrine, and physical factors interact to produce the shape of the immature skeleton places.[426] During the embryonic period (i.e., 1 week after conception to the end of the second month of gestation), morphogenesis occurs.[452] An interactive cascade of events (i.e., epigenesis) unfolds, producing a shape. The molecular basis of this complex process is being elucidated.[480] Activation of genes involved in specifying shape may control the synthesis and release of morphogens, such as the growth factors (Table 6-1), the spatial distribution of which defines the body plan.[95,436,496] At 8 weeks of gestation, vascular invasion occurs at the midshaft of the humerus in association with endochondral bone formation; this marks the end of the embryonic period and the beginning of the fetal period.

Primary centers of ossification appear rapidly at other sites. In long bones, chondrocyte hypertrophy

TABLE 6-1. Growth Factors

FACTOR	EFFECTS
TGF-β superfamily	
TGF-β1 (CIF-A)	Upregulate bone and cartilage components of types I, II, III, V, VI, and X collagen; fibronectin, osteopontin, osteonectin, thromospondin, proteoglycans, alkaline phosphatase
TGF-β2 (CIF-B)	
BMP-2 through BMP-7	
BMP-3 (osteogenin)	Down regulate metalloproteinases, osteoclasts
BMP-1 (OP-1)	Indefinite effect on chondrocytes
	Osteoclasts lead to or promote upregulation of TGF-β
FGF	
Acidic (aFGF) and basic (bFGF)	Upregulate endothelial cell and chondrocyte replication and neovascularization
Insulin-like growth factors	
Somatomedins	In skeletal growth, mediate many growth-promoting effects of growth hormone
	Upregulate the incorporation of sulfate into proteoglycan
PDGF	
A and B chains	Potent mitogen for cells of connective origin
	TGF-β leads to or promotes upregulation of PDGF-B, which leads to or promotes upreglation of protooncogenes MYC, FOS

BMP, bone morphogenetic proteins; CIF, cartilage-inducing factor; FGF, fibroblast growth factors; OP, osteogenic protein; PDGF, platelet-derived growth factor; TGF, transforming growth factor.

and death and osseous replacement advance toward both ends, leaving the cartilaginous growth plates or physes, which continue to function as endochondral bone generators until adolescence. Bone formation in the cartilaginous epiphyses occurs in the secondary centers of ossification, many of which do not appear until after birth. The timing of endochondral bone formation in various anatomic sites can be useful in establishing biologic or bone age.[216]

The fine structures of bone and cartilage have certain similarities. Both have well-defined cell populations and a characteristic extracellular matrix, and collagen is an important constituent of the matrices of both tissues (Table 6-2).[83,111] Class 1 collagens (i.e., types I, II, III, V and XI) are the banded, fiber-forming collagens. The fibrillar collagens consist of three parallel protein chains, called α-chains, that are organized into triple helices. The α-chains differ in their primary amino acid sequences, total amino acid compositions, and degrees of glycosylation.[83,111] In bone, the matrix is largely type I collagen, which is organized to allow nucleation and the growth of hydroxyapatite crystals at a finite number of sites.[207] The type I collagen consists of two α1(I)-chains and one α2(I)-chain. Type II collagen is the major collagen of cartilage matrix. It consists of three identical α1(II)-chains.

Class 2 collagens (i.e., types IX and XII) do not form aggregates alone but rather bind to the other collagens in forming fibrils. Class 3 collagens (i.e., types IV, VI, VII and X) form fibrous structures separate from the banded collagen fibers. Class 4 collagen includes types VIII and XIII, whose function is being investigated.

Several noncollagenous proteins are not so abundant as collagen, but they may be important in the regulation of mineralization.[91,92,403] These proteins are proteoglycans, phosphoproteins, and osteocalcin, which binds calcium through an α-carboxyglutamic acid moiety.

The cell types of osseous tissue are osteoblasts, osteocytes, and osteoclasts. It appears that osteoblasts are derived from mesenchymal osteoprogenitor cells. Osteoblasts are large, active cells that elaborate the matrix for bone formation. Osteoblasts that become surrounded by matrix and eventually become ossified bone persist in the form of osteocytes. Osteoclasts are multinucleated cells, originating from hematopoietic tissues, that are responsible for bone resorption.[506]

Bone is a dynamic tissue, and its turnover results from a fairly close coupling of resorption and formation. The net effect of these processes in the normal immature skeleton is an increase in mass throughout the period of growth. Bone tissue remodeling or turnover is a complex phenomenon mediated by the variety of metabolic and endocrine factors presented in this chapter. Turnover is important in skeletal homeostasis, fracture healing, and bone graft incorporation.[191,436]

There are three types of cartilage in the body: hyaline (e.g., articular cartilage, growth plates), fibrocartilage (i.e., menisci), and elastic cartilage (i.e., ear

TABLE 6-2 Collagen Types

TYPES OF COLLAGEN	TISSUES
Class 1: Fiber-Forming Collagens	
Type I α1(I)$_2$α2(I)	Skin, tendon, ligament, bone, cornea
Gene for α1[I] = *COL1A1* on chromosome 17	
Gene for α2[I] = *COL1A2* on chromosome 7	
Type II α1(II)$_3$	Cartilage, nucleus pulposus
Gene for α1(II) = COL2A1 on Chromosome 12	
Type III α1(III)$_3$	Skin and a variety of connective tissues with type I
Type V α1(V)α2(V)α3(V)	Fetal and vascular tissues
Type XI	Cartilage
Class 2: Fibril-Associated Collagens	
Type IX	Cartilage
Type XII	Ligament, tendon, perichondrium, periosteum
Class 3: Independent Fiber Systems	
Type IV	Basement membranes
Type VI	In cartilaginous and noncartilaginous connective tissues
Type VII	Anchoring fibrils
Type X	Hypertrophic chondrocytes during endochondral ossification
Class 4: Unknown Fiber Forms and Functions	
Type VIII	
Type XIII	

cartilage). All cartilages have an extracellular matrix consisting of collagen and proteoglycan; the matrix is particularly well defined in hyaline cartilage. Proteoglycan occurs in several macromolecular forms consisting of long-chain sugar polymers (i.e., chondroitin sulfates and keratin sulfate) attached to a core protein. Large numbers of proteoglycans form hydrophilic, highly electronegative aggregates along a filament of hyaluronic acid and are crucial to the structure of the cartilaginous mass. Collagen and proteoglycan are synthesized by chondrocytes.

Different types of cartilage have different compositions. Articular cartilage is aneural, alymphatic, and avascular. The property of resisting vascular invasion is important to the function of physeal cartilage. Growth plates or physes are specialized hyaline cartilaginous structures responsible for bone growth.[73] In long bones, a physis becomes radiographically distinct at either end with the appearance of the secondary center of ossification. In round and flat bones, the growth plate is a roughly spherical structure and is never visualized as a distinct radiolucency. The growth characteristics of physeal regions are endowed during the embryonic period but are subject to a variety of postnatal modifications, including metabolic factors and physical force.[452]

A longitudinal section of a growth plate reveals several zones.[73] On the epiphyseal side of the growth plate is the resting zone, which seems to participate in storing lipids and other materials. The proliferative zone contains the dividing cells of the growth plate. In the hypertrophic zone, the flattened cells of the proliferative zone enlarge and become spherical to ellipsoid. On the metaphyseal side is the zone of provisional calcification and formation of the primary spongiosa. The blood supply to the growth plate is dual, with epiphyseal vessels supporting the zone of growth and the metaphyseal vessels supporting ossification. In the lower hypertrophic zone, matrix vesicles, membrane-bound particles that contain calcific materials, are formed by the chondrocytes and are deposited in the longitudinal septa, presumably as a prerequisite for bone formation.[413,528] Neutral protease and pyrophosphatase activity located in this region lower the concentration of inhibitors of calcification and allow ossification to proceed.[164] A mini–growth plate beneath the articular cartilage enables the epiphysis to enlarge during growth, but rather than ossifying at maturity, it remains cartilaginous and may be subject to stimulation even after maturity.

Cartilage proliferation and growth plate function throughout the body are subject to control by several humoral factors.[2,496] Most notable are growth hormone and the somatomedins (see Table 6-1). Early experimental studies showed that growth was at least partially regulated by growth hormone by demonstrating that administration of pituitary extracts to hypophysectomized rats caused a significant proliferative response in growth plates.[130] Subsequent experiments demonstrated that the relation between administration of growth hormone and the phenomenon of epiphyseal growth was indirect and that it was mediated by somatomedins, materials synthesized in the liver in response to the administration of the pituitary preparation.[385]

Somatomedins are a group of short-chain polypeptides that affect DNA synthesis in the growth plate chondrocytes and enhance amino acid transport, RNA synthesis, and synthesis of proteoglycan and collagen.[496] Sensitivity to somatomedins is reduced in cartilage from older persons and in cartilage from early embryonic tissues, and it is postulated that these materials are less important for growth in early development. The growth plate chondrocytes also demonstrate sensitivity to basic fibroblast growth factor.[497,499]

Numerous other factors are important in growth plate regulation. Nutrition and insulin regulate growth plate function. Protein in the diet exerts a positive control over the somatomedins. Excess glucocorticoids appear to suppress growth by inhibiting protein synthesis in cartilage and by interfering with somatomedin production and action. Estrogens decrease somatomedin production; androgens increase growth, but not through the somatomedin system. Similarly, increased levels of thyroxine increase growth, but it is not clear whether this effect is mediated through growth hormone and the somatomedins.[193]

The regulation of bone formation is equal in complexity to that of cartilage proliferation. In the immature skeleton, under normal physiologic conditions, the two are linked at the physis, and many of the humoral factors discussed influence osseous and cartilaginous tissue.[91,253,426,431,461,505] Bone formation is also controlled by serum concentration of ions, such as calcium and phosphate, which contribute to the mineral phase; by the hormones (e.g., parathyroid hormone, calcitonin) that regulate these ions; and by other factors such as prostaglandin E_2, osteoclast-activating factor, and forms of transforming growth factor-β.[47,95,403]

Excess glucocorticoids inhibit bone formation in a complex manner. Glucocorticoid excess is associated with decreased calcium and phosphate levels and with inhibition of matrix synthesis.[482] Insulin is associated with an increase in bone formation.[92] Although in vitro, direct, anabolic effects on bone have been demonstrated, in vivo effects may be mediated by interactions with somatomedins and nutrition. Conversely, defects in early fracture healing have been documented in experimental diabetes.[158] Thyroid hormones are necessary for normal turnover of bone. Thyroid hormone increases osteoclastic bone resorption, but it is also associated with increased growth, possibly mediated through the somatomedins.

Androgens and estrogens affect skeletal growth and net bone formation. Testosterone causes an increase in growth plate activity, but estrogens appear to be inhibitory. The action on bone is less clear. In the growing skeleton, testosterone seems to increase skeletal mass (possibly on the basis of androgen-induced increase in muscle mass), but estrogen appears to stabilize the skeleton or at least to have an antiosteoporotic effect in postmenopausal women.

Prostaglandin E_2 is a potent stimulator of bone resorption.[47] Perhaps because of the combination of bone resorption and formation, bone synthesis may also be stimulated in the immature skeleton. Cyanotic infants treated with prostaglandin E_2 to maintain the patency of the ductus arteriosus have had increased periosteal bone formation.[158,504] Osteoclast-activating factor is elaborated by lymphocytes and may have a role in the formation of hematopoietic marrow.[403]

The physiology of parathyroid hormone (PTH), vitamin D, and calcitonin is fully discussed later in this chapter. At this point, it is sufficient to indicate that calcium levels are normally maintained constant by the body; phosphate levels vary more with intake but are also defended. Vitamin D exists in a variety of forms. It stimulates the transport of calcium and phosphate across the intestine and can stimulate bone resorption. PTH in response to low serum calcium levels stimulates osteoclastic resorption of bone, mediated through osteoblasts.[506] PTH increases the renal tubular reabsorption of calcium and decreases that of phosphate. Calcitonin has the reverse effect, promoting the movement of calcium and phosphate into bone. However, at least in humans, its importance does not seem to be as great as that of PTH.

Physical factors are important in regulating bone formation.[98,138] Two laws define the effect of load on proliferating cartilage and bone.[351] The Hueter-Volkmann principle states that growth plates exhibit increased growth in response to tension and decreased growth in response to compression.[246] Wolff's law states that osseous tissue remodels in response to the stress placed across it.[527] An example of compressive inhibition of growth according to the Hueter-Volkmann principle is the decreased growth anticipated from the concavity of the kyphotic spine in untreated Scheuermann disease. An example of bone remodeling according to Wolff's law is the arrangement of the trabeculae in the femoral neck. The basis of these laws at the cellular level is gradually being elucidated.[74,213] Experimental data link the mechanical force to a class of cell receptors, called integrins, that transduce the force to changes in the cytoskeleton and presumably ultimately to the genome.[514]

Although all the factors previously described play a role in the development and function of the skeletal system, genetic determinants expressed through the biology of the cell, even in postnatal life, may be the critical unifying factor. The concentrations of the enzymes necessary for normal differentiation of the skeleton, the number and availability of hormone receptors on chondrocytes and bone cells, the production of hormones, the transport systems for calcium and phosphate, and the synthetic systems for vitamin D may be genetically determined and, in normal populations, may ultimately dictate variations in the size, thickness, and shape of bones. In persons whose skeletal morphology falls outside the normal range and who are regarded as displaying metabolic bone disease, genetic errors may be the primary or accessory cause of the development of a stereotypical syndrome. In the pediatric population, in whom acquired disorders are less common, genetic causes should not be overlooked.

The following sections contain discussions of pathologic states and specific disorders often grouped as metabolic bone diseases. They are classified according to whether the primary abnormality is mainly in the mineral phase, in the organic phase, in the endocrine system, or in an indeterminate site.

MINERAL PHASE

Excluding the rachitic syndromes, most bone diseases of children in which disorders of calcium and phosphorus metabolism play a significant role are genetic (e.g., pseudohypoparathyroidism, hypophosphatasia, hyperphosphatasia) or iatrogenic (e.g., corticosteroid-induced osteopenia, anticonvulsant rickets). True metabolic bone diseases, as seen in adults, are rare in children, and disorders such as hyperparathyroidism and milk alkali syndrome are so infrequently seen in the pediatric population that they are rarely mentioned. A discussion of metabolic bone disease in children is largely confined to the subjects of rickets and renal osteodystrophy. To appreciate the aberrations seen in these two still prevalent disorders, a brief review of calcium and phosphorus balance and homeostasis is essential.

Calcium and Phosphorus Homeostasis

With the exception of the small but important amount of protein-bound and ionic calcium in the serum and extracellular space, most of the body's calcium is stored in the bones and is held in the form of hydroxyapatite, a salt with the generic formula $Ca_{10}(PO_4)_6(OH)_2$, which is composed of the very tiny crystals embedded in the collagen fibers of the cortical and cancellous bone.[31,238,346,521] The small size of the crystals ($5 \times 10 \times 20$ nm) provides an enormous surface area, and this factor, combined with the reactivity of the crystal surface and the hydration shell that surrounds it, allows a vast and rapid exchange process with the extracellular fluid. This process converts the mechanically solid structure of bone to a highly interactive reservoir for calcium, phosphorus, and other ions.[346,401] In disorders such as rickets and renal osteodystrophy, the depleted extracellular compartment of calcium can be replenished from the bone compartment, although at the expense of the strength and integrity of the skeleton.

In analyzing the homeostatic mechanisms that control the metabolism of calcium and phosphorus, three truths become evident. These principles underlie all internal shifts, and it is necessary to understand them fully to comprehend the causes and mechanisms of the rachitic syndromes.

First, a principle of inorganic chemistry states that the salt $CaHPO_4$ is not freely soluble in water. At the pH of body fluids, calcium and phosphate concentrations in the serum exceed the critical solubility product and are presumed to be held in solution by an elaborate inhibitor system. This metastable state allows the deposition of hydroxyapatite during bone formation with minimal expenditure of energy and simultaneously makes the body potentially susceptible to possible ectopic calcification and ossification as a result of increments in either or both of these materials.

Second, a principle of physiology states that the irritability, conductivity, and contractility of smooth and skeletal muscle and the irritability and conductivity of nervous tissue are inversely proportional to the calcium ion concentration. The equation for cardiac muscle is the reverse: a direct proportionality. Calcium also is an intracellular messenger, and it may be fundamental to biologic function in differential cellular organelle function.[252,409,528] The concentration of calcium in each of these compartments is a fine balance and, under certain circumstances, an exquisite one, and minimal decreases in ionic calcium concentration can lead to tetany, convulsions, or diastolic death. Conversely, increases in the concentration of calcium can lead to muscle weakness, somnolence, and ventricular fibrillation. It is essential for the body to guard the concentration of ionized calcium, and many of the mechanisms described are designed to protect against such disasters.[181,408]

Third, a principle of biochemistry states that diffusion of calcium across a cellular barrier cannot take place without a transport system. The discoveries of the components of this transport system have constituted some of the major scientific accomplishments of the 20th century and have greatly altered our approaches to the treatment of rachitic syndromes.

The transport of calcium across a gut cell occurs during absorption of calcium from the lumen of the gastrointestinal tract, across the renal tubular cell to the peritubular space in the process of tubular reabsorption of calcium, or across a bone cell in the process of crystal lysis, which occurs during bone resorption.[65,137,181,346,401] Although some evidence suggests that the mechanisms for these three processes differ somewhat, they all involve the action of the active form of vitamin D and PTH and are inhibited by an increase in the concentration of cytosol phosphate.[20,21,226,401] The principal and best-defined model is transport across the gut cell.

The gut cell at the site of absorption of calcium (i.e., distal duodenum and proximal jejunum) has a surface receptor for PTH. The circulating level of PTH is increased in response to a decrease in the serum level of ionized calcium. The circulating hormone binds to the receptor and activates an intracellular mechanism in which ATP is converted to cyclic AMP by the action of adenylcylase (Fig. 6-1). Cyclic AMP has two effects. It renders the cell membrane more permeable to ionic calcium, presumably by altering the charge on the membrane, and it induces the mitochondria, which are intracellular storehouses for calcium, to release their calcium. Both actions markedly increase the intracellular concentration of calcium but do not promote transport to the extracellular space.

At this point, the active form of vitamin D, 1,25-dihydroxyvitamin D_3 or calcitriol, acts intranuclearly to enhance the transcription from DNA of a messenger RNA that codes for the synthesis of calcium transport factor or binding protein.[266] This low-molecular-weight protein is capable of binding and transporting calcium across the cell into the pericellular space and the extracellular fluid (Fig. 6-2).[156,196,308,487,488] PTH and vitamin D work independently but not completely so. Increased concentrations of PTH are partly responsible for the increased rate of synthesis of 1,25-dihydroxyvitamin D from 25-hydroxyvitamin D. The action of the active form of vitamin D is essential to the system, but the role of PTH is less important.[20,98,221,360] This explains why the vitamin D–deficient state is more serious than hypoparathyroidism.

The role of phosphate in the calcium transport system has only recently been understood. Increases in the cytosol concentration of phosphate, such as those that occur with chronic renal failure, turn off the system and act at the level of the renal tubule to decrease the synthesis of the potent vitamin D.[55] Presumably as a protective action against exceeding the critical solubility product for calcium acid phosphate (first principle), high levels of phosphate prevent absorption of phosphate from the gastrointestinal tract, prevent reabsorption of calcium from the renal tubules, and probably prevent lysis of bone crystal. High levels of phosphate do not protect against the osteoclastic resorption of the skeleton associated with excessive concentrations of PTH.

A review of the process by which the ingested or synthesized provitamins D are converted into the active material necessary for transport of calcium can aid in the understanding of calcium homeostasis and the development of the rachitic syndromes.[266] The provitamins D consist of ergosterol ingested in the form of animal fats and 7-dehydrocholesterol synthesized in the liver (Fig. 6-3).[31,137] Both sterols are metabolically inactive, are transported in the serum by a special transport protein, and are stored in the skin.[221] In the presence of ultraviolet light at a wavelength of about

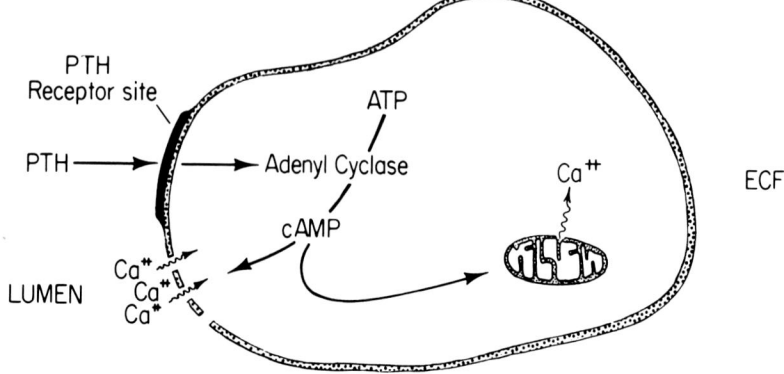

FIGURE 6-1. Action of parathyroid hormone (PTH) in calcium transport in the gut cell. Circulating PTH binds to the receptor site on the cell membrane and activates an adenylcyclase system that induces the synthesis of cyclic adenosine monophosphate (AMP) from adenesine triphosphate (ATP). Cyclic AMP (cAMP) acts to render the cell membrane more permeable to calcium ions and to induce the mitochondria to release calcium. Both of these actions fill the cytosol with ionized calcium (Ca^{++}). (ECF, extracellular fluid.)

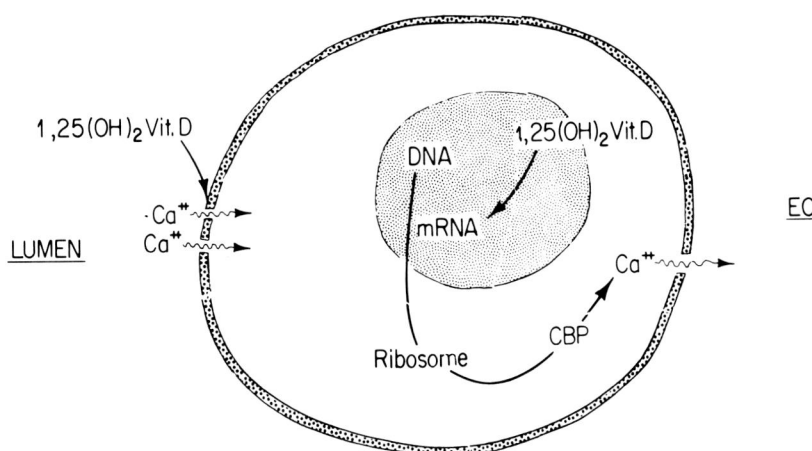

FIGURE 6-2. Actions of vitamin D on intracellular transport of calcium by the gut cell. The active hormone derived from ingested or synthesized vitamin D, 1,25-dihydroxyvitamin D (1,25(OH)$_2$Vit. D), acts intranuclearly to enhance transcription of messenger RNA for the synthesis of a calcium-binding protein (CBP), a low-molecular-weight protein that is material in the transport of calcium ion across the cell membrane. As for most sterols, 1,25-dihydroxyvitamin D exerts a *nonspecific* effect on the cell membrane to render it more permeable for the transport of the ionized calcium (Ca^{++}). (ECF, extracellular fluid.)

315 nm, a chemical conversion opens a bond on the first ring. The structures are activated to form calciferol (i.e., vitamin D$_2$) and cholecalciferol (i.e., vitamin D$_3$), respectively (see Fig. 6-3).[31,44] The compounds are then transported to the liver, in which, in the presence of an appropriate hydrolase, they are converted to the first polar metabolite, 25-hydroxyvitamin D (Fig. 6-4). In experimental circumstances, the latter material has been found to be more active than the parent compounds and acts considerably more rapidly.[59–61,261,307]

The final and most critical conversion occurs in the kidney. In the presence of specific hydrolases and a number of biochemical cofactors, 25-hydroxyvitamin D is converted to 24,25-dihydroxyvitamin D or 1,25-dihydroxyvitamin D. The former acts as a balance hormone, probably with only limited action on gut, kidney, and bone. The latter serves as the potent transport promoter for the three cellular sites (Fig. 6-5).[98,240,241] The generic name of 1,25-dihydroxyvitamin D$_3$ is calcitriol. The conditions that seem to dictate which of the two polar metabolites is synthesized have been established. The data suggest that a low serum calcium level and a high PTH level favor conversion to the 1,25 analog, and a high serum calcium level, a higher serum phosphate level, and a low PTH level favor formation of the less potent 24,25-dihydroxyvitamin D (see Fig. 6-5).[68,98,138,189,411] The protective action of the level of serum phosphate on the calcium absorptive mechanisms. A high concentration of phosphate appears to shunt the 25-hydroxyvitamin D into the less active 24,25-dihydroxy form and away from the more active 1,25-dihydroxy form.

In understanding calcium homeostasis, it is important to review some aspects of PTH metabolism and action. PTH is elaborated by the normal glands almost entirely in response to the serum concentration of ionized calcium.[181,401] Magnesium plays a role in release of the hormone, but the synthetic response is directed by a negative-feedback system with calcium only.[9,22,401] The lower the serum level, the more PTH is synthesized and elaborated. PTH acts with 1,25-dihy-

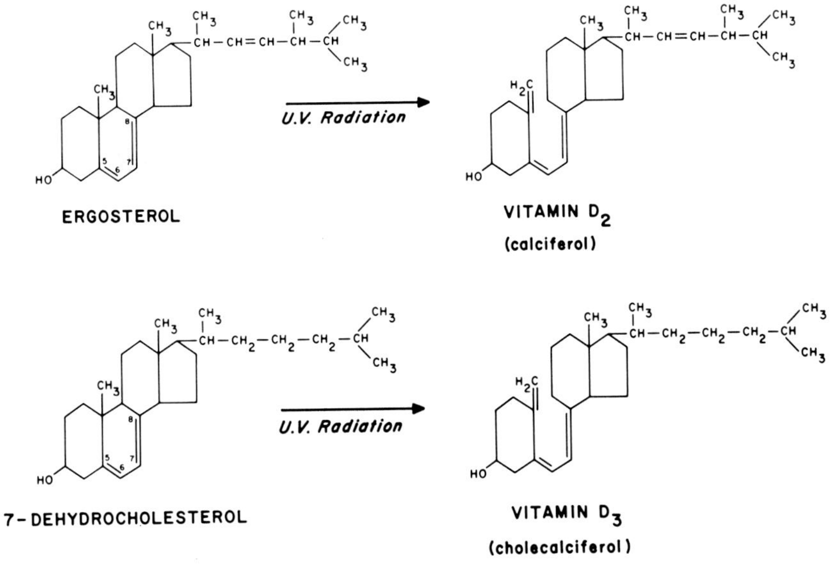

FIGURE 6-3. Provitamins ergosterol and 7-dehydrocholesterol are stored in the skin and activated by ultraviolet radiation to vitamins D$_2$ and D$_3$, respectively, by opening a bond in the first ring.

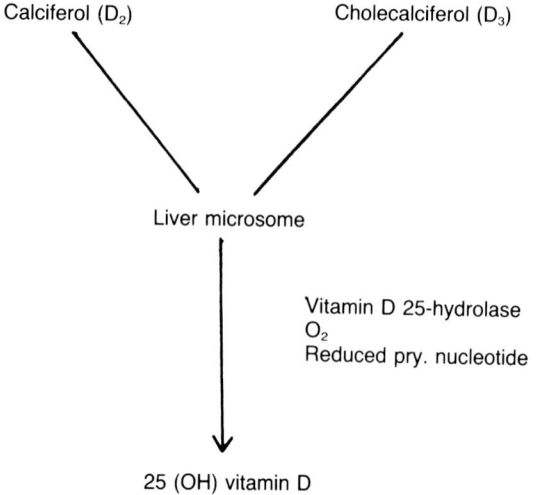

FIGURE 6-4. The first conversion of vitamin D takes place in the liver, where a specific enzyme, vitamin D 25-hydrolase, acts on the molecules to form 25-hydroxyvitamin D, a more active form of the sterol.

droxyvitamin D to facilitate cellular calcium transport in absorption from the gut, reabsorption from the renal tubule, and lysis of hydroxyapatite crystal.[20,22,401] PTH acts independently of vitamin D to activate the osteoclast population to resorb bone; this action and the other three mentioned tend to flood the extracellular space and serum with ionized calcium, correcting the deficit that initiated the demand.[22,226] Such activity puts the patient at risk of exceeding the critical solubility product for calcium and phosphate. Another action of PTH (also probably independent of vitamin D) is to diminish markedly the tubular reabsorption of phosphate. This causes a phosphate diabetes and eliminates, at least partially, the threat posed by the increased concentration of ionized calcium.[22,55,408]

In considering the actual handling of calcium and phosphorus by the intact mammalian system, it should be apparent that there are three sites of cell-mediated transport, particularly for calcium—the gut cell, the renal tubule, and bone—and that the transport taking place at these sites is mediated by the synergistic action of at least two hormones exogenous to the cell: PTH and 1,25-dihydroxyvitamin D. Both hormones are at least partially controlled by negative feedback to the concentrations of calcium. Both also appear to be inhibited at the level of the cell by hyperphosphatemia. Two other actions of PTH, which are independent of vitamin D and uninhibited by hyperphosphatemia, are osteoclastic resorption of bone and decreased tubular reabsorption of phosphate.

Because of the tight control exerted by the calcium transport system on calcium absorption from the gastrointestinal tract, it is difficult to define a minimum daily requirement for balance.[44,181,354] Most people on a well-balanced diet ingest approximately 1.0 g of calcium per day, but if a person does not eat or drink dairy products regularly, this value may drop considerably (Fig. 6-6). If a person is in neutral balance for calcium, less than 200 mg of the ingested 1.0 g is absorbed; the remainder passes out in the feces.

In addition to vitamin D and PTH, other factors operating in the gastrointestinal tract significantly affect the absorption of calcium. The first factor is pH.[250] All calcium salts are more soluble in acid media, and the ingested ionized calcium is no exception. Loss of the normal contribution of acid from the stomach reduces the solubility of the calcium salts and decreases absorption of the ionized cation. The second factor is also a function of solubility; $CaHPO_4$ is not freely soluble at the pH of body solutions, even in the acidic medium of the upper gastrointestinal tract. A diet rich in phosphate may decrease the absorption of calcium by binding the cation to HPO_4^{2-} and precipi-

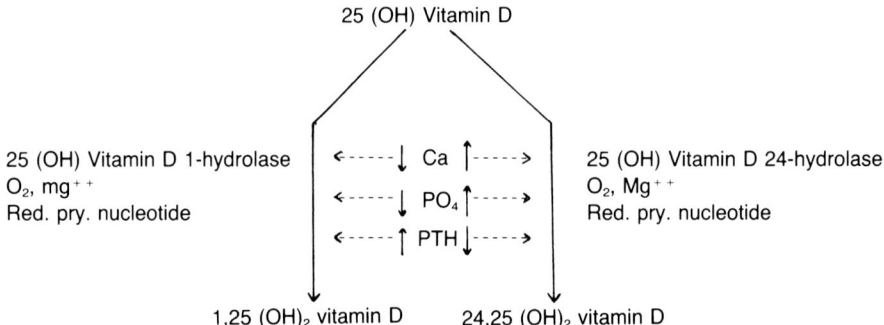

FIGURE 6-5. The second conversion of vitamin D takes place in the kidney, where at least two pathways have been described. The *maintenance* pathway (when the need is minimal, as defined by a normal calcium and phophorus and a low parathyroid hormone [PTH]) occurs in the presence of a specific enzyme (25-hydroxyvitamin D 24-hydrolase) and results in the less active 24,25-dihydroxyvitamin D. If calcium transport is required as signaled by the presence of a low serum calcium and phosphorus and a high PTH level), the body converts the 25-hydroxyvitamin D to the much more active form, 1,25-dihydroxyvitamin D.

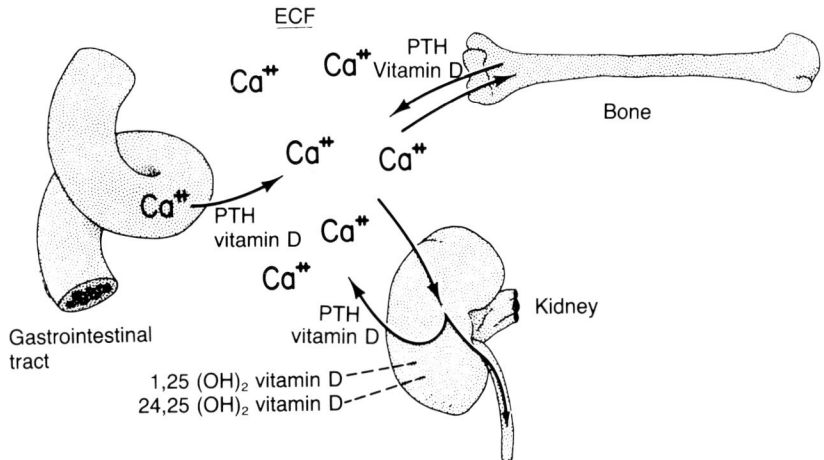

FIGURE 6-6. Calcium kinetics in the normocalcemic state. The synergistic actions of vitamin D and parathyroid hormone (PTH) appear to be necessary for the transport of calcium ions across the gut wall. Depending on the need for increased transport, 25-hydroxyvitamin D is converted to 24,25- or 1,25-dihydroxyvitamin D.

tating most of the ingested calcium as insoluble material.[29,346]

Ionic calcium can be chelated by some organic materials with a high affinity for the element. Although these materials may remain soluble, they cannot be absorbed.[29] The materials that bind calcium in this manner include phytate, oxalate, and citrate, and excesses of these substances in the diet may markedly reduce the absorption of calcium.[29,80,346,524] Calcium in the presence of a free fatty acid forms an insoluble soap that cannot be absorbed.[29,150] Disorders of the biliary or enteric tracts associated with steatorrhea are likely to reduce the absorption of calcium, because it forms an insoluble compound and because ingested fat-soluble vitamin D is less likely to be absorbed under these circumstances.[500]

Absorption of phosphorus occurs somewhat lower in the gastrointestinal tract than that of calcium and probably requires some cellular action (Fig. 6-7).[181,343,346] The action, however, is not selective, and there is not much control exerted by the endogenous or exogenous systems, because most of the phosphorus presenting to the cell in the ionized form (mostly as $H_2PO_4^-$ or HPO_4^{2-}) is absorbed. Approximately 2 g of phosphorus are ingested daily by people on a normal diet; more than three fourths of this amount are absorbed and eventually excreted in the urine. The only additional conditions in the gastrointestinal tract that exert any influence on the absorption of phosphate are high concentrations of calcium and the presence of beryllium, an unusual enteric constituent, or aluminum, which is much more common because of the use of $Al(OH)_3$ in many antacid preparations.[181,343,346] Aluminum phosphate is a relatively insoluble material, and its formation markedly reduces the rate of absorption of phosphate.

A balance diagram for calcium is shown in Figure 6-6. The absorption of calcium from the gastrointestinal tract, reabsorption of calcium from the renal tubule, and bone-blood exchange are the three major components of the calcium control system. All are under the control of the potent 1,25-dihydroxyvitamin D and PTH synergistic transport system. If calcium concentrations diminish (e.g., in a deficiency state for calcium or vitamin D), the response in the intact person is brisk and highly effective (Fig. 6-8). The lowered serum calcium level stimulates the production of PTH, which activates the synthesis of 1,25-dihydroxyvitamin

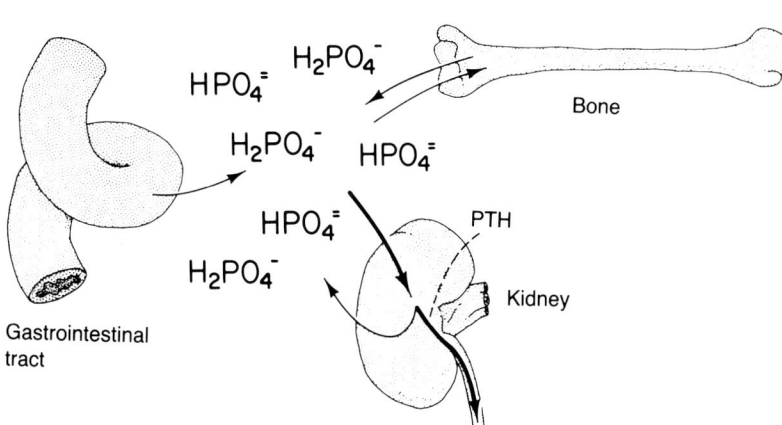

FIGURE 6-7. Diagrammatic representation of phosphate kinetics. Phosphate (PO_4) is absorbed lower in the gastrointestinal tract than calcium is and is freely transported across the gut cell to enter the extracellular space, in which it represents a major buffer system. Transport into and out of the bone is passive and related to the kinetics of the formation and breakdown of hydroxyapatite crystals. Tubular reabsorption of phosphate, however, is highly variable, with reabsorption ranging from almost 100% to less than 50%. The principal factor in decreasing tubular reabsorption of phosphate is parathyroid hormone (PTH).

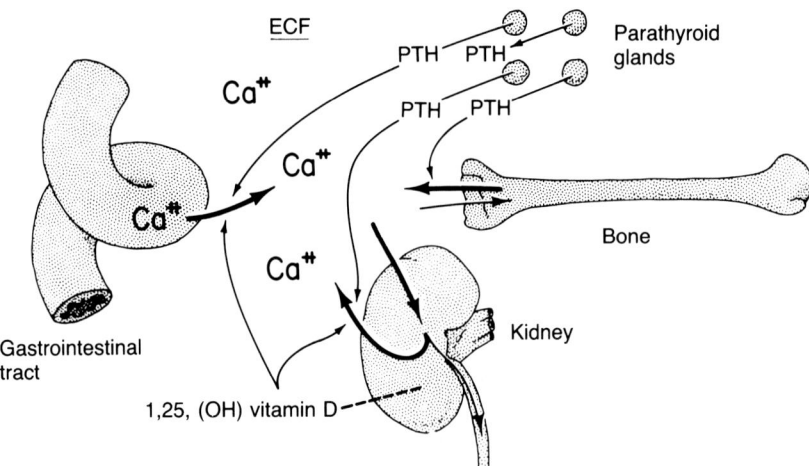

FIGURE 6-8. Calcium kinetics in the hypocalcemic state. A reduced concentration of calcium ion in the extracellular fluid (ECF) signals the parathyroid glands to release more of the potent hormone, which then acts at the level of the gut cell, renal tubule, and bone to increase transport of calcium and rapidly replenish the body fluids with calcium. An increase in parathyroid hormone (PTH) favors the synthesis of 1,25-dihydroxyvitamin D in the kidney and acts to promote phosphate diuresis by markedly diminishing the tubular reabsorption of phosphate.

D. Together, the two agents act to increase calcium absorption from the gut, tubular reabsorption of filtered calcium in the kidney, and resorption of bone. (Bone resorption occurs by lysis of the crystalline apatite and by osteoclastic resorption.) Any excess phosphate that appears as a result of the breakdown of bone is, under the influence of excess PTH, rapidly excreted by the kidney by means of a marked decrease in the tubular reabsorption of phosphate. In this manner, short-term calcium deficits, even if profound, may be rapidly corrected by a highly effective balance system.

The system in humans that counteracts hypercalcemia is not as efficient as the system that responds to hypocalcemia (Fig. 6-9). The principal mechanism of control is to turn off PTH action and vitamin D metabolism, but there is also a mechanism for lowering serum calcium, which, at least in humans, is not very effective. The hormone calcitonin mediates this mechanism. In avian species, calcitonin is very potent in this role. In mammals, calcitonin elicits only a limited response. Moreover, the autogenous calcitonin secreted by the C cells of the thyroid gland is not adequate to counteract a significant calcium overload, acutely or chronically.[338,401,408] If exogenous calcitonin is added (even from a different species), it may be effective in reducing hypercalcemia. This effect suggests that the calcitonin receptors, particularly on the bone cell, are operative but that the autogenous supply or release under control of the response feedback loop is inadequate. The major action of endogenous or exogenous calcitonin is at the level of bone. Numerous studies have demonstrated that calcitonin decreases the number of osteoclasts and the activity of the remaining osteoclasts.[21,28,338] This action reduces the rate of bone breakdown. Such a reduction in bone breakdown seems to be precisely that which is desired in Paget disease, and calcitonin has been used extensively in the treatment of this disease. The actions of calcitonin on the enteric tract and the renal cell remain far less well defined.

Rickets and Osteomalacia

The earliest descriptions of the syndrome of rickets appeared in the English literature around 1650, sug-

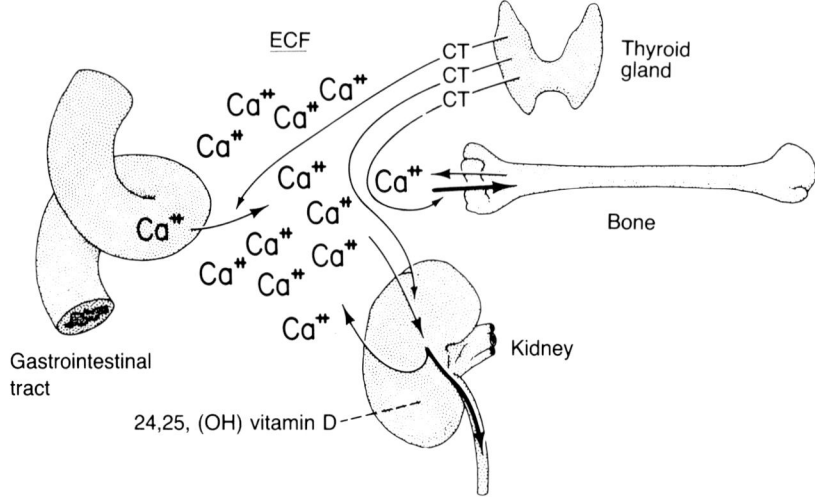

FIGURE 6-9. Calcium kinetics in the hypercalcemic state. Increased concentrations of calcium in the extracellular fluid (ECF) can cause release of calcitonin from the C cells of the thyroid gland (the ultimobranchial body in avian species), which acts to diminish calcium concentration principally by stabilizing the osteoclast and decreasing its action on the bone. Hypercalcemia and a low concentration of parathyroid hormone (PTH) act independently to diminish the synthesis of 1,25-dihydroxyvitamin D and decrease transport of calcium in the gut cell, tubule, and bone. The mechanism is not effective in humans.

gesting that the disease is an ancient one.[208,518] The history of discovery of the causes of the disorder is a fascinating saga of medical detective work and should be reviewed by the interested reader.[181,311,346]

Although there are numerous etiologic pathways, all the disease states grouped under the term rickets have as their pathogenic mechanism a relative decrease in calcium, phosphorus, or both, which is of such magnitude that it interferes with the processes of epiphyseal growth and normal mineralization of the skeleton of the growing child. The counterpart of these disorders in the adult, called osteomalacia, lacks the factor of growth abnormality, but the effects on the bones are identical. When rickets or osteomalacia occurs in patients with chronic renal failure, it has additional features that affect the skeleton; it is then known as renal osteodystrophy.

Despite the rather extensive list of possible causes of rickets and osteomalacia, the clinical presentation, histologic abnormality, radiographic changes, and some of the chemical abnormalities are virtually identical. All patients with rickets show a striking similarity to one another, and the disease, regardless of cause, is stereotypical in presentation.

Clinical Manifestations

Children with rickets are described as apathetic and irritable, often with a short attention span and seeming indifference. They are content to sit for long periods and, as observed frequently in earlier texts, often assume a Buddha posture.[453,455] The height of a child with rickets is often under the third percentile, although the weight may be normal or higher than for age-matched normal cohorts.[364,474]

In younger children with florid disease, a rather remarkable constellation of characteristic signs may be demonstrated. Children with rickets show flattening of the skull, prominence of the frontal bones (i.e., frontal bossing), enlargement of the cartilaginous components of the suture lines (i.e., caput quadratum or hot-cross-bun skull), delayed dentition, enamel defects, and frequent and severe carious lesions in the teeth.[256] Examination of the chest is likely to show enlargement of the costal cartilages (i.e., rachitic rosary), indentation of the lower ribs where the diaphragm inserts (i.e., Harrison groove), and occasionally pectus carinatum.[256,370,453] Children often have respiratory infections, and in earlier days, pneumonia was a common cause of morbidity and mortality.

The spine commonly is affected in the rachitic child, most characteristically with a long smooth dorsal kyphosis, known as the rachitic catback; occasionally slight to moderate scoliosis of limited progression exists. Abdominal distention is common (i.e., rachitic pot belly), and diarrhea and constipation have been described.

Children with florid rickets may have weak musculature of the abdomen (contributing to the potbelly appearance) and of the extremities, which sometimes appears flaccid.[437,451,507] Abductor weakness and a lurching gait are prominent features in some children who are walkers, and the onset of walking is often delayed.

The extremities are most profoundly affected in rickets and cause the child to be brought to the orthopaedist. Ligamentous laxity is common. The long bones are often somewhat shortened and deformed, usually with bowing abnormalities in the lower extremities and varus deformities of the humeri and forearms. Because of the cupping and flaring of the epiphyseometaphyseal regions, the elbows, wrists, knees, and ankles appear enlarged on physical examination. Fractures occur frequently. Slipped capital femoral epiphyses are rarely seen in patients with vitamin D–deficient or D–resistant rickets but are commonly seen in cases of renal osteodystrophy.[179,210,321,329] Mehls and colleagues think that epiphyseal slippage in renal osteodystrophy results more from the associated hyperparathyroidism and metaphyseal resorption and failure than from the widening of the growth plate.[329] This, together with the increasing availability of chronic dialysis pending renal transplantation, increases the population at risk for epiphyseal slippage at the proximal femur and at other anatomic locations.[489]

These changes are characteristic of children with severe and florid disease, usually caused by vitamin D deficiency. The changes are rarely seen in the United States but may be prevalent in other areas of the world.[209,289,336,363,434] The findings usually are subtle or vague.[429] The child with rickets is irritable and inattentive. He or she is short, has slightly thickened wrists or ankles, and possibly has bowing of one or both tibias. The diagnostic challenge is much greater with these limited findings.

Histologic Changes

The osseous and epiphyseal changes in the rachitic skeleton are striking.[152–155,256] The cortices are thinned and often show areas of increased resorption.[195,256] The quantity of medullary bone is decreased, and the trabeculae are thin and irregularly shaped. The feature that most significantly helps to establish the diagnosis is the presence of a layer of unmineralized bone (osteoid seam) surrounding a mineralized segment (Fig. 6-10).[25,195,257,316,367] This failure to mineralize newly formed bone appears most prominently in the spicules of the medulla and can be highlighted by appropriate staining techniques.[316] Although the find-

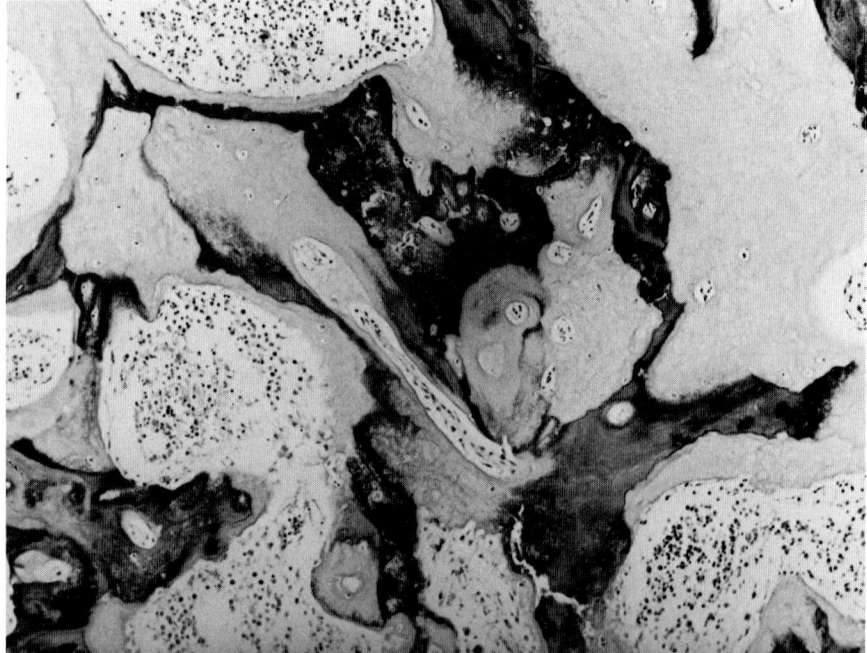

FIGURE 6-10. Histologic appearance of trabecular bone in a patient with rickets. The trabeculae are smaller than normal, but the striking feature is the presence of large masses of unmineralized osteoid surrounding central portions of irregularly mineralized bone. These osteoid seams are not pathognomonic, but when they are as wide as shown in this figure, they are diagnostic of rickets and osteomalacia. The darker-staining central portions of the bone are mineralized, and the lighter outer portions are osteoid. (von Kossa stain; original magnification ×350).

ing is not pathognomonic (i.e., also occurs in hyperparathyroidism, fibrous dysplasia, and some bone tumors), wide osteoid seams are characteristic of rickets and osteomalacia. Bone morphometricians can often establish the diagnosis with certainty on the basis of a properly studied iliac crest biopsy.[25,195,321,405] Extensive focal collections of osteoid may be seen in specific locations of the skeleton that correspond to the Looser lines; this finding is pathognomonic of the disease.[256,346]

Histologic alterations in the epiphyseal plate seen in rickets are equally striking and are diagnostic. With the exception of hypophosphatasia and to a lesser extent the milder forms of metaphyseal dysostosis (Schmid type), no other syndrome produces changes remotely resembling rickets. The resting and proliferative zones of the rachitic physeal plate are relatively normal in appearance, although some researchers have described a shortening of the columns in the region of the proliferative zone.[154,155] The maturation zone, however, shows a gross distortion (Fig. 6-11). The normally orderly columnation is usurped by a disorderly increase in the hypertrophic zone, with only a small amount of intervening matrix.[154,155,256] The plate is enlarged in its width, presumably because of the softening of the structure with limited resistance to the mechanical forces acting on it, and more characteristically, in its axial height, by as much as 5 to 15 times normal.[155,256,372]

The zone of provisional calcification in patients with rickets is poorly defined, with only a few of the defective bars between the almost nonexistent columns of chondrocytes showing the deposition of mineral.[153] Tongues of viable cartilage without evidence of active endochondral replacement descend far into the

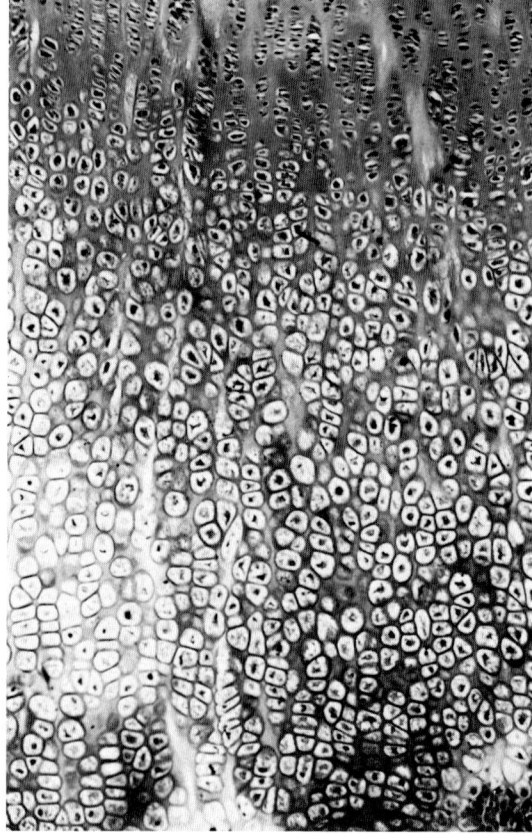

FIGURE 6-11. Histologic appearance of the epiphyseal plate in rickets. The resting and proliferative zones are relatively normal, but there is an extensive and pathognomic alteration in the maturation zone, which shows a loss of columnization, a marked increase in the axial height of the zone, and a profligate profusion of the cells. The zone of provisional calcification is poorly calcified and irregular. (Safranin-O, fast green, iron hematroxylin stain; original magnification ×100).

metaphyseal regions.[247,288] The blood supply of the physes is altered. The zone of primary spongiosa shows only limited bone formation. The few spicules of bone that form are poorly mineralized or nonmineralized and have wide osteoid seams.[256]

Radiographic Changes

When the clinician has knowledge of the altered histology, it is simple to define the radiographic changes observed in children with rickets.[389,479] The decreased bone mass of the skeletal system can be translated into osteopenia, with thin cortices and smaller trabeculae.[87,181,418,471] However, the irregular mineralization of bone, causing the histologic finding of osteoid seams, creates an indistinct image on radiographs, and the cortical and trabecular markings are often described as fuzzy or coarse and irregular.[175,464,471] The appearance of the physis or growth plate is the most remarkable feature and is virtually pathognomonic (Figs. 6-12 and 6-13).[87] The normally curvilinear or almost transverse, well-defined line on a radiography often shows irregular cupping and widening. In-

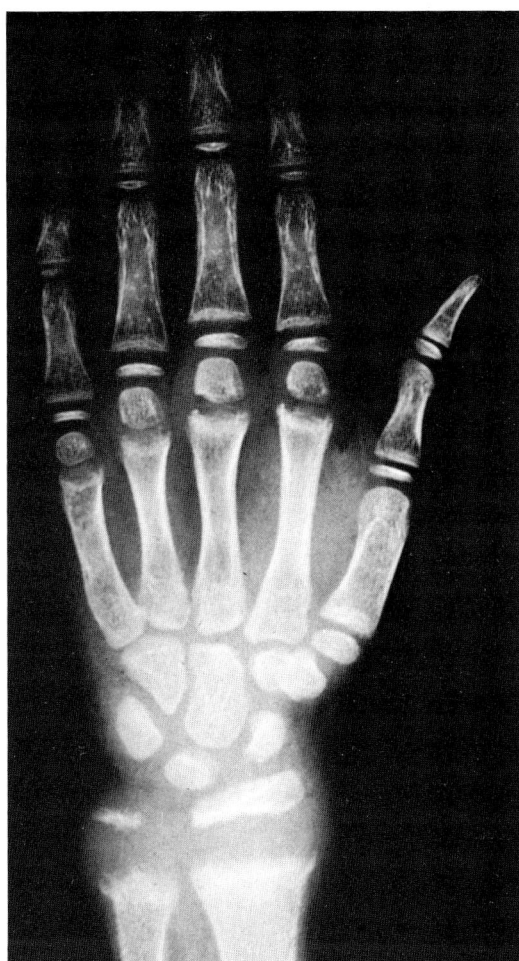

FIGURE 6-13. Changes in the epiphyseal plates of the wrist and hand are seen in this radiograph of an 8-year-old child with florid rickets. The distal radial and ulnar epiphyseal lines are markedly increased in axial height and show cupping; the zone of provisional calcification is absent. The changes in the slower-growing physes of the more distally placed bones are less marked, emphasizing the fact that rickets is a disease of the growing skeleton (in contrast to osteomalacia), and if the physeal regions grow slowly, the findings are much less prominent.

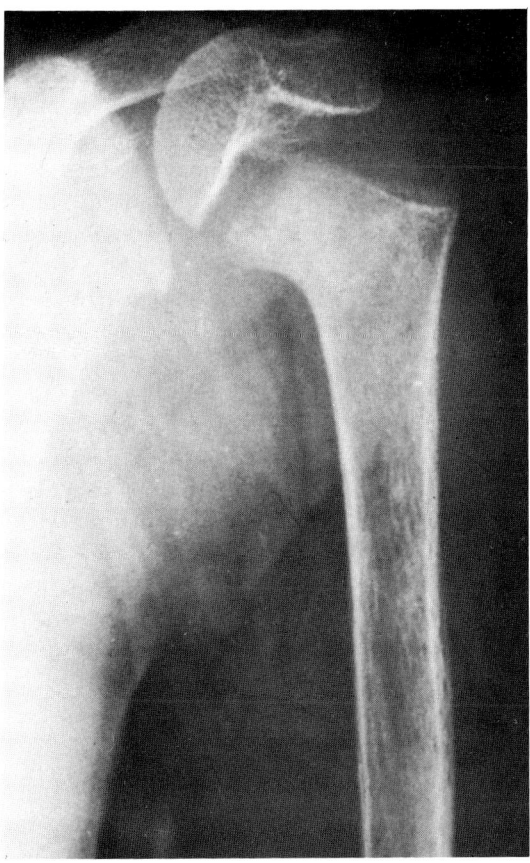

FIGURE 6-12. Radiographic appearance of rachitic changes in the humerus of an 11-year-old girl with florid vitamin D–resistant rickets. Notice the thin and indistinct cortices and the fuzzy, poorly defined trabeculae. The axial height of the epiphyseal plate is markedly increased, and the zone of provisional calcification is almost completely absent.

variably, the axial height of the line is markedly increased.[87,181,311] The zone of provisional calcification, which is ordinarily a thin, dense, white line on the radiograph, appears indistinct or is absent.[389,471] The primary spongiosa of the metaphysis is often even more osteopenic than the remainder of the bones, giving a washed out appearance to the juxtaepiphyseal region.[256,418,471,472]

In children with rickets, the most significant finding among the bone changes are the Looser lines, also known as umbauzonen or Milkman pseudofractures (Fig. 6-14). These localized collections of osteoid appear as ribbon-like linear radiolucent lines, transverse to the long axis of the bone, often not extending completely across the bone and preferring the concave sides of the long bones, medial femoral neck, ischial and pubic rami, ribs, clavicles, and axillary borders

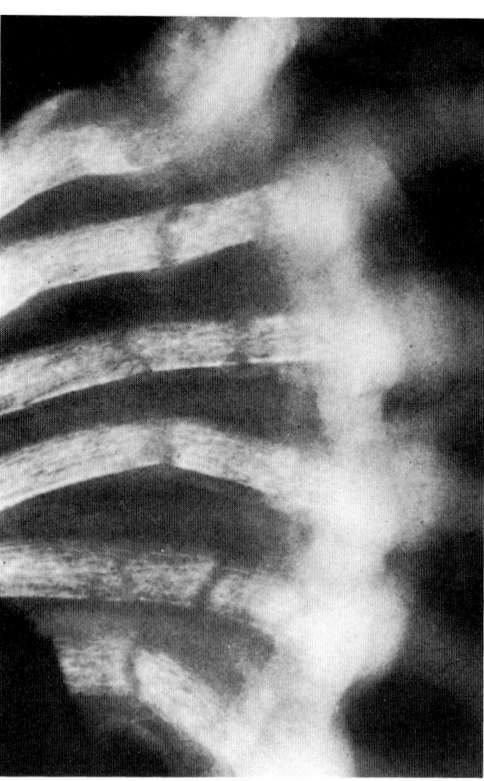

FIGURE 6-14. Looser lines seen in the rib cage of a child with florid rickets. These transverse radiolucent lines, which resemble incomplete fractures, are localized accumulations of osteoid of unknown cause. They are pathognomonic for rickets and osteomalacia.

of the scapulas. Though not true fractures, the Looser lines represent areas of weakening of the bone and may become complete transverse fractures, sometimes with only minor trauma.[236] Looser lines occur in 20% of the patients with rickets of all types but are more common in the vitamin D–resistant and renal osteodystrophic groups.[472]

Radiographic changes in patients with florid rickets are extensive and virtually unmistakable. However, in mild cases, there may be minimal or no changes, which makes the diagnosis more difficult. Bone scanning is sometimes helpful, because there may be patchy increased activity over the shafts of the long bones, ribs, and skull and especially at the sites of Looser lines.[375,450] It is appropriate to consider the first-order laboratory tests for calcium, phosphorus, and alkaline phosphatase in suspected metabolic bone disease. After obtaining the history and performing a physical examination, the physician customarily orders radiographs and analysis of the serum calcium, phosphorus, and alkaline phosphatase levels. Although changes may be subtle, this approach usually detects an abnormality (Table 6-3) that establishes the diagnosis or merits proceeding with further testing and obtaining appropriate consultation.

Causes

Numerous factors are involved in the pathogenesis of rickets (Table 6-4). The symptoms, physical findings, and radiographic alterations rarely provide clues to the cause of the disease, with the exception of renal osteodystrophy. Most patients present for evaluation with a remarkably stereotypical pattern.

In general, the changes associated with nutritional rickets appear earlier and are milder that those seen with vitamin D–resistant disease.[429] Changes occurring with gastrointestinal diseases often are consistent with the stigmata of those disorders. Patients with chronic renal disease also have findings consistent with severe secondary hyperparathyroidism and may radiographically display ectopic calcification, ossification, and occasionally osteosclerosis. To understand the manifestations of the different types of rickets and how to differentiate them and to plan treatment, it is essential to consider their pathogenesis.

Deficiency rickets primarily include vitamin D–deficient rickets, possibly chronic calcium deficiency,[382] phosphate deficiency (a rare cause),[256] and the presence of chelators in the diet.[25,181,346,458,525] All forms are rare in the United States, except in children subjected to highly atypical diets[34,161,227] or in infants born prematurely.[67,90,98,123,206,367] The model for the pathogenesis of deficiency rickets (except rickets resulting from primary hypophosphatemia) is shown in Figure 6-15.[181] The patient's intake of vitamin D is inadequate, and an insufficient quantity of 1,25-dihydroxyvitamin D is synthesized by the kidney. The result is diminished absorption of calcium from the gastrointestinal tract and resultant hypocalcemia, which promotes the release of PTH. Release of PTH partially restores the serum calcium to normal but causes a marked decrease in phosphate reabsorption in the kidney. The combination of low serum calcium, mild secondary hyperparathyroidism, and hypophosphatemia produces the syndrome of classic or vitamin D–deficient rickets. Children with this disorder usually have low to low-normal serum calcium levels, low serum levels of phosphorus, elevated levels of serum alkaline phosphatase, elevated PTH levels, low concentrations of 25-hydroxyvitamin D and 1,25-dihydroxyvitamin D, diminished levels of urinary calcium, and markedly diminished tubular reabsorption of phosphate (see Table 6-3).[24,181,200,311,346,400]

GASTROINTESTINAL RICKETS. The gastrointestinal causes of rickets are more common in most settings in the United States today than those associated with deficiency states. Gastric rickets, an unusual sequel to ulcer surgery and the dumping syndrome, is rare in children, but hepatic and small bowel problems are considerably more common and probably

TABLE 6-3 Chemical Findings in Various Forms of Rickets

	SERUM						URINE		MISCELLANEOUS SERUM AND URINE VALUES
TYPE OF RICKETS	Ca^{2+}	P	Alk Phos	PTH	25(OH) Vit D	1,25(OH)$_2$ Vit D	% TRP	Ca^{2+}	
Vitamin D–deficient rickets	↓ or →	↓	↑	↑	↓	↓	↑	↓	
Dietary phosphate deficiency	→	↓	↑	→	→	→	→	→	
Gastrointestinal rickets	↓	↓	↑	↑	↓	↓ or →	↓	↓	↓ Absorption from gastrointestinal tract
Vitamin D–resistant rickets									Amino acids, sugar, water, base in urine
I. Phosphate diabetes	→	↓↓		→	→	→	↓↓	→	
II. Reduced 1,25(OH)$_2$ vitamin D production	↓	↓	↑	↑	→	↓↓	↓	↓	
III. End-organ insensitivity	↓	↓	↑	↑	↑ or →	↑ or →	↓	↓	
IV. Renal tubular acidosis	↓	↓	↑	↑	↑ or →	↑ or →	↓	↑	Na ↓, K ↓, Cl ↑; acidosis alkaline urine
Renal osteodystrophy	↓	↑	↑	↑↑	↓↓	↓↓	?	↓↓	BUN ↑

↑, increased; ↓, decreased; →, unchanged or normal; Alk Phos, alkaline phosphatase; BUN, blood urea nitrogen; Ca, calcium; Cl, chloride; K, potassium; Na, sodium; P, phosphate; PTH, parathyroid hormone; TRP, tubular reabsorption of phosphate; Vit D, vitamin D forms.

TABLE 6-4 Causes of Rickets and Osteomalacia

Deficiency Diseases
Vitamin D deficiency
Chelators in the diet
Phosphorus deficiency

Gastrointestinal Disorders
Gastric rickets
Hepatobiliary disease
Enteric disorders

Vitamin D–Resistant Rickets (Acquired or Genetic)
Phosphate diabetes
Decrease in 1,25-dihydroxyvitamin D production
End-organ insensitivity
Renal tubular acidosis

Unusual Forms of Rickets
Rickets with fibrous dysplasia
Rickets with neurofibromatosis
Rickets with soft tissue and bone tumors
Rickets with anticonvulsant medication

Renal Osteodystrophy

account for most of the acquired forms of the disease seen in pediatric practice.[102,136,163] The hepatic causes are principally disorders in which there is an obstructive jaundice or a significant interference with the production of bile salts.[27,359] Without the emulsification action of these salts, fat accumulates in the feces and causes a significant interference with the absorption of fat-soluble vitamin D and, if free fatty acids are present, with the precipitation of the ingested calcium ions as insoluble soaps.[280,304] If hepatic damage is sufficient, the synthesis of 25-hydroxyvitamin D is reduced.[31,131,233]

In the enteric forms of rickets, injury to the gut wall caused by such disorders as the malabsorption syndrome,[359,492] gluten-sensitive enteropathy,[312,350] Crohn disease, chronic ulcerative colitis, sarcoidosis, and tuberculosis and by surgical bypass procedures[104,181,343,359,532] decreases the rate of absorption of vitamin D and calcium. If the factors of steatorrhea and rapid transit are added, there may be a profound decrease in the extracellular compartment of calcium and the development of mild to moderately severe rickets.[186,200] The mechanism by which these disorders produce rickets is not unlike that shown in Figure 6-15 for classic vitamin D–deficiency disease, except that the causes of the decrease in gastrointestinal

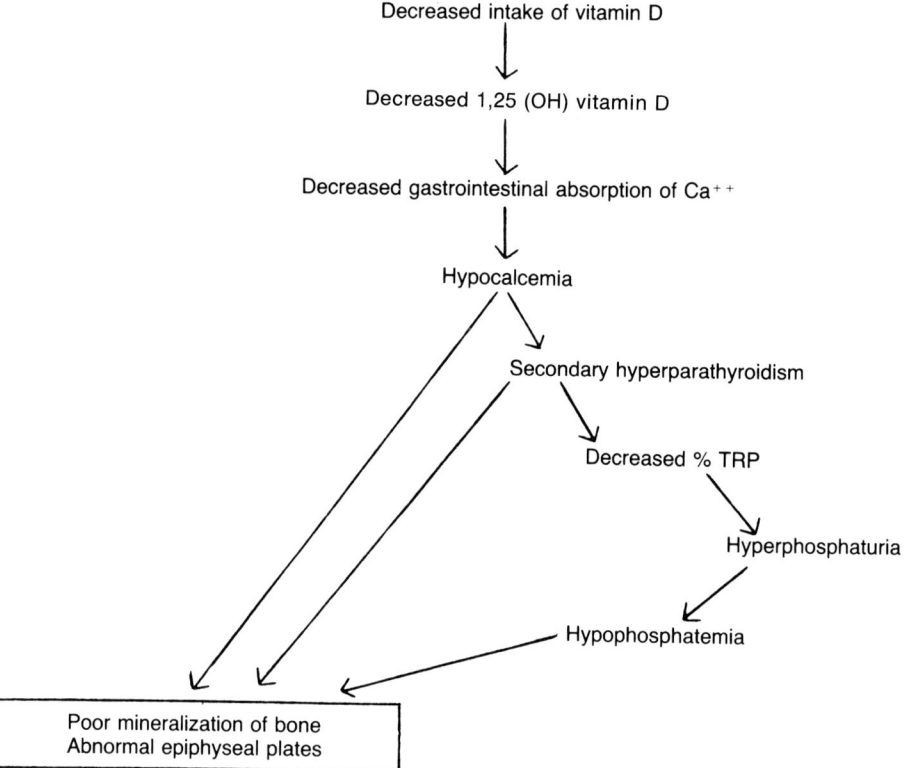

FIGURE 6-15. Mechanism of development of vitamin D–deficient rickets. A diminished intake of vitamin D causes a decreased synthesis of the potent 1,25-dihydroxyvitamin D, which causes a reduction in the absorption of calcium from the gastrointestinal tract. This progression leads to hypocalcemia, which causes a secondary hyperparathyroidism, and a reduced tubular reabsorption of phosphate (TRP), which lowers the serum phosphate. The reduced concentrations of calcium and phosphorus and the secondary hyperparathyroidism cause the clinical, histologic, and radiographic manifestations of rickets and osteomalacia.

absorption of calcium are those just cited. Beyond that level, the disorder progresses in a manner similar to that shown in the illustration. Chemically, the patients are found to be hypocalcemic, hypophosphatemic, hyperphosphatasic, and hypocalciuric, and they demonstrate elevated levels of PTH and variable concentrations of 25-hydroxyvitamin D and 1,25-dihydroxyvitamin D (depending on the amount of interference with the absorption of the vitamin).[231] These patients commonly have test results that show altered hepatic function and diminished absorptive capacity by the gut wall, and abnormalities are discovered on endoscopic and imaging studies designed to elucidate the nature of the disease process in the small bowel (see Table 6-4).

VITAMIN D–RESISTANT RICKETS. Vitamin D–resistant rickets may be acquired or genetic in origin and have a wide distribution of patterns, many of which are eponymically and, less commonly, biochemically distinct.[8,33,84,85,142,149,150,173,181,190,225,227,298,306,311,346,370,381,530] Historically, patients with these diseases were first differentiated on the basis of their resistance to the ordinary treatment doses of vitamin D and were found to have abnormal urinary excretory patterns for phosphate, sugar, amino acids, water, fixed base, bicarbonate, and some unusual materials such as ketone bodies (i.e., Lowe syndrome) and glycine (i.e., superglycine syndrome).[101,145,306] Others were found to have deposition of crystals of cystine in the liver, bone marrow,

and anterior chamber of the eye (i.e., Lignac-Fanconi syndrome)[33,54] or the presence of pure renal tubular acidosis (i.e., Butler-Albright syndrome).[348,349,415,441] Although it is historically correct and sometimes valuable to categorize vitamin D–resistant rickets in this way, there are only four basic pathogenic mechanisms operative, and all the syndromes result from one or two of these mechanisms.[217,254] Grouping the syndromes according to pathogenic mechanisms is a much sounder system, because it better directs the plan of treatment.

There are four types of vitamin D–resistant rickets: phosphate diabetes (i.e., failure of the reabsorptive mechanism for phosphate); failure of production of 1,25-dihydroxyvitamin D (i.e., vitamin D–dependent rickets); end-organ insensitivity to 1,25-dihydroxyvitamin D; and renal tubular acidosis.

In patients with phosphate diabetes, the defect principally lies in the renal tubule and is characterized by a failure to resorb phosphate filtered by the glomerulus.[25,254,370] Although there may be other resorptive defects for glucose,[145,190,298,311] amino acids,[173,190,224] or even water and fixed base[293,311] and an impairment of vitamin D synthesis in some cases,[254] the main cause of rachitic disease is probably hyperphosphaturia and profound hypophosphatemia.[254,513] After comparing the mechanism for vitamin D–deficient rickets (see Fig. 6-15), it should be apparent that children with phosphate diabetes rickets absorb vitamin D normally, make an adequate amount of 1,25-dihydroxyvitamin

D, absorb calcium normally from the gastrointestinal tract, and have no mild secondary hyperparathyroidism. However, they become rachitic because of a vast decrease in phosphate available for mineralization of the skeleton.[219] The same mechanism is operative in the rare patient who develops a dietary hypophosphatemia. The chemical findings in this group of patients are unique in that the calcium, PTH, and 25-hydroxyvitamin D and 1,25-dihydroxyvitamin D levels are often normal or only slightly lowered, but the serum level of inorganic phosphate is markedly reduced and the rate of tubular reabsorption of phosphate is often less than 50% (see Table 6-3).[127,311,370] Treatment of this group of patients with excessive amounts of vitamin D is of little value, and to achieve even a partial cure, fairly large doses of neutral phosphate must be added to the diet often.[97,170,184,303,323]

Patients who synthesize inadequate amounts of the potent 1,25-dihydroxyvitamin D are similarly resistant to standard doses of the vitamin, because they are less able to convert 25-hydroxyvitamin D to 1,25-dihydroxyvitamin D (see Fig. 6-15).[439,502] Biochemically, they show all the manifestations of the vitamin D–deficient group, except that their 25-hydroxyvitamin D levels may be normal, but their concentrations of 1,25-dihydroxyvitamin D are remarkably diminished (see Table 6-3).[439] Treatment of this group is best achieved by the addition of exogenous 1,25-dihydroxyvitamin D, which, if the syndrome has been correctly diagnosed, should be curative.[39,141,168,502]

The patients who have end-organ insensitivity are similar to those in the second group, because they ingest adequate amounts of vitamin D but, instead of a block to synthesis, they produce both polar metabolites, 25-hydroxyvitamin D and 1,25-dihydroxyvitamin D, in ample quantities. The problem appears to lie with the gut cell, which displays a relative insensitivity to autogenous 1,25-dihydroxyvitamin D.[77,464] Despite adequate amounts of the active D vitamins, the gut cell is unable to synthesize the transport system, and the movement of calcium is sharply reduced. These patients develop hypocalcemia, secondary hyperparathyroidism, hypophosphatemia, reduced urinary calcium, and reduced tubular reabsorption of phosphate, but the values for 25-hydroxyvitamin D and 1,25-dihydroxyvitamin D are normal or, in many cases, elevated (see Table 6-3).[77] Management of patients with end-organ insensitivity is difficult. In some patients, the insensitivity is relative and can be overcome by increased amounts of exogenous 1,25-dihydroxyvitamin D (still below the level of toxicity).[77] In other patients, calcium infusions may present a temporary solution but have limited application in long-term management.[112]

The fourth form of vitamin D–resistant rickets, renal tubular acidosis, is a misnomer because it is not directly related to vitamin D but is the result of an acquired or genetic error in renal handling of fixed base and bicarbonate.[165,166,348,414,441] In one form, the kidney is unable to establish a hydrogen ion gradient and therefore must excrete fixed base, including sodium and calcium.[349] In another form of renal tubular acidosis, the failure of the tubule to resorb bicarbonate causes a loss of fixed base as a cation.[349] Regardless of cause, the patient develops renal tubular acidosis, characterized chemically by a hyperchloremic, hyponatremic, hypokalemic acidosis with an alkaline urine (see Table 6-3).[36,324,349,415,438,441] In many patients with a broader lesion, resorption of phosphate is also impaired, heightening the degree of metabolic bone disease. In some, because of the increased movement of calcium through the collecting system at an alkaline pH (and failure of citrate production), renal calcinosis can be severe and can lead to renal failure.[36,114,181,250,311]

Because of the pathogenesis of these syndromes, the use of vitamin D in other than low doses is usually contraindicated. The treatment of choice is correction of the metabolic abnormality by alkalization. For most patients, this rectifies the metabolic disturbance.[124,324]

UNUSUAL FORMS OF RICKETS. Several unusual forms of rickets deserve attention. Three are types of vitamin D–resistant rickets and are defined in terms of the disease state and in terms of the associated syndrome. For example, severe rickets may be a concomitant finding in patients with neurofibromatosis[311,432,478] or fibrous dysplasia.[144,220,287,325,483] The cause or relation to either syndrome is unknown. Rickets may also occur in certain patients with benign or even low-grade malignant soft tissue tumors or, less frequently, with bone tumors of the fibrous series.[26,128,342,391] Production of an anti vitamin D factor or a phosphaturic agent by the lesion has been postulated, primarily on the basis of the almost immediate reversal of the metabolic and radiographic alteration with resection of the tumor and prompt return of the metabolic problem with recurrence of the lesion.[373] One report partially characterized such a factor.[89]

Another unusual form is rickets associated with anticonvulsant medication. For more than 15 years, scientists and clinicians have observed that patients who receive almost any anticonvulsant medication may develop a mild chemical (and occasionally osseous) rickets.[18,64,87,100,121,146,182,347,507] Although the disorder is reversible with administration of vitamin D, it represents a major problem, partly because it is difficult to diagnose by standard means and, more important, because the irritability of the central nervous system is inversely proportional to calcium ion concentration (i.e., second principle).[296,526] As the concentration of calcium falls in relation to the use of anticonvulsant medication, the patient may not respond to medication and have more convulsions. The biochemical defect in these patients appears to result from a mild injury to the hepatic cell that alters the microsomal enzyme system sufficiently to decrease the concentration of 25-hydroxyvitamin D.[146,202,219,347] Diagnosis is based on the findings of classic vitamin D deficiency in a child who is receiving anticonvulsant medication. The concentrations of 25-hydroxyvitamin D are usually sharply reduced. The goal of treatment is to increase vitamin D and, if possible, to reduce the levels of the anticonvulsant drugs.[239] One report emphasized that the relation between the administration of anticonvulsant medication and the occurrence of rickets in an otherwise healthy population is not a simple one.[494]

Renal Osteodystrophy

The constellation of clinical problems associated with chronic renal failure affects most of the organ systems and produces moderate to severe impairment of these systems. The skeletal system shares in these disabilities to an extraordinary degree; it is affected by osteoporosis, osteomyelitis, and gout associated with chronic debilitating illness and the problems associated with attempts at management (e.g., corticosteroid-induced osteoporosis, osteonecrosis, dialysis osteomalacia, arthropathy), and errors in calcium and phosphorus homeostasis.[301,310]

In the years that preceded the period of aggressive therapy of chronic renal disease, the prognosis for survival of patients with renal failure was so poor that the osseous manifestations were considered a medical curiosity, worthy only of emergency treatment for fractures and other acute changes but of little importance to the overall picture. During the past three decades, this pattern has changed radically. With dialysis systems and renal transplantation, patients with chronic renal disease can live considerably longer and can be expected to participate in activities that require a competent skeleton. Management of the whole patient now demands careful attention to the problems of the skeletal system and a thorough understanding of their pathogenesis.[58,366]

PATHOPHYSIOLOGY. The pathophysiologic events that lead to the syndrome of renal osteodystrophy are illustrated in Figure 6-16. Damage to the glomerulus causes retention of phosphate, producing hyperphosphatemia.[211,346] Concomitant tubular injury leads to a reduction in the production of 1,25-dihydroxyvitamin D.[31,72,139,311,322,371] Hyperphosphatemic suppression of 1,25-dihydroxyvitamin D synthesis and reduced tubular mass conspire to offer only a small fraction of the potent principle to the gut cell.[419] The increased concentration of phosphate in the cytosol reduces the absorption of calcium in the gut to virtually zero. Balance studies have shown that more calcium is excreted in the feces than is ingested in the diet, suggesting intestinal secretion of the mineral. All these factors conspire to produce profound hypocalcemia.[69,72,106,264,271,275,466,467]

If it were not for the acidosis characteristic of chronic renal disease, which makes more soluble the small quantity of available calcium salts, the level of calcium in the serum would lead to severe neural, motor, and cardiac disorders in many patients. The negative-feedback system that causes elaboration of PTH in response to decreases in serum calcium is unimpaired by chronic renal failure, and, within a short period, marked secondary hyperparathyroidism occurs, usually in the form of a clear cell hyperplasia of all four glands.[52,224,311,371,468] The increased elaboration of PTH is ineffective in increasing gastrointestinal absorption or renal tubular reabsorption because of the absence of vitamin D and the presence of increased phosphate. The principal action of the increased PTH is on the skeleton.[256] The syndrome that occurs includes rickets (associated with the reduced concentration of calcium in the body fluids) and osteitis fibrosa, a severe lysis of the skeleton from overproduction of PTH.[78,256,371]

For reasons not fully understood, 20% of patients with renal osteodystrophy also have osteosclerosis, most frequently in the spine, but sometimes affecting the long bones as well, which is characterized histologically by an increase in the numbers of trabeculae rather than an increased mineral accretion in the osteoid of the rachitic bone or repair of the destructive lesions associated with chronic hyperparathyroidism.[116,214,269,290,516]

Patients with chronic renal disease are hypophosphatemic, and even when there is reduced pH, which shifts the solubility product, they depend on a lowered serum calcium to avoid precipitation of the relatively insoluble $CaHPO_4$. If for any reason, such as spontaneous improvement, dietary indiscretions, or dialysis factors, calcium rises to near-normal levels, the calcium salts may be precipitated in a variety of ectopic sites. The principal findings in this unfortunate group of patients depend on the sites of deposition of the salts, but calcification or ossification of the corneas and conjunctivae (red eyes of renal failure),[1,49,50,390,397] skin, muscular coats of the major arteries and arterioles,[12,192,310,369,425] and periarticular soft tissues is the typical pattern encountered.[369,390]

The four pathophysiologic entities—rickets and osteomalacia, osteitis fibrosa (secondary hyperparathyroidism), osteosclerosis, and ectopic calcification or ossification—comprise the syndrome of renal osteodystrophy.[361] Frequently associated with this syndrome are the side effects of treatment (e.g., dialysis,

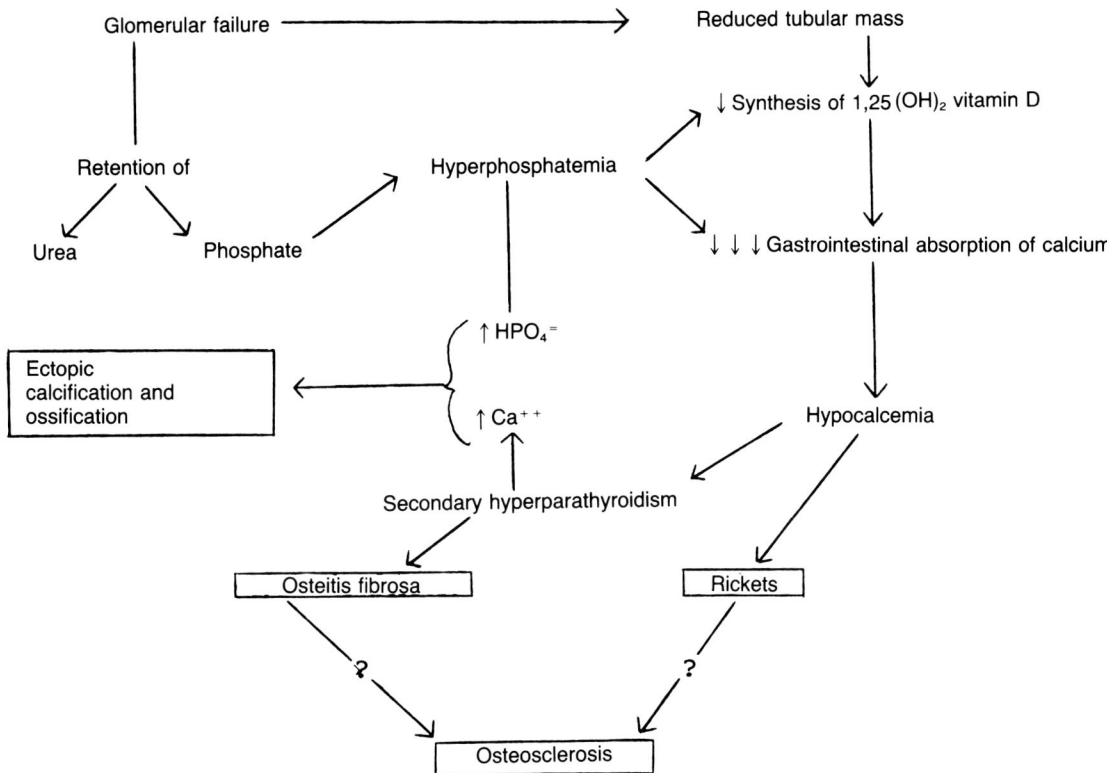

FIGURE 6-16. Mechanism of development of the chemical and bony changes in renal osteodystrophy. Reduced renal function and glomerular failure cause retention of urea and phosphate, leading to hyperphosphatemia, which, along with a reduction in tubular mass, causes a profound reduction in the synthesis of 1,25-hydroxyvitamin D. This condition, plus the direct effect of increased concentrations of phosphate in the serum, reduces the gastrointestinal absorption of calcium and causes a profound hypocalcemia and severe secondary hyperparathyroidism. These changes produce the clinical syndromes of rickets and osteitis fibrosa. For unknown reasons, 20% of the patients with this combination of chemical abnormalities also have an osteosclerosis. Because the phosphate concentration is chronically increased, an occasional increment in the serum calcium can lead to rapid ectopic calcification and ossification in the conjuctivae, skin, blood vessels, and periarticular regions.

steroid treatment), infections, and pathologic fractures.

The pediatric patient with renal osteodystrophy is almost always shorter than his or her peers and is slow in reaching milestones and exhibiting age-related phenomena, such as appearance of secondary centers of ossification or signs of sexual maturation.[244] Older terms for the disorder, such as renal infantilism or renal nanism, are reflections of this retardation, which is considerably more marked in these patients than in patients with rickets of other causes.

CLINICAL MANIFESTATIONS. The patient with chronic renal failure may have all the features of rickets and exhibit bone tenderness and skeletal fragility.[132,244,256,371,466] Fractures occur frequently with minor trauma and are very disabling. The presence of calcification in the conjunctivae and skin can produce significant irritation and itching. The periarticular calcification and ossification can cause severe limitation and pain in one or several joints (Fig. 6-17). The gait is disturbed, sometimes because of rickets-associated ligamentous laxity and muscular weakness and because of slipped femoral epiphyses that can occur from alterations in the mechanics and physiology of the proximal femurs (Fig. 6-18).[179,210,316,329] Slippage of epiphyses at other anatomic sites has been described.[329,489] The profound hyperparathyroidism seen in renal osteodystrophy and the consequent resorption of metaphyseal regions, combined with the chronicity of this entity because of modern medical management, provide the basis for the common occurrence of slipped epiphyses.[329] Although hyperparathyroidism does exist with vitamin D–deficient or vitamin D–resistant rickets, it is less profound in patients with these entities than in patients with renal osteodystrophy. Moreover, the time for medical correction of these conditions is relatively short, and slipped epiphyses are rarely seen in vitamin D–deficient or vitamin D–resistant rickets.

The radiographic changes seen in renal dystrophy are also unique in that the findings of rickets (indistin-

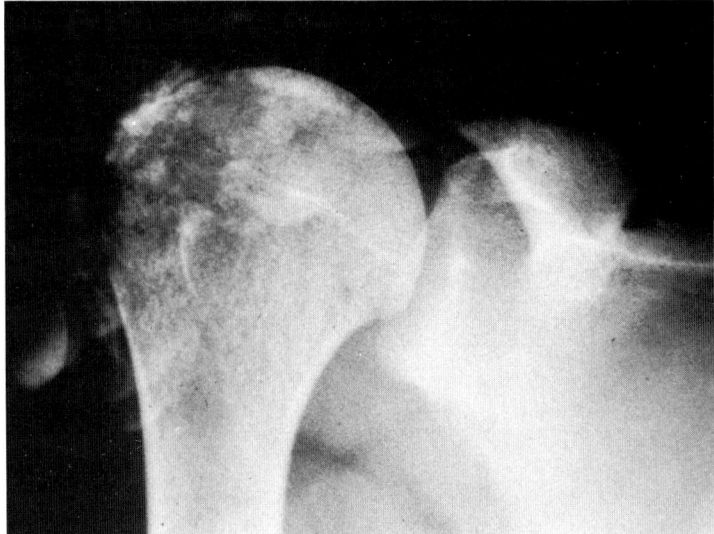

FIGURE 6-17. Radiograph of the shoulder of a young patient with renal osteodystrophy, shows extensive calcification in the deltoid muscle, which has caused severe limitation of movement. Because of the radiographic projection, most of the calcification projects over the humeral head.

guishable from those associated with other causes) may be overshadowed by the changes of osteitis fibrosa.[13,116,132,135,162,214,244,516] "Salt and pepper" skull, absence of the lamina dura on dental films, loss of cortical outline of the outer centimeter of the clavicles,[17,63] subperiosteal resorption of the ulnas[285] and terminal tufts of the distal phalanges,[416,476,477] and rarefaction and subperiosteal resorption of the medial proximal tibias may dominate the picture (Fig. 6-19).[284,477]

In severe and long-standing cases of renal osteodystrophy, brown tumors, appearing as large, oval or round rarefactions with indistinct margins, which sometimes thin and expand the cortex and provide the sites of pathologic fractures, may be present in the pelvis or long bones (Fig. 6-20). These may suggest to the unwary examiner the presence of a primary bone tumor or metastatic disease such as lymphoma or leukemia.[256] Areas of sclerosis are occasionally seen next to the areas of rarefaction. This is most common in the spine, in which the alternating areas look like the stripes of a rugger jersey, but a similar pattern is seen occasionally in the long bones. Ectopic calcification and ossification are frequently observed on routine radiographs and, particularly in the pediatric age group, are helpful in establishing the diagnosis.

The biochemical alterations in patients with chronic renal disease and osteodystrophy reflect the general state of the disturbances in renal and osseous physiology. Blood urea nitrogen (BUN), creatinine, and uric acid levels are elevated, and acidosis and hypoalbuminemia usually are detected. The calcium concentration is almost invariably low (usually less than 8.0 mg/dL), and the serum inorganic phosphate level is elevated (greater than 5 mg/dL). The alkaline phosphatase and PTH levels are increased commensurate with the extent of the disease. Concentrations of 25-

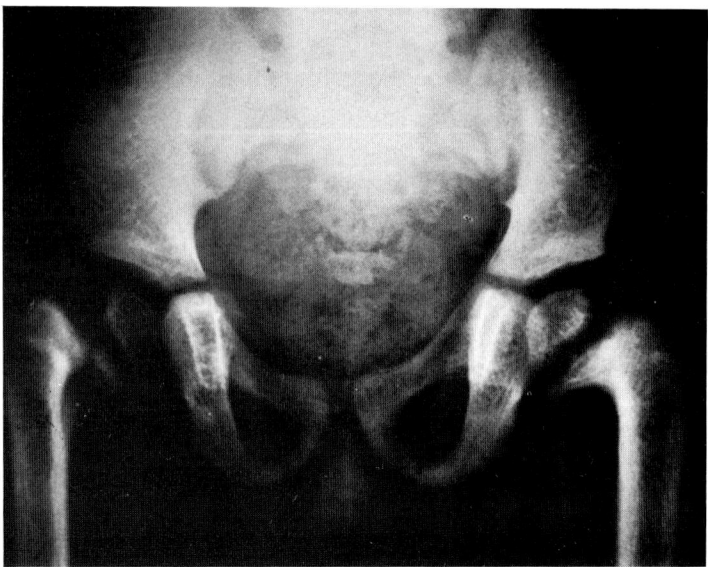

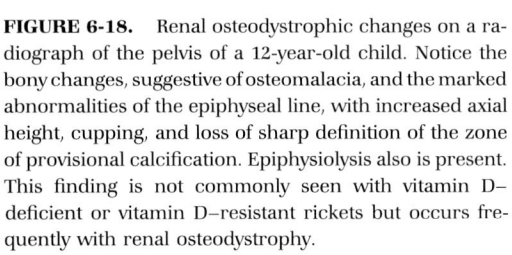

FIGURE 6-18. Renal osteodystrophic changes on a radiograph of the pelvis of a 12-year-old child. Notice the bony changes, suggestive of osteomalacia, and the marked abnormalities of the epiphyseal line, with increased axial height, cupping, and loss of sharp definition of the zone of provisional calcification. Epiphysiolysis also is present. This finding is not commonly seen with vitamin D–deficient or vitamin D–resistant rickets but occurs frequently with renal osteodystrophy.

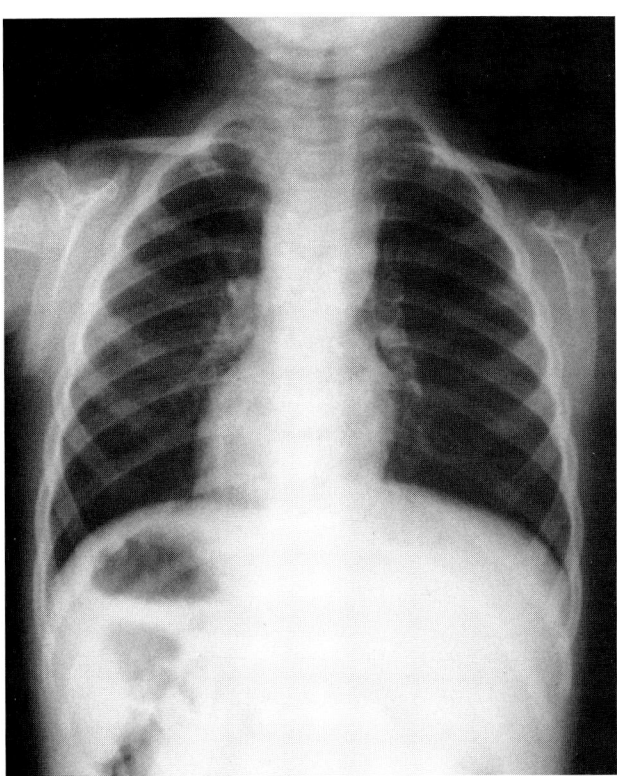

FIGURE 6-19. The radiographic changes of hyperparathyroidism are seen in this patient with renal osteodystrophy. Notice the resorption at the distal ends of the clavicles.

hydroxyvitamin D and 1,25-dihydroxyvitamin D are always diminished, and urinary calcium is low, although fecal calcium is increased (see Table 6-3).

Management

The orthopaedist's role in the diagnosis and treatment for the many disorders associated with rickets and renal osteodystrophy has shifted considerably with the understanding of the basic science of these entities. Pediatric orthopaedic surgeons and pediatricians continue to be the principal diagnosticians dealing with children who have findings suggesting rachitic disease. The various forms of rickets should continue to be important elements of the differential diagnosis in children who present for evaluation with a bowed extremity, repeated fractures, abnormalities of the spine, gait disturbances, diminished height, and failure to thrive. Radiography, radionuclide imaging, and measurements of BUN, creatinine, calcium, phosphorus, alkaline phosphatase, 25-hydroxyvitamin D, 1,25-dihydroxyvitamin D, PTH, and a variety of urinary measurements, including calcium, are invaluable aids in establishing the diagnosis of rickets and in categorizing according to precise cause. The physician begins with history and physical. Radiographs of the knee, including the most active growth plates in the

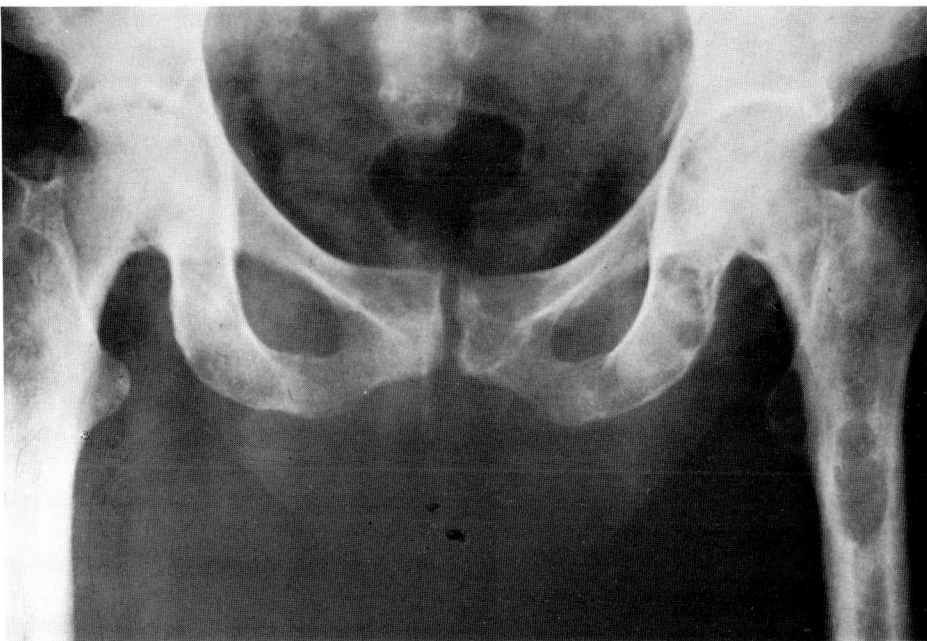

FIGURE 6-20. Radiograph of the pelvis of a patient with renal osteodystrophy shows the marked changes of secondary hyperparathyroidism. Several brown tumors are seen in the femoral shafts and ischial rami. These appear as expanded destructive lesions, resembling primary or metastatic bone tumors.

body, the distal femoral and proximal tibial physes, are useful as a screen. Serum calcium, phosphorus, and alkaline phosphatase levels are customarily determined as part of this initial evaluation. Additional radiographic studies and the chemical studies suggested in Table 6-3 may then be pursued to a diagnosis. If the pediatric orthopaedist is making the diagnosis, communication with the primary pediatrician is appropriate, after which further consultation may be obtained with specialists in pediatric nephrology or gastroenterology.

Determination of the change in skeletal morphology associated with metabolic bone disease is guided by general principles and specifically designed to address the pathophysiology of the subcategory of illness and the needs of the individual patient. Management of the underlying metabolic disturbance is always the necessary first step, because it alone may be curative, the general health status of the individual depends on it, and orthopaedic intervention without it will prove disappointing. However, will management of the metabolic disturbance alone be sufficient to address the skeletal abnormality? Generally, the extent of remodeling that is likely to occur depends on the growth remaining after correction of the abnormal physiology. There are no definitive data about the change in morphology with bracing. Because of the wider experience with children's fractures, remodeling in this setting tends to be appreciated under the heading of clinical judgment. The problem in metabolic bone disease in childhood is more complicated. The underlying pathophysiology may be improved but not actually rendered normal; growth, the basis for remodeling, may itself be abnormal; and the biomechanical properties of the bone may be particularly adversely affected when the child is most ill, making fixation difficult if operative intervention is undertaken. Every clinical situation requires individual analysis.

In its various forms, rickets tends to manifest in infancy or early childhood. The pediatrician, pediatric endocrinologist, nephrologist, or gastroenterologist addresses the altered physiology with the use of agents such as vitamin D, 1,25-dihydroxyvitamin D, calcium infusions, neutral phosphate solutions, and other dietary and pharmacologic interventions. It is usually possible to achieve a cure for many rickets patients, with expectations of normal growth and lifestyle.[58] In fractures and rickets in very-low-birth-weight infants, improved enteral intake is the major intervention, with orthopaedic intervention largely a matter of occasional splinting and observation.[278] Similarly, deficiency rickets, gastrointestinal rickets, and vitamin D–resistant rickets in infancy or early childhood usually respond to the correction of the metabolic abnormality. However, remodeling of skeletal deformity even in childhood rickets is not necessarily universal, and intervention may be required, particularly in cases of vitamin D–resistant rickets.[303,465] Fractures in childhood require appropriate management. Vigilance for uncommon subsequent physeal disturbances is still appropriate. In the multiply handicapped patient during adolescence, the existence of vitamin D deficiency as the basis of underlying fractures needs to be considered.[294]

Angular and rotatory deformities of the lower extremities in metabolic bone disease need to be interpreted with a perspective of natural history. Salenius and Vankka[433] described the physiologic development of the tibiofemoral angle starting at 15 degrees of varus at birth, becoming neutral at 18 months of age, proceeding to valgus of approximately 10 degrees, and achieving physiologic valgus at 7 years of age. This general progression is associated with an internal tibial torsion, which also tends to change to an external torsion over early childhood.[463] The extant alignment at the time of occurrence of the metabolic bone disease is usually accentuated.[277] Rickets occurring within the first year of life usually leads to a pronounced genu varum and internal tibial torsion. With correction of the metabolic abnormality, return to the pattern described by Salenius and Vankka is anticipated. If this is not the case, coordination of care between the pediatric orthopaedic surgeon and the physician making the metabolic adjustments is important to ensure that metabolic response is appropriate. After that is ascertained, the issue of bracing arises.

Using bracing, presumably employing the Hueter-Volkmann principle intelligently, to change the morphology of the skeleton usually generates some controversy. For physiologic alignment changes, there is little need to brace, and what in the past had been interpreted as a response to brace treatment is generally regarded as the progress of normal development.[433,463] For metabolic problems, the pediatric orthopaedist can observe for some relatively arbitrary period. If the malalignment fails to improve in the face of metabolic correction, bracing to counteract the deformity should be considered. Although uncommon in rickets, refractory cases may require surgery.[427] Full-length standing radiographs in anteroposterior and lateral planes are essential to establish the deviations in the mechanical axis.[368] The sites of the deviations can be established and the plan for osteotomy or osteotomies devised with tracings. In early childhood rickets, fixation that does not affect the growth plates is particularly important. Plates have been advocated.[427] Before employing plates, the osseous tissue quality must be corrected by the metabolic intervention, or the screws tend to lose purchase. Intramedullary fixation is generally easier to employ when there are multiple deviations in the mechanical axis necessitating multiple osteotomies or the quality of the osseous tissue cannot be rendered normal, as in osteogenesis imperfecta and in some types of rickets.[177]

Management of renal osteodystrophy is more complicated and involves management of the primary disorder by dialysis or renal transplantation and control of the calcium and phosphate levels by appropriate drug treatment and infusions.[123,176] Occasionally, parathyroidectomy is necessary to control the hyperparathyroidism, particularly in patients with tertiary hyperparathyroidism.[167,176] Administration of vitamin D must be carried out with considerable care to avoid the complications of ectopic ossification and calcification.[371] Intravenous infusion of 1,25-dihydroxyvitamin D has been advocated in some refractory cases of osteitis fibrosa.[15]

As with rickets, the orthopaedic manifestations include fractures, growth disturbances and angular malalignments. Only some of these resolve with improvement in metabolic status.[366] Site-specific fracture management is important. The incidence of fractures should decrease with correction of the metabolic disturbances. Slipped epiphyses are common in renal osteodystrophy at the proximal femur, distal femur, distal tibia, and forearm.[329,366,489] Correction of the metabolic status is always the first step to restore the overall physiologic status of the patient and improve the quality of the bone. At sites other than the proximal femur, some period of observation is logical for the remodeling considerations previously discussed and subsequent corrective osteotomy if remodeling is not occurring. Slipped capital femoral epiphysis in renal osteodystrophy is perhaps more controversial. Although some of the general principles governing idiopathic slipped capital femoral epiphyses also apply, the questions of fixation and bilaterality have advocates of different approaches.[117] Because these slips in renal osteodystrophy can occur in patients younger than 10 years of age, methods of fixation that can allow growth rather than promoting growth plate closure merit consideration.[218] In adolescence, after correction of the metabolism, fixation to promote growth plate closure can be performed.[358,366] In some cases of metabolic bone problems, fixation may not be possible to promote growth plate closure, and bone peg epiphyseodesis should be performed.[118]

The mechanism of growth disturbance is not completely defined. In addition to the overall physiologic status of the patient, disturbance in the growth factor control of physes has been implicated. Somatomedin disturbance and disturbance in the bone morphogenetic proteins and osteogenic proteins may also occur.[10] Because the major production site of one of the osteogenic proteins is the kidneys, renal failure could interfere with its production. The problem of growth disturbance in renal osteodystrophy even after treatment with transplantation must still be solved.

Because renal osteodystrophy tends to occur in later childhood and because there is a physiologic valgus at that point in development, genu valgum is frequently encountered and may persist even though metabolic abnormalities are corrected.[366] The principles applied in genu varum can be followed in this condition. Observation during the period of medical management is prudent. Failure to improve over months in the face of medical improvement should prompt consideration of bracing. Persistence is appropriately treated surgically. The deviations in mechanical axis are established with full-length radiographs.[368] Valgus occurring through the distal femur is common in patients with renal osteodystrophy and may be treated with stapling toward the end of growth. The amount of overgrowth from the lateral aspect of the growth plate required for correction may be determined from the Green-Anderson growth charts.[277] Stapling of the medial aspect of growth plate may be enacted at the time indicated. If this option cannot be enacted because of insufficient growth remaining, metaphyseal osteotomies may be required using staple or blade plate fixation.[177] An alternative approach is to perform a gradual angular correction with an external fixator.[469]

Hypophosphatasia

In some classification systems, hypophosphatasia is included with deficiency states of calcium and vitamin D, renal tubular disorders, and renal glomerular disorders (renal osteodystrophy) as a cause of rickets. Although there are some clinical and roentgenographic similarities, hypophosphatasia has a different pathophysiology from that of rickets. The link should be recognized, but differentiation of hypophosphatasia from rickets and osteomalacia must also be made.

Hypophosphatasia was described as early as 1929, but it was subsequently differentiated from the rachitic syndromes by Rathbun in 1948.[248,412] It has since been documented as resulting from a genetic error in the synthesis of alkaline phosphatase by bone, leukocytes, intestinal mucosa, and kidney.[412,456] Hypophosphatasia is transmitted as an autosomal recessive trait.[326,519] Asymptomatic heterozygotes may be readily identified by a decrease in serum and leukocyte alkaline phosphatase and, as in patients with clinical disease, by the presence of large concentrations of phosphoethanolamine in the urine.

Patients affected with hypophosphatasia usually show the changes early in life.[188,326,412] The principal findings in those with the fully developed syndrome are growth retardation, failure to thrive, irritability, fever, vomiting, constipation, and signs of increased intracranial pressure.[326] Craniosynostosis is a common finding in infants, and the cranial bones may be poorly ossified. Suture lines may be enlarged and bear a close resemblance to craniotabes. As in rickets, dentition may be markedly delayed, and the teeth develop extensive caries.[386] Examination of the extremities and thorax is likely to show enlargement of the metaphyseal areas adjacent to the joints, bowing and knock-knee deformities, prominent costochondral junctions, and kyphosis. Milder forms of the disorder in which the onset of symptoms is delayed have been described and may not be clinically evident until adolescence or adult life.[42,53,519] Manifestations include fractures after minor trauma, poor fracture healing with laboratory study abnormalities, and the radiographic appearance of osteomalacia.[14]

Radiographic studies of the patient affected with hypophosphatasia show generalized osteopenia, most marked in the calvarium and metaphyseal regions of the long bones.[125] The bones may be bowed, and the epiphyseal-metaphyseal areas may show a peculiar cupped or wedge-shaped deformity, principally affecting the center of the physis, with irregular notches at the margins (Fig. 6-21).[125] This is similar to the radiographic appearance of rickets. The epiphyseal centers are somewhat delayed in appearance but normal in outline. Histologic studies show large quantities of unmineralized osteoid in the bones, particularly in regions of active growth and in the region of the synostotic sutures.[326] As in rickets, the epiphyseal cartilages are irregular, with lengthening of the columns and diminished vascular invasion and mineralization.[42,412]

The cause of hypophosphatasia is believed to be a decreased production of alkaline phosphatase, presumably because of an error in DNA coding by the cells that ordinarily produce the enzyme.[283,326] Because the enzyme is necessary for the maturation of the primary spongiosa of the developing epiphyseal plate, the deformities that develop in affected patients are largely evident in the skeleton, in which they mimic the change of rickets. Synthesis of bone is probably unimpaired, but because of the relative absence of alkaline phosphatase, the mineralization process is inadequate, and large quantities of osteoid are produced. Diagnosis is based on the finding of a uniformly low concentration of serum alkaline phosphatase with usually normal values for calcium, 25-hydroxyvitamin D, 1,25-dihydroxyvitamin D, and PTH.[42,53,187,248,326] Some severely affected children may have marked hypercalcemia, thought to be caused by hypersensitivity to vitamin D.[187] An unusual feature of the disease is the increased serum concentration and excessive urinary excretion of phosphoethanolamine.[187,212,327,412] The significance of this finding, which is not specific to hypophosphatasia, is still unexplained.[297]

Children or adults with mild forms of hypophosphatasia are often shorter in stature than their peers but have limited symptoms or signs.[14,519] Those with florid disease at birth present major problems in management. Increased intracranial pressure, hypercalcemia, renal failure, and overwhelming infections may cause considerable threat to life. The mortality rate for the infantile form of hypophosphatasia is 50% to 70%.[188] If the child survives, considerable skeletal deformity and disability occur; most of these patients are dwarfed. The fractures common in these patients heal very slowly.[14,255]

There is no definitive therapy. In theory, diseases with an enzyme deficiency as the underlying cause may ultimately be treated by introduction of the appropriate gene into a stem cell population, but practical application is still in the future. Vitamin D in large doses has provided some benefit that was reversed with withdrawal of the medication.[187] Pathologic fracture in hypophosphatasia (as in metabolic and endo-

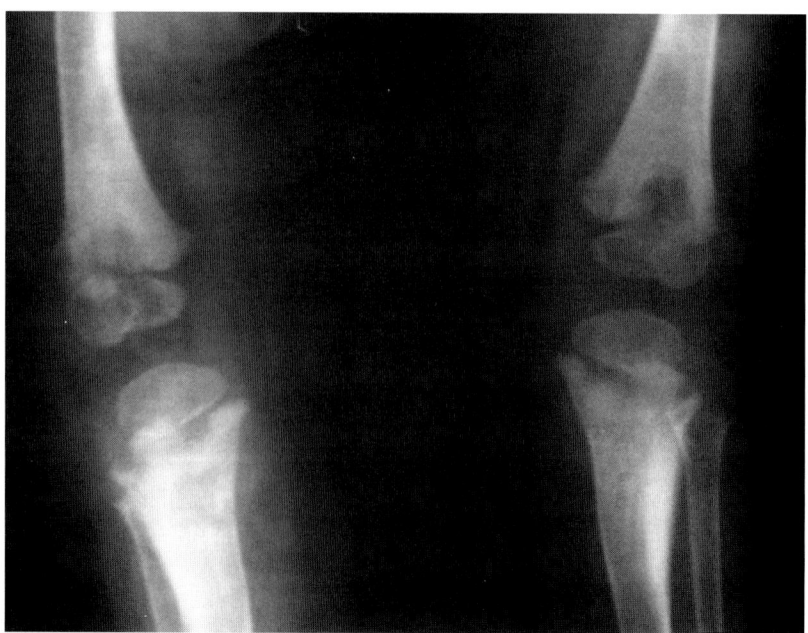

FIGURE 6-21. The central cup- or wedge-shaped ossification defects of the central physes are particularly prominent at the distal femurs in a patient with hypophosphatasia.

crine entities with bone of poor mechanical quality) may be a difficult problem for the orthopaedist. In the pediatric patient with the severe form of hypophosphatasia, the dilemmas bear a resemblance to those encountered in osteogenesis imperfecta. Intramedullary fixation can be undertaken, attempting to avoid growth plate injury. In the adult patient, intramedullary fixation and bone grafting may be indicated.[14,108]

Parathyroid Disorders

Primary disorders of calcium homeostasis, except for rickets and renal osteodystrophy, are not common in children. Although it is unlikely that the pediatric orthopaedist is the first practitioner to see patients with parathyroid disorders, it is worthwhile for him or her to be aware of several such entities.

HYPERPARATHYROIDISM. An increased level of PTH in renal failure was previously discussed. In chronic renal failure, the hyperparathyroidism is secondary or tertiary. Secondary hyperparathyroidism is compensatory for the hypocalcemia and remains reversible with correction of the underlying renal failure. Tertiary hyperparathyroidism is also compensatory originally but, because of the long-standing stimulation of the parathyroid glands, becomes autonomous even with correction of the renal failure. In primary hyperparathyroidism, autonomous hyperfunction of the glands occurs not as a compensation to any antecedent stimulus, and hypercalcemia itself is the basis for the presenting symptoms.[23,48,56] In the clinical situation, because of the diffuse effects of the disturbance in calcium homeostasis, the symptoms at first are bewildering. If the mnemonic device, "stones, bones, and abdominal groans," is remembered, the bewildering complaints become explicable on the basis of hypercalcemia. The critical solubility product of calcium and phosphorus is exceeded; precipitation in the urinary tract leads to renal calculi and colic. The induced osteoclastic resorption of bone causes skeletal pain. Smooth muscle action in the gut is inhibited by hypercalcemia. Abdominal pain, constipation, and weight loss follow. The irritability and conductivity of nervous tissue are decreased by hypercalcemia. Aberrations of mental status and ultimately lethargy and obtundation ensue. Hypertension is frequently present.

The radiographic features of primary hyperparathyroidism are similar to those of secondary hyperparathyroidism. There is generalized osteopenia and cortical thinning. Resorption is particularly severe at the terminal tufts of the distal phalanges and the distal clavicles (see Fig. 6-19).

The classic laboratory findings in patients with hyperparathyroidism are elevated serum calcium, decreased serum phosphorus, and elevated alkaline phosphatase levels.[56] Unfortunately, these values can be normal despite an elevated PTH level. Further testing may be required in difficult situations to establish the diagnosis. These tests include a urinary clearance study to clarify a decreased percentage of tubular reabsorption of phosphate, measurement of urinary cyclic AMP, and assaying directly for serum PTH.

Treatment is directed toward correcting the underlying cause of hyperparathyroidism. For adenomas and hyperplasia, treatment is usually surgical.[126] Preliminary metabolic management may be required. Although fractures can occur and need to be managed by customary principles, there should be pediatric endocrinologic management of the hypercalcemia.[406,475]

HYPOPARATHYROIDISM. The manifestations of hypoparathyroidism are recognized more easily by the disturbance of calcium homeostasis than by the skeletal changes.[76] The principles of calcium homeostasis previously discussed logically explain the symptoms and signs that are seen. Irritability of nervous and muscle tissue is high because the serum calcium is low.[520] Tetany, paresthesias, and alteration in mental status may be seen. If hypocalcemia occurs early in development, mental retardation may result. If it occurs later, mood changes may be seen. The Chvostek and Trousseau signs are used to elicit the tetany and spasm.

Radiographic findings in patients with hypoparathyroidism include increased density of the long bones and skull. Soft tissue calcifications, including the basal ganglia, may also be seen.

Laboratory changes include a decrease in total and serum ionized calcium and elevated serum phosphorus. As with all calcium measurements, hypocalcemia must be interpreted with the serum albumin concentration, because decreased albumin necessarily leads to decreased bound serum calcium and total serum calcium.

Treatment for hypoparathyroidism is endocrine related rather than orthopaedic.[30] The principal treatment agent is vitamin D. Vitamin D and PTH work synergistically to facilitate the transport of calcium across the gut, by the renal tubule, and from the bone. Vitamin D is capable of exerting its effect at each of these sites. Considerably higher than physiologic (i.e., pharmacologic) doses of vitamin D are required. Management must be carried out very carefully to avoid vitamin D toxicity.

PSEUDOHYPOPARATHYROIDISM. Pseudohypoparathyroidism is related to endocrine and genetic factors more than to orthopaedic factors.[7,515] Skeletal changes are present, however, and the disorder represents an unusual but important form of metabolic bone disease that is associated with end-organ insensitivity. The characteristics of pseudohypoparathyroidism are mental retardation, short stature, central nervous system irritability, and tetany. Radiographs may reveal soft tissue calcifications that are especially common in the basal ganglia. Hand films demonstrate shortening of the fourth and fifth metacarpals (Fig. 6-22). Brachydactyly can be seen as part of many syndromes.[490] The workup is usually coordinated with genetic and pediatric endocrine services. Biochemical findings include a low serum calcium and a high serum inorganic phosphorus concentration. The laboratory finding most helpful in the diagnosis is the failure of a phosphate diuresis after administration of PTH (Ellsworth-Howard test).

Pseudohypoparathyroidism is a genetic disorder in which production of PTH is normal, but the cells that serve as the target for the hormone are unresponsive.[157,174,205,314,515] There may be several different types of defects causing the lack of response. A sex-linked dominant mode of transmission with variable penetrance seems to be operative. Heterogeneity is possible, and other modes of transmission have been suggested.

A similar syndrome has been described in which affected patients demonstrate all the clinical stigmata of pseudohypoparathyroidism but show no chemical alterations. This disorder, also genetic and presumably a variant, is pseudopseudohypoparathyroidism.

Hypercalcemia

In addition to the hypercalcemia associated with hyperparathyroid states, there are several other causes of hypercalcemia in childhood.[133,180] These causes are relatively rare and are more frequently based on endocrine disorders than on metabolic bone disease. These entities are often of considerable importance, and despite their rarity in orthopaedic practice, a brief review is necessary.

Hypervitaminosis D can cause a profound and occasionally life-threatening hypercalcemia. Vitamin D and the potent 1-hydroxyvitamin D and 1,25-dihydroxyvitamin D are used in the treatment of rickets, osteomalacia, and hypoparathyroidism. Despite the clear need of the patient, it is possible to overdose with these drugs, especially with potent analogs, and the resultant hypercalcemia causes a picture similar to that described in the section on primary hyperparathyroidism. Treatment consists of lowering the serum calcium. Vitamin D administration should be stopped, and the patient should be promptly treated by diuresis, which is usually accomplished by administration of large volumes of saline and furosemide. Replacement of urinary losses of water, sodium, and potassium is often necessary, and these should be carefully monitored. Although sodium phosphate infusions were advocated at one time, they are now contraindicated, because a reconsideration of the calcium homeostasis mechanism indicates that such an infusion is likely to cause precipitation of calcium acid phosphate. Administration of oral phosphate in a nonabsorbable preparation binds calcium in the intestinal lumen and decreases absorption. Glucocorticoids can diminish calcium absorption and decrease tubular reabsorption.

Hypercalcemia is associated with some neoplasms, although more frequently in adults than in children.[353,394] The mechanisms postulated are multiple. Direct invasion of bone by massive metastases can produce hypercalcemia. Some tumors tend to produce agents that act in a manner similar to PTH or prostaglandins and cause significant increases in the resorption of bone and sometimes profound hypercalcemia.[47] Treatment begins as just described for hypervitaminosis D. In some case of malignant disease, treatment with mithramycin, a chemotherapeutic agent that interferes with osteoclastic resorption, may be justified.

Hypercalcemia arising during periods of immobilization has been reported, more often in adults than

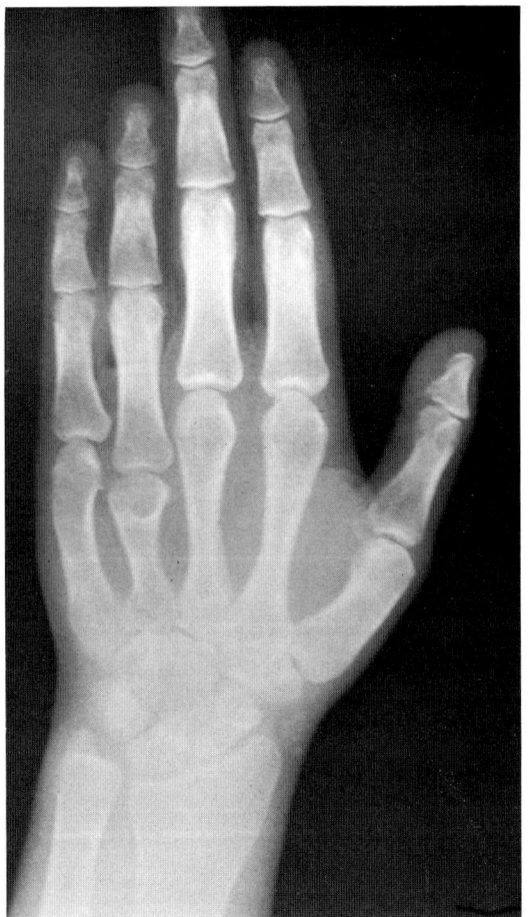

FIGURE 6-22. Radiograph of the hand of a patient with pseudohypoparathyroidism. Notice the shortened fourth and fifth metacarpals.

in children.[251,273,292,335,384] Disuse osteoporosis is not an unusual consequence of immobilization but is almost never associated with hypercalcemia. Children placed on prolonged bed rest in traction or casts can rarely develop a florid hypercalcemia, with lethargy, obtundation, abdominal symptoms, and urinary calculi.[384] However, hypercalcemia must be considered in the differential diagnosis in immobilization situations. Treatment is as described for hypervitaminosis D.

Idiopathic hypercalcemia of childhood is a rare condition, seen more often in Great Britain than in the United States. The disorder is probably a series of heterogeneous syndromes. One of the more common syndromes, Williams syndrome, is characterized by a peculiar elfin facies with a small mandible and upturned nose.[522] Cardiovascular anomalies, such as supravalvular aortic stenosis, have been reported in addition to mental retardation. The multiple anomalies suggest an in utero mesenchymal defect, but the relation of the abnormality in calcium handling to the other defects is not clear. Williams syndrome should be differentiated from the idiopathic hypercalcemia that was first described in Great Britain and thought to result from hypervitaminosis D secondary to overzealous supplementation.

Heavy Metal Intoxication

Heavy metal poisoning is usually not considered among the metabolic bone diseases of children. The manifestations of lead intoxication, which is the most common variety of metal poisoning, are more frequently neurologic and gastrointestinal than osseous.[99] However, the pediatric orthopaedist may be presented with certain radiographic findings that should be recognized.[286]

Lead can be stored in the metaphyses, where bone is being rapidly laid down by growth plates. The radiographic appearance is characteristically broad bands of markedly increased radiodensity in the metaphyseal area, adjacent to the epiphyseal plates (Fig. 6-23). Normally, the metaphyseal region in growing children may appear slightly more dense than in adults, but the radiodensity in most cases of lead intoxication is far beyond the normal range. In a few cases, the radiographic results are negative or equivocal. Lead lines in the gums and hematologic and chemical findings establish the diagnosis.[157]

ORGANIC PHASE

Although differentiation of the mineral phase from the organic phase of bone metabolism is simplistic and neglects interactions between the two phases, the classification is useful for discussing physiology and differentiating clinical syndromes. Mineral homeostasis was discussed earlier in this chapter. The diseases of the organic phase are introduced by a brief review of the cellular and organic aspects of bone physiology.

Bone Physiology

Bone is a specialized form of connective tissue with several important roles. It is rigid, provides form, and

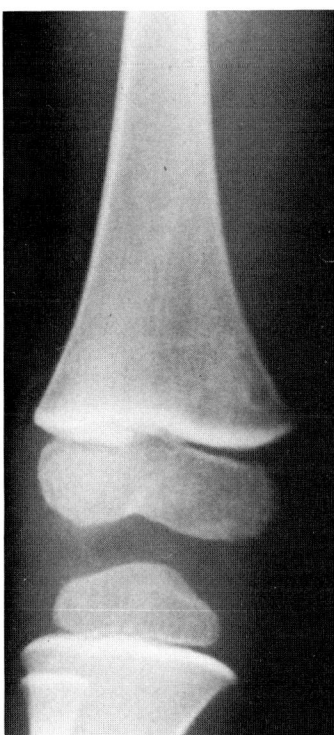
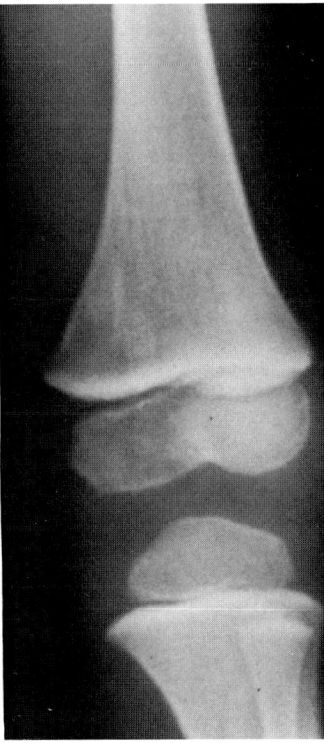

FIGURE 6-23. Radiograph of the knee of a patient with lead poisoning. Notice the broad, radiodense metaphyseal lines. Lead has accumulated at the site of bone formation.

contributes to structural stability. Bone is the primary body store for calcium and phosphorus and also serves as an envelope for the blood-forming marrow elements. When injured, bone normally heals with its native tissue rather than scar. In the child, the modeling process accounts for growth and continued reshaping of the bones.[122] In the adult, although the shape of the bones in general remains unchanged, the tissue undergoes continued internal remodeling, in which bone cells are responsible for continued resorption and formation, resulting in the replacement of old bone by new bone.[194,410]

Bone is a composite material. Based on dry weight, 77% is inorganic, primary hydroxyapatite. The remaining 23% is organic, and almost 90% of this is in the form of collagen. The remaining noncollagenous organic material consists of phospholipids, other glycoproteins, and proteoglycans. The collagen molecules within the fibers are highly ordered, with the fibrillar arrangement consisting of a three-quarter stagger.[207] There is an 8% overlap that produces hole zones essential to the deposition of hydroxyapatite crystals and the linkage to the noncollagenous proteins within and in juxtaposition to the collagen fibers. The biomechanical properties of bone in part result from the organic and inorganic components. Bone is anisotropic; the collagen molecules and fibrils, haversian systems, and trabeculae are not randomly oriented. Their orientation ensures that the biomechanical properties of the materials composing the tissue are maximized.

The collagen molecule is a macromolecule made up of three polypeptide chains, each of about 1000 amino acids arranged in a triple helix.[160,242,365] One third of the amino acids are glycine, and 20% to 30% are proline or hydroxyproline. Thirteen different types of collagen have been described.[83,242,291,365] The list is still growing (see Table 6-2). Type I collagen, the most common, is found in bone, tendon, and skin. Type II is the predominant form in cartilage.

The individual chains of collagen are synthesized in the rough endoplasmic reticulum and assembled into a triple helix intracellularly before extrusion. Several posttranslational changes occur, including hydroxylation of some of the proline and lysine residues and glycosylation of some of the hydroxylysine residues. The hydroxyproline residues make the triple helix more heat stable, and the hydroxylysine residues are important in the development of cross-links. After translocation to the extracellular space, portions of the amino- and carboxy-terminal nonhelical portions of the procollagen molecule are cleaved, and the collagen molecules aggregate to form fibrils, where additional reactions occur to produce stable intramolecular and intermolecular cross-linkages. Interspersed around the collagen molecules are the other noncollagenous proteins.

After collagen production, some still poorly defined events occur that render the bone matrix (i.e., osteoid) mineralizable. Under appropriate conditions, including the presence of adequate amounts of calcium and phosphorus and the production of alkaline phosphatase by the cells, the hydroxyapatite crystals are deposited within the collagen fiber. Many aspects of the mineralization process still are not clear.[66,83,229,413] Some investigators have suggested that the process results primarily from physicochemical phenomena that occur because of the specific nature of collagen and noncollagenous organic structure. Others have suggested that mineralization begins as an energy-dependent intracellular process that requires the presence of one or more vitamin D metabolites. Proteoglycans also may play a significant role in the process.[81]

The process is not completed with the end of mineralization. Because of incompletely understood signals, bone as an organ responds to stress according to Wolff's law. After mineralization, bone may undergo partial resorption with subsequent new formation, possibly in a different location, for the purpose of producing bone that is more appropriately oriented to resist stress. This action depends on combined osteoclastic and osteoblastic activity.[506] Its mediation at the cellular level may occur by mechanical transduction across the cell membrane and through the cytoskeleton, ultimately affecting the genome.[514]

Advances in the knowledge of collagen biochemistry, physiology of mineralization, and cellular processes responsible for bone cell differentiation and function have led to a better understanding of many metabolic bone diseases. Defects in the mineralization process are numerous and may lead to the rachitic diseases previously discussed. There are many sites for disturbances in collagen production; some of these defects have been identified in diseases such as osteogenesis imperfecta, the Ehlers-Danlos syndromes, and some skeletal dysplasias.[111] Problems with bone cell differentiation, function, or both have been found in osteopetrosis and idiopathic juvenile osteoporosis. As additional metabolic and biochemical abnormalities are identified in these diseases, greater insight will be gained regarding pathogenesis, and more effective forms of treatment will evolve.

Osteogenesis Imperfecta

Osteogenesis imperfecta has traditionally been categorized as a heritable disorder of connective tissue affecting the bone and soft tissue; studies have also revealed a number of metabolic abnormalities.[328] The disease was probably first described by Malebranche[309] in 1674, and since then, it has been discussed under at least 40 different names or eponyms, some of the more common of which are Lobstein disease,[302] Vrolik disease,[509] van der Hoeve disease, fragilitas ossium, osteomalacia congenita, and osteoporosis fetalis.[94,305,447,529] Advances in collagen biochemistry and electron microscopy and the results of genetic, epidemiologic, and dental studies support the concept that osteogenesis imperfecta is a series of syndromes representing classes of molecular defects, each with a reasonably well-defined clinical pattern.[185,447,448] Most types of osteogenesis imperfecta have been linked to mutations in type I collagen.[111]

Clinical Manifestations

The nature and severity of the clinical features depend on the type of osteogenesis imperfecta.[43,111,447] General features include the characteristic fragility of bone, short stature, scoliosis, defective dentinogenesis of deciduous or permanent teeth or both, middle ear deafness, laxity of ligaments, and blue sclerae and tympanic membranes. Many patients have misshapen skulls with a wide intertemporal measurements and small, triangular faces. The bones are gracile and diffusely osteopenic, with thin cortices and an attenuated trabecular pattern. The long bones have narrow diaphyses, and bowing and fractures are common. The fracture healing process is undisturbed in terms of sequence of events, but the new bone has the same deficient biomechanical characteristics. Fractures may occur at any age, and the age of occurrence is one basis for classification. In the milder forms of osteogenesis imperfecta, the incidence of fractures decreases with age.

The pelvis in osteogenesis imperfecta may have a trefoil shape, and protrusio acetabuli is common, presumably because of repeated fractures. A softened base of the skull may lead to platybasia and potential neurologic sequelae. Dentinogenesis imperfecta results in soft, translucent, and brownish teeth. The teeth are affected in a nonuniform manner; the primary and secondary teeth may be involved to a greater or lesser degree. The osteopenic vertebrae may fracture easily, resulting in a flattened or biconcave shape. The laxity of the ligaments results in hypermobile joints and an increased incidence of joint dislocation. Inguinal, umbilical, and diaphragmatic hernias are common. The skin is thin, translucent, and easily distensible. Although increased vascular fragility is common, major arterial or aortic aneurysms are rarely encountered. The differential diagnosis includes juvenile osteoporosis, nonaccidental injury,[148] and rarely, a malignancy such as leukemia. The severity of involvement ranges from a crushed stillborn fetus, in the most severe cases, to an infant with multiple or unusual fractures[151] or severe postnatal deformities to the almost symptom-free adult.[407] The adult, on careful clinical evaluation, reveals a history of occasional fracture and mild osteopenia, and the family history may be contributory.

The issue of discerning nonaccidental injury from osteogenesis imperfecta can arise. Because a given, single fracture may occur in nonaccidental injury or osteogenesis imperfecta, it is hazardous to exclude osteogenesis imperfecta by the radiographic pattern alone.[148] Conversely, multiple fractures at different stages of healing, posterior rib fractures, and metaphyseal corner fractures are highly specific for nonaccidental injury.[93,276] The history is extremely helpful. Fractures from child abuse occur most frequently in children younger than 3 years of age.[93] If the physician is caring for a patient who is not yet ambulatory and has multiple fractures, the data would imply a severe type of osteogenesis imperfecta, which is usually diagnosed with fractures at birth. It is possible for a child with a mild form of osteogenesis imperfecta to become ambulatory and sustain a fracture with relatively mild trauma. A positive family history and signs such as abnormal dentition or blue sclerae or a systemic osteopenia revealed by radiography may be helpful in this situation.

Culture of dermal fibroblasts for characterization of the type I collagen may be part of the workup, but the molecular basis for the entire spectrum of osteogenesis imperfecta has not been established.[111] The matching of a child's type I collagen with a previously described molecular abnormality may establish the diagnosis of osteogenesis imperfecta, but not matching does not necessarily exclude osteogenesis imperfecta in problem situations. The combination of history, physical examination, and radiographic pattern remains of paramount significance. Fractures and rickets can occur in very-low-birth-weight infants, but the setting of a birth weight less than 1500 g, hospitalization, biochemical abnormalities, and subsequent resolution with development are key features of this syndrome.[278] Fractures can occur in primary hyperparathyroidism, but there are biochemical abnormalities in this setting.[406,475] A patient with Menkes kinky hair syndrome can present with metaphyseal corner fractures, but presentation is more likely in the setting of a newborn male (X-linked recessive trait) with failure to thrive and the sparse, kinky hair, giving the syndrome its name.[281] "Overdiagnosis of child abuse is a tragedy, but an incorrect diagnosis of osteogenesis imperfecta may put a child's life at risk."[93]

The inheritance of osteogenesis imperfecta was once thought to be autosomal dominant. The fact that there was considerable variability of phenotypic expression in different members of a kindred led to the concept of variable penetrance and expressivity.[529] Investigations of multiple kindreds led some investigators to conclude there was a high rate of spontaneous mutation, but others emphasize the need for a careful history, physical examination, and metabolic studies and collagen typing to detect subclinical involvement in some patients in a pedigree.

Classification

It is not surprising that numerous classifications have been proposed for osteogenesis imperfecta. Looser used the terms congenita and tarda to differentiate what he thought were different forms of the disease based on when the first fractures occurred applying congenita only to intrauterine fractures.[305] Seedorff used this definition of congenita but divided tarda into gravis (i.e., fractures occurring at birth or within the first year of life) and levis (i.e., fractures occurring after one year).[440] Bauze used deformity of the femurs as a guide to differentiate the clinical types.[43]

The classification most widely accepted is the Sillence classification. The Sillence classification of osteogenesis imperfecta takes into account multiple features of this entity to provide some order to the wide heterogeneity.[447,448] This classification provides the framework to which the molecular biologic information is being added.[111] Sillence proposed a numeric classification, types I to IV, with several modifiers. Types I and IV were thought to be transmitted by an autosomal dominant mode and types II and III by an autosomal recessive mode. Dental findings were used to further subtype (i.e., A without and B with dentinogenesis imperfecta). Sillence also recognized several pedigrees that seemed to have an X-linked inheritance pattern, although these were not included in the classification that he has proposed (Table 6-5).

Type I osteogenesis imperfecta is the common mild form. The molecular basis for this is a 50% reduction in the production of type I collagen.[111] Overall morphology may be normal or nearly so, with fractures occurring in later childhood and decreasing toward adolescence. Type II is lethal in the perinatal period, with many of the mutations occurring in the glycine residues of type I collagen. Type III osteogenesis imperfecta is the severe form, with fractures occurring at birth. The molecular basis for this type of osteogenesis imperfecta has not been as fully characterized as it has been for the other types. Types II and III are not difficult to diagnose clinically, but correlation of these clinical entities with molecular defects expands our knowledge of bone physiology and ultimately may provide more effective forms of treatment. Type IV is a moderately severe form of osteogenesis imperfecta, with glycine point mutations in type I collagen. Clinically, this type has great variation, overlapping types I and III, and it may represent a heterogeneous group of patients who do not readily fit into the other categories. A molecular characterization of this group aids in establishing the diagnosis of osteogenesis imperfecta and typing it in problematic situations.

Orthopaedic management for type I osteogenesis imperfecta is customary fracture management. Management for types III and IV includes issues about adaptive equipment, rehabilitation, intramedullary rodding, and scoliosis management. This approach also points to another problem. The Sillence classification, which has been and remains the most helpful classification for the geneticist in ordering the many features of this entity, may be less helpful for the pediatric orthopaedist consulted in the perinatal period and confronted by concerned parents with questions about musculoskeletal prognosis.

Shapiro advanced a congenita-tarda classification in trying to address this issue.[442] In this classification scheme, congenita implies that fractures occurred in utero or at birth. The congenita group is further subdivided into A (i.e., crumpled femurs and ribs) and B (i.e., normal bone contours but with fractures). The tarda group is also divided into A (i.e., fractures before walking) and B (i.e., fractures after walking). At follow-up, the congenita A group had a high mortality rate (94%). The congenita B mortality rate was only 8%; 59%

TABLE 6-5 Osteogenesis Imperfecta Classification

TYPE	INHERITANCE	CLINICAL FEATURES
I	Autosomal dominant	Bone fragility, blue sclerae, onset of fractures after birth (most preschool age). Type A, without dentinogenesis imperfecta; type B, with dentinogenesis imperfecta
II	Autosomal recessive	Lethal in perinatal period, dark blue sclerae, concertina femurs, beaded ribs
III	Autosomal recessive	Fractures at birth, progressive deformity, normal sclerae and hearing
IV	Autosomal dominant	Bone fragility, normal sclerae, normal hearing. Type A, without dentinogenesis imperfecta; type B, with dentinogenesis imperfecta

Data from Sillence DO. Osteogenesis imperfecta: an expanding panorama of variance. Clin Orthop 1981;159:11, and Sillence DO, Senn A, Danks DM. Genetic heterogeneity in osteogenesis imperfecta. J Med Genet 1979;16:101.

were in wheelchairs, and 33% were ambulatory. In the tarda A group, 33% were in wheelchairs, and 67% were ambulatory. In the tarda B group, 100% were ambulatory. Most intramedullary rodding was performed in the congenita B and tarda A groups.

The problems of the Sillence classification for the pediatric orthopaedist do not obviate its usefulness and general acceptance, and it is the classification employed for the remainder of the discussion.

The radiographic features of osteogenesis imperfecta patients depend on the disease type, but they must be interpreted with the history and physical examination results to establish the type (Figs. 6-24 through 6-27).[159,447,448] Findings may or may not be obvious at birth, depending on the type. In almost every case, some degree of generalized osteopenia can be detected. In type II and to a certain extent in type III, the femurs have a crumpled "concertina" appearance. A similar deformity, presumably caused by previous fractures, may or may not be seen early in type I. Later in childhood, the long bones in type I appear slender and gracile, with thin cortices and deformities resulting from multiple fractures. In type III, in later childhood, the bones are often short, and children may be classified as dwarfs. The head is misshapen, and the skull exhibits wormian bones. The vertebrae may show evidence of multiple fractures, with resultant platyspondylia and sometimes with severe scoliosis. In severe cases, the metaphyses may appear cystic, a finding occasionally present at birth but more often developing during infancy or childhood.

The histologic changes in the bones of patients with osteogenesis imperfecta have been the subject of considerable investigation, and researchers vary in their descriptions of them, in part reflecting the heterogeneity of the entity. Toward the more severe end of the spectrum of osteogenesis imperfecta, fairly uniform agreement exists about the nature of the bone, which often appears woven and only occasionally exhibits a lamellar pattern. The cortices are thin, with poorly developed haversian systems, and the trabeculae in the metaphyses are markedly attenuated. Several investigators have observed a hypercellularity, with increased numbers of osteocytes per unit area or volume of bone.[120] No change occurs in the osteoclast population. The collagen fibers of the cornea and skin share in the disturbance and have a looser arrangement and thinner fibers. Histologic study of the epiphyseal and articular cartilages have failed to show an abnormality. Ultrastructural studies confirm the

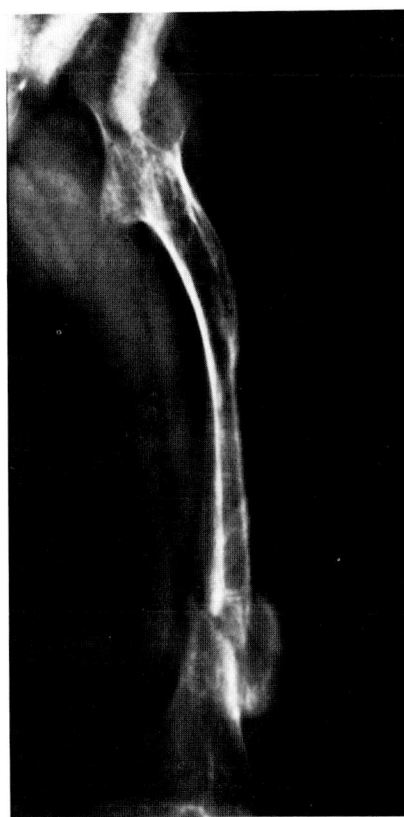

FIGURE 6-24. Radiograph of a patient with osteogenesis imperfecta, type I. The patient had blue sclerae. Fractures began soon after birth, with resulting deformity.

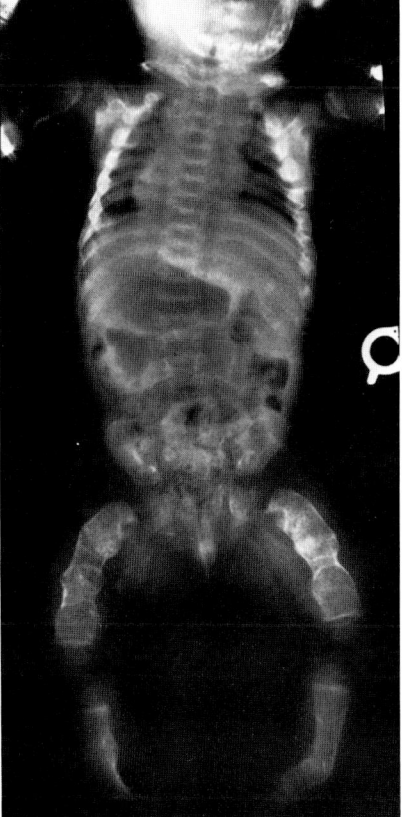

FIGURE 6-25. Child with osteogenesis imperfecta, type II. Notice the concertina-like appearance of the femurs and the beading of the ribs.

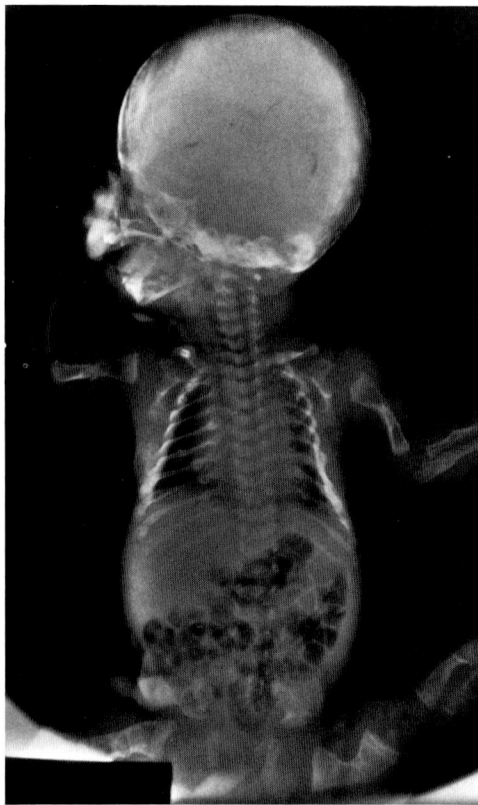

FIGURE 6-26. Child with osteogenesis imperfecta, type III. Fractures were present at birth; progressive deformity occurred with further development.

more random arrangement of the collagen fibers of the bone (and other sites) and the thinner fiber diameters. The osteoblasts contain excessive concentrations of glycogen. In type II osteogenesis imperfecta, chondrogenesis at the growth plates is normal, with the skeletal dysmorphology arising from abnormal endochondral ossification on the metaphyseal side of the physis, failure of the ring of LaCroix, and multiple fractures with axial and angular distortion.[317]

The techniques of molecular biology have demonstrated abnormalities in type I collagen as the basis for at least some types of osteogenesis imperfecta.[111] Elucidation of this cause required much classical investigative work to provide the pertinent information on which to build the molecular search. Biochemical studies of osteogenesis imperfecta patients have shown that the calcium, phosphorus, magnesium, vitamin D, and PTH levels are within normal limits. Subsequent research began to reveal abnormalities in collagen.[454,495] In normal bones, the collagen is almost entirely type I, although in fetal tissues and in very young infants, some of the collagen is in the form of type III or V. This finding diminishes with age; in most older children, only type I can be recognized. In lethal osteogenesis imperfecta, a considerable increase in the concentration of types III and V and a marked variation in cross-linking were found.[392] Changes in the various types of osteogenesis imperfecta were documented to include an increase in collagen hydroxylysine residues in bone, a decrease in hydroxylysinonorleucine in skin collagen, and abnormalities of α1- and α2-polypeptides in cultured skin fibroblasts.[41,185,380,383] With an improved classification system of the heterogeneity in osteogenesis and expanding techniques in molecular biology, increasingly precise abnormalities in type I collagen are being correlated with the clinical syndromes and with entities such as the Ehlers-Danlos syndromes and skeletal dysplasias.[111,172]

Not all the clinical manifestations nor all the subtypes of osteogenesis imperfecta may be directly linked to collagen abnormalities, and other metabolic disturbances may at least be contributory.[120,140,503] Increased sweating, heat intolerance, increased body temperature, and resting tachycardia and tachypnea have been described. Although this finding suggested the possibility of hyperthyroidism, increased serum thyroxine levels have been an inconsistent finding. Hyperthermia during anesthesia has been reported, and occasionally a patient manifests true malignant hyperthermia. The serum inorganic pyrophosphate concentrations can be increased, and studies of leukocyte metabolism suggest an uncoupling of oxidative phos-

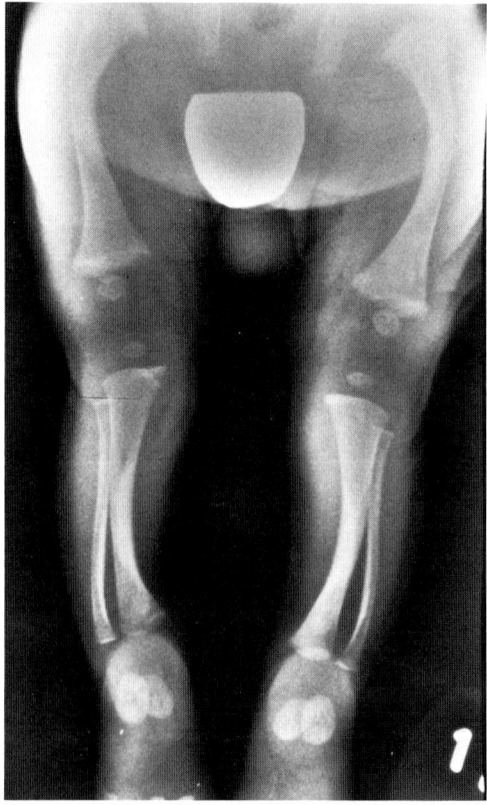

FIGURE 6-27. Patient with osteogenesis imperfecta, type IV. The patient had normal sclerae. The femurs and tibias are bowed. The type IV phenotype, when severe, can overlap with that of type III.

phorylation. Platelet function studies have demonstrated defects in adhesion and clot retraction.

Management

Treatment depends on the type of osteogenesis imperfecta. Type I osteogenesis, at least in its milder forms, may have little impact on the patient, and the role of the pediatric orthopaedic surgeon may be limited to conventional fracture care. Type II, lethal perinatal osteogenesis imperfecta, has some degree of variability. In the most severe cases, very early death occurs before pediatric orthopaedic intervention. Types III and IV represent the greatest challenges.

Several systemic treatment modalities have been attempted, but medical management remains ineffective, experimental, or still theoretical. Investigators have used calcium, vitamin C, vitamin D, fluoride, calcitonin, diphosphonates, and magnesium without benefit.[115] An early report on the efficacy of (3-amino-1-hydroxypropylidene)-1,1-biphosphonate has been made.[245] The theoretical possibilities of molecular treatments for specific types of osteogenesis imperfecta loom on the horizon.[111] Stimulating production of type I collagen in type I osteogenesis imperfecta or correcting the point mutations in certain cases of types II or IV should, in theory, cure the disease, but achieving this in practice remains a goal for the future.

Orthopaedic management of even the severe types III and IV osteogenesis imperfecta can be important in fracture prevention, fracture management, and function.[110,272,337,344,399,421] As with any heterogeneous condition, controversies about the efficacy of any specific treatment abound. It does seem worthwhile to proceed with an aggressive program of exercises, standing with bracing, working to develop ambulatory potential, and proceeding with appropriate seating, including wheelchair locomotion if required.[204]

The treatment for fractures in osteogenesis imperfecta is sometimes difficult because of the patient's ligamentous laxity, structural abnormalities of the bones, and frequency of multiple fractures with even minor or no trauma. Fractures heal readily, often with exuberant callus, but the callus formed in response to the fracture is identical in structure with the rest of the skeleton; it is plastic and easily deformed by forces associated with weight bearing or the action of muscles across the fracture site. As a result, uncontrollable deformities or shortening often occur during or after the treatment phase, which contribute to the crippling and disability experienced by patients with severe forms of the disease.

Closed treatment methods usually are employed. Use of lightweight polypropylene splints or braces may prove helpful in getting the child to bear weight soon to avoid the compounding problems of immobilization. Devices such as a parapodium may help a child to acquire an upright posture. Vacuum pants have been described for this purpose.[295] If management by closed means proves difficult, treatment with internal fixation may be enacted. Intramedullary fixation is superior to plates and screws, which tend to dislodge from the weakened bones.

The issue about the optimal age for operation has attracted different opinions. Ryoppy, Alberty, and Kaitila advocated proceeding as early as 6 weeks of age.[430] The criteria for this decision were recurrent fractures with appropriate care, progressive deformation, a cycle of immobilization leading to further weakening, and humanitarian reasons. Solid devices were used, anticipating a change to elongating devices. It was thought that this approach decreased the incidence of refracture and aided function. The insertion of solid rods percutaneously after closed osteoclasis has been reported.[331,430,446]

The alternative, which has been more frequently elected, has been to accept deformity or treat deformity with closed methods as possible in the course of early fracture management, get the child to the approximate age of 5 years, and proceed with corrective osteotomies of larger bones. The method of multiple corrective osteotomies with intramedullary fixation for the lower and upper extremities has been accepted for managing recurrent fractures with deformity and maintaining function.[457,493,523] Such procedures have been done with solid rods, employing exchanges as the child grew. The introduction of the elongating Bailey-Dubow rod seemed to provide a solution but also generated problems such as disconnection of the T-piece from the rods. Crimping the T-piece seems to provide an effective although incomplete solution. Nevertheless, the Bailey-Dubow rods seem to be a method of intramedullary fixation that diminishes the rate of reoperation, with a complication rate similar to that of non-elongating rods (Fig. 6-28).[199,357,393] Other alternatives are closed osteoclasis, with subsequent management using methods such as skin traction, pneumatic splints, or casting.[345]

Fractures in the milder types of osteogenesis imperfecta may present some problems with different options for solution. In the very mild forms, customary fracture management may apply. In more severe forms, recurrent fracture and subsequent bowing may be seen, especially at the femurs or tibias. There is no absolute rule on which to base intervention with intramedullary rodding in these situations. The risk-benefit analysis should consider recurrent fracture (i.e., two to three fractures being an arbitrary but practical limit before surgery) and deformity versus possible injury to the blood supply and physeal regions of the growing ends of long bones.

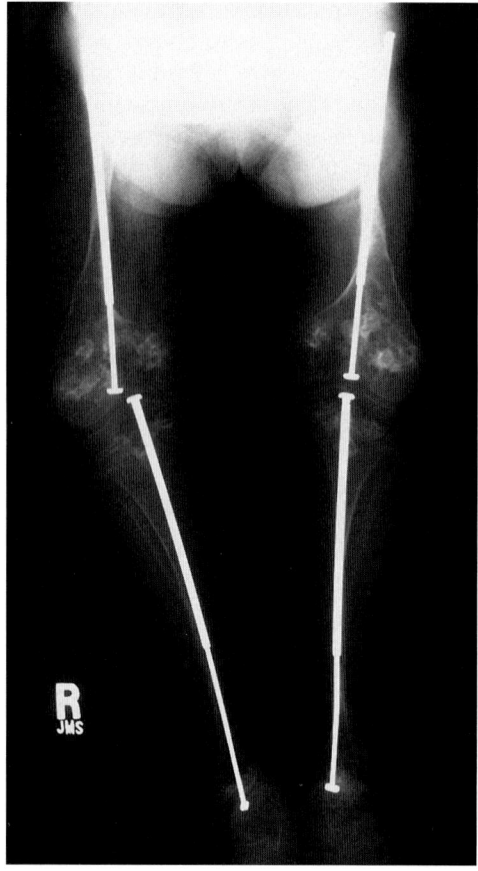

FIGURE 6-28. Radiograph of a patient with osteogenesis imperfecta, type III, after insertion of Bailey-Dubow rods.

One of the most difficult disorders to treat in osteogenesis imperfecta and in other disorders with osteopenia is scoliosis. The curves tend to advance relentlessly, and bracing is ineffective in controlling the progression of the deformity. Internal fixation is considerably hampered by the poor quality of the bone. Newer methods of segmental instrumentation are changing the approach to scoliosis in osteogenesis imperfecta and other diseases with osteopenia.[232] Curves may be fused early (at 40 degrees) to halt the relentless progression.[232] This should help in maintaining function and preventing respiratory complications.

Idiopathic Juvenile Osteoporosis

It is important to clarify any confusion regarding the terminology of metabolic bone disease. Osteopenia is a nonspecific term, indicating a reduction in bone mass as determined by radiographic study or by special techniques such as computed tomographic analysis or absorption photometry. Within this category, there are four diagnostic groups, based in part on the pathology and special studies of tissue, such as histology and bone morphometric analysis. These groups are osteoporosis, in which the bone is normal in appearance and structure but reduced in amount; osteomalacia, in which the bone matrix is laid down normally but is not properly mineralized; osteitis fibrosa, in which the bone is resorbed rapidly as a result of excessive PTH; and malignant disease, in which the bone is replaced and at times actively resorbed by local deposits of malignant cells. When radiographic examination reveals decreased bone mass, it is essential to view the process initially as osteopenia, rather than to make a more specific diagnosis such as osteoporosis and seek to define its cause among the various syndromes within the four broad categories defined.

Idiopathic juvenile osteoporosis is a rare, self-limited disorder of unknown cause that affects previously healthy children.[70,105] Since it was first described, at least 45 patients have been reported, but much remains to be learned about its cause and pathophysiology.[143,262,263,279,491] Although one series reported several patients who had symptoms before 5 years of age, the age of onset of symptoms is usually between 8 and 14 years, and resolution usually occurs spontaneously within 2 to 4 years after onset or after puberty. Idiopathic juvenile osteoporosis must be differentiated from other osteopenic conditions affecting children, especially from osteogenesis imperfecta, hematologic malignancies, thyrotoxicosis, and Cushing disease. The diagnosis of idiopathic juvenile osteoporosis is made by the positive identification of features of this disease and by ruling out the other diseases with similar manifestations.

Idiopathic juvenile osteoporosis is initially characterized by bone and joint pain, followed by an arrest of growth, various degrees of osteopenia, vertebral body collapse, and metaphyseal fractures (Figs. 6-29 and 6-30). The disease may be limited to the spine. When long bones are involved, bone loss is generalized but usually more marked at the metaphyses. The diaphyses, affected to a lesser degree, are not as thin and narrow as in osteogenesis imperfecta. Prolonged disuse may exaggerate and enhance this picture.

The pathophysiology of idiopathic juvenile osteoporosis is obscure.[171,197,223] Symptoms usually resolve after puberty, which suggests that the disease is endocrine in origin. Biochemical measurements of these patients are difficult to interpret because of the extraordinarily rapid alterations in metabolism that occur just before puberty. Serum calcium and phosphorus levels are normal. Alkaline phosphatase and urinary hydroxyproline levels are normal or slightly above normal. Metabolic studies have shown these patients to be in a negative calcium balance initially and in a positive calcium balance during recovery. Intestinal calcium absorption is abnormally low, and hypercalciuria may exist. Normal 25-hydroxyvitamin D levels with very low 1,25-dihydroxyvitamin D levels

ORGANIC PHASE **171**

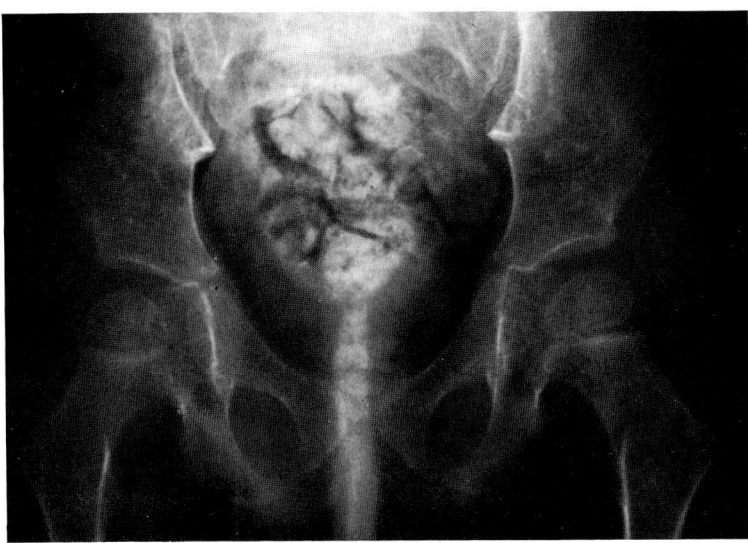

FIGURE 6-29. Child with juvenile osteoporosis. The osteoporosis affects the pelvis and the femurs.

have been reported.[315] Few data regarding PTH levels are available.

Microradiographic and histomorphometric studies of bone biopsies of patients with idiopathic juvenile osteoporosis have been confusing.[105] Increased resorbing surfaces have been demonstrated with microradiographic techniques, but the rates of formation were not evaluated. A normal osteoclast population with a decrease in the number of osteoblasts has been reported, suggesting a defect in bone formation. Other evidence suggests increased resorption and increased formation or a combined high turnover state. One serious problem with these studies is sampling error. The osteopenic changes are most marked in the metaphyseal regions, but the biopsies are obtained from the iliac crests.

Because the cause and pathophysiology of idiopathic juvenile osteoporosis are poorly understood, it is not surprising that effective treatment remains ill defined. It is not clear whether any of these regimens can favorably alter the natural history. A greater awareness of idiopathic juvenile osteoporosis using careful metabolic studies before and after treatment should help to elucidate the pathophysiology of this rare but interesting disease.

The pediatric orthopaedic surgeon sees patients with idiopathic juvenile osteoporosis for the spinal deformity (i.e., kyphosis) and pain, which may be present especially at the outset of the disease. He or she must be aware of the stage of workup for the patient so that the differential diagnosis has been excluded and idiopathic juvenile osteoporosis has been established. In this setting, antikyphotic bracing has been recommended.[260] It is initiated at 23 hours each day for approximately 1 year and then tapered consistent with maintaining a normal kyphosis and relief of symptoms. Because this is a relatively small group of patients with a tendency toward improvement, the efficacy of bracing can be questioned, but residual deformity without bracing has been described.[260]

Although osteoporosis secondary to disuse is not idiopathic, it is mentioned for two reasons. First, the lack of stress across osseous tissue can affect the balance between absorption and formation, causing a

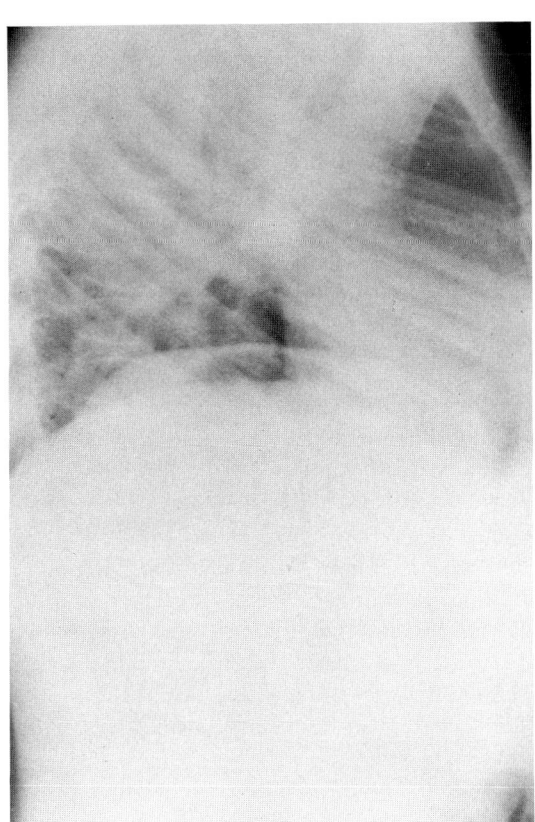

FIGURE 6-30. Juvenile osteoporosis. This lateral radiograph of the spine shows the typical biconcave appearance of the vertebrae.

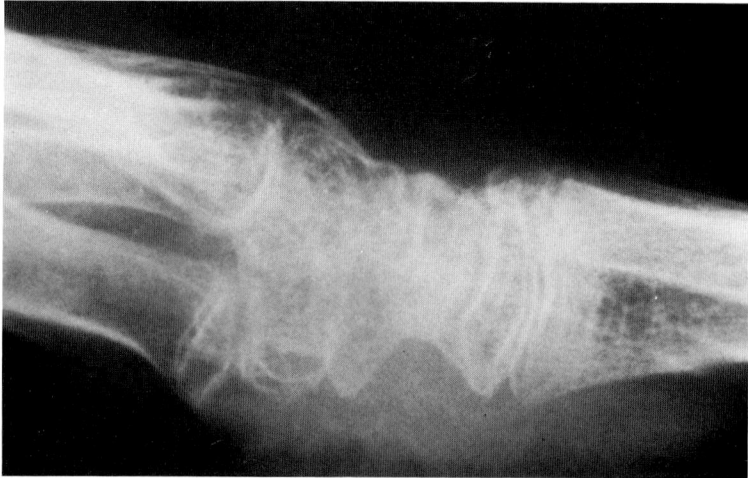

FIGURE 6-31. Disuse atrophy of the wrist and distal forearm after cast immobilization.

net decrease in bone mass (Fig. 6-31). Although the precise link between mechanical force and cell physiology is unknown, such a link may play a role in the development of osteoporoses of unknown cause.[74,514] Second, disuse atrophy has practical consequences in pediatric orthopaedics. After prolonged cast immobilization, children often show some degree of osteoporosis, with resultant weakening of the skeleton. This phenomenon is accentuated in children with neuromuscular diseases. A gradual return to activity is important in fracture rehabilitation in patients with neuromuscular diseases, including functional polypropylene bracing to avoid vicious cycles of increased fragility followed by recurrent fracture after removal of immobilizing devices.

Osteopetrosis

Osteopetrosis is an unusual disorder of the skeletal system in which, because of a failure of osteoclastic and chondroclastic resorption, the bones become exceedingly dense. The marrow spaces and foraminal openings are encroached on by the unresorbed masses of dense bone, and these features, plus the fragility of the pathologic bone, dominate the clinical picture.[313,332] Three clinically distinct forms of osteopetrosis are now recognized.[443] The infantile malignant form is transmitted as an autosomal recessive trait and is fatal within the first several years of life without treatment. An intermediate form, also transmitted in an autosomal recessive pattern, exists, appears within the first decade of life, and does not follow a malignant course. The patient with the autosomal dominant type has a normal life expectancy but many orthopaedic problems. The autosomal dominant form was first described by Albers-Schonberg (i.e., Albers-Schonberg disease).[5] Other names applied to both forms of the disease are marble bone disease and osteosclerosis fragilis generalisata.[45,228,235] Although generally considered a primary disorder of bone metabolism with diminished bone resorption due to an osteoclast defect, studies indicate that osteopetrosis may more appropriately be considered an immune disorder resulting from a thymic defect that leads to the osteoclast abnormality.[333]

The autosomal recessive malignant form of osteopetrosis is manifested in infancy with thick, poorly remodeled, dense bones and poor development of the medullary canal.[444] The child generally shows a failure to thrive, myelophthisic anemia and thrombocytopenia, hepatosplenomegaly, lymphadenopathy, spontaneous bruising, abnormal bleeding, and multiple fractures. Because of the abnormal bone modeling process, the neural foramina in the skull become small, causing neural encroachment and optic, oculomotor, and facial palsies. There are no reports of any person with untreated autosomal recessive malignant osteopetrosis surviving more than 20 years; death usually occurs from overwhelming infection or hemorrhage.

The autosomal recessive intermediate form of osteopetrosis tends to be diagnosed in later childhood after a fracture.[443] In retrospect, some of the features of the malignant form, such as anemia, dental anomalies, or disproportion, can be identified in milder presentations in this condition.

Radiographically, the bones are overly dense in osteopetrosis patients (Figs. 6-32 and 6-33). There may be transverse bands in the metaphyseal regions and longitudinal striations in the shafts. The metaphyseal regions, particularly in the proximal humerus and distal femur, may develop a flask-shaped configuration. The pelvis may appear as a bone within a bone, and the sclerotic vertebrae may have a rugger jersey appearance.

The autosomal dominant form of osteopetrosis is much more benign, and the general health and life span of the patient are usually unaffected. Mild anemia may be present; facial palsies and deafness can occur but are not necessarily features of this form of os-

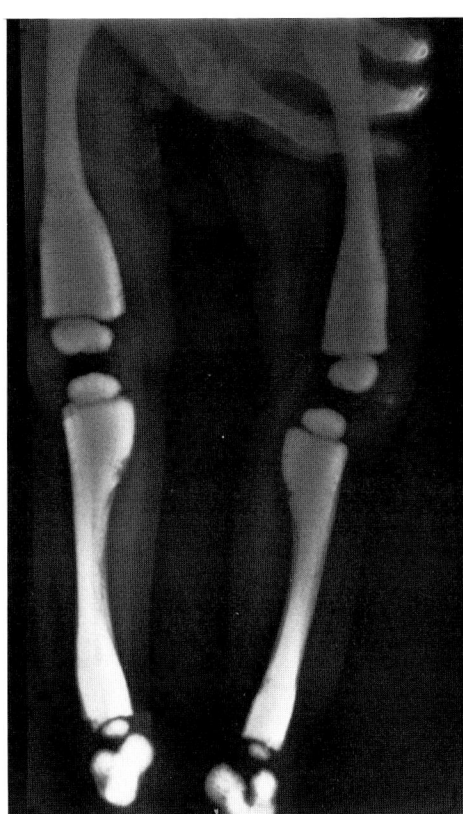

FIGURE 6-32. Patient with osteopetrosis and generalized increased density of the bones.

teopetrosis. Fractures and subsequent deformities such as coxa vara are common.

The histology of the osteopetrotic bone shows that, in addition to thickened trabeculae and cortices, tongues of cartilage bars persist at the sites of endochondral bone formation and may project far into the metaphysis and even into the diaphysis.[282,444] The persistence of cartilage bars, normally resorbed by osteoclastic action in the zone of primary spongiosa, is a characteristic of rickets and osteopetrosis, but in osteopetrosis, the cartilage bars are calcified, and their central portions undergo osseous metaplasia. The bone is relatively hypocellular, with a paucity of osteoblasts and almost complete absence of osteoclasts. The subperiosteal new bone is in part nonlamellar, suggesting that intramembranous bone formation is also abnormal, but it is less well defined than the abnormality in endochondral bone formation. Kinetic data for calcium in osteopetrotic rats and humans have shown a low accretion rate and a dramatically reduced resorption rate.[79,147,378,387,511] These observations suggest a defect in bone cell differentiation and function, the most obvious of which involves the osteoclast.[318]

The classic experiments of Walker demonstrated that osteopetrosis in mice was reversible with parabiosis or marrow transplants.[510-512] Several studies of osteopetrotic rodents and humans have revealed the role of a thymic defect in this disease. Osteopetrotic mice of the *op* strain have precocious thymic atrophy. Milhaud and colleagues found that the cell mitogens concanavalin A and phytohemagglutinin have little effect on tritiated thymidine incorporation in thymic cells from osteopetrotic rats, and several other immune defects have been demonstrated in these rodent models.[319,334] In some strains, parenteral administration of bone marrow or transplantation of thymic tissue from normal litter mates appears to correct the bone abnormalities, but in other strains, splenic or thymic lymphocytes alone may cure the disease.[237,512]

Systemic treatment is an issue for the autosomal recessive malignant form. High-dose 1,25-dihydroxyvitamin D_3 coupled with a low-calcium diet has been

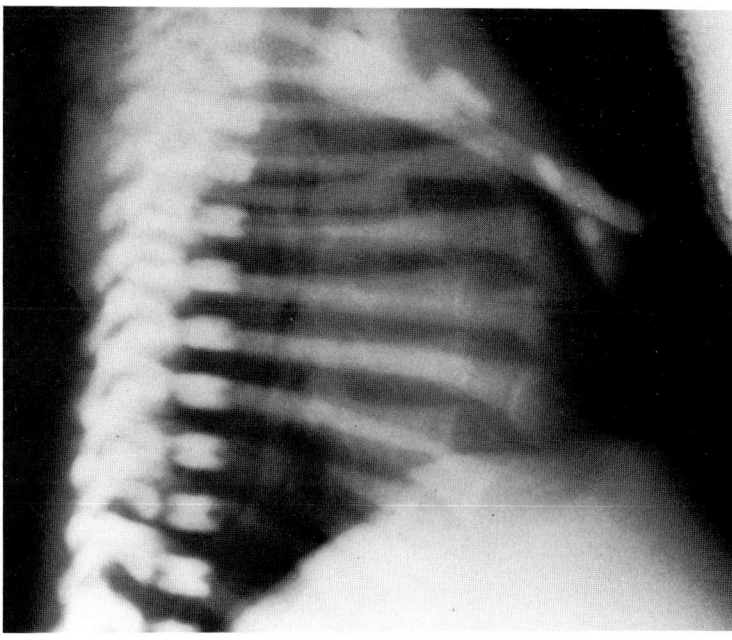

FIGURE 6-33. Patient with osteopetrosis. The increased bone density is also present in the vertebrae. In some patients, an alternating pattern of density is seen, producing a rugger jersey spine.

employed because of its ability to simulate osteoclasts and bone resorption.[443] The autosomal recessive malignant form of osteopetrosis has been successfully treated by allogeneic bone marrow transplantation from HLA-identical siblings or by marrow ablation with cyclophosphamide and total body irradiation or busulfan, followed by marrow transplantation from an HLA-mismatched donor.[37,38,107,267,445,459] These studies represent significant progress in the treatment of this disease and provide further insight into the origin of the osteoclast.

The pediatric orthopaedic concerns about osteopetrosis are numerous.[443] Transverse fractures with minimal displacement occur in the infantile malignant form and may be difficult to recognize. Without immobilization, abundant callus can occur in the healing phase. Fractures in the intermediate recessive and dominant forms are common and mandate conventional treatment. Although healing does occur, the time to healing can be prolonged.[332] Coxa vara and long bone deformity can result during the course of multiple fractures. Both are amenable to corrective osteotomy.[332,443] Intramedullary fixation is desirable but can be difficult because of the hardness of the bone and compromise of the marrow space. Osteomyelitis is common because of the diminished vascularity and immune response. This problem is most common in the mandible but also can be seen in the long bones. Back pain is frequently encountered in the benign dominant form of osteopetrosis and responds to rest, including bracing and antiinflammatory medication.

Periosteal Reaction and Soft Tissue Calcification and Ossification

Numerous metabolic, inflammatory, traumatic, neoplastic, and idiopathic disorders of the infant's or child's skeleton may produce symptoms of localized or diffuse periosteal new bone formation on radiographic study.[3,481] Unlike that of adults, the child's periosteum is easily stimulated to form new bone, and depending on the nature of the process, new bone formation may be diffuse and may cause considerable disability. Three of these disorders—hypervitaminosis A, Caffey disease, and scurvy—are discussed later in this chapter, but a brief history and chronologic differential for the various syndromes are first provided.

TABLE 6-6   Causes of Periosteal Reaction and Cortical Thickening in Infancy and Early Childhood

ENTITY	PEAK AGE AT DETECTION	CHARACTERISTICS
Physiologic periosteal reaction of newborn	1–6 mo	Thin, even periosteal reaction symmetric along femora, tibiae, humeri
Congenital or Genetic		
Menkes kinky hair syndrome	Newborn	Failure to thrive; X-linked defective copper absorption; male; sparse, kinky hair; central nervous system degeneration, metaphyseal fractures and periosteal reaction confused with abuse and rickets
Engelmann-Camurati disease	4–6 y	Autosomal dominant; progressive midshaft thickening of long bones; waddling gait; normal laboratory findings, except slight elevation of alkaline phosphatase
Infective		
Osteomyelitis	Any age	Classic bacterial osteomyelitis with lytic or blastic changes at metaphysis and periosteal reaction as disease progresses; elevated erythrocyte sedimentation rate (ESR); viral and fungal types exist; *Salmonella* osteomyelitis in sickle cell disease may begin at diaphysis, ESR not elevated
Congenital syphilis	>3 mo (severe spirochetal infection can cause fetal loss)	Many manifestations possible; osteochondritis with metaphyseal lytic lesions; diaphyseal osteitis; periostitis; positive serology for syphilis
Inflammatory		
Juvenile chronic arthritis	5–10 y	Periarticular reaction at phalanges, metacarpals, and metatarsals

(continued)

TABLE 6-6 (Continued)

ENTITY	PEAK AGE AT DETECTION	CHARACTERISTICS
Traumatic		
Accidental or nonaccidental injury	Any age	Accidental injury should result in local reaction consistent with age-appropriate activities (i.e., single tibial reaction 7–10 days after injury in a child who is walking); nonaccidental injury can result in multiple areas of periosteal reaction inconsistent with age-appropriate activities.
Burns	Weeks to months following burn	Usually a local response but can have elements of hypertrophic osteoarthropathy
Metabolic		
Hypertrophic osteoarthropathy	Any age	Usually associated with physiologic abnormality in pulmonary, cardiac, or gastrointestinal systems; tibial, fibular, radial, ulnar diaphyseal, and metaphyseal involvement; clubbing
Hypervitaminosis A	>9 mo	Periosteal reaction in long bones, typically ulnas and metatarsals, epiphyseal and metaphyseal ossification abnormalities and physeal lesions possible; elevation of serum vitamin A level
Scurvy	>9 mo	Epiphyseal and metaphyseal changes most prominent around knees with associated subperiosteal hemorrhages; abnormal vitamin C levels in serum or blood
Hyperphosphatemia	Associated with tumoral calcinosis; 2nd and 3rd decades of life but reported in childhood and infancy	Periostitis in tubular bones; calcified soft tissue masses; elevated serum phosphorus level
Healing phase of rickets	After treatment of rickets	Periosteal reaction adjacent to healing growth plates
Prostaglandin-induced hyperostosis	After weeks of prostaglandin E_1 administration to maintain ductus patency in congenital heart disease	Symmetric, diffuse periosteal reaction in long bones and ribs; elevated alkaline phosphatase level
Neoplastic		
Acute leukemia	2–5 y	Diffuse osteopenia, metaphyseal rarefactions; commonly, symmetric periosteal reaction in long bones
Metastatic neuroblastoma, retinoblastoma	Similar to leukemia, with presentations <2	Similar to leukemia
Idiopathic		
Caffey disease	6 wk–6 mo	Mandible, asymmetric involvement of clavicle, scapula, ribs, or tubular bones without associated lytic lesions; elevated alkaline phosphatase level and ESR

The salient features of periosteal reaction or cortical thickening in infancy or early childhood are recorded in Table 6-6. Physiologic periosteal reaction of the newborn is most prominent from 1 to 6 months of life. This condition is usually an incidental finding on radiographs obtained for other reasons. The periosteal reaction is thin, even, and symmetric, occurring along the femur, tibia, and humerus on both sides. Periosteal reaction can be seen in Menkes kinky hair syndrome, an X-linked recessive disorder producing defective copper absorption.[281] Although the radiographic pattern with metaphyseal spurs and adjacent periosteal reaction may suggest abuse or healing rickets, the typical child is a male neonate with profound failure to thrive and progressive central nervous system degeneration in addition to the characteristic hair after which the entity is named.

In Engelmann-Camurati disease, autosomal dominant in transmission, the progressive cortical thickening of the long bones is customarily seen at 4 to 6 years of age in association with a waddling gait resulting from progressive neuromuscular degeneration.[355]

Infection can occur at any age; in bacterial osteomyelitis, the periosteal reaction is usually associated with lytic and blastic metaphyseal changes. Congenital syphilis rarely is manifested in children younger than 3 months of age. Severe spirochetal infection may lead to fetal loss; survivors may develop early or late childhood lesions in rather protean manifestations. However, during infancy, a periosteal reaction resulting from syphilis usually occurs with metaphyseal lesions.[417]

A periosteal reaction resulting from trauma can occur at any age; the features differentiating accidental trauma from nonaccidental trauma were discussed previously. Periosteal new bone can be associated with burns.[169] Metabolic conditions can cause a periosteal reaction in a variety of settings. Hypervitaminosis A and scurvy appear usually no earlier than 9 months of age.

The neoplastic conditions that can result in the periosteal reaction in early childhood are leukemia, neuroblastoma, and retinoblastoma. Diffuse periosteal reaction associated with leukemias most often appears in children older than 2 years of age. Neuroblastoma and retinoblastoma can have similar radiographic appearances and may be seen earlier.

Although the peak occurrence of Caffey disease is 6 weeks to 6 months of age, it can occur before 6 weeks. Periosteal new bone formation before 6 weeks is consistent with infection, trauma, or Caffey disease.[93,148,276]

Caffey Disease

Infantile cortical hyperostosis, or Caffey disease, is a disorder of unknown cause affecting the skeleton and contiguous myofascial tissues.[51,86,88,462] It is characterized by a febrile illness with hyperirritability, swelling of soft tissues, and cortical thickening of bone.[377] The bones of the jaw and forearm are the most common sites, but occasionally, the lesion is diffuse. The average age of onset is usually younger than 9 weeks of age, and several cases in which the disease began in utero have been described.

The child with Caffey disease may be febrile. The sedimentation rate and serum level of alkaline phosphatase are often elevated, but cultures and serologic studies fail to show an infectious agent. Radiographs reveal a periosteal reaction involving any bone except the vertebrae and phalanges. Caffey makes the point that involvement of a single bone, with the exception of the mandible, suggests trauma. Mandibular involvement is characteristic (Fig. 6-34). In the extremities, the ulna is most frequently involved (Fig. 6-35).

Pathologic study of the involved tissue of patients with Caffey disease has failed to define a specific alteration, although hyperplasia of collagen fibers and fibrinoid degeneration have been seen. A case report described the absence of cortical bone at the diaphyses, which were entirely cancellous.[377] Most patients recover spontaneously, but for some, the severity of the disease requires short periods of corticosteroids to reduce the morbidity. Occasionally, a patient develops a chronic syndrome that persists into late childhood. The possibility of coexistent infection should be considered.[57]

Hypervitaminosis A

Overdosage with vitamin A can be acute or chronic.[183,198,299] Vitamin A is a necessary constituent in the synthesis of visual pigments, but it is also required in appropriate amounts for membrane stability. Excess or deficiency may lead to rupture of lysosomal

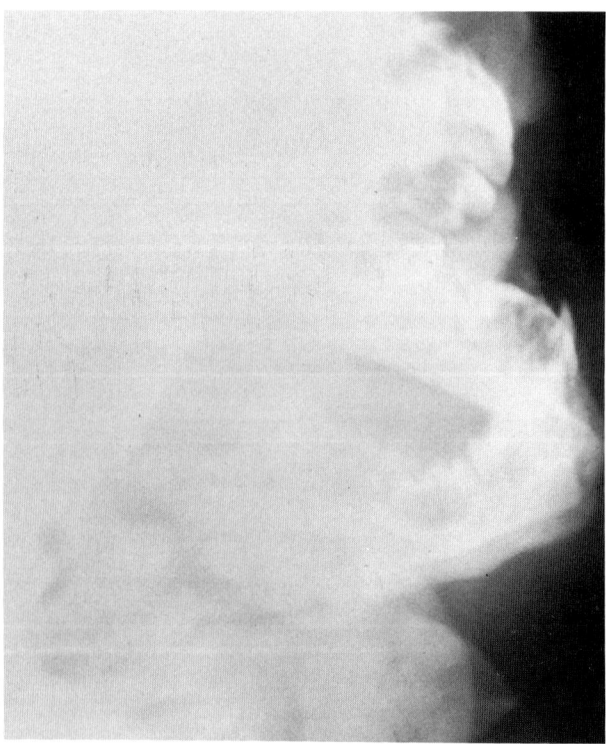

FIGURE 6-34. This oblique view of the mandible of a patient with Caffey disease demonstrates the characteristic periosteal reaction.

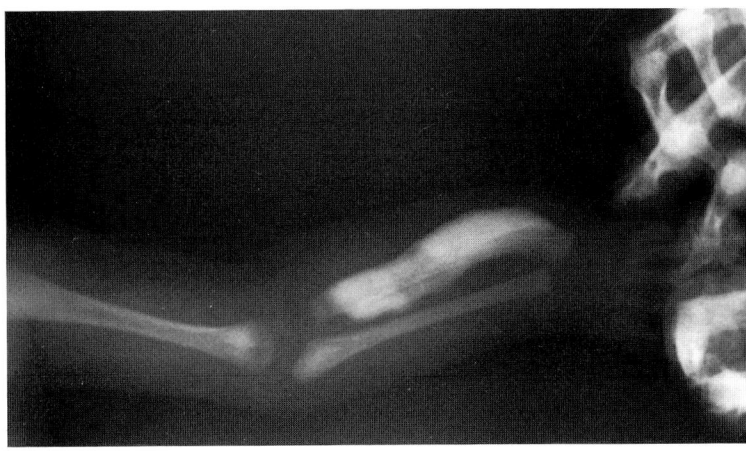

FIGURE 6-35. The ulna is the most frequently involved bone in the extremities of patients with Caffey disease.

membranes. Vitamin A participates in the biology of epithelium, and in excess, it causes a proliferation of basal cells and hyperkeratinization. Acute vitamin A intoxication causes increased intracranial pressure, vomiting, and lethargy. Several weeks or months of chronic overingestion (if the child survives) leads to a syndrome characterized by pruritus, skin lesions, failure to thrive, and muscle and bone tenderness. Radiographs in this later phase show the periosteal reaction in many of the long bones. Epiphyseal and metaphyseal ossification abnormalities occur with central physeal lesions. Hypercalcemia may be present, and serum vitamin A levels are elevated. Histologic study of the bones shows an increase in resorptive surfaces, suggesting that the combination of resorption and formation has been accelerated to a hypermetabolic state.

Scurvy

Scurvy, the pathologic state associated with a deficiency of vitamin C, is perhaps the best understood metabolic disease and is certainly the most preventable.[40] All the clinical and pathologic manifestations of scurvy are based on the now well-defined role of ascorbic acid in the synthesis of collagen. In the course of synthesis of collagen, a necessary step is the hydroxylation of the amino acids, proline and lysine, to hydroxyproline and hydroxylysine, both active participants in the intramolecular and intermolecular crosslinks that stabilize collagen. The hydroxylation step takes place early in the synthetic process and requires ferrous iron, oxygen, α-ketoglutarate, and ascorbic acid. In the absence of ascorbate (neither humans nor guinea pigs can synthesize vitamin C), the step cannot occur, and the collagen that is synthesized is defective. If the mother's intake of vitamin C is adequate during pregnancy, the infant usually does not manifest the disease for several months (i.e., late onset), even if there is dietary insufficiency. Breast-feeding by a mother who has an adequate supply of vitamin C is usually sufficient to prevent scurvy.

The pathologic process that results from inadequate intake of vitamin C is characterized by production of collagen fibers of poor quality; all the body's systems are affected. Blood vessels become excessively permeable and rupture readily, normal bone formation is reduced, and bone that forms lacks tensile strength and has a defective structural arrangement.

Clinically, children with scurvy appear undernourished, apathetic, and irritable. They show generalized weakness, poor wound healing, petechial hemorrhages, ecchymoses, and bone pain that often leads to pseudoparalysis.

Radiographic findings in the skeleton of patients with scurvy may be seen in any of the long bones but are most prominent around the knees (Fig. 6-36). Bone density is diminished, and the cortices are markedly thinned. An area of marked radiolucency, which causes the zone of provisional calcification at the physeometaphyseal junction to stand out in bold relief (i.e., white line of Fraenkel), is observed in the metaphysis. Brittleness of the zone of provisional calcification may lead to fractures and marginal spurs (i.e., Pelken sign). A zone of radiolucency forms beneath this zone, and separation may occur. The epiphyseal nucleus is also markedly radiolucent, but the calcification front of the cartilage is unaffected, producing an appearance of ringed epiphyses (i.e., Wimberger sign). Subperiosteal hemorrhages occur, lifting the periosteum and causing pain and pseudoparalysis. These areas calcify with treatment and have the appearance of periosteal new bone.

Laboratory studies may help to differentiate scurvy from other possible entities, most notably sepsis. A fasting serum vitamin C level can be obtained if scurvy is being considered. This can be difficult to interpret. Ascorbic acid concentration in the buffy coat of blood is thought to be a better measure. A nonspecific aminoaciduria also exists in case of scurvy. Treat-

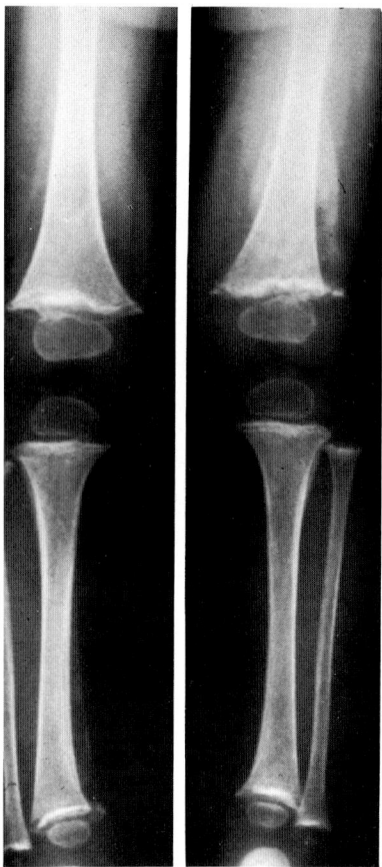

FIGURE 6-36. Patient with scurvy, early in treatment. The subperiosteal hemorrhage, especially on the left femur, has begun to ossify. The white lines of Fraenkel can still be seen at the distal femurs.

ment is replacement of the deficient ascorbic acid. Minimal daily requirements are 30 mg for infants and 50 mg for adults. Therapeutic dosages may be 200 mg or higher.

Calcification of Soft Tissues

Calcification or ossification in the soft tissues can represent diagnostic and therapeutic problems. Cutaneous calcification may be secondary to injury, to disturbance in calcium and phosphorus metabolism, or to unknown factors. This calcification may be called calcinosis universalis or calcinosis cutis circumscripta.[249] True ossification of cutaneous osteomatosis has been reported, although rarely in the pediatric age group.[299] If these entities are caused by a metabolic disturbance, treatment is directed toward rectifying the underlying problem. For idiopathic types of soft tissue calcification, such as that associated with collagen vascular diseases, no specific treatment exists, and removal of symptomatic deposits may be indicated.

Tumoral calcinosis consists of lobulated calcified soft tissue masses adjacent to joints.[215,234,352] Although it usually is seen in the second and third decades of life, it can be seen in infants and children. The serum phosphorus level is sometimes elevated. A defect in phosphorus transport or metabolism has been implicated but not established as the cause of the tumoral calcinosis.[340] The differential diagnosis includes collagen vascular diseases, hyperparathyroidism, and hypervitaminosis D, which must be excluded by history, physical examination, and laboratory data. Excision of the lesions surgically has not been entirely satisfactory because of the possibilities of skin ulceration or recurrence.[19,215] Treatment of tumoral calcinosis in adults has been successfully accomplished medically with phosphorus deprivation.[274,352] Reports of tumoral calcinosis in children and infants have been made.[19,215,234,423] The best treatment in this age group remains open to some judgment. Use of phosphorus deprivation in the immature skeleton, at least in theory, would be rachitogenic, and excision of symptomatic lesions may be the logical course.[19,234,423] However, successful medical treatment has been reported for a 6-year-old child using aluminum hydroxide antacid administration to bind phosphate and dietary phosphate restriction over the course of 6 months.[215] An initial medical approach appears justified, even for a patient with a skeletally immature skeleton. A pediatric orthopaedist and a pediatric nephrologist or gastroenterologist make a logical team to balance the ongoing calcium and phosphorus needs of the skeleton with a restriction sufficient to affect the lesions favorably. If these somewhat conflicting goals cannot be met, excision may be indicated.[19,234,423]

Ossification in the deeper soft tissues may represent fibrodysplasia ossificans progressiva (i.e., myositis ossificans progressiva) or myositis ossificans circumscripta or traumatica. Fibrodysplasia ossificans is a genetic condition.[109,268] Digital abnormalities are present at birth; the most common are underdevelopment of the great toes and short, abnormal first metatarsals. Hearing loss, premature baldness, and mental retardation can be additional clinical features of this entity. Although the cause is undefined, one possibility is an abnormal modulation of pluripotential fibroblasts into osteoblasts. There is no satisfactory treatment. Excision alone does not halt progressive ossification and limitation of the range of motion of joints. The effect of adjunctive metabolic treatments is difficult to assess. Respiratory failure with chest wall constriction may be terminal.

In myositis ossificans circumscripta, there is usually a clear history of trauma or an associated condition such as neurologic or thermal injury, in which case the entity is usually called myositis ossificans traumatica.[169,201,339] In spontaneous myositis ossificans circumscripta without a clear history of trauma or associated condition, the entity may be called pseudomalignant myositis.[362] Spontaneous myositis ossificans circumscripta is uncommon but has been reported in early childhood.[376] The history of the patient with myositis ossificans traumatica usually facilitates the radiographic differentiation from malignant processes. The ossification is more mature at the surface peripheral to the underlying bone, with an intervening space without osseous tissue. Although the periosteum as a source of the ossification has been considered, pluripotential fibroblasts modulating into osteoblasts may also be the source of myositis ossificans traumatica.

In myositis ossificans traumatica, spontaneous resolution can occur with only observation. When there is limitation of the joint range of motion (particularly associated with burns and head injuries), resection of a traumatically induced myositis may be undertaken during the quiescent phase, after it is certain that it is no longer growing or spontaneously resolving.[169,201] Adjunctive regimens such as irradiation[32] are not indicated in children, but antiinflammatory programs have been used.[339] Occasionally, differentiating pseudomalignant myositis from malignant conditions may prove difficult, necessitating biopsy, and this is best coordinated with the pathologist who is reviewing all features of the case in interpreting the histology.

Connective Tissue Syndromes

Marfan Syndrome

The Marfan syndrome is a genetic disorder of connective tissue, and like osteogenesis imperfecta and Ehlers-Danlos syndrome, it has some degree of heterogeneity. The mode of inheritance is thought to be autosomal dominant transmission.[328,398] Common findings are in the skeletal, ocular, and cardiovascular systems. The skeleton shows arachnodactyly (i.e., abnormally long and slender digits), dolichostenomelia (i.e., long, narrow limbs), pectus deformities, and scoliosis. In the cardiovascular system, aortic regurgitation, aortic dilatation, aneurysms, and mitral valve prolapse can occur. Ocular findings are myopia and superior displacement of the lens (compare with homocystinuria).

Marfan syndrome has been classified into four more or less distinct types: asthenic, nonasthenic, contractural, and hypermobile. Cardiac manifestations are particularly pronounced in the asthenic type. In contractural Marfan syndrome, the joints have a decreased range of motion. In the hypermobile type, joint motion is increased (compare with Ehlers-Danlos syndrome, type III).

The Marfan syndrome has been linked to a fibrillin gene on chromosome 15, as has ectopia lentis; congenital contractural arachnodactyly has been linked to a fibrillin gene on chromosome 5.[501] These findings make possible the diagnosis of the Marfan syndrome on the basis of genetic linkage and analysis. However, the diagnosis is still established by a combination of findings in two of the three affected systems (i.e., ocular, cardiac, and musculoskeletal) and a positive family history.[398] Although genetic analysis usually establishes the diagnosis, the pediatric orthopaedist frequently participates in this process because of the musculoskeletal findings. The ratio of upper segment (i.e., head to pubic symphysis) to lower segment (i.e., pubic symphysis to plantar surface) is calculated. In the normal mature skeleton, this ratio is 0.93. (Tables are required to calculate the normal ratio at various points in growth.) Because of the dolichostenomelia, in the Marfan syndrome, this ratio is decreased to 0.85 or less.[270] Steinberg described the thumb sign. The thumb is grasped in a clenched fist.[473] In the Marfan syndrome, because of the arachnodactyly, the thumb protrudes past the ulnar border of the hand.

Although the radiographic findings for patients with the Marfan syndrome are fairly typical for this disorder, no single sign is pathognomonic because of variable expressivity in this syndrome and considerable overlap with the normal population Arachnodactyly can easily be defined by radiographic examination because of the long, slender phalanges, metatarsals, and metacarpals and the increased ratio of length to width of the second to fifth metacarpals (Fig. 6-37). The lengths of the second through fifth metacarpals are divided by the widths of respective diaphyses, and the ratios are averaged. Positive arachnodactyly is defined as a ratio greater than 8.8 in males and greater than 9.4 in females.[371] These findings may also be seen in minimally affected persons, who have no other manifestations of the disease.

Scoliosis may occur and is relatively indistinguishable from that in other patients, but in some, the vertebral height is notably increased (Fig. 6-38). Bone density is normal compared with the osteopenia seen in homocystinuria. The curve pattern frequently is single right thoracic or double right thoracic and left lumbar.[341] The thoracic curve is most commonly lordoscoliotic. The thoracolumbar junction is prone to kyphosis, probably because of the underlying ligamentous laxity.[11]

It is important for the orthopaedist who sees undiagnosed patients with the Marfan phenotype to consider it when treating sprains and other injuries associated with the altered ligamentous structure or scoliosis. The potential for serious ocular abnormalities and life-threatening cardiac abnormalities exists with the musculoskeletal problems. The potential car-

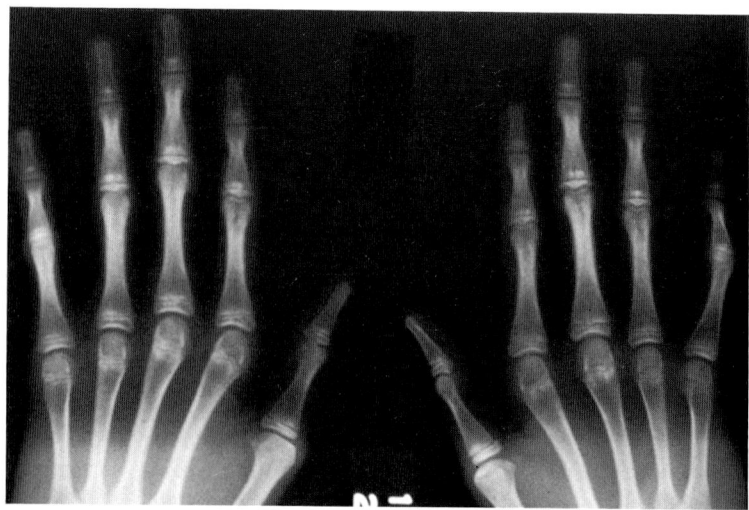

FIGURE 6-37. Hands showing arachnodactyly. Notice the long, thin metacarpals and phalanges.

diac problems are aortic and mitral vavular disease and aortic aneurysm. After the diagnosis of the Marfan syndrome has been considered and workup pursued, electrocardiogram and echocardiogram are customarily obtained. If the echocardiogram reveals positive findings, the cardiology service should participate in the patient's care. Scoliosis should be aggressively treated. The treatment guidelines follow those for idiopathic scoliosis. Curves greater than 50 degrees require surgery.[422] The cardiac status is important at this juncture. Vavular disease requires antibiotic prophylaxis, with the specific recommendations varying among cardiology services.

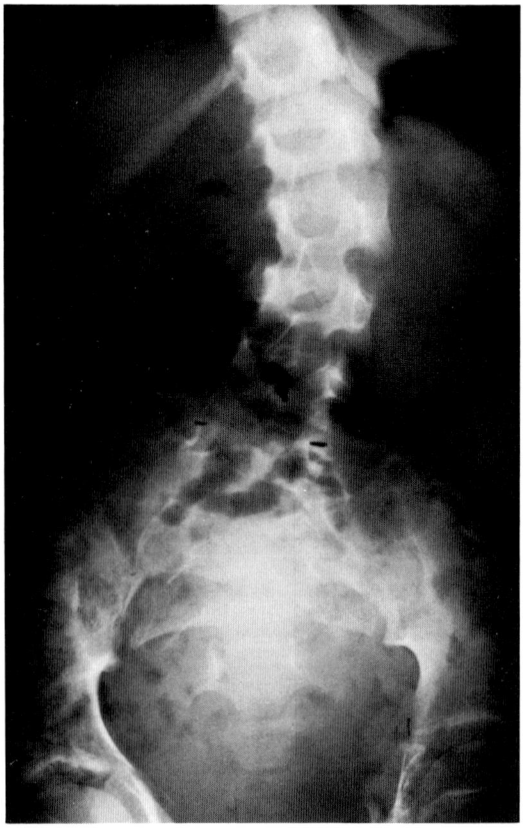

Ehlers-Danlos Syndrome

Ehlers-Danlos syndrome (EDS) once was considered to be a single genetically induced entity characterized by hyperextensibility of the skin, joint hypermobility, easy bruisability, soft tissue and bony fragility, calcification of soft tissues, and various degrees of osteopenia. The syndrome was thought to result from a single error but to have variable expressivity. It has been established that EDS is a family of disorders embracing a large variety of defects in collagen metabolism.[83] At least 13 types of EDS have been identified, and the groups are now considered to comprise the most common heritable disorder of connective tissue.[111] The genetic basis for types I, II, and III does not seem to reflect a difference in the type I or III collagens, which are in skin and ligaments, and presumably is expressed in other collagens or noncollagenous proteins in the matrix. Type VII EDS does have abnormalities in type I collagen similar to the abnormality found in type IV osteogenesis imperfecta (OI), but the two syndromes are distinct.[111] Type VII EDS has multiple joint dislocations but no clinical bone fragility, whereas type IV OI has joint hypermobility but no instability and the bone fragility characteristic of OI.

The orthopaedic manifestations of EDS vary with the type but may also be considered collectively.[4,46] This has practical significance for the pediatric orthopaedic surgeon because, as in those with Marfan syndrome, these patients may present to the pediatric orthopae-

FIGURE 6-38. Patient with Marfan syndrome. Scoliosis is obvious. The bone quality is normal, unlike the osteopenia seen in homocystinuria.

dist without a previous diagnosis. Consideration of the diagnosis of EDS may then prompt further consultation, such as genetics and dermatology, leading to a diagnosis, subtyping, and a clearer definition of the associated conditions. The general orthopaedic conditions include joint hypermobility, joint instability,[35,404] arthralgias, and scoliosis. Scoliosis is particularly common in types III and VI EDS. As in the Marfan syndrome, treatment generally proceeds along guidelines for idiopathic scoliosis, with an awareness of associated conditions and particularly cautious monitoring of the response to bracing.

In EDS I, the gravis variety, joint hypermobility and skin hyperextensibility dominate the picture. The skin, although hyperextensible, is not lax and returns to its original configuration. Areas of recurrent bruising cause accumulation of pigment (Fig. 6-39). Subcutaneous calcified nodules may be present in these regions and may be seen on radiographs. EDS I is transmitted as an autosomal dominant trait.

In EDS II, the mitis variety, the manifestations are similar to those in EDS I but milder. The transmission pattern is also autosomal dominant.

In EDS type III, also known as benign familial hypermobility, joint hypermobility is present, but scar formation is normal, unlike the situation in EDS I and II. The inheritance pattern is autosomal dominant. There is not a clinical laboratory test to establish a diagnosis of EDS III, which is made on the basis of history (including family history) and physical examination. It is worthwhile for the orthopaedist to consider this diagnosis for a patient with instability of multiple joints. In such a setting, successful surgical reconstruction may be difficult, and fusion ultimately may be required.[4] Cardiac evaluation for the possibility of a floppy mitral valve may be desirable.

EDS type IV is the vascular or ecchymotic type and can be further subtyped. It results from abnormalities in type III collagen, the type required for vascular integrity. Autosomal dominant and recessive modes of transmission have been described. The clinical findings are thin skin, usually normal joint mobility, and visceral rupture.

In EDS V, the skin hyperextensibility is similar to that of EDS II but with less marked joint mobility and skin fragility. Its transmission is considered to be X-linked.

EDS type VI is the most clearly biochemically characterized syndrome. Patients with this ocular-scoliotic type of EDS have relative decreases in the concentrations of lysine hydroxylase and therefore have deficient concentrations of hydroxylysine in their collagen.[388] Because lysine hydroxylation is a posttranslational modification of the collagen necessary for normal cross-links, the collagen fibers are loosely organized and more soluble. As with most enzymatically based genetic diseases, transmission occurs as an autosomal recessive trait. Ocular fragility and scoliosis are present.

EDS type VII, arthrochalasis multiplex congenita, is notable for extreme joint laxity. Three subtypes with abnormalities in type I collagen metabolism have been identified.[111] Developmental dysplasia of the hip is common.[35] Autosomal dominant and recessive modes of transmission exist.

In EDS VIII, the usual stigmata are present, but progressive periodontal disease is a distinguishing feature. The biochemical defect is unknown. Inheritance is as an autosomal dominant trait.

Homocystinuria

Cysteine ($SHCH_2CH[NH_2]COOH$) is not an essential amino acid; it is synthesized from methionine and serine. Cystine or dicysteine is the disulfide resulting from the oxidation of two cysteine moieties. The homolog homocysteine ($SHCH_2CH_2CH[NH_2]COOH$) contains an additional methyl group compared with

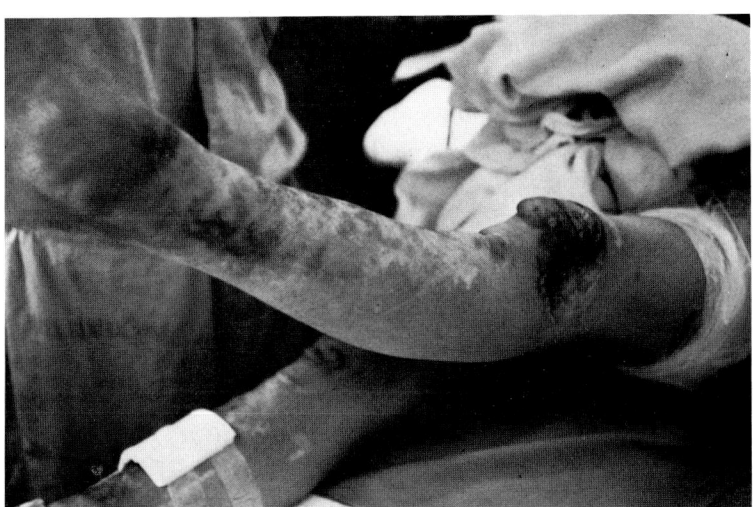

FIGURE 6-39. Patient with Ehlers-Danlos syndrome, type I. The knees and pretibial regions have been subjected to recurrent injury and have accumulated heme pigmentation. (Courtesy of Michael G. Ehrlich, M.D., Providence, RI.)

cysteine. Homocystine is the disulfide from two homocysteine groups. Homocysteine is an intermediary metabolite in the production of cysteine from methionine. There are three enzymatic steps in this pathway for which defects have been described that lead to the accumulation of homocysteine and homocystine in the blood and homocystine in the urine.[178,203]

Type I homocystinuria has a phenotype similar to the Marfan syndrome.[71] Patients with homocystinuria are tall with long limbs and may have arachnodactyly and scoliosis. Dislocation of the lens is common, but unlike that seen in the Marfan syndrome, the displacement is inferior. Osteoporosis is a marked feature of type I homocystinuria, but in the Marfan syndrome, bone quality is normal. Vertebral osteoporosis may be present in homocystinuria, producing biconcavity and flattening of vertebral bodies. Florid arachnodactyly and scoliosis are more common in the Marfan syndrome, and the vertebral bodies are normal or excessively tall. Widening of epiphyses and metaphyses of long bones is more typically seen in homocystinuria. Another notable feature of type I homocystinuria is an abnormality in clotting, which leads to venous and arterial thromboembolic episodes.[62]

The biochemical defect in type I homocystinuria is thought to be a deficiency of cystathionine synthetase, which normally catalyzes the chemical union of homocysteine and serine to form cystathionine. The enzyme uses pyridoxine (vitamin B_6) as a cofactor. Blood levels of methionine are increased in patients with this metabolic error. Screening marfanoid patients for homocystine in the urine with the cyanide nitroprusside test can differentiate type I homocystinuria from the phenotypically similar Marfan syndrome. Some degree of mental retardation may affect patients with homocystinuria.[75]

Types II and III homocystinuria are biochemically distinct, because the errors cause blocks at other points. Blood levels of methionine are normal. The other stigmata, such as skeletal changes and thromboses, are absent.

Treatment for homocystinuria depends on the type. In type I, the typical course is methionine restriction and pyridoxine supplementation. This may also have the beneficial effect of preventing thromboses.[62] For types II and III, methionine restriction is harmful. Treatment with cofactors also varies for the other types. Vitamin B_{12} is suggested in the management of type II, and folic acid is used for type III.

As with all inborn errors of metabolism, homocystinuria may reveal other physiologic aspects. Hyperhomocysteinemia is an independent risk factor for vascular disease.[103] It may have a role in the generation of neural tube defects.[470] The role of folate, B_6, and B_{12} in treating hyperhomocysteinemia and its sequelae is evolving.

ENDOCRINOPATHIES AND CONDITIONS WITH INDEFINITE PATHOPHYSIOLOGY

Although the spectrum of disorders of the endocrine glands can manifest symptoms in several ways, alterations in the rate of growth and skeletal morphology are common in children. The pediatrician usually detects the problem and then consults the orthopaedist; it is essential that he or she be aware of the nature and significance of these disorders. Although skeletal growth has been discussed extensively in another chapter, some salient features of the growth process are germane to endocrine physiology are briefly reviewed here.

Several parameters are useful in assessing growth: height, sitting height, arm span, head circumference, and body weight.[484,486] These factors must be interpreted in relation to chronologic and biologic age. Because of difficulties in interpretation, investigators have advocated increasingly sophisticated means of assessment.[82,485] Nevertheless, the factors are appropriate in the primary study of the patient. All parameters must be interpreted according to cross-sectional distributions in the general population or, if possible, longitudinally in the individual over time. The latter approach is especially useful in determining whether a borderline value is actually pathologic for a given patient.

Examples of different growth patterns are shown in Figures 6-40 through 6-43. The child whose curve continues to fall below the normal percentiles is much more likely to have a hormonal problem than the child whose curve stays on a constant low percentile. Placement in the third percentile and below in absolute height raises suspicion, and when combined with a commensurate decrease in growth velocity, such an abnormality warrants further investigation.

Several features of morphometry and growth can be assessed in a crude manner without consulting the standard charts. The first of these is the ratio or percentage of sitting height relative to total height. At birth, the ratio should approximate 70%. (This value also can be expressed as a ratio of upper segment [i.e., head to pubic symphysis] to lower segment [i.e., pubic symphysis to plantar surface] and should equal 1.69.) By 3 years of age, the sitting height should constitute 57% of total height, and in adolescence, the value should be 52%. As a rough approximation, 25 cm of growth can be expected in the first year of life, 10 cm in the second year, 6 cm in the third year, 6 cm in the fourth year, and 5 cm annually thereafter, with a spurt at the beginning of adolescence. The velocity of growth throughout childhood has been the subject of extensive analytic study and is a far more sensitive

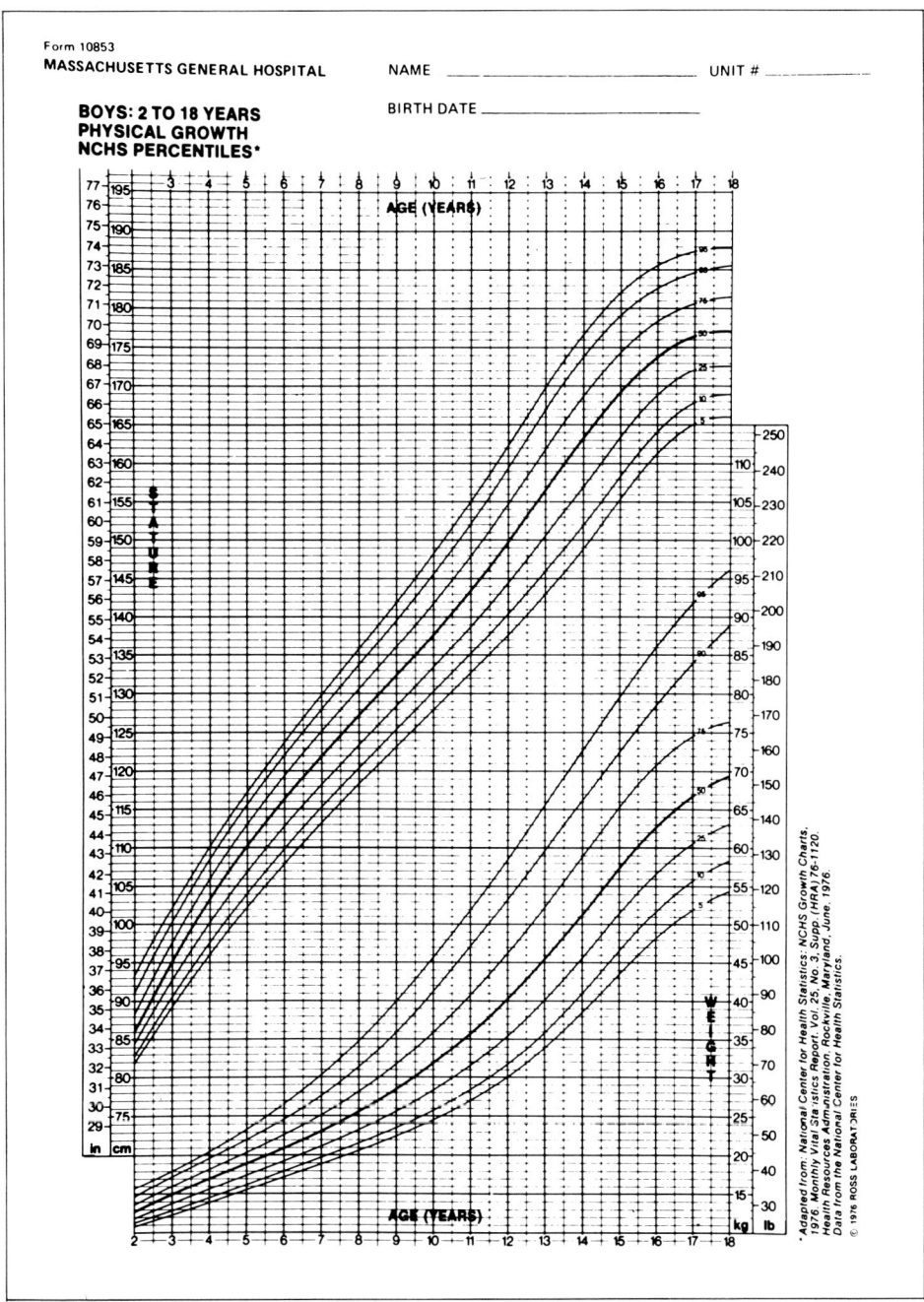

FIGURE 6-40. Normal growth charts of boys, 2 to 18 years of age.

indicator than absolute stature in the detection of a problem (see Fig. 6-43).

Correlating these parameters relative to some index of maturity is an important issue, and Tanner and associates have devoted much effort to this.[484,486] Because any stage of development is a combination of anatomic and physiologic changes and this combination may be different for each person, any single parameter for a person compared with standard parameters may not accurately reflect that person's maturity. A combination of physical and radiographic criteria may have to be invoked. For most orthopaedic applications, radiographs of the left wrist and hand for bone age in children 2 years of age and older are the customary index of age, but the orthopaedist must be aware that there are limitations to this method.[216,485] These include interobserver variability in determining the bone age, variation in the correlation of growth with bone age among different genetic populations, and a relatively large standard deviation in the correlation within a population during the growth spurt.

The initial diagnostic approach for patients suspected of having an endocrine-related growth problem should include a careful history of pattern of

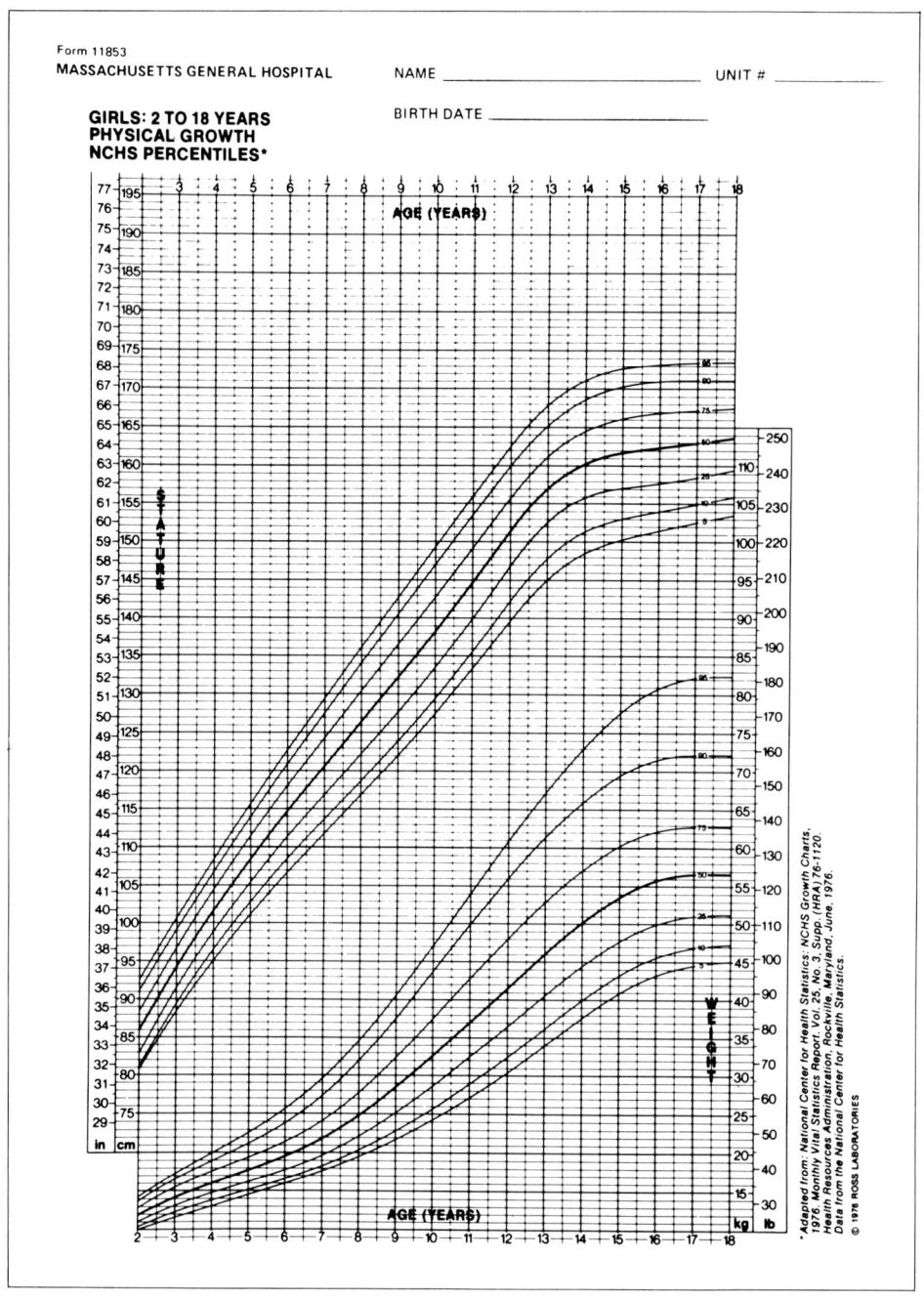

FIGURE 6-41. Normal growth charts of girls, 2 to 18 years of age.

growth, familial history, and history of associated gastrointestinal, renal, and neurologic signs or symptoms. Endocrine disturbances should be evaluated. Menarcheal history is important in the female. In addition to a general physical examination, the growth patterns previously described must be measured accurately. Breast development and the age of appearance of and the extent of development of axillary and pubic hair and gonads should be assessed. Routine laboratory studies should include complete blood count, urinalysis, glucose, BUN, creatinine, electrolytes, calcium, phosphorus, and alkaline phosphatase levels and a left wrist and hand radiographic examination for bone age. Additional laboratory studies may be necessary in the pursuit of specific entities.

Normal Variant Short Stature

By definition, normal variant short stature (NVSS) involves a current and predicted height below the third percentile, a birth weight greater than 2.5 kg, no apparent organic cause for growth retardation, and a normal serum level of growth hormone (tested with pharmacologic provocation).[428] NVSS has tentatively been

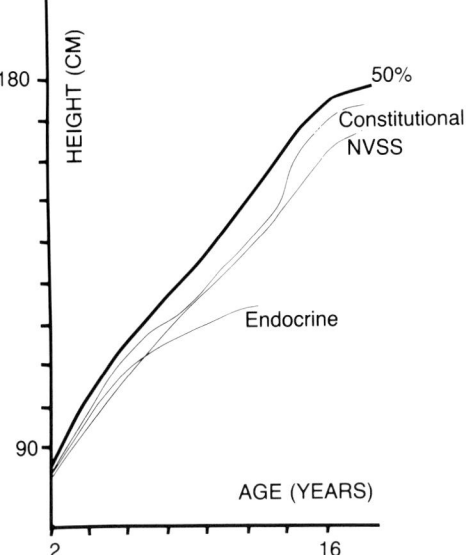

FIGURE 6-42. Different patterns of growth disturbance. The normal 50th percentile serves as a reference. In the endocrine disturbance, a progressive falloff in growth occurs. Constitutional growth delay starts normally, falls off over the first few years of life, and finally regains its earlier percentile level. Normal variant short stature (NVSS) remains at a constant but low (third or less) percentile.

further classified, but the significance of this is yet to be established. Practically speaking, 85% of short-statured persons fall into this category, for which no specific cause can be established. A slightly different category of short stature is described by the term constitutional growth delay. In this situation, there is normal early growth, followed by a deceleration during the first 2 years, with subsequent reestablishment of a normal pattern. As with NVSS, no metabolic or endo-

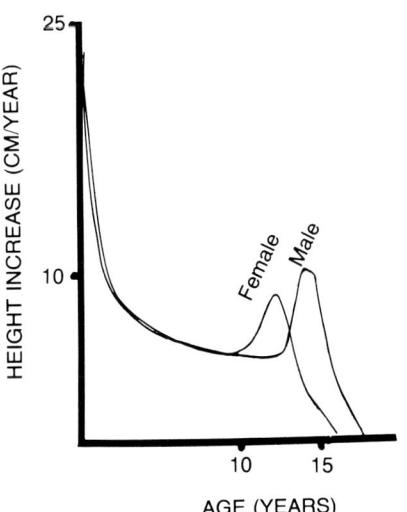

FIGURE 6-43. Growth velocity curves. Plotted in this manner, changes in growth rates frequently can be detected early. (Adapted from Tanner JM, Whitehouse RH, Takaishi M. Standards from birth to maturity for height, weight, height velocity, and weight velocity: British children, 1965. Arch Dis Child 1966;41:454.)

crine abnormality can be established. This growth pattern is clear in retrospect but causes concern at the time of presentation; a workup is recommended to rule out other problems. The differential diagnosis includes other conditions (discussed in subsequent sections) that cause short stature.

Treatment is usually a matter of explanation and reassurance. One report suggested a possible role for growth hormone as therapy for a subgroup of this population; however, while growth hormone supplies remain limited, the use of this agent has not been universally advocated.[428] The role of nutrition as a cause of NVSS has yet to be fully evaluated, and improving dietary intake of proteins and other important constituents remains the principal method of management.[119]

Growth Hormone Deficiency and Hypopituitarism

Deficiency of growth hormone leads to progressive inhibition of linear growth and maturation.[320,402] Birth weight and height are usually normal in children with this disorder. Typically, the deviations begin to become evident after the first year of life. Deficiency of growth hormone may or may not be associated with other deficiencies of hypothalamic releasing factors or other pituitary hormones, including, from the anterior portion, human growth hormone, adrenocorticotropin (ACTH), thyroid-stimulating hormone (TSH), follicle-stimulating hormone, prolactin or lactogenic hormone, luteinizing hormone, or testicular interstitial cell–stimulating hormone; from the middle portion, melanocyte-stimulating hormone; and from the posterior portion, antidiuretic hormone (ADH) and oxytocin.[238,424] The clinical manifestations of growth hormone deficiency can be narrow, affecting only growth, or diffuse, with a broad range of additional abnormalities. Deficiencies of ACTH and TSH can be recognized by appropriate biochemical tests, but deficiencies of gonadotropins usually cannot be diagnosed until the age at which puberty would otherwise be expected. The basic clinical manifestation is progressive retardation in growth and maturation (Fig. 6-44).

When growth hormone deficiency is suspected on clinical grounds, laboratory testing is essential.[300] The studies available are one-time assay tests, with results varying according to stress and alterations in response to chemical and pharmacologic manipulation. The first major investigative effort is an exercise test in which growth hormone levels are measured by radioimmunoassay during walking. Resting values are usually below 5 ng/mL; minimum peak values are in the 7 to 12 ng/mL range. If the exercise test result is normal, the production of growth hormone is considered adequate. If it is abnormal, a pharmacologic stress

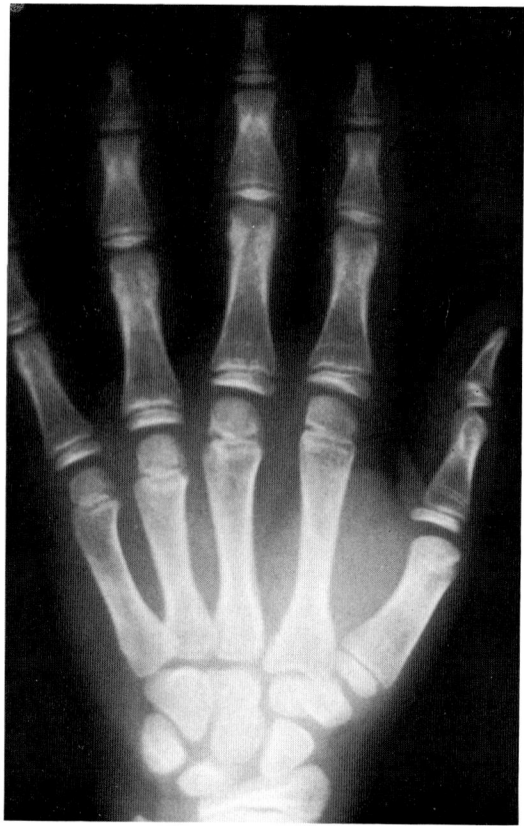

FIGURE 6-44. Patient with panhypopituitarism. The patient had retarded height and maturation. The bone age was 11 years; the chronologic age was 20 years.

test can be performed. Several protocols have been advanced, including insulin-induced hypoglycemia, arginine infusion, and an L-dopa–propranolol test.[96] If the rise in growth hormone is still inadequate and thyroid function is normal, growth hormone deficiency has been confirmed.

The underlying cause of growth hormone deficiency may be idiopathic: previous head injury; psychosocial problems, including malnutrition and neglect; and intracranial tumor.[395,396] It is particularly important to rule out the presence of a craniopharyngioma by thorough neurologic examination, visual field studies, fundoscopic examination, skull radiographs, and computed tomography.

The differential diagnosis of growth hormone–deficient short stature includes several entities. In NVSS, the patient continues to grow at a constant but low level, but in constitutional growth delay, there is a return to a higher growth curve without intervention. Although delayed puberty may be difficult to differentiate from growth hormone deficiency, maturity milestones, once established, continue to appear at a normal rate. A growth hormone assay may be helpful in making these differential diagnoses. At times, children with one of the gastrointestinal or renal diseases mentioned in previous sections may present for evaluation because of growth retardation, but the general initial workup reveals the presence of such disease. Disorders associated with chromosomal abnormalities should be considered. Turner syndrome usually has many other stigmata, but an XO/XX mosaic may be more difficult to differentiate. Hypothyroidism and gonadal dysfunction also must be included in the differential diagnosis.

Treatment for growth hormone deficiency must start with the exclusion and correction of the psychosocial causes of the deficiency, because in these cases, the response to growth hormone administration is suboptimal. In other cases, human growth hormone administration is the treatment of choice.[460] If growth hormone deficiency is associated with other hormonal deficiencies, replacement treatment for these factors must be included in the therapeutic regimen. The response to growth hormone in these selected cases is usually dramatic. Unfortunately, a few patients develop antibodies to the hormone, and its value is markedly diminished.

Hypothyroidism

The manifestations of a deficiency in thyroid hormone depend on age. In the newborn period, hypothyroidism manifests itself as cretinism; the infant is described as sluggish and shows increasingly short stature and developmental delay, immature facies, a broad flat nasal bridge, and coarse hair. The child often manifests constipation, severe feeding problems, persistence of jaundice, a protruding tongue, and a protuberant abdomen with an umbilical hernia. Mental development is retarded, and if recognition and treatment are delayed, irreparable nervous system damage may occur.

In the older child, manifestations usually more closely resemble those seen in adults with hypothyroidism. Changes in facial appearance are less commonly seen. Retardation of growth is characteristic, and radiographically, the secondary centers of ossification appear late and show a peculiar fragmentation that may be misinterpreted as evidence of osteonecrosis.[420] Lethargy, changes in personality, and poor school performance may be the presenting features. Slipped capital femoral epiphyses may be seen.[517] In untreated cases, slippage may not be seen until the child is older; because it can also occur during the treatment for hypothyroidism as the bone age advances, vigilance is important (Fig. 6-45).[533] In some children with mild hypothyroidism, retarded linear growth and delayed skeletal maturation may be the only manifestations.

Specific laboratory studies for hypothyroidism include measurement of thyroid hormones and TSH. Additional thyroid studies may be necessary to define

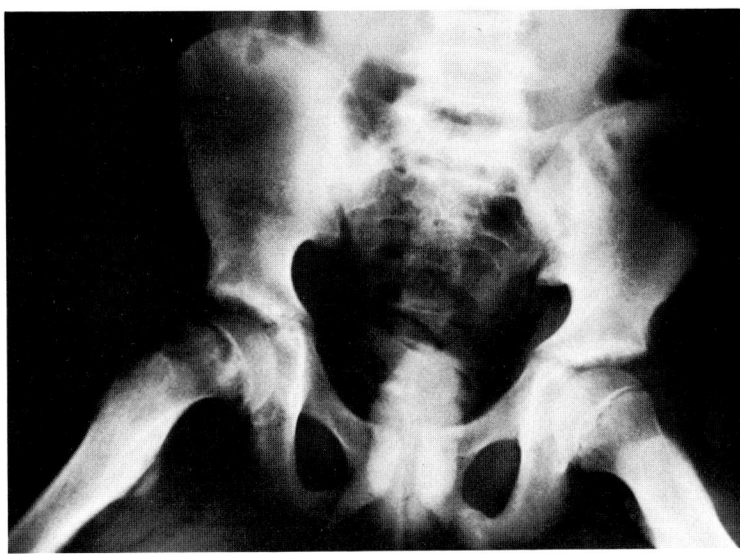

FIGURE 6-45. Slipped capital femoral epiphysis in a boy being treated for hypothyroidism. The patient's chronologic age was 13 years, 11 months, and his bone age was 12 years, 6 months.

the precise locus of the hypothyroidism. Normal values must be interpreted in terms of age. In the case of growth retardation, a growth hormone assay must also be performed. However, the serum growth hormone level usually does not rise, even in response to the provocative tests, until the hypothyroidism has been corrected. Bone age is typically delayed to a more severe degree than in other endocrinopathies, affecting maturation. Delay in the appearance of secondary centers involves all epiphyses. For congenital hypothyroidism, a knee film is more useful than a wrist film (Fig. 6-46). The distal femoral secondary center of ossification that should be present at term is absent. Occasionally, irregularities in ossification give a stippled appearance to the secondary centers. In the proximal femur, this may impart a Perthes-like radiographic appearance, but both proximal femurs are symmetrically involved (Fig. 6-47). One study found a group of Perthes patients to be generally euthyroid but to have a moderate elevation of free thyroxine, suggesting a disturbance in chondrocyte maturation in this disease.[356]

Treatment for hypothyroidism is replacement with an appropriate dosage of thyroid hormone, a therapy that requires fine tuning to avoid acceleration in bone maturation and premature closure of epiphyseal plates. Even with appropriate treatment, evidence indicates that juvenile-acquired hypothyroidism results in a permanent height deficit relative to the duration of hypothyroidism before treatment.[420]

Gonadal Abnormalities and Sex Steroids

Some of the effects of sex steroids on growth and turnover were discussed in the early part of this chapter. The manner by which these hormones act is still not completely clear, but according to theory, specific receptors for these steroids are on the membrane or in the cytoplasm of the target cells.[265,449] No receptors for androgens or estrogens have been identified in chondrocytes from the epiphyseal plate, unlike the specific receptors for somatomedins.[498]

Despite the absence of specific binding sites, two major effects of sex steroids on the skeleton have been

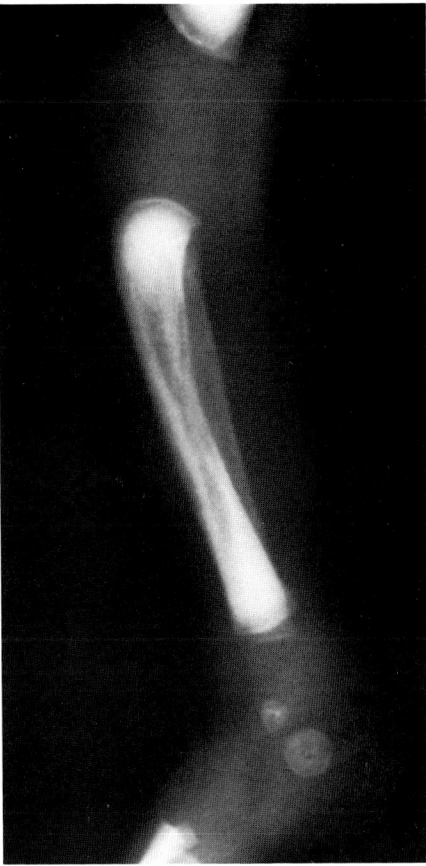

FIGURE 6-46. Child with congenital hypothyroidism at term. The distal femoral secondary center should be ossified but is absent.

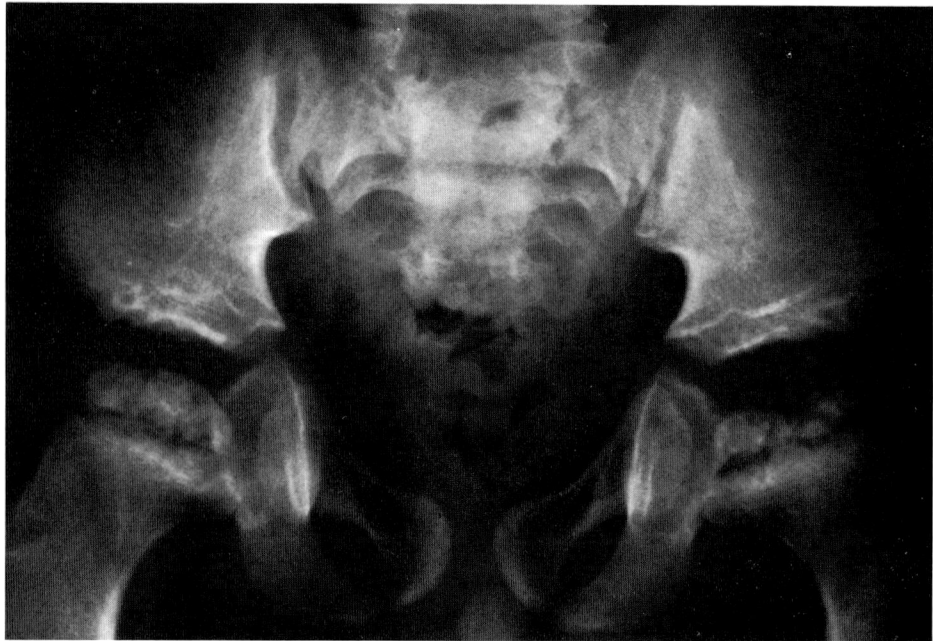

FIGURE 6-47. Patient with later-onset hypothyroidism. A Perthes-like pattern can be seen in the femoral epiphyses, but both are at a similar stage of fragmentation.

identified: promotion of maturation and an increase in the rate of growth. The typical early finding in syndromes associated with sexual precocity is accelerated growth. At first, the child is taller than his or her peer population according to chronologic age. Later, the acceleration of maturation predominates, and if untreated, the patient ultimately suffers a growth impairment compared with his or her peer group. As an example, an increased concentration of testosterone in childhood results in virilization and in initially increased epiphyseal growth. With advancing time, the plate closes prematurely, and ultimately, the child is shorter in stature than his peers. Conversely, in humans and animals, early castration initially slows the rate of growth but materially increases the length of time until epiphyseal closure; the eunuch often is taller than the average child. Estrogens also promote maturational changes in the epiphysis, but because cell proliferation and matrix production are often retarded, the person with an abundance of estrogen may be considerably shorter.

Sex steroids are also produced by the adrenal cortex. They may be especially important for females, because they are converted to testosterone activity and may initiate the adolescent growth spurt.

It is evident from the forgoing facts that the syndromes associated with precocious puberty and adrenal hyperplasia must be considered in the differential diagnosis of disturbances of growth or premature skeletal maturation, and the abnormalities associated with decreased gonadal function such as Turner syndrome or Prader-Willi syndrome must be considered in the differential diagnosis of delayed skeletal maturation.

Glucocorticoid-Related Abnormalities

The abnormalities in the skeleton associated with alterations in adrenal glucocorticoid production are encountered considerably less frequently in children than in adults. However, Cushing syndrome occurs (Fig. 6-48), and the musculoskeletal abnormalities of Addison disease have also been reported.[258,531] Iatrogenic problems secondary to the administration of steroids for asthma, neoplasms, immunosuppression, and other diseases are more common in childhood.

Although no definite receptor for glucocorticoids has been found in epiphyseal chondrocytes, the effects of these agents on the growing skeleton are profound. Proteoglycan and collagen synthesis are sharply decreased, and chondrocyte differentiation in the zone of growth is impaired. An excess of glucocorticoids may exert an effect through suppression of growth hormone synthesis or somatomedin production. Corticoids also inhibit calcium absorption, although based on this factor alone, rickets must be rare.

Of greatest concern is the action of glucocorticoids on the skeleton itself, because sustained high doses produce profound and usually irreversible osteopenia, even after the drug is discontinued. However, a study of adults demonstrated that 1,25-dihydroxyvitamin D_3 and calcium used prophylactically prevented corticosteroid-related bone loss in the lumbar spine.[435] Children on corticosteroids may exhibit

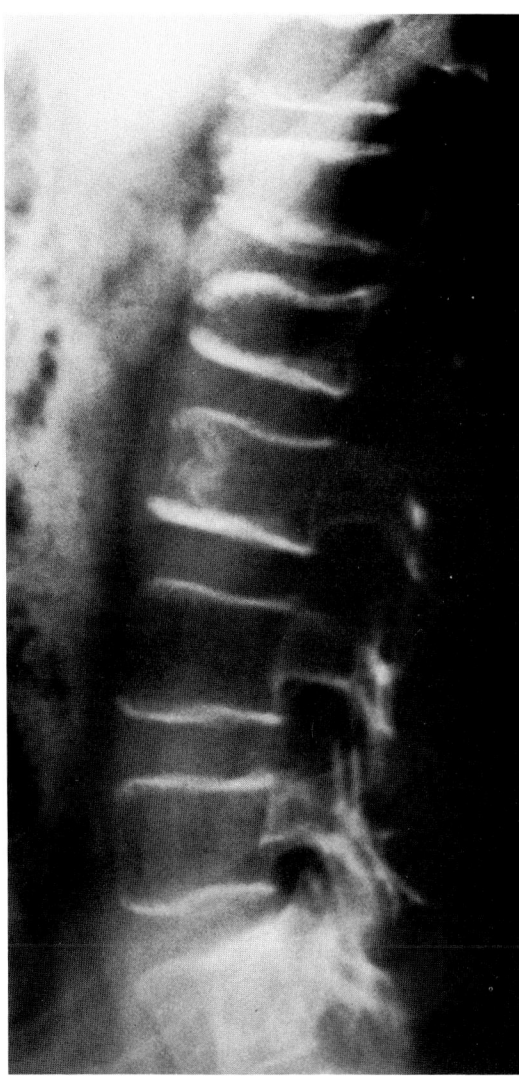

FIGURE 6-48. Cushing syndrome in an adolescent. There is marked steroid-induced osteoporosis.

fairly severe osteoporosis, often with compression fractures of the vertebrae. The possibility of osteonecrosis occurring in 6% to 25% of children receiving prolonged therapy with high doses of corticosteroids is significant; it is a major cause of disability. Unfortunately, there is no absolutely safe dosage of glucocorticoids for children. The agents should be used only when absolutely necessary and at the lowest possible dosage consistent with clinical well-being.

Fibrous Dysplasia

Fibrous dysplasia (i.e., osteitis fibrosa cystica disseminata) is a disease of unknown cause that produces sites in one, several, or many bones, in which the normal medullary mix of osseous and marrow elements are replaced by what appears to be benign neoplastic fibrous tissue.[129,222,230] Fibrous dysplasia is a difficult entity to classify. It can be classified under neoplasms and is covered fully in that chapter in this text. The intriguing but incompletely understood association with multiple endocrine problems warrants mention in a chapter on metabolic bone disease of the immature skeleton. Fibrous tissue undergoes ossification by a form of intramembranous bone formation, without apparent conversion of the fibroblasts to osteoblasts; the bone produced consists of small, irregular, purposeless, and often poorly mineralized trabeculae. The disease process is most active during growth, showing considerable activity on bone scan and causing internal scalloping of the cortices, weakening of the bone, and pathologic fracture. It often persists into adult life. Fibrous dysplasia occasionally may be associated with significant endocrine disturbances, which can dominate the picture.[6] The relation between the fibrous lesions of the marrow space and the endocrine disturbances is obscure.

The clinical manifestations of fibrous dysplasia may vary greatly.[129] The lesions may be isolated (i.e., monostotic) or found in several bones on one side of the skeleton or scattered throughout the skeleton (i.e., polyostotic). Solitary lesions are rarely accompanied by endocrine problems or are of concern to the patient unless fracture supervenes. At the opposite end of the spectrum are the cases in which the lesions are polyostotic and widely disseminated. The patient may display multiple sites of skeletal involvement with severe distortion of the normal bony configuration and facial appearance as a result of asymmetric enlargement of the facial bones (i.e., hemihypertrophy cranii). The patients with florid disease suffer frequent fractures, particularly at sites such as the pelvic rami and necks of femurs. Lesions in the necks of femurs may cause progressive coxa vara, leading to the shepherd's crook deformity.

Radiologic findings in patients with fibrous dysplasia vary somewhat, depending on the bone involved and the site, but the bone usually is expanded at the site. The cortices are thinned but intact and scalloped from within. The area of the lesion shows few trabecular markings, and instead, the fibrous tissue and small bony spicules (below the resolution of the x-ray beam) project a ground-glass consistency. In florid cases of fibrous dysplasia, deformities and other sequelae of old fractures are evident. Skin abnormalities are frequently seen in the more florid types of polyostotic fibrous dysplasia. These lesions are macular and light brown (café-au-lait spots). They often have an irregular border (i.e., "coast of Maine"), unlike similar lesions with a smooth border (i.e., "coast of California") seen in neurofibromatosis.

The associated endocrine problems that occur in patients with fibrous dysplasia raise the suspicion that fibrous dysplasia itself may have an endocrine cause, but this has never been proved. The endocrinopathies

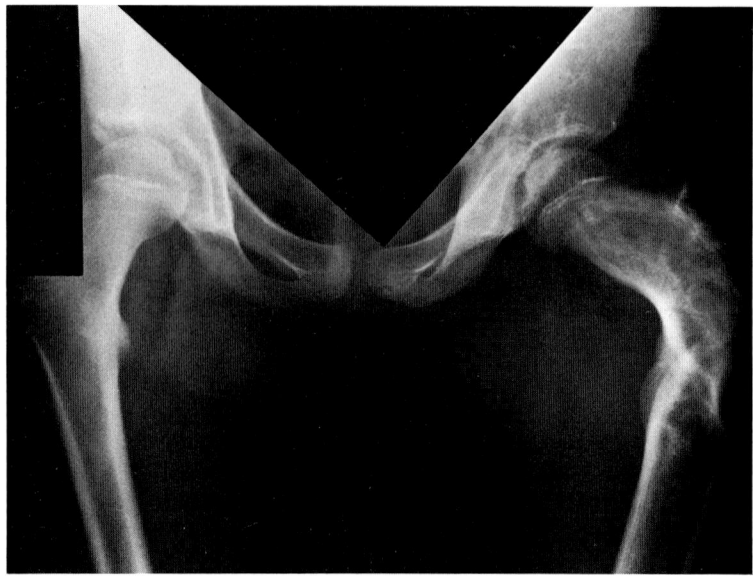

FIGURE 6-49. A patient with fibrous dysplasia has a shepherd's crook deformity of the left hip.

that occur with fibrous dysplasia are not common but are dramatic in presentation. About 1 of 30 patients with polyostotic dysplasia shows a marked precocious puberty (i.e., Albright syndrome), which is thought to be gonadal in origin. Secondary sex characteristics may be apparent by 1 year of age and menses by 2 years. The disorder is much more common among females than males. In some patients, a very severe form of vitamin D–resistant rickets may be present, and in others, a high degree of hyperthyroidism or Cushing syndrome may occur. These lesions are difficult to treat, and each requires careful study to assess the extent of the process and the endocrine abnormality.

The natural history of fibrous dysplasia is variable.[222] If multiple lesions become obvious during early childhood, the skeleton deformity may become severe. Localized lesions that manifest in adolescence are less likely to cause problems.

Treatment for fibrous dysplasia consists of surgical intervention at the site in which the lesion has caused or is likely to cause pathologic fracture. Deformity at the proximal femur may be particularly difficult to treat (Fig. 6-49). Generous osteotomies may be required in this location to move the femoral neck out of the considerable varus. As in other diseases with bone of poor quality, intramedullary fixation is preferable to plates and screws, which tend to cut out from such bone.[16] The Zickel nail has been advocated as an intramedullary device to fix the dysplastic femoral neck after osteotomy.[113] Intramedullary devices with interlocking technology are an apparent solution to this problem, although reports describing this application are not yet in the literature. The issue of the best graft or bone-inducing agent or synthetic in this condition also awaits definitive data. Bone grafting in fibrous dysplasia is challenging. Autografts tend to be replaced with fibrous tissue, reflecting the poorly understood pathogenesis of the condition. Allografted bone usually is more slowly revascularized than autografted bone.[134,243,379,508] The persistence of an allograft on a clinical radiograph may not correlate with increased biomechanical strength. Nevertheless, the use of allografts applied to fibrous dysplasia raises interesting possibilities, which await further investigation before definitive recommendations can be made.[259]

References

1. Abrams JD. Corneal and other findings in patients on intermittent dialysis for renal failure. Proc R Soc Lond 1966;59:533.
2. Adamson LF, Anast CS. Amino acid, potassium, and sulfate transport and incorporation by embryonic chick cartilage: the mechanism of the stimulatory effects of serum. Biochim Biophys Acta 1966;121:10.
3. Aegerter E, Kirkpatrick J. Orthopaedic diseases. Philadelphia: WB Saunders, 1975:440.
4. Ainsworth SR, Aulicino PL. A survey of patients with Ehlers-Danlos syndrome. Clin Orthop 1993;286:250.
5. Albers-Schonberg H. Eine bisher nicht beschriebene Allgemeinerkrankung skelettes im Rontgenbild. Forschr Geb Rontgenstr 1907;11:261.
6. Albin J, Wu R. Abnormal hypothalamic-pituitary function in polyostotic fibrous dysplasia. Clin Endocrinol 1981;14:435.
7. Albright F, Burnett C, Smith P, et al. Pseudohypoparathyroidism—an example of "Seabright-Bantam syndrome." Report of three cases. Endocrinology 1942;30:922.
8. Albright F, Butler AM, Bloomberg E. Rickets resistant to vitamin D therapy. Am J Dis Child 1937;54:529.
9. Albright F, Reifenstein EC. The parathyroid glands and metabolic bone disease. Baltimore: Williams & Wilikins, 1948.
10. Alper J. Boning up: newly isolated proteins heal bad breaks. Science 1994;263:324.
11. Amis J, Herring JA. Iatrogenic kyphosis: a complication of Harrington instrumentation in Marfan's syndrome. J Bone Joint Surg [Am] 1984;66:460.

12. Andersen DH, Schlesinger ER. Renal hyperparathyroidism with calcification of the arteries in infancy. Am J Dis Child 1942;63:102.
13. Andersen J, Neilsen HJ. Renal osteodystrophy in non-dialysed patients with chronic renal failure. Acta Radiol 1980;21:803.
14. Anderton JM. Orthopaedic problems in adult hypophosphatasia: a report of two cases. J Bone Joint Surg [Br] 1979;61:82.
15. Andress DL, Norris KC, Coburn JW, et al. Intravenous calcitriol in the treatment of refractory osteitis fibrosa of chronic renal failure. N Engl J Med 1989;321:274.
16. Andrisano A, Soncini G, Calderoni PP, Stilli S. Critical review of infantile fibrous dysplasia: surgical treatment. J Pediatr Orthop 1991;11:478.
17. Anton HC. Thinning of the clavicular cortex in adults under the age of 45 in osteomalacia and hyperparathyroidism. Clin Radiol 1979;30:307.
18. Aponte CJ, Petrelli MP. Anticonvulsants and vitamin D metabolism. JAMA 1973;225:1248.
19. Aprin H, Sinha A. Tumoral calcinosis. Report of a case in a one-year-old child. Clin Orthop 1984;185:83.
20. Arnaud C, Fischer J, Rasmussen H. The role of the parathyroids in the phosphaturia of vitamin D deficiency. J Clin Invest 1964;43:1256.
21. Arnaud C, Tsao HS, Littledike T. Calcium homeostasis, parathyroid hormone and calcitonin: preliminary report. Mayo Clin Proc 1970;45:125.
22. Arnaud CD, Tenenhouse AM, Rasmussen H. Parathyroid hormone. Annu Rev Physiol 1967;29:349.
23. Arnaud SB, Goldsmith RS, Stickler GB, et al. Serum parathyroid hormone and blood minerals: interrelationships in normal children. Pediatr Res 1973;7:485.
24. Arnaud SB, Stickler GB, Haworth JC. Serum 25-hydroxyvitamin D in infantile rickets. Pediatrics 1976;57:221.
25. Arnstein AR, Frame B, Frost HM. Recent progress in osteomalacia and rickets. Ann Intern Med 1967;67:1296.
26. Asnes RS, Berdon WE, Bassett VA. Hypophosphatemic rickets in an adolescent cured by excision of a non-ossifying fibroma. Clin Pediatr 1981;20:646.
27. Atkinson M, Nordin BEC, Sherlock S. Malabsorption and bone disease in prolonged obstructive jaundice. Q J Med 1956;25:299.
28. Austen LA, Heath H. Calcitonin: physiology and pathophysiology. N Engl J Med 1981;304:269.
29. Avioli LV. Intestinal absorption of calcium. Arch Intern Med 1972;129:345.
30. Avioli LV. The therapeutic approach to hypoparathyroidism. Am J Dis Child 1974;57:34.
31. Avioli LV, Haddad JG. Progress in endocrinology and metabolism. Vitamin D: current concepts. Metab Clin Exp 1973;22:507.
32. Ayers DC, Evarts CM, Parkinson JR. The prevention of heterotopic ossification in high risk patients by low-dose radiation therapy after total hip arthroplasty. J Bone Joint Surg [Am] 1986;68:1423.
33. Baar HS, Bickel H. Cystine storage disease with aminoaciduria and dwarfism. Part 8. Morbid anatomy, histology, and pathogenesis of Lignac-Fanconi disease. Acta Paediatr Scand Suppl 1952;90:171.
34. Backrach S, Fisher J, Parks JS. An outbreak of vitamin D–deficiency rickets in a susceptible population. Pediatrics 1979;64:871.
35. Badelon O, Bensahel H, Csukonyi Z, Chaumien J-P. Congenital dislocation of the hip in Ehlers-Danlos syndrome. Clin Orthop 1990;255:138.
36. Baines GH, Barclay JA, Cooke WT. Nephrocalcinosis associated with hyperchloremia and low plasma bicarbonate. Q J Med 1945;14:113.
37. Ballet JJ, Griscelli C. Lymphoid cell transplantation in human osteopetrosis. In: Horton JE, Tarpley TM, Davis WF, eds. Mechanisms of localized bone loss: proceedings of the First Scientific Evaluation Workshop on localized bone loss. Washington, DC: Information Retrieval, 1978:399.
38. Ballet JJ, Griscelli C, Coutris C, et al. Bone marrow transplantation in osteopetrosis. Lancet 1977;2:1137.
39. Balsan S, Garabedian M. 1,25-Dihydroxyvitamin D_3 and 1,alpha-hydroxyvitamin D_3 in children: biologic and therapeutic effects in nutritional rickets and different types of vitamin D resistance. Pediatr Res 1975;9:586.
40. Banks SW. Bone changes in acute and chronic scurvy: an experimental study. J Bone Joint Surg [Am] 1943;25:553.
41. Barsh GS, David KE, Byers PH. Type I osteogenesis imperfecta: a nonfunctional allele for pro alpha (I) chains for type I procollagen. Proc Natl Acad Sci U S A 1982;79:3838.
42. Bartter FC. Hypophosphatasia. In: Stanbury JB, Wyngaarden JB, Fredrickson DS, eds. The metabolic basis of inherited disease. 2nd ed. New York: McGraw-Hill, 1966.
43. Bauze RJ, Smith R, Francis MJO. A new look at osteogenesis imperfecta. J Bone Joint Surg [Br] 1975;57:2.
44. Beal VA. Calcium and phosphorus in infancy. J Am Diet Assoc 1968;53:450.
45. Beighton P, Hamersma H. The orthopaedic implications of the sclerosing bone dysplasias. South Afr Med J 1980;11:600.
46. Beighton P, Horan F. Orthopaedic aspects of the Ehlers-Danlos syndrome. J Bone Joint Surg [Br] 1969;51:444.
47. Bennett A, Harvey W. Prostaglandins in orthopaedics. J Bone Joint Surg [Br] 1981;63:152.
48. Bergman L, Hagberg S. Primary hyperparathyroidism in a child investigated by determination of ultrafiltrable calcium. Am J Dis Child 1993.
49. Berlyne GM. Microcrystalline conjunctival calcification in renal failure. A useful sign. Lancet 1968;2:366.
50. Berlyne GM, Shaw AG. Red eyes in renal failure. Lancet 1967;1:4.
51. Bernstein RM, Zaleske DJ. Familial aspects of Caffey's disease: a report of a family and review of the English literature. Am J Orthop 1995;24.
52. Berson SA, Yalow RS. Parathyroid hormone in plasma in adenomatous hyperparathyroidism, uremia, and bronchogenic carcinoma. Science 1966;154:907.
53. Bethune JD, Dent CD. Hypophosphatasia in the adult. Am J Med 1960;28:615.
54. Bickel H, Baar HS, Astley R, et al. Cystine storage disease with aminoaciduria and dwarfism. Acta Paediatr Scand Suppl 1952;90:1.
55. Bijovet OLM. Kidney function in calcium and phosphate metabolism. In: Avioli LV, Krane SM, eds. Metabolic bone disease. New York: Academic Press, 1977:49.
56. Bjernulf A, Hall K, Sjogren I, et al. Primary hyperparathyroidism in children. Acta Paediatr Scand 1970;59:249.
57. Blasier RB, Aronson DD. Infantile cortical hyperostosis with osteomyelitis of the humerus. J Pediatr Orthop 1985;5:222.
58. Blockey NJ, Murphy AV, Mocan H. Management of rachitic deformities in children with chronic renal failure. J Bone Joint Surg [Br] 1986;68:791.
59. Blunt JW, DeLuca HF. The synthesis of 25-hydroxycholecalciferol. A biologically active metabolite of vitamin D_3. Biochemistry 1969;8:671.
60. Blunt JW, DeLuca HF, Schnoes HK. 25-Hydroxycholecalciferol. A biologically active metabolite of vitamin D_3. Biochemistry 1968;7:3317.
61. Blunt JW, Tanaka Y, DeLuca HF. The biological activity of 25-hydroxycholecalciferol. A metabolite of vitamin D_3. Proc Natl Acad Sci U S A 1968;61:1503.
62. Boers GHJ, Smals AGH, Trijbels FJM, et al. Heterozygosity

for homocystinuria in premature peripheral and cerebral occlusive arterial disease. N Engl J Med 1985;313:709.
63. Bonavita JA, Dalinka MK. Shoulder erosions in renal osteodystrophy. Skeletal Radiol 1980;5:105.
64. Borgstedt AP, Bryson MF, Young LW, Forbes GB. Long-term administration of anti-epileptic drugs and the development of rickets. J Pediatr 1972;81:9.
65. Borle AB. Membrane transfer of calcium. Clin Orthop 1967;52:267.
66. Boskey AL. Current concepts of the physiology and biochemistry of calcification. Clin Orthop 1981;157:225.
67. Bosley AR, Verrier-Jones ER, Campbell MJ. Aetiological factors in rickets of prematurity. Arch Dis Child 1980;55:683.
68. Boyle IT, Gray RW, DeLuca HF. Regulation by calcium of in vivo synthesis of 1,25-dihydroxycholecalciferol and 21,25-dihydroxycholecalciferol. Proc Natl Acad Sci U S A 1971;68:2131.
69. Brautbar N, Kleemna CR. Disordered divalent ion metabolism in kidney disease: comments on pathogenesis and treatment. Adv Nephrol 1979;8:179.
70. Brenton DP, Dent CE. Idiopathic osteoporosis. In: Bickel H, Stern J, eds. Inborn errors of calcium and bone metabolism. Baltimore: University Park Press, 1976.
71. Brenton DP, Dow CJ, James JIP, et al. Homocystinuria and Marfan's syndrome. J Bone Joint Surg [Br] 1972;54:277.
72. Brickman AS, Coburn JW, Norman AW. Action of 1,25-dihydroxycholecalciferol, a potent kidney-produced metabolite of vitamin D_3 in uremic man. N Engl J Med 1972;287:891.
73. Brighton CT. Longitudinal bone growth: the growth plate and its dysfunctions. In: Griffin PP, ed. Instructional course lectures XXXVI. Park Ridge, IL: American Academy of Orthopaedic Surgeons, 1987:3.
74. Brighton CT, Strafford B, Gross SB, et al. The proliferative and synthetic response of isolated calvarial bone cells of rats to cyclic biaxial mechanical strain. J Bone Joint Surg [Am] 1991;73:320.
75. Brill PW, Mitty JA, Gaull GE. Homocystinuria due to cystathionine synthetase deficiency: clinical roentgenologic correlations. AJR Am J Roentgenol 1974;121:45.
76. Bronsky D, Kiamko RT, Waldstein S. Familial idiopathic hyperparathyroidism. Am J Med 1974;57:34.
77. Brooks MH, Bell NH, Love L, et al. Vitamin D–dependent rickets, type II. Resistance of target organs to 1,25-dihydroxyvitamin D. N Engl J Med 1978;298:996.
78. Brown DJ, Dawborn JK, Thomas DP, et al. Assessment of osteodystrophy in patients with chronic renal failure. Aust N Z J Med 1982;12:250.
79. Brown DM. Pathogenesis of osteopetrosis: a comparison of human and animal spectra. Pediatr Res 1971;5:181.
80. Bruce HM, Callow RK. Cereals and rickets. The role of inositalhexaphosphoric acid. Biochem J 1934;28:517.
81. Buckwalter JA. Proteoglycan structure in calcifying cartilage. Clin Orthop 1982;172:207.
82. Bunch WH, Dvonch VM. Pitfalls in the assessment of skeletal immaturity: an anthropologic case study. J Pediatr Orthop 1983;3:220.
83. Burgeson RE, Nimni ME. Collagen types: molecular structure and tissue distribution. Clin Orthop 1992;282:250.
84. Burnett CH, Dent CE, Harper C, Warland BJ. Vitamin D–resistant rickets: analysis of twenty-four pedigrees with hereditary and sporadic cases. Am J Med 1964;36:222.
85. Butler AM, Wilson JL, Farber S. Dehydration and acidosis with calcification at renal tubules. J Pediatr 1936;8:489.
86. Caffey J. Infantile cortical hyperostosis: a review of the clinical and radiographic features. Proc R Soc Lond 1957;50:347.
87. Caffey J. Pediatric x-ray diagnosis. 5th ed. Chicago: Year Book Medical Publishers, 1967.
88. Caffey J. Pediatric x-ray diagnosis, Chicago: Year Book Medical Publishers, 1972.
89. Cai Q, Hodgson SF, Kao PC, et al. Brief report: inhibition of renal phosphate transport by a tumor product in a patient with oncogenic osteomalacia. N Engl J Med 1994;330:1645.
90. Callenback JC, Sheehan MB, Abramson SJ, Hall RT. Etiologic factors in rickets of very low birthweight infants. J Pediatr 1981;98:800.
91. Canalis E. Effect of growth factors on bone cell replication and differentiation. Clin Orthop 1985;193:246.
92. Canalis EM, Dietrich JW, Maina DM, Raisz LG. Hormonal control of bone collagen synthesis in vitro: effects of insulin and glucagon. Endocrinology 1977;100:668.
93. Carty HML. Fractures caused by child abuse. J Bone Joint Surg [Br] 1993;75:849.
94. Castells S, Colbert C, Chakrabarti C, et al. Therapy of osteogenesis imperfecta with synthetic salmon calcitonin. J Pediatr 1979;95:807.
95. Centrella M, McCarthy TL, Canalis E. Transforming growth factor-beta and remodeling of bone. J Bone Joint Surg [Am] 1991;73:1418.
96. Chaknakjian ZH, Marks JF, Fink CW. Effect of levodopa (L-dopa) on serum growth hormone in children with short stature. Pediatr Res 1973;7:71.
97. Chan JC, Bartter FC. Hypophosphatemic rickets: effect of 1,alpha,25-hydroxyvitamin D_3 on growth and mineral metabolism. Pediatrics 1979;64:448.
98. Cheeney RW. Current clinical applications of vitamin D metabolite research. Clin Orthop 1981;161:285.
99. Chisholm JJ Jr. Increased lead absorption and lead poisoning. In: Behrman RE, Vaughan VC, III, eds. Nelson's textbook of pediatrics. 12th ed. Philadelphia: WB Saunders, 1983.
100. Christiansen C, Kristensen M, Rodbro P. Latent osteomalacia in epileptic patients on anticonvulsants. Br Med J 1972;3:738.
101. Chutorian A, Rowland LP. Lowe's syndrome. Neurology 1966;16:115.
102. Clark CG, Crooks J, Dawson AA. Disordered calcium metabolism after Polya partial gastrectomy. Lancet 1964;1:734.
103. Clarke R, Daly L, Robinson K, et al. Hyperhomocyteinemia: an independent risk factor for vascular disease. N Engl J Med 1991;324:1149.
104. Clayton BE, Cotton DA. A study of malabsorption after resection of the entire jejunum and the proximal half of the ileum. Gut 1961;2:18.
105. Cloutier MD, Hayles AB, Riggs BL, et al. Juvenile osteoporosis: report of a case including a description of some metabolic and microradiographic studies. Pediatrics 1967;40:649.
106. Coburn JW, Popovtzer MM, Massry SG, et al. The physicochemical state and renal handling of divalent ions in chronic renal failure. Arch Intern Med 1969;124:302.
107. Coccia BF, Krivit W, Cervenka J. Successful bone marrow transplantation for infantile osteopetrosis. N Engl J Med 1980;302:701.
108. Coe JD, Murphy WA, Whyte MP. Management of femoral fractures and pseudofractures in adult hypophosphatasia. J Bone Joint Surg [Am] 1986;68:981.
109. Cohen RB, Hahn GV, Tabas JA, et al. The natural history of heterotopic ossification in patients who have fibrodysplasia ossificans progressiva. J Bone Joint Surg [Am] 1993;75:215.
110. Cole NL, Goldberg MH, Loftus M, et al. . Surgical management of patients with osteogenesis imperfecta. J Oral Maxillofac Surg 1982;40:578.
111. Cole WG. Etiology and pathogenesis of heritable connective tissue diseases. J Pediatr Orthop 1993;13:392.
112. Colombo JP, Donath A. The effect of calcium infusions on renal handling of amino acids in hypophosphatemic vitamin D–resistant rickets. Acta Paediatr Scand 1975;64:703.

113. Connolly JF. Shepherd's crook deformities of polyostotic dysplasia treated by osteotomy and Zickel nail fixation. Clin Orthop 1977;123:22.
114. Cooke RE, Kleeman CR. Distal tubular dysfunction with renal calcification. Yale J Biol Med 1950;23:199.
115. Cowell HR, Ray S. Talipes equinovarus and syndrome identification. Contemp Orthop 1984;9:51.
116. Craven JD. Renal glomerular osteodystrophy. Clin Radiol 1964;15:210.
117. Crawford AH. Current concepts review. Slipped capital femoral epiphysis. J Bone Joint Surg [Am] 1988;70:1422.
118. Crawford AH. Correspondence. J Bone Joint Surg [Am] 1990;72:632.
119. Crawford JD. Meat, potatoes, and growth hormone. N Engl J Med 1981;305:163.
120. Cropp GJ, Meyers DN. Physiological evidence of hypermetabolism in osteogenesis imperfecta. Pediatrics 1972;49:375.
121. Crosley CJ, Chee C, Berman PH. Rickets associated with long-term anticonvulsant therapy in a pediatric outpatient population. Pediatrics 1975;56:52.
122. Cruess RL. Physiology of bone formation and resorption. In: Cruess RL, ed. The musculoskeletal system. New York: Churchill Livingstone, 1982;
123. Crutchlow WP, David DS, Whitsell J. Multiple skeletal complications in a case of chronic renal failure treated by kidney homotransplantation. Am J Med 1971;50:390.
124. Cunningham J, Fraher LJ, Clemens TL, et al. Chronic acidosis with metabolic bone disease. Effect of alkali on bone morphology and vitamin D metabolism. Am J Med 1982;73:199.
125. Currarino G, Neuhauser EBD, Reyersback GC, et al. Hypophosphatasia. AJR Am J Roentgenol 1957;78:392.
126. Cutler RE, Reiss E, Ackerman LV. Familial hyperparathyroidism. N Engl J Med 1964;270:859.
127. Dancaster CP, Jackson WPU. Familial vitamin D–resistant rickets. Arch Dis Child 1957;34:383.
128. Daniels RA, Weisenfeld I. Tumorous phosphaturic osteomalacia. Report of a case associated with multiple hemangiomas of bone. Am J Med 1967;67:155.
129. Danon M, Crawford JD. The McCune-Albright syndrome. Ergeb Inn Med Kinderheilkd 1987;55:81.
130. Daughaday WH, Reeeder C. Synchronous activation of DNA synthesis in hypophysectomized rat cartilage by growth hormone. J Lab Clin Med 1968;68:357.
131. Daum F, Rosen JF, Roginsky M, Cohen MI, Finberg L. 25-Hydroxycholecalciferol in the management of rickets associated with extrahepatic biliary atresia. J Pediatr 1976;88:1041.
132. David DS. Calcium metabolism in renal failure. Am J Med 1975;58:48.
133. David NJ, Verner JV, Engel FL. The diagnostic spectrum of hypercalcemia. Am J Med 1962;33:88.
134. De Boer HH. The history of bone grafts. Clin Orthop 1988;226:292.
135. Debnam JW, Bates ML, Kopelman RC, et al. Radiological/pathological correlations in uremic bone disease. Radiology 1977;125:653.
136. Deller DJ, Begley MD. Calcium metabolism and the bones after partial gastrectomy. I. Clinical features and radiology of the bones. Aust Ann Med 1963;12:282.
137. DeLuca HF. Vitamin D: new horizons. Clin Orthop 1971;78:423.
138. DeLuca HF. Parathyroid hormone as a trophic hormone for 1,25-dihydroxyvitamin D_3, the metabolically active form of vitamin D. N Engl J Med 1972;287:250.
139. DeLuca HF. The biochemical basis of renal osteodystrophy and post-menopausal osteoporosis: a view from the vitamin D system. Curr Med Res Opin 1981;7:279.
140. Delvin EE, Glorieux FH, Lopez E. In vitro sulfate turnover in osteogenesis imperfecta congenita and tarda. Am J Med Genet 1979;4:349.
141. Delvin EE, Glorieux FH, Marie PJ, Pettifor JM. Vitamin D dependency: replacement therapy with calcitriol? J Pediatr 1981;99:26.
142. Dent CE. Rickets and osteomalacia from renal tubule defects. J Bone Joint Surg [Br] 1952;34:266.
143. Dent CE. Idiopathic juvenile osteoporosis. Birth Defects 1969;5:134.
144. Dent CE, Gertner JM. Hypophosphatemic osteomalacia in fibrous dysplasia. Q J Med 1976;45:411.
145. Dent CE, Harris H. Hereditary forms of rickets and osteomalacia. J Bone Joint Surg [Br] 1956;38:204.
146. Dent CE, Richens A, Rowe DJF, Stamp TCB. Osteomalacia with long-term anticonvulsant therapy in epilepsy. Br Med J 1970;4:69.
147. Dent CE, Smellie JM, Watson L. Studies in osteopetrosis. Arch Dis Child 1965;40:7.
148. Dent JA, Paterson CR. Fractures in early childhood: osteogenesis imperfecta or child abuse. J Pediatr Orthop 1991;11:184.
149. DeToni G. Remarks on the relations between renal rickets (renal dwarfism) and renal diabetes. Acta Paediatr Scand 1933;16:479.
150. DeToni G. Renal rickets with phospho-gluco-amino renal diabetes. Ann Paediatr 1956;187:42.
151. DiCesare PE, Sew-Hoy A, Krom W. Bilateral isolated olecranon fractures in an infant as presentation of osteogenesis imperfecta. Orthopedics 1992;15:741.
152. Dodds GS, Cameron HC. Studies on experimental rickets in rats. I. Structural modifications of the epiphyseal cartilages in the tibia and other bones. Am J Anat 1934;55:135.
153. Dodds GS, Cameron HC. Studies on experimental rickets in rats. II. The healing process in the head of the tibia and other bones. Am J Pathol 1938;14:273.
154. Dodds GS, Cameron HC. Studies on experimental rickets in rats. III. The behavior and rate of cartilage remnants in the rachitic metaphysis. Am J Pathol 1939;15:723.
155. Dodds GS, Cameron HC. Studies on experimental rickets in rats. IV. The relation of rickets to growth, with special reference to the bones. Am J Pathol 1943;19:169.
156. Drescher D, DeLuca HF. Vitamin D stimulated calcium binding protein from rat intestinal mucosa. Purification and some properties. Biochemistry 1971;10:2302.
157. Drezner M, Neelon FA, Lebovitz HE. Pseudohypoparathyroidism type II. A possible defect in the reception of the cyclic AMP signal. N Engl J Med 1973;289:1056.
158. Drvaric DM, Parks WJ, Wyly JB, et al. Prostaglandin-induced hyperostosis. Clin Orthop 1989;246:300.
159. Duffrin H, Sundaram M. Radiologic case study: osteogenesis imperfecta. Orthopedics 1987;10:1304.
160. Dunker AK, Zaleske DJ. Stereochemical considerations for constructing alpha-helical protein bundles with particular application to membrane proteins. Biochem J 1977;163:45.
161. Dwyer JT, Dietz WH, Hass G, Suskind R. Risk of nutritional rickets among vegetarian children. Am J Dis Child 1979;133:134.
162. Eastwood JB. Renal osteodystrophy—a radiological review. Crit Rev Diagn Imaging 1977;9:77.
163. Eddy RL. Metabolic bone disease after gastrectomy. Am J Med 1971;50:442.
164. Ehrlich MG, Armstrong AL, Neuman RG, et al. Patterns of proteoglycan degradation by a neutral protease from human growth-plate epiphyseal cartilage. J Bone Joint Surg [Am] 1982;64:1350.
165. Elkinton JR. Renal acidosis. Am J Med 1960;28:165.
166. Elkinton JR, Huth EJ, Webster GD Jr, McCance RA. The renal

167. Esselstyn CB Jr, Popowniak KL. Parathyroid surgery in treatment of renal osteodystrophy and tertiary hyperparathyroidism. Surg Clin North Am 1971;51:1211.
168. Etches P, Pickering D, Smith R. Cystinotic rickets with vitamin D metabolites. Arch Dis Child 1993;
169. Evans EB. Musculoskeletal changes complicating burns. In: Epps CH Jr, ed. Complications in orthopaedic surgery. 2nd ed. Philadelphia: JB Lippincott, 1986:1307.
170. Evans GA, Arulanantham K, Gage J. Primary hypophosphatemic rickets. Effect of ral phosphate and vitamin D on growth and surgical treatment. J Bone Joint Surg [Am] 1980;62:1130.
171. Evans RA, Dunstan CR, Hills E. Bone metabolism in idiopathic juvenile osteoporosis: a case report. Calcif Tissue Int 1983;35:5.
172. Eyre DR, Upton M, Shapiro F, et al. Non-expression of cartilage type II collagen in a case of human achondrogenesis (Langer-Saldino variant). Trans Orthop Res Soc 1986;11:459.
173. Fanconi G. Der fruhinfantile nephrotisch-glykosurische Zwergwuchs mit hypophosphatamishcer Rachitis. Jahrb Kinderheilkd 1936;147:299.
174. Farfel Z, Brickman AS, Kaslow HR, et al. Defect of receptor-cyclase coupling protein in pseudohypoparathyroidism. N Engl J Med 1980;303:237.
175. Feist JH. The biologic basis of radiologic findings in bone disease. Recognition and interpretation of abnormal bone architecture. Radiol Clin North Am 1970;8:183.
176. Felts HJ, Whitley JE, Anderson DD, et al. Medical and surgical treatment of azotemic osteodystrophy. Ann Intern Med 1965;62:1272.
177. Ferris B, Walker C, Jackson A, Kirwan E. The orthopaedic management of hypophosphataemic rickets. J Pediatr Orthop 1991;11:367.
178. Finkelstein JD. Methionine metabolism in mammals: the biochemical basis for homocystinuria. Metab Clin Exp 1974;23:387.
179. Floman Y, Yosipovitch Z, Licht A, Viskoper RJ. Bilateral slipped upper femoral epiphysis: a rare manifestation of renal osteodystrophy. Case report with discussion of its pathogenesis. Isr J Med Sci 1975;11:15.
180. Forbes GB, Cafarelli C, Manning J. Vitamin D and infantile hypercalcemia. Pediatrics 1968;42:203.
181. Fourman P, Royer P. Calcium metabolism and bone. 2nd ed. Philadelphia: FA Davis, 1968:
182. Frame B. Hypocalcemia and osteomalacia associated with anticonvulsant therapy. Ann Intern Med 1971;74:294.
183. Frame B, Jackson CE, Reynolds WA, et al. Hypercalcemia and skeletal effects in chronic hypervitaminosis and skeletal effects in chronic hypervitaminosis A. Ann Intern Med 1974;80:44.
184. Frame B, Smith RW Jr, Fleming JL, Manson G. Oral phosphates in vitamin D–refractory rickets and osteomalacia. Am J Dis Child 1963;106:147.
185. Francis MJO, Bauze RJ, Smith R. Osteogenesis imperfecta: a new classification. Birth Defects 1985;11:99.
186. Franck WA, Hoffman GS, Davis JS, et al. Osteomalacia and weakness complicating jejunoileal bypass. J Rheumatol 1979;6:51.
187. Fraser D. Hypophosphatasia. Am J Med 1957;22:730.
188. Fraser D, Yendt ER, Christie FHE. Metabolic abnormalities in hypophosphatasia. Lancet 1955;1:286.
189. Fraser DR, Kodicek E. Regulation of 25-hydroxycholecalciferol-1-hydrolase activity in kidney by parathyroid hormone. Nature 1973;241:163.
190. Fraser DR, Salter RB. The diagnosis and management of the various types of rickets. Pediatr Clin North Am 1958;26:417.
191. Friedlaender GE. Current concepts review. Bone grafts. J Bone Joint Surg [Am] 1987;69:786.
192. Friedman SA, Novack S, Thomson GE. Arterial calcification and gangrene in uremia. N Engl J Med 1969;280:1392.
193. Froesch ER, Zapf J, Audhya TK, Ben-Porath E, Segen BJ, Gibson KD. Non-suppressible insulin-like activity and thyroid hormones: major pituitary-dependent sulfation factors for chick embyro cartilage. Proc Natl Acad Sci U S A 1976;73:2904.
194. Frost HM. Mathematical elements of lamellar bone remodeling. Springfield, IL: Charles C Thomas, 1964:
195. Frost HM. Bone dynamics in osteoporosis and osteomalacia. Springfield, IL: Charles C Thomas, 1966.
196. Fullmer CS, Wasserman RH. Bovine intestinal calcium-binding proteins (CaBP): purification and some properties. Fed Proc 1972;31:693.
197. Gallagher CJ, Riggs BL, Eisman J. Intestinal calcium absorption and serum vitamin D metabolites in normal subjects and osteoporotic patients. J Clin Invest 1979;64:729.
198. Gamble JG, Ip SC. Hypervitaminosis A in a child from megadosing. J Pediatr Orthop 1985;5:219.
199. Gamble JG, Strudwick WJ, Rinsky LA, Bleck EE. Complications of intramedullary rods in osteogenesis imperfecta: Bailey-Dubow rods versus nonelongating rods. J Pediatr Orthop 1988;8:645.
200. Garabedian M, Vainsel M, Mallet E, et al. Circulating vitamin D–metabolite concentrations in children with nutritional rickets. J Pediatr 1983;103:381.
201. Garland DE, Hanscom DA, Keenan MA, et al. Resection of heterotopic ossification in the adult with head trauma. J Bone Joint Surg [Am] 1985;67:1261.
202. Gascon-Barre M, Cote MG. Influence of phenobarbital and diphenylhydantoin on the healing of rickets in the rat. Calcif Tissue Res 1978;25:93.
203. Gaull G, Sturman JA, Schaffner F. Homocystinuria due to cystathionine synthase deficiency enzymatic and ultrastructural studies. J Pediatr 1974;84:381.
204. Gerber LH, Binder H, Weintrob J, et al. Rehabilitation of children and infants with osteogenesis imperfecta. Clin Orthop 1990;251:254.
205. Glass EJ, Barr DGD. Transient neonatal hyperparathyroidism secondary to maternal pseudohypoparathyroidism. Arch Dis Child 1981;56:555.
206. Glass EJ, Hume R, Hendry GMA, et al. Plasma alkaline phosphatase activity in rickets of prematurity. Arch Dis Child 1982;57:373.
207. Glimcher MJ, Krane SM. The organization and structure of bone and the mechanism of calcification. In: Ramachandran GN, Gould BS, eds. Treatise on collagen. New York: Academic Press, 1968.
208. Glisson R. De rachitide sive marbo puerili qui vulgo The Rickets Dicitur Tracttatus. Adscitis in operis societatem Georgio Bate et Ahasuero Regemortero. London: G Du-Gardi, 1650.
209. Goel KM, Sweet EM, Logan RW, et al. Florid and subclinical rickets among immigrant children in Glasgow. Lancet 1976;1:1141.
210. Goldman AB, Lane JM, Salvati E. Slipped capital femoral epiphyses complicating renal osteodystrophy: a report of three cases. Radiology 1978;126:33.
211. Goldman R, Basset SH, Duncan GB. Phosphorus excretion in renal failure. J Clin Invest 1954;33:1623.
212. Goyer RA. Ethanolamine phosphate excretion in a family with hypophosphatasia. Arch Dis Child 1963;38:205.
213. Greco F, DePalma L, Speddia N, Mannarini M. Growth plate cartilage metabolic response to mechanical stress. J Pediatr Orthop 1989;9:520.

214. Greenfield GB. Roentgen appearance of bone and soft-tissue changes in chronic renal disease. AJR Am J Roentgenol 1972;116:749.
215. Gregosiewicz A, Warda E. Tumoral calcinosis: successful medical treatment. J Bone Joint Surg [Am] 1989;71:1244.
216. Greulich WW, Pyle SI. Radiographic atlas of skeletal development of the hand and wrist. 2nd ed. Stanford: Stanford University Press, 1959.
217. Habener JF, Mahaffey JE. Osteomalacia and disorders of vitamin D metabolism. Annu Rev Med 1978;29:327.
218. Hagglund G, Bylander B, Hansson LI, Selvik G. Bone growth after fixing slipped femoral epiphyses: brief report. J Bone Joint Surg [Br] 1988;70:845.
219. Hahn TJ, Scharp CR, Halstead LR, et al. Parathyroid hormone status and renal responsiveness in familial hypophosphatemic rickets. J Clin Endocrinol Metab 1975;41:926.
220. Halvorsen S, Aas K. Renal tubular defects in fibrous dysplasia of the bones. Report of two cases. Acta Paediatr Scand 1961;50:297.
221. Harmeyer J, DeLuca HF. Calcium-binding protein and calcium absorption after vitamin D administration. Arch Biochem Biophys 1969;133:247.
222. Harris WH, Dudley HR, Barry RJ. The natural history of fibrous dysplasia. J Bone Joint Surg [Am] 1962;44:207.
223. Harris WH, Heaney RP. Skeletal renewal and metabolic bone disease. N Engl J Med 1969;280:193.
224. Harrison HE. The varieties of rickets and osteomalacia associated with hypophosphatemia. Clin Orthop 1957;9:61.
225. Harrison HE, Harrison HC. The effect of acidosis upon the renal tubular absorption of phosphate. Am J Physiol 1941;134:781.
226. Harrison HE, Harrison HC. The interaction of vitamin D and parathyroid hormone on calcium, phosphorus and magnesium homeostasis in the rat. Metab Clin Exp 1964;13:952.
227. Harrison HE, Harrison HC. Rickets then and now. J Pediatr 1975;87:1144.
228. Hasenhuttl K. Osteopetrosis. Review of the literature on comparative studies on a case with a 24-year follow-up. J Bone Joint Surg [Am] 1962;44:359.
229. Hay ED. Embryonic induction and tissue interaction. International Congress Series No. 432:126. Amsterdam: Excerpta Medica, 1978.
230. Henry A. Monostotic fibrous dysplasia. J Bone Joint Surg [Br] 1969;51:300.
231. Hepner GW, Jowsey J, Arnaud C, et al. Osteomalacia and celiac disease: response to 25-hydroxyvitamin D. Am J Med 1965;65:1015.
232. Herring JA. Indications, patient selection, and evaluation in pediatric orthopedics. In: Luque ER, ed. Segmental spinal instrumentation. Thorofare, NJ: Slack, 1984:64.
233. Heubi JE, Tsang RC, Steichen JJ, et al. 1,25-Dihydroxy-vitamin D_3 in childhood hepatic osteodystrophy. J Pediatr 1979;94:977.
234. Heydemann JS, McCarthy RE. Tumoral calcinosis in a child. J Pediatr Orthop 1988;8:474.
235. Hinkel CL, Beiler DD. Osteopetrosis in adults. AJR Am J Roentgenol 1955;74:46.
236. Hodkinson HM. Fracture of the femur as a presentation of osteomalacia. Gerontol Clin 1971;13:189.
237. Hofer M, Hirschel B, Kirschner P, et al. Brief report: disseminated osteomyelitis from *Mycobacterium ulcerans* after a snakebite. N Engl J Med 1993;328:1007.
238. Hoffman WS. The biochemistry of clinical medicine. 4th ed. Chicago: Year Book Medical Publishers, 1970.
239. Hoikka V, Savolainen K, Karjalainen P, et al. Treatment of osteomalacia in institutionalized epileptic patients on long-term anticonvulsant therapy. Ann Clin Res 1982;14:72.
240. Holick MF, Schnoes HK, DeLuca HF, et al. Isolation and identification of 24,25-hydroxycholecalciferol, a metabolite of D_3 made in the kidney. Biochemistry 1972;11:4251.
241. Holick MF, Schnoes HK, DeLuca HF, et al. Isolation and identification of 1,24-dihydroxycholecalciferol. A metabolite of vitamin D active in intestine. Biochemistry 1971;10:2799.
242. Hollister DW, Byers PH, Holbrook KA. Genetic disorders of collagen metabolism. Adv Hum Genet 1982;12:1.
243. Hopp SG, Dahners LE, Gilbert JA. A study of the mechanical strength of long bone defects treated with various bone autograft substitutes: an experimental investigation in the rabbit. J Orthop Res 1989;7:579.
244. Hsu AC, Kooh SW, Fraser D, et al. Renal osteodystrophy in children with chronic renal failure: an unexpectedly common and incapacitating complication. Pediatrics 1982;70:742.
245. Huaux JP, Lokietek W. Is APD a promising drug in the treatment of severe osteogenesis imperfecta? J Pediatr Orthop 1988;8:71.
246. Hueter C. Anatomische Studien an den Extremitatengelenken Neugebornener und Erwachsener. Virchows Arch 1862;25:572.
247. Huffer WE, Lacey DL. Studies on the pathogenesis of avian rickets. II. Necrosis of perforating epiphyseal vessels during recovery from rickets caused by vitamin D_3 deficiency. Am J Pathol 1982;109:302.
248. Huhne R, Schonfeld H. Eine eigenartige Wachtumsstorung im Kindeslater. Monatsschr Kinderheilkd 1929;42:267.
249. Hurwitz S. Clinical pediatric dermatology. Philadelphia: WB Saunders, 1981:185.
250. Huth EJ, Webster GD Jr, Elkinton JR. Renal excretion of hydrogen ion in renal tubular acidosis. III. An attempt to detect latent cases in a family; comments on nosology, genetics, and etiology of primary disease. Am J Med 1960;29:586.
251. Hyman LR, Boner G, Thomas JC, et al. Immobilization hypercalcemia. Am J Dis Child 1972;124:723.
252. Iannotti JP, Brighton CT, Stambough JL, Storey BT. Calcium flux and endogenous calcium content in isolated mammalian growth-plate chondrocytes, hyaline-cartilage chondrocytes, and hepatocytes. J Bone Joint Surg [Am] 1985;67:113.
253. Ibbotson KJ, Twardzik DR, D'Souza SM, et al. Stimulation of bone resorption in vitro by synthetic transforming growth factor-alpha. Science 1985;228:1007.
254. Isogna KL, Broadus AD, Gertner JM. Impaired phosphorus conservation and 1,25 dihydroxyvitamin D generation during phosphorus deprivation in familial hypophosphatemic rickets. J Clin Invest 1983;71:1562.
255. Jacobson DP, McClain EJ. Hypophosphatasia in monozygotic twins. A case report. J Bone Joint Surg [Am] 1967;49:377.
256. Jaffe HL. Metabolic, degenerative, and inflammatory diseases of bones and joints. Philadelphia: Lea & Febiger, 1972:381.
257. Jaworski ZFG. Pathophysiology, diagnosis, and treatment of osteomalacia. Orthop Clin North Am 1972;3:623.
258. Jennings AS, Liddle TW, Orth DN. Results of treating childhood Cushing's disease with pituitary irradiation. N Engl J Med 1977;297:957.
259. Jofe MH, Gebhardt MC, Tomford WW, Mankin HJ. Reconstruction for defects of the proximal part of the femur using allograft arthroplasty. J Bone Joint Surg [Am] 1988;70:507.
260. Jones ET, Hensinger RN. Spinal deformity in idiopathic juvenile osteoporosis. Spine 1981;6:1.
261. Jones G, Schnoes HK, DeLuca HF. Isolation and identification of 1,25 dihydroxy vitamin D_2. Biochemistry 1975;14:1250.
262. Jowsey J. Metabolic diseases of bone. Philadelphia: WB Saunders, 1977.
263. Jowsey J, Johnson KA. Juvenile osteoporosis. Bone findings in seven patients. J Pediatr 1972;81:511.
264. Juttman JR, Hagenouw-Taal JC, Lameyer LD, et al. Intestinal calcium absorption, serum phosphate, and parathyroid hor-

mone in patients with chronic renal failure and osteodystrophy before and during hemodialysis. Calcif Tissue Res 1978;26:119.
265. Kan K, Cruess RL, Posner B, et al. Receptor proteins for steroid and peptide hormones at the epiphyseal line. Trans Orthop Res Soc 1981;6:110.
266. Kanis JA. Vitamin D metabolism and its clinical application. J Bone Joint Surg [Br] 1982;64:542.
267. Kaplan FS, August CS, Fallon MD, et al. Successful treatment of infantile malignant osteopetrosis by bone-marrow transplantation. J Bone Joint Surg [Am] 1988;70:617.
268. Kaplan FS, Tabas JA, Gannon F, et al. The histopathology of fibrodysplasia ossificans progressiva. J Bone Joint Surg [Am] 1993;75:220.
269. Kaye M, Pritchard JE, Halpenny GW, et al. Bone disease in chronic renal failure with particular reference to osteosclerosis. Medicine (Baltimore) 1960;39:157.
270. Keech MR, Wendt VE, Reed RC, et al. Family studies of the Marfan syndrome. J Chronic Dis 1966;19:57.
271. Kessner DM, Epstein FH. Effect of renal insufficiency on gastrointestinal transport of calcium. Am J Physiol 1965;209:141.
272. King JD, Bobechko WP. Osteogenesis imperfecta. An orthopaedic description and surgical review. J Bone Joint Surg [Br] 1971;53:72.
273. King LR, Knowles HC, McLaurin RL. Calcium, phosphorus, and magnesium metabolism following head injury. Ann Surg 1973;177:126.
274. Kirk TS, Simon MA. Tumoral calcinosis: report of a case with successful medical management. J Bone Joint Surg [Am] 1981;63:1167.
275. Kleeman CR, Massry SG, Coburn JW, et al. Calcium and phosphorus metabolism and bone disease in uremia. Clin Orthop 1970;68:210.
276. Kleinman PK, Blackbourne BD, Marks SC, Karellas A, Belanger PL. Radiologic contributions to the investigation and prosecution of cases of fatal infant abuse. N Engl J Med 1989;320:507.
277. Kling TF Jr. Angular deformities of the lower limbs in children. Orthop Clin North Am 1987;18:513.
278. Koo WWK, Sherman R, Succop P, et al. Fractures and rickets in very low birth weight infants: conservative management and outcome. J Pediatr Orthop 1989;9:326.
279. Kooh SW, Cumming WA, Fraser D, et al. Transient childhood osteoporosis of unknown cause. Amsterdam: Excerpta Medica, 1973.
280. Kooh SW, Jones G, Reilly BJ, Fraser D. Pathogenesis of rickets in chronic hepatobiliary disease in children. J Pediatr 1979;94:870.
281. Kozlowki K, McCrossin R. Early osseous abnormalities in Menkes' kinky hair syndrome. Pediatr Radiol 1980;8:191.
282. Kramer B, Yuska H, Steiner MM. Marble bones. II. Chemical analysis of bone. Am J Dis Child 1939;57:1044.
283. Kretchmer N, Stone M, Bauer C. Hereditary enzymatic effects as illustrated by hypophosphatasia. Ann N Y Acad Sci 1958;75:279.
284. Kricun ME, Resnick D. Patellofemoral abnormalities in renal osteodystrophy. Radiology 1982;143:667.
285. Kricun ME, Resnick D. Elbow abnormalities in renal osteodystrophy. AJR Am J Roentgenol 1983;140:577.
286. Kumar S, Shahabuddin S, Haboubi N, et al. Angiogenesis factor from human myocardial infarcts. Lancet 1983;II:364.
287. Kunin AS. Polyostotic fibrous dysplasia with hypophosphatemia: a metabolic study. Metab Clin Exp 1962;11:978.
288. Lacey DL, Huffer WE. Studies on the pathogenesis of avian rickets. I. Changes in epiphyseal and metaphyseal vessels in hypocalcemic and hypophosphatemic rickets. Am J Pathol 1982;109:288.
289. Laditan AA, Adeniyi A. Rickets in Nigerian children—response to vitamin D. J Trop Med Hyg 1975;78:206.
290. Lalli AF, Lapides J. Osteosclerosis occurring in renal disease. AJR Am J Roentgenol 1963;93:924.
291. Lane JM, Suda M, von der Mark K, et al. Immunofluorescent localization of structural collagen types in endochondral fracture repair. J Orthop Res 1986;4:318.
292. Lawrence GD, Loeffler RG, Martin LG, et al. Immobilization hypercalcemia. J Bone Joint Surg [Am] 1973;55:87.
293. Leaf A. The syndrome of osteomalacia, renal glycosuria, aminoaciduria, and increased phosphate clearance (the Fanconi syndrome). In: Stanbury JB, Wyngaarden JB, Fredrickson DS, eds. The metabolic basis of inherited disease. 2nd ed. New York: McGraw-Hill, 1966.
294. Lee JJK, Lyne ED, Kleerekoper M, Logan MS, Belfi RA. Disorders of bone metabolism in severely handicapped children and young adults. Clin Orthop 1989;245:297.
295. Letts M, Monson R, Weber K. The prevention of recurrent fractures of the lower extremities in severe osteogenesis imperfecta using vacuum pants: a preliminary report in four patients. J Pediatr Orthop 1988;8:454.
296. Liakakos D, Papadopoulos Z, Vlachos P, et al. Serum alkaline phosphatase and urinary hydroxyproline values in children receiving phenobarbital with an without vitamin D. J Pediatr 1975;87:291.
297. Licata AA, Radfar N, Bartner FC. The urinary excretion of phosphoethanolamine in diseases other than hypophosphatasia. Am J Med 1978;64:133.
298. Lightwood R, Payne WW, Black JA. Infantile renal acidosis. Pediatrics 1953;12:628.
299. Lim MO, Mukherjee AB, Hansen JW. Dysplastic cutaneous osteomatosis. Arch Dermatol 1981;117:797.
300. Lin T, Tucci JR. Provocation tests of growth hormone release. Ann Intern Med 1974;80:464.
301. Liu SH, Chu HI. Studies of calcium and phosphorus with special reference to pathogenesis and effects of dihydrotachysterol (AT10) and iron. Medicine (Baltimore) 1943;22:103.
302. Lobstein JF. De la fragilite des os, ou de l'osteopsathyrose. Traite de l'anatomie pathologique. vol 2. Paris: Levrault FG, 1833.
303. Loeffler RD, Sherman FC. The effect of treatment on growth and deformity in hypophosphatemic vitamin D–resistant rickets. Clin Orthop 1982;162:4.
304. Long RG, Wills MR. Hepatic dystrophy. Br J Hosp Med 1978;20:312.
305. Looser E. Zur Kenntnis der Osteogenesis imperfecta congenita et tarda. Mitt Grenzbiet Med Chir 1906;15:161.
306. Lowe CU, Terrey M, MacLachlan EA. Organic aciduria, decreased from renal ammonia production, hydrophthalmos, and mental retardation. Am J Dis Child 1952;83:164.
307. Lund J, DeLuca HF. Biologically active metabolite of vitamin D from bone, liver and blood serum. J Lipid Res 1966;7:739.
308. MacGregor RR, Hamilton JW, Cohn DV. The induction of calcium-binding protein biosynthesis in intestine by vitamin D_3. Biochim Biophys Acta 1970;222:482.
309. Malebranche N. Traite de la recherche de la verite. Liv. 2, Chap. 7. Paris, 1674.
310. Mallick NP, Berlyne GM. Arterial calcification after vitamin D therapy in hyperphosphatemic renal failure. Lancet 1968;2:1316.
311. Mankin HJ. Review article: rickets, osteomalacia, and renal osteodystrophy. J Bone Joint Surg [Am] 1974;56:101.
312. Mann JG, Brown WR, Kern F. The subtle and variable expressions of gluten-induced enteropathy (adult celiac disease, nontropical sprue). Am J Med 1970;48:357.

313. Manzke E, Gruber HE, Hines RW, et al. Skeletal remodeling and bone-related hormones in two adults with increased bone mass. Metab Clin Exp 1982;31:25.
314. Marcus R, Wilber JF, Aurbach GD. Parathyroid hormone–sensitive adenyl cyclase from the renal cortex of a patient with pseudohypoparathyroidism. J Clin Endocrinol Metab 1971;33:537.
315. Marder HK, Tsang RC, Hug G, et al. Calcitriol deficiency in idiopathic juvenile osteoporosis in the young. J Bone Joint Surg [Br] 1980;62:417.
316. Marie PJ, Pettifor JM, Ross FP, Glorieux FH. Histological osteomalacia due to dietary deficiency in children. N Engl J Med 1982;307:584.
317. Marion MJ, Gannon FH, Fallon MD, Mennuti MT, Lodato RF, Kaplan FS. Skeletal dysplasia in perinatal lethal osteogenesis imperfecta. Clin Orthop 1993;293:327.
318. Marks SC. Pathogenesis of osteopetrosis in the rat: reduced bone resorption due to reduced osteoclast function. Am J Anat 1973;138:165.
319. Marks SC, Walker DG. The hematogenous origin of osteoclasts: experimental evidence from osteopetrotic (microphthmic) mice treated with spleen cells from beige mouse donors. Am J Anat 1981;161:1.
320. Marshall WA. Human growth hormone and its disorders. London: Academic Press, 1977.
321. Martin W, Riddervold HO. Epiphysiolysis in rickets. Va Med Q 1980;107:566.
322. Mason RS, Lissner D, Wilkinson M, et al. Vitamin D metabolites and their relationship to azotemic osteodystrophy. Clin Endocrinol 1980;13:375.
323. Mason RS, Rohl RG, Lissner D, Posen S. Vitamin D metabolism in hypophosphatemic rickets. Am J Dis Child 1982;136:909.
324. Mautalen C, Montoreano R, LaBarrere C. Early skeletal effect of alkali therapy upon the osteomalacia of renal tubular acidosis. J Clin Endocrinol Metab 1976;42:875.
325. McArthur RG, Hayles AG, Lambert PW. Albright's syndrome with rickets. Mayo Clin Proc 1979;54:313.
326. McCane RA, Fairweathr DVI, Barrett AM, et al. Genetic, clinical, biochemical, and pathological features of hypophosphatasia. Q J Med 1956;25:523.
327. McCane RA, Morrison AB, Dent CD. The excretion of phosphoethanolamine in hypophosphatasia. Lancet 1955;1:131.
328. McKusick VA. Heritable disorders of connective tissues. 4th ed. St. Louis: CV Mosby, 1972.
329. Mehls O, Ritz E, Krempien B, et al. Slipped epiphyses in renal osteodystrophy. Arch Dis Child 1975;50:545.
330. Meinhardt H. A boundary model for pattern formation in vertebrate limbs. J Embryol Exp Morphol 1983;76:115.
331. Middleton RWD, Frost RB. Percutaneous intramedullary rod interchange in osteogenesis imperfecta. J Bone Joint Surg [Br] 1987;69:429.
332. Milgram JW, Jasty M. Osteopetrosis. J Bone Joint Surg [Am] 1982;64:912.
333. Milhaud G, Labat ML. Osteopetrosis reconsidered as a curable immune disorder. Biomedicine 1979;30:71.
334. Milhaud G, Labat ML, Parant M, et al. Immunologic defect and its correction in the osteopetrotic mutant rat. Proc Natl Acad Sci U S A 1977;74:339.
335. Millard FJC, Nassim JR, Woollen JW. Urinary calcium excretion after immobilization and spinal fusion in adolescents. Arch Dis Child 1970;45:399.
336. Miller CG, Chutkin W. Vitamin D–deficiency rickets in Jamaican children. Arch Dis Child 1976;51:214.
337. Miller EA. Observation on the surgical management of osteogenesis imperfecta. Clin Orthop 1981;159:154.
338. Minkin C, Talmage RV. A study in secretion and function of thyrocalcitonin in normal rats. In: Talmage RV, Balanger LF, eds. Parathyroid hormone and thyrocalcitonin (calcitonin). Amsterdam: Excerpta Medica Foundation, 1968.
339. Mital MA, Garber JE, Stinson JT. Ectopic bone formation in children and adolescents with head injuries: its management. J Pediatr Orthop 1987;7:83.
340. Mitnick PD, Goldfarb S, Slatopolsky E, et al. Calcium and phosphorus metabolism in tumoral calcinosis. Ann Intern Med 1980;92:482.
341. Moe JH, Winter RB, Bradford DS, Lonstein JE. Scoliosis in Marfan's syndrome. In: Scoliosis and Other Spinal Deformities. Philadelphia: WB Saunders, 1978:315.
342. Moncrieff MW, Brenton DP, Arthur LJ. Case of tumor rickets. Arch Dis Child 1978;53:740.
343. Moore JH, Tyler C. Studies on the intestinal absorption and excretion of calcium and phosphorus in the pig. Part 2. The intestinal absorption and excretion of radioactive calcium and phosphorus. Br J Nutr 1955;9:81.
344. Morefield WG, Miller GR. Aftermath of osteogenesis imperfecta: a disease in adulthood. J Bone Joint Surg [Am] 1980;62:113.
345. Morel G, Houghton GR. Pneumatic trouser splints in the treatment of severe osteogenesis imperfecta. Acta Orthop Scand 1982;53:547.
346. Morgan B. Osteomalacia, renal osteodystrophy, and osteoporosis. Springfield, IL: Charles C Thomas, 1973.
347. Morijiri Y, Sato T. Factors causing rickets in institutionalized handicapped children on anticonvulsant therapy. Arch Dis Child 1981;56:446.
348. Morris RC. Renal tubular acidosis. Mechanisms, classification, and implication. N Engl J Med 1969;281:1405.
349. Morris RC, Sebastian A, McSherry E. Renal acidosis. Kidney Int 1972;1:322.
350. Moss AJ, Waterhouse C, Terry R. Gluten-sensitive enteropathy with osteomalacia without steatorrhea. N Engl J Med 1965;272:825.
351. Moss ML. The design of bones. In: Owen R, Goodfellow J, Bullough P, eds. Scientific foundations of orthopaedics and traumatology. Philadelphia: WB Saunders, 1980:59.
352. Mozaffarian G, Lafferty FW, Pearson OH. Treatment of tumoral calcinosis with phosphorus deprivation. Ann Intern Med 1972;741:745.
353. Muggia F, Heineman HO. Hypercalcemia associated with neoplastic disease. Ann Intern Med 1970;73:281.
354. National Academy of Sciences National Research Council. Food and Nutrition Board recommended dietary allowances, publication 1694. 7th ed. Washington, DC: National Academy of Sciences, National Research Council, 1968.
355. Naveh Y, Kaftori JK, Alan V, et al. Progressive diaphyseal dysplasia: genetics and clinical and radiographic manifestations. Pediatrics 1984;74:399.
356. Neidel J, Boddenberg B, Zander D, Schicha H, Rutt J, Hackenbroch MH. Thyroid function in Legg-Calve-Perthes disease: cross-sectional and longitudinal study. J Pediatr Orthop 1993;13:592.
357. Nicholas RW, James P. Telescoping intramedullary stabilization of the lower extremities for severe osteogenesis imperfecta. J Pediatr Orthop 1990;10:219.
358. Nixon JR, Douglas JF. Bilateral slipping of the upper femoral epiphysis in end-stage renal failure. J Bone Joint Surg [Br] 1980;62:18.
359. Nordin BEC. Effect of malabsorption syndrome on calcium metabolism. Proc R Soc Lond 1961;54:497.
360. Norman AW. Evidence for a new kidney-produced hormone 1,25-dihydroxy-cholecalciferol, the proposed biologically active form of vitamin D. Am J Clin Nutr 1971;24:1346.

361. Norman ME, Mazur AT, Borden S, et al. Early diagnosis of juvenile renal osteodystrophy. J Pediatr 1980;97:226.
362. Ogilvie-Harris DJ, Fornasier VL. Pseudomalignant myositis ossificans: heterotopic new-bone formation without a history of trauma. J Bone Joint Surg [Am] 1980;62:1274.
363. Ohara-May J, Widdowson EM. Diets and living conditions of Asian boys in Coventry with and without signs of rickets. Br J Nutr 1976;36:23.
364. Olin A, Creasman C, Shapiro F. Free physeal transplantation in the rabbit: an experimental approach to focal lesions. J Bone Joint Surg [Am] 1984;66:7.
365. Olsen BR, Ninomiya Y, Gordon MK. A new dimension in the extracellular matrix. Third International Conference on the Chemistry and Biology of Mineralized Tissues. Program and Abstracts 1988;60.
366. Oppenheim WL, Salusky IB, Kaplan D, Fine RN. Renal osteodystrophy in children. In: Castells S, Finberg L, eds. Metabolic bone disease in children. New York: Marcel Dekker, 1990;197.
367. Oppenheimer SJ, Snodgrass GJ. Neonatal rickets. Histopathology and quantitative bone changes. Arch Dis Child 1980;55:945.
368. Paley D, Tetsworth K. Mechanical axis deviation of the lower limbs. Clin Orthop 1992;280:65.
369. Parfitt AM. Soft-tissue calcification in uremia. Arch Intern Med 1969;124:544.
370. Parfitt AM. Hypophosphatemic vitamin D–refractory rickets and osteomalacia. Orthop Clin North Am 1972;3:653.
371. Parfitt AM. Renal osteodystrophy. Orthop Clin North Am 1972;3:681.
372. Park EA. Observations on the pathology of rickets with particular reference to the changes at the cartilage shaft junctions of the growing bones. Bull N Y Acad Med 1939;14:495.
373. Parker MS, Klein I, Haussler MR, Mentz DH. Tumor-induced osteomalacia. Evidence of a surgically correctable alteration in vitamin D metabolism. JAMA 1981;245:492.
374. Parrish JG. Heritable disorders of connective tissue. Proc R Soc Med 1960;53:515.
375. Paul PD, Lloyd DJ, Smith FW. The role of bone scanning in neonatal rickets. Pediatr Radiol 1983;13:89.
376. Pazzaglia UE, Beluffi G, Colombo A, et al. Myositis ossificans in the newborn. J Bone Joint Surg [Am] 1986;68:456.
377. Pazzaglia UE, Byers P, Beluffi G, et al. Pathology of infantile cortical hyperostosis (Caffey's disease). J Bone Joint Surg [Am] 1985;67:1417.
378. Pearce L. Hereditary osteopetrosis of the rabbit. III. Pathological observations: skeletal abnormalities. J Exp Med 1950;92:591.
379. Pelker RR, McKay J Jr, Troiano N, et al. Allograft incorporation: a biomechanical evaluation in a rat model. J Orthop Res 1989;7:585.
380. Peltonen L, Palotie A, Prockop DJ. A defect in the structure of type I procollagen in a patient who had osteogenesis imperfecta: excessive mannose in the COOH-terminal peptide. Proc Natl Acad Sci U S A 1980;77:6179.
381. Perry W, Stamp TC. Hereditary hypophosphatemic rickets with autosomal recessive inheritance and severe osteosclerosis. J Bone Joint Surg [Br] 1978;60:430.
382. Pettifor JM, Ross P, Wang J, et al. Rickets in children of rural origin in South Africa: is low dietary calcium a factor? J Pediatr 1978;92:320.
383. Pettinen RP, Lichtenstein JR, Martin GR, et al. Abnormal collagen metabolism in cultured cells in osteogenesis imperfecta. Proc Natl Acad Sci U S A 1975;72:586.
384. Pezeshki C, Brooker AF Jr. Immobilization hypercalcemia. J Bone Joint Surg [Am] 1977;59:971.
385. Phillips LS, Vassilopoulos-Sellin R. Somatomedins. N Engl J Med 1980;302:371.
386. Pimstone B, Eissenberg E, Silverman S. Hypophosphatasia: genetic and dental studies. Ann Intern Med 1966;65:722.
387. Pinchus JB, Gittleman IF, Kramer B. Juvenile osteopetrosis: metabolic studies in two cases and further observations on the composition of the bones in this disease. Am J Dis Child 1947;73:458.
388. Pinnell SR, Krane SM, Kenzora JE, et al. A hereditary disorder of connective tissue: hydroxylysine-deficient collagen disease. N Engl J Med 1972;386:1013.
389. Pitt MJ. Rachitic and osteomalacia syndromes. Radiol Clin North Am 1981;19:581.
390. Platt R, Owen TK. Renal dwarfism associated with calcification of arteries and skin. Lancet 1934;2:135.
391. Pollack JA, Schiller AL, Crawford JD. Rickets and myopathy cured by removal of a nonossifying fibroma of bone. Pediatrics 1973;52:364.
392. Pope FM, Nicholls AC, Eggleton C, et al. Osteogenesis imperfecta (lethal) bones contain types III and V collagen. J Clin Pathol 1980;33:534.
393. Porat S, Heller E, Seidman DS, Meyer S. Functional results of operation in osteogenesis imperfecta: elongating and nonelongating rods. J Pediatr Orthop 1991;11:200.
394. Powell D, Singer FR, Murray TM, et al. Nonparathyroid humoral hypercalcemia in patients with neoplastic diseases. N Engl J Med 1973;289:176.
395. Powell GF, Brasil JA, Blizzard RM. Functional deprivation and growth retardation simulating idiopathic hypopituitarism. I. Clinical evaluation of the syndrome. N Engl J Med 1967;276:1271.
396. Powell GF, Brasil JA, Ruiti S, et al. Emotional deprivation and growth retardation simulating idiopathic hypopituitarism. II. Endocrinologic evaluation of the syndrome. N Engl J Med 1967;276:1279.
397. Putkonen T, Wangel GA. Renal hyperparathyroidism with metastatic calcification of the skin. Dermatologica 1959;118:127.
398. Pyeritz RE, McKusick VA. The Marfan syndrome: diagnosis and management. N Engl J Med 1979;300:772.
399. Quisling RW, Moore GR, Jahrsdoefer RA. Osteogenesis imperfecta. Arch Otolaryngol 1979;105:207.
400. Raghuramulu N, Reddy V. Serum 25-hydroxy vitamin D levels in malnourished children with rickets. Arch Dis Child 1980;55:285.
401. Raisz LG. Bone metabolism and calcium regulation. In: Avioli LV, Krane SM, eds. Metabolic bone disease. New York: Academic Press, 1978.
402. Raisz LG, Kream B. Hormonal control of skeletal growth. Annu Rev Physiol 1981;43:225.
403. Raisz LG, Kream BE. Regulation of bone formation. N Engl J Med 1983;309:29.
404. Rames RD, Strecker WB. Recurrent elbow dislocations in a patient with Ehlers-Danlos syndrome. Orthopedics 1991;14:705.
405. Ramser JR, Villaneuva AR, Frost HM. Cortical bone dynamics in osteomalacia, measured by tetracycline bone labeling. Clin Orthop 1966;49:89.
406. Randall C, Lauchlan SC. Parathyroid hyperplasia in an infant. Am J Dis Child 1963;105:364.
407. Rao S, Patel A, Schildhauer T. Osteogenesis imperfecta as a differential diagnosis of pathologic burst fractures of the spine. Clin Orthop 1993;289:113.
408. Rasmussen H. Ionic and hormonal control of calcium homeostasis. Am J Med 1971;50:567.
409. Rasmussen H. The calcium messenger system. N Engl J Med 1986;314:1094.
410. Rasmussen H, Bordier P. The cellular basis of metabolic bone disease. N Engl J Med 1973;289:25.

411. Rasmussen H, Wong M, Bikle D, Goodman DBP. Hormonal control of 25-hydroxycholecalciferol to 1,25-dihydroxycholecalciferol. J Clin Invest 1972;51:2502.
412. Rathbun JC. Hypophosphatasia. Am J Dis Child 1948;75:822.
413. Reinholt FP, Hjerpe A, Jansson K, et al. Stereological studies on the epiphyseal growth plate in low phosphate, vitamin D–deficiency rickets with special reference to the distribution of matrix vesicles. Calcif Tissue Int 1984;36:95.
414. Relman AS. Renal acidosis and renal excretion of acid in health and disease. Adv Intern Med 1964;12:295.
415. Relman AS, Levinsky NG. Kidney disease: acquired tubular disorders with special reference to disturbances of concentration and dilution and of acid-base regulation. Annu Rev Med 1961;12:932.
416. Resnick D, Deftos LJ, Partemore JG. Renal osteodystrophy: magnification radiography of target sites of absorption. AJR Am J Roentgenol 1981;136:711.
417. Resnick D, Niwayama G. Osteomyelitis, septic arthritis, and soft tissue infection: the organisms. In: Resnick D, Niwayama G, eds. Diagnosis of bone and joint disorders. 2nd ed. Philadelphia: WB Saunders, 1988:2647.
418. Reynolds WA, Karo JJ. Radiologic diagnosis of metabolic bone disease. Orthop Clin North Am 1972;3:521.
419. Ritz E, Malluche HJ, Krempien B, et al. Pathogenesis of renal osteodystrophy: roles of phosphate and skeletal resistance to PTH. Adv Exp Med Biol 1978;103:423.
420. Rivkees S, Bode HH, Crawford JD. Long-term growth in juvenile acquired hypothyroidism: the failure to achieve normal adult stature. N Engl J Med 1988;318:599.
421. Roberts JM, Solomons CC. Management of pregnancy in osteogenesis imperfecta. Obstet Gynecol 1975;45:168.
422. Robins PR, Moe JH, Winter RB. Scoliosis in Marfan's syndrome. J Bone Joint Surg [Am] 1975;57:358.
423. Rodriguez-Peralto JL, Lopez-Barea F, Torres A, et al. Tumoral calcinosis in two infants. Clin Orthop 1989;242:272.
424. Root AW, Bongiovanni AM, Eberlai WR. Diagnosis and management of growth retardation with special reference to the problem of hypopituitarism. J Pediatr 1971;78:737.
425. Rosen H, Friedman SA, Raizner AE, et al. Azotemic arteriopathy. Am Heart J 1972;84:250.
426. Rosier RN. Orthopaedic basic science: update. Orthopedics 1987;10:1793.
427. Rubinovitch M, Said SE, Glorieux FH, et al. Principles and results of corrective lower limb osteotomies for patients with vitamin D–resistant hypophosphatemic rickets. Clin Orthop 1988;237:264.
428. Rudman D, Kutner MH, Blackston RD, et al. Children with normal variant short stature: treatment with human growth hormone for six months. N Engl J Med 1981;305:123.
429. Rudolf M, Arulanatham K, Greenstein RM. Unsuspected nutritional rickets. Pediatrics 1993;
430. Ryoppy S, Alberty A, Kaitila I. Early semiclosed intramedullary stabilization in osteogenesis imperfecta. J Pediatr Orthop 1987;7:139.
431. Sadowski H, Shuai K, Darnell JE Jr, Gilman MZ. A common nuclear signal transduction pathway activated by growth factor and cytokine receptors. Science 1993;261:1739.
432. Salassa RM, Jowsey J, Arnaud CD. Hypophosphatemic osteomalacia associated with "nonendocrine" tumors. N Engl J Med 1970;283:65.
433. Salenius P, Vankka E. The development of the tibio-femoral angle in children. J Bone Joint Surg [Am] 1975;57:259.
434. Salimpour R. Rickets in Tehran. Study of 200 cases. Arch Dis Child 1975;50:63.
435. Sambrook P, Birmingham J, Kelly P, et al. Prevention of corticosteroid osteoporosis. A comparison of calcium, calcitriol, and calcitonin. N Engl J Med 1993;328:1747.
436. Sandberg MM, Aro HT, Vuorio EI. Gene expression during bone repair. Clin Orthop 1993;289:292.
437. Schott GD, Wills MR. Muscle weakness in osteomalacia. Lancet 1976;1:626.
438. Schreiner GE, Smith LH, Kye LH. Renal hyperchloremic acidosis. Familial occurrence of nephrocalcinosis with hyperchloremia and low serum bicarbonate. Am J Med 1953;15:122.
439. Scriver CR, Reade TM, DeLuca HF, Hamstra AJ. Serum 1,25-dihydroxy vitamin D levels in normal subjects and in patients with hereditary rickets or bone disease. N Engl J Med 1978;299:976.
440. Seedorff KS. Osteogenesis imperfecta: a study of clinical features and heredity based on 55 Danish families comprising 180 affected persons. Copenhagen: Ejnar Munksgaard, 1949.
441. Seldin DW, Wilson JD. Renal tubular acidosis. In: Stanbury JB, Wyngaarden JB, Fredrickson DS, eds. The metabolic basis of inherited disease. 2nd ed. New York: McGraw-Hill, 1966:1230.
442. Shapiro F. Consequences of an osteogenesis imperfecta diagnosis for survival and ambulation. J Pediatr Orthop 1985;5:456.
443. Shapiro F. Osteopetrosis: current clinical considerations. Clin Orthop 1993;294:34.
444. Shapiro F, Glimcher MJ, Holtrop ME, et al. Human osteopetrosis. A histological, ultrastructural, and biochemical study. J Bone Joint Surg [Am] 1980;62:384.
445. Sieff CA, Levinsky RJ, Rogers DW, et al. Allogeneic bone-marrow transplantation in infantile malignant osteopetrosis. Lancet 1983;1:437.
446. Sijbrandij S. Percutaneous nailing in the management of osteogenesis imperfecta. Int Orthop 1990;14:195.
447. Sillence DO. Osteogenesis imperfecta: an expanding panorama of variance. Clin Orthop 1981;159:11.
448. Sillence DO, Senn A, Danks DM. Genetic heterogeneity in osteogenesis imperfecta. J Med Genet 1979;16:101.
449. Simpson JL. Disorders of sexual differentiation: etiology and clinical delineation. New York: Academic Press, 1976.
450. Singh BN, Spies SM, Mehta SP, et al. Unusual bone scan presentation in osteomalacia: symmetrical uptake—a suggestive sign. Clin Nucl Med 1978;3:292.
451. Skaria J, Katiyar BC, Srivastava TP, Dube B. Myopathy and neuropathy associated with osteomalacia. Acta Neurol Scand 1975;51:37.
452. Sledge CB, Zaleske DJ. Developmental anatomy of joints. In: Resnick D, Niwayama G, eds. Diagnosis of bone and joint disorders. 2nd ed. Philadelphia: WB Saunders, 1988:604.
453. Smith R. The pathophysiology and management of rickets. Orthop Clin North Am 1972;3:601.
454. Smith R, Francis MJO, Bauze RJ. Osteogenesis imperfecta: a clinical and biochemical study of a generalized connective tissue disorder. Q J Med 1975;44:555.
455. Smith R, Stern G. Muscular weakness in osteomalacia and hyperparathyroidism. J Neurol Sci 1969;8:511.
456. Sobel EH, Clark LC, Fox RP, et al. Rickets: deficiency of "alkaline" phosphatase activity and premature loss of teeth in childhood. Pediatrics 1953;11:309.
457. Sofield HA, Millar EA. Fragmentation, realignment, and intramedullary rod fixation of deformities of the long bones in children. A ten-year appraisal. J Bone Joint Surg [Am] 1959;41:1371.
458. Sognen E. Calcium-binding substances and intestinal absorption. Acta Pharmacol Toxicol 1964;21(Suppl1):1.
459. Sorell M, Kapoor N, Kirkperuch C. Marrow transplantation for juvenile osteopetrosis. Am J Med 1981;70:1280.
460. Soyka LF, Bode HH, Crawford JD, et al. Effectiveness of long

term human growth therapy for short stature in children with human growth hormone deficiency. J Clin Endocrinol Metab 1970;30:1.
461. Sporn M, Roberts AB, Wakefield LM, Assoian RK. Transforming growth factor-beta: biological function and chemical structure. Science 1986;233:532.
462. Staheli LT, Church CC, Ward BH. Infantile cortical hyperostosis (Caffey's disease). JAMA 1968;203:96.
463. Staheli LT, Corbett M, Wyss C, King H. Lower-extremity rotational problems in children. J Bone Joint Surg [Am] 1985;67:39.
464. Stamp TCB, Baker LR. Recessive hypophosphatemic rickets and possible etiology of the vitamin D–resistant syndrome. Arch Dis Child 1976;51:360.
465. Stamp WG, Whitesides TE, Field MH, Scheer GE. Treatment of vitamin D–resistant rickets. A long-term evaluation of its effectiveness. J Bone Joint Surg [Am] 1964;46:965.
466. Stanbury SW. Bone disease in uremia. Am J Med 1968;44:714.
467. Stanbury SW, Lamb GA. Metabolic studies of renal osteodystrophy. I. Calcium, phosphorus, and nitrogen metabolism in rickets, osteomalacia, and hyperparathyroidism complicating uremia and in the osteomalacia of the adult Fanconi syndrome. Medicine (Baltimore) 1962;41:1.
468. Stanbury SW, Lamb GA. Parathyroid function in chronic renal failure. A statistical survey of the plasma biochemistry in azotaemic renal osteodystrophy. Q J Med 1966;35:1.
469. Stanitski DF. Treatment of deformity secondary to metabolic bone disease with Ilizarov technique. Clin Orthop 1994;301:38.
470. Steegers-Theunissen RPM, Boers GHJ, Trijbels FJM, Eskes TKAB. Neural-tube defects and derangement of homocysteine metabolism. N Engl J Med 1991;324:199.
471. Steinbach HG, Noetzli M. Roentgen appearance of the skeleton in osteomalacia and rickets. AJR Am J Roentgenol 1964;91:955.
472. Steinbach HL, Kolb FO, Gilfillan R. Mechanism of production of pseudofractures in osteomalacia (Milkman's syndrome). Radiology 1954;62:388.
473. Steinberg I. A simple screening test for the Marfan syndrome. AJR Am J Roentgenol 1966;97:118.
474. Streeter GL. Developmental horizons in human embryos. IV. A review of the histogenesis of cartilage and bone. Contrib Embryol 1949;33:149.
475. Stuart C, Aceto T Jr, Kuhn JP, Terplan K. Intrauterine hyperparathyroidism. Postmortem findings in two cases. Am J Dis Child 1979;133:67.
476. Sundaram M, Joyce PF, Shields JB, et al. Terminal phalangeal tufts: earliest site of renal osteodystrophy findings in hemodialysis patients. AJR Am J Roentgenol 1981;136:363.
477. Sundaram M, Wolverson MK, Heiberg E, et al. Erosive azotemic osteodystrophy. AJR Am J Roentgenol 1981;136:363.
478. Swann GF. Pathogenesis of bone lesions in neurofibromatosis. Br J Radiol 1954;27:623.
479. Swischuk LE, Hayden CK. Rickets: a roentgenographic scheme for diagnosis. Pediatr Radiol 1979;8:203.
480. Tabin CJ. Retinoids, homeoboxes, and growth factors: toward molecular models for limb development. Cell 1991;66:199.
481. Talab YA, Mallouh A. Hyperostosis with hyperphosphatemia: a case report and review of the literature. J Pediatr Orthop 1988;8:338.
482. Tam CS, Wilson DR, Hitchman AJ, Harrison JE. Protective effect of vitamin D_2 on bone apposition from the inhibitory action of hydrocortisone in rats. Calcif Tissue Int 1981;33:167.
483. Tanaka T, Swann S. A case of McCune-Albright syndrome with hyperthyroidism and vitamin D–resistant rickets. Helv Paediatr Acta 1977;32:263.
484. Tanner JM, Goldstein H, Whitehouse RH. Standards for children's height at ages 2 to 9 years allowing for height of parents. Arch Dis Child 1970;45:755.
485. Tanner JM, Whitehouse RH, Marshall WA, et al. Assessment of skeletal maturity and predition of adult height (TW2 method). London: Academic Press, 1975.
486. Tanner JM, Whitehouse RH, Takaishi M. Standards from birth to maturity for height, weight, height velocity, and weight velocity: British children, 1965. Arch Dis Child 1966;41:454.
487. Taylor AM. Intestinal vitamin D–induced calcium-binding protein: time course of immunocytological localization following 1,25-dihydroxyvitamin D_3. J Histochem Cytochem 1983;31:426.
488. Taylor AM, Wasserman RH. Vitamin D–induced calcium binding protein: comparative aspects in kidney and intestine. Am J Physiol 1972;223:110.
489. Tebor GB, Ehrlich MG, Herrin J. Slippage of the distal tibial epiphysis. J Pediatr Orthop 1983;3:211.
490. Temtamy SA, McKusick VA. Brachydactyly as part of syndromes. In: Bergsma D, ed. The genetics of hand malformations. New York: Alan R Liss, 1978:227.
491. Teotia M, Teotia S, Singh RK. Idiopathic juvenile osteoporosis. Am J Dis Child 1979;133:894.
492. Thompson GR, Lewis B, Booth CC. Absorption of vitamin D_3–^3H in control subjects and patients with intestinal malabsorption. J Clin Invest 1966;45:94.
493. Tiley F, Albright JA. Osteogenesis imperfecta: treatment by multiple osteotomy and intradmedullary rod insertion. J Bone Joint Surg [Am] 1973;55:701.
494. Timperlake RW, Cook SD, Thomas KA, et al. Effects of anticonvulsant drug therapy on bone mineral density in a pediatric population. J Pediatr Orthop 1988;8:467.
495. Trelstad RL, Rubin D, Gross J. Osteogenesis imperfecta congenita. Evidence for a generalized molecular disorder of collagen. Lab Invest 1977;36:501.
496. Trippel SB. Basic science of the growth plate. Curr Opin Orthop 1990;1:279.
497. Trippel SB, Chernausek SD, Van Wyk JJ, et al. Demonstration of type I and type II somatomedin receptors on bovine growth plate chondrocytes. J Orthop Res 1988;6:817.
498. Trippel SB, Van Wyk JJ, Mankin HJ. Localization of somatomedin-C binding to bovine growth-plate chondrocytes in situ. J Bone Joint Surg [Am] 1986;68:897.
499. Trippel SB, Wroblewski J, Makower A-M, et al. Regulation of growth-plate chondrocytes by insulin-like growth-factor I and basic fibroblast growth factor. J Bone Joint Surg [Am] 1993;75:177.
500. Tryfus H. Hepatic rickets. Ann Paediatr 1959;192:81.
501. Tsipouras P, Del Mastro R, Sarfarazi M, et al. Genetic linkage of the Marfan syndrome, ectopia lentis, and congenital contractural arachnodactyly to the fibrillin genes on chromosomes 15 and 5. N Engl J Med 1992;326:905.
502. Tsuchiya Y, Matsuo N, Cho H, et al. Vitamin D and vitamin D dependency. Contrib Nephrol 1980;22:80.
503. Turkainen J. Altered glycosaminoglycan production in cultured osteogenesis imperfecta skin fibroblasts. Biochem J 1983;213:171.
504. Ueda K, Saito A, Nakano H, et al. Cortical hyperostosis following long-term administration of prostaglandin E in infants with cyanotic congenital heart disease. J Pediatr 1980;97:834.
505. Urist MR, DeLange RJ, Finerman GAM. Bone cell differentiation and growth factors. Science 1983;220:680.
506. Vaes G. Cellular biology and biochemical mechanism of bone resorption: a review of recent developments on the formation, activation, and mode of action of osteoclasts. Clin Orthop 1988;231:239.
507. Villareale ME, Chiroff RT, Bergstrom WH, et al. Bone changes induced by diphenylhydantoin in chicks on a controlled vitamin D intake. J Bone Joint Surg [Am] 1978;60:911.

508. Virolainen P, Vuorio E, Aro HT. Gene expression at graft-host interfaces of cortical bone allografts and autografts. Clin Orthop 1993;297:144.
509. Vrolik W. Tabulae ad illustradam embryogenesin hominis et mammalium, tam naturalem quam abnormen. Amsterdam: GMP Londonck, 1949.
510. Walker DG. Osteopetrosis cured by temporary parabiosis. Science 1973;180:875.
511. Walker DG. Experimental osteopetrosis. Clin Orthop 1973;97:158.
512. Walker DG. Bone resorption restored in osteopetrotic mice by transplants of normal bone marrow and spleen cells. Science 1975;190:784.
513. Walton J. Familial hypophosphatemic rickets: a delineation of its subdivisions and pathogenesis. Clin Pediatr 1976;15:1007.
514. Wang N, Butler JP, Ingber DE. Mechanotransduction across the cell surface and through the cytoskeleton. Science 1993;260:1124.
515. Weinberg AG, Stone RT. Autosomal dominant inheritance in Albright's hereditary osteodystrophy. J Pediatr 1971;79:997.
516. Weller M, Edeiken J, Hodes PJ. Renal osteodystrophy. AJR 1968;104:354.
517. Wells D, King JD, Roe TF, Kaufman FR. Review of slipped capital femoral epiphysis associated with endocrine disease. J Pediatr Orthop 1993;13:610.
518. Whistler D. Disputatio Medica Inauguralis de Morbo puerili Anglorum quem patrio idiomate indigenae vocant the rickets. London: Wilhemi, Christiani, Boxii, 1645.
519. Whyte MP, Teitelbaum SI, Murphy WA. Adult hypophosphatasia. Clinical, laboratory, and genetic investigation of a large kindred with review of the literature. Medicine (Baltimore) 1979;58:329.
520. Whyte MP, Weldon W. Idiopathic hypoparathyroidism presenting with seizures during infancy: X-linked recessive inheritance in a large Missouri kindred. J Pediatr 1981;99:608.
521. Widdowson EM, McCance RA. The metabolism of calcium, phosphorus, magnesium and strontium. Pediatr Clin North Am 1965;12:595.
522. Williams JCP, Baratt-Boyes BG, Lowe JB. Supravavular aortic stenosis. Circulation 1961;24:1311.
523. Williams PF. Fragmentation and rodding in osteogenesis imperfecta. J Bone Joint Surg [Br] 1965;47:23.
524. Wills MR, Phillips JB, Day RC, Bateman EC. Phytic acid and nutritional rickets in immigrants. Lancet 1972;1:771.
525. Winnacker JL, Yeager H, Saunders RB, et al. Rickets in children receiving anticonvulsant drugs. Biochemical and hormonal markers. Am J Dis Child 1977;131:286.
526. Winters RW, Graham JB, Williams TF, et al. A genetic study of familial hypophosphatasia and vitamin D–resistant rickets with a review of the literature. Medicine (Baltimore) 1958;37:97.
527. Wolff J. Das Gesetz der Transformation de Knochen. Berlin: Hirschwald, 1892.
528. Wuthier RE. A review of the primary mechanism of endochondral calcification with special emphasis on the role of cells, mitochondria and matrix vessicles. Clin Orthop 1982;169:219.
529. Wynne-Davis R, Gormley J. Clinical and genetic patterns in osteogenesis imperfecta. Clin Orthop 1981;159:26.
530. Yong JM. Cause of raised serum alkaline phosphatase after partial gastrectomy and in other malabsorption states. Lancet 1966;1:1132.
531. Zaleske DJ, Bode HH, Benz R, Krishnamoorthy KS. Association of sciatica-like pain and Addison's disease. A case report. J Bone Joint Surg [Am] 1984;66:297.
532. Zerwekh JE, Glass K, Jowsey J, et al. A unique form of osteomalacia associated with end-organ refractoriness to 1,25-dihydroxyvitamin D and apparent defective synthesis of 25-hydroxyvitamin D. J Clin Endocrinol Metab 1979;49:171.
533. Zubrow AB, Lane JW, Parks JS. Slipped capital femoral epiphysis occurring during treatment for hypothyroidism. J Bone Joint Surg [Am] 1978;60:256.

Chapter 7

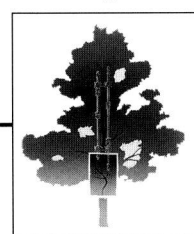

The Osteochondrodysplasias

George S. Bassett

Achondroplasia
　Clinical Features
　Growth and Development
　Radiographic Features
　Medical Considerations
　Orthopaedic Implications
Hypochondroplasia
　Clinical Features
　Radiographic Features
　Orthopaedic Implications
Metatropic Dysplasia
　Clinical Features
　Radiographic Features
　Medical Considerations
　Orthopaedic Implications
Chondroectodermal Dysplasia
　Clinical Features
　Radiographic Features
　Orthopaedic Implications
Diastrophic Dysplasia
　Clinical Features
　Radiographic Features
　Medical Considerations
　Orthopaedic Implications
Kniest Dysplasia
　Clinical Features
　Radiographic Features
　Medical Considerations
　Orthopaedic Implications
Spondyloepiphyseal Dysplasia Congenita
　Clinical Features
　Radiographic Features
　Medical Considerations
　Orthopaedic Implications

Spondyloepiphyseal Dysplasia Tarda
　Clinical Features
　Radiographic Features
　Orthopaedic Implications
Pseudoachondroplastic Dysplasia
　Clinical Features
　Radiographic Features
　Orthopaedic Implications
Multiple Epiphyseal Dysplasia
　Clinical Features
　Radiographic Features
　Orthopaedic Implications
Chondrodysplasia Punctata
　Clinical Features
　Radiographic Features
　Medical Considerations
　Orthopaedic Implications
Metaphyseal Chondrodysplasia
　Clinical Features
　Radiographic Features
　Medical Considerations
　Orthopaedic Implications
Dyschondrosteosis
　Clinical Features
　Radiographic Features
　Orthopaedic Implications
Cleidocranial Dysplasia
　Clinical Features
　Radiographic Features
　Orthopaedic Implications
Larsen Syndrome
　Clinical Features
　Radiographic Features
　Orthopaedic Implications

The skeletal dysplasias, more appropriately called osteochondrodysplasias, are a group of disorders characterized by an intrinsic abnormality in the growth and remodeling of cartilage and bone.[11,14] These generalized disturbances in the development of the skeleton affect the skull, spine, and extremities in various degrees. The resulting alterations in the size and shape of the limbs and trunk frequently are associated with disproportionately short stature (i.e., dwarfism) if the standing height falls below the third percentile for age.

The osteochondrodysplasias are a heterogeneous group of disorders, and most are heritable. More than 160 types are distinguishable by clinical, genetic, and radiographic criteria. Many of these conditions also have distinct histologic, biochemical, and molecular biologic defects. Apart from the clearly recognizable dysplasias, a myriad of intrinsic skeletal dysplasias of unclassified types exist. As a group, the incidence of these disorders, including lethal forms, is 1 in 3000 to 5000 births.[1,4]

The nomenclature traditionally used for skeletal dysplasias is a combination of terms derived from a variety of sources. Some names originate from descriptive Greek terminology (e.g., metatropic dysplasia, diastrophic dysplasia), and some reflect the name of the physician credited with the first description of the disorder (e.g., Kniest dysplasia, Larsen syndrome). Other names are based on the radiographically determined region of the skeleton involved, such as multiple epiphyseal dysplasia, metaphyseal chondrodysplasia, or spondyloepiphyseal dysplasia. However, these radiographic distinctions do not necessarily reflect the extent of histologic involvement. For instance, alterations of chondrocytes are seen in the physeal and metaphyseal regions of patients with multiple epiphyseal dysplasia in addition to the obvious epiphyseal involvement. Additional terms such as rhizomelic (proximal), mesomelic (middle), and acromelic (distal) are used to describe the segment of the limb with the greatest involvement. These terms refer to the arm, forearm, and hand or to the thigh, leg, and foot regions, respectively.

Dwarfing conditions frequently are referred to as short-limb or short-trunk types, according to whether trunk or limbs are more extensively involved. Achondroplasia, hypochondroplasia, and the metaphyseal chondrodysplasias are considered short-limb dwarfing conditions, based on their clinical appearances. The extremities are disproportionately short compared with the trunk. The sitting height of these persons is within normal range. In contrast, short-trunk dwarfing conditions produce greater shortening of the spine relative to the limbs. Kniest syndrome, metatropic dysplasia, and the spondyloepiphyseal dysplasias are in this category. However, the broad designations of short-trunk and short-limb disproportions may not reflect accurately the severity or frequency of clinical problems that the patient experiences. For instance, persons with pseudoachondroplasia have greater limb involvement (ie, short-limb dwarfism) but may have significant atlantoaxial instability associated with neurologic sequelae. The most common disabling problem that the achondroplastic dwarf encounters throughout life is lumbar spinal stenosis, although it is not reflected in the descriptive designation of short-limb disproportionate dwarf.

The diversity of the skeletal dysplasias and the heterogeneity that may exist within a specific disorder have made classification difficult. The most widely accepted divisions and nomenclature are based on the International Classification of Osteochondrodysplasias, revised in 1991 by the International Working Group on Constitutional Diseases of Bone (Appendix 7-1).[2] The classification sought to facilitate the recognition of specific disorders by grouping morphologically similar entities by roentgenographic criteria alone. Previous attempts to use clinical and pathologic criteria in addition to roentgenographic criteria led to many inconsistencies. This chapter deals with several of the more commonly encountered osteochondrodysplasias, most of which are considered dwarfing conditions.

Establishing an accurate diagnosis for many of the skeletal dysplasias frequently necessitates consultation with a geneticist knowledgeable in the osteochondrodysplasias. Many of these disorders have specific subtypes with variable clinical manifestations and patterns of genetic transmission. For example, there are autosomal recessive, X-linked dominant, and X-linked recessive forms of chondrodysplasia punctata. These differentiations are difficult for most orthopaedic surgeons to make. The specific orthopaedic deformities identified and their natural history are different for many of the osteochondrodysplasias.

Without a proper diagnosis, the total care of the patient may be compromised. Care includes accurate genetic counseling and the recognition and treatment of musculoskeletal abnormalities and other intrinsic medical problems. The tools used for evaluating these patients, including a careful history and physical examination, are not unique. However, there is particular emphasis on the family history and an understanding of what is normal development for each of these dysplasias. Appropriate radiographs must be obtained and properly evaluated.[5]

Identifying the body region that is disproportionately shortened is clinically and radiographically feasible. When difficulties arise, published standards of the clinical parameters of trunk height and extremity lengths are useful for analysis. For example, lower segment and trunk disproportions can be evaluated by comparing the ratio of sitting (trunk) to standing heights with the ratios presented in tables of proportionate children.[6] In some cases, determining whether a rhizomelic or mesomelic condition exists is facilitated by making a comparison with radiographic standards of measured bone lengths and ratios for upper and lower extremities.[9,13]

Advances made in the fields of biochemistry and molecular biology have been applied to the study of the osteochondrodysplasias. For many of these disorders, specific protein defects have been identified, and the defect has been localized to the chromosome and loci (see Appendix 7-1; see Chap. 5).

An important resource for short stature individuals is the Little People of America (LPA). This national organization addresses the social, physical, and medical needs of its constituency. Monthly meetings are sponsored by local chapters found in most major cities. The LPA also holds annual regional and national conventions. The Dwarf Athletic Association of America (DAAA), a member of the U.S. Olympic Committee and U.S. Organization of Disabled Athletes, promotes athletic participation in a wide range of athletic events for short stature individuals at the local, national, and international levels.

ACHONDROPLASIA

The most common type of short-limb disproportionate dwarfism is achondroplasia, with an estimated incidence of 1 in 20,000 to 50,000 live births. The term achondroplasia, implying absent cartilage formation, was first used by Parrot in 1878 to differentiate patients with this condition from rachitic patients with proportionate short stature.[63] Although the word achondroplasia is inaccurate from a histopathologic perspective, its use is universal and accepted by the International Working Group on Constitutional Diseases of Bone.[2]

The genetics of achondroplasia is well established. A single gene is responsible and is transmitted as an autosomal dominant trait. At least 80% of cases are the result of a random new mutation. In sporadic cases, a paternal age older than 36 years is a common factor.[85] Most parents of achondroplastic offspring are of average size and have no family history of dwarfing conditions. The risk of producing a second affected child is almost negligible. However, the achondroplastic patient has a 50% chance of transmitting this gene to each child. Average-sized siblings have no increased risk of producing an achondroplastic child. When both parents are achondroplastic, 50% of their children receive a single mutated gene from one parent, 25% receive a mutated gene from each parent (homozygous), and 25% are unaffected. Homozygous achondroplasia is ordinarily fatal in the first few months of life. The specific gene responsible for achondroplasia has has been mapped to the fourth chromosome (4p16.3), which excludes the locus for type II collagen on chromosome 12.[28]

The primary defect found in achondroplastic dwarfs presumably is abnormal endochondral bone formation. Periosteal and intramembranous ossification is normal. Reports of histologic studies are conflicting, possibly because of differences in biopsy sites and in the ages of the patients. Biopsies of the iliac crest and other regions of appositional growth, such as the fibular head, appear normal histologically. Glycosaminoglycan determinations are normal for iliac crests and fibular growth plates.[42,44,54,65,68,71]

The normal periosteal and appositional bone growth combined with slowed endochondral ossification helps to explain many of the observed clinical and radiographic characteristics of persons with achondroplasia. The iliac crest apophyses (i.e., appositional growth) are almost normal, giving rise to large, square iliac wings. Endochondral growth at the triradiate cartilage is abnormal, resulting in horizontal acetabular roofs. The tubular bones are short and broad, reflecting normal periosteal growth in the presence of abnormal endochondral physeal growth. One explanation given for the discrepancy in length between the fibula and the tibia is the presence of normal appositional growth at the ends of the fibula.[68] The quantitative differences in longitudinal bone growth giving rise to a rhizomelic pattern of shortening cannot be explained histologically.[71]

Clinical Features

Achondroplasia is recognizable at birth as a disproportionate short-limb dwarfing condition. Characteristics include an enlarged neurocranium with frontal bossing, flattening of the nasal bridge, midface hypoplasia (including the maxilla), and relative prominence of the mandible. The trunk length is normal, with flattening of the anteroposterior dimension of the chest. There is flaring of the lower ribs in infancy, with noticeable protuberance of the abdomen. Before walking, an achondroplastic child has a kyphosis centered at the thoracolumbar junction and lordosis in the interscapular thoracic region. This kyphosis, which is related to ligamentous laxity and hypotonia, resolves spontaneously to a large extent after independent ambulation begins. At this stage, an exaggerated lumbar lordosis with forward rotation of the pelvis develops, and the spinal deformity is associated with hip flexion contractures and a prominent abdomen and buttocks.

The extremity involvement is rhizomelic, with the proximal segments more severely involved than the middle or distal segments. The shoulders appear broad because of normal clavicular development (i.e., membranous bone) and well-developed musculature. The bulky muscle mass with excessive skin, adipose tissue, and deep creases contributes to the appearance of short, broad extremities. Typically, there is loss of full extension of the elbow, ranging from 15 to 30 degrees. This lack of extension is not a flexion contracture; it is a result of abnormal development of the joint itself. Posterolateral dislocation of the radial heads may occur, contributing to loss of full extension of the elbow and mild limitation of supination. A "trident" hand is common and is characterized by a persistent space between the long and ring fingers when approximation of the patient's finger is attempted in full extension. Typically, the fingertips of achondroplastic persons reach to the level of the hips, which causes difficulty with hygiene and dressing.

The lower extremities of achondroplastic dwarfs are characterized by rhizomelic shortening, hip flexion contractures, marked ligamentous laxity with external rotation of the extremity, and genu recurvatum before walking age. Congenital hip dysplasia has not been reported. Angular deformities are common after walking begins. There is pronounced bowing of the tibia, frequently resulting in significant genu varum and some degree of ankle varus deformity (Fig. 7-1). A valgus alignment sometimes occurs, but it usually resolves. A rapidly progressive valgus deformity secondary to ligamentous laxity occasionally develops. Most achondroplastic dwarfs have a waddling gait and manifest a circumduction motion of the hips and lower extremities during attempted running.

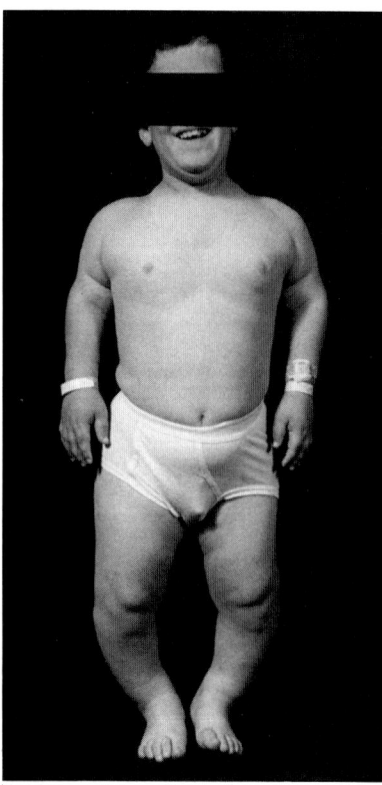

FIGURE 7-1. A 14-year-old achondroplastic dwarf. Typical features include normal trunk height with rhizomelic shortening and genu varum.

Growth and Development

Speech and language development are normal in achondroplastic infants, but motor milestones are frequently delayed. These clinical impressions have been confirmed by the use of standardized cognitive and psychomotor tests.[39] Head control and independent sitting, standing, and ambulation may lag 3 to 6 months behind age-matched, average-sized children.[80] Traditionally, the significant motor delays observed in this group of patients have been related to several causes, including the enlarged neurocranium, arrested hydrocephalus, hypotonia, ligamentous laxity, and the mechanical disadvantage of shortened limbs with a relatively normal-sized trunk. Studies have found an association of the narrowed foramen magnum with abnormalities of somatosensory evoked potentials and lower psychomotor developmental indices.[39] Standard growth curves have been developed for head circumference and for standing and sitting heights of those with achondroplasia.[43,57] Sitting height, a reflection of trunk length, is within normal limits for males and females. Standing height is below the third percentile for both sexes, a reflection of lower extremity shortening. The mean adult standing height for men is 132 cm (52 in), and that for women is 125 cm (49 in).[43]

Radiographic Features

In the neonatal period, radiographs of the skeleton, including the skull, spine, and extremities, reveal characteristic features of achondroplastic dwarfs.[48] A lateral radiograph of the skull demonstrates midface hypoplasia, an enlarged calvaria, frontal prominence, and shortening of the base of the skull, which is formed by endochondral ossification. The size of the foramen magnum is diminished and is measured most accurately by computed tomography (CT).[38,84] There is a distinct narrowing of the interpedicular distances from proximal to distal in the lumbar spine (Fig. 7-2). The sagittal view reveals shortening of the pedicles and vertebral bodies, with significant posterior scalloping (Fig. 7-3). Before walking age, various degrees of thoracolumbar kyphosis exist. Occasionally, this kyphosis is associated with anterior wedging of the 12th thoracic or 1st lumbar vertebral body. After walking age, kyphosis generally improves, and an exaggerated lumbar lordosis develops. The inclination of the sacrum becomes increasingly horizontal. Scoliosis of more than 20 degrees develops in some patients.[3,7,20,85]

The pelvis in persons with achondroplastic dwarfism is typically broad and short, and the ilium has a square appearance. The sacrosciatic notch is short, and the acetabular roof is horizontal (Fig. 7-4). True coxa vara is not present, but because there is

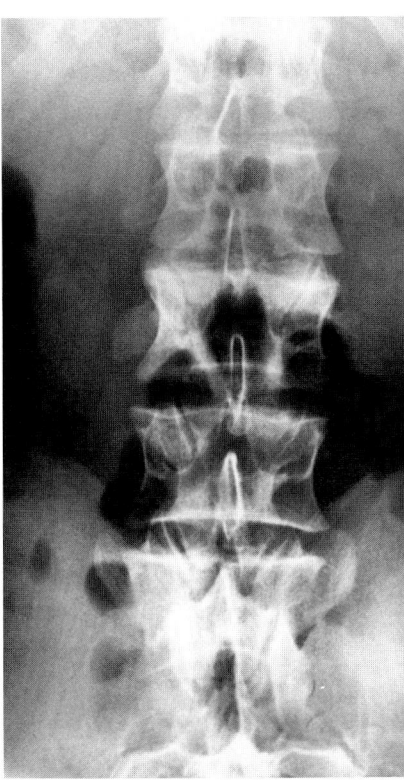

FIGURE 7-2. A 27-year-old achondroplastic dwarf. Notice the progressive interpedicular narrowing of the lumbar spine.

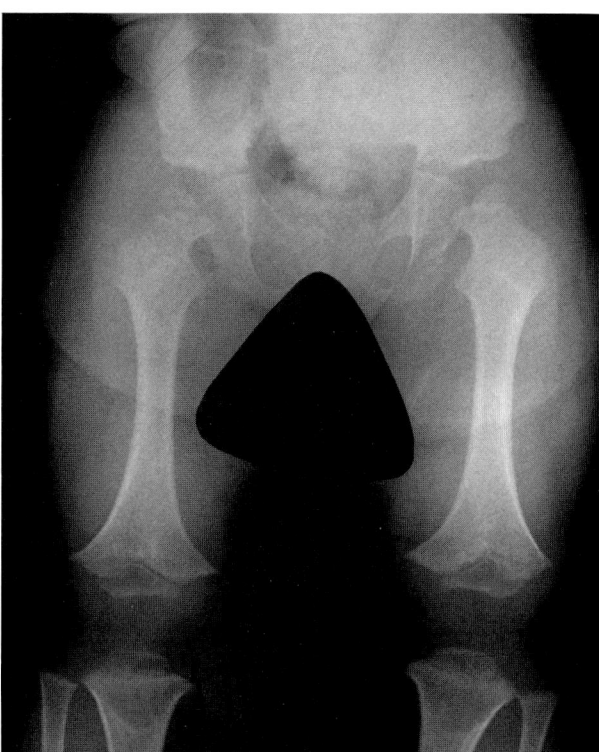

FIGURE 7-4. An 18-month-old achondroplastic dwarf. Typical findings include square iliac crests, horizontal acetabular roofs, small sacrosciatic notches, radiolucent areas in the proximal femur, and an inverted-V–shaped distal femoral physis.

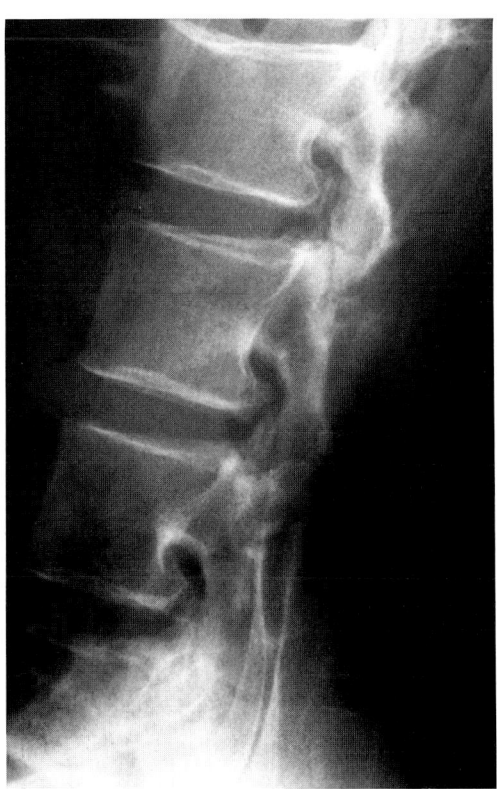

FIGURE 7-3. A 27-year-old achondroplastic dwarf. The radiograph shows marked foraminal stenosis, scalloping of the posterior vertebral bodies, and short, broad pedicles.

normal appositional growth, the greater trochanter is overgrown with respect to the femoral head and short femoral neck. The long bones have metaphyseal flaring and are short and thick. During the first year, the proximal metaphyses of the femur and the humerus have oval areas of radiolucency. Sites of major muscle attachments, such as the deltoid and patellar tendon tuberosity, are especially prominent. The distal femoral physes have an inverted-V configuration in childhood (see Fig. 7-4). Bowing, if present, usually involves the tibia more than the femur. The fibulas typically grow longer than the tibias. The upper extremities are characterized by marked shortening of the humeri, and radial head dislocation frequently occurs. The proximal and middle phalanges of the hand are broader, with greater shortening than the distal phalanges or metacarpals.

Medical Considerations

Weight control is a lifelong problem for achondroplastic dwarfs.[72] Obesity typically begins in early childhood and is common in all age groups. Early nutritional counseling and dietary modification is often required in childhood.[36] Maxillary hypoplasia leads to dental crowding and malocclusion, often requiring orthodontic treatment.

Recurrent otitis media is common in achondroplastic children. Poor drainage of the eustachian tubes results from underdevelopment of the midface and relative hypertrophy of the tonsils and adenoids. Because hearing deficits may result from chronic middle ear infections, early recognition and treatment are required. Research has identified a high incidence of conductive hearing losses and evidence of a primary ossicular chain dysplasia in achondroplasia.[55,67] Speech problems caused by tongue thrust are common but often resolve spontaneously by school age.

Chest wall diameters are narrowed in achondroplasia. As a consequence, pulmonary function, particularly vital capacity, is reduced, averaging 68% for affected females and 72% for affected males compared with normally proportioned individuals.[75,76] Infants and children with achondroplasia are at increased risk for respiratory complications, such as pneumonia, cyanotic spells, or apnea, compared with the general population. These problems have many causes, including upper airway obstruction, a small chest wall, and neurogenic effects from brain stem compression at the level of the foramen magnum.[59,70]

In achondroplastic dwarfs, abnormal development of the base of the skull, which is formed by endochondral ossification, results in a foramen magnum that is smaller than in nonachondroplastic individuals. In average-sized individuals, the most rapid growth of the foramen magnum occurs during the first 18 months of life, with completion of growth by 5 years of age. In persons with achondroplasia, the foramen magnum is smaller at birth and does not show the anticipated dramatic enlargement during infancy and childhood. The foramen magnum of an adult achondroplastic individual approximates the overall dimensions of a nonachondroplastic 2-year-old child. In addition to the growth retardation related to alterations of endochondral ossification, abnormal development and premature fusion of the posterior synchondroses has been identified, affecting the transverse diameter to a greater extent than the sagittal dimension.[37,38]

Narrowing of the foramen magnum may result in a variety of neurologic problems in the first several years of life. Numerous examples of cervicomedullary compression have been reported, with symptoms of respiratory insufficiency, apnea, cyanotic episodes, feeding problems, quadriparesis, and sudden death (Fig. 7-5).[33,34,64,70,86,87] Autopsy studies have found examples of obvious constriction at the foramen magnum level and evidence of gliosis of the brain stem secondary to chronic compression.[34,64] Somatosensory evoked potential (SSEP) abnormalities have been reported for 44% of neurologically intact achondroplastic dwarfs and are probably related to brain stem compression

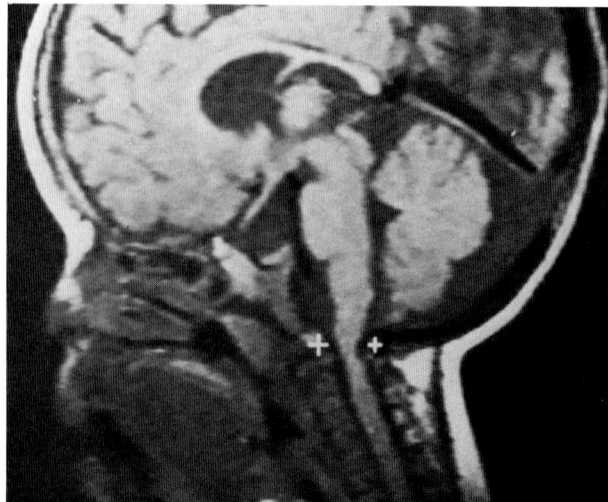

FIGURE 7-5. A 14-year-old achondroplastic dwarf. The magnetic resonance image demonstrates cervicomedullary compression at the foramen magnum.

at the level of the foramen magnum.[39,58] Perhaps the hypotonia observed in the first 2 years of life is a reflection of chronic brain stem compression in some children.[39,87] Given the incidence and potential severity of neurologic symptoms associated with foramen magnum stenosis, a baseline magnetic resonance image (MRI) and SSEP evaluation are strongly recommended in infancy.

Significant improvement of severe neurologic symptoms has been reported for many patients after foramen magnum decompression.[19,22,59,86,87] However, serious complications may follow occipital decompression, and prophylactic surgery is not recommended unless there are signs and symptoms of neurologic compromise due to a narrowed foramen magnum. Cranial enlargement coupled with poor head control places the achondroplastic infant at risk for extension injuries. Parents need to be apprised of their need to cradle the child's head during lifting and other changes of position until satisfactory head control is achieved.

The head circumference is enlarged in achondroplastic dwarfs. Medical imaging techniques, including cerebral angiography, venography, pneumoencephalography, CT, and cisternography, have failed to establish a single cause of neurocranial enlargement. Examples of true megaloencephaly, dilated ventricles without hydrocephalus, and communicating and noncommunicating forms of hydrocephalus have been observed in achondroplastic dwarfs.[23,66,86] For most patients, there is no evidence of a cerebrospinal fluid block in the subarachnoid or ventricular spaces. Several investigators have produced evidence implicating increased intracranial venous pressure in the cause of hydrocephalus, secondary to significant stenosis of the jugular foramen.[66,74,86] The mild ventricular enlargement usually is not associated with signs of increased intracranial pressure. It is thought that this enlargement represents arrested hydrocephalus, and in most patients, shunting is not required. Ventricoperitoneal shunts are indicated for patients with rapidly progressive head enlargement beyond the norms established for achondroplasia or for patients with increased intracranial pressure or neurologic signs and symptoms.

The use of growth hormone in dwarfing conditions is extremely controversial. Although growth hormone is an important regulator of longitudinal growth through promotion of chondrocyte proliferation, there is no evidence suggesting that achondroplastic individuals are growth hormone deficient. Nevertheless, the appeal of pharmacologically stimulating linear growth has led several centers to prospectively evaluate the use of recombinant human growth hormone in achondroplasia. Modest increases in growth velocity have occurred in some patients, particularly those with the lowest growth velocities before treatment. However, the results are preliminary, involving a limited number of skeletally immature patients. Long-term studies of a sufficient number of patients are needed to evaluate the results statistically. It is unknown whether the ultimate height of an achondroplastic patient will be significantly increased with growth hormone therapy or the primary effect will be earlier maturation and the cessation of longitudinal growth.[41,45,60,61] Recombinant growth hormone use should be limited to centers with approved investigational protocols.

The mortality rates for achondroplastic individuals are increased for all age groups. For children younger than 4 years of age, sudden death was the most common cause and brain stem compression was identified in one half. For the 5- to 24-year-old age group, central nervous system and respiratory abnormalities accounted for one half of the mortalities. Cardiovascular problems were the most frequent cause of death for the 25- to 54-year-old age group.[35]

Orthopaedic Implications

Spinal deformities are the most common and potentially disabling problem for the achondroplastic dwarf. The spinal canal is developmentally narrowed, particularly in the lower lumbar segments.[20,46,48,50,52] Stenosis of the spinal canal and intervertebral foramen is secondary to short, thickened pedicles, interpedicular narrowing, thickened laminae, and inferior facets.[31,50,53] Additional factors, such as intervertebral disc herniation, degenerative spondylolysis, excessive lumbar lordosis, or anterior wedging of the vertebral bodies from a thoracolumbar kyphosis, narrow the canal further.

Measurements of the subarachnoid fluid space in achondroplastic adults reveals depths averaging less than 1.5 mm dorsally, ventrally, and laterally.[82]

The symptoms of spinal stenosis include low back pain, leg pain, dysesthesia, paresthesia, paraparesis, incontinence, and neurogenic claudication. Initially, the claudication manifests as vague symptoms of aching or tiredness of the lower extremities induced by walking or standing. These complaints are alleviated by flattening the lordosis through squatting or forward flexion. Frequently, the symptoms slowly progress, with a sensation of numbness or tingling and eventual weakness. Walking tolerance is diminished, necessitating frequent stops to alleviate pain. Symptoms of lower extremity radiculopathy from nerve root compression or cauda equina syndrome occur in more than 50% of achondroplastic dwarfs.[27,46,56] The incidence of low back pain appears to be even higher. The mean age of onset of back or lower extremity symptoms is 26 years, with one third of the patients symptomatic by 15 years of age.[77,78] However, paraplegia resulting from a thoracolumbar stenosis has been reported in a 7-month-old achondroplastic infant.[32] Patients with significant thoracolumbar kyphosis have been found as adults to have a higher incidence and severity of symptomatic spinal stenosis compared with achondroplastic individuals without abnormal kyphosis.[47] These symptoms include sensory deficits, posterior column dysfunction, and lower motor neuron and upper motor neuron signs.

Treatment for neurologic symptoms depends on their duration and severity. The cross-sectional anatomy of the canal can be evaluated noninvasively by CT (Fig. 7-6). Before surgical decompression of the stenotic lumbar spine, MRI is usually indicated to determine whether associated disc herniations exist and

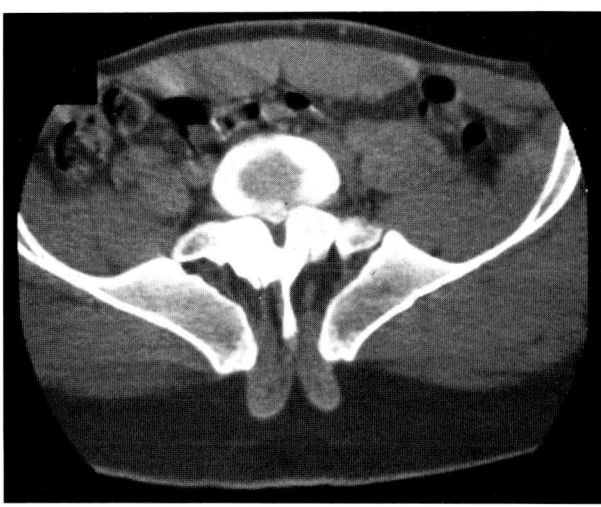

FIGURE 7-6. A 22-year-old achondroplastic dwarf. The computed tomographic scan of L5–S1 demonstrates marked stenosis.

the proximal level of compression. If necessary, myelography is typically accomplished by way of a cisternal puncture and demonstrates pooling of dye between intervening disc spaces in the concave posterior portion of the vertebral bodies.[79] Weight reduction is an important element in surgical and nonsurgical treatment of achondroplastic patients. Attempts to relieve the signs and symptoms of spinal stenosis through reversal of hyperlordosis by pelvic tilt exercises or stretching of hip flexion contractures have had unpredictable results. Bracing the patient in flexion has had some success, but the patient's mobility is compromised, and additional problems are created for accomplishing the tasks of personal hygiene and activities of daily living. Consideration has been given to intertrochanteric extension osteotomy of the femur to reduce lordosis and hip flexion contractures. However, the results of this procedure have not been reported for sufficient numbers of patients with satisfactory long-term follow-up.

Surgical treatment for lumbar spinal stenosis in cauda equina syndrome consists of wide, multilevel laminectomies extending to the pedicles and lateral recesses with foraminotomies. Extradural removal of herniated disc material is performed as necessary. The length of decompression usually extends from the lower thoracic spine to the sacrum to prevent recurrent symptoms. Maintaining the integrity of the facet joints is necessary to prevent postlaminectomy instability. However, the thickened inferior facet usually encroaches on the canal, necessitating undercutting and removal of the medial portion of the inferior facet. Instability rarely results from the wide decompression. However, if instability does occur, anterior fusion may be necessary. A solid posterolateral fusion is difficult to achieve after wide laminectomy because of the diminutive size of the transverse processes.

Achondroplastic patients with symptoms of intermittent claudication or disc herniation are more likely to have symptomatic relief after surgery than patients with chronic persistent signs. Some patients have significant generalized stenosis involving the cervical and thoracic spine as well, precluding an optimal result. The reported results of decompression for lumbar spinal stenosis and cauda equina syndrome have varied.[3,52,56,69] Improvement after surgery has been temporary for many patients, requiring reoperation to widen or lengthen the decompression. The results of less than 100 achondroplastic patients undergoing laminectomy have been reported in the literature, and fewer than one half of these have improved with surgical intervention. However, most had what is considered inadequate decompression by current standards: decompressions that are too short or too narrow (midline). Although some of these patients have developed hypertrophic scarring at the site of the initial decompression, many have developed compression adjacent to the level of surgery. Current recommendations regarding the extent of the initial surgery include decompression three levels cephalad to the myelographic block or proximal extent of compression demonstrated by MRI, distally to the second sacral level, and laterally at least to the facet joints. This often entails decompression of ten segments or more.[69] The results of this more extensive approach have been encouraging, with greater relief of symptoms and fewer recurrences.[77,78]

Unfortunately, progressive neurologic loss has occurred in some patients after surgery, with the development of incontinence or permanent paralysis. The virtual lack of subarachnoid fluid space precludes the traditional techniques of laminectomy using sublaminar rongeurs if dural injury such as tears are to be avoided. High-speed, well-cooled burs are used to thin the lamina to the anterior cortex, followed by careful piecemeal removal of the remaining lamina with thin curets or cervical punches is recommended.[51,82]

Thoracolumbar kyphosis is the most common anatomic deformity of the spine seen in achondroplastic persons. In one large series, thoracolumbar kyphosis was confirmed in 35% of the achondroplastic individuals examined. This deformity occurred in 94% of those younger than 1 year of age, 39% of those between 2 and 5 years, 11% of those between 5 and 10 years, and 35% of those older than than 20 years of age.[47] Some degree of kyphosis is anticipated to occur in almost all children before walking age and is usually recognized when children first begin to sit. Typically, the kyphosis is severe at the thoracolumbar junction, with lordosis of the thoracic spine proximal to the gibbus in the sitting position. The kyphosis may not reduce completely in the prone position. Many factors have been implicated in the cause of the kyphosis, including an enlarged neurocranium, hypotonia, ligamentous laxity, and hip flexion contractures.

In most patients (as many as 90% in one series), spontaneous improvement of this kyphosis usually occurs when independent ambulation begins.[7] My colleagues and I have observed spontaneous improvement of kyphosis measuring more than 80 degrees before walking age in several patients. Other researchers have reported similar findings (Fig. 7-7).[40] However, some degree of kyphosis persists in 15% to 35% of adult achondroplastic dwarfs.[20,46,47,85] Commonly, there is anterior wedging of the apical vertebra at the 12th thoracic or first lumbar level. The gibbus may be extensive, measuring greater than 100 degrees in some patients (Fig. 7-8).[3,81] Patients may be asymptomatic, although more commonly, they have symptoms of spinal stenosis, including low back pain, radiculopathy, claudication, or paraparesis that may develop acutely.

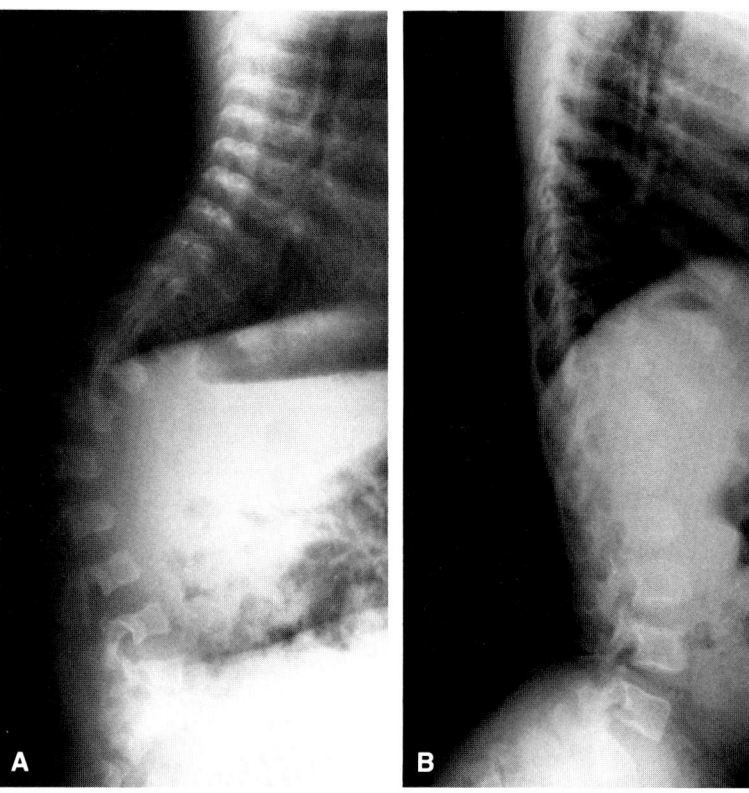

FIGURE 7-7. Example of achondroplasia and improvement of thoracolumbar kyphosis with growth and development. **(A)** Sitting lateral radiograph demonstrates 80-degree kyphosis, vertical orientation of the sacrum, and thoracic lordosis proximally at 9 months of age. **(B)** Kyphosis spontaneously reduced after walking began (3.5 years of age). The sacrum is horizontal, with increased lumbar lordosis.

Although kyphosis correlates strongly with neurologic symptoms, the magnitude of the neurologic involvement is not necessarily related to the size of the deformity.[46,47,51]

Treatment for kyphosis generally consists of observation of the child who has not begun to walk, because spontaneous resolution frequently occurs. If wedging of the apical vertebra persists after independent ambulation begins, the use of an extension-type thoracolumbosacral orthosis may be considered.[73] If the kyphosis fails to reduce, combined anterior and posterior fusions should be recommended for many patients to prevent further progression and neurologic compromise. Candidates for surgery include patients with persistent wedging of the apical kyphotic vertebra and those with a thoracolumbar kyphosis measuring greater than 30 degrees at 5 years of age.[81] If the kyphosis results in a neurologic deficit such as paraplegia, laminectomy alone is not indicated, because it can further destabilize the spine. Treatment should consist of anterior cord decompression with strut grafting and posterior fusion. Postoperatively, the patient is immobilized in a hyperextension cast.

Posterior instrumentation generally is not recommended because the canal size is already narrowed. Any instrumentation placed in the canal, such as hooks or sublaminar wires, is contraindicated because of the marked stenosis and lack of subarachnoid fluid space.[81,82] Studies have revealed a greater than 50% incidence of intraoperative changes in the SSEP during instrumentation, even with the use of spinous process wiring techniques that do not encroach on the canal.[81] Neurologic improvement varies after decompression and fusion.

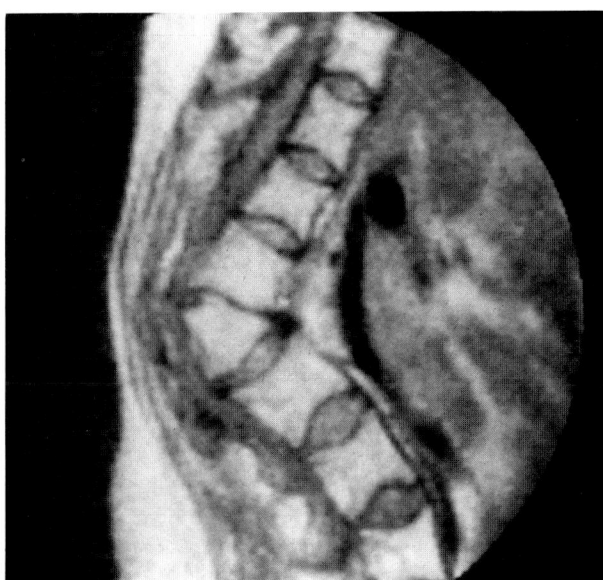

FIGURE 7-8. A 40-year-old achondroplastic dwarf. The magnetic resonance image demonstrates severe kyphosis with apical wedging in a patient with progressive paralysis.

The incidence of kyphoscoliosis may be as high as 33% to 50% in adult achondroplastic dwarfs.[20,46] However, the curve magnitude is generally mild, measuring less than 30 degrees at maturity. Primary treatment for scoliosis is rarely necessary.

Lower extremity problems are the other major concern for the orthopaedist involved in the care of achondroplastic dwarfs. In general, hip dysplasia and coxa vara do not occur in achondroplastic dwarfs, although mild overgrowth of the greater trochanter does.[7,16,20,48] The epiphyseal cartilage is not significantly involved. Femoral head deformity is uncommon, and hip joint congruity is well maintained. Premature osteoarthritis is not a typical feature of achondroplasia, and if hip pain is present, it probably is caused by a pathologic condition of the lumbar spine.

Genu varum occurs frequently, affecting at least half of all achondroplastic dwarfs.[7,20] The more rapid growth of the fibula compared with that of the tibia has been implicated as the cause of tibia vara.[68] However, in one study, no correlation between the magnitude of the tibial-fibular discrepancy and the degree of genu varum could be determined.[57] Some patients develop a valgus deformity of the knee despite the elongated fibula. Other factors implicated include ligamentous laxity and obesity. Osteoarthritis of the knee is observed rarely in adults, despite the prevalence of severe genu varum deformities. This may reflect the functional limitations of spinal stenosis, which affects many adult achondroplasts. In achondroplastic dwarfs, prophylactic realignment of the lower extremities to prevent osteoarthritis is not warranted, although many patients or their parents seek surgical correction for cosmetic reasons. However, in many patients, symptoms develop requiring treatment that are related to a progressive varus deformity, including progressive ligamentous laxity of the knee and pain in the lower extremities. Frequently, gaping of the lateral compartment or lateral translation of the tibia on the femur can be seen during stance phase. Bracing has not been effective in controlling genu varum and has been implicated in the development of peroneal nerve palsies.[20]

Two alternatives exist for surgical correction of genu varum. Standard treatment consists of proximal tibiofibular osteotomies for the extremities requiring immediate correction of symptomatic or rapidly progressing deformities. The osteotomies may be performed through small incisions without internal fixation, with long-leg cast immobilization for 6 weeks. When evaluating postoperative radiographs, the surgeon must achieve realignment of the hip-knee-ankle mechanical axis at the osteotomy site rather than through stressing the ligaments of the knee. The other surgical alternative for selected patients is proximal and distal fibular epiphyseodesis. Correction is achieved with the remaining growth of the tibia over time. Indications include symptoms that do not require immediate correction in a patient between the ages of 7 and 10 years. In my opinion, this procedure is rarely indicated as an isolated procedure. Proximal fibular epiphyseodesis may be warranted in conjunction with proximal tibiofibular osteotomy in a younger child with severe genu varum to prevent recurrent deformity.

Limb lengthening of the upper and lower extremities for achondroplastic individuals is being promoted, primarily in Europe. With the newer techniques of distraction and external fixation, gains in the length of the lower extremities in excess of 30 cm are being achieved over the femoral and tibial segments, followed by upper extremity (humeral) lengthenings. A variety of techniques have been promoted, including gradual distraction of the osteotomy callous (i.e., callotasis) or epiphyseal plates (i.e., chondrodiatasis) using monolateral frames or Ilizarov ring fixators for lengthening. Different sequences for the lower extremity lengthenings have been proposed, including staged ipsilateral femorotibial lengthenings, staged bilateral femoral and tibial lengthenings, and staged femoral–contralateral tibial lengthenings. The advantages and disadvantages of each of these sequences are promulgated by their advocates.

These extensive lengthenings in achondroplastic patients have been accomplished with fewer complications than encountered for patients with congenital limb deficiencies such as congenital short femur or fibular hemimelia. Nevertheless, multiple problems persist during these six-segment lengthenings, with the potential for major complications. Neurologic injury, most commonly footdrop, has been reported in as many as 35% of short stature patients undergoing extended limb lengthening procedures.[24] Pain, vascular compromise, soft tissue contractures, loss of motion, knee subluxation, infection, angular deformity, premature or delayed consolidation, psychologic changes, and death have been reported. Controversy still exists about the advisability of limb lengthening in dwarfs because of the prolonged duration of treatment required, the magnitude and multitude of potential complications, and the paucity of information about the long-term effects of this procedure on adjacent articulations. Social, psychologic, physical, functional, and economic factors must be carefully considered.[18,21,24–26,29,30,49,62,83] If lengthenings are to be performed, simultaneous correction of any existing angular deformities such as genu varum also should be performed. Villarrubias has developed a method by which the lumbar hyperlordosis is simultaneously corrected during femoral lengthening.[83] It is unknown whether this reduction of the lumbar hyperlordosis will decrease the incidence of spinal stenosis for this group of patients.

As advocacy groups for their constituencies, the LPA and DAAA are generally opposed to these procedures as a means solely to increase an individual's stature. Philosophically, these organizations emphasize the positive aspects of their constituents' abilities and lives rather than viewing the issue of short stature as a disability. Experienced and sensitive health care providers should avoid the term "normal," substituting the term "average" when addressing height issues with patients with dwarfing conditions or their families.

HYPOCHONDROPLASIA

Hypochondroplasia is a separate osteochondrodysplasia characterized by mild short-limb dwarfism. It was first reported in the English literature by Beals in 1969.[88] Generally, the diagnosis is not made before the child is 2 years of age. Patients with severe involvement may share many features with those with achondroplasia. Less affected patients may attain an adult height up to 152 cm (60 in) and have an almost normal clinical appearance.[85,88,90,93]

Transmitted as an autosomal dominant trait, hypochondroplasia does not represent a milder expression of the same gene mutation responsible for achondroplasia; these are genetically distinct entities.[72,85] Most new cases of hypochondroplasia represent sporadic mutations, and unlike achondroplasia, no significant paternal age has been reported.

The treatment of short stature with recombinant human growth hormone in children with hypochondroplasia has produced various results. In one series of 31 children treated for as long as 3 years, increases in growth velocity were observed during the first year of treatment, diminishing over the next 2 years. Considerable variability in clinical response occurred in this series.[89] Other investigators have identified a strong linkage of the insulin-like growth factor 1 gene (IGF1) locus at chromosome 12q23 to a subgroup of patients with hypochondroplasia. Twenty children with clinically and radiographically similar forms of hypochondroplasia were treated with recombinant human growth hormone. One group with proportionate increases in lower extremity and spinal growth were heterozygous for the IGF1 gene, but the other group, with homozygous involvement at this locus, demonstrated an accentuation of the body disproportion with growth hormone therapy.[92] The implications of these studies should be emphasized. These phenotypically similar subgroups of hypochondroplasia appear to have different genetic defects, and the response to any attempts at growth enhancement medically may be different. This is likely to be true for many of the osteochondrodysplasias, especially those with apparently wide clinical heterogeneity. Moreover, the long-term outcomes for recombinant human growth hormone therapy are unknown. The decreased growth velocities with time of these patients may indicate that the primary effect of growth hormone therapy is an acceleration of skeletal maturation and that significant increases in stature at the end of growth may not occur. If increases in overall height are obtained at the expense of greater body disproportions, the outcome may not be favorable.

Clinical Features

The diminished height of persons with hypochondroplasia results primarily from a shortening of the lower limb segments; measurement of the trunk height is almost normal. The limb shortening of the upper and lower extremities is symmetric, not exhibiting the marked rhizomelic pattern of achondroplasia. Except for mild frontal bossing, the facial appearance is normal, lacking the midface hypoplasia and nasal bridge depression seen in those with achondroplasia. Head circumference generally is reported to be normal, although investigators in one study documented the presence of macrocephaly at birth in 66% of patients in their series.[88,91,93] Patients with hypochondroplasia have less extensive lumbar lordosis and abdominal protuberance than patients with achondroplasia. Trident hand defects, scoliosis, and thoracolumbar kyphosis are also infrequently seen in hypochondroplasia patients, although mild joint laxity persists. Significant genu varum occurs in fewer than 10% of these patients.[85]

One series compared the incidence of symptomatic spinal stenosis in achondroplasia with that found in hypochondroplasia. Eighty-nine percent of achondroplastic patients were symptomatic compared with 33% of hypochondroplastic patients. The symptoms were milder in hypochondroplasia patients, and no neurologic deficits were observed. Approximately 10% of these patients may have mental retardation of mild degree.

Radiographic Features

Radiographic findings vary from mild involvement to an appearance similar to achondroplasia in the more severely affected hypochondroplasia patient. Specific primary and secondary criteria have been proposed for the radiographic diagnosis of hypochondroplasia. The primary criteria include narrowed lumbar inter-

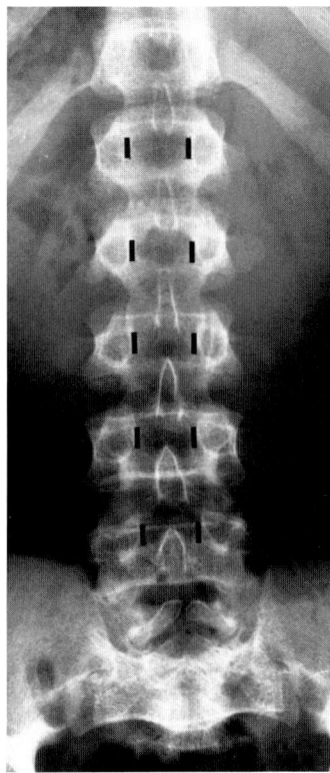

FIGURE 7-9. A 17-year-old patient with hypochondroplasia has mild interpedicular narrowing of the lumbar spine.

pedicular distances (Fig. 7-9); short, square iliac crests with short, broad femoral necks; mild metaphyseal flaring and shortening of the long tubular bones; and mild brachydactyly. Shortening of the lumbar pedicles, concavity of the posterior vertebral bodies, elongation of the distal fibula, shortening of the distal ulna, and elongation of the ulnar styloid were considered secondary criteria.[91]

Orthopaedic Implications

The skeletal abnormalities seen in hypochondroplasia patients usually are mild and rarely require surgical intervention. If present, genu varum is usually mild and ordinarily does not require realignment osteotomy. Symptoms of spinal stenosis may be present but generally are less severe than those experienced by achondroplastic patients. Unless significant neurologic deficits affect the patient, treatment should be conservative.

METATROPIC DYSPLASIA

Metatropic dysplasia is a rare skeletal dysplasia characterized by a change in body proportions with growth. Because of the short limbs and relatively long trunk during infancy, this condition often has been confused with achondroplasia. With growth, a severe kyphoscoliosis typically develops, resulting in a marked shortening of the trunk and an apparent reversal in body proportions. This short-trunk dwarfism may resemble Morquio disease clinically. In 1966, Maroteaux and associates differentiated this dysplasia from other disorders and suggested the name "metatropic," from the Greek word "metatropos," meaning changing patterns.[95,96]

Metatropic dysplasia is be transmitted as an autosomal dominant trait.[94]

Clinical Features

In addition to the change of body proportions from short-limb to short-trunk dwarfism with growth, many patients with metatropic dysplasia have a small tail-like appendage overlying the lower sacrum. The head and face of these patients have a normal appearance, which differentiates them from patients with achondroplasia. The limbs are significantly short, with bulbous enlargement of the joints and restricted motion. Severe angular deformities ordinarily do not occur. With time, the kyphoscoliosis that is usually present at birth progresses, causing a noticeable deformity of the trunk. Many children die of respiratory failure in infancy. Patients who survive to adulthood have significant cardiorespiratory difficulties secondary to their spinal deformities. Typical adult height varies between 110 and 120 cm (43–47 in).[97]

Radiographic Features

Spinal involvement in infants with metatropic dysplasia is characterized by marked platyspondyly. There is apparent widening of the disc spaces, because ossification of the vertebral bodies is delayed (Fig. 7-10). As ossification proceeds during growth, the platyspondyly becomes less marked. Kyphoscoliosis, typically present early in life, progresses, leading to further wedging of the vertebrae. Odontoid hypoplasia with atlantoaxial instability has been reported. In one series of 12 patients, odontoid hypoplasia affected all patients, and atlantoaxial instability demonstrated by lateral flexion-extension radiographs was detected in 6 (50%).[98] The long bones have marked flaring of the metaphyseal regions and significant shortening, giving them a dumbbell shape (Fig. 7-11). The fibulas typically are longer than the tibias, and mild genu varum may result. Frequently, the femoral necks are irregularly ossified. The epiphyses also have delayed ossification, and joint incongruity may result; premature osteoarthritis of major weight-bearing joints is a common sequela. The iliac crests are broad and square, with deep, horizontal acetabular roofs and beaking of the lateral margins. Protrusio acetabuli may be observed.

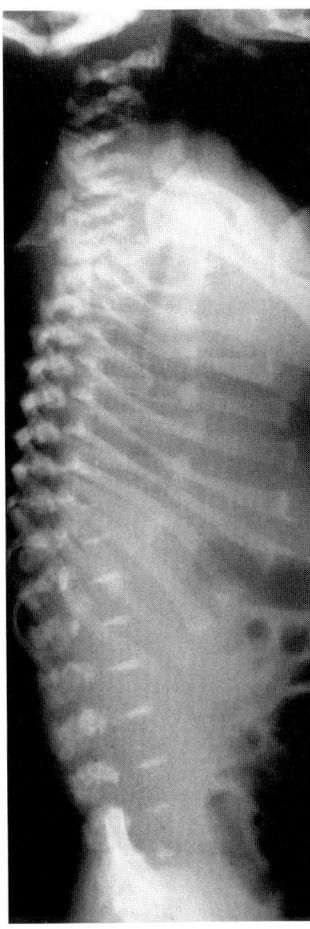

FIGURE 7-10. Newborn with metatropic dysplasia. Notice the marked platyspondyly with delayed ossification of the vertebral bodies. The metaphyses of the ribs are flared. (Courtesy of Judy Hall, M.D., Vancouver, British Columbia.)

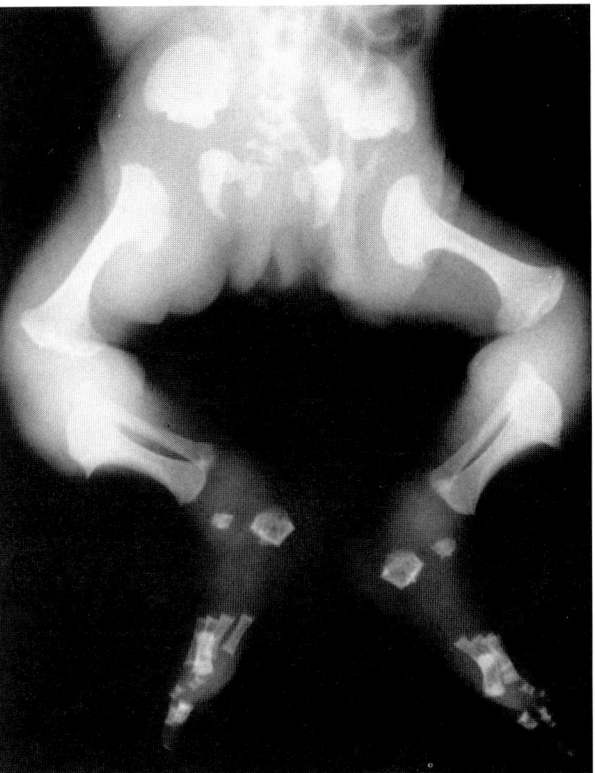

FIGURE 7-11. Newborn with metatrophic dysplasia. There is marked flaring of the metaphyses and significant shortening leading to a dumbell-shaped appearance. The iliac crests are broad and square, with deep acetabular roofs.

Medical Considerations

Many infants have severe respiratory difficulties that are frequently life threatening. One significant component is the small thorax, which may be further compromised by the early development of spinal deformities. Restrictive and obstructive changes have been identified during pulmonary function testing. However, respiratory compromise may also have a neurologic basis. A high incidence of C1–C2 abnormalities occur in metatropic dysplasia, which may lead to myelopathic changes. Ventriculomegaly has also been identified in 25% of patients evaluated by CT scans in one series. Symptomatic hydrocephalus occurred in one patient and required shunting.[98]

Orthopaedic Implications

Stability of the upper cervical spine in patients with metatropic dysplasia should be evaluated periodically with lateral flexion-extension radiographs. In the growing child, I recommend repeating these films every 3 or 4 years unless clinical symptoms or signs warrant otherwise. Traditionally, an atlantodens interval greater than 5 mm indicates instability, although many of these patients are asymptomatic. For the apparently asymptomatic patient with radiographic evidence of instability, I recommend obtaining a flexion-extension MRI to evaluate for cord compression. An atlantoaxial instability greater than 5 mm may require posterior surgical stabilization if there are neurologic signs and symptoms or evidence of cord compression demonstrated by MRI. I recommend prophylactic fusion for an atlantoaxial instability of 8 mm or more, even if the patient is asymptomatic. Several patients with dwarfing conditions and chronic instability of this magnitude declined surgical stabilization and have subsequently become quadriplegic after falls or motor vehicle accidents. Fusion to the occiput may be necessary if congenital anomalies or a large synchondrosis involve the posterior ring of the body of the first cervical vertebra.

Scoliosis or kyphosis may progress rapidly during the first 5 years of life. These curves are typically rigid and, with progression, have been associated with cardiopulmonary failure. Quadriplegia has been associated with severe kyphosis. For curves smaller than 40 degrees, brace treatment should be instituted. However, if progression occurs despite bracing, early surgical intervention must be considered. Preoperative pulmonary function studies also should be considered. Fusion in situ with external mobilization is generally preferable to spinal instrumentation for these rigid kyphoscoliotic curves. Halo traction has been found to be a safe and effective means of obtaining and maintaining curve correction.[3]

CHONDROECTODERMAL DYSPLASIA

Chondroectodermal dysplasia, also known as Ellis–van Creveld syndrome, was first described by the two named authors in 1940.[99] This rare disorder is characterized by short-limb disproportionate dwarfism, polydactyly, dysplasia of fingernails and toenails, dental deficiencies, and congenital heart disease. Transmitted as an autosomal recessive trait, chondroectodermal dysplasia is most commonly seen among the Amish of Lancaster County, Pennsylvania. The incidence in this group is reported to be at least 5 per 1000 births. Thirteen percent of the Amish of Lancaster County are estimated to be heterozygous carriers of the gene responsible for chondroectodermal dysplasia.[102]

Clinical Features

One third of infants with chondroectodermal dysplasia are stillborn or die of cardiorespiratory causes in the first 2 weeks of life.[102] Congenital heart disease, including a single atrium or atrial septal defects, is common. Malformations involving the thoracic cage or cartilage of the bronchial tree have been implicated in other deaths. Genital anomalies include epispadias, hypospadias, and undescended testes.

These short-limb disproportionate dwarfs are characterized by acromesomelia, with the forearms, hands, legs, and feet involved to a greater extent than the proximal limb segments.[100] Postaxial polydactyly of the hands is universal, occasionally involving the feet as well. Syndactyly of digits also may occur. The middle and distal phalanges are disproportionately short compared with the proximal phalanges. This discrepancy may lead to difficulties with full hand closure. The nails of the fingers and toes are dysplastic.[105]

Characteristically, a valgus alignment of the knees frequently progresses, producing a marked deformity (Fig. 7-12). In severe cases, the patient appears to have significant knee flexion contractures. However, in most instances, this is an illusion. On careful examination, it is apparent that the patient walks with the femur and tibia externally rotated. The plane of the knee may be externally rotated as much as 45 degrees in conjunction with the marked valgus alignment. The medial collateral ligaments are frequently lax, and the

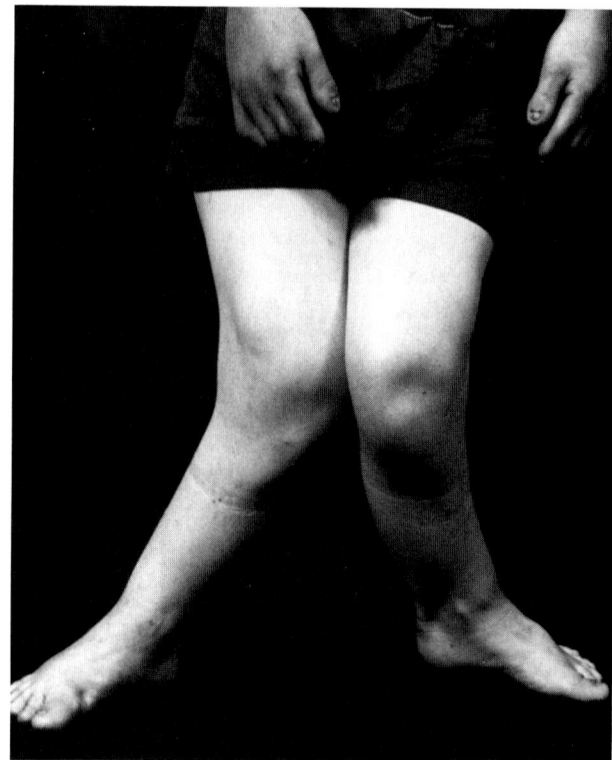

FIGURE 7-12. A 12-year-old patient with chondroectodermal dysplasia has a severe genu valgum deformity with superolateral patellar dislocation. The knees are externally rotated. Notice the dysplastic fingernails.

patella is dislocated superolaterally. Spinal deformities and dislocated hips have rarely been reported. Premature eruption of teeth may occur at birth; oligodontia and other dental abnormalities are common. The upper lip is short, often with a pseudocleft of the midline. Multiple frenula are also typical.

Radiographic Features

Cone epiphyses are usually present in the middle phalanges of patients with chondroectodermal dysplasia. Typically, the capitate and hamate bones are fused (Fig. 7-13). The bones of the forearm are disproportionately short, with hypoplasia of the proximal radius and distal ulna. The radial head may be dislocated.

The pelvis has a characteristic configuration, including small iliac crests and sciatic notches, with a peculiar, distally directed spike of bone originating from the inner pelvis at the triradiate cartilage. The hip joints are congruous. However, the femoral necks are generally expanded and in valgus position. There is growth failure of the lateral portion of the proximal tibial epiphysis. The epiphyseal disturbance of the proximal tibia leads to a valgus deformity of the knee. In severe cases of chondroectodermal dysplasia, there is relative overgrowth of the medial femoral condyles, and the patella is dislocated. An exostosis is commonly

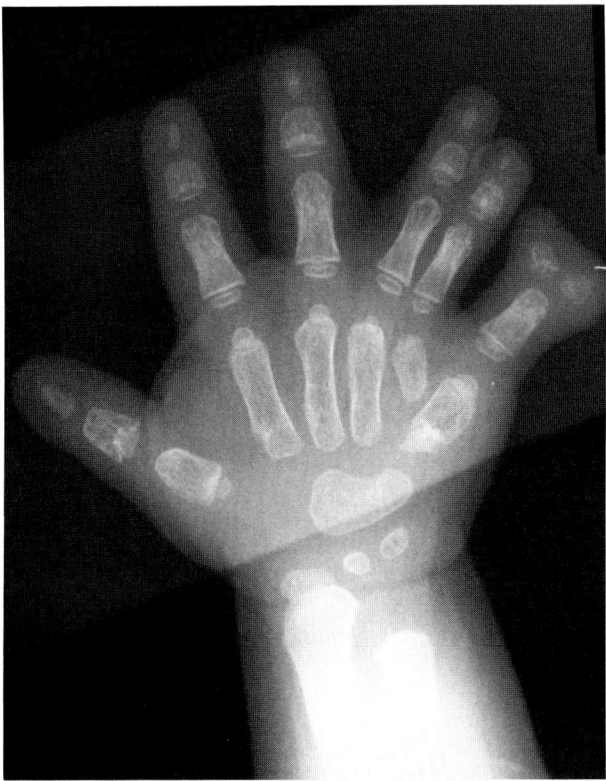

FIGURE 7-13. A 6-month-old patient with chondroectodermal dysplasia. Notice the postaxial polydactyly with syndactyly, disproportionate shortening of middle and distal phalanges, cone epiphyses of the middle phalanges, and fusion of the capitate and hamate bones.

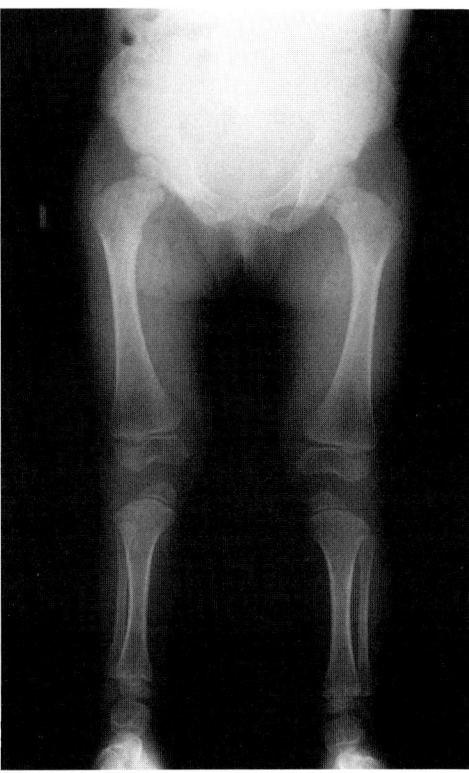

FIGURE 7-14. A 6-month-old patient with chondroectodermal dysplasia. There is mesomelic shortening with a growth disturbance of the lateral tibial epiphysis and early genu valgum deformity. The fibulas are disproportionately short.

observed that arises from the proximal medial tibial metaphysis. The fibulas are disproportionately short compared with the tibias (Fig. 7-14). The spine is generally normal.

Orthopaedic Implications

Excision of the postaxial digits and release of syndactyls are indicated for most patients with chondroectodermal dysplasia, if their cardiac status is stable. Generally, no additional treatment is required for the upper extremities. Progressive genu valgum deformities usually require surgical intervention. Brace treatment has not been effective in preventing progression. Realignment osteotomy should be considered for valgus deformities of more than 15 to 20 degrees on standing lower extremity radiographs. A valgus deformity of 45 degrees may exist in severe cases.

Careful preoperative planning must consider all components of the deformity, which may include an increased femoral neck-shaft angle, distal medial femoral condylar overgrowth, lateral tibial epiphyseal depression, external rotation of the knee and ankle, and lateral patellar dislocation. For a successful outcome, there should be restoration of a normal mechanical axis through the hip, knee, and ankle. At the completion of treatment, the joint surfaces of the knee and ankle should be perpendicular to the mechanical axis and any malrotation corrected. This may require simultaneous multilevel osteotomies with angular, rotatory, and translatory corrections.[103,104] For instance, realignment may include a varus rotation osteotomy of the hip to normalize the valgus neck-shaft angle and to rotate the distal femur internally. Internal rotation up to 45 degrees may be required to correct the externally rotated knee axis. A varus supracondylar osteotomy may be necessary if there is excessive medial femoral condylar overgrowth contributing to the genu valgum deformity. A varus–internal rotation osteotomy of the proximal tibia usually is required to correct the typical valgus–external rotation deformity arising from the marked depression of the lateral tibial epiphysis. Internal or external fixators may be used, depending on the functional needs of the patient and the preference of the surgeon. For these complex deformities, the use of ring fixators with translational hinges allows three-dimensional correction of deformities with simultaneous angulation, translation, rotation performed acutely in the operating room or gradually during the postoperative period. However, these multilevel, multiplanar deformities necessitate complex frames if this method is to be used and should only be used by the experienced surgeon.

For less severe cases, satisfactory realignment of the lower extremity may be accomplished by a single proximal tibiofibular osteotomy. One useful method available is an oblique osteotomy of the proximal tibia. Beginning below the tibial tubercle, an oblique metaphyseal osteotomy is completed, directed posterosuperiorly. With medial rotation of the distal fragment, simultaneous correction of the external rotation and valgus is accomplished.[101,106]

In patients with chondroectodermal dysplasia, valgus deformity may recur after proximal tibiofibular osteotomy because of the continued growth disturbance of the lateral proximal tibial epiphysis. This recurrence is a distinct possibility in the young patient in whom osteotomies are required early for rapidly progressive deformities; continued follow-up until skeletal maturity is required for these patients. Alternatively, proximal medial tibial epiphyseodesis may be considered at the time of tibial osteotomy to prevent a recurrent valgus deformity.

DIASTROPHIC DYSPLASIA

Diastrophic dysplasia is a rare type of skeletal dysplasia characterized by extreme short-limb dwarfism with specific hand, foot, and ear abnormalities. Typically, severe spinal deformities develop, and significant flexion contractures are present. In 1960, Lamy and Maroteaux differentiated this disorder from other dwarfing conditions and suggested the name diastrophic dwarfism, based on the geologic term, meaning to twist.[117] The preferred term is diastrophic dysplasia.[2] Diastrophic dysplasia is transmitted as an autosomal recessive trait; parents of a child with this condition have a 25% chance of conceiving another similarly affected child. Multipoint linkage analysis has determined the genetic locus for diastrophic dysplasia to the distal long arm of chromosome 5 (5q31-q34).[109] Prenatal diagnosis has been made by ultrasound.[108]

Histologic, histochemical, and ultrastructural studies of cartilage in children with diastrophic dysplasia have revealed decreased numbers of atypical chondrocytes with evidence of degeneration, fibrotic foci and abnormally large collagen fibrils in the intercellular matrix. Whether a specific defect of type II collagen exists in this disorder is controversial.[15,119,124]

Clinical Features

Persons with diastrophic dysplasia are characterized by extreme short stature with micromelia; the mean height for diastrophic adults is 118 cm (46 in; Fig. 7-15).[112] There is usually no adolescent growth spurt at the onset of puberty. Some patients die in infancy of respiratory failure, but most have a normal life span unless there are cardiopulmonary sequelae from severe scoliosis or quadriplegia secondary to cervical kyphosis. Diastrophic dysplasia is recognizable at birth. The head is normocephalic, and the facial appearance is characteristic, with a narrow nasal bridge, broadened midnose, and flared nostrils. There is a

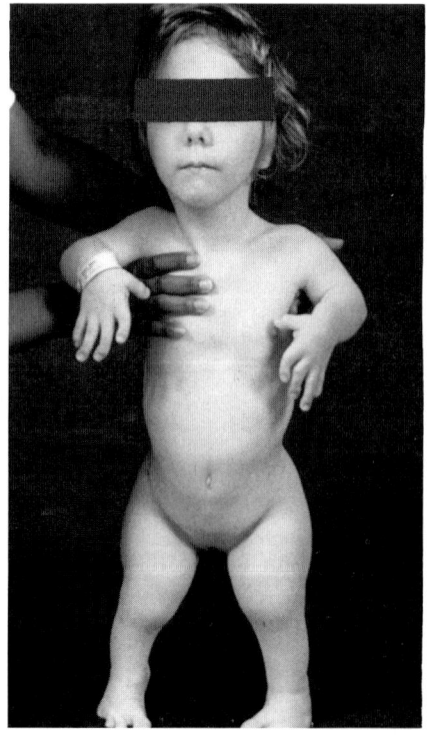
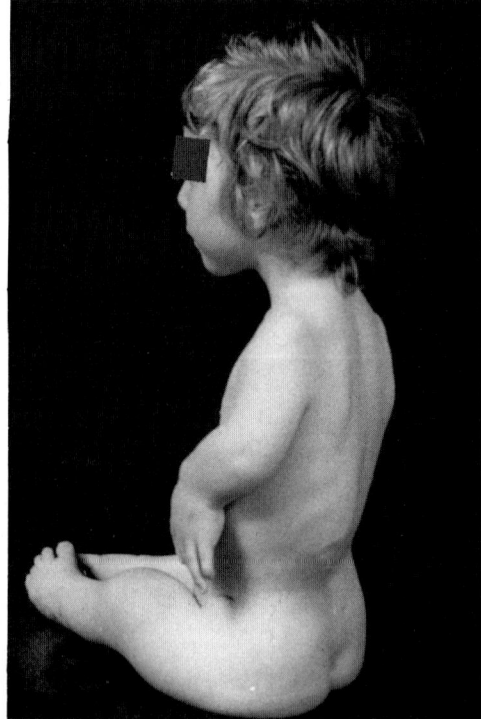

FIGURE 7-15. A 7-year-old patient with diastrophic dysplasia. Typical features include a normal head, micromelia, hitchhiker thumb, flexion contractures, kyphoscoliosis, and clubfeet.

circumoral fullness with a broad mouth. The face is long and the jaw square. Cleft palate is reported in 59% of affected persons. A peculiar ear deformity develops in more than 80% of patients. Swelling of the pinnae begins within the first 6 weeks of life but is not present at birth. Typically, this swelling appears by 3 weeks of age and has an acute inflammatory appearance for several weeks. The pinnae become hard and thickened, and the cartilage usually deforms and calcifies, giving rise to the "cauliflower ear." Hearing impairment secondary to stenosis of the external auditory canal has affected some persons.[126]

Specific abnormalities of the hands and feet are almost universal in persons with diastrophic dysplasia. Symphalangism of the proximal interphalangeal joints of the fingers and the "hitchhiker thumb" are characteristic. The thumbs are abducted and hypermobile, with a disproportionately shortened first metacarpal. The hands are broad and short and frequently are ulnarly deviated. Rigid bilateral equinovarus deformities of the feet are typical and are extremely resistant to cast treatment. The extremities are shortened, and a rhizomelic pattern exits. The functional length of the upper and lower limbs is further compromised by severe flexion contractures of the elbows, hips, and knees. An increased fixed lumbar lordosis develops secondary to the lower extremity contractures. Marked limitation of motion occurs in major joints. Spinal deformities are often severe, and progressive thoracic kyphoscoliosis or cervical kyphosis frequently occurs. Primary cardiac and renal abnormalities are not typical of this disorder. These patients have normal intelligence and a characteristic voice that is soft and hoarse.

Another group has been designated as having a diastrophic variant. These persons lack certain of the characteristic features or have less severe involvement than those with classic diastrophic dysplasia. Several clinical and radiographic studies comparing these two groups have been reported. A variability in the phenotypic expression was found to occur even among siblings of persons with diastrophic dysplasia. Histologic differences have not been identified in the iliac crest growth plate biopsies.[12] These studies suggest that the diastrophic variant disorder does not represent a distinct skeletal dysplasia but represents a milder phenotypic form of diastrophic dysplasia.[113,116]

Radiographic Features

The skull in persons affected with diastrophic dysplasia is normal in size and configuration, although intracranial calcifications occasionally are evident.[111,126] These calcifications should be differentiated from the radiodensities visible on the lateral skull radiographs from superimposition of the calcified pinnae of ears.

However, calcification of the pinnae is not limited to those with diastrophic dysplasia but is observed in several systemic diseases such as diabetes mellitus, ochronosis, acromegaly, and Addison's disease.[118] The thoracic cage is small, with relatively normal clavicles. The ribs are short, and premature ossification of the costal cartilages occurs.

Generally, the vertebral bodies in those with diastrophic dysplasia show minimal irregularities before the development of spinal deformities. With progressive kyphoscoliosis, wedging of the vertebrae may be seen. The congenital segmentation abnormalities reported in several series are associated with progressive spinal deformity.[125,126] Kyphosis, scoliosis, or kyphoscoliosis of the thoracic or thoracolumbar spine occurs in more than 80% of patients and frequently develops into a severe progressive structural curve.[121,125] There is an exaggerated lumbar lordosis with horizontal inclination of the sacrum and frequently a posterior wedging of the fifth lumbar vertebral body. The increased lumbar lordosis appears to develop secondary to severe flexion contractures of the hips and knees. The interpedicular distance often narrows distally at the fourth or fifth lumbar vertebral level.[107] However, the laminae and facets are not thickened, and there is rarely significant bulging of the anulus fibrosus posteriorly into the canal. Symptoms of spinal stenosis usually do not occur in diastrophic dysplasia.

Cervical kyphosis is a common finding in persons with diastrophic dysplasia (Fig. 7-16). The apical vertebra at the third, fourth, or fifth cervical vertebra often appears hypoplastic and wedged. With the development of increasing cervical kyphosis, the odontoid process lies parallel with the occipital condyles at the base of the skull. However, despite the altered relation between the occiput and the first and second cervical vertebrae, atlantoaxial instability has only been reported in one individual.[122] Spina bifida occulta typically occurs over various levels of the middle to lower cervical spine and also has been reported in the lumbar spine.[107,109]

The long bones are short and broad, with marked flaring of the metaphyses. A rhizomelic pattern of shortening is present in upper and lower extremities. The epiphyseal centers of ossification for all major joints are delayed in appearing. After ossification occurs, epiphyseal deformity is obvious, with flattening and irregularity. The metaphyseal-epiphyseal regions appear expanded compared with the length of the diaphyses, giving rise to a bulbous appearance of the joint. The ulna usually is shorter, with resultant ulnar deviation of the hands. In the lower extremities, a valgus deformity of the knee develops and is often associated with a subluxated or dislocated patella. Significant valgus angulation of the ankle does not occur despite a shortened fibula.

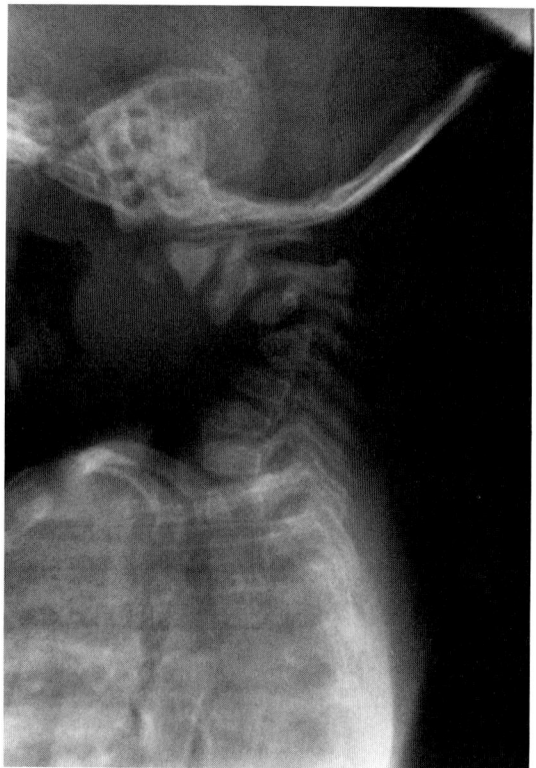

FIGURE 7-16. A 10-month-old patient with diastrophic dysplasia, as seen on flexion lateral cervical spine radiograph. There is severe kyphosis with instability at C2–C3 and C3–C4. The apical vertebrae are hypoplastic and wedged. Notice the horizontal orientation of the odontoid in flexion.

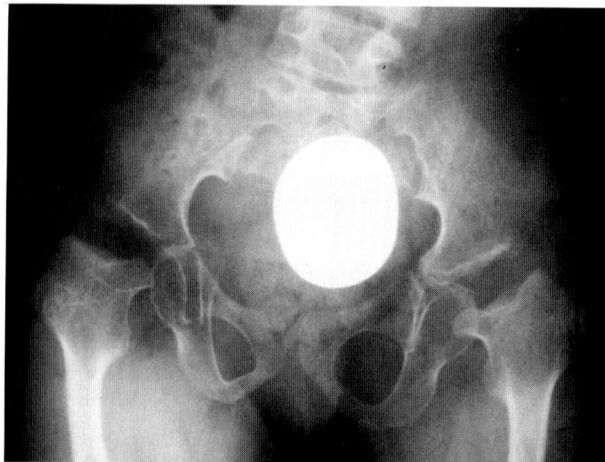

FIGURE 7-17. A 3-year-old patient with diastrophic dysplasia. Notice the bilateral hip deformities with a central saucer-shaped defect of ossification and subluxation.

All tubular bones of the hands and feet of those with diastrophic dysplasia are short and broad, with greater involvement of the metacarpals. The thumb metacarpophalangeal joint is typically subluxated or dislocated, giving rise to the "hitchhiker" deformity. The carpal and tarsal centers of ossification for the hands and feet appear early but are irregular in appearance. Severe equinovarus foot deformities are almost universal. The pelvis is mildly flared, and a prominent notch is commonly seen above the acetabulum. The capital femoral epiphyses are markedly delayed in appearing. With ossification, a central saucer-shaped defect in the capital femoral epiphysis remains unossified (Fig. 7-17). This results in a broad, flattened femoral head with a short neck that is poorly contained by the acetabulum. Hip dislocation or osteoarthritis is a common sequela of coxa vara and severe incongruity. Bilateral hip dislocations developed in 22% of patients in one reported series.[126]

Medical Considerations

Early comprehensive medical attention must be given to the diastrophic infant with respiratory difficulties. These problems may be compounded by a cleft palate, because aspiration with feeding may occur. Although surgical repair of the cleft palate is usually necessary, it should not be performed without careful assessment of the cervical spine, because of the high incidence of kyphosis and instability.

Orthopaedic Implications

When confronted with the multiple problems observed in patients with diastrophic dysplasia, such as spinal deformities, limited joint motion with contractures, severe clubfoot abnormalities, and a predisposition for early osteoarthritis, treatment priorities must be established. Cervical kyphosis has been reported in as many as one third of individuals with diastrophic dysplasia and is frequently associated with instability. This is a major concern because of the risk of quadriplegia from progressive kyphosis, especially during intubation for patients undergoing general anesthesia.[114,121] (Fig. 7-18). The cervical kyphosis usually develops during the first 2 years of life. Of the four patients with cervical kyphosis reported in one series, quadriplegia developed in one, a 7-year-old patient whose kyphosis measured greater than 100 degrees. Cervical kyphosis measuring from 40 to 82 degrees in three other patients younger than 4 years of age resolved completely.[107] Two of these patients were placed in a Milwaukee brace for associated scoliosis.

If cervical kyphosis is present, lateral flexion-extension cervical spine radiographs should be obtained to assess stability at the apex of the kyphosis. If there are neurologic symptoms or signs, magnetic resonance imaging is useful for evaluating possible cord compression.[115] Additional information may be gained by obtaining MRI scans in flexion and extension positions.

Treatment depends on the magnitude of the kyphosis and whether instability or neurologic compro-

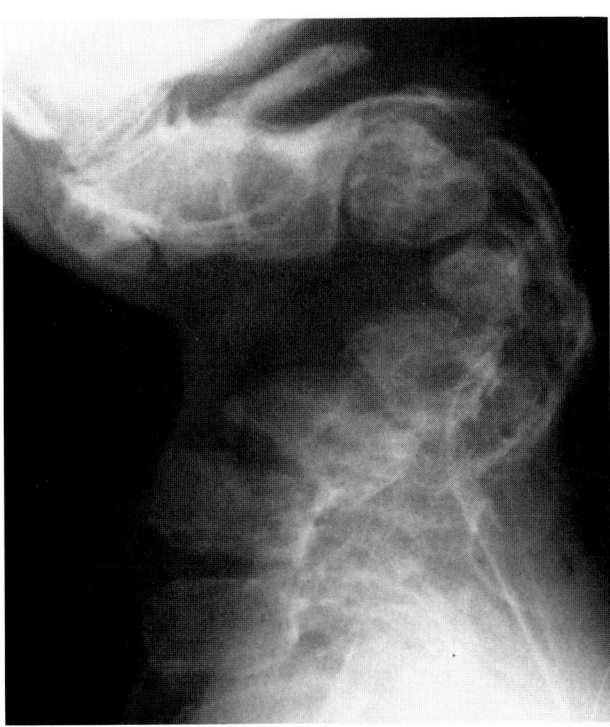

FIGURE 7-18. A 16-year-old patient with diastrophic dysplasia. Untreated cervical kyphosis resulted in quadriplegia.

mise is present. If there is no instability associated with the kyphosis in the neurologically normal child, a nonoperative approach consisting of observation or bracing is prudent, with the expectation that the kyphosis will improve in many of these patients. However, if significant flexion instability exists or the kyphosis progresses, bracing is indicated. The most useful orthosis in my experience is a modified Milwaukee brace. If there is no improvement with a trial of bracing or there is evidence of neurologic compromise, surgical intervention is warranted. Posterior fusion techniques may be successfully used for patients with cervical kyphosis and instability without neurologic deficits. This generally necessitates halo-vest immobilization and may be used in children as young as 18 months if multiple pins are used.

If there is neurologic involvement, operative intervention generally requires anterior decompression and fusion in conjunction with a posterior fusion because of the kyphotic deformity. Halo-vest immobilization is extremely useful in these patients. Care must be taken during posterior exposure because midline cervical spina bifida occulta is common. During induction of anesthesia, fiberoptic intubation is often required because of the short neck and associated kyphosis.

Thoracolumbar spinal deformities, including kyphosis, scoliosis, or kyphoscoliosis, occur frequently in diastrophic dysplasia. In one series of 36 patients, 83% had evidence of spinal deformities.[125] Scoliosis was identified in 37% of 102 diastrophic dwarfs from Finland. Thirteen of these patients had deformities in excess of 50 degrees.[121] In both series, the diastrophic dwarfs developing severe curves usually had early signs of deformity by 2 to 4 years of age. However, other children have curves that are small and relatively flexible. Nevertheless, curve progression is common, and if left untreated, kyphoscoliosis of more than 100 degrees may occur.[107,110,121,125] These deformities are typically rigid, rotated, and sharply angular. Because of the poor outcome for many of these untreated curves, early orthotic management with a Milwaukee brace should be strongly considered while the curves are small. If orthotic management is started early, control of the spinal deformity is frequently successful for several years. Most spinal growth is usually completed by age 10 years in diastrophic dysplasia. However, if the curve progresses despite bracing, surgical intervention is indicated, even in the young patient. If the kyphosis is more than 50 degrees, anterior fusion should be strongly considered in conjunction with the posterior fusion. Although posterior instrumentation has been used successfully in some patients, attempted correction of kyphoscoliotic deformities with instrumentation has been associated with neurologic compromise in large, rigid curves.[110,125] Serious consideration should be given to anteroposterior fusion in situ with postoperative immobilization as a safer alternative to intraoperative distraction for large deformities.[107] Fortunately, symptoms referable to spinal stenosis are quite uncommon for diastrophic dwarfs.[121]

Rigid foot deformities are a frequent occurrence in diastrophic dysplasia. In a series of 102 patients, metatarsus adductus with hindfoot valgus affected 43%, equinovarus deformities affected 37%, and equinus affected 8%.[123] These abnormalities, especially the clubfoot deformities, are usually rigid and resistant to cast correction. Cast treatment is further compromised by the extreme shortening and bulkiness of the leg and thigh. Although some children obtain satisfactory improvement of an equinovarus deformity with casting, many require posteromedial releases. In one series, 26 of 51 patients underwent surgery to correct the foot deformity.[126] These releases tend to be technically difficult because of the size, rigidity, and configuration of the foot. It is best to wait until the child is at least 1 year of age before surgery is performed. Unfortunately, complete correction of the equinus and varus deformity is often not achieved. Consideration may be given to talectomy or talar decancellation and manipulating the foot into a plantargrade position (ie, Verebelyi-Ogston procedure). These options would be considered salvage procedures but may be the only choices available to correct a severe, rigid foot deformity. The cervical spine must be evaluated thoroughly before administration of general anesthesia.

Progressive hip deformities are a significant concern in diastrophic dysplasia patients, because progressive dislocation or incongruity and premature osteoarthritis commonly occur. Unfortunately, the lack of motion of the hips and knees with flexion contractures approaching 45 degrees in many patients hinders conventional treatment for dysplasia. The capital femoral epiphyses are late to ossify and poorly contained by the acetabula. Deformities with flattening, extrusion, hinge abduction, and dislocations commonly occur. Early surgical intervention with pelvic or femoral osteotomies to contain the unossified femoral head is usually precluded because of joint stiffness and because of the necessity to treat the other significant skeletal abnormalities.

Attention should be directed toward gaining and maintaining a range of motion of the hip, knee, and ankle that is as functional as possible. In some instances, this may require judicious soft tissue releases of these joints. However, it must be recognized that the limited motion is a reflection of extraarticular contractures and of intraarticular deformities. The amount of correction hoped for through releases frequently is unable to be obtained. If significant symptomatic deformity of the femoral head develops, a valgus-extension intertrochanteric osteotomy may be considered in patients with a functional range of motion of the hip. However, the acetabulum must be sufficient to contain the redirected femoral head, or dislocation could occur. Hip arthrography should be performed preoperatively to assess these variables. In selected patients, simultaneous femoral and pelvic osteotomies may be successfully performed.

For the severely symptomatic adult patients, the osteotomies are not feasible, leaving total hip arthroplasty as the only alternative. These arthroplasties are complex, frequently requiring custom components, simultaneous osteotomy of the proximal femur, acetabular bone grafting, and major soft tissue releases. In a series of 15 cementless hip arthroplasties in 10 patients, the total complication rate was 25%, including two intraoperative fractures and two femoral nerve palsies.[120]

KNIEST DYSPLASIA

Kniest dysplasia, named for the physician who first described a patient with this disorder in 1952, has been previously confused with metatropic dysplasia.[127] However, based on clinical, radiographic, and histologic differences, Kniest dysplasia is considered a separate, distinct osteochondrodysplasia.[97] It is characterized by disproportionate short-trunk dwarfism, kyphoscoliosis, atypical facial appearance, and significant joint stiffness and contractures, including the hands. Myopia, cleft palate, and hearing losses commonly occur. This condition is transmitted as an autosomal dominant trait, and most cases are the result of a new mutation. Defects in type II collagen have been identified in this disorder secondary to a processing defect of the C-propeptide.[130]

Clinical Features

Recognition of Kniest dysplasia may be delayed until early childhood in patients with very mild involvement. However, most patients have features identifiable at birth, including short stature, short limbs with joint enlargement, stiffness, and facial abnormalities. Dislocated hips and clubfoot deformities are seen occasionally. Inguinal or umbilical hernias are common. By 1 year of age, contractures of the elbows, hips, and knees are evident. Motor development is delayed, probably because of joint stiffness and contractures. These children ordinarily do not have neurologic deficits, and they have normal intelligence. By the time the child is 3 years of age, all the usual manifestations of Kniest dysplasia are evident.[131,132] The face is round, with a depressed midface and prominent eyes and forehead. Cleft palate is found in at least 50% of patients. Severe myopia and retinal detachment may develop.

There is significant disproportionate short-trunk dwarfism and rhizomelic involvement of the extremities. The thorax is short and broad. The short stature is further compounded by thoracic kyphoscoliosis, exaggerated lumbar lordosis, and significant hip-knee flexion contractures. Adult height ranges from 106 to 145 cm (42–57 in).[132] The elbows, wrists, knees, and ankles are enlarged and prominent. Typically, the fingers are stiff, resulting in a poor grasp. The metacarpophalangeal joints usually are extended, and flexion contractures of the proximal interphalangeal joints are present.

Radiographic Features

Osteoporosis of the spine and extremities, present from birth, exists throughout life of the person with Kniest dysplasia.[97,128,131] The skull is normal, but abnormalities of the odontoid have been observed, ranging from hypoplasia to enlargement and persistence of the neurocentral synchondrosis.[17,128] Occipitoatloid or atlantoaxial instability may occur.[129] Platyspondyly or hypoplasia of cervical vertebrae is common. Coronal clefts of the vertebral bodies may remain until the child is 1 year of age. Anterior wedging and generalized platyspondyly with elongation and kyphoscoliosis are common in the thoracic and lumbar spine. The interpedicular distances often appear widened because of the platyspondyly (Fig. 7-19). The actual interpedicular distance is normal, although it appears widened with respect to the decreased height of the vertebral body. The long tubular bones are shortened, with rhizomelic involvement. The metaphyses are flared, and the epiphyses, once ossified, are large and deformed.

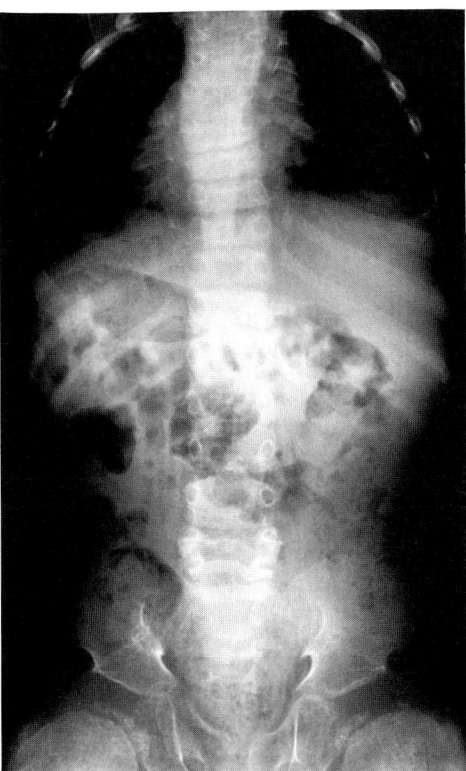

FIGURE 7-19. A 4-year-old patient with Kniest dysplasia. Generalized osteoporosis with platyspondyly, mild thoracic scoliosis, and interpedicular widening are apparent. The thorax is normal, and the pelvis is small, with marked broadening of the femoral neck and delayed femoral head ossification.

Valgus deformities of the lower limbs typically occur (Fig. 7-20).

The pelvis is characteristic, with short and broad iliac crests, hypoplastic and vertically oriented pubic rami, and small, insufficient acetabula. The femoral heads ossify in late childhood and are typically deformed and subluxated. The femoral necks are broad and expanded. Significant changes of premature osteoarthritis develop early. Peculiar flocculent calcifications are observed in the epiphyseal and metaphyseal regions, especially about the hip and knees.[97,128] Similarly, radiodensities may be identified on spinal radiographs. Hand involvement is significant, with generalized osteoporosis and narrowing of the intercarpal and phalangeal joints of the fingers and thumbs. The tubular bones are mildly shortened, with widening of the medullary canal. Epiphyseal irregularities with soft tissue swelling of the metacarpophalangeal and interphalangeal joints occur.

Radiographically, the dumbbell-shaped long bones of patients with Kniest dysplasia resemble those seen in metatropic dysplasia, but they are not as severely involved. The vertebrae in metatropic dysplasia are flattened and elongated significantly, lacking vertical clefts. The spinal deformity is usually more severe in metatropic dysplasia than in Kniest dysplasia. The

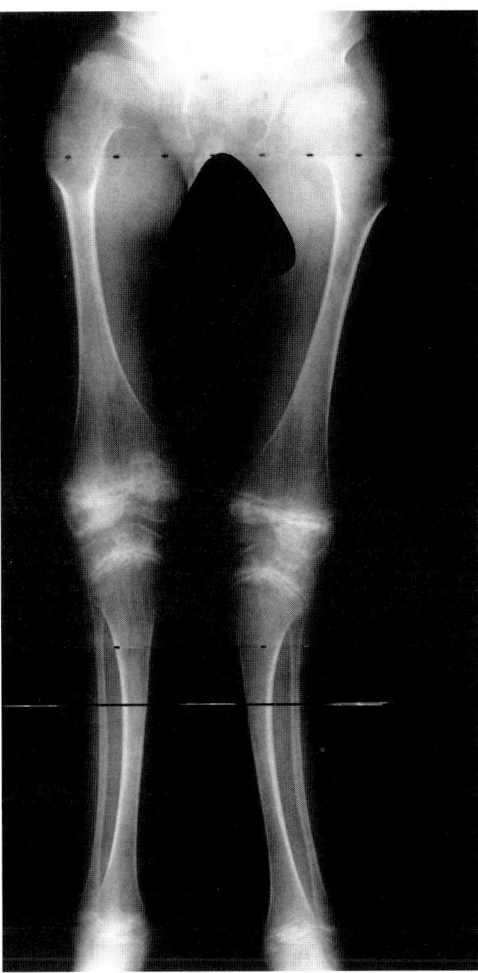

FIGURE 7-20. A 12-year-old patient with Kniest dysplasia. There is expansion of the ends of the long bones, with flocculent calcifications within the eiphyseal and metaphyseal regions. Angular deformities and intraarticular incongruities are evident.

thoracic cage in Kniest dysplasia is normal or broad compared with the long, narrow thorax of metatropic dysplasia.[132] Generally, skeletal involvement in metatropic dysplasia is more severe than that seen in Kniest dysplasia.

Medical Considerations

In Kniest dysplasia patients, severe respiratory distress and recurrent infections during infancy may be associated with tracheomalacia and cleft palate. Hearing losses have occurred often and appear to be related to chronic otitis media. Prompt recognition and appropriate treatment for respiratory infections are required. Frequent ophthalmologic examinations are essential to identify retinal detachment and myopia.

Orthopaedic Implications

Assessment of upper cervical instability is essential, and if significant instability exists, posterior spinal stabilization is required. The guidelines for obtaining flexion-extension lateral radiographs and indications for surgical stabilization are similar to those discussed previously for metatropic dysplasia. Thoracolumbar kyphosis and thoracic kyphoscoliosis are not unusual in persons with Kniest dysplasia. These deformities usually are less severe than those seen in metatropic dysplasia, and surgical treatment is required less frequently.

The major orthopaedic problems in Kniest dysplasia patients are limited joint motion and contractures. Early involvement in a physical and occupational therapy program is recommended to gain and maintain motion, especially in the metacarpophalangeal joints, proximal interphalangeal joints, hips, knees, and ankles. Patients with Kniest dysplasia are predisposed to symptoms of early osteoarthritis, especially in the weight-bearing joints. If significant valgus deformity of the knees or ankles exists, a realignment osteotomy may be considered.

Unfortunately, in Kniest dysplasia patients, symptomatic osteoarthritis of the hip is common in the second or third decade of life. If conservative measures fail to relieve the symptoms of osteoarthritis, surgical reconstruction may be indicated. If hip joint congruity is improved with adduction of the hip, a valgus intertrochanteric osteotomy may be considered. Abduction of the femur frequently produces hinge abduction. Arthrography facilitates preoperative planning. If the hip flexes to 90 degrees, adding 20 to 25 degrees of extension to the osteotomy reduces the contracture and improves the gait pattern. However, if there is insufficient flexion, the addition of an extension component to the osteotomy may interfere with sitting and stair-climbing ability. Often, motion is so limited that an osteotomy is precluded, leaving total hip arthroplasty as the only reasonable alternative for severely symptomatic hips in adults.

Treatment of clubfoot deformities should be initiated in infancy with manipulation and casting. However, these deformities may be resistant, and surgical release is frequently necessary. Some patients with Kniest dysplasia have significant pain at the first metatarsophalangeal joint because of a dorsal bunion or hallux rigidus. If shoe modifications fail, resectional arthroplasty, cheilectomy, or arthrodesis in extension may be recommended.

SPONDYLOEPIPHYSEAL DYSPLASIA CONGENITA

Spondyloepiphyseal dysplasia (SED) is a descriptive term for a group of disorders with primary involvement of the vertebrae and epiphyseal centers resulting in a short-trunk disproportionate dwarfism.[140] Other generalized dysplasias with significant vertebral involvement affect the metaphyseal region of the long bones rather than the epiphyseal region. These are generically described by the term spondylometaphyseal dysplasia (SMD).[138] An even more uncommon group of disorders, called spondylepimetaphyseal dysplasia (SEMD) or spondylometepiphyseal dysplasia (SMED), based on the location of the most extensive radiographic changes, have been identified as well.[133] The clinical and radiographic differences among the various spondylodysplasias are frequently age related and not distinguishable at birth. The clinical heterogeneity and variable inheritance patterns that exist for these disorders emphasize the need for referral to a geneticist who is knowledgeable in the osteochondrodysplasias.[136]

Spondyloepiphyseal dysplasia congenita (SED congenita) is a specific disorder that is readily differentiated from other SEDs, including chondrodysplasia punctata, Morquio disease, pseudoachondroplasia, SED tarda, and the SEMD, SMD, or SMED variants. Although this disorder is transmitted as an autosomal dominant trait, most cases are sporadic, the result of a new mutation. The primary defect of SED congenita has been linked to a mutation of the type II collagen gene locus, COl2A1, on chromosome 12.[134,137,139] This same mutation has not been identified for SMD or SEMD. Histopathologic studies of growth zones have not revealed a consistent pattern of involvement, perhaps reflecting the heterogeneity of the SED.[141,143]

Clinical Features

The diagnosis of SED congenita may be made at birth. Newborn infants are short, with disproportionate involvement of the trunk. Head circumference is normal, but the face is flat, with wide-set eyes. A cleft palate is common. The neck is short, and a pectus carinatum deformity occurs in combination with a barrel-shaped chest. Increased lumbar lordosis and associated hip flexion contractures are observed, even in the newborn period. The abdomen is protuberant. The hands and feet are relatively normal in length, in striking contrast to the extreme shortness of the proximal and middle segments of the limbs. Talipes equinovarus deformities are not unusual. Valgus alignment of the knees commonly develops, and genu varum also may occur. Thoracic scoliosis may become evident in adolescence (Fig. 7-21). SED congenita has been confused clinically with Morquio disease. However, these two disorders are readily distinguishable by radiographic differences and by the presence of corneal opacities, cardiac involvement, and urinary excretion of keratosulfate in the patient with Morquio disease.

Traditionally, two groups of SED congenita have been defined, differentiated by the severity of the coxa vara and the magnitude of skeletal involvement. The

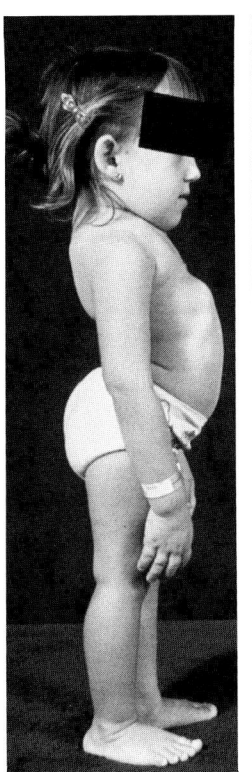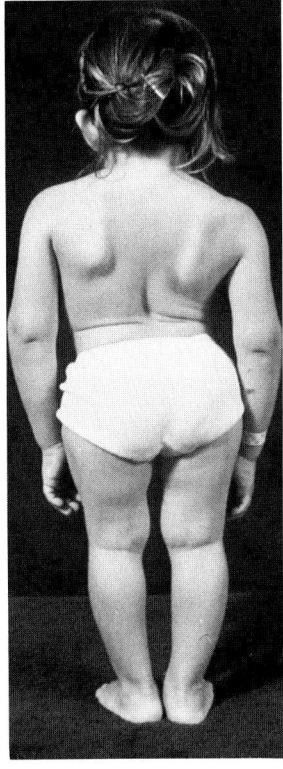

FIGURE 7-21. An 11-year-old patient with spondyloepiphyseal dysplasia congenita. Severe dwarfism is the result of a short neck and trunk, pectus carinatum, thoracic scoliosis, exaggerated lumbar lordosis, and hip flexion deformities.

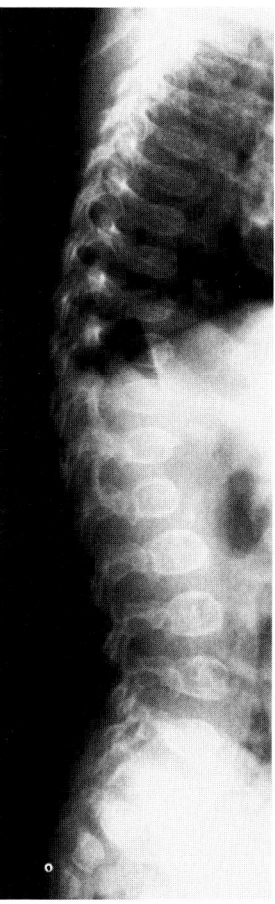

FIGURE 7-22. An 18-month-old patient with spondyloepiphyseal dysplasia congenita. Notice the generalized platyspondyly with anterior tongue-like projections of the thoracic spine and oval lumbar vertebrae secondary to posterior wedging.

distinction between those with severe coxa vara and those with only mild involvement usually is not possible until the patient is 3 or 4 years of age.[142] Those patients with SED congenita and mild coxa vara fall just below the third percentile in height. The adult height of those with severe coxa vara ranges between 90 and 120 cm (35–50 in).[112,140] However, this differentiation into two types is rather arbitrary. Most geneticists recognize SED congenita as a specific, single disorder with heterogeneic involvement.

Radiographic Features

The development of ossification centers is delayed in those with SED congenita. The epiphyseal centers of the femoral head, knee, calcaneus, and talus usually are not present at birth. There are various degrees of platyspondyly, with posterior wedging of vertebral bodies giving rise to oval or pear-shaped vertebrae (Fig. 7-22). In adolescents and young adults, end plate irregularities and narrowed intervertebral disc spaces become obvious with an increased anteroposterior diameter of the vertebral bodies. Lumbar lordosis is usually exaggerated. Progressive kyphoscoliosis may develop in late childhood. Odontoid hypoplasia or os odontoideum leading to atlantoaxial instability is common. Flexion-extension lateral cervical radiographs may reveal anterior, posterior, or combined anterior and posterior instability.

In patients with SED congenita, the iliac crests are short and small, with horizontal acetabular roofs and delayed ossification of the pubis. Ossification of the capital femoral epiphysis is usually delayed, and coxa vara of varying severity is almost universal (Fig. 7-23). In patients with severe coxa vara, progressive varus deformity may occur, leading to discontinuity of the femoral neck and proximal migration of the greater trochanter. At times, the coxa vara may be associated with progressive dislocation if ligamentous laxity exists. The delayed ossification of the femoral head predisposes the hip to deformation, with flattening, lateral extrusion, hinge abduction, and premature osteoarthritis.

The ossification centers of the distal femur and proximal tibia are also delayed, associated with flattening and irregularity of the articular surface. Genu valgum is common and often associated with the overgrowth of the medial femoral condyle. Genu varum is rare. The metaphyses of the long tubular bones may show mild flaring and irregular ossification from alter-

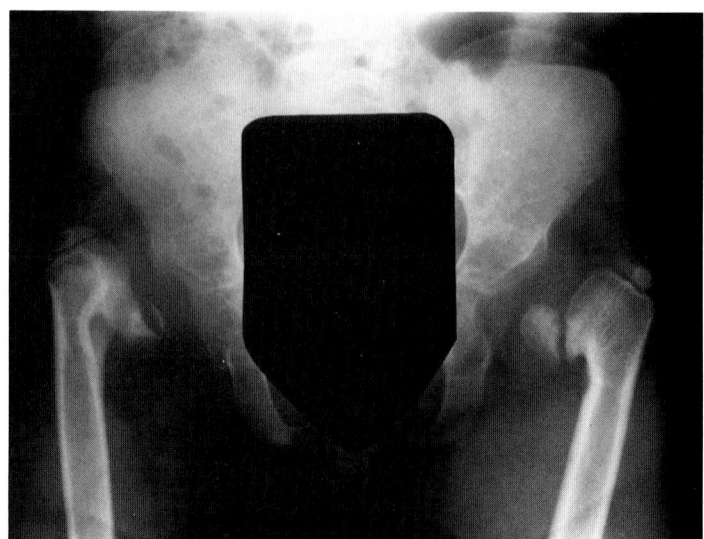

FIGURE 7-23. A 6-year-old patient with spondyloepiphyseal dysplasia congenita. Notice the severe coxa vara with delayed ossification of the capital femoral epiphyses.

ations in endochondral bone formation. The short tubular bones of the hands and feet show minimal broadening and shortening, in contrast to that seen in pseudoachondroplastic dysplasia. Ossification of carpal and tarsal centers usually is delayed. In contrast, the radiographic manifestations of Morquio disease include wide flaring of the ilia, no delay in pubic ossification, shallow acetabula, coxa valga, and severe involvement of the hands and feet.

Medical Considerations

Respiratory difficulties may develop in infancy related to the small thorax, but most of these children survive. Severe myopia or retinal detachment has been found in more than 50% of patients in some series.[140] Congenital cataracts are not characteristic of persons with SED congenita. Regular ophthalmologic examination is necessary to identify pathologic retinal conditions early and treat them appropriately.

Orthopaedic Implications

Odontoid hypoplasia or os odontoideum is commonly seen in patients with SED congenita and may lead to atlantoaxial instability.[8,135] Cervical myelopathy may result from the instability. Symptoms include delayed motor development, decreased endurance, and alterations in respiration. Throughout the growth and development of these patients, careful neurologic assessments must be performed. Lateral flexion-extension cervical radiographs should be obtained every 3 to 4 years until skeletal maturity. In some instances, plain radiographs may be difficult to interpret. Lateral flexion-extension tomograms or cineradiography may facilitate the evaluation of instability. With flexion, an atlantodens interval of greater than 5 mm is indicative of instability, although the patient is often asymptomatic. However, many patients with odontoid hypoplasia are stable in flexion, but on extension, they demonstrate significant posterior subluxation of the atlas on the axis. The anterior ring of the atlas frequency slides posteriorly over the body of the second cervical vertebra. An os odontoideum can significantly narrow the spinal canal (Fig. 7-24).

In some patients, combined anterior and posterior instability is demonstrated radiographically. Magnetic resonance imaging of the atlantoaxial region in flexion and extension is useful to delineate cord compression. Posterior atlantoaxial fusion is indicated for patients with clinical signs or symptoms of myelopathy, for asymptomatic patients with MRI evidence of cord compression, or prophylactically for patients with atlantoaxial instability of 8 mm or more. Fusion to the occiput frequently is required because of the small size of the posterior ring of the atlas or a large midline synchondrosis. Halo-cast immobilization is preferable to wiring techniques, and decortication is completed carefully with a high-speed dental bur. In cases of extension instability, posterior wiring techniques may overreduce the atlas on the axis, leading to iatrogenic injury to the upper cervical cord. This must be avoided.

Scoliosis or kyphoscoliosis in SED congenita patients was reported in 14 of 17 patients in one series.[142] Single- and double-curve patterns have been described. The thoracic kyphosis may be severe, measuring as much as 130 degrees.[3] Paraplegia has resulted from severe, rigid deformities.[142] These spinal deformities ordinarily develop in late childhood or early adolescence. In the skeletally immature patient with scoliosis of 40 degrees or less, the initial treatment should be a brace. Patients with curves that progress despite brace treatment or that are more than 50 degrees should be considered as candidates for surgical stabilization. In contrast to achondroplasia, there is no sig-

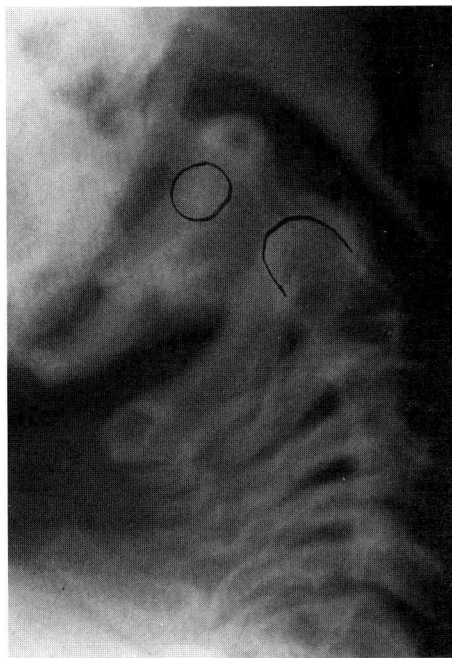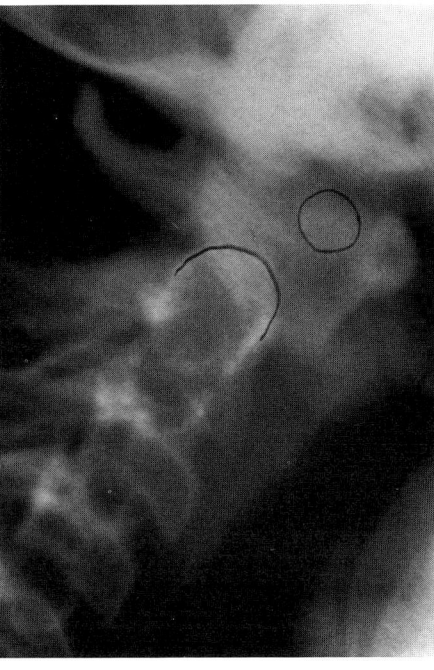

FIGURE 7-24. A 10-year-old patient with spondyloepiphyseal dysplasia congenita. Flexion-extension lateral cervical spine radiographs reveal posterior instability associated with an os odontoideum.

nificant spinal stenosis in SED congenita. Posterior instrumentation systems may be used judiciously to obtain and maintain correction. However, for severe deformities, combined anteroposterior surgery using halo-dependent traction has been a valuable adjunct.

Treatment of hip deformity is often necessary in the patient with severe SED congenita. If the femoral neck-shaft angle is 100 degrees or less, a valgus intertrochanteric osteotomy should be considered to prevent progressive varus deformity or discontinuity of the femoral neck. The neck-shaft angle should be corrected to at least 140 degrees at the time of surgery to prevent recurrent deformity. Simultaneous extension of the distal fragment with the valgus osteotomy decreases the flexion deformity of the hip and may improve the excessive lumbar lordosis. For patients with coxa vara and femoral head deformity leading to subluxation or hinge abduction, reconstructive measures frequently are indicated because of hip pain or decreased walking tolerance. These patients are predisposed to premature osteoarthritis. Hip arthrography often reveals improved congruity with adduction and flexion of the femur. In contrast, for patients with deformation of the femoral head, abduction of the femur frequently increases the incongruity.

The procedure of choice for symptomatic patients is the valgus-extension intertrochanteric osteotomy. In the completely dislocated hip, reconstruction may be feasible with a combination of open reduction, valgus intertrochanteric, and pelvic osteotomies, provided there is a satisfactory range of motion and continuity of the femoral neck. In my experience, a Chiari osteotomy or shelf augmentation has been required given the severe acetabular deficiency present with these dislocated hips.

If surgery is contemplated, consideration must be given to the alignment of the whole lower extremity and not just the hip. Most patients with SED congenita have a valgus deformity of their knees and ankles in addition to the coxa vara deformity. Typically, simultaneous multilevel osteotomies of the hip, knees, and ankles are required for lower extremity realignment, according to the principles previously outlined.[103,104] Patients with valgus deformities of the knee frequently have knee pain and increased laxity of the medial collateral ligament. A varus supracondylar osteotomy should be considered for patients with symptomatic knees or severe valgus deformities. Unlike patients with achondroplasia, patients with SED congenita or the other variants are at high risk for the development of osteoarthritis in adulthood. Normalization of lower extremity malalignment may delay the onset of degenerative changes, but long-term outcome studies have not been reported. Total joint replacement may be considered for carefully selected adult patients with SED congenita with symptomatic osteoarthritis. However, these are difficult procedures, often requiring simultaneous corrective osteotomies and custom components.

SPONDYLOEPIPHYSEAL DYSPLASIA TARDA

Spondyloepiphyseal dysplasia tarda (SED tarda) is a generalized skeletal dysplasia affecting primarily the spine and the epiphyses of the larger, more proximally located joints. As its name implies, clinical manifestations are late in onset. Some patients show mild growth retardation in childhood, and others go unrecognized until the adolescent years, when hip pain or scoliosis develops. SED tarda is transmitted as an X-linked condition, which at times has shown milder manifestations in females. Linkage studies have established that the *SEDL* locus lies on the distal part of the short arm of the X chromosome (Xp22).[147]

Clinical Features

Children with SED tarda are normal at birth, developing clinical manifestations of trunk or hip involvement after 4 years of age. There is mild disproportionate trunk shortening, but many patients achieve an adult height of more than 153 cm (60 in).[144,145] True dwarfism may not result, but scoliosis or increased dorsal kyphosis with an exaggerated lumbar lordosis may develop. Scoliosis may become quite severe, requiring active treatment. Patients may have symptoms of back pain or stiffness. Angular deformities of the lower extremities are not ordinarily seen. Typically, patients develop hip pain and stiffness in the first or second decade and are referred to an orthopaedist because of suspected bilateral Perthes disease. Progressive osteoarthritis of the hips or knees that becomes symptomatic by early adulthood is sometimes seen.[146]

Radiographic Features

Epiphyseal involvement in the patient with SED tarda is primarily in the shoulders, hips, and knees symmetrically. For the weight-bearing joints of the lower extremities, delayed ossification predisposes to joint deformation and premature osteoarthritis. Changes in the hip may mimic bilateral Perthes disease (Fig. 7-25).[157] There are various degrees of coxa magna, flattening, extrusion, and subluxation. There is acetabular involvement as well, and the acetabula frequently are insufficient to contain the abnormal femoral heads. Epiphyseal enlargement and flattening of the femoral condyles with deformation of the apposing tibial articulations are also seen. Genu varum or genu valgum deformities may occur but generally are mild. Involvement of the distal tibial epiphysis is usually less extensive. The hands and feet are minimally affected.

Atlantoaxial instability may occur secondary to odontoid hypoplasia or to an os odontoideum. Assessment of the upper cervical spine should include lateral flexion-extension radiographs. Instability may occur in flexion, in extension, or in both planes. Platyspondyly of some degree affects the rest of the spine (see Fig. 7-25); however, the thoracic spine typically is in-

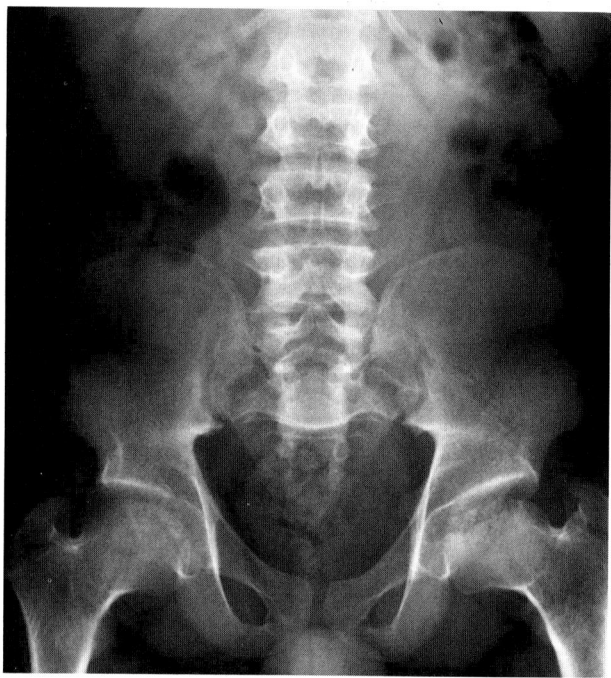

FIGURE 7-25. A 19-year-old patient with spondyloepiphyseal dysplasia tarda. Mild platyspondyly is present with symmetric ossification irregularities of both femoral heads, mimicking Perthes disease.

volved to a greater extent. Anterior wedging or beaking may be present. In the X-linked recessive type of SED tarda, there is typically a mound of bone in the central and posterior portions of the superior and inferior end plates of the vertebral bodies. This frequently is associated with sclerosis in the region of the end plate with disc-space narrowing. These changes are seen on lateral radiographs and are not features of the autosomal dominant or recessive type of SED tarda. Scoliosis is common and may progress, requiring treatment.

Orthopaedic Implications

Guidelines for treating SED tarda patients for scoliosis are similar to those recommended for adolescent idiopathic scoliosis. Bracing should be used for curves approaching 30 degrees in the skeletally immature patient. Occasionally, the scoliosis may be severe enough to require posterior spinal fusion.[145] In patients with atlantoaxial instability, strong consideration should be given to posterior stabilization. External immobilization with a halo vest or cast is preferred, especially for patients with instability in extension. Posterior wiring of the atlas on the axis may result in overreduction of the first cervical vertebra and lead to neurologic injury. This is particularly hazardous if an os odontoideum is associated with the extension instability.

Osteoarthritis of the hip is a common sequela of SED tarda. Symptoms may develop as early as the second decade, requiring surgical intervention. A valgus or valgus-extension intertrochanteric osteotomy frequently improves the congruity of the hip. This procedure is particularly useful for the patient with flattening of the femoral head, narrowing of the weight-bearing articulation, or hinge abduction. Coxa magna may be evident in many patients, and acetabular augmentation may be useful if the acetabulum is insufficient to contain the enlarged femoral head. Preoperative arthrography is extremely useful for assessing hip joint congruity and the extent of the femoral head covered by the acetabular articular cartilage. Ultimately, total hip arthroplasty may be indicated for individuals with significant degenerative changes. Realignment osteotomies rarely are required for knees and ankles in SED tarda patients.

PSEUDOACHONDROPLASTIC DYSPLASIA

Pseudoachondroplastic dysplasia is a heterogeneous group of disorders that generically are a form of SED. However, pseudoachondroplastic dysplasia is a distinct dwarfing condition readily differentiated from SED congenita or tarda. Pseudoachondroplasia, as originally described in 1959 by Maroteaux and Lamy, is characterized by moderate to severe epiphyseal-metaphyseal changes and spinal involvement transmitted as an autosomal dominant trait.[154] Four subtypes have been proposed: two dominant groups (types I and III) and two recessive groups (types II and IV). These are further differentiated by the severity of skeletal involvement, with type I having the mildest changes and type IV the most severe changes.[10,149,150] The validity of these four subtypes is open to dispute. Most cases of pseudoachondroplastic dysplasia are autosomal dominant. The gene for the autosomal dominant form of pseudoachondroplasia has been mapped to chromosome 19.

Microscopic studies of cartilage from patients with the Maroteaux and Lamy type of pseudoachondroplastic dysplasia (type III) have revealed distinct abnormalities. Light microscopy reveals disordered cell columns with a clumping of chondrocytes and cytoplasmic inclusions. Ultrastructural and histochemical examination of hyaline cartilage, fibrocartilage, and physeal cartilage reveals an accumulation of inclusions within the rough endoplasmic reticulum and alterations in the proteoglycans responsible for glycosaminoglycan aggregates.[15,148,155] These changes are similar to those observed for multiple epiphyseal dysplasia, suggesting a common pathogenesis. Linkage studies have excluded gene defects for type II collagen (COL2A1) and proteoglycan link protein (CRTL1) in pseudoachondroplasia.[151]

Clinical Features

Pseudoachondroplastic dysplasia, one of the more common skeletal dysplasias, generally is not recognizable at birth. Growth retardation rarely is observed before the child is 2 or 3 years of age, at which time the rhizomelic shortening of the extremities becomes evident. Short-limb disproportionate dwarfism develops, with adult height ranging from 106 to 130 cm (42–51 in).[152] The face and head have a normal appearance in contrast to that seen in achondroplasia. The trunk is normal, except for an exaggerated lumbar lordosis (Fig. 7-26). Scoliosis may occur, but these curves are rarely severe enough to require surgical intervention. Thoracolumbar kyphosis is less common in patients with pseudoachondroplastic dysplasia than in those with achondroplasia and rarely progresses to a severe gibbus deformity. Marked ligamentous laxity of all joints is common, but the hands and feet are involved to a greater extent than is observed in SED. The short, broad digits have a stubby appearance, lacking normal proximal to distal tapering. Pes planus often occurs. Varus or valgus deformities of the knees

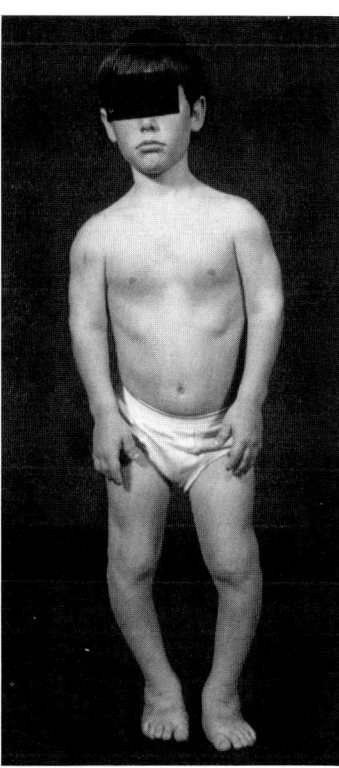

FIGURE 7-26. A 12-year-old patient with pseudoachondroplastic dysplasia. The head and trunk are normal, but there is rhizomelic shortening of the extremities. The hands and feet are short and broad.

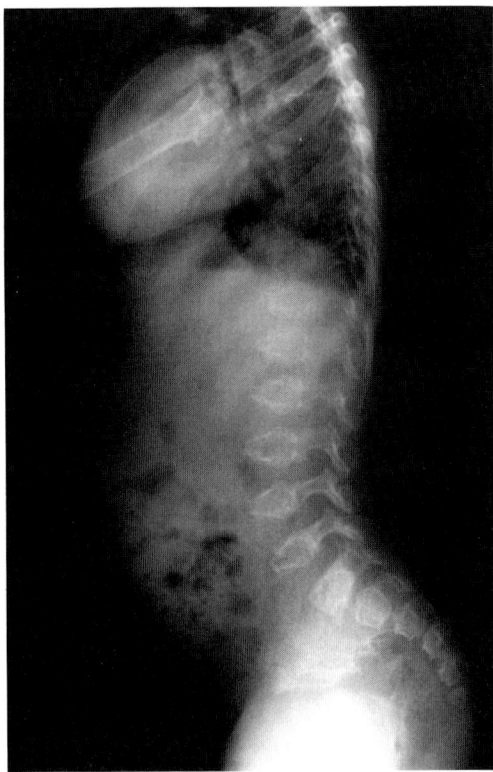

FIGURE 7-27. A 3-year-old patient with pseudoachondroplastic dysplasia has platyspondyly with anterior beaking.

occur frequently and result from osseous changes and marked ligamentous laxity. Some patients develop a windswept appearance from unilateral genu varum with contralateral genu valgum alignment. Windswept deformities are usually associated with pelvic obliquity and may lead to scoliosis.[7,153] Significant flexion contractures are uncommon in the absence of osteoarthritis.

Radiographic Features

The skull in patients with pseudoachondroplastic dysplasia is normal radiographically. Platyspondyly is generally mild, with oval vertebral bodies. In some patients, delayed ossification in the region of the attachment of the anulus produces anterior beaking of the vertebral bodies (Fig. 7-27). Unlike the achondroplastic spine, interpedicular distances are not narrowed in the lumbar spine. Scoliosis or thoracolumbar kyphosis may develop. Odontoid hypoplasia with atlantoaxial instability has been reported.[8,153] The generalized ligamentous laxity in these patients may be an additional predisposing factor in the development of instability.

Epiphyseal and metaphyseal changes characterize the long bone involvement in pseudoachondroplastic dysplasia. There is rhizomelic shortening, with flaring of the metaphyses and delayed ossification of the epiphyses. Epiphyseal involvement results in deformation of articular surfaces with subsequent incongruity and premature osteoarthritis. Weight-bearing joints are affected most severely (Fig. 7-28).

In patients with pseudoachondroplastic dysplasia, early deformation of the femoral head may be evidenced early by a "sagging rope" sign and may occur before adolescence.[156] As ossification progresses, the abnormalities of the femoral heads may resemble bilateral Perthes disease, as in multiple epiphyseal dysplasia.[157] The acetabulum poorly contains the enlarged, flattened femoral head. Subluxation and hinge

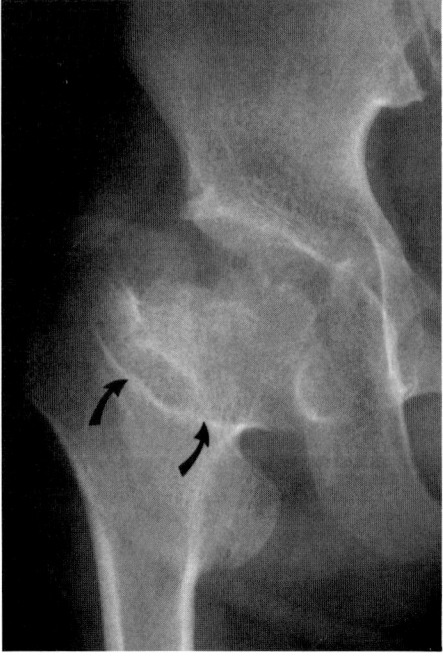
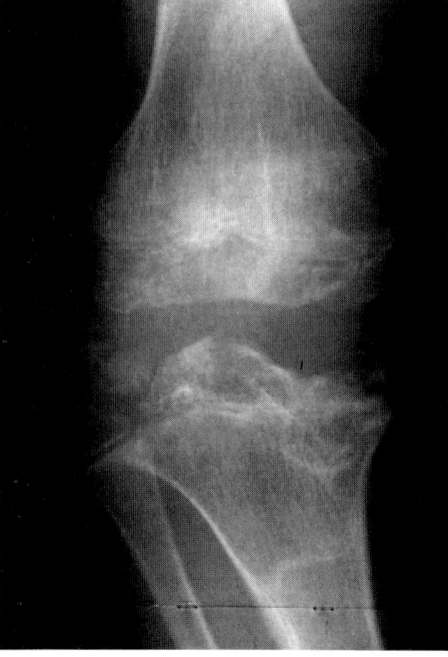

FIGURE 7-28. A 14-year-old patient with pseudoachondroplastic dysplasia. There is delayed ossification of the capital femoral epiphysis, trochanteric overgrowth, and a sagging rope sign, indicative of femoral head deformity. The genu varum is associated with flattening of the femoral condyles and delayed ossification.

abduction may develop, but dislocation infrequently occurs. Subluxation is accentuated in cases of adduction alignment of the femur, as found in patients with a windswept deformity.

Carpal and tarsal bones have delayed maturation. The tubular bones of the hands and feet are short and broad, with irregular epiphyses and flattened metaphyses. Pes planus is common.

Orthopaedic Implications

All patients with pseudoachondroplastic dysplasia require assessment of the upper cervical spine for instability. Myelopathy may develop from chronic compression of the cervical cord because of atlantoaxial instability. Symptoms may range from decreased endurance to quadriplegia. Flexion-extension lateral radiographs should be obtained for all patients initially. In addition to a careful history and physical examination, it is advisable to repeat these radiographs every 3 or 4 years until skeletal maturity to detect possible progressive instability. Obtaining a lateral flexion-extension MRI is advisable for patients with instability of more than 5 mm. Posterior atlantoaxial arthrodesis is indicated for patients with signs or symptoms of myelopathy and prophylactically for asymptomatic patients with an atlantodens interval of more than 8 mm.

Angular deformities of the lower extremities are a significant problem in persons with pseudoachondroplastic dysplasia. These include varus, valgus, and recurvatum deformities. Bracing has not been beneficial for prevention or correction of malalignment. Unlike achondroplastic patients, in whom genu varum is readily correctable by a proximal tibial osteotomy, varus deformity of the lower limb in pseudoachondroplastic dysplasia patients may require supracondylar and proximal tibial osteotomies for satisfactory restoration of alignment. The achondroplastic patient has minimal femoral bowing, but the pseudoachondroplastic patient usually has femoral and tibial involvement. As for any patient with lower extremity malalignment, properly obtained standing anteroposterior and lateral radiographs of the entire lower extremity are necessary to document the location and severity of the clinical deformity. Is the deformity in the femur, the tibia, through the knee because of ligamentous laxity, or a combination of these factors?[103,104] A useful technique for assessing complex deformities is to obtain a supine long radiograph with the patient's knees apposed and the legs crossed. This radiograph eliminates potential ligamentous laxity and is useful for demonstrating the anatomic location of the bowing, showing whether it is predominantly tibial or tibial and femoral (Fig. 7-29).

The goal of treatment is restoration of the mechanical axis of the lower extremity with the plane of the femoral condyles parallel with the floor. For pa-

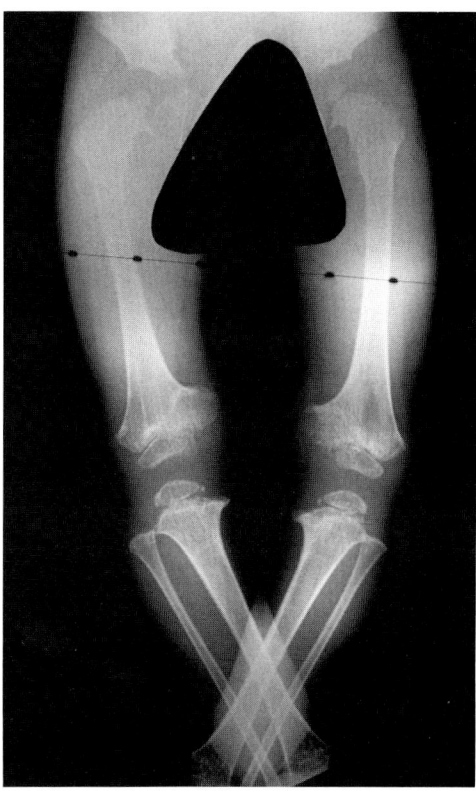

FIGURE 7-29. A 3-year-old patient with pseudoachondroplastic dysplasia. The supine cross-leg radiograph reveals that the varus deformity involves the femurs and the tibias. A proximal tibial osteotomy can improve the alignment of the extremity, but the femoral condyles will still be in varus.

tients with significant valgus deformity of the knee, a varus supracondylar osteotomy can achieve satisfactory realignment. A combination of osteotomies often is required for pseudoachondroplastic patients with windswept deformities, including the hip, knee, and ankle. A variety of internal or external fixation techniques are available, depending on the needs of the patient and the experience and preference of the surgeon. If external cast immobilization is used, care must be taken at surgery to ensure that realignment is achieved at the osteotomy site rather than through the lax ligaments of the knee; otherwise, undercorrection may occur. Arthrography is often beneficial at the time of surgery to determine proper alignment, because ossification of the epiphyses is delayed. Unfortunately, the deformity in the growing child frequently recurs and is further compounded by marked ligamentous laxity. Osteoarthritis of the hips and knees is a common sequela of the deformation that occurs in the growing patient, and many adults with pseudoachondroplasia ultimately require total joint arthroplasty. These are difficult procedures in these patients because of the size of the bones, angular deformities, and ligamentous laxity.

Valgus-extension intertrochanteric osteotomy has been a useful procedure for those pseudoachondroplastic dysplasia patients in whom there is subluxation or hinge abduction. Prerequisites include satisfactory motion and improved congruity, as proved by preliminary hip arthrography with the hip adducted. In addition to improving the congruity of the weight-bearing articulation, the function of the hip abductors is improved by valgus osteotomy. Occasionally, in addition to femoral osteotomy, pelvic reconstruction is recommended to increase the coverage of the femoral head. By the time reconstruction is necessary, the hips of these patients usually are not concentrically reduced. Innominate osteotomies are contraindicated. Shelf augmentations or Chiari osteotomies increase the size of the acetabulum and are considered the procedures of choice.

MULTIPLE EPIPHYSEAL DYSPLASIA

Multiple epiphyseal dysplasia (MED) is one of the most common osteochondrodysplasias and is characterized by disturbance of normal ossification involving many epiphyses. This is a distinct disorder that is readily differentiated from other epiphyseal dysplasias, such as chondrodysplasia punctata and hereditary arthroophthalmopathy (Stickler syndrome). Historically, a milder form of MED, described by Ribbing, has been differentiated from the more severe form, the Fairbank type.[158,167,169] All levels of severity may be present within a kindred, and in most patients, the involvement is symmetric but often is not uniform in every anatomic location. This uneven involvement makes a division into two types arbitrary, because the changes in many patients lie along the continuum between the Ribbing and the Fairbank types.

MED usually is transmitted as an autosomal dominant trait, although autosomal recessive transmission has been reported occasionally.[10] Histologic, ultrastructural, and biochemical studies have shown a disturbance of endochondral ossification in the epiphyseal region, as the name of this disorder indicates, and in the physeal region. Intracytoplasmic inclusions have been identified in the cartilage cells, representing dilatations of the rough endoplasmic reticulum that contain large accumulations of the core protein of proteoglycans. These changes are similar, although less severe, than those described for pseudoachondroplastic dysplasia, suggesting a common pathogenesis.[15,160,170]

Clinical Features

Most patients with MED are referred to orthopaedic surgeons for complaints of lower extremity joint pain, restricted motion, or gait disturbances. The joints appear prominent with symmetric involvement. The hips, knees, and ankles are affected primarily. Angular deformities, including coxa vara, genu varum, and genu valgum, may be associated with flexion contractures. The digits of the hands and feet may be noticeably shortened. Symptoms may develop in late childhood, adolescence, or early adult life. Usually, some diminution in stature occurs, although typically, it is not severe. The adult standing height ranges from 145 to 170 cm (57–67 in) because of disproportionate limb shortening. The spine is minimally involved and usually not symptomatic. The face and head are normal.

Radiographic Features

The principal radiographic changes occur in the epiphyses of the tubular bones, although some physeal irregularities may occur in patients with MED. Typically, joint involvement is symmetric. Spinal involvement, if present, consists of mild end plate irregularities of the thoracic vertebrae. Kyphosis or scoliosis is not a characteristic feature of MED. The epiphyseal centers of ossification are usually delayed in their appearance. After ossification begins, it is irregular or mottled, gradually improving with time. Frequently, the epiphyses appear fragmented, a reflection of multiple separate centers of ossification that eventually coalesce. However, flattening and deformation of joint surfaces occur, leading to premature osteoarthritis.

Joint deformities in MED patients result from growth factors and mechanical factors. Histologic examination reveals abnormal growth and maturation of cartilage and bone. The delayed ossification appears to leave the growing epiphyseal cartilage relatively unsupported, predisposing it to progressive deformation with loading forces. Angular deformities such as genu valgum occur secondary to asymmetric physeal growth. Significant malalignment also alters mechanical forces across the joint and may lead to deformity and premature osteoarthritis.

Upper extremity involvement may be minimal or severe, with significant flattening and irregularities of the epiphyses of the proximal humerus, elbow, and wrist joints. The distal ulna commonly is longer than the radius, leading to subluxation. The tubular bones of the hands often are shortened, with maximal involvement of the middle and distal phalanges. The ossification centers of the carpal bones are small, irregular, and delayed in appearance. Carpal length to width ratios are abnormal in most persons with MED.[161,162,163]

The hips frequently are most severely involved in patients with MED. The capital femoral epiphyses are late in appearing. After ossification begins, these epiphyses are small, irregular, or fragmented. If a sagging rope sign is present, deformation of the femoral head is likely.[156] This sign is often observed before significant ossification of the capital femoral epiphysis

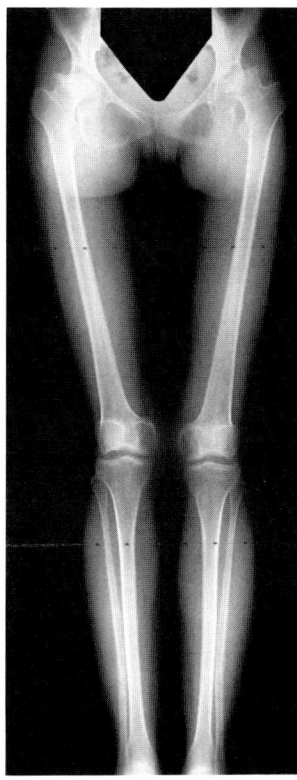

FIGURE 7-30. A 22-year-old patient with multiple epiphyseal dysplasia has severe, symmetric involvement of the hips, knees, and ankles. The femoral heads are deformed, with cystic changes and poor acetabular coverage. The femoral condyles are flattened, with shallow intercondylar notches.

bilateral Perthes disease.[159] However, bilateral Perthes disease is rarely symmetric, and cystic changes, not observed in those with MED, are usually seen in the metaphyseal regions. Acetabular changes, ranging from irregular ossification to severe dysplasia or protrusio acetabuli, may be observed in those affected with MED. The acetabulum is not primarily affected in Perthes disease.[157] A skeletal survey should be obtained for patients with bilateral Perthes disease to rule out a generalized dysplasia (Fig. 7-30). Anteroposterior radiographs of the knees and ankles are the most useful tools for this evaluation. Changes in the distal femoral epiphysis may be subtle, but normal standards for epiphyseal height and width have been reported.[162,168]

Avascular necrosis of the femoral head may be associated with MED. These changes usually occur unilaterally, resulting in an asymmetric appearance of the hip. Sequential radiographs show a progression of the Perthes-like changes superimposed on the irregular ossification of MED. These changes include increased density, followed by resorption and the subsequent reparative phase of creeping substitution and reossification. Subchondral fracture lines (i.e., crescent sign), collapse, and extrusion also may occur (Fig. 7-31).[165]

Bone scintigraphy and MRI may be useful in the early stage of avascular necrosis if the changes are not readily apparent on plain radiographs because of the ossification abnormalities of MED. However, bone scintigrams may be difficult to interpret, because the distribution of activity parallels areas of irregular ossification. If a photopenic area is observed that corresponds to a region of ossification of the femoral head, avascular necrosis exists. The most useful imaging technique for necrosis seen in patients with MED is MRI. Areas of bone infarction in the capital femoral epiphysis lose their positive signal (Fig. 7-32).[165,166]

is seen. At this stage, hip arthrography often demonstrates a mild mushroom-shaped femoral head with various degrees of flattening or extrusion. A progressive deformity usually develops, such as coxa vara, subluxation, hinge abduction, and premature osteoarthritis. The femoral necks are broad and short.[171]

Many patients are referred to the orthopaedist for

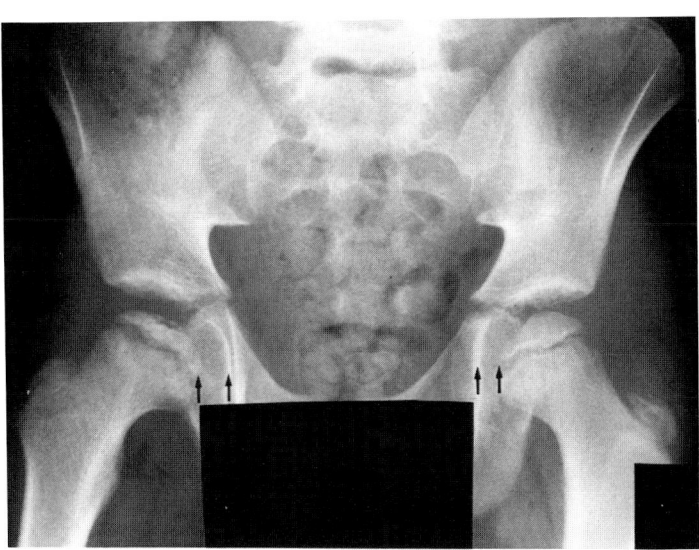

FIGURE 7-31. An 8-year-old patient with multiple epiphyseal dysplasia. Notice the avascular necrosis of the right hip superimposed on multiple epiphyseal dysplasia. There is apparent lateral displacement (Waldenström sign) and a crescent sign.

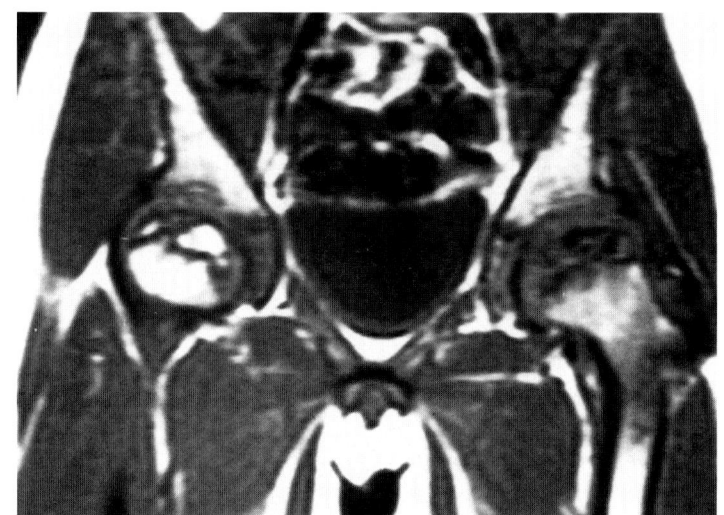

FIGURE 7-32. A 7-year-old patient with multiple epiphyseal dysplasia. The magnetic resonance image demonstrates the loss of positive signal in the left hip, indicative of avascular necrosis.

The knees are often severely affected in patients with MED. The femoral condyles are usually flattened and rectangular, with a shallow intercondylar notch (see Fig. 7-30). The appearance may mimic severe osteochondritis dissecans.[163] Typically, there is increased genu valgum, although varus deformities also may occur. A valgus deformity of the ankle with irregular articular surfaces is common. The talus usually is affected to a greater extent than the distal tibial articulation.

Orthopaedic Implications

The challenge of MED for the orthopaedic surgeon is the almost inevitable premature osteoarthritis. Patients with incongruity of the articular surfaces of major joints at the end of skeletal growth are at greatest risk. Significant symptoms of pain, limitation of motion, and gait disturbance may develop as early as the second or third decade of life for patients with severe involvement. Less involved patients with relatively congruous articular surfaces at maturity are still susceptible to premature osteoarthritis, but it occurs at a later age. It appears that, apart from the obvious mechanical factors leading to osteoarthritis, the articular cartilage is imperfect and is unable to withstand the normal cyclical loading of major joints, particularly in the lower extremities.[161,171]

Unfortunately, many patients presenting for evaluation and treatment have significant incongruity of articular surfaces and degenerative changes. For these "late" cases, total joint arthroplasty may be the only reasonable treatment option. The femoral head frequently deforms in children and adolescents, becoming mushroom-shaped with subsequent subluxation. Realignment osteotomies may be considered if there is a satisfactory range of motion and no significant degenerative changes.

Careful preoperative planning is essential and usually should include arthrography. Hip arthrograms typically reveal medial pooling of dye, indicative of subluxation or incongruity.

Abduction of the hip usually does not improve concentricity, and hinge abduction may be documented. In contrast, congruity of the hip often is improved with adduction of the femur. In this instance, if there is satisfactory acetabular coverage, a valgus intertrochanteric osteotomy should be considered to prevent further instability and deformity and to relieve pain. This osteotomy also has the advantage of lengthening the abductor moment arm because the hip usually is in mild varus with trochanteric overgrowth. Redirectional acetabular osteotomies, such as the Salter or Pemberton procedures, are not warranted because some degree of incongruity is usually present. The femoral head is frequently too large for the acetabulum, and mere redirection does not adequately contain the femoral head.

Shelf augmentation, as described for the treatment of Legg-Perthes disease may play a role in the treatment of hip of early deformities in the epiphyseal dysplasias.[164,172] Conceptually, the shelf procedure is an excellent method of containment of the mushroom-shaped femoral head and may prevent significant subluxation, hinge-abduction, and severe incongruity. However, there are no reported series involving sufficient numbers of patients with adequate long-term follow-up to know whether this procedure can alter the natural history of this disorder.

If avascular necrosis is superimposed on MED, the hip usually becomes painful early, and further limitation of motion is evident, particularly abduction and internal rotation. The combination of avascular necrosis and MED leads to a worse prognosis than either condition alone. Initial treatment involves decreasing the symptoms of synovitis and includes bed rest, traction, and judicious physical therapy, as in Perthes disease. Containment of the femoral head by abduction bracing should be considered for the child 8 years of age or younger. After the pain has resolved and motion has been regained from these conservative measures, hip arthrography should be performed to document and assess the adequacy of containment and concentricity in abduction. If the congruity is poor, an abduction brace should not be used. Surgical containment by varus intertrochanteric osteotomy is contraindicated, because of the preexisting coxa vara. As an alternative to abduction bracing, the shelf procedure may be considered as an alternative means of containing the femoral head.[164,172]

Valgus deformity of the knees or ankles may be corrected by realignment osteotomy and should be strongly considered for the symptomatic patient with MED. For excessive valgus alignment of the knee, careful preoperative assessment is necessary to determine the proper site of osteotomy in the distal femur or the proximal tibia. Traditionally, valgus deformities of the knee are treated by supracondylar osteotomies. However, for many patients, the plane of motion of the knee joint is parallel with the floor in the standing position despite mild increases in the valgus orientation of the femoral shaft. Although a varus supracondylar osteotomy could improve the clinical appearance of the extremity, the femoral condyles would be in varus, increasing the weight-bearing forces through the lateral compartment of the knee. The valgus deformity is often greater on the tibial side than the femoral side. In this instance, a proximal tibiofibular osteotomy is preferred to realign the lower extremity. Recurrent deformity may occur in the growing child because of asymmetric physeal and epiphyseal growth. Realignment osteotomies are usually performed closer to skeletal maturity unless progressive deformity or significant symptoms develop in childhood requiring earlier intervention.

CHONDRODYSPLASIA PUNCTATA

Chondrodysplasia punctata is the name given to a heterogeneic group of disorders characterized by multiple punctate calcifications in infancy. The stippling is best visualized on newborn radiographs and generally disappears by 1 or 2 years of age.[173,179] The many skeletal manifestations of this osteochondrodysplasia frequently are associated with skin, facial, ocular, and cardiac abnormalities.[178] Spranger initially described two distinct forms of chondrodysplasia punctata: the Conradi-Hunermann form and a severe rhizomelic form.[192,193] Four additional subtypes are recognized: X-linked dominant, X-linked recessive, Sheffield, and tibia-metacarpal types.[176,177,181,186,187,190,191,192,194,195]

Stippled calcifications on a radiograph of a newborn are not a specific indication of chondrodysplasia punctata. These calcifications are present in many conditions, including the Zellweger syndrome (i.e., cerebrohepatorenal syndrome), generalized gangliosidosis, Smith-Lemli-Opitz syndrome, intrauterine infections such as rubella, various chromosomal abnormalities (i.e., trisomy 18 and 21), vitamin K enzymatic deficiencies, and hypothyroidism.[10,175,188,189,190] A syndrome similar to chondrodysplasia punctata has been described in infants born to mothers who have ingested warfarin sodium or Dilantin during pregnancy and in infants with the fetal alcohol syndrome.[180,182,195]

The most common type of chondrodysplasia punctata is the Conradi-Hunermann form, transmitted as an autosomal dominant trait. However, most cases are thought to be the result of a spontaneous mutation. A wide variation of clinical expression exists. Some patients die in infancy from severe involvement, but patients with the mildest form may go unrecognized unless radiographs are obtained in infancy before disappearance of the stippling. The possible existence of a mild unrecognized form of chondrodysplasia in a relative often complicates the process of differentiating between a spontaneous mutation and an autosomal dominant transmission.

The second major subtype of chondrodysplasia is the recessive rhizomelic form, which has been linked to an inborn error of peroxisome metabolism. A deficiency of the dihydroxyacetone-phosphate acyltransferase has been identified.[98] This disorder typically has been fatal in the first year of life, although several infants have survived beyond 1 year despite a multiplicity of severe medical problems.[194]

Clinical Features

Patients with the Conradi-Hunermann form of chondrodysplasia punctata have a prominent forehead, wide-set eyes, flattening of the malar region, depressed nasal bridge, and a bifid nasal tip. Congenital cataracts are present in as many as one fifth of these patients. Alopecia is commonly seen, along with ichthyosiform skin changes. Cardiac lesions may be present, and patients with severe involvement may have mental retardation.[108]

For the rhizomelic form, microcephaly, growth retardation, severe psychomotor delay, feeding difficulties, spasticity, and large joint contractures predominate. Additional findings include a high incidence of congenital cataracts (72%), and optic nerve hypoplasia or sensorineural deafness may be present. Frequently, the facial features for the rhizomelic form differ in that the nasal bridge is typically well formed and the nasal tip is bulbous. These patients usually die of respiratory causes or complications of seizures during the first year of life.[193,194]

Prenatal diagnosis has been made by amniocentesis through the measurement of plasmalogen biosynthesis and phytanic acid oxidation activity.[184]

Skeletal abnormalities include short-limb dwarfism, limb length discrepancy, coxa vara, flexion contractures, and significant spinal deformities such as atlantoaxial instability, congenital scoliosis, and kyphosis. Clubfoot and calcaneovalgus foot deformities have been described.

Radiographic Features

The characteristic punctate calcifications are radiographically observable at birth and usually disappear by 1 year of age. The stippling variously affects the hyaline cartilage of epiphyses, carpal bones, and pelvis (Fig. 7-33). Calcifications also may be observed along the vertebral column and in extraskeletal locations such as the trachea and larynx. Unilateral or bilateral coxa vara frequently is associated with asymmetric shortening of the femur (Fig. 7-34). Lateral radiographs in infancy reveal coronal clefts in the vertebral bodies, representing separate anterior and posterior centers of ossification. The appearance of secondary centers of ossification, particularly the capital femoral epiphyses, often is delayed. This may lead to flattening or deformation, and in patients with milder involvement, it may result in a radiographic appearance similar to that of a person with epiphyseal dysplasia. Congenital hemivertebrae or congenital unilateral bars typically give rise to early progressive spinal deformities. Odon-

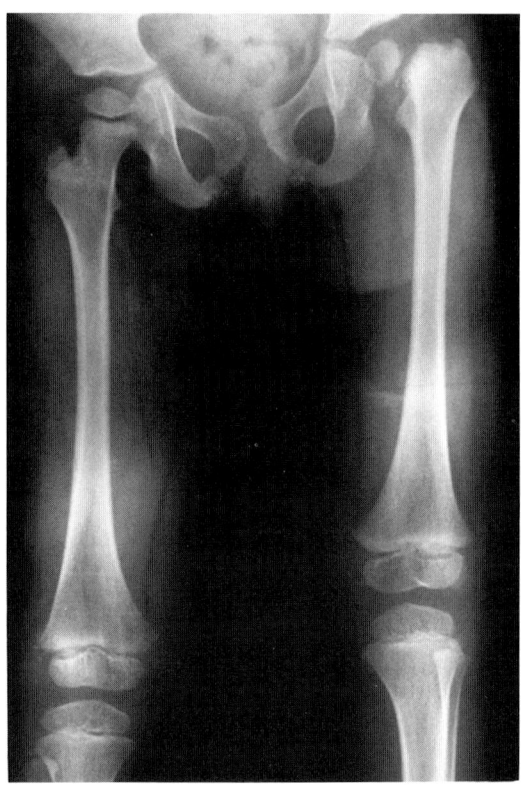

FIGURE 7-34. A 2-year-old patient with chondrodysplasia punctata. Notice the unilateral coxa vara, femoral shortening, and persistent calcific stippling in the ischial region and the knee.

toid hypoplasia, os odontoideum, and instability have been reported. Skeletal involvement in the rhizomelic form of chondrodysplasia punctata is typically symmetric but more severe, involving epiphyses and metaphyses. Severe upper and lower extremity rhizomelic shortening is present with significant metaphyseal flaring or cupping.[17,174,185,193]

Medical Considerations

Ophthalmologic consultation and examination for congenital cataracts are essential for patients with chondrodysplasia punctata. Optic atrophy has been reported as well. The possibility of renal abnormalities and congenital heart disease requires careful medical assessment. The clinical heterogeneity of this group of disorders, various inheritance patterns, and the multitude of possible causes of stippled epiphyses necessitate consultation with a geneticist knowledgeable about the osteochondrodysplasias.

Orthopaedic Implications

Spinal deformities are the most common skeletal problem observed in chondrodysplasia punctata patients. Possible abnormalities of the upper cervical spine with atlantoaxial instability must be assessed by means of lateral flexion-extension radiographs. If

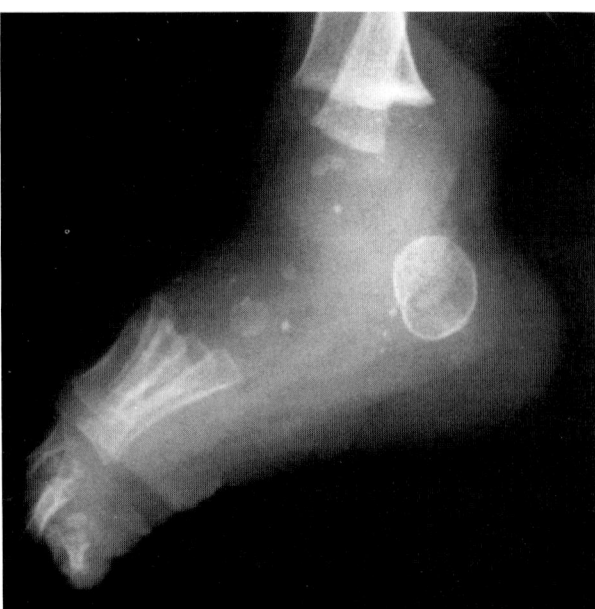

FIGURE 7-33. A 5-month-old patient with chondrodysplasia punctata. Notice the characteristic calcific stippling of the tarsal bones and distal tibial-fibular epiphyses.

significant instability is present, posterior atlantoaxial fusion may be indicated, as previously discussed for SED. Scoliosis or kyphosis secondary to congenital vertebral anomalies is also common. Many patients require stabilization during the first 1 or 2 years of life for a rapidly progressive curve, but others do not have significant progression until adolescence. Bracing is not indicated for these congenital curves.

Lower extremity abnormalities include coxa vara, limb length discrepancies, and flexion contractures. Most flexion contractures are not severe enough to require surgical intervention and are well maintained with stretching exercises. Valgus intertrochanteric osteotomy should be considered for patients with significant coxa vara, evidenced by a neck-shaft angle of less than 100 degrees or persistent ossification defect of the femoral neck. Limb length inequality is not treated by epiphyseodesis, because these patients are already below the third percentile for height. Discrepancies of more than 3 to 4 cm may occur, and lengthening may be considered. The typical prerequisites for lengthenings must be adhered to, including satisfactory range of motion and a stable, congruous joint at both ends of the bone to be lengthened. If the coxa vara is severe, causing deformity or instability of the hip, femoral lengthening should not be performed.

METAPHYSEAL CHONDRODYSPLASIA

Metaphyseal chondrodysplasia is the preferred term given to a heterogeneous group of intrinsic dysplasias characterized by radiographic changes in the metaphyses of the short and long tubular bones with normal epiphyses. This category includes the more common Schmid and McKusick types of metaphyseal dysplasia, metaphyseal chondrodysplasia with malabsorption and neutropenia, and the extremely rare metaphyseal chondrodysplasias described by Jansen, Pena, Spahr, and others.[10] Although previously called metaphyseal dysostoses, the metaphysis does not represent the site of greatest involvement histologically. The defect appears to lie in the proliferative and hypertrophic zones of the physis.

The alteration in endochondral ossification is a consequence of abnormalities in the chondrocytes in cartilage matrix. Light microscopy reveals cell clusters or nests rather than normal columnization.[12,196,205] Ultrastructural studies reveal that there is an accumulation of granular precipitates in the cisternae of the rough-surfaced endoplasmic reticulum.[196,204]

Clinical Features

Schmid Type

The Schmid-type metaphyseal chondrodysplasia is one of the more frequently observed metaphyseal dysplasias.[207] These patients are typically referred for evaluation of short stature, leg pains, bowed legs, increased lordosis, and waddling gait.[206] Many patients initially have been considered to have vitamin D–resistant rickets. This confusion has led to the inappropriate administration of vitamin D to some patients.[197,198] Schmid-type metaphyseal chondrodysplasia is transmitted as an autosomal dominant trait, and affected patients appear clinically normal at birth. Throughout life, the head and face remain unaffected, and apart from an increased lumbar lordosis or mild expansion of the costochondral junctions, the spine and thorax have a normal appearance. Compared with other skeletal dysplasias, the overall diminution in height is mild, with most patients attaining a standing height of 150 cm (59 in). Upper extremity involvement is mild, evidenced by swelling of the wrist, flexion contractures of the elbows, and mild shortening. The lower extremities are involved to a greater extent and are responsible for the diminished standing height. Varus deformities affect the knees and ankles, with bowing visible in the thigh and the leg.

McKusick Type

McKusick identified a distinct metaphyseal dysplasia, originally called cartilage-hair hypoplasia, as a common cause of dwarfing among the Old Order Amish of North America and the Finnish. The incidence among the Amish is estimated at 1 or 2 per 1000 live births and 1 per 23,000 in Finland.[200,205] Although frequent in these two populations, this skeletal dysplasia is less commonly observed in other population groups than the Schmid type. McKusick-type metaphyseal chondrodysplasia is transmitted as an autosomal recessive trait, and patients with this disorder have light-colored, sparse hair. Microscopically, the hair is smaller in diameter than normal hair and often lacks pigmentation.[208]

These patients have a predisposition to intestinal malabsorption, megacolon, and viral infections, particularly chickenpox, because of an alteration of cellular immunity.[205,210] Patients are at increased risk for developing various malignancies. Anemia frequently occurs in childhood.[201]

Disproportionate short stature usually occurs to a greater degree in the McKusick type than in the Schmid type, with adult height ranging from 106 to 147 cm (42–58 in). Growth curves have been established for this disorder.[203] The fingers also are involved to a greater extent than in the Schmid type, with excessive mobility of the fingers and wrist joints. Most have some degree of generalized ligamentous laxity and a limitation of full elbow extension.[201] Genu varum is generally mild compared with that of the Schmid type. Distal fibular overgrowth appears to predispose patients with McKusick-type metaphyseal chondrodysplasia to varus ankle deformities. Chest wall involvement may resemble rickets, with enlargement of the costochondral junctions (i.e., rachitic rosary) and symmetric depression of the lower rib cage at the site of attachment of the diaphragm (i.e., Harrison grooves). Pectus excavatum is common (Fig. 7-35).

Radiographic Features

Schmid Type

Spinal changes occur infrequently in patients with Schmid-type metaphyseal chondrodysplasia. Atlantoaxial instability and mild thoracic scoliosis have been reported.[3] Radiographic changes characteristically occur at the metaphyseal regions of tubular bones, including the hands and feet. The metaphyses are widened and scalloped. Lines of provisional calcification are present but irregular. Radiolucent cysts may project into the metaphysis from the physis, representing unossified islands of cartilage. Some widening of the physis occurs, especially medially at the distal femur and proximal tibia, but not to the extent that is observed in rickets. The structure and density of the bones are otherwise normal. The long bones are shortened, and bowing is accentuated. Varus deformities of the hips and ankles are common.[199]

Several investigators have observed radiographic improvement of the metaphyseal lesions after prolonged immobilization or recumbency. The increased physeal widening normalizes with healing of the metaphyseal cysts, and the lines of provisional calcifications assume a regular appearance. However, when weight bearing is resumed, the metaphyseal changes recur. It appears that weight bearing may play a role in the development of varus deformities of the lower extremities in patients with metaphyseal chondrodysplasia.[197,198,206,209]

McKusick Type

In cases of cartilage-hair hypoplasia, greater shortening occurs in the long bones than in the Schmid type. Coxa vara is less common and less severe. Bilateral hip dislocations occurred in three patients and Legg-Perthes in two of the 108 Finnish patients reported.[201] Involvement of the metaphyses of the knee is more uniform, in contrast to the medial asymmetry found in the Schmid type. Genu varum, when present, tends to be mild (Fig. 7-36). Distal fibular

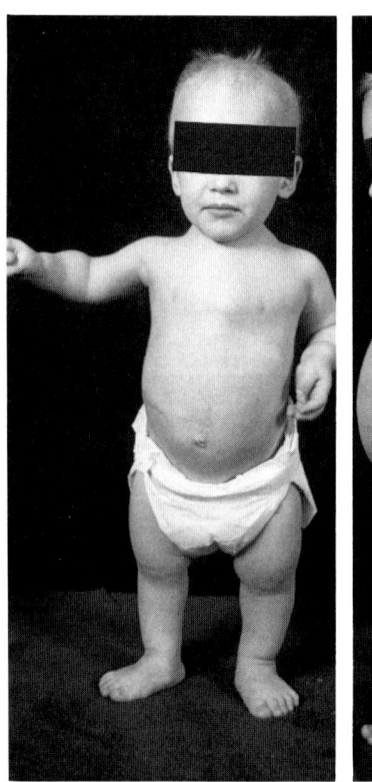
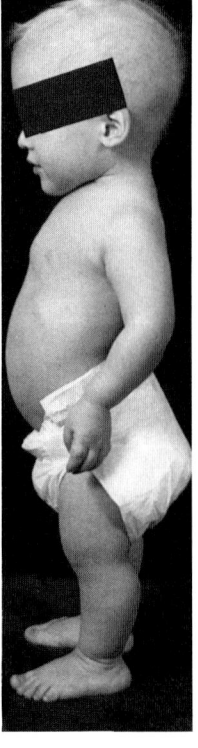

FIGURE 7-35. An 18-month-old patient with McKusick-type metaphyseal chondrodysplasia. Notice the characteristic light, sparse hair, disproportionate short stature, pectus excavatum, Harrison grooves, and varus deformities of the lower extremities. Mild increased lumbar lordosis, flexion contractures of the elbows, and expansion of the wrists are also part of the deformity.

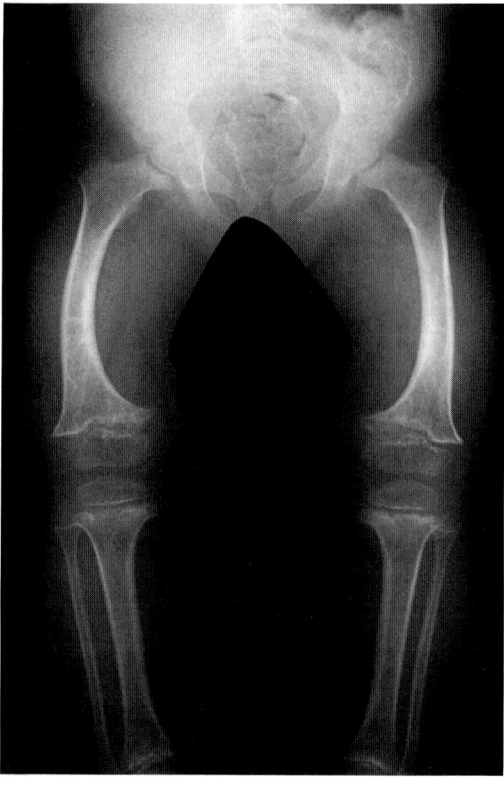

FIGURE 7-36. A 4-year-old patient with McKusick-type metaphyseal chondrodysplasia. The pelvis is normal, apart from the silver clips from surgical treatment of megacolon. Mild coxa vara, bowing of the femurs and tibias with metaphyseal expansion, and irregular zones of provisional calcification are evident.

overgrowth frequently results in a varus deformity of the ankle. Atlantoaxial instability also has been reported in McKusick-type metaphyseal chondrodysplasia.[8] Radiographic changes in the thorax, including metaphyseal changes at the costochondral junctions of the ribs, Harrison grooves, and a prominent sternum, occur in two thirds of the patients.[201] The height of the lumbar vertebral bodies is increased out of proportion to their width, an appearance referred to as columnization of the vertebrae.[205] Caudal widening of the interpedicular distance does occur but is less than normal. Mild scoliosis affects as many as one fourth of these individuals, and exaggerated lumbar lordosis occurs in virtually all.[201,202]

Medical Considerations

The metaphyseal chondrodysplasia must be differentiated from disturbances of vitamin D metabolism if unnecessary pharmacologic intervention is to be avoided. Vitamin D therapy is ineffective for the treatment of metaphyseal chondrodysplasia.[205,206] Apart from the radiographic differences, biochemical abnormalities are not found in Schmid-type or McKusick-type metaphyseal chondrodysplasia.

Immunologic abnormalities have been found in more than one half of the patients with cartilage-hair hypoplasia. These patients are more susceptible to infections in childhood with a predisposition to severe varicella. These patients are at higher risk for malignancy including skin carcinomas, lymphomas, and sarcomas. Childhood anemia has been reported in 79% of children affected with cartilage-hair hypoplasia and was severe enough to warrant transfusion in 16%. Signs and symptoms of intestinal malabsorption and megacolon often develop in these patients.[201] Pediatric consultation is advisable.

Orthopaedic Implications

All patients with McKusick-type metaphyseal chondrodysplasia should be evaluated for possible atlantoaxial instability by lateral flexion-extension radiographs. If instability is more than 5 mm, a lateral flexion-extension MRI should be obtained to evaluate possible cord compression. If there is cord compromise, posterior atlantoaxial arthrodesis is indicated. Prophylactic fusion is warranted for the asymptomatic patient with instability measuring 8 mm or greater. In general, spinal deformities are mild and do not require active intervention. The coxa vara rarely requires corrective osteotomy. The genu varum present in infancy usually improves with growth during the first decade. Premature osteoarthritis is not common, because the epiphyses are normal and the residual varus deformities ordinarily are mild. Rarely, the genu varum does not improve, and surgery may be required for progressive varus deformity or pain. If surgical intervention is warranted clinically, a proximal tibiofibular osteotomy corrects simultaneously the varus deformity that is present at the knee and the ankle. Patients with McKusick-type metaphyseal chondrodysplasia occasionally require operative intervention for varus deformity of the ankle. In these instances, if the genu varum deformity is minimal, a supramalleolar osteotomy is preferred.

DYSCHONDROSTEOSIS

Dyschondrosteosis, first described by Léri and Weill, is characterized by a Madelung deformity of the wrist, mesomelic shortening of the upper and lower extremities, and autosomal dominant transmission with variable penetrance.[211,217,218] Controversy exists about whether the Madelung deformity, if bilateral, is an isolated abnormality separate from a generalized skeletal dysplasia.[214,216] The Madelung deformity has been associated with Turner syndrome and is common in patients with multiple hereditary exostoses (i.e., diaphyseal aclasis) or Ollier disease.[211] Premature closure of the ulnar-volar portion of the distal radial epiphysis may produce a similar deformity, although the most cases are unilateral. Langer concluded that bilateral Madelung deformities do not exist apart from dyschondrosteosis unless some other cause is present.[216] Felman and Kirkpatrick suggest that a diagnosis of dyschondrosteosis, a generalized skeletal dysplasia, should not be made for patients with bilateral Madelung deformities who are above the 25th percentile in height (i.e., not short-statured) unless there are other family members who have typical dyschondrosteosis.[214] However, some patients with dyschondrosteosis do not necessarily have the Madelung deformity; in these cases, the shortening of the radius and ulna is almost equal.[211]

Clinical Features

A definite diagnosis of dyschondrosteosis generally cannot be made until late childhood or adolescence, when the wrist deformity or short stature becomes obvious. Standing height is typically only mildly affected, with adult height ranging from 135 to 170 cm (53–70 in).[215] Disproportionate shortening of the limbs with mesomelic involvement occurs. The Madelung deformity, as evidenced by dorsal prominence of the ulnar head, dorsolateral bowing of the radius with shortening and volar subluxation of the wrist occasionally becomes painful during adolescence. Typically, there is limitation of the motion of the wrist and elbow, including pronation and supination. Lower limb changes are usually less severe, although asymmetric shortening of the tibia and fibula may occur, leading to mild angular deformities such as genu varum or valgus inclination of the ankle.[211]

Radiographic Features

A skeletal survey of a patient with dyschondrosteosis reveals minimal bony abnormalities in addition to the changes found in the radius, ulna, tibia, and fibula. In the presence of a clinical Madelung deformity, there is shortening and bowing of the radius with failure in the development of the ulnar aspect of the distal radial epiphysis. There is an abnormal ulnar and volar tilt of the distal radial articular surfaces. The distal radial epiphysis is triangular. The ulna is also disproportionately shortened, although usually not to the extent that the radius is shortened. The ulnar head is dislocated dorsally, and the carpal bones are wedged between the ends of the radius and the ulna (Fig. 7-37).[216] In patients with less severe involvement, the shortening of the radius and ulna may be more symmetric, although still disproportionate compared with the remainder of the extremity. The shafts may be thickened, with minimal bowing and subluxation of the wrist.[211] The Madelung deformity associated with multiple hereditary exostoses or Ollier disease is typified by excessive shortening of the ulna in comparison with the radius and the presence of multiple cartilaginous lesions identified on skeletal survey.

There is disproportionate shortening of the tibia and fibula with respect to the femur seen in patients with dyschondrosteosis. Epiphyseal and metaphyseal changes are absent, except for the occasional presence of an exostosis involving the proximal medial tibial metaphysis. The fibula may be excessively long compared with the tibia and occasionally has been associated with genu varum. However, valgus deformity of the ankle mortise has been observed when there is asymmetric shortening of the fibula.[183] Other mild, specific skeletal changes have been identified, including hypoplasia of the capital humeral epiphysis, cubitus valgus, coxa valga, and shortening of the metacarpals.

Orthopaedic Implications

Patients with dyschondrosteosis may require surgical intervention because of chronic wrist pain related to a severe Madelung deformity. For many patients, a period of protection with a lightweight wrist splint and administration of antiinflammatory agents alleviates the discomfort. If pain persists, surgical reconstruction may be considered. This requires a realignment osteotomy of the distal radius in combination with shortening of the distal ulna.[212,213] Alternatively, Vickers and Nielsen reported the results of prophylactic physiolysis (i.e., Langenskiold procedure) of the ulnar-volar distal radial physis in adolescents. Results were favorable if surgery was performed before significant deformities developed.[219]

CLEIDOCRANIAL DYSPLASIA

Cleidocranial dysplasia is an autosomal dominant disorder primarily involving bones formed by intramembranous ossification, such as the facial bones, cranium, and clavicles. The vertebral column and appendicular skeleton also are affected, indicating a disturbance of endochondral ossification as well. Marie and Sainton reported their observations of four patients in 1898 and named this disorder cleidocranial dysostosis. They described the now classic findings of increased transverse enlargement of the cranial vault, retarded ossification of the fontanelles, disturbances of dentition, hypoplasia-aplasia of the clavicles, and hereditary transmission of these malformations.[220] The

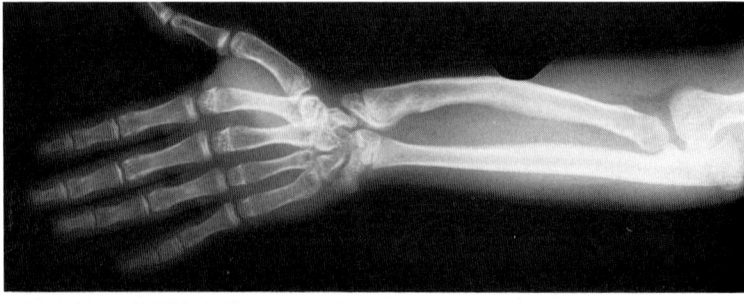
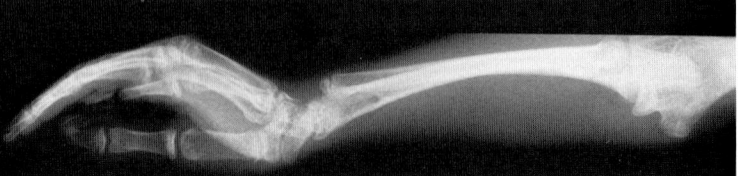

FIGURE 7-37. A 13-year-old patient with dyschondrosteosis has typical Madelung deformity.

preferred term is cleidocranial dysplasia, in recognition that a generalized disturbance of bone growth and development is present in this disorder. A specific chromosomal abnormality (8q22) was identified in one kindred.[221]

Clinical Features

Somatic development is altered, with evidence of growth retardation and slightly retarded skeletal maturation, in cleidocranial dysplasia. Stature is diminished with most male patients, ranging between the 5th and 50th percentile, and in female patients, falling below the 5th percentile.[225] Craniofacial abnormalities are numerous. In the calvaria, there is a marked delay of maturation as manifested by a severe reduction of calcification of all bones. For the newborn infant with cleidocranial dysplasia, development of the skull approximates that of a 20-week gestational age fetus. Midline defects in the sutures persist, in addition to biparietal cranial enlargement, frontal bossing, hypertelorism, midface hypoplasia, mandibular prognathism, and a highly arched palate. Nasal bone development is virtually absent along with absent or diminished paranasal sinuses.[227,228] Dental abnormalities are universal, including delayed or absent eruption of permanent teeth, defective formation, and supernumerary teeth. However, formation and maturation of primary teeth is normal.[226]

Those patients with absence of all or a significant portion of the clavicle have excessive shoulder mobility. Many are able to completely appose the shoulders anteriorly (Fig. 7-38). Palpable defects of the clavicles are present. Hand abnormalities include short, tapered fingers and thumb, with relative elongation of the second metacarpal. Clinodactyly of the fifth finger may be present as well.[224] The thorax is narrow and sloping, commonly associated with pectus excavatum. Scoliosis may develop in many patients, and syringomyelia has been reported.[222] Developmental coxa vara is a frequent problem for patients with cleidocranial dysplasia.[229]

Radiographic Features

Typically, patients with cleidocranial dysplasia have delayed closure at the sagittal and metopic sutures. The anterior fontanelle may remain open into adulthood. Other cranial findings include wormian bones, lateral bulging of the parietal bones, and calvarial thickening and sclerosis. An abnormal inclination of the clivus and foramen magnum have also been described.[224,228] Abnormalities of the clavicle include complete absence, hypoplasia, and most commonly, absence of the central portion of the clavicle with rudimentary medial and lateral portions remaining.

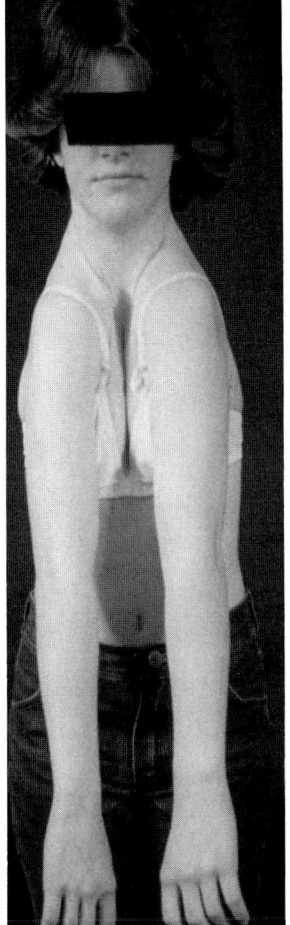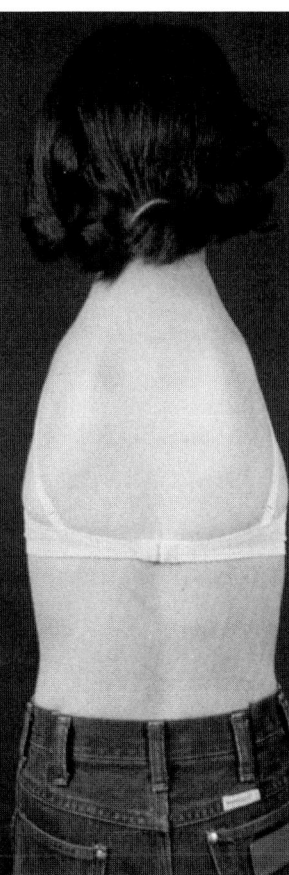

FIGURE 7-38. A 16-year-old patient with cleidocranial dysplasia has excessive shoulder mobility.

A remodeling defect of the sternal head with persistent flaring rather than the normal tubular configuration has been observed.[223,224] The clavicular defects frequently are associated with "drooping" ribs (Fig. 7-39). Many spinal abnormalities occur and appear to be related to abnormal development of ossification centers. Neural arch defects in the cervical thoracic spine occurred in 68% of patients and lumbar spondylolysis in 24% of patients in one series.[224] Posterior wedging of thoracic vertebrae is common. Scoliosis may develop, and in some instances, it is secondary to hemivertebrae formation.

In patients with cleidocranial dysplasia, the pelvis is typically involved, with hypoplasia of the iliac crest and delayed or absent ossification of the pubic symphysis. Hip abnormalities are common, such as unilateral or bilateral coxa vara, coxa valga, and shortening and broadening of the femoral head and neck (Fig. 7-40). A distinctive lateral notching of the capital femoral epiphysis may be found in some children.[224] The capital femoral epiphyses may be ossified at birth. In these

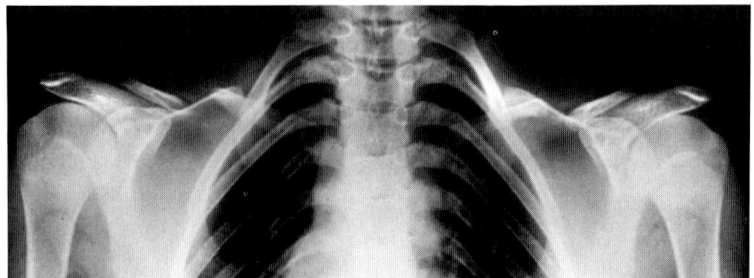

FIGURE 7-39. A 16-year-old patient with cleidocranial dysplasia. Notice the bilateral central defects of the clavicles and drooping ribs.

instances, the femoral neck is not ossified, and the physis appears excessively widened.[17] However, discontinuity of the femoral head and neck does not occur.

Hand abnormalities include shortening of the middle phalanges with cone epiphyses, pointed terminal tufts of the distal phalanges, accessory epiphyses at the base of the second or fifth metacarpals, broad, shortened first metacarpals, and clinodactyly.[224,225]

Orthopaedic Implications

Surgical intervention is not required for the clavicular defect found in patients with cleidocranial dysplasia. These deformities are asymptomatic, and attempts to reconstruct the clavicle are not recommended. Bone grafting is not indicated, as in congenital pseudarthrosis of the clavicle.

A valgus intertrochanteric osteotomy should be performed for progressive coxa vara or for a varus deformity of 100 degrees or less in the growing child. A femoral neck-shaft angle of greater than 140 degrees is desirable and is associated with significant improvement of acetabular dysplasia in children.[229] For patients with significant coxa vara and trochanteric overgrowth at maturity, trochanteric advancement may be considered to improve a Trendelenburg gait.

LARSEN SYNDROME

Larsen and associates described in six patients the constellation of findings that constitute Larsen syndrome.[231] This disorder is a true skeletal dysplasia, involving the face, spine, and appendicular skeleton. It is transmitted primarily as an autosomal dominant trait, but autosomal recessive transmission also has been observed.[10]

Clinical Features

Typical facial features have been described, including ocular hypertelorism, depression of the nasal bridge with flattening of the midface, and a prominent forehead. A cleft palate or abnormality of the uvula also may be present. Radial head dislocations usually are associated with cubitus varus, a loss of extension, and diminished pronation or supination. The fingers are cylindrical rather than tapering, and the distal phalanx of the thumb is spatulate. Scoliosis may affect the tho-

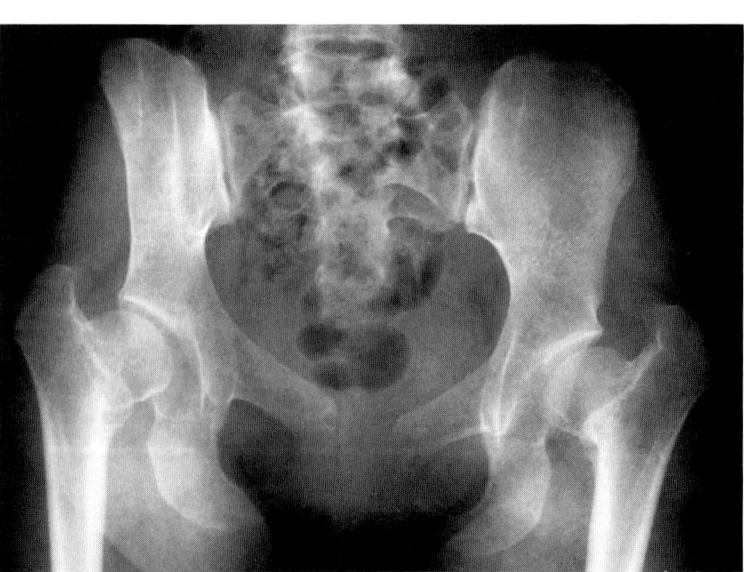

FIGURE 7-40. A 23-year-old patient with cleidocranial dysplasia. Notice the bilateral coxa vara, failure of ossification of the symphysis pubis, and hypoplasia of the iliac crest.

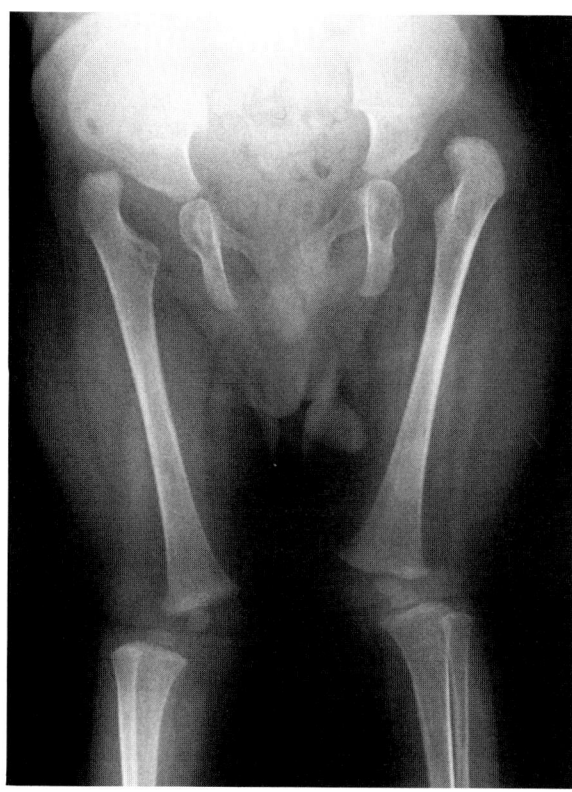

FIGURE 7-41. A 9-month-old patient with Larsen syndrome has bilateral dislocated hips and knees.

racic or lumbar spine. Increased lumbar lordosis is a common finding, a result of bilateral hip dislocations. Other lower extremity problems include anterior dislocation of the knee, evidenced by hyperextension deformity, and severe equinovarus or equinovalgus deformities of the feet. Hydrocephalus has been reported in one kindred, affecting two of three involved siblings.[235] Hearing impairment has also been described.

Radiographic Features

Dislocations of the hips, the knees, and the radial heads occur most frequently in Larsen syndrome (Fig. 7-41). However, dislocations also have been described in the shoulder, the carpometacarpal joint of the thumb, the patella, the metatarsocuneiform joints, and the wrists.[230,233,235] Hand abnormalities may occur, including loss of the normal distal tapering of the phalanges (giving a cylindrical appearance), delta phalanx of the thumb, shortened metacarpals, and pseudoepiphyses at the base of the second metacarpal. Characteristically, the carpal bone has multiple ossification centers. In addition to severe equinovarus or equinovalgus deformities, fusion of the embryonic centers for the calcaneus is delayed (Fig. 7-42).[235] Abnormal ossification of the cuboid also has been reported.[233]

Congenital defects of the cervical, thoracic, and lumbar spine occur frequently in patients with Larsen syndrome.[230-235] Deformities of the cervical spine are most common, including vertebral body hypoplasia, posterior element dysraphism, spondylolysis, and segmentation abnormalities. Severe cervical kyphosis may result and has been associated with significant neurologic alterations. (Fig. 7-43).[232,234] Thoracic scoliosis is usually secondary to congenital abnormalities, including hemivertebrae, wedged vertebrae, and posterior element anomalies. Similarly, scoliosis or spondylolysis may occur in the lumbar spine. Spinal dysraphism is observed frequently in the lumbar and sacral spine, although myelomeningoceles have not been reported.[230,231,233]

Orthopaedic Implications

Orthopaedic surgeons should avoid the tendency to diagnose Larsen syndrome in any child with multiple dislocations unless the characteristic facies and other osseous anomalies are present. Hip, knee, and foot deformities usually resist conservative treatment in these patients. Reduction of the knee dislocations should be completed before treatment of the hips, because at least 45 degrees of knee flexion is desirable to relax the hamstrings to maintain the reduction of the hip. If a hyperextension deformity or subluxation of the knee is present, manipulative casting may be

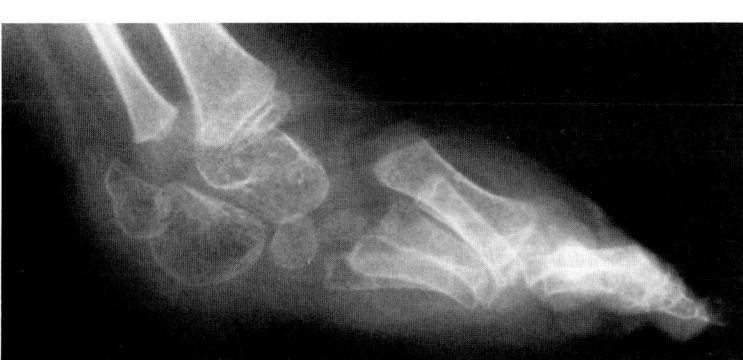

FIGURE 7-42. A 2-year-old patient with Larsen syndrome has severe equinovarus deformity. Two ossification centers of the calcaneus persist.

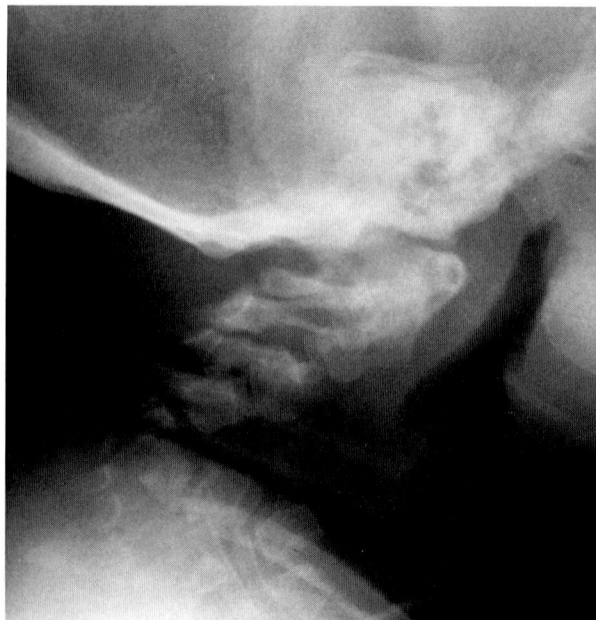

FIGURE 7-43. An 18-month-old patient with Larsen syndrome has severe cervical kyphosis secondary to vertebral body hypoplasia and spinal dysraphism.

initiated in the newborn. However, if the knee is dislocated, open reduction generally is required to achieve a satisfactory result. The surgical procedure for reduction includes V-Y lengthening of the quadriceps mechanism, transverse anterior capsulotomy, and release of the collateral ligaments, if necessary, to achieve 90 degrees of flexion. After reduction of the knee is accomplished and motion is regained, reduction of the hip dislocation should be considered. In general, this requires open reduction using standard techniques and may require femoral shortening to facilitate reduction. If not corrected by manipulative casting, equinovarus foot deformities are treated by posteromedial releases.

The high incidence of cervical spine abnormalities in patients with Larsen syndrome necessitates careful evaluation of the cervical spine at first presentation and before administration of any anesthetic agent. Potential instability should be assessed by lateral flexion-extension radiographs. Cervical kyphosis has been implicated as the cause of generalized hypotonia from birth, quadriplegia, and sudden death of patients with Larsen syndrome.[230,234] Patients with mild cervical kyphosis associated with hypoplasia of a vertebral body should be observed. These patients usually do not have significant instability, and progressive kyphosis is infrequently seen.

Surgical stabilization is indicated for Larsen syndrome patients with the most severe cervical kyphosis or instability. Posterior fusion may not be sufficient for patients with severe kyphosis or large dysraphic segments. In these circumstances, staged anteroposterior fusion should be considered.

References
General

1. Andersen P. Prevalence of lethal chondrodysplasias in Denmark. Am J Med Genet 1989;32:484.
2. Beighton P, Giedion ZA, Gorlin R, et al. International classification of osteochondrodysplasias. Am J Med Genet 1992; 44:223.
3. Bethem D, Winter RB, Lutter L, et al. Spinal disorders of dwarfism. Review of the literature and report of eighty cases. J Bone Joint Surg [Am] 1981;63:1412.
4. Erik P Jr, Hauge M. Congenital generalized bone dysplasias: a clinical, radiological, and epidemiological survey. J Med Genet 1989;27:37.
5. Hall B. Approach to skeletal dysplasia. Pediatr Clin North Am 1992;39:279.
6. Hensinger RN. Standards in pediatric orthopaedics. Tables, charts, and graphs illustrating growth. New York: Raven Press, 1986.
7. Kopits SE. Orthopaedic complications of dwarfism. Clin Orthop 1976;114:153.
8. Kopits SE, Perovic MN, McKusick VA, et al. Congenital atlantoaxial dislocations in various forms of dwarfism. Proceedings of the American Academy of Orthopaedic Surgeons, Washington, DC, 1972. J Bone Joint Surg [Am] 1972;54:1349.
9. Marsh MM. Linear growth of long bones of the extremities from infancy through adolescence. Am J Dis Child 1955; 89:725.
10. McKusick VA. Mendelian inheritance in man. Catalogue of autosomal dominant, autosomal recessive, and X-linked phenotypes. 10th ed. Baltimore: Johns Hopkins University Press, 1992.
11. Rimoin DL. The chondrodystrophies. Adv Hum Genet 1974;5:1.
12. Rimoin DL, Silberberg R, Hollister DW. Chondro-osseous pathology in the chondrodystrophies. Clin Orthop 1976;114:137.
13. Robinow M, Chumlea WC. Standards for limb bone length ratios in children. Radiology 1982;143:433.
14. Sillence DO, Horton WA, Rimoin DL. Morphologic studies in skeletal dysplasias. Am J Pathol 1979;96:813.
15. Stanescu V, Stanescu R, Maroteaux P. Pathogenic mechanisms in osteochondrodysplasias. J Bone Joint Surg [Am] 1984; 66:817.
16. Stelling FH. The hip in heritable conditions of connective tissue. Clin Orthop 1973;90:33.
17. Wynne-Davies R, Hall CM, Apley AG. Atlas of skeletal dysplasias. New York: Churchill Livingstone, 1985.

Achondroplasia

18. Aldegheri R, Trivella G, Renzi-Brivio L, et al. Lengthening of the lower limbs in achondroplastic patients. A comparative study of four techniques. J Bone Joint Surg [Br] 1988;70:69.
19. Aryanpur J, Hurko O, Francomano C, et al. Craniocervical decompression for cervicomedullary compression in pediatric patients with achondroplasia. J Neurosurg 1990;73:375.
20. Bailey JA. Orthopaedic aspects of achondroplasia. J Bone Joint Surg [Am] 1970;52:1285.
21. Bell DF, Boyer MI, Armstrong PF. The use of the Ilizarov technique in the correction of limb deformities associated with skeletal dysplasia. J Pediatr Orthop 1992;12:283.

22. Carson B, Winfield J, Wang H, et al. Surgical management of cervico-medullary compression in achondroplastic patients. In: Nicoletti B, ed. Human achondroplasia: a multidisciplinary approach. New York: Plenum Press, 1986:207.
23. Cohen ME, Rosenthal AD, Matson DD. Neurological abnormalities in achondroplastic children. J Pediatr 1967;71:367.
24. Correll J. Surgical correction of short stature in skeletal dysplasias. Acta Paediatr Scand 1991;377:143.
25. DeBastiani G, Aldegheri R, Brivio LB, et al. Chondrodiatasis—controlled symmetrical distraction of the epiphyseal plate: limb lengthening in children. J Bone Joint Surg [Br] 1986;68:550.
26. DeBastiani G, Aldegheri R, Renzi-Brivio L, et al. Limb lengthening by callus distraction (callotasis). J Pediatr Orthop 1987;7:129.
27. Fortuna A, Ferrante L, Santoro. Narrowing of the thoracolumbar spinal canal in achondroplasia. J Neurosurg Sci 1989;33:185.
28. Francomano CA, Le P-L, Pyeritz RE. Molecular genetic studies in achondroplasia. In: Nicoletti B, ed. New York: Plenum Press, 1986:53.
29. Ganel A, Horoszowski H, Kamhin M, et al. Leg lengthening in achondroplastic children. Clin Orthop 1979;144:194.
30. Ganel A, Israel A, Horoszowski H. Fatal complication of femoral elongation in an achondroplastic dwarf. A case report. Clin Orthop 1984;185:69.
31. Giglio GC, Passariello R, Pagnotta G, et al. Anatomy of the lumbar spine in achondroplasia. In: Nicoletti B, ed. Human achondroplasia: a multi-disciplinary approach. New York: Plenum Press, 1986:227.
32. Hahn YS, Engelhard HH, Naidich T. Paraplegia resulting from thoracolumbar stenosis in a seven-month-old achondroplastic dwarf. Pediatr Neurosci 1989;15:39.
33. Hecht JT, Butler IJ. Neurologic morbidity associated with achondroplasia. J Child Neurol 1990;5:84.
34. Hecht JT, Butler IJ, Scott CI. Long-term neurological sequelae in achondroplasia. Eur J Pediatr 1984;143:58.
35. Hecht JT, Francomano CA, Horton WA, et al. Mortality in achondroplasia. Am J Hum Genet 1987;41:454.
36. Hecht JT, Hood OJ, Schwartz RJ, et al. Obesity in achondroplasia. Am J Med Genet 1988;31:597.
37. Hecht JT, Horton WA, Reid CS, et al. Growth of the foramen magnum in achondroplasia. Am J Med Genet 1989;32:528.
38. Hecht JT, Nelson FW, Butler IJ, et al. Computerized tomography of the foramen magnum: achondroplastic values compared to normal standards. Am J Med Genet 1986;20:355.
39. Hecht JT, Thompson NM, Weir T, et al. Cognitive and motor skills in achondroplastic infants: neurologic and respiratory correlates. Am J Med Genet 1991;41:208.
40. Herring jA. Kyphosis in an achondroplastic dwarf. J Pediatr Orthop 1983;3:250.
41. Horton WA, Hecht JT, Hood OJ, et al. Growth hormone therapy in achondroplasia. Am J Med Genet 1992;42:667.
42. Horton WA, Hood OJ. Growth plate cartilage studies in achondroplasia. In: Nicoletti B, ed. Human achondroplasia: a multi-disciplinary approach. New York: Plenum Press, 1986:81.
43. Horton WA, Rotter JI, Rimoin DL, et al. Standard growth curves for achondroplasia. J Pediatr 1978;93:435.
44. Ippolito E, Maynard JA, Mickelson MR, et al. Histochemical and ultrastructural study of the growth plate in achondroplasia. In: Nicoletti B, ed. Human achondroplasia: a multidisciplinary approach. New York: Plenum Press, 1986:61.
45. Isaksson OGP, Lindahl A, Nilsson A, et al. Action of growth hormone: current views. Acta Paediatr Scand Suppl 1988;343:12.
46. Kahanovitz N, Rimoin DL, Sillence DO. The clinical spectrum of lumbar spine disease in achondroplasia. Spine 1982;7:137.
47. Kopits SE. Thoracolumbar kyphosis and lumbosacral hyperlordosis in achondroplastic children. In: Nicoletti B, ed. Human achondroplasia: a multi-disciplinary approach. New York: Plenum Press, 1986:241.
48. Langer LO Jr, Baumann PA, Gorlin RJ. Achondroplasia. Am J Roentgenol 1967;100:12.
49. Lavini F, Renzi-Brivio L, DeBastiani G. Psychologic, vascular, and physiologic aspects of lower limb lengthening in achondroplastics. Clin Orthop 1990;250:138.
50. Lonstein JE. Anatomy of the lumbar spine canal. In: Nicoletti B, ed. Human achondroplasia: a multi-disciplinary approach. New York: Plenum Press, 1986:219.
51. Lonstein JE. Treatment of kyphosis and lumbar stenosis in achondroplasia. In: Nicoletti B, ed. Human achondroplasia: a multi-disciplinary approach. New York: Plenum Press, 1986:283
52. Lutter LD, Langer LO. Neurological symptoms in achondroplastic dwarfs—surgical treatment. J Bone Joint Surg [Am] 1977;59:87.
53. Lutter LD, Lonstein JE, Winter RB, et al. Anatomy of the achondroplastic lumbar canal. Clin Orthop 1977;126:139.
54. Maynard JA, Ippolito EG, Ponseti IV, et al. Histochemistry and ultrastructure of the growth plate in achondroplasia. J Bone Joint Surg [Am] 1981;63:969.
55. McDonald JM, Seipp WS, Gordon EM, et al. Audiologic findings in achondroplasia. In: Nicoletti B, ed. Human achondroplasia: a multi-disciplinary approach. New York: Plenum Press, 1986:143.
56. Morgan DF, Young RF. Spinal neurological complications of achondroplasia. Results of surgical treatment. J Neurosurg 1980;52:463.
57. Nehme A-ME, Riseborough EJ, Tredwell SJ. Skeletal growth and development of the achondroplastic dwarf. Clin Orthop 1976;116:8.
58. Nelson FW, Goldie WD, Hecht JT, et al. Short-latency somatosensory evoked potentials in the management of patients with achondroplasia. Neurology 1984;34:1053.
59. Nelson FW, Hecht JT, Horton WA, et al. Neurologic basis of respiratory complications in achondroplasia. An Neurol 1988;24:89.
60. Nilsson A, Isgaard J, Lindahl A, et al. Regulation by growth hormone of number of chondrocytes containing IGF-I in rat growth plate. Science 1986;233:571.
61. Nishi Y, Kaliyama M, Miyagawa S, et al. Growth hormone therapy in achondroplasia. Acta Endocrinol 1993;5:394.
62. Paley D. Current techniques of limb lengthening. J Pediatr Orthop 1988;8:73.
63. Parrot JM. Sur les malformations achondroplasiques et le Dieu Ptah. Bull Soc Antropol 1878;1:296.
64. Pauli RM, Scott CI, Wassman ER Jr, et al. Apnea and sudden unexpected death in infants with achondroplasia. J Pediatr 1984;104:342.
65. Pedrini-Mille A, Pedrini V. Proteoglycans and glycosaminoglycans of human achondroplastic cartilage. J Bone Joint Surg [Am] 1982;64:39.
66. Pierre-Kahn A, Hirsch JF, Renier D, et al. Hydrocephalus and achondroplasia: a study of 25 observations. Childs Brain 1980;7:205.
67. Pinelli V, Masi R, Partipilo P, et al. Otologic impairments in achondroplasia: a nosologic assessment. In: Nicoletti B, ed. Human achondroplasia: a multi-disciplinary approach. New York: Plenum Press, 1986:149.
68. Ponseti IV. Skeletal growth in achondroplasia. J Bone Joint Surg [Am] 1970;52:701.
69. Pyeritz RE, Sack GH Jr, Udvarhelyi GB. Thoracolumbosacral laminectomy in achondroplasia: long term results in 22 patients. Am J Med Genet 1987;28:433.

70. Reid CS, Pyeritz RE, Kopits SE, et al. Cervicomedullary compression in young patients with achondroplasia: value of comprehensive neurologic and respiratory evaluation. J Pediatr 1987;110:522.
71. Rimoin DI, Hughes GN, Kaufman RL, et al. Endochondral ossification in achondroplastic dwarfism. N Engl J Med 1970;283:728.
72. Scott CI Jr. Achondroplastic and hypochondroplastic dwarfism. Clin Orthop 1976;114:18.
73. Siebens AA, Kirby N, Hungerford D. Orthotic correction of sitting abnormality in achondroplastic children. In: Nicoletti B, ed. Human achondroplasia: a multi-disciplinary approach. New York: Plenum Press, 1986:313.
74. Steinbok P, Hall J, Flodmark O. Hydrocephalus in achondroplasia: the possible role of intracranial venous hypertension. J Neurosurg 1989;71:42.
75. Stokes DC, Pyeritz RE, Wise RA, et al. Spirometry and chest wall dimensions in achondroplasia. Chest 1988;93:364.
76. Stokes DC, Wohl ME, Wise RA, et al. The lungs and airways in achondroplasia. Do little people have little lungs? Chest 1988;98:145.
77. Streeten E, Uematsu S, Hurko O, et al. Extended laminectomy for spinal stenosis in achondroplasia. In: Nicoletti B, ed. Human achondroplasia: a multi-disciplinary approach. New York: Plenum Press, 1986:261.
78. Streeten E, Uematsu S, Hurko O, et al. Extended laminectomy for spinal stenosis in achondroplasia. Basic Life Sci 1988;48:261.
79. Suss RA, Udvarhelyi GB, Wang G, et al. Myelography in achondroplasia: value of a lateral C1-2 puncture and non-ionic, water soluble contrast medium. Radiology 1983;149:159.
80. Todorov AB, Scott CI Jr, Warren AE, et al. Developmental screening tests in achondroplastic children. Am J Med Genet 1981;9:19.
81. Tolo VT. Surgical treatment of kyphosis in achondroplasia. In: Nicoletti B, ed. Human achondroplasia: a multi-disciplinary approach. New York: Plenum Press, 1986:257.
82. Uematsu S. Wang H, Hurko O, et al. The subarachnoid fluid space in achondroplastic spinal stenosis: the surgical implication. In: Nicoletti B, ed. Human achondroplasia: a multi-disciplinary approach. New York: Plenum Press, 1986:275.
83. Vilarrubias JM, Ginebreda I, Jimeno E. Lengthening of the lower limbs and correction of hyperlordosis in achondroplasia. Clin Orthop 1990;250:143.
84. Wang H, Rosenbaum AE, Reid CS, et al. Pediatric patients with achondroplasia: CT evaluation of the craniocervical junction. Radiology 1987;164:515.
85. Wynne-Davies R, Walsh K, Gormley J. Achondroplasia and hypochondroplasia. Clinical variation and spinal stenosis. J Bone Joint Surg [Br] 1981;63:508.
86. Yamada H, Nakamura S, Tajima M, et al. Neurological manifestations of pediatric achondroplasia. J Neurosurg 1981;54:49.
87. Yang SS, Corbett DP, Brough AJ, et al. Upper cervical myelopathy in achondroplasia. Am J Clin Pathol 1977;68:68.

Hypochondroplasia

88. Beals RK. Hypochondroplasia. A report of five kindreds. J Bone Joint Surg [Am] 1969;51:728.
89. Bridges NA, Hindmarsh PC, Brook CG. Growth of children with hypochondroplasia treated with growth hormone for up to three years. Horm Res 1991;36(Suppl 1):56.
90. Fasanelli S. Hypochondroplasia: radiological diagnosis and differential diagnosis. In: Nicoletti B, ed. Human achondroplasia: a multi-disciplinary approach. New York: Plenum Press, 1986:163.
91. Hall BD, Spranger J. Hypochondroplasia: clinical and radiological aspects in 39 cases. Radiology 1979;133:95.
92. Mullis PE, Patel MS, Brickell PM, et al. Growth characteristics and response to growth hormone therapy in patients with hypochondroplasia: genetic linkage of the insulin-like growth factor I gene at chromosome 12q23 to the disease in a subgroup of these patients. Clin Endocrinol 1991;34:265.
93. Oberklaid F, Danks DM, Jensen F, et al. Achondroplasia and hypochondroplasia. Comments on frequency, mutation rate, and radiological features in skull and spine. J Med Genet 1979;16:140.

Metatropic Dysplasia

94. Beck M, Roubechek M, Rogers JG, et al. Heterogeneity of metatropic dysplasia. Eur J Pediatr 1983;140:231.
95. Boden SA, Kaplan FS, Fallon MD, et al. Metatropic dwarfism. J Bone Joint Surg [Am] 1987;69:174.
96. Maroteaux P, Spranger JW, Wiedemann H-R. Der Metatrophische Zwergwuchs. Arch Kinder 1966;173:211.
97. Rimoin DL, Siggers DC, Lachman RS, et al. Metatropic dwarfism, the Kniest syndrome, and the pseudoachondroplastic dysplasias. Clin Orthop 1976;114:70.
98. Shohat M, Lachman R, Rimoin DL. Odontoid hypoplasia with vertebral subluxation and ventriculomegaly in metatropic dysplasia. J Pediatr 1989;114:239.

Chondroectodermal Dysplasia

99. Ellis RWB, van Creveld S. A syndrome characterized by ectodermal dysplasia, polydactyly, chondrodysplasia, and congenital morbus cordia. Arch Dis Child 1940;15:65.
100. Kaitila II, Leisti JT, Rimoin DL. Mesomelic skeletal dysplasias. Clin Orthop 1976;114:94.
101. Kruse RK, Bowen JR, Heithoff S. Oblique tibial osteotomy in the correction of tibial deformity in children. J Pediatr Orthop 1989;9:476.
102. McKusick VA, Egeland JA, Eldridge R, et al. Dwarfism in the Amish. I. The Ellis-van Creveld syndrome. Bull Johns Hopkins Hosp 1964;115:306.
103. Paley D, Tetsworth K. Mechanical axis deviation of the lower limbs: preoperative planning of uniapical angular deformities of the femur or tibia. Clin Orthop 1992;280:48.
104. Paley D, Tetsworth K. Mechanical axis deviation of the lower limbs: preoperative planning of multiapical frontal plane angular and bowing deformities of the femur and tibia. Clin Orthop 1992;280:65.
105. Pinelli G, Cottafava F, Senes FM, et al. Ellis-van Creveld syndrome: description of four cases. Orthopaedic aspects. Ital J Orthop Traumatol 1990;16:113.
106. Rab GT. Oblique tibial osteotomy for Blount's disease (tibia vara). J Pediatr Orthop 1988;8:715.

Diastrophic Dysplasia

107. Bethem D, Winter RB, Lutter L. Disorders of the spine in diastrophic dwarfism. J Bone Joint Surg [Am] 1980;62:529.
108. Gembruch U, Niesen M, Kehrberg H, et al. Diastrophic dysplasia: a specific prenatal diagnosis by ultrasound. Prenat Diagn 1988;8:539.
109. Haestbacka J, Kaitila I, Sistonen P, et al. A linkage map spanning the locus for diastrophic dysplasia (DTD). Genomics 1991;4:968.
110. Herring J. The spinal disorders in diastrophic dwarfism. J Bone Joint Surg [Am] 1978;60:177.
111. Hollister DW, Lachman RS. Diastrophic dwarfism. Clin Orthop 1976;114:61.

112. Horton WA, Hall JG, Scott CI, et al. Growth curves for height for diastrophic dysplasia, spondyloepiphyseal dysplasia congenita, and pseudoachondroplasia. Am J Dis Child 1982;136:316.
113. Horton WA, Rimoin DL, Lachman RS, et al. The phenotypic variability of diastrophic dysplasia. J Pediatr 1978;93:609.
114. Kash IJ, Sane SM, Samaha FJ, et al. Cervical cord compression in diastrophic dwarfism. J Pediatr 1974;78:862.
115. Krecak J, Starshak RJ. Cervical kyphosis in diastrophic dwarfism: CT and MRI findings. Pediatr Radiol 1987;17:321.
116. Lachman R, Sillence D, Rimoin D, et al. Diastrophic dysplasia: the death of a variant. Radiology 1981;140:79
117. Lamy M, Maroteaux P. Le nanisme diastrophique. Presse Med 1960;68:1977.
118. McKusick VA, Goodman RM. Pinnal calcification: observations in systemic disease not associated with disorded calcium metabolism. JAMA 1962;179:230.
119. Murray LW, Hollister DW, Rimoin DL. Diastrophic dysplasia: evidence against a defect of type II collagen. Matrix 1989;9:459.
120. Peltonen JI, Hoikka V, Poussa M, et al. Cementless hip arthroplasty in diastrophic dysplasia. J Arthroplasty 1992; 7(Suppl):369.
121. Poussa M, Merikanto J, Ryoeppy S, et al. The spine in diastrophic dysplasia. Spine 1991;16:881.
122. Richards BS. Atlanto-axial instability in diastrophic dysplasia. A case report. J Bone Joint Surg [Am] 1991;73:614.
123. Ryoeppy S, Poussa M, Merikanto J, et al. Foot deformities in diastrophic dysplasia. An analysis of 102 patients. J Bone Joint Surg 1992;74:441.
124. Shapiro F. Light and electron microscopic abnormalities in diastrophic dysplasia growth cartilage. Calcif Tissue Int 1992;51:324.
125. Tolo VT, Kopits SE. Spinal deformity in diastrophic dysplasia. Orthop Trans 1983;7:31.
126. Walker BA, Scott CI, Hall JG, et al. Diastrophic dwarfism. Medicine (Baltimore) 1972;51:41.

Kniest Dysplasia

127. Kniest W. Zur Abgrenzung der Dyostotosis Enchondralis von der Chondrodystrophie. Z Kinder 1952;70:633.
128. Lachman RS, Rimoin DL, Hollister DW, et al. The Kniest syndrome. AJR 1975;123:805.
129. Merrill KD, Schmidt TL. Occipitoatlantal instability in a child with Kniest syndrome. J Pediatr 1990;116:596.
130. Poole AR, Pidoux I, Reiner A, et al. Kniest dysplasia is characterized by an apparent abnormal processing of the C-propeptide of type II collagen resulting in imperfect fibril assembly. J Clin Invest 1988;81:579.
131. Siggers DC, Rimoin DL, Dorst JP, et al. The Kniest syndrome. Birth Defects 1974;10:193.
132. Spranger JW, Maroteaux P. Kniest disease. Birth Defects 1974;10:50.

Spondyloepiphyseal Dysplasia Congenita

133. Anderson CE, Sillence DO, Lachman RS, et al. Spondylomet-epiphyseal dysplasia, Strudwick type. Am J Med Genet 1982;13:243
134. Cole WG, Hall RK, Rogers JG. The clinical features of spondyloepiphyseal dysplasia congenita resulting from the substitution of glycine 997 by serine in the alpha 1(II) chain of type II collagen. J Med Genet 1993;30:27.
135. Fielding JW, Hensinger RN, Hawkins RJ. Os odontoideum. J Bone Joint Surg [Am] 1980;62:376.
136. Harrod MJ, Friedman JM, Currarino G, et al. Genetic heterogeneity in spondyloepiphyseal dysplasia congenita. Am J Med Genet 1984;18:311.
137. Horton WA, Campbell D, Machado MA, et al. Type II collagen screening in the human chondrodysplasias. Am J Med Genet 1989;34:579.
138. Maroteaux P, Spranger J. The spondylometaphyseal dysplasias. A tentative classification. Pediatr Radiol 1991;21:293.
139. Murray LW, Bautista J, James PL, et al. Type II collagen defects in the chondrodysplasias. I. Spondyloepiphyseal dysplasias. Am J Med Genet 1989;45:5.
140. Spranger JW, Langer LO Jr. Spondyloepiphyseal dysplasia congenita. Radiology 1970;94:313.
141. Williams B, Cranley RE. Morphologic observations on four cases of SED congenita. Birth Defects 1974;10:75.
142. Wynne-Davies R, Hall C. Two clinical variants of spondyloepiphysial dysplasia congenita. J Bone Joint Surg [Br] 1982;64:435.
143. Yang SS, Chen H, Williams P, et al. Spondyloepiphyseal dysplasia congenita: a comparative study of chondrocyte inclusions. Arch Pathol Lab Med 1980;104:208.

Spondyloepiphyseal Dysplasia Tarda

144. Barber KE, Gow PJ, Mayo KM. A family with multiple musculoskeletal abnormalities. Am Rheum Dis 1984;43:275.
145. Diamond LS. A family study of spondyloepiphyseal dysplasia. J Bone Joint Surg [Am] 1970;52:1587.
146. Kaibara N, Takagishi K, Katsuki I. Spondyloepiphyseal dysplasia tarda with progressive arthropathy. Skeletal Radiol 1983;10:13.
147. Pinelli G, Cottafava F, Senes FM. Spondyloepiphyseal dysplasia tarda: linkage with genetic markers from the distal short arm of the X chromosome. Hum Genet 1988;81:61.

Pseudoachondroplastic Dysplasia

148. Cooper RR, Ponseti IV, Maynard JA. Pseudoachondroplastic dwarfism. A rough-surfaced endoplasmic reticulum storage disorder. J Bone Joint Surg [Am] 1973;55:475.
149. Hall JG. Pseudoachondroplasia. Birth Defects 1975;1:187.
150. Hall JG, Bailey JA, Dorst JP, et al. Pseudoachondroplastic SED, recessive Maroteaux-Lamy type. Birth Defects 1969;5:254.
151. Hecht JT, Blanton SH, Wang Y, et al. Exclusion of human proteoglycan link protein (CRTL1) and type II collagen (COL2A1) genes in pseudoachondroplasia. Am J Med Genet 1992;44:420.
152. Horton WA, Hall JG, Scott CI, et al. Growth curves for height for diastrophic dysplasia, spondyloepiphyseal dysplasia congenita, and pseudoachondroplasia. Am J Dis Child 1982; 136:316.
153. Kopits SE, Lindstrom JA, McKusik VA. Pseudoachondroplastic dysplasia: pathodynamics and management. Birth Defects 1974;10:341.
154. Maroteaux P, Lamy M. Les formes pseudo-achondroplastique des dysplasies spondylo-epiphysaries. Presse Med 1959; 67:383.
155. Pedrini-Mille A, Maynard JA, Pedrini VA. Pseudoachondroplasia: biochemical and histochemical studies of cartilage. J Bone Joint Surg [Am] 1984;66:1408.

Multiple Epiphyseal Dysplasia

156. Apley AG, Wientroub S. The sagging rope sign in Perthes' disease and allied disorders. J Bone Joint Surg [Br] 1981;63:43.
157. Crossan JF, Wynne-Davies R, Fulford GE. Bilateral failure of the capital femoral epiphysis: bilateral Perthes disease, multi-

ple epiphyseal dysplasia, pseudoachondroplasia, and spondyloepiphyseal dysplasia congenita and tarda. J Pediatr Orthop 1983;3:297.
158. Fairbank T. Dysplasia epiphysialis multiplex. Br J Surg 1947;34:325.
159. Griffiths HE, Witherow PJ. Perthes disease and multiple epiphyseal dysplasia. Postgrad Med J 1977;53:464.
160. Hunt DD, Ponseti IV, Pedrini-Mille A, et al. Multiple epiphyseal dysplasia in two siblings. J Bone Joint Surg [Am] 1967;49:1611.
161. Ingram RR. The shoulder in multiple epiphyseal dysplasia. J Bone Joint Surg [Br] 1991;73:277.
162. Ingram RR. Early diagnosis of multiple epiphyseal dysplasia. J Pediatr Orthop 1992;12:241.
163. Jacobs PA. Dysplasia epiphysialis multiplex. Clin Orthop 1968;58:117.
164. Kruse RW, Guille JT, Bowen JR. Shelf arthroplasty in patients who have Legg-Calve-Perthes disease. A study of long-term results. J Bone Joint Surg [Am] 1991;73:1338.
165. MacKenzie WG, Bassett GS, Mandell GA, et al. Avascular necrosis of the hip in multiple epiphyseal dysplasia. J Pediatr Orthop 1989;9:666.
166. Mandell GA, MacKenzie WG, Scott CI Jr, et al. Identification of avascular necrosis in the dysplastic proximal femoral epiphysis. Skeletal Radiol 1989;18:273.
167. Ribbing S. Studien uber Hereditare. Multiple Epiphysenstorungen. Acta Radiol 1937;(Suppl):34.
168. Schlesinger AE, Poznanski AK, Pudlowski RM, et al. Distal femoral epiphyses: normal standards for thickness and application to bone dysplasias. Radiology 1986;159:515.
169. Spranger J. The epiphyseal dysplasias. Clin Orthop 1976;114:46.
170. Stanescu R, Stanescu V, Muriel MP, et al. Multiple epiphyseal dysplasia, Fairbank type: morphologic and biochemical study of cartilage. Am J Med Genet 1993;45:501.
171. Treble NJ, Jensen FO, Bankier A, et al. Development of the hip in multiple epiphyseal dysplasia. Natural history and susceptibility to premature osteoarthritis. J Bone Joint Surg [Br] 1990;72:1061.
172. Willett K, Hudson I, Catterall A. Lateral shelf acetabuloplasty: an operation for older children with Perthes' disease. J Pediatr Orthop 1992;12:563.

Chondrodysplasia Punctata

173. Andersen PE, Justesen P. Chondrodysplasia punctata: report of two cases. Skeletal Radiol 1987;16:223.
174. Bethem D. Os odontoideum in chondrodystrophia calcificans congenita. A case report. J Bone Joint Surg [Am] 1982;64:1385.
175. Borg SA, Fitzer PM, Young LY. Roentgenologic aspects of adult cretinism. AJR 1975;123:820.
176. Burck U. Mesomelic dysplasia with punctate epiphyseal calcifications. Eur J Pediatr 1982;138:67.
177. Curry CJR, Magenis RE, Brown M, et al. Inherited chondrodysplasia punctata due to a deletion of the terminal short arm of an X-chromosome. N Engl J Med 1984;311:1010.
178. Fairbank HAT. Dysplasia epiphysealis punctata. Symptoms: stippled epiphyses, chondrodystrophia calcificans congenita (Hunermann). J Bone Joint Surg [Br] 1949;31:114.
179. Gilbert EF, Opitz JM, Spranger JW, et al. Chondrodysplasia punctata—rhizomelic form, pathologic and radiographic studies of three infants. Eur J Pediatr 1976;123:89.
180. Hanson JW, Smith DW. The fetal hydantoin syndrome. J Pediatr 1975;87:285.
181. Happle R. X-linked dominant chondrodysplasia punctata. Hum Genet 1979;53:65.
182. Harrod MJ, Sherrod PS. Warfarin embryopathy in siblings. Obstet Gynecol 1981;57:673.
183. Heymans HSA, Oorthuys JWE, Nelck G, et al. Rhizomelic chondrodysplasia punctata: another peroxisomal disorder. N Engl J Med 1985;313:187.
184. Hoefler S, Hoefler G, Moser AB, et al. Prenatal diagnosis of rhizomelic chondrodysplasia punctata. Prenat Diagn 1988;8:571.
185. Lawrence JJ, Schlesinger AE, Kozlowski K, et al. Unusual radiographic manifestations of chondrodysplasia punctata. Skeletal Radiol 1989;18:15.
186. Manzke H, Christophers E, Wiedemann H-R. Dominant sex-linked inherited chondrodysplasia punctata: a distinct type of chondrodysplasia punctata. Clin Genet 1980;17:97.
187. Mueller RF, PM Crowle, Jones RAK, et al. X-linked dominant chondrodysplasia punctata. Am J Med Genet 1985;20:137.
188. Pauli RM, Lian JB, Mosher DF, et al. Association of congenital deficiency of multiple vitamin K-dependent coagulation factors and the phenotype of the warfarin embryopathy: clues to the mechanism of teratogenicity of coumarin derivatives. Am J Med Genet 1987;41:566.
189. Pike MG, Applegarth DA, Dunn HG, et al. Congenital rubella syndrome associated with calcific epiphyseal stippling and peroxisomal dysfunction. J Pediatr 1990;116:88.
190. Rittler M, Menger H, Spranger J. Chondrodysplasia punctata, tibia-metacarpal (MT) type. Am J Med Genet 1990;37:200.
191. Sheffield LJ, Halliday JL, Danks DM, et al. Clinical, radiologic, and biochemical classification of chondrodysplasia punctata. Am J Med Genet 1989;45(Suppl A):A64.
192. Silengo MC, Luzzatti L, Silverman FN. Clinical and genetic aspects of Conradi-Hunermann disease: a report of three familial cases and review of the literature. J Pediatr 1980;97:911.
193. Spranger JW, Opitz JM, Bidder U. Heterogeneity of chondrodysplasia punctata. Humangenetik 1971;11:190.
194. Wardinsky TD, Pagon RA, Powell BR, et al. Rhizomelic chondrodysplasia punctata and survival beyond one year: a review of the literature and five case reports. Clin Genet 1990;38:84.
195. Wulfsberg EA, Curtis J, Jayne CH. Chondrodysplasia punctata: a boy with X-linked recessive chondrodysplasia punctata due to an inherited X-Y translocation with a current classification of these disorders. Am J Med Genet 1992;43:823

Metaphyseal Chondrodysplasia

196. Cooper RR, Ponseti IV. Metaphyseal dysostosis: description of an ultrastructural defect in the epiphyseal plate chondrocytes. Case report. J Bone Joint Surg [Am] 1973;55:485.
197. Dent CE, Normano ICS. Metaphyseal dysostosis, type Schmid. Arch Dis Child 1958;39:444.
198. Evans R, Caffey J. Metaphyseal dysostosis resembling vitamin D–refractory rickets. Am J Dis Child 1958;95:640.
199. Kozlowski K. Metaphyseal and spondylometaphyseal chondrodysplasias. Clin Orthop 1976;114:83.
200. Maekitie O. Cartilage-hair hypoplasia in Finland: epidemiological and genetic aspects of 107 patients. J Med Genet 1992;29:652.
201. Maekitie O, Kaitila I. Cartilage-hair hypoplasia—clinical manifestations in 108 Finnish patients. Eur J Pediatr 1993;152:211.
202. Maekitie O, Marttinen E, Kaitila I. Skeletal growth in cartilage-hair hypoplasia. A radiologic study of 82 patients. Pediatr Radiol 1992;22:434.
203. Maekitie O, Perheentupa J, Kaitila I. Growth in cartilage-hair hypoplasia. Pediatr Res 1992;31:176.
204. Maynard J, Ippolito EG, Ponseti IV, et al. Histochemistry and ultrastructure of the growth plate in metaphyseal dysostosis: further observations on the structure of the cartilage matrix. J Pediatr Orthop 1981;1:161.

205. McKusick VA, Eldridge R, Hostetler JA, et al. Dwarfism in the Amish. II. Cartilage-hair hypoplasia. Bull Johns Hopkins Hosp 1965;116:285.
206. Rosenbloom AL, Smith DW. The natural history of metaphyseal dysostosis. J Pediatr 1965;66:857.
207. Schmid F. Beitrag zur Dysostis enchondrolic Metaphysaria. Monatsschr Kinderheilkd 1949;97:393.
208. Vander-Burgt I, Haraldsson A, Oosterwijk JC, et al. Cartilage hair hypoplasia, metaphyseal chondrodysplasia type McKusick: description of seven patients and review of the literature. Am J Med Genet 1991;41:371.
209. Wasylenko MJ, Wedge JH, Houston CS. Metaphyseal chondrodysplasia, Schmid type. A defect of ultrastructural metabolism: case report. J Bone Joint Surg [Am] 1980;62:660.
210. Wilson WG, Aylsworth AS, Folds JD, et al. Cartilage-hair hypoplasia (metaphyseal chondrodysplasia, type McKusick) with combined immune deficiency: variable expression and development of immunologic functions in sibs. Birth Defects 1978;4(Suppl 6A):117.

Dyschondrosteosis

211. Dawe C, Wynne-Davies R, Fulford GE. Clinical variation in dyschondrosteosis: a report on 13 individuals in 8 families. J Bone Joint Surg [Br] 1982;64:377.
212. Dobyns JH. Madelung's deformity. In: Green DP, ed. Operative hand surgery. New York: Churchill Livingstone, 1982:425.
213. Fagg PS. Wrist pain in the Madelung's deformity of dyschondrosteosis. J Hand Surg [Br] 1988;13:11.
214. Felman AH, Kirkpatrick JA. Dyschondrosteoses: mesomelic dwarfism of Leri and Weill. Am J Dis Child 1970;120:329.
215. Kaitila II, Leisti JT, Rimoin DL. Mesomelic skeletal dysplasias. Clin Orthop 1976;114:94.
216. Langer LO Jr. Dyschondrosteosis, a heritable bone dysplasia with characteristic roentgenographic features. AJR 1965;95:178.
217. Léri A, Weill J: Une affection congenitable et symmetrique du developpement asseux: la dyschondrosteose. Bull Soc Med Hosp Paris 1929;53:1491.
218. Mohan V, Gupta RP, Helmi K, et al. Leri-Weill syndrome (dyschondrosteosis): a family study. J Hand Surg [Br] 1988;13:16.
219. Vickers D, Nielsen G. Madelung deformity: surgical prophylaxis (physiolysis) during the late growth period by resection of the dyschondrosteosis lesion. J Hand Surg [Br] 1992;17:401.

Cleidocranial Dysplasia

220. Bick EM, Marie P, Sainton P. The classic: on hereditary cleidocranial dysostosis. Clin Orthop 1968;58:5.
221. Brueton LA, Reeve A, Ellis R, et al. Apparent cleidocranial dysplasia associated with abnormalities of 8q22 in three individuals. Am J Med Genet 1992;43:612.
222. Dore DD, MacEwen GD, Boulos MI. Cleidocranial dysostosis and syringomyelia: review of the literature and case report. Clin Orthop 1987;214:229.
223. Eventov I, Reider-Grosswasser I, Weiss S, et al. Cleidocranial dysplasia. A family study. Clin Radiol 1979;30:323.
224. Jarvis JL, Keats TE. Cleidocranial dysostosis: a review of 40 new cases. AJR 1974;121:5.
225. Jensen BL. Somatic development in cleidocranial dysplasia. Am J Med Genet 1990;35:69.
226. Jensen BL, Kreiborg S. Development of the dentition in cleidocranial dysplasia. J Oral Pathol Med 1990;19:89.
227. Jensen BL, Kreiborg S. Development of the skull in infants with cleidocranial dysplasia. J Craniofac Genet Dev Biol 1993;13:89.
228. Jensen BL, Kreiborg S. Craniofacial abnormalities in 52 school-age and adult patients with cleidocranial dysplasia. J Craniofac Genet Dev Biol 1993;13:98.
229. Richie MF, Johnston CE II. Management of developmental coxa vara in cleidocranial dysostosis. Pediatr Orthop 1989;12:1001.

Larsen Syndrome

230. Bowen JR, Ortega K, Ray S, et al. Spinal deformities in Larsen syndrome. Clin Orthop 1985;197:159.
231. Larsen LJ, Schottstaedt ER, Bost FC. Multiple congenital dislocations associated with characteristic facial abnormality. J Pediatr 1950;37:574.
232. Micheli LJ, Hall JE, Watts HG. Spinal instability in Larsen syndrome: report of three cases. J Bone Joint Surg [Am] 1976;58:562.
233. Oki T, Terashima Y, Murachi S, et al. Clinical features and treatment of joint dislocations in Larsen's syndrome: report of three cases in one family. Clin Orthop 1976;119:206.
234. Roach JW, Birch JG, Johnston CE, et al. The cervical spine in Larsen's syndrome. Presented at the Scoliosis Research Society, Vancouver, BC, 1987.
235. Steel HH, Kohl EJ. Multiple congenital dislocations associated with other skeletal anomalies (Larsen's syndrome) in three siblings. J Bone Joint Surg [Am] 1972;54:75.

APPENDIX 7-1 Classification of Osteochondrodysplasias of the International Working Group on Constitutional Diseases of Bone

OSTEOCHONDRODYSPLASIAS	INHERITANCE PATTERN	CHROMOSOME	GENE	PROTEIN
A. Defects of the tubular and flat bones and axial skeleton				
1. Achondroplasia group				
Thanatophoric dysplasia	AD			
Thanatophoric dysplasia, straight femur and cloverleaf skull type	AD			
Achondroplasia	AD	4p16.3		
Hypochondroplasia	AD			
2. Achondrogenesis				
Type IA	AR			
Type IB	AR			
3. Spondylodysplastic group (perinatally lethal)				
San Diego type	Sp			
Torrance type	Sp			
Luton type	Sp			
4. Metatropic dysplasia group				
Fibrochondrogenesis	AR			
Schneckenbecken dysplasia	AR			
Metatropic dysplasia	AD			
5. Short rib (SR) dysplasia group (with or without polydactyly[P])				
SR(P) type I Saldino-Noonan	AR			
SR(P) type II Majewski	AR			
SR(P) type III Verma-Naumoff	AR			
SR(P) type IV Beemer-Langer	AR			
Asphyxiating thoracic dysplasia	AR			
Ellis–van Creveld dysplasia	AR			
6. Atelosteogenesis/diastrophic dysplasia group				
Boomerang dysplasia	Sp			
Atelosteogenesis type 1	Sp			
Atelosteogenesis type 2 (de la Chapelle)	AR			
Omodysplasia I (Maroteaux)	AD			
Omodysplasia II (Borochowitz)	AR			
Otopalatodigital syndrome type 2	XLR			
Diastrophic dysplasia	AR	5q31-q34		
Pseudodiastrophic dysplasia	AR			
7. Kniest-Stickler dysplasia group				
Dyssegmental dysplasia, Silverman-Handmaker type	AR			
Dyssegmental dysplasia, Rolland-Desbuquois type	AR			
Kniest dysplasia	AD			
Otospondylomegaepiphyseal dysplasia	AR			
Stickler dysplasia (heterogeneous, some not linked to COL2A1)	AD	12q13.1-q13.3	COL2A1	Type II collagen
8. Spondyloepiphyseal dysplasia congenita group				
Langer-Saldino dysplasia (achondrogenesis type II)	AD	12q13.1-q13.3	COL2A1	Type II collagen

(continued)

APPENDIX 7-1 Continued

OSTEOCHONDRODYSPLASIAS	INHERITANCE PATTERN	CHROMOSOME	GENE	PROTEIN
Hypochondrogenesis	AD	12q13.1-q13.3	COL2A1	Type II collagen
Spondyloepiphyseal dysplasia congenita	AD	12q13.1-q13.3	COL2A1	Type II collagen
9. Other spondyloepimetaphyseal dysplasias				
X-linked spondyloepiphyseal dysplasia tarda	XLD	Xp22	SEDL	
Other late-onset spondyloepi-(meta)-physeal dysplasias (i.e., Namaqua-land, Irapa)				
Progressive pseudorheumatoid dysplasia	AR			
Dyggve-Melchior-Clausen dysplasia	AR			
Wolcott-Rallison dysplasia	AR			
Immunoosseous dysplasia	AR			
Pseudachondroplasia	AD	19		
Opsismodysplasia	AR			
10. Dysostosis multiplex group				
Mucopolysaccharidosis IH	AR	4p16.3	IDA	α-Iduronidase
Mucopolysaccharidosis IS	AR	4q16.3	IDA	α-Iduronidase
Mucopolysaccharidosis II	XLR	Xq27.3-q28	IDS	Iduronate-2-sulfatase
Mucopolysaccharidosis IIIA	AR			Heparan sulfate sulfatase
Mucopolysaccharidosis IIIB	AR			N-Ac-α-D-glucosaminidase
Mucopolysaccharidosis IIIC	AR			Ac-CoA: α-glucosaminidase-N-Acetyltransferase
Mucopolysaccharidosis IIID	AR	12q14	GNS	N-Ac-glucosamine-6-sulfate-sulfatase
Mucopolysaccharidosis IVA	AR			Galactosamine-6-sulfatase
Mucopolysaccharidosis IVB	AR	3p21-p14.2	GLBI	β-Galactosidase
Mucopolysaccharidosis VI	AR	5q13.3	ARSB	Arylsulfatase B
Mucopolysaccharidosis VII	AR	7q21.11	GUSB	β-Glucoronidase
Fucosidosis	AR	1p34	FUCA	α-Fucosidase
α-Mannosidosis	AR	19p13.2-q12	MANB	α-Mannosidase
β-Mannosidosis	AR	4	MNB	β-Mannosidase
Aspartylglucosaminuria	AR	4q23-q27	AGA	Aspartylglucosaminidase
GM$_1$ gangliosidosis, several forms	AR	3p21-p14.2	GLB1	β-Galactosidase
Sialidosis, several forms	AR	6p21.3	NEU	α-Neuraminidase
Sialic storage disease	AR			
Galactosialidosis, several forms	AR	20q13.1	GSL	Neur/Gal expressive protein
Mucosulfatidosis	AR			Multiple sulfatases
Mucolipidosis II	AR	4q21-q23		N-Ac-Gluc-Phosphotransferase
Mucolipidosis III	AR	4q21-q23		N-Ac-Gluc-Phosphotransferase
Mucolipidosis IV	AR			
11. Spondylometaphyseal dysplasias				
Spondylometaphyseal dysplasia, Kozlowski type	AD			
Spondylometaphyseal dysplasia, corner fracture type (Sutcliffe)	AD			
Spondyloenchondrodysplasia	AR			
12. Epiphyseal dysplasias				
Multiple epiphyseal dysplasia, Fairbanks or Ribbing types	AD			

(continued)

***APPENDIX 7-1**   Continued*

OSTEOCHONDRODYSPLASIAS	INHERITANCE PATTERN	CHROMOSOME	GENE	PROTEIN
13. Chondrodysplasia punctata (stippled epiphyses) group				
Rhizomelic type	AR			Peroxisome
Conradi-Hünermann type	XLD	Xq28	*CPXD*	
X-linked recessive type	XLR	Xpter-p22.32	*CPXR*	
MT type (tibial-metacarpal type)	Sp			
Others, including CHILD syndrome, Zellweger syndrome; warfarin embryopathy, chromosomal abnormalities; fetal alcohol syndrome				
14. Metaphyseal dysplasias				
Jansen type	AD			
Schmid type	AD			
Spahr type	AR			
McKusick type (CHH)	AR			
Metaphyseal anadysplasia	XLR?			
Shwachman type	AR			
Adenosine deaminase deficiency	AR	20q13.11	*ADA*	
15. Brachyrachia (short spine dysplasia)				
Brachyolmia, several types				
16. Mesomelic dysplasias				
Dyschondrosteosis	AD			
Langer type	AR			
Nievergelt type	AD			
Robinow type	AD			
17. Acro/acromesomelic dysplasias				
Acromicric dysplasia	Sp			
Geleophysic dysplasia	AR			
Acrodysostosis	AD			
Trichorhinophalangeal dysplasia type 1	AD	8q24.12	*TQPS1*	
Trichorhinophalangeal dysplasia type 2	AD	8q24.11-q24.13	*TQPS2*	
Saldino-Mainzer dysplasia	AR			
Pseudohypoparathyroidism, several types	AD AR? XLD?			
Cranioectodermal dysplasia	AR			
Acromesomelic dysplasia	AR			
Grebe dysplasia	AR			
18. Dysplasias with significant (but not exclusive) membraneous bone involvement				
Cleidocranial dysplasia	AD			
Osteodysplasty, Melnick-Needles	XLD			
19. Bent bone dysplasia group				
Campomelic dysplasia	AR		*CMD1*	
Kyphomelic dysplasia	AR			
Stüve-Wiedemann dysplasia	AR			
20. Multiple dislocations with dysplasias				
Larsen syndrome	AD			
Desbuquois syndrome	AR			

(continued)

APPENDIX 7-1 Continued

OSTEOCHONDRODYSPLASIAS	INHERITANCE PATTERN	CHROMOSOME	GENE	PROTEIN
Spondyloepimetaphyseal dysplasia with joint laxity	AR			
21. Osteodysplastic primordial dwarfism group				
Type 1	AR			
Type 2	AR			
22. Dysplasias with decreased bone density				
Osteogenesis imperfecta, several types	AD	17q21.31-q22.05	COL1A1	Collagen type I
	AD	7q21.3-22.1	COL1A2	Collagen type I
	AR			
Osteoporosis with pseudoglioma	AR			
Idiopathic juvenile osteoporosis	Sp			
Bruck syndrome	AR			
Homocystinuria	AR	21q22.3	CBS	Cystathionine-β-synthase
Singleton-Merten syndrome	Sp			
Geroderma osteodysplastica	AR			
Menkes syndrome	XLR	Xq12.q13	MNK	
23. Dysplasias with defective mineralization				
Hypophosphatasia	AD	1p36.1p34	ALPL	Alkaline phosphatase
Hypophosphatemic rickets	XR			
Pseudodeficiency rickets, several types	AR			
Neonatal hyperparathyroidism	AR			
24. Dysplasias with increased bone density				
Osteopetrosis				
a. Precocious type	AR			
b. Delayed type	AD			
c. Intermediate type	AR			
d. With renal tubular acidosis	AR	8q22	CA2	Carbonic anhydrase II
Dysosteosclerosis	AR			
Pycnodysostosis	AR			
Osteosclerosis, Stanescu type	AD			
Axial osteosclerosis, including				
a. Osteomesopycnosis	AD			
b. With bamboo hair (Netherton syndrome)	AR			
c. Trichothiodystrophy	AR			
Osteopoikilosis	AD			
Melorheostosis	Sp			
Osteopathia striata	Sp			
Osteopathia striata with cranial sclerosis	AD			
Diaphyseal dysplasia, Camurati-Engelmann	AD			
Craniodiaphyseal dysplasia	AD			
	AR			
Lenz-Majewski dysplasia	Sp			
Craniometadiaphyseal dysplasia	Sp			
Endosteal hyperostoses				
a. Van Buchem disease	AR			
b. Sclerosteosis	AR			

(continued)

APPENDIX 7-1 Continued

OSTEOCHONDRODYSPLASIAS	INHERITANCE PATTERN	CHROMOSOME	GENE	PROTEIN
c. Worth disease	AD			
d. With cerebellar hypoplasia	AR			
Pachydermoperiostosis	AD			
Frontometaphyseal dysplasia	XLR			
Craniometaphyseal dysplasia				
a. Severe type	AR			
b. Mild type	AD			
Pyle (disease) dysplasia	AR			
Osteoectasia with hyperphosphatasia	AR			
Oculodentoosseous dysplasia				
a. Severe type	AR			
b. Mild type	AD			
Familial infantile cortical hyperostosis, Caffey	AD			
B. Disorganized development of cartilaginous and fibrous components of the skeleton				
Dysplasia epiphysealis hemimelica	Sp			
Multiple cartilaginous exostoses	AD	8q23-q24.1		
Enchondromatosis (Ollier)	Sp			
Enchondromatosis with hemangioma (Maffucci)	Sp			
Metachondromatosis	AD			
Osteoglophonic dysplasia	Sp			
Fibrous dysplasia (Jaffe-Lichtenstein)	Sp			
Fibrous dysplasia with pigmentary skin changes and precocious puberty (McCune-Albright)	Sp			
Cherubism	AD			
Myofibromatosis (generalized fibromatosis)	AR			
C. Idiopathic Osteolyses				
1. Predominantly phalangeal				
Hereditary acrosteolysis, several forms				
Hajdu-Cheney type	AD			
2. Predominantly carpal or tarsal				
Carpal-tarsal osteolysis with nephropathy	AD			
Francois syndrome (dermochondrocorneal dystrophy)	AR			
3. Multicentric				
Winchester syndrome	AR			
Torg type	AR			
Mandibuloacral dysplasia	AR			
4. Other				
Familial expansile osteolysis	AD			

AD, Autosomal dominant; AR, autosomal recessive; XLD, X-linked dominant; XLR, X-linked recessive; Sp, sporadic.

Adapted from Beighton P, Giedion ZA, Gorlin R, et al. International classification of osteochondroplasias. Am J Med Genet 1992;44:223.

Chapter 8

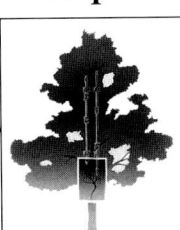

Syndromes of Orthopaedic Importance

Michael J. Goldberg

Neurofibromatosis
   Nonorthopaedic Manifestations
   Orthopaedic Manifestations
Proteus Syndrome
Arthrogryposis
   Arthrogryposis Multiplex Congenita
   Other Forms of Arthrogryposis
Down Syndrome
Fetal Alcohol Syndrome
Nail-Patella Syndrome
De Lange Syndrome
Familial Dysautonomia
Rubinstein-Taybi Syndrome
Progeria
Russell-Silver Dwarfism
Turner Syndrome
Noonan Syndrome
Prader-Willi Syndrome
Beckwith-Wiedemann Syndrome
Stickler Syndrome
VACTERLS and VATER Association
Goldenhar Syndrome
Trichorhinophalangeal Syndrome
Mucopolysaccharidoses
   Morquio Syndrome

The word syndrome is derived from a Greek word that means to run together. When several relatively uncommon anomalies occur in the same individual, it may be nothing more than coincidence. However, if they all result from the same cause or occur in the same pattern in other children, that particular combination of birth defects is called a syndrome. A syndrome should be suspected if a characteristic orthopaedic malformation (e.g., radial clubhand) is encountered, if all four extremities are affected, if limb deformities are symmetric, if there are several associated nonorthopaedic anomalies, or if there is a familiar dysmorphic face.[1,4] Children who have syndromes look more like each other than they do their parents.

The evaluation of a child for a syndrome always includes a family history, a systems review, and a search for minor dysmorphic features, such as abnormal palm creases or abnormal shape of digits or toes. These may not be of immediate orthopaedic significance, but they are the clues to look further.

Syndrome identification may not promote a basic understanding of the pathogenic mechanisms. Syndromes may arise from a single genetic defect, a chromosomal defect, an environmental teratogen, or a combination of genetic and environmental factors.[1,3,5] Physicians should not mistakenly assume that phenotypically different patients have distinct or separate disorders. What may initially appear to be a separate syndrome because of certain phenotypic features may represent mutations of the same gene; the mutation can occur in a different position along the gene. For example, the four clinical types of osteogenesis imperfecta described by Sillence (see Chap. 6) all represent defects in the construction of type I collagen and the two genes responsible: COL1A1 and COL1A2. Similarly, Duchenne muscular dystrophy and Becker muscular dystrophy are the result of mutations in the dystrophin gene. The severity of the disorder is the result of the size of the gene defect and where along the reading frame the mutation occurs.[187]

The care of children with syndromes always involves multiple specialists.[2,6] Discussions of the risk of subsequent pregnancies is in the realm of the genetic counselor. For parents, naming the condition often implies that it is then treatable or curable. This, sadly, is not the case. The importance of understanding syndromes is recognizing that associated medical abnormalities may adversely influence orthopaedic outcomes and may influence surgical timing and management.

NEUROFIBROMATOSIS

Neurofibromatosis (NF) is the most common single-gene disorder in humans, affecting 1 of 3000 newborns.[34,55,57] The gene for NF1 (i.e., von Recklinghausen disease) has been mapped to the long arm of chromosome 17 (17q11.2).[30,62,69] The *NF1* gene has been cloned and is an exceptionally large gene, with three smaller genes contained within a large intron. At least one of these smaller genes encodes for a protein neurofibrin, which is similar to the GTPase-activating proteins.[32] Although the exact function of these proteins is unknown, it seems to be important in downregulating the activity of the products of *RAS* oncogenes. The *NF1* gene can be considered a tumor-suppressor gene that interacts with a cellular protooncogene. Some of the clinical manifestations of NF reflect a balance of oncogene and suppressor gene behavior. Despite the rapid progress in molecular biology, the precise pathogenic mechanisms remain unknown.

NF is a neural crest disorder. Cells from the neural crest migrate to become pigmented cells of the skin, parts of the brain, spinal cord, peripheral nerves, and adrenals. The interactions between cells derived from the neural crest and nerve growth factors have been implicated in the pathogenesis, but the pathobiology needs clarification.

NF is an autosomal dominant disorder with 100% penetrance, but one half of the cases are sporadic mutations and are associated with an older than average paternal age. There have been various classifications and subgroupings of this disorder. In the most important schemes, classic von Recklinghausen disease, peripheral NF, or NF1 accounts for 85% of all cases. Central NF (NF2) is characterized by bilateral acoustic neuromas and a paucity of peripheral findings.

The most renowned patient with NF, Joseph Merrick, called the Elephant Man, probably did not have this diagnosis and better fits Proteus syndrome.[28]

Nonorthopaedic Manifestations

The clinical manifestations are diverse, and variations in severity occur even in monozygotic twins.[35,55,57] Chil-

dren may look normal at birth, but 50% of patients eventually develop serious musculoskeletal problems.[19] The diagnosis of NF1 requires that the person have two or more of the following features[53]:

- At least six café-au-lait spots, larger than 5 mm in diameter for children and larger than 15 mm for adults
- Two neurofibromas or a single plexiform neurofibroma
- Freckling in the axillae or inguinal region
- An optical glioma
- At least two Lisch nodules (i.e., hamartoma of the iris)
- A distinctive osseous lesion, such as vertebral scalloping or cortical thinning
- A first-degree relative with NF1

Cutaneous Markings

Café-au-lait spots are discrete, tan spots (Fig. 8-1). They may take up to 1 year to appear and then the numbers and size steadily increase. Although six

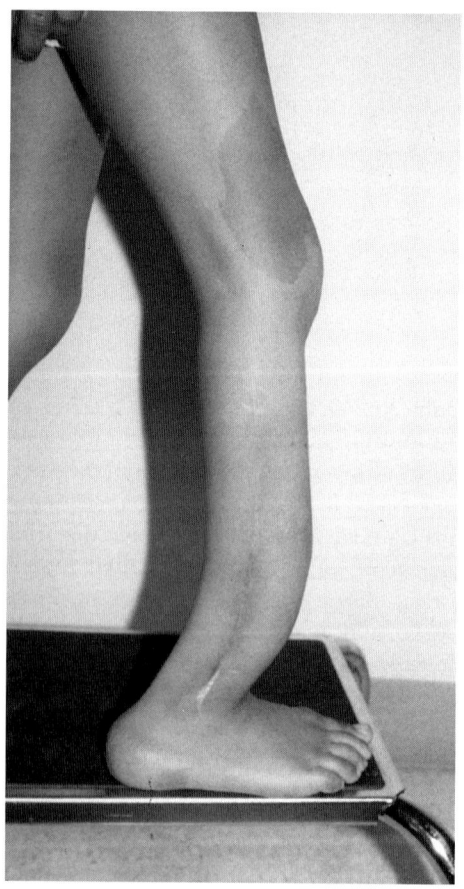

FIGURE 8-1. Neurofibromatosis in a 6-year-old child. Notice the large café au lait spot on the thigh and the anterior bowed tibia typical of pseudarthrosis. Prior surgery was unsuccessful. (From Goldberg MJ. The dysmorphic child: an orthopaedic perspective. New York: Raven Press, 1987.)

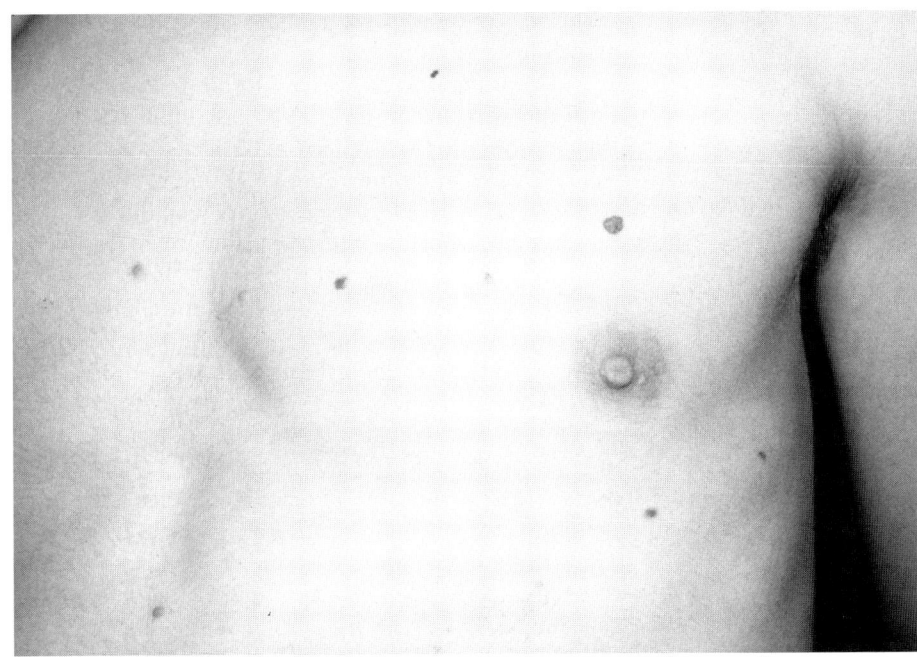

FIGURE 8-2. Neurofibromatosis in a 14-year-old patient. Cutaneous neurofibromas make their appearance with the onset of puberty. (From Goldberg MJ. The dysmorphic child: an orthopaedic perspective. New York: Raven Press, 1987.)

smooth-edged café-au-lait spots larger than 1 cm classically are a requirement, there exists great variation in the number of café-au-lait spots, their shape, and their size.

Axillary and inguinal freckling is common and serves as a good diagnostic markers, because such freckling is exceptionally rare except in people with NF.

Hyperpigmented nevi are dark brown areas that commonly are sensitive to touch. They typically overlie a deeper plexiform neurofibroma.

Neurofibroma

The two types of neurofibromas are different in their anatomic configuration and in clinical morbidity. The most common is the cutaneous neurofibroma, composed of benign Schwann cells and fibrous connective tissue (Fig. 8-2). They may occur anywhere but are usually just below the skin. They may not be detectable until 10 years of age, and with puberty, there is a rapid increase in their number. When many are grouped together on the skin, it is known as a fibroma molluscum. Rarely is there a neurologic deficit associated with this type of peripheral neurofibroma.

Plexiform neurofibromas are usually present at birth and are highly infiltrative in the surrounding tissues. The overlying skin is often darkly pigmented. They are highly vascular, and plexiform neurofibromas lead to limb gigantism, facial disfigurement, and invasion of the neuroaxis (Figs. 8-3 and 8-4). There is no effective management of plexiform neurofibroma. Their vascularity and infiltrative nature make complete extirpation almost impossible, with a substantial risk of uncontrollable hemorrhage and neurologic deficit. Although speculative, the use of angiogenesis inhibitors, such as interferon-α, over a prolonged period may be beneficial.[25,26]

Orthopaedic Manifestations

There are many skeletal manifestations, but the presence of an unusual scoliosis, nonunion of a long bone, overgrowth of a part, or a curious bone lesion seen

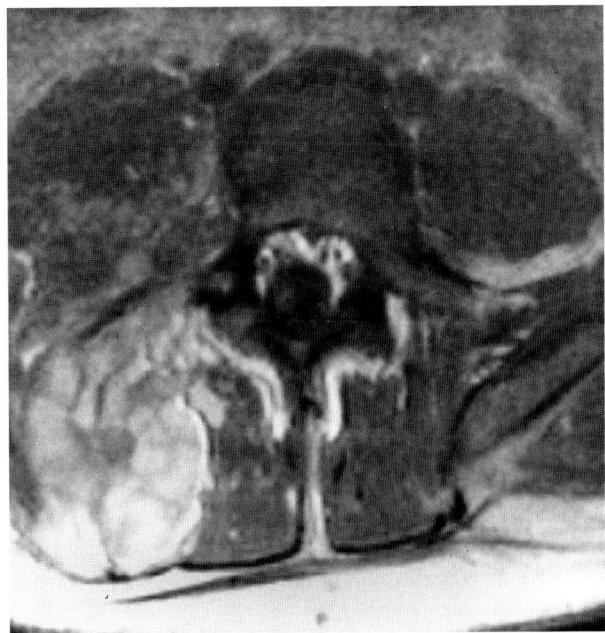

FIGURE 8-3. Neurofibromatosis in a 16-year-old patient. The magnetic resonance image at the level of L4–L5 demonstrates a large plexiform neurofibroma that invades the neural axis. It extends from the level of L3 to the sacrum.

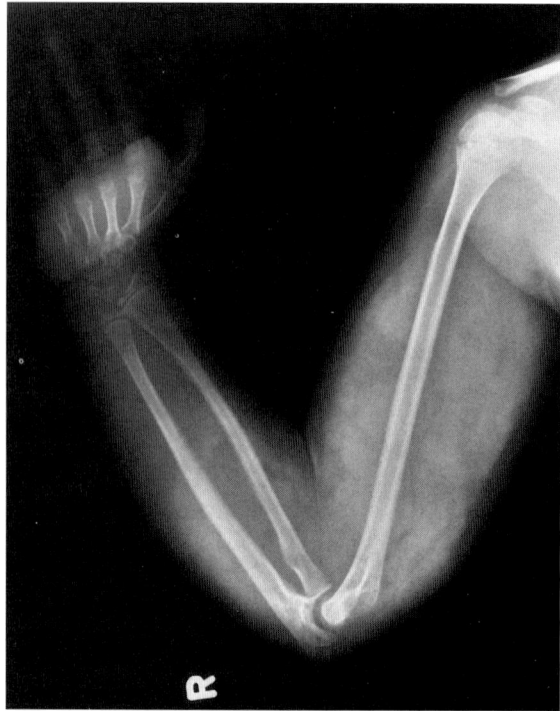

FIGURE 8-4. Neurofibromatosis in a 10-year-old patient. Hypertrophy affects the arm from the shoulder to the fingertips, the major component is soft tissue. Nodular densities throughout the upper arm are consistent with a plexiform neurofibroma. Notice the lack of skeletal overgrowth and some attenuation of the radius and ulna from external compression by the neurofibroma. (From Goldberg MJ. The dysmorphic child: an orthopaedic perspective. New York: Raven Press, 1987.)

on x-ray films should alert the physician to consider a diagnosis of NF.[19]

Scoliosis is common, and although there is no standard curve pattern, curves tend to fall into two behavioral patterns: a dystrophic curve and an idiopathic curve. The dystrophic scoliotic curve is a short, sharp, single thoracic curve typically involving four to six segments (Fig. 8-5).[7,15,19,20,27,37,59,66] It is associated with distortion of the ribs and vertebrae. The onset is early in childhood, and it is relentlessly progressive. The most important risk factors for progression are an early age of onset, a high Cobb angle at the first visit, and an apical vertebrae that is severely rotated, scalloped, and located in the middle to lower thoracic area.[27] The combination of curve progression and vertebral malformation mimics congenital scoliosis in appearance and behavior. Dystrophic curves are refractive to brace treatment. Sagittal plane deformities may occur, including an angular kyphosis (i.e., gibbus) and a scoliosis that has so much rotation that curve progression is more obvious on the lateral than on the anterior posterior roentgenogram.[27] In those with angular kyphosis, there is a risk of paraplegia. It is difficult to surgically stabilize dystrophic curves;[13,33,58] nevertheless, prompt surgical stabilization is recommended for those with risk factors and early progression.[27]

Most curves in NF resemble idiopathic scoliosis curves. Their relation to NF is not understood, and their precise incidence debated. These curves can be managed like any other idiopathic curve.

There are several vertebral abnormalities evident on radiographs. These include scalloping of the posterior body, enlargement of the neural foramina, and defective pedicles occasionally with a completely dislocated vertebral body.[18,36,56,67,68] Such findings may mean that there is a dumbbell-shaped neurofibroma in the spinal canal extending out through a neural foramina. In NF patients, the dura behaves similar to the dura in patients with a connective tissue disorder, and dural ectasia is common, with pseudomeningoceles protruding through the neural foramina (Fig. 8-6).[12,16,22,23] The incidence of anterolateral meningoceles was underestimated until asymptomatic patients were screened with magnetic resonance imaging (MRI).[24,60]

The erosion of the pedicles may lead to spinal instability, especially in the cervical spine. MRI and

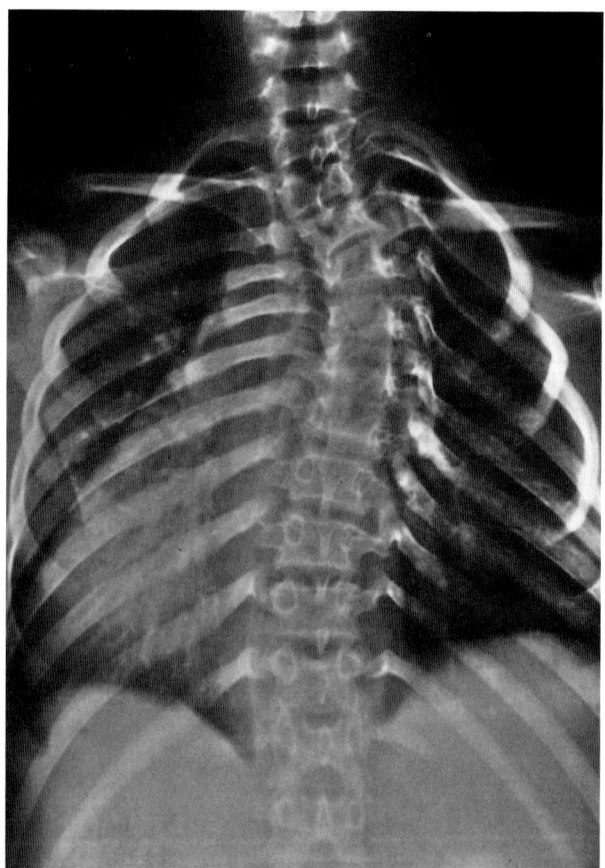

FIGURE 8-5. Neurofibromatosis in a 14-year-old patient. The dystrophic curve is produced by a short-segment scoliosis. Ribboned ribs show cystic irregularities. (From Goldberg MJ. The dysmorphic child: an orthopaedic perspective. New York: Raven Press, 1987.)

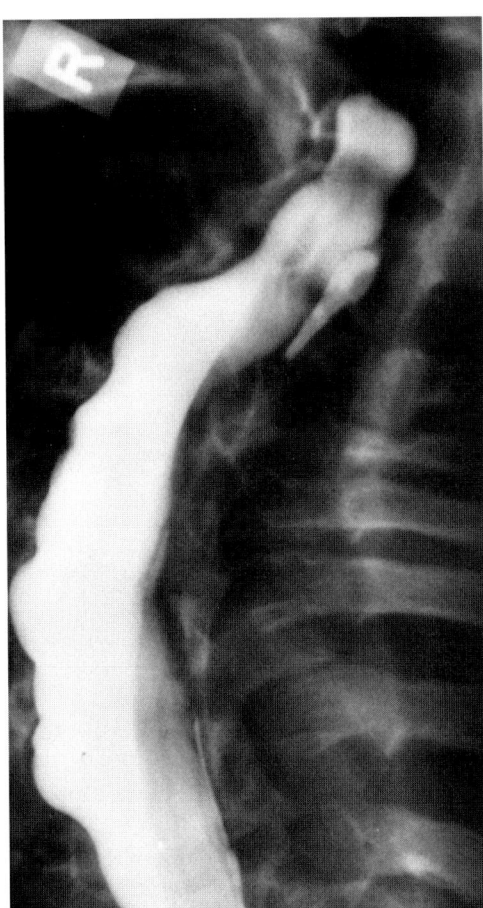

FIGURE 8-6. Myelogram of a young adult with neurofibromatosis and scoliosis with pseudomeningoceles and dural ectasia.

Patients with NF often exhibit overgrowth, ranging from a single digit to an entire limb and from mild anisomelia to massive gigantism. Any child with focal gigantism, such as macrodactyly, is best thought of as having NF until proven otherwise. When NF is compared with the more symmetric idiopathic hemihypertrophy, there is disproportional overgrowth involving the skin and subcutaneous tissue more than bone (see Fig. 8-4).

There are several curious roentgenographic lesions seen in the skeletons of those with NF (Fig. 8-9).[24] These may vary from a benign scalloping of the cortex, to cystic lesions in long bones looking much like nonossifying fibromas, to permeative bone destruction; some patients have a combination of lesions. NF can mimic benign and malignant bone lesions.[40,42,44] Roentgenograms of the pelvis usually show various degrees of coxa valga, but for as many as 20% of patients, there is radiographic evidence of protrusio acetabuli.[37,47]

About 5% of patients with NF eventually develop a malignancy, although this figure may be too high if

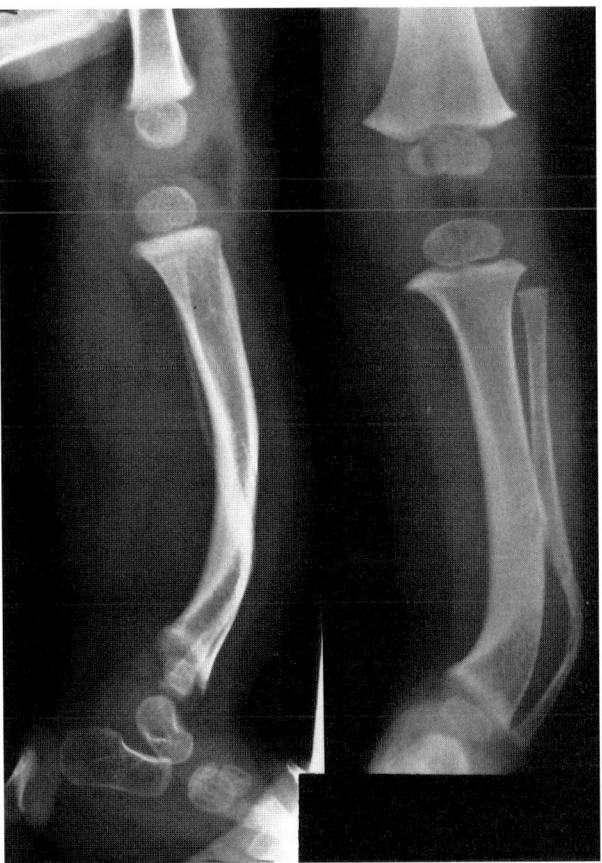

FIGURE 8-7. Neurofibromatosis in a 1-year-old patient. The anterolateral bow of the tibia and fibula warrant concern for impending fracture and pseudarthrosis. (From Goldberg MJ. The dysmorphic child: an orthopaedic perspective. New York: Raven Press, 1987.)

computed tomography (CT) scans are helpful preoperatively to delineate the presence of defective vertebrae or dural abnormalities and assist in choosing the spinal instrumentation system. The goal of surgery in dystrophic curves is spinal stabilization and markedly deformed spines with large dural outpocketing and foraminal neurofibroma are reasonably best fused in situ.

Pseudarthrosis of a long bone is typically associated with NF.[19] It usually affects the tibia, with a characteristic anterolateral bow obvious in infancy (Fig. 8-7).[51,52] Fracture follows, with spontaneous union unlikely and surgical union a challenge. A combination of careful but modest resection of the pseudarthrosis site, near-perfect alignment of the tibia, and intramedullary rod fixation, crossing the ankle joint, seems to offer the best results.[9,10] The precise mechanism is unknown, and neurofibromas have not been found at the pseudarthrosis site. The pseudarthrosis process may affect the ulna,[11,21,46,54] radius,[29,38,39,49] femur, or clavicle,[8] and in each instance, there follows a progressive nonunion, with bone loss and difficulty achieving union with treatment (Fig. 8-8).

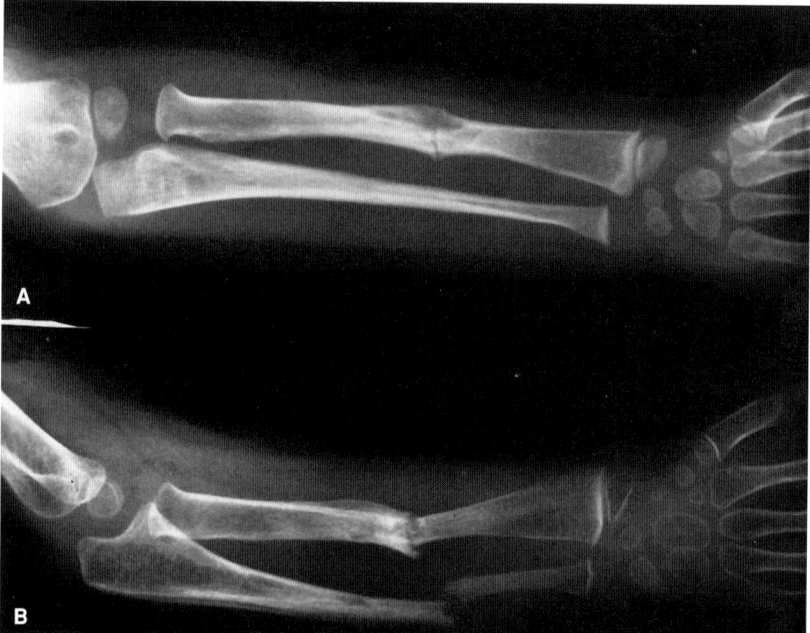

FIGURE 8-8. Neurofibromatosis in a 3-year-old patient. The radiograph shows progressive pseudarthrosis of the radius and ulna after a pathologic fracture. (**A**) Fracture through the cystic lesion of the radius and thinning of the midulna. (**B**) After 10 months of cast immobilization, pseudarthrosis affects the radius and ulna. (From Goldberg MJ. The dysmorphic child: an orthopaedic perspective. New York: Raven Press, 1987.)

the number of undiagnosed cases of NF are taken into account.[14,48,61,64] The tumor is usually a central nervous system lesion: an optic nerve glioma, acoustic neuroma, or astrocytoma.[43] There is a risk of malignant degeneration of a neurofibroma to a neurofibrosarcoma; this process can occur in a central or peripheral neurofibroma.[17,31,50,63] Molecular biology studies of degenerated neurofibroma have revealed that alterations in the *P53* gene, an important tumor-suppressor gene located on the short arm of chromosome 17, is critical to the progression of a neurofibroma to neurofibrosarcoma. The discovery has not yet been clinically applied. There is a propensity for children with neurofibroma to develop other malignancies, such as Wilms tumors or rhabdomyosarcomas.

There are other important manifestations of NF. Affected children are short but tend to have large heads. About 50% have an intellectual handicap that varies from frank mental retardation to problems with school performance. Hypertension, on the basis of renal artery stenosis or pheochromocytoma, is reported regularly, as is a curious type of metabolic bone disease similar to hypophosphatemic osteomalacia.[41,65] Lisch nodules are melanocytic hamartomas projecting from the surface of the iris and easily visualized by slit lamp examination. They occur in 100% of patients with NF who are older than 20 years of age, but they also are important in the diagnosis of children, because they are more likely to be found in young patients than neurofibromas.[45]

Specific management of the characteristic orthopaedic deformities such as scoliosis and pseudarthrosis is discussed elsewhere in this book. Treatment often requires specialized pediatric orthopaedists to achieve good outcomes. Nevertheless, the common orthopaedic manifestations of NF, including scoliosis, limb overgrowth, pseudarthrosis, and curious radiographic appearances of lesions, enable the initial diagnosis to be made if the syndrome is kept in mind.

PROTEUS SYNDROME

The Proteus syndrome is named after the ancient Greek demigod who could change appearance and assume different shapes. The progressive nature of the deformities seen in this syndrome can lead to grotesque overgrowth, facial disfigurement, angular malformation, and severe scoliosis.[86,90] John Merrick, called the Elephant Man, is thought to have had this syndrome, rather than NF.[75,87] This clarification is important for the syndromologist and for parents of children with NF whose strong emotional feelings may be attached to the theatrical presentation of *Elephant Man*.[78]

The signs of Proteus syndrome overlap those other hamartomatous overgrowth conditions, such as idiopathic hemihypertrophy, Klippel-Trenaunay syndrome, Maffucci syndrome, and NF.[74] It is a bizarre array of abnormalities that include hemihypertrophy, macrodactyly, and partial gigantism of the hands, feet, or both.[72,81,82,84] In most children with macrodactyly, it is an isolated deformity involving a single finger or toe.

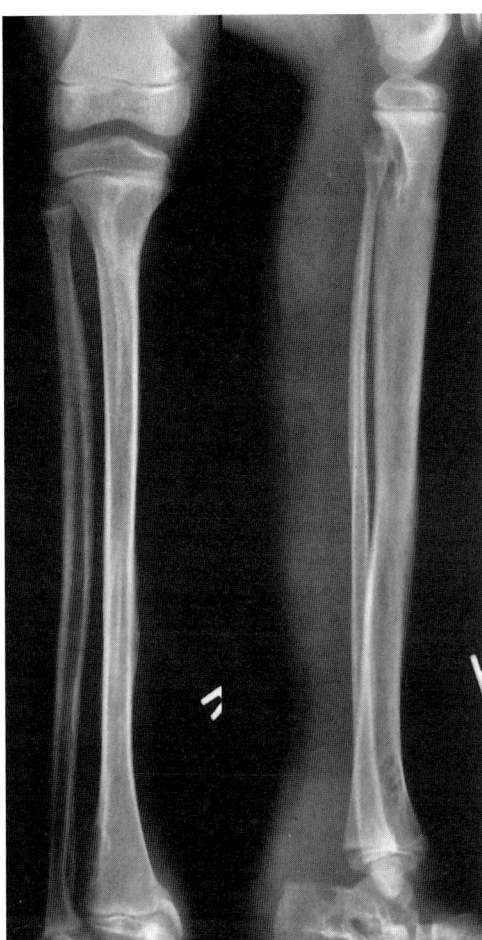

FIGURE 8-9. Neurofibromatosis in a 10-year-old patient. The radiograph shows an array of cystic and scalloped skeletal lesions in the tibia and os calcis of right leg. Some of the lesions are characteristic of neurofibromatosis. Other lesions, occurring in isolation, can mimic benign fibrous tumors. Scalloped cortical erosion at the upper end of the femur, permeative bone destruction in the region of the os calcis, and metaphyseal cystic lesions are other features. (From Goldberg MJ. The dysmorphic child: an orthopaedic perspective. New York: Raven Press, 1987.)

When more than one digit is involved, its immediate neighbor is also affected. Digital involvement in the hand favors the sensory distribution of the median nerve.[1] The index is the most frequently affected finger, followed by the long finger and the thumb. It is the second toe that is most commonly macrodactylous. The regional sensory nerve is greatly increased in size, taking a tortuous route through the fatty tissue. The precise relation between the hypertrophied nerve and the macrodactyly is unknown. When macrodactyly affects nonadjacent toes or fingers or opposite extremities, it is almost always Proteus syndrome. There is a characteristic thickening and deep furrowing of the skin on the palms of the hands and soles of the feet. The array of cutaneous manifestations include hemangiomas and pigmented nevi of various intensities and subcutaneous lipomas (Fig. 8-10). Varicosities are present although true arteriovenous malformations are rare. There are cranial hyperostoses, and occasionally exostosis of the hands and feet.

Several orthopaedic deformities are difficult to manage, including focal and regional gigantism, scoliosis, and kyphosis.[77,85] Rather large vertebral bodies, known as megaspondylodysplasia, are present.[71] Angular malformations of the lower extremities, especially genu valgum, are common. Because the genu valgum is often associated with restricted range of motion, joint stiffness, flexion contractures, and joint pain, it is postulated that an intraarticular growth disturbance contributes to the angular malformation. Roentgenographic hip abnormalities are frequently discovered in asymptomatic patients, but acetabular dysplasia and late developmental dysplasia of the hip often prove troublesome. Deformities in the hindfoot are frequent and are usually heel valgus, but congenital equinovarus and "Z-foot" deformities have also been described.[74,85]

Not all of these signs are present in any one patient.[73,76,88] There are many incomplete cases. The key to diagnosis is worsening of existing features and the appearance of new ones. A schema developed by Hotamisligil may be used to assist in diagnosis.[80] This rating scale assigns points based on various clinical findings, including macrodactyly, hemihypertrophy, thickening of the skin, lipomas, subcutaneous tumors, verrucae, epidermal nevus, and macrocephaly.

Although a common enough syndrome for every large children's service to have a patient or two, most of the literature consists of case reports. Precise surgical recommendations have no assurance of predictable outcomes. Macrodactyly is managed by ablation rather than debulking, but the results even for isolated nonsyndromic macrodactyly are poor. Anisomelia has been managed with epiphyseodesis, although limb lengthening may be considered. Osteotomies have been used to correct angular malformations and bone surgery to correct foot deformity. This approach must be tempered by the observation that rapid recurrence of deformity after corrective surgery or sudden overgrowth of the operative limb have been reported. It raises the possibility that abnormal amounts of localized growth factors are present and somehow contribute to the pathogenesis of this disease.[77] The cause and inheritance pattern are uncertain, although autosomal dominance is suggested from a few case reports.[70,76,79] The life expectancy is unknown.[89] Patients between the ages of 9 months and 29 years have been reported. Functional ability depends on the severity of the limb deformity and the presence of a brain or other intracranial abnormalities.[83,84]

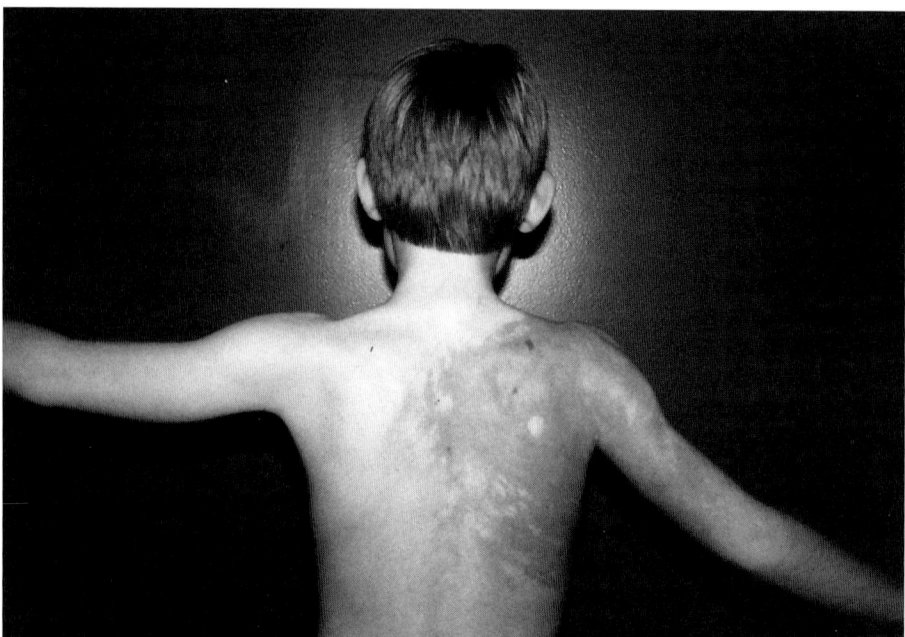

FIGURE 8-10. Proteus syndrome. Notice the cutaneous markings, large hemangioma of the shoulder, and lightly pigmented area on the back. There is some atrophy of the shoulder and arm muscles and a fixed contracture of the elbow.

ARTHROGRYPOSIS

Arthrogryposis represents a group of about 150 syndromes, all of which have in common obvious joint contractures that are present at birth. Arthrogryposis has come to be used as a noun referring to a specific disease and as an adjective, arthrogrypotic, referring to rigid joint contractures. When children with multiple congenital joint contractures are studied, it becomes apparent that there are distinct disorders with different clinical courses, prognoses, genetics, causes, and pathologic processes.[103,111] There is, nevertheless, considerable overlap, and as more of the molecular genetics is known, individual syndromes will be renamed and reclassified. From a purely clinical point of view and with the goal trying to find what syndrome may be present, a simple classification schema is useful[103]:

I. Arthrogryposis involving all four extremities. This includes arthrogryposis multiplex congenita, Larsen syndrome, and Pena-Shokier, with more or less total body involvement.
II. Arthrogryposis that predominantly or exclusively involves the hands and feet. These are the distal arthrogryposes. Because facial involvement is common in this group, Freeman-Sheldon whistling face is included.
III. Pterygia syndromes in which identifiable skin webs cross the flexion aspects of the knees, elbows and other joints. Multiple pterygias and popliteal pterygia fit in this group.

It is perhaps easiest to address the other syndromes if arthrogryposis multiplex congenita (amyoplasia) is first defined.

Arthrogryposis Multiplex Congenita

Arthrogryposis multiplex congenita is the best known of the multiple congenital contracture syndromes.[109,121] In the original description in 1841, Adolf Wilhelm Otto referred to his patient as a "human wonder with curved limbs."[115] Although attempts have been made to change the name arthrogryposis multiplex congenita to multiple congenital contractures or amyoplasia, the popularity of arthrogryposis remains. Regardless of nosology, rather strict criteria for diagnosis can be established.[103]

Manifestations and Diagnosis

The limbs are striking in appearance and position (Fig. 8-11). They are featureless and tubular. Normal skin creases are lacking, but there may be deep dimples over the joints. Muscle mass is reduced, although in infancy, there is often abundant subcutaneous tissue. Typically, the shoulders are adducted and internally rotated, the elbow more often extended than flexed, and the wrist flexed severely, with ulnar deviation. The fingers are flexed, clutching the thumb. In the lower extremities, the hips are flexed, abducted, and externally rotated; the knees are typically in extension, although flexion is possible; and clubfeet are the

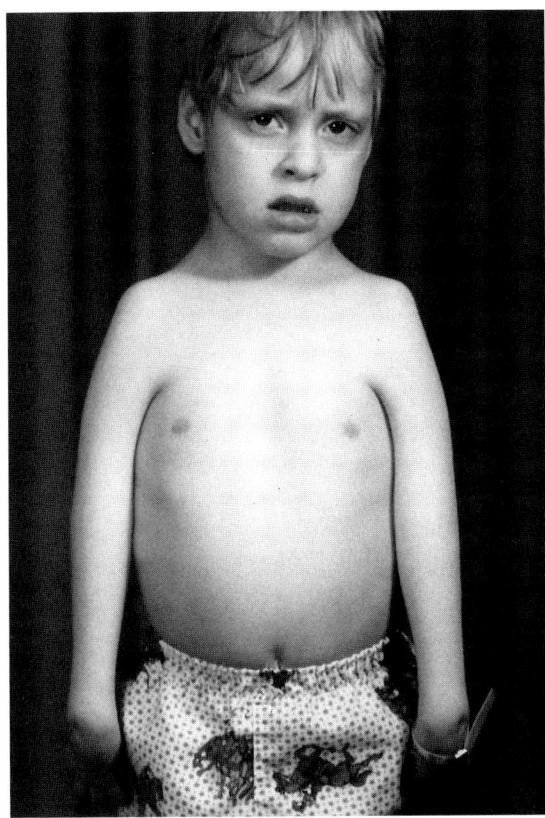

FIGURE 8-11. Arthrogryposis multiplex congentia. The picture shows the classic limb position and fusiform limbs lacking flexion creases.

rule. Joint motion is restricted. The condition is pain free, with a firm, inelastic block to movement beyond a very limited range. In two thirds of the patients, all four limbs are affected equally, but in one third, lower limb deformities predominate, and only on rare occasions do the upper extremities predominate. Deformities tend to be more severe and more rigid distally. The hips may be dislocated unilaterally or bilaterally.

The viscera usually are spared malformations, although gastroschisis has been reported. As a consequence of the general muscle weakness, there is a 15% incidence of inguinal hernia. Major feeding difficulties due to a stiff jaw and an immobile tongue are frequently encountered in infancy and lead to respiratory infections and failure to thrive.[119]

The face is not particularly dysmorphic. A few subtle features, such as narrowing of the face, link the appearance of those with this syndrome to each other (see Fig. 8-11).

Intelligence is normal and the natural ability for these patients to learn substitution techniques enhances even small gains obtained from surgery or physical therapy. There is, however, a strong association between initial feeding difficulties and subsequent language development, which should not be mistaken for retardation.[119]

If a child meets the criteria of characteristic limb position, normal intelligence, no visceral abnormalities, no dysmorphic face, and a negative family history, it is reasonable to make the diagnosis of arthrogryposis multiplex congenita. Otherwise, another syndrome must be searched for.

The cause is unknown. Classic arthrogryposis multiplex congenita is not a genetic disorder. Affected individuals have reproduced only normal children. A second affected child has not been reported in any family. There is, however, an increased incidence of classic arthrogryposis affecting only one of identical twins.[110,127] The development of arthrogryposis may be influenced by an adverse intrauterine factor or the twinning process itself. Teratogens have been suggested, but none are proven despite the multiple animal models that lend support to that theory.[102,108,118,121,124] The event seems to be entirely sporadic, although some epidemics occurred in the 1960s.[130]

Clinical examination remains best for establishing a diagnosis. Roentgenograms show a loss of subcutaneous fat and muscle. Radiographs reveal that the joints are normal and that changes are adaptive and acquired over time as a consequence of fixed position (Fig. 8-12). Electromyograms and muscle biopsies are of questionable diagnostic value. They have been used to separate neuropathic from myopathic arthrogryposis, but the clinical implications of such distinctions are not clear. A diagnosis of arthrogryposis can be suspected when prenatal ultrasound detects an absence of fetal movement, especially if seen in combination with polyhydramnios.[102]

Histologic analysis discloses a small muscle mass with fibrosis and fat between the muscle fibers. Myopathic and neuropathic features often are found in the same muscle biopsy specimen. The periarticular soft tissue structures are fibrotic, and in essence, there is a fibrous ankylosis.

The number of anterior horn cells (α motor neurons) in the spinal cord is decreased, without an increase in the number of microglial cells.[92,97,117] The pattern of motor neuron loss in specific spinal cord segments correlates with the peripheral deformities and the affected muscles, suggesting a primary central nervous system disorder as important in the cause.[95]

Despite every large medical center having treated patients with arthrogryposis and despite the epidemics, the natural history and long-term outcomes are not well known.[96,99] There is a paucity of descriptions of adults in the literature. Some contractures seem to worsen with age, and the joint becomes stiffer. No new joints become involved. Scoliosis develops in about one third of the patients. At least 25% of affected

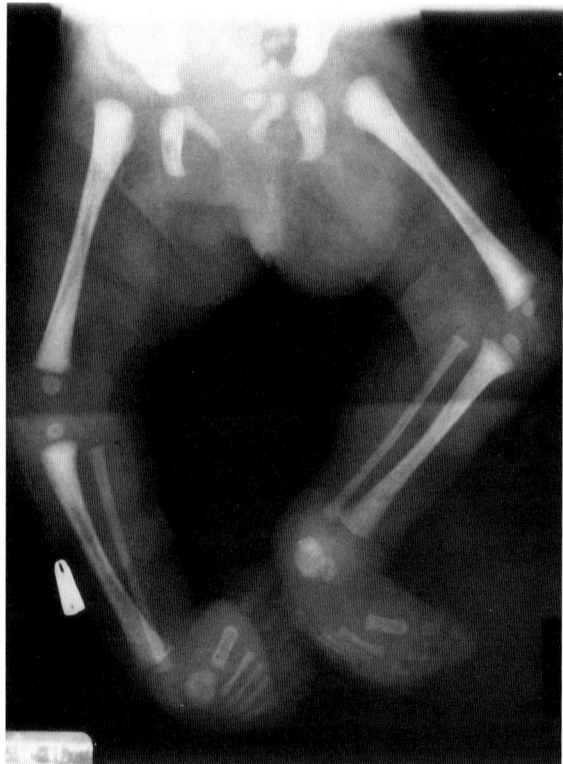

FIGURE 8-12. Arthrogryposis multiplex congenita at birth. Features include club feet, knee flexion deformity, and dislocated right hip. The articular surfaces are normal. Adaptive changes occur as a consequence of the fixed position. (From Goldberg MJ. The dysmorphic child: an orthopaedic perspective. New York: Raven Press, 1987.)

patients are nonambulators, and many others are limited household walkers.[112] As a rule, those with arthrogryposis who are very weak as infants stay weak, and those who appear stronger as infants stay strong. Adult dependency seems to be related to education and coping skills more than to the magnitude of joint contractures. Early family counseling is important.

Treatment

Each joint presents unique opportunities for orthopaedic intervention, but at times, an overview of the totally involved patient must be borne in mind. The overall goals are lower limb alignment and stability for ambulation and upper extremity motion for self care.[103,107,126] Outcomes seem better if joint surgery is done early, before adaptive intraarticular changes, but it is not uncommon to correct one joint and delay correction of another. Correcting the joints simultaneously or prematurely may jeopardize the overall success.[121]

It is important to think about how one contracture relates to another. In general, articular surgery is done early, and osteotomies are performed closer to the completion of growth. It is important to promote early motion and avoid casts if possible. Long-term bracing and other assistive devices are the rule.

Joint contractures make the birthing process difficult, and neonatal fractures may result.[100] Only after a thorough search for diaphyseal fractures should physical therapy begin in the nursery.[116] Mobilization of the joint and realignment is best accomplished by early and frequent range of motion exercises and splinting of the joint in a position of function with a removable orthotic.[116,121] When started in infancy and continued at home throughout their first year of life, a therapeutic range of motion program may be expected to improve the joint contractures and increase the passive range of motion. The active range of motion does not improve very much.[121] Fractures may accompany an overly vigorous program.

About two thirds of patients have developmental dysplasia of the hip or frank dislocation (see Fig. 8-12).[114,120,121,123] At birth, the hips are flexed and abducted. Although hip motion does improve with physical therapy, gait is significantly affected by hip contractures, and release of soft tissue contractures early may be needed, especially if there is a significant flexion deformity. The most effective treatment for dislocation of the hip is unknown. Closed methods rarely succeed.[120,128] Studies of children with untreated dislocated hips concluded that those with bilateral dislocations frequently had satisfactory range of motion, their hips did not prevent them from walking, although rarely, about the community, and pain was uncommon.[114,123,128] Those with unilateral dislocations fared less well. More were limited to the household with walkers, and although scoliosis was present in most patients, it was worse and more frequent in those with unilateral dislocations.[121]

In both groups, limitation of ambulation results more from the severe involvement of all four extremities than from the dislocated hips.[121] The recommendation that a unilateral dislocated hip be reduced and bilateral ones left alone has had considerable support in the literature.[114,120,121,128] Because hip surgery was often delayed until the knees were mobilized, the reduction did not occur until 1 year of age. Initial reports, however, of early open reduction of unilateral and bilateral dislocated hips through a medial adductor approach are promising, and the reduced period of immobilization has improved postoperative range of motion of hips and knees.[123]

Although the classic description of the knees is that they are hyperextended, most are in flexion (see Fig. 8-12).[106,121,122,125] The precise plane of motion is often difficult to determine, and although physical therapy is recommended, medial lateral instability may result. Hyperextension deformity responds better to physical therapy than do flexion deformities. If the flexion deformity remains more than 30 degrees, ambulation is precluded because of the associated overall muscle weakness, especially of the quadriceps and gluteus maximus. Sometime before 2 years of age, soft tissue surgery, including posterior capsulotomy may be considered. Supracondylar osteotomies of the femur are recommended toward the end of growth.[121,122,125] A knee hyperextension deformity should be treated before the hip. The knee initially does well with physical therapy and orthosis, but the promising early results are often disappointing over time, with surgery often needed later. Late osteoarthritis seems more common in those with persistent hyperextension.

A severe and resistant clubfoot is characteristic (see Fig. 8-12).[105,121,132] It is rare for the arthrogrypotic clubfoot to respond to physical therapy and casts. An extensive circumferential release with resection of the tendon insertions is necessary, including surgery on the plantar aspect of the foot. Surgery for the clubfoot is usually done at about 1 year of age or later. In the child with multiple affected joints, the knees are usually mobilized first, dislocated hips are then reduced, and the clubfoot is corrected. Primary talectomy has been recommended because of the high incidence of failed soft tissue surgery.[104,113] Salvage talectomy is an alternative. As a teenager, triple arthrodesis is often needed. The treatment goal is to create a plantigrade braced foot. A vertical talus is an unusual foot deformity in arthrogryposis multiplex congenita, and if encountered, the physician must think of the distal arthrogryposes or pterygia syndromes.

The physician should never think of an individual joint in the upper extremity, but only the whole arm.[94,129] Analysis needs to include each hand alone and how the two hands work together as an effective functional unit. Although timing of surgery in the upper extremity is controversial, surgical interventions are usually postponed until a thorough functional assessment can be made. There are two key goals in treatment of the upper extremities: self-help skills, such as feeding and toileting, and mobility skills, such as pushing out of a chair and use of crutches.

The shoulder is usually satisfactory without treatment. For the elbow, it is ideal to achieve flexion to 90 degrees from the fixed extended position. The fibrotic joint capsule and the weak muscles make the prospect of achieving active elbow flexion unlikely. Passive elbow flexion to a right angle is a prerequisite for considering a tendon transfer for active elbow flexion. Restoration of elbow motion by capsulotomy and triceps lengthening has had only fair success, diminishing the likelihood for success when an arthrogrypotic muscle is used to motor the joint.[101] The triceps brachii and pectoralis have been the most frequently tried, and success has been fair at best.[91,129] Distal humeral osteotomy, designed to place the elbow into flexion and correct some of the shoulder internal rotation deformity, may be performed toward the end of the first decade.[128,129] It is designed to improve hand to mouth function. Care must be taken not to excessively externally rotate the distal humerus. The hand and wrist is usually flexed and ulna deviated, but variations within this pattern exists.[93,131] In general, the ulna side digits are more involved. Proximal interphalangeal flexion deformities rarely respond to physical therapy or surgery. The thumb is flexed and adducted into the palm and responds better to surgery than do the other digits.

Approximately one third of patients develop scoliosis.[98] It is a neuromuscular curve instead of a congenital curve. It is C-shaped, often with hyperlordosis, and responds poorly to orthoses. Indications for surgery are similar to those for other neuromuscular scoliosis.

Other Forms of Arthrogryposis

Larsen syndrome, distal arthrogryposis, Freeman-Sheldon syndrome, and the pterygia syndromes have joint contractures, dislocations, and deformities that are similar to classic arthrogryposis multiplex congenita, but they also have several distinctive features.

Larsen Syndrome

The essential features of Larsen syndrome are multiple congenital dislocations of large joints, a characteristic flat face, and ligamentous laxity (Fig. 8-13).[138]

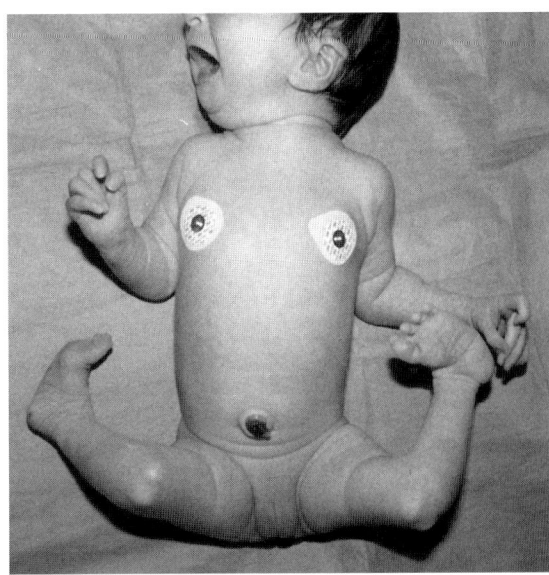

FIGURE 8-13. Larsen syndrome in a 1-week-old patient who has bilateral dislocated knees and clubfeet. (From Goldberg MJ. The dysmorphic child: an orthopaedic perspective. New York, Raven Press, 1987.)

It is rare, but several large series have been reported. The cause is unknown. It is autosomal dominant in some families, but other families suggest an autosomal recessive inheritance pattern.[134,140,144] Autosomal recessive inheritance may have the more severe phenotype. The biochemical defect is unknown.

The clinical features include a face that is flattened, especially when observed in profile; some hypertelorism; and a broad forehead. Dislocation of multiple joints appears in a characteristic pattern that includes bilateral dislocated knees, with the tibia anterior on the femur; bilateral dislocated hips; bilateral dislocated elbows; and bilateral clubfeet.[135,137,139,143,145] The physician should think of this syndrome whenever dislocated knees are detected. The ligaments are lax or entirely absent. The ligamentous laxity is often so substantial that Larsen syndrome may be confused with Ehlers-Danlos syndrome. The children have normal intelligence. The prognosis is generally good with aggressive orthopaedic treatment if the child survives the first year of life. The mortality figures for the first year may be as high as 40%. During the neonatal period, the cartilage supporting structure of the larynx and trachea is soft, and there may be alarming elasticity of the thoracic cage at the costochondral junction, leading to respiratory failure and death. Congenital cardiac septal defects and acquired lesions of the mitral valve and aorta, similar to those found in Marfan syndrome, further complicate medical and anesthesia management.[136]

On x-ray films, the knees are dislocated, with the tibia anterior to the femur.[139] Arthrograms show a small or absent suprapatellar pouch, absent cruciate ligaments, and a misaligned patella (Fig. 8-14). The elbows have complex dislocations: radial-humeral, ulnar-humeral, and radial-ulnar. Radial-ulnar synostosis is common and usually associated with ulnar-humeral dislocation (Fig. 8-15B). A spheroid ossicle frequently occurs anterior to the elbow joint; its origin is unknown. There is an increased number of carpal centers (Fig. 8-15A), extra ossification centers in the foot, and a curious double ossification pattern of the calcaneus (Fig. 8-15C). Abnormal cervical spine segmentation is typical with instability, a complication often associated with myelopathy.

The primary goal is to achieve knee stability, but lax ligaments are the major obstacle. Reduction usually requires surgery, but often the knee remains unstable because of a deficiency of the anterior cruciate ligament. Long-term orthoses are often needed. Successful anterior cruciate ligament reconstruction with synthetic ligaments has not been reported. It is important to perform knee surgery early, certainly before correcting the dislocated hip or clubfeet.[139,142] Although most knees do not respond to attempts at manipulation and cast correction, it has been traditional to try

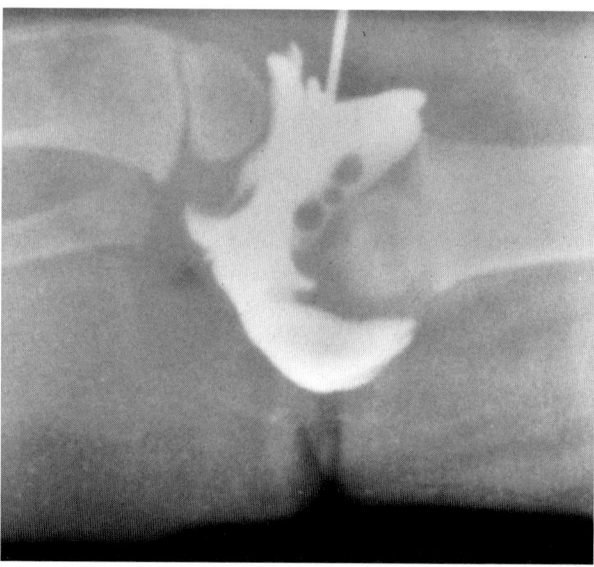

FIGURE 8-14. Larsen syndrome in a 5-month-old patient. The arthrogram of a knee shows anterior dislocation of the tibia on the femur and no suprapatellar pouch.

this approach initially. Too vigorous manipulations result in distal femoral metaphyseal-physeal fractures. If the commonly associated pulmonary problems permit, surgery may be undertaken as early as 3 to 4 months of age. Cautious restoration of the range of motion (gaining full extension is often a problem) while guarding against redisclocation by using a flexion splint or brace often delays addressing the hips until 1 years of age.

The hips are dislocated, often despite a rather normal-appearing acetabulum. There is a sensation of good range of motion, although the hip may prove to be irreducible. After the knee deformity has been corrected, unilateral hip dislocations are treated. Because of the problems with difficult reductions, redislocations, and the seemingly paradoxical excellent range of motion of the dislocated hips, it is reasonable to leave bilateral dislocated hips alone.

The clubfeet can be managed in a cast until the knee deformity is corrected. Some feet can be corrected with serial plasters, but long-term results suggest less residual deformity when the foot is treated surgically.[139] The foot may need to be braced to control ankle instability.

Despite the dislocations of the elbow or shoulder, the arms remain functional and rarely require treatment. Crutches or walkers can be used despite the dislocations.

Although scoliosis is common, the major concern is structural abnormalities of the cervical vertebrae.[133,141] There are combinations of synostosis and instability, and a cervical kyphosis and forward subluxation may result in quadriplegia and death. Stabilization early may be needed, although when done in very young children, considerable technical problems may be encountered.

Anesthesia complications are common. The mobile infolding arytenoid cartilage creates airway difficulties.[146] The anesthesiologist should be aware of possible cervical spine instability, and a preoperative lateral film is recommended.

With aggressive orthopaedic treatment, the prognosis for children with Larsen syndrome is generally good. Management, however, calls for careful monitoring of cardiorespiratory status in the first year and of the spine throughout life.

Distal Arthrogryposis

Children with distal arthrogryposis have characteristic fixed hand contractures and foot deformities, but the major large joints of the arms and legs are spared.[148,151,155] Craniofacial abnormalities are often associated, which has caused distal arthrogryposis to be separated into several eponymic syndromes, a situation that leads to confusion.[150] The cardinal features of distal arthrogryposis are the hand deformity with ulna deviation of the fingers at the metacarpophalangeal joint, flexion deformities at the proximal interphalangeal and metacarpophalangeal joints, and a cup-like palm with a single palmar crease (Fig. 8-16). The thumb is flexed and adducted, with a web at its base.[156] Distal arthrogryposis is common and it is often seen in hand clinic, where it often is incorrectly called multiple camptodactyly.

The inheritance pattern of distal arthrogryposis is autosomal dominant, but there may be considerable variation in families that leads to missing the diagnosis.[149,150,152,156]

Although the hand deformity is characteristic and constant, the feet may be clubbed, have stiff metatarsus adductus, or on occasion, have a vertical talus. The major joints in the upper and the lower extremity are otherwise normal, although a minor knee flexion deformity may be found. Intelligence is normal. The associated craniofacial anomalies are cleft lip or cleft palate, and in those families, the syndrome of distal arthrogryposis may have an eponymous name.[153,154] Roentgenograms show normal bony architecture, and

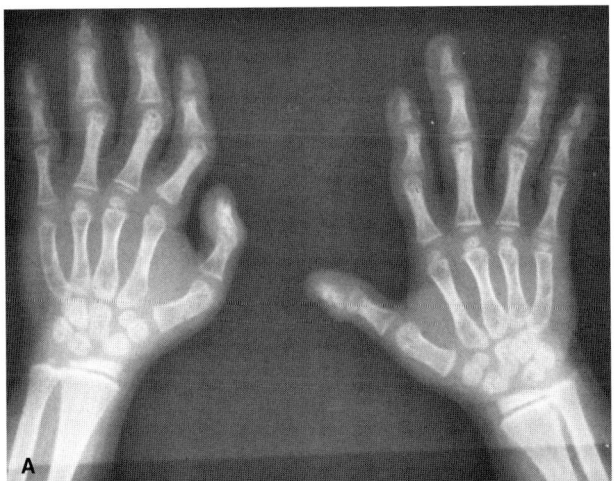
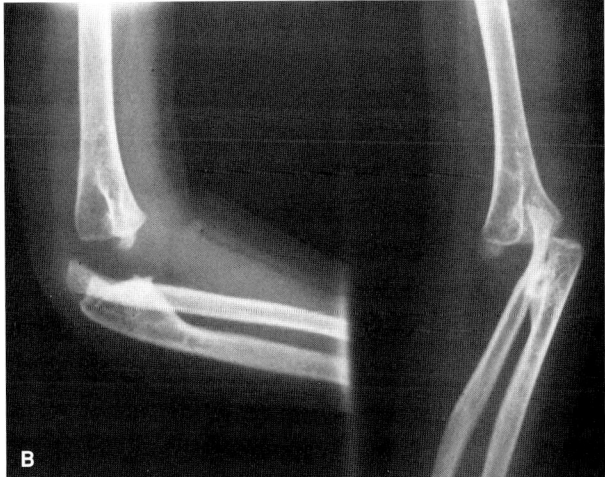
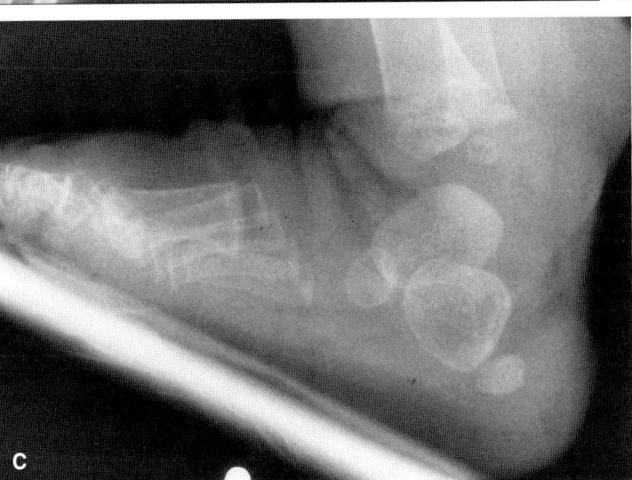

FIGURE 8-15. A 4-year-old patient with Larsen syndrome. Characteristic roentgenograms (**A**) The hands show an increased number of carpal centers and interphalangeal joint subluxations. (**B**) The elbows, demonstrate total dislocation but full functional ability. (**A** and **B** from Goldberg MJ. The dysmorphic child: an orthopaedic perspective. New York: Raven Press, 1987.) (**C**) The foot has an abnormal os calcis containing two ossification centers.

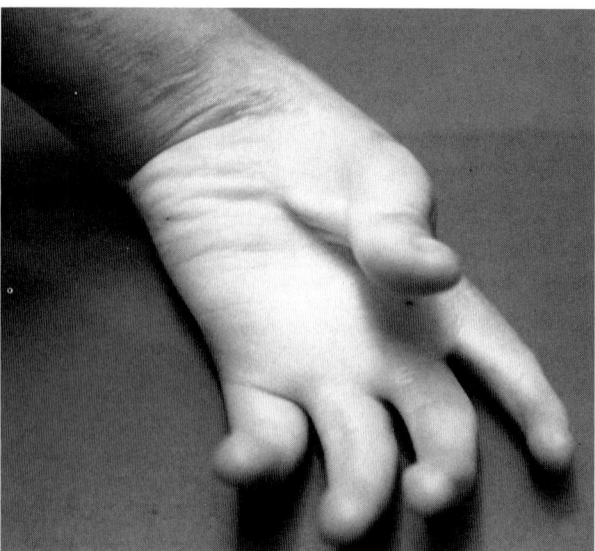

FIGURE 8-16. Distal arthrogryposis. Characteristic hand is the result of ulnar deviation at the metacarpophalangeal (MCP) joints. Notice the deeply cupped palm and webbing of the MCP joint of the thumb.

only with persistence of deformities in the hand and feet are articular changes detected. This syndrome can be diagnosed prenatally in families that are at risk by detecting the unchanged position and lack of motion of the hands in contrast to the normal activity of the large uninvolved joints.[147]

Overall, the child does well with physical therapy. The hands function well because the shoulders, elbows, and wrists are normal. Thumb surgery to lengthen the flexor pollicis longus and rebalance the extensor is the most common surgery. The feet more frequently require surgery, although many clubfeet can be corrected with manipulation and serial casts. The outcome of treatment of clubfoot is better in this syndrome than for other arthrogrypotic clubfeet.

Freeman-Sheldon Syndrome

Freeman-Sheldon syndrome is often combined with distal arthrogryposis because of the similar hand and foot deformities. However, the associated anomalies and a variable inheritance makes Freeman-Sheldon a distinct syndrome. It is recognized by its most characteristic feature, a "whistling face." The original name craniocarpotarsal dystrophy is misleading.[160,168] This syndrome is usually sporadic, although there is evidence of autosomal dominant and autosomal recessive inheritance.[157,163,170] Clinically, the distinguishing feature is the face (Fig. 8-17). The eyes are deeply set. The cheeks are fleshy, and pursed lips simulate whistling. There is a small mouth and a curious H-shaped dimple in the chin. The hands demonstrate the classic distal arthrogryposis pattern described earlier.[159,163,166]

The foot deformity is clubfeet in 80% and vertical talus in the remainder (Fig. 8-18). The feet are rigid.[159,163,166]

Scoliosis is common.[163,166] It was initially not recognized as a common feature, but it affects more than one half of the patients. The onset is in the first decade. It is often severe, with a left thoracic pattern reported regularly. The vertebrae are normally shaped.

Associated other contractures include flexion deformities of the elbow and knee, decreased shoulder range of motion, decreased neck range of motion, and dislocated hips. Each of these contractures is difficult to manage, characteristic of an arthrogrypotic syndrome. The radiographic features are adaptive changes to the skeleton over time.[165] The buccinator muscle is hypoplastic, and electromyograms and muscle biopsies are identical to the peripheral muscle studies in classic arthrogryposis multiplex congenita.[167]

During infancy, dysphagia and aspiration lead to failure to thrive and death. Surgery to permit adequate mouth opening for feeding may be necessary.[164] If the children survive the neonatal period, they do well and have normal intelligence.

The hands need early physical and occupational therapy, but there is less spontaneous improvement than seen with the other distal arthrogryposis syndromes. Thumb surgery is common.[169] It is important to do hand surgery early, especially if there is decreased shoulder or elbow motion. The clubfoot and vertical talus deformities are resistant to nonoperative measures. Scoliosis is often rigid and resistant to bracing.

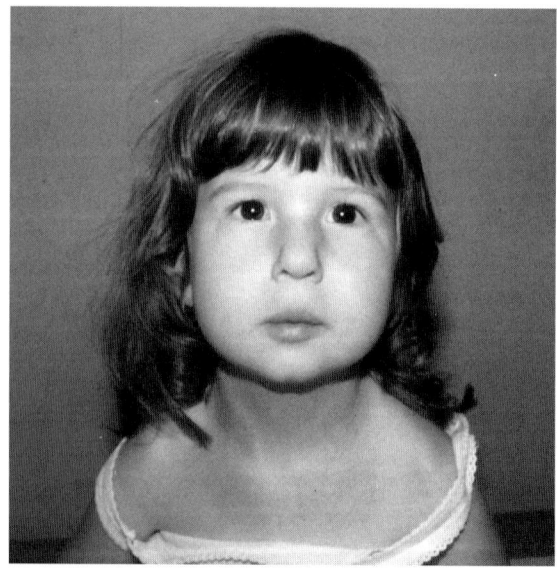

FIGURE 8-17. Freeman-Sheldon syndrome in a 3-year-old patient. Notice the small chin and mouth, long philtrum, puffy cheeks, deeply set eyes, and small chin cleft. (From Goldberg MJ. The dysmorphic child: an orthopaedic perspective. New York: Raven Press, 1987.)

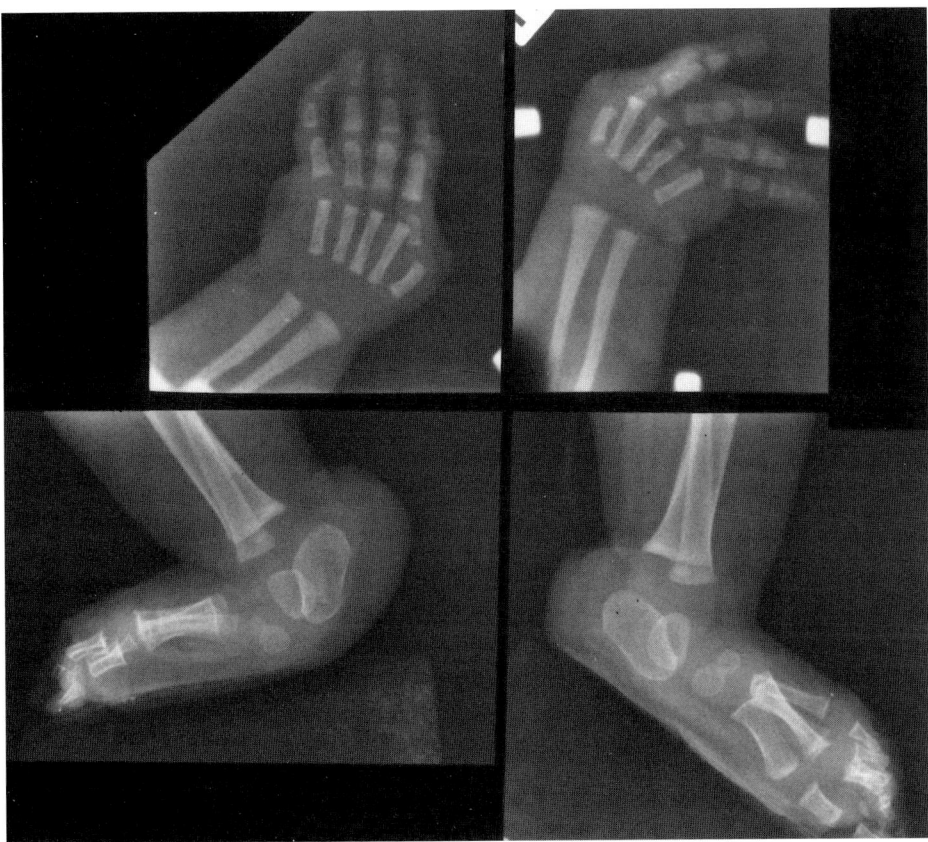

FIGURE 8-18. Freeman-Sheldon syndrome in a 5-year-old patient. Radiographs of the hands demonstrate ulnar deviation at the metacarpophalangeal joint, typical of a distal arthrogryposis syndrome. The feet show bilateral congenital vertical tali. All other joints in this patient were normal. (From Goldberg MJ. The dysmorphic child: an orthopaedic perspective. New York: Raven Press, 1987.)

When surgery is undertaken, the anesthesiologist must be alerted about the small mouth and inflexible neck, which may make intubation difficult. Anesthesia complications are common, some the result of abnormalities related to the laryngeal cartilages.[158,161,162,164]

Pterygia Syndromes

Pterygium comes from a Greek word meaning little wing. A pterygium is a web. It can be seen as an isolated malformation in some syndromes, such as the pterygium colli in the neck of patients with Klippel-Feil syndrome.

There are two clinically important pterygia syndromes: multiple pterygium syndrome and popliteal pterygia syndrome.[178] Several pterygium syndromes are lethal, with the affected patients not surviving pregnancy or the newborn period.[174,175] The web syndromes are separated genetically as autosomal recessive (i.e., lethal pterygium syndrome and multiple pterygium) and autosomal dominant (i.e., popliteal pterygium).[179] However, they often overlap. Lethal pterygium syndrome may be diagnosed prenatally by detecting hydrops and cystic hygroma colli.[181] It has been suggested that there is a jugular lymphatic obstruction in the embryo and a loss of muscle without central nervous system involvement, quite unlike classic arthrogryposis multiplex congenita.[186] There has also been some suggestion of abnormally fragile collagen in pterygia syndrome, but the exact molecular defects have not been established.

Multiple pterygia syndrome (i.e., Escobar syndrome) is characterized by a web across every flexion crease in the extremities, most prominently across the popliteal space, the elbow, and in the axilla (Fig. 8-19).[185,188] There also are webs across the neck laterally and anteriorly from sternum to the chin, drawing the facial features down. The fingers are webbed. The webs can be obvious, but if they are not, the affected children can look very much like those with arthrogryposis multiplex congenita. The two features that differentiate this syndrome from classic arthrogryposis are vertical talus and congenital spine deformity. The vertical talus is fairly constant in multiple pterygium syndrome and can only be managed surgically. Circumferential release and prolonged protection, as in managing any arthrogrypotic foot deformity, is necessary. The spine deformity is significant, with multiple segmentation abnormalities and a lordoscoliosis (Figs. 8-20 and 8-21).[190] The lordoscoliosis may be substantial enough to interfere with trunk and chest growth, leading to respiratory death during the first or second year of life (see Fig. 8-21). Mobility depends much on the magnitude of the lower extremity webs and the remaining joint motion, with many patients limited to wheelchair for locomotion. The children

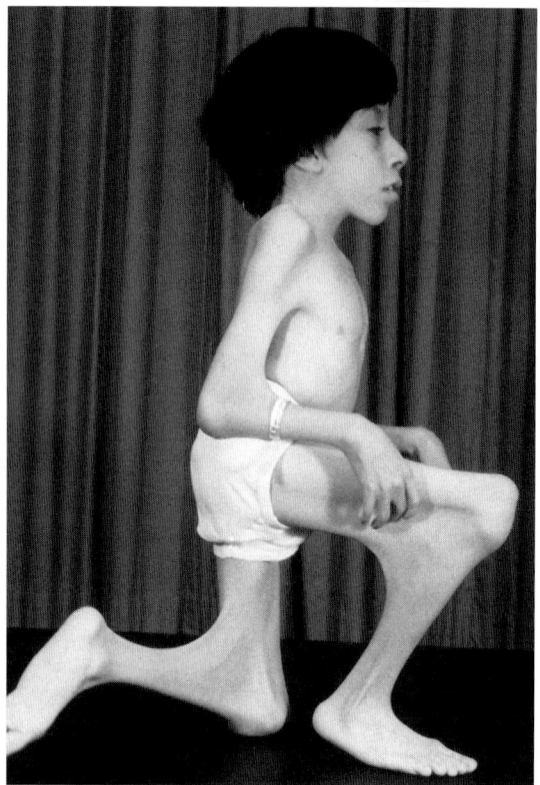

FIGURE 8-19. Multiple pterygium syndrome in a 12-year-old patient. Antecubital webs fix the elbows, and popliteal webs prevent ambulation. The patient had normal intelligence and became a college graduate. (From Goldberg MJ. The dysmorphic child: an orthopaedic perspective. New York: Raven Press, 1987.)

thought. For example, mild webs in joints of the upper extremity may be found in patients with popliteal pterygium syndrome. Adaptive changes in the joints occur over time. Radiographically, the patella becomes elongated and the femoral condyles flattened as a result of knee flexion deformity.

From a management perspective, the determining factors are the magnitude of scoliosis and the size of the web crossing the knee. The thoracic vertebral dysplasia, thoracic lordosis, and the small chest impairs lung development, resulting in early death in those with multiple pterygium syndrome. For the longer-term survivor, management of the spine deformity is identical to those with nonsyndromic congenital scoliosis. Preoperative evaluation of intraspinal contents by MRI and ultrasound of the kidney are indicated. Correction of deformity is unlikely, and the

have normal intelligence and efforts for their independence should be maximized. Surgery is rarely needed for the upper extremities.

Popliteal pterygium syndrome (i.e., fascial-genital-popliteal syndrome) has recognizable features in the face, the genitals, and the knee.[176,177,182,183,187] The features include a cleft lip and palate, lip pits, and intraoral adhesions.[184,191] A fibrous band crosses the perineum and distorts the genitalia.[173] A popliteal web is usually present bilaterally.[187] It runs from thigh to ankle, resulting in a severe knee flexion deformity. Tibia hypoplasia may be associated. Within the popliteal web is a superficial fibrous band over which lies a tent of muscle running from the os calcis to the ischium and known in the older literature as a calcaneoischiadicus muscle. The popliteal artery and vein are usually deep, but the sciatic nerve is superficial in the web, just underneath the fibrous band (Fig. 8-22).

There is a distinctive foot abnormality in this syndrome: a bifid great toenail and syndactyly of the lesser toes.

Although the original cases of multiple and popliteal pterygium syndromes were clearly defined, there is more phenotypic variation in both than originally

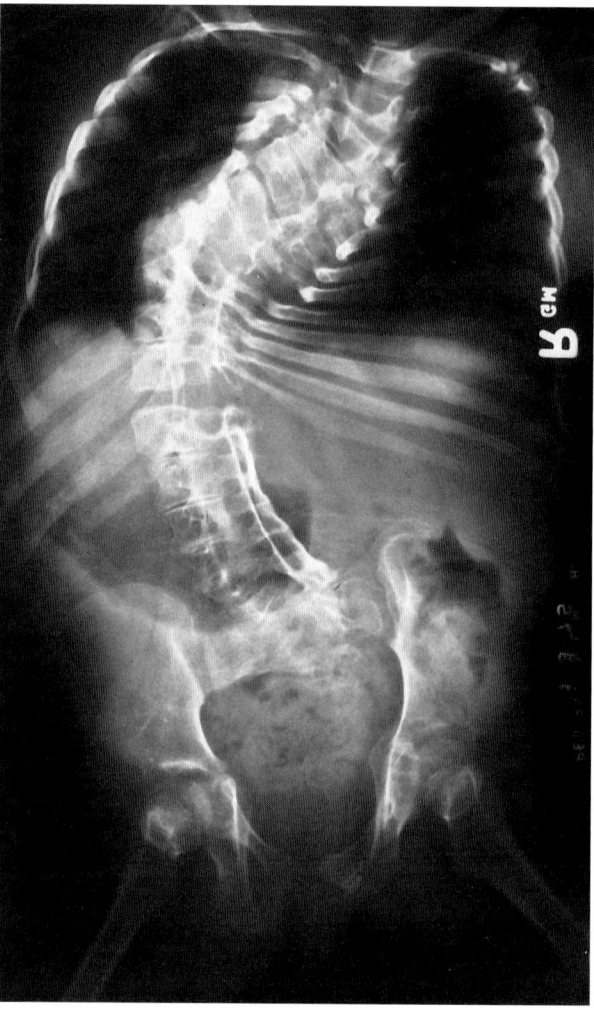

FIGURE 8-20. Multiple pterygium syndrome in a 13-year-old patient. Radiograph shows severe scoliosis, vertebral abnormalities, and an unsegmented bar from T9 to T12 and from L1 to S1, with an apparent gap between the bars. (From Goldberg MJ. The dysmorphic child: an orthopaedic perspective. New York: Raven Press, 1987.)

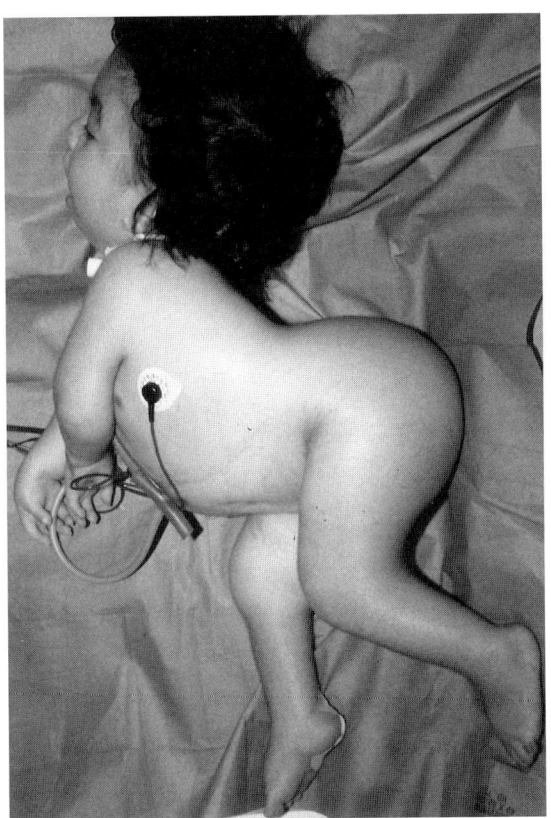

FIGURE 8-21. Multiple pterygium syndrome. Severe limitation of trunk growth was caused by vertebral fusions and lordoscoliosis. Death occurred at 24 months of age because of respiratory failure.

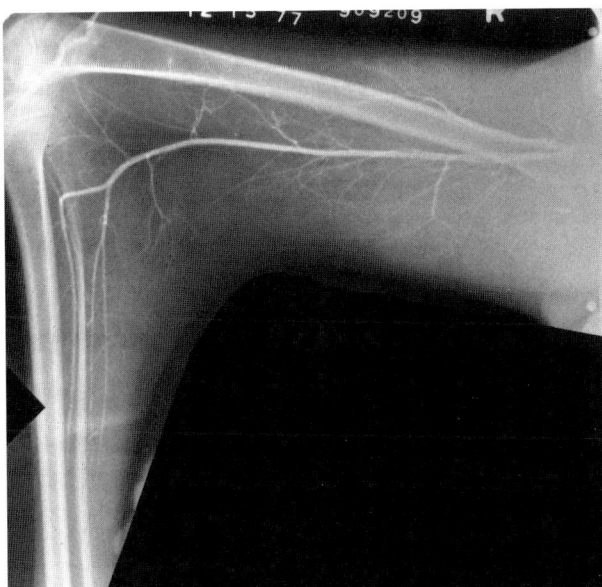

FIGURE 8-22. Popliteal pterygium in a 13-year-old patient. Arteriogram shows that the popliteal artery has been drawn up from its normal position. At the margin of the web is the sciatic nerve. (From Goldberg MJ. The dysmorphic child: an orthopaedic overview. New York: Raven Press, 1987.)

decision for early fusion must balance the factors of curve progression and limiting spine growth.

The knee is the joint that limits mobility in both syndromes and is the joint that most determines future ambulatory potential.[171,172,180,187] Traditionally, treatment of the knee begins with physical therapy, but its effectiveness is doubtful. Early popliteal web surgery is recommended before the onset of too-great adaptive changes in the articular surfaces and before further vascular shortening. There is a high recurrence rate despite braces. Femoral shortening and extension osteotomy are usually postponed until after maturity, but if almost full knee extension cannot be achieved at surgery, even if during infancy or childhood, femoral shortening can be considered.[189] The indications for and the success of gradual distraction techniques have yet to be demonstrated.

DOWN SYNDROME

Down syndrome is the most common and perhaps the most readily recognizable malformation in humans (Fig. 8-23).[203] Complete trisomy 21 accounts for 95% of the cases, with 2% mosaics and 3% translocations. The overall risk is 1 per 660 live births, and the incidence is closely related to maternal age. If the mother is younger than 30 years of age, the risk is 1 of 5000 live births, and if the mother is older than 35 years of age, the incidence rises to 1 in 250. Analysis of patients with translocations indicates that the critical region necessary for Down syndrome resides in part of the long arm of chromosome 21. Many of the classic phenotypic features, such as the characteristic facies, hand anomalies, congenital heart disease, and some aspects of the mental retardation result from the duplication of a single band, 21q22.2-22.3.[195] All the features of Down syndrome occur in the normal population, but they do so at a much lower incidence and are not grouped together.

There is a remarkable array of orthopaedic manifestations in those with Down syndrome. Some 10% of people with Down syndrome show an increased atlantodens interval on lateral spine films (Fig. 8-24A).[209,218,219,224,229] The implications of this have been overstated and understated, because study populations have been uncontrolled, adult and pediatric, and institutionalized and community members, and the roentgenographic techniques have varied from standard lateral to flexion-extension. The normal excursion of C1 during neck motion in patients with Down syndrome is unknown, and whether an increased atlantodens interval truly represents instability is not certain.[218,231] This lack of information is complicated by the broad array of other abnormalities in the upper cervical spine, including instability at occiput–C1,[202,211,227,229] odontoid dysplasia (Fig.

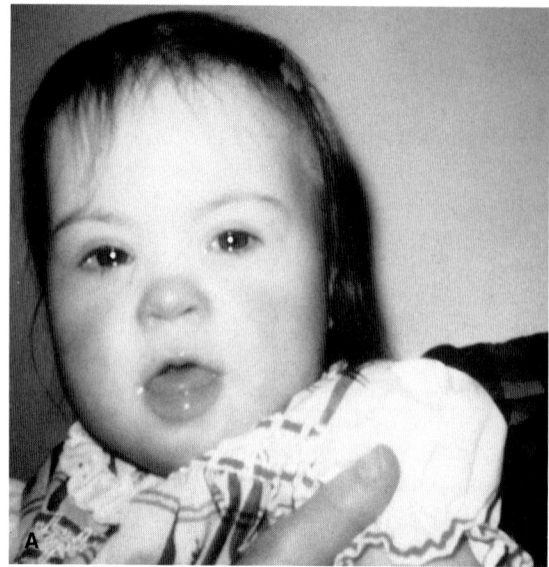 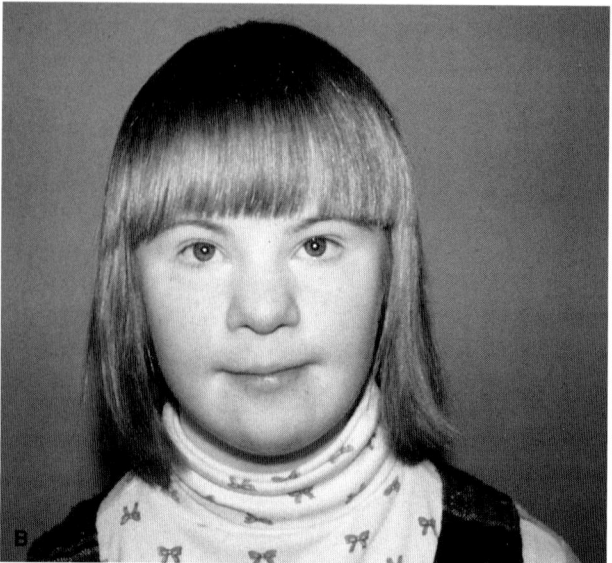

FIGURE 8-23. Down syndrome. The child has the characteristic face, with upward-slanting eyes, epicanthal folds, open mouth of early childhood, and flattened profile. (**A**) At 1 year of age. (Courtesy of Murray Feingold, M.D., Boston, MA.) (**B**) At 10 years of age. (From Goldberg MJ. The dysmorphic child: an orthopaedic perspective. New York: Raven Press, 1987.)

8-24C),[215,218] laminal defects at C1 (Fig. 8-24B),[210] spondylolisthesis (Fig. 8-24D), and precocious arthritis in the midcervical region (Fig. 8-24E).[201,228] Although routine screening radiographs often disclose these cervical spine abnormalities, roentgenograms are not reliable in predicting myelopathy.[197,215,217,220,224,231] Details of managing the cervical spine in Down syndrome are found in Chapter 21.

About one half the patients with Down syndrome have scoliosis, with an idiopathic pattern in 99%.[1,199] Congenital scoliosis is rare. Scoliosis is five times more likely to be detected in a severely retarded institutionalized population than in an ambulatory setting, which suggests confounding variables of detection and neuromuscular factors. Management by orthoses is as successful as in adolescents not affected by Down syndrome.

Surveys suggest an incidence of spondylolisthesis of about 6%, with the lumbar spine at L4–L5 and L5–S1 being most commonly involved. The condition may occur in the cervical spine.

The pelvis of an infant with Down syndrome has a diagnostic roentgenographic appearance characterized by flat acetabula and flared iliac wings. Before chromosome analysis, measurement of pelvic x-ray angles proved to be exceptionally accurate in diagnosing Down syndrome in the newborn.[196] Congenital dislocated hips are rare, but progressive dysplasia may begin during later childhood. This loss of acetabular containment and the inherent capsular laxity may lead to an acute or gradual complete dislocation (Fig. 8-25A, B). Although the onset of acetabular dysplasia is in late childhood, it can be progressive even after maturity, leading to adult dislocations (Fig. 8-25C, D).[206,222,225] As an adult, hip instability and developmental dysplasia of the hip leads to functional disability, interfering with walking and reducing independent mobility. Reconstruction during childhood includes femoral and acetabular osteotomies and careful imbrication of the redundant capsule is always required.[192,194,204,264] There are no good solutions for postmature onset of developmental dysplasia of the hip or long-standing dislocation in the adult.

Slipped capital femoral epiphyses are reported in all Down syndrome series, although the precise incidence is unknown (Fig. 8-26).[199,213] There appears to be a higher than expected risk for avascular necrosis. The reasons are not clear, but the factors include an increased number of acute slips and more late diagnoses. It is tempting to speculate about an association with the hypothyroid state, which is common in Down syndrome.

The configuration of the knee is that of genu valgum with a subluxed and dislocated patella (Fig. 8-27).[200] Repair of patellar instability is to be undertaken with caution and adherence to strict indications, such as impairment of ambulation or fixed knee flexion deformity. Recurrence is common, but fortunately, most knees do not need surgery; one survey indicated no more than 5% of the Down population.[200] However, there are few long-term studies of people with Down syndrome. Despite the fact that these people are living longer and have moved from institutions into the community, recommendations regarding management of

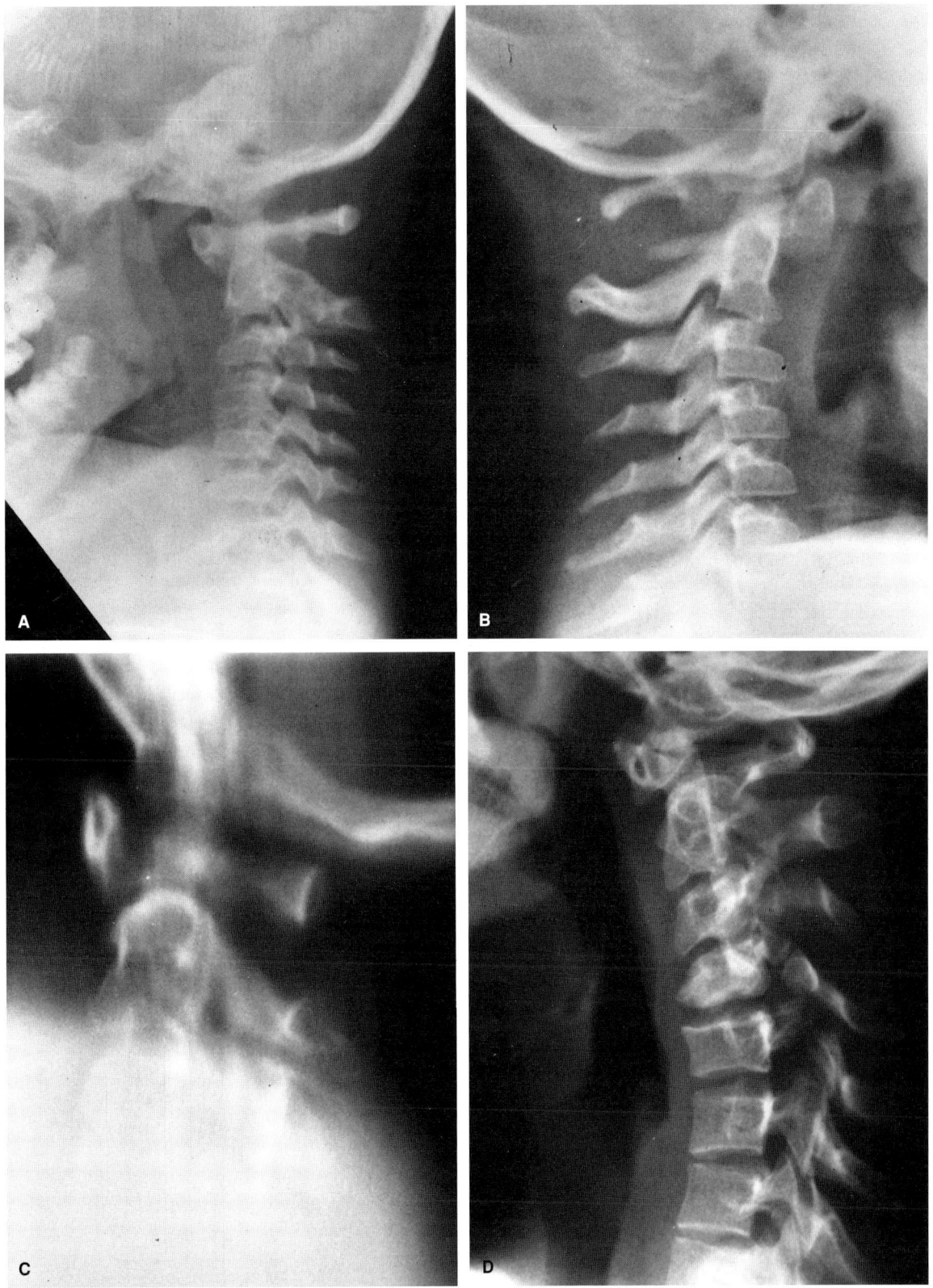

FIGURE 8-24. Cervical spine abnormalities in a patient with Down Syndrome. (**A**) Atlantodens instability at 8 years of age. (**B**) Hypoplastic posterior elements of C1 at 3 years of age. (**C**) Os odontoidium and increased atlantodens interval at 14 years of age. (**D**) Midcervical spondylolysis at 16 years of age. (**E**) Precocious osteoarthritis of the midcervical spine at 40 years of age. (From Goldberg MJ. The dysmorphic child: an orthopaedic perspective. New York: Raven Press, 1987.) *(continued)*

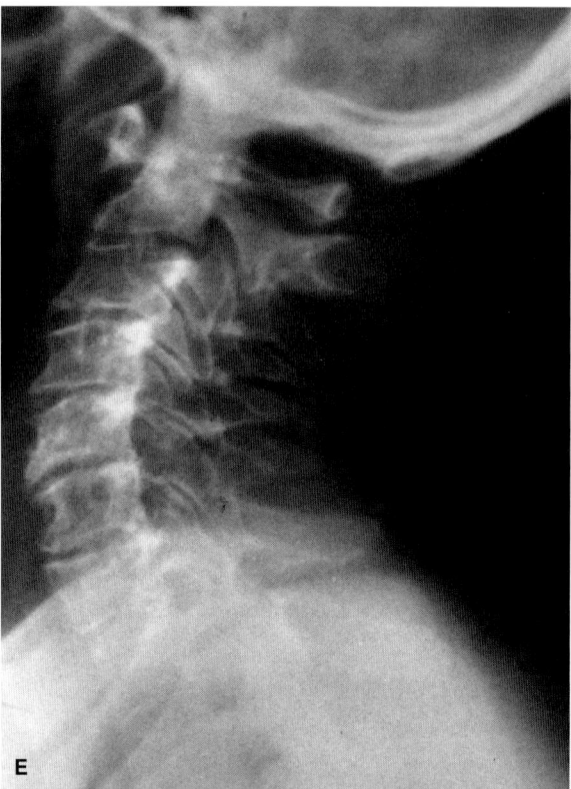

FIGURE 8-24 (*Continued*)

the unstable patella in childhood cannot be made with any certainty.

The characteristic appearance of the feet in childhood is one of an asymptomatic flexible planovalgus shape, with an increased space between the great and second toes. In many, hallux valgus develops in adolescence, and in adulthood, bunions may become quite symptomatic. There is no evidence that prophylactic orthotics are beneficial in childhood. Repair of hallux valgus and bunion may be needed as a late adolescence or young adulthood. Because of the hindfoot valgus, pronation, and external tibial torsion, the forces that produce bunions are obvious, and fusion of the first metatarsophalangeal joint should be considered. Because maintaining mobility in adults with Down syndrome is exceedingly important, any foot impairment must be treated.

The upper extremities in children with Down syndrome have characteristic findings, such as a simian crease and clinodactyly of the small finger, but these features have no clinical significance.[193]

A polyarticular arthropathy occurs in about 10% of those with Down syndrome.[205,212,226] Whether this is true juvenile rheumatoid arthritis or a unique inflammatory arthritis due to genetic or immune defects is unknown; the natural history is not documented. Delayed diagnosis is common. Nonsteroidal antiinflammatory drugs have been the mainstay of treatment. Foot symptoms are exceptionally frequent with the onset of polyarthropathy (Fig. 8-28).

Short stature is a cardinal feature; the average for male adults is 155 cm (61 in), and the average for female adults is 145 cm (57 in).[198] Prenatal diagnosis of Down syndrome by ultrasound has included detecting a short femur and humerus, but its reliability is questioned.[214,223,230] Milestones are delayed, with most children not walking until 2 to 3 years of age. The classic gait pattern is broad based, toed out, and waddling.[216,221] Ligamentous laxity and marked joint hypermobility are evident; the children are able to assume the most intriguing sitting postures. This ligamentous laxity was thought to predispose them to orthopaedic pathology such as C1–C2 instability and dislocated hips and patellae, but confirmation is lacking.[197,208] Attempts at relating standardized tests for ligamentous laxity (e.g., finger or elbow hyperextension) with the incidence of C1–C2 or other joint subluxation have failed to show a correlation.[197,208]

The general features of Down syndrome are well known. There is a characteristic flattened face. Mental retardation is typical, but performance is far better than expected from standard IQ testing. Congenital heart disease occurs in about one half of patients and is usually a septal defect (e.g., arteriovenous communis, ventricular septal defect). Duodenal atresia is found regularly. Leukemia occurs in about 1%.[1,3,5] There is a high incidence of endocrinopathies, hypothyroidism in particular.[1,3,5] Infections are common, although the precise molecular mechanism not apparent.[5] The appearance of premature aging is obvious, and there often is an early-onset Alzheimer disease.[207]

The natural history of those with Down syndrome has changed in the last few decades. Longevity has increased because of the aggressive surgical approach to congenital heart disease, chemotherapy for leukemia, and antibiotics for infection. Survival into the sixties is common. About 1 of 5 persons with Down syndrome has a musculoskeletal problem. Many, however, are merely x-ray abnormalities or curious physical findings. These patients often have excellent functional performance despite the abnormalities. There is a paucity of well-documented, long-term orthopaedic studies. Treatment programs must balance functional performance with physical and x-ray findings.

FETAL ALCOHOL SYNDROME

Fetal alcohol syndrome is a pattern of malformations originally delineated in children of alcoholic mothers. The full-blown syndrome is usually only seen in children of chronic alcoholics who drink throughout

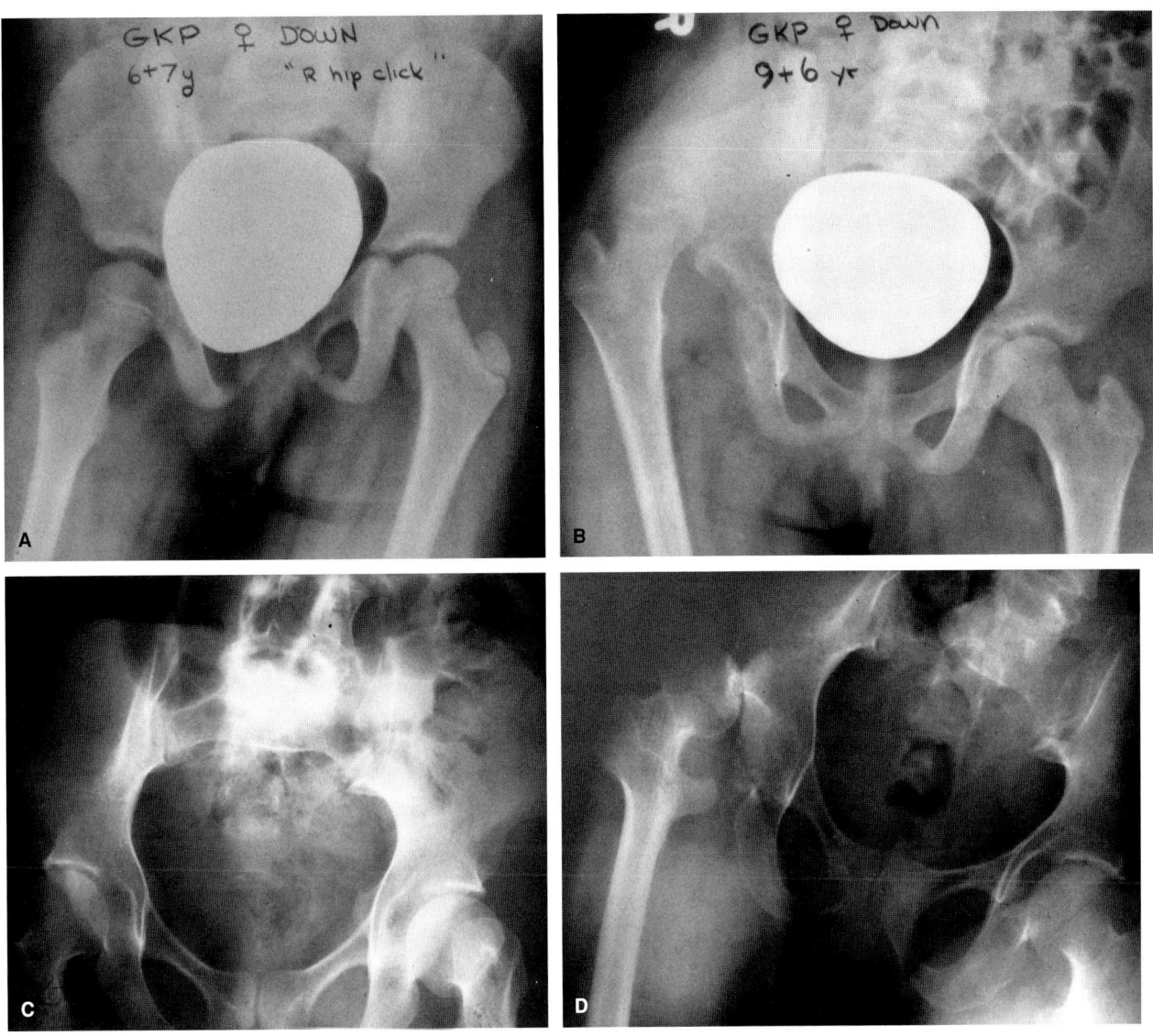

FIGURE 8-25. Down syndrome patient with late-onset developmental dysplasia of the hip and dislocation. (A) Standing roentgenogram of the pelvis at 6.5 years of age. (B) At 9.5 years of age, the patient suddenly refused to walk because of hip dislocation. (From Goldberg MJ. The dysmorphic child: an orthopaedic perspective. New York: Raven Press, 1987.) (C) Pelvic radiograph of a 31-year-old man with Down syndrome. (D) Three years later, dislocation of right hip occurred. (From Hresko MT, McCarthy JC, Goldberg MJ. Hip disease in adults with Down syndrome. J Bone Joint Surg 1993;75B:604.)

pregnancy. Lesser manifestations of the syndrome, known as fetal alcohol effects, may be related to more moderate alcohol ingestion.[237] Although the risk to alcoholic mothers is known, there is substantial difference of opinion about the effects of moderate alcohol use during pregnancy.[238,242,248] Alcohol is considered a teratogen, the most likely one for a mother to encounter.[247] The overall incidence of full-blown fetal alcohol syndrome is 0.33 per 1000 live births.[232,244] For an alcoholic mother, there is a 30% risk for fetal alcohol syndrome in her child. The precise mechanism by which alcohol induces the dysmorphic features is unknown, but the condition is preventable. In 1991, the cost for caring for children with fetal alcohol syndrome was estimated to be $250 million.[232]

A cardinal clinical feature is disturbed growth; the children have intrauterine growth retardation, small weight, and small length at birth, and these limitations remain despite good nutrition during childhood (Fig. 8-29).[250,252] Their smallness and a loss of fat suggest a search for endocrine dysfunction; the patients often look similar to those who are growth hormone deficient. The second cardinal feature is disturbed central nervous system development. Many children with fetal alcohol syndrome are found in cerebral palsy clinics. The typical child has a small head, a small brain, and

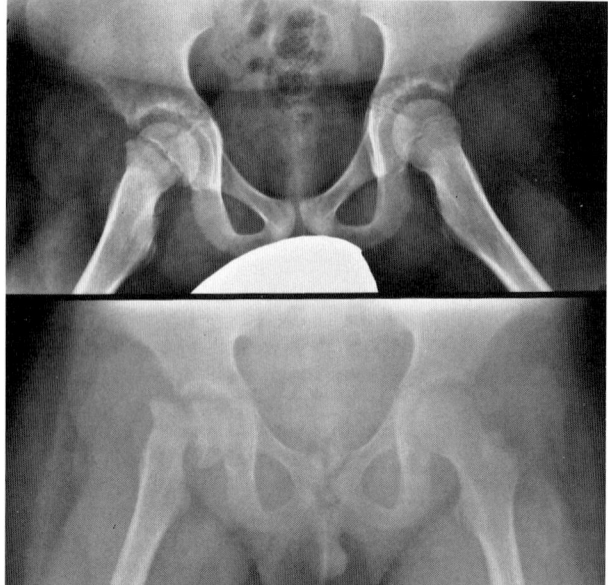

FIGURE 8-26. Effects of Down syndrome in a 12-year-old boy with 4 months of knee pain. The grade I slipped capital femoral epiphysis progressed to a total slip while the patient was undergoing preoperative evaluation and bed rest. (From Goldberg MJ. The dysmorphic child: an orthopaedic perspective. New York: Raven Press, 1987.)

delayed motor milestones. Accomplishing fine motor skills is also delayed. Hypotonia is present early but many develop spasticity later. The typical face has three characteristic features: short palpebral fissures (i.e., the eyes appear small), a flat philtrum (i.e., no groove below the nose), and a thin upper lip (see Fig. 8-29).[233,249]

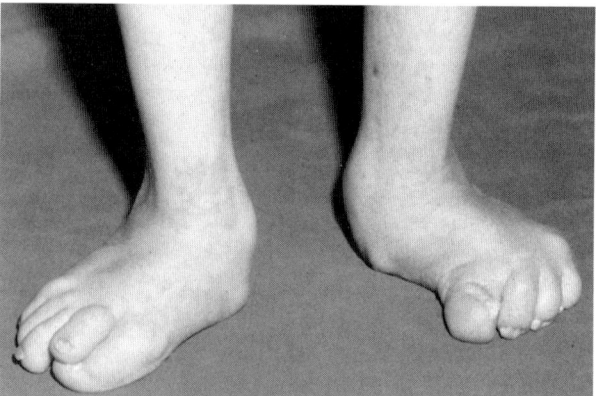

FIGURE 8-28. Polyarthritis of Down syndrome and valgus feet led to significant deformity in a 16-year-old patient. (From Goldberg MJ. The dysmorphic child: an orthopaedic perspective. New York: Raven Press, 1987.)

About 50% have an orthopaedic abnormality, but most are not disabling.[235,254,255] At birth, the range of motion is restricted, especially of the hands and feet, and occasionally, these contractures are fixed. The contractures typically respond well to physical therapy, although residual stiffness in the proximal interphalangeal joints may remain. Clubfoot is common, and about 10% have developmental dysplasia of the hip. The clubfoot is usually not rigid.[240] Cervical spine fusions, usually involving C2 and C3, may be indicated by radiographs.[236,245,246,251,253,255] These may resemble the picture seen in Klippel-Feil syndrome, but there are usually none of the other findings associated with that syndrome. Synostoses are also common in the upper extremity, with fusions involving the radial-ulnar articulation and the carpal bones, all without disabil-

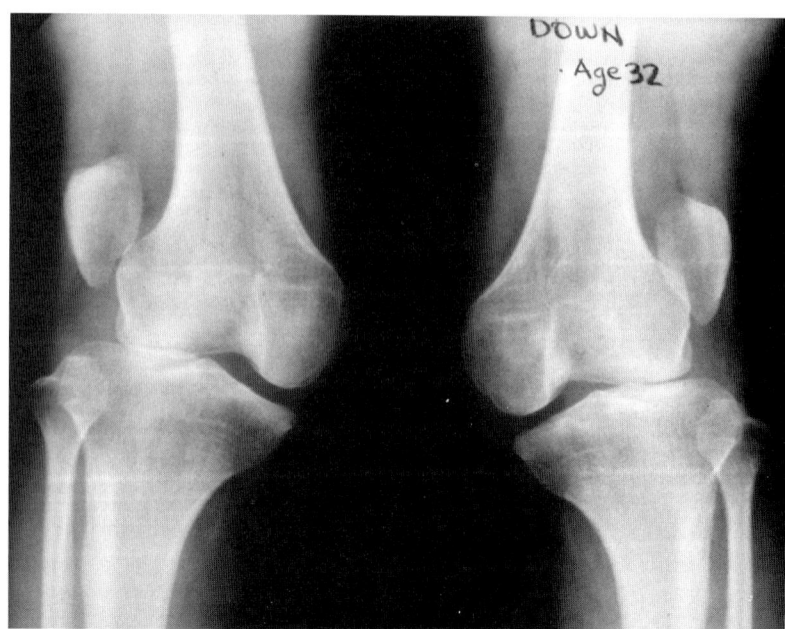

FIGURE 8-27. Down syndrome effects in a 32-year-old patient. The radiograph shows bilateral dislocated patellae and an oblique orientation of the joint line. The patient is fully ambulatory, but before standing, must manually reduce the patellae to the midline. (From Goldberg MJ. The dysmorphic child: an orthopaedic perspective. New York: Raven Press, 1987.)

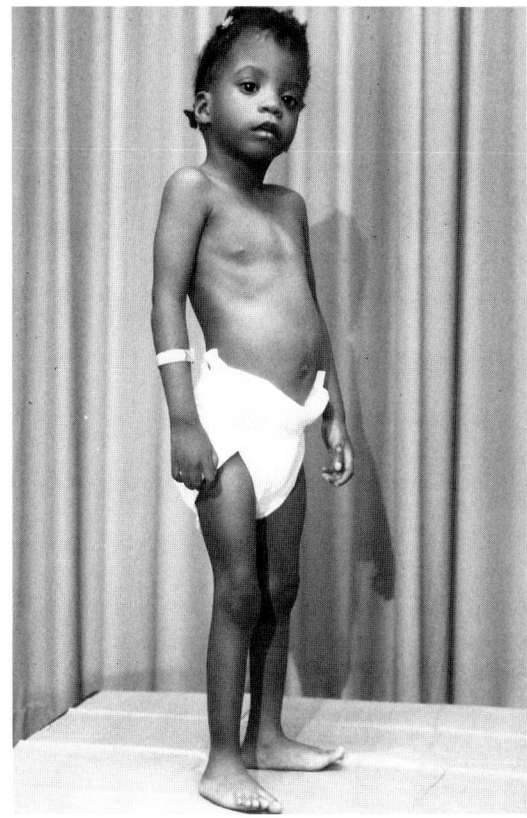

FIGURE 8-29. The 3-year-old patient is small and has the characteristic face of fetal alcohol syndrome. (From Goldberg MJ. The dysmorphic child: an orthopaedic perspective. New York: Raven Press, 1987.)

ity.[236,241,251] Stippled epiphyses may be seen in the lower extremities and rarely in the upper extremities.[243] Case reports link neural tube defects and fetal alcohol syndrome.[234,239]

The future for children with fetal alcohol is dim despite placement out of the alcoholic home. Intellect remains retarded, with little catch up. It is imperative for Social Services Departments to be involved early.

NAIL-PATELLA SYNDROME

Children with nail-patella syndrome have a quartet of findings that include nail dysplasia, patellar hypoplasia, elbow dysplasia, and iliac horns.[256] This is an autosomal dominant disorder, with the gene located on chromosome 9, next to the ABO blood groups. There is great variability in expression, even within a single family pedigree.

The most prominent feature is the dystrophic nails (Fig. 8-30A). The nail may be completely absent, hypoplastic, or show grooves and distortions in its surface.[249,257] The thumb is more involved than the small finger, and the ulnar border more involved than the radial. The hands are often very symmetric, and fingernails are more involved than toenails.

The second cardinal feature is hypoplastic patellae.[260] They are quite small but may be entirely absent (see Fig. 8-30B). They are unstable and may be found in a position of fixed dislocation. The patellar abnormality highlights the total knee dysplasia, with an abnormal femoral condyle and a curious septum running from the patella to the intercondylar groove (septum interarticularis), dividing the knee into two compartments. Abnormalities in varus and valgus alignment occur with valgus more commonly because of the small, flat lateral femoral condyle.[260]

The third feature is a dislocated radial head (see Fig. 8-30C).[260,267] The elbow joint is dysplastic, with abnormalities in the lateral humeral condyle, mimicking in many ways the dysplasia of the knee. The trochlea is large and the capitellum hypoplastic, creating an asymmetric shape that may predispose the radial head to dislocation.

The fourth and pathognomonic feature is iliac horns: bony exostoses on the posterior surface of the ilium (Fig. 8-30D).[258] They are asymptomatic and require no treatment.

There are other important orthopaedic findings:

- Short stature, with the children falling between the 3rd and 10th percentiles
- Shoulder girdle dysplasia that represents curious x-ray features and not any significant functional disability[265]
- Foot deformity that is common and often severe, frequently the chief presenting complaint of children with nail-patella syndrome, more so than nail or patella problems.[260,261] Deformities include variations of stiff calcaneal valgus, metatarsus adductus, and clubfeet.
- Restricted range of motion and contractures affect several large joints, including knee flexion deformities and external rotation contracture of the hip. When these contractures are severe and accompanied by stiff clubfeet, the diagnosis may be mistaken for arthrogryposis multiplex congenita.
- Madelung deformity[256,262]
- Spondylolysis[263]
- In some adults, inflammatory arthropathy[266]

The most important nonorthopaedic condition is kidney failure. The nephropathy of nail-patella syndrome causes significant morbidity, affecting the patient's longevity.[259,264]

Disability and presenting complaints are different at different ages. During childhood, it is foot deformity; during adolescence and young adulthood, it is problems with the knees; and in the older adult, it is renal failure.

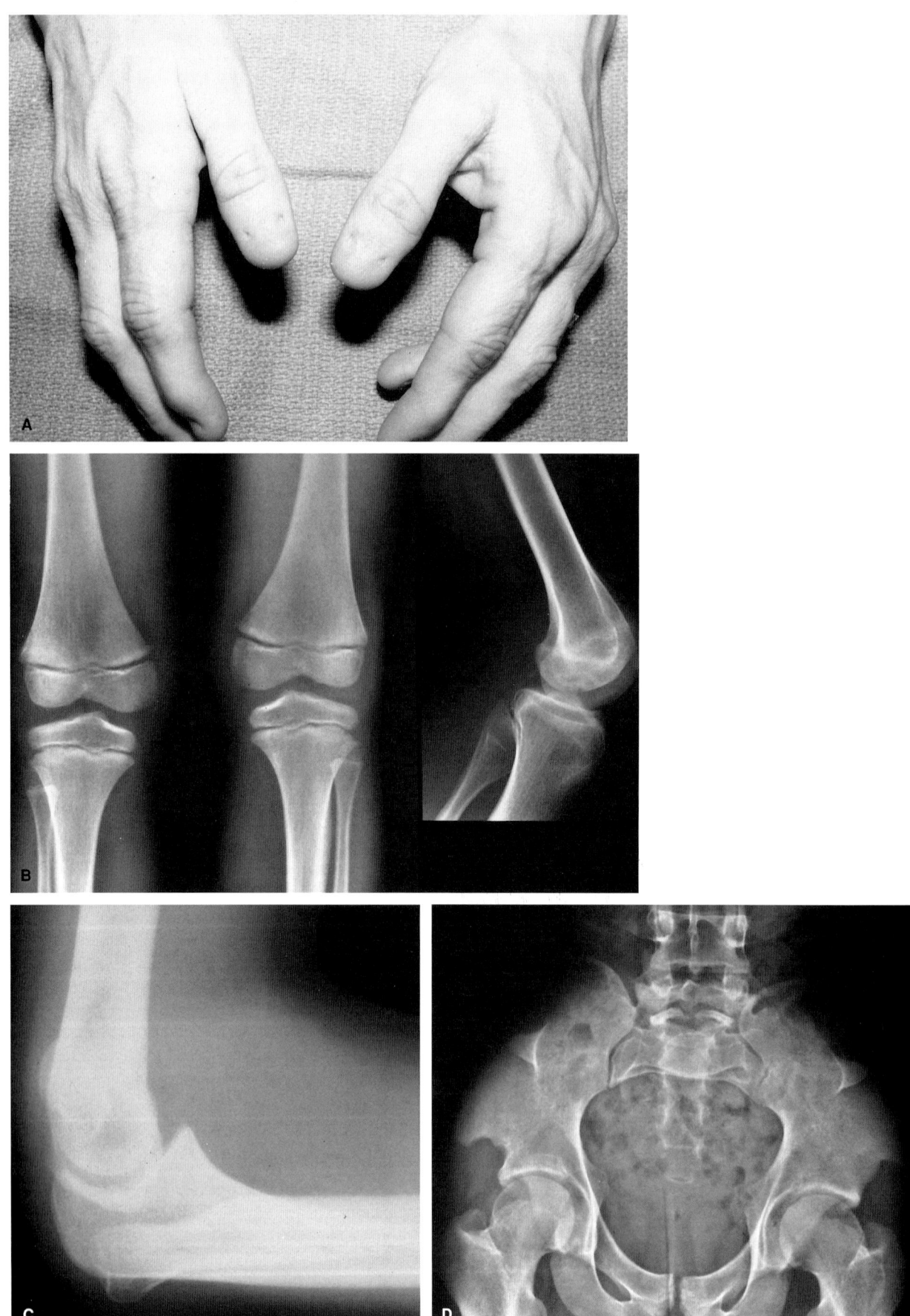

FIGURE 8-30. Nail-patella syndrome. The classic quartet of features consists of (**A**) dystrophic nails, (**B**) absent patellae (notice the region of osteochondritis dissecans on the lateral film), (**C**) posterior dislocation of the radial head, and (**D**) iliac horns.

The nails require no treatment. The knee disability is variable and related to the magnitude of quadriceps dysfunction and the dislocated patella. Poor femoral condyles challenge achieving patella stability. As a rule, limited soft tissue or capsular releases are ineffective, but combined proximal and distal patella realignments have an overall favorable outcome.[260] A contracted and fibrotic quadriceps may result in a knee extension contracture, and in such cases, quadricepsplasty is indicated along with the patella realignment. More commonly, an associated knee flexion deformity may requires hamstring release and posterior capsulotomy, although the results have been inconsistent.[260] Residual deformity, which is usually flexion or rotational, is managed by femoral osteotomy toward the end of the first decade. Osteochondritis dissecans of the femoral condyle is relatively common (see Fig. 8-30B). The intraarticular septum makes arthroscopic management difficult, but the septum can be removed arthroscopically.

Attempts to relocate the radial head typically fail. Excision of the radial head does improve symptoms arising from the prominent lateral bump, but the range of motion is rarely improved. Radial head excision is indicated only occasionally.[260]

The foot deformity may be significant, and clubfoot almost always requires circumferential release to improve the position.[260]

DE LANGE SYNDROME

The exceptionally characteristic face of a child with growth retardation makes the clinical diagnosis of de Lange syndrome reasonably reliable.[275] The syndrome itself is only clinically defined, with the precise genetics unknown. Affected people do not reproduce. Duplication of or deletion of the chromosome band 3q25-29 produces a phenotype similar to de Lange.[280,282] In these instances, the mother is always the transmitting parent, suggesting genomic imprinting. The syndrome is relatively common, occurring 1 in 10,000 live births, and it is possible to make a prenatal diagnosis by ultrasound.[268,274] Except for the mental retardation and the occasional ulnar dysgenesis, there are no serious orthopaedic or visceral malformations associated with the syndrome.[272,275]

The face is immediately recognizable: downturned corners of the mouth, single eyebrow, elongated philtrum, and long eyelashes (Fig. 8-31).[272,278] The small size begins with intrauterine growth retardation. Children remain small, with a delayed skeletal age. The mortality rate in the first year of life is high because of defective swallowing mechanisms,[284] gastroesophageal reflux,[269] aspiration, and respiratory infections. If the children survive their first year, they usually do well, but the long-term outcome is not well known. Almost all walk, but their milestones are delayed. There is retarded mentation, but the added features of no speech and no interactions cause major disability.[277] Self-multilating behavior can be an obstacle to orthopaedic care.[273,286]

Most have mild orthopaedic deformities of the upper extremities (Fig. 8-32).[270,271,274,276,279,281,283] They form a curious constellation of a small hand, a proximally placed thumb, clinodactyly of the small finger, and decreased elbow motion, usually caused by a dislocated radial head. This combination rarely causes any

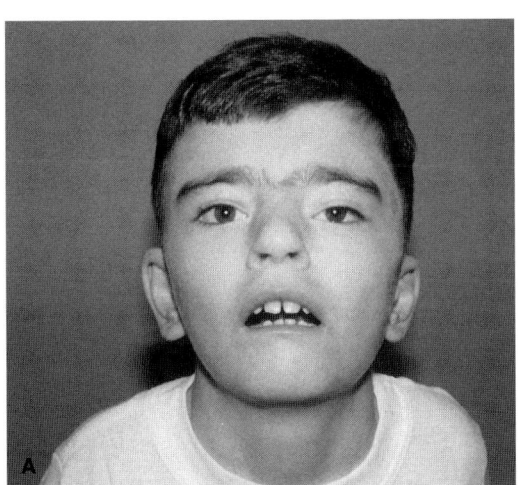
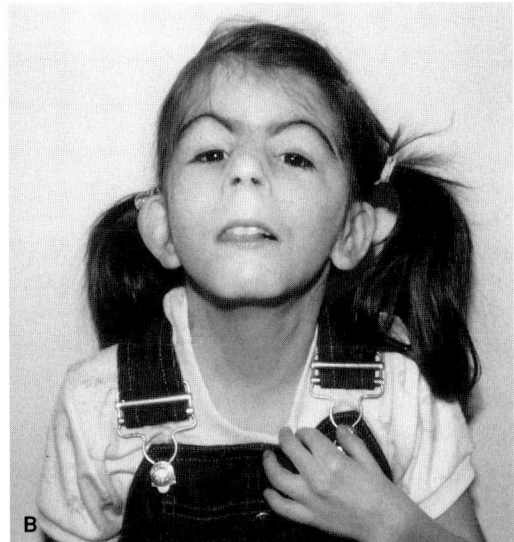

FIGURE 8-31. Cornelia de Lange syndrome. Notice the classic facial features of heavy eyebrows meeting in the midline, upturned nose, downturned corners of the mouth, and long eyelashes in (**A**) a 13-year-old boy and (**B**) a 7-year-old girl. (From Goldberg MJ. The dysmorphic child: An orthopedic perspective. New York: Raven Press, 1987.)

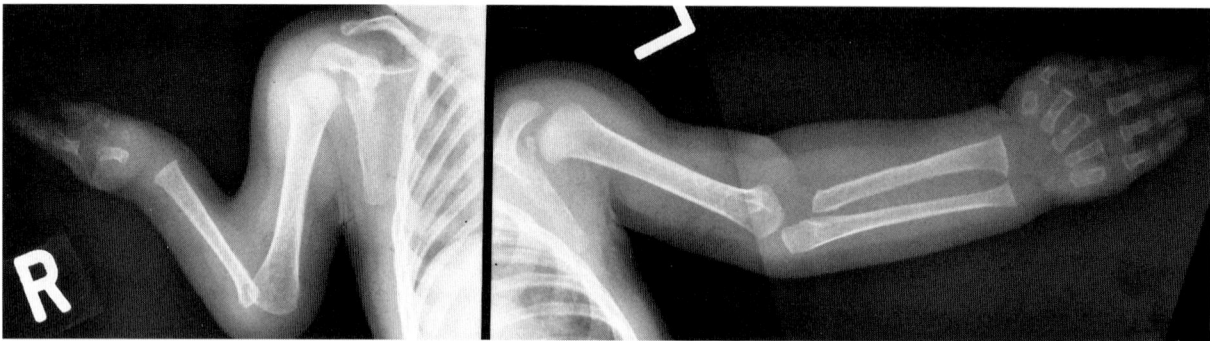

FIGURE 8-32. Cornelia de Lange syndrome in a child demonstrating a severely affected upper extremity on her right side (i.e., absent ulna and fingers) and a mildly affected arm on her left (i.e., short thumb and dysplasia of proximal radius). (From Goldberg MJ. The dysmorphic child: an orthopaedic perspective. New York: Raven Press, 1987.)

disability. Some patients, however, have severe deformities of the upper extremity in the form of an absent ulna and a monodigital hand, a condition that can be be unilateral or bilateral (see Fig. 8-32).

The lower extremities are usually spared. Tight heel cords and other cerebral palsy–like contractures are seen occasionally. Syndactyly of the toes is fairly constant. Aplasia of the tibia has been reported rarely. There is possibly a higher incidence of Legg-Perthes disease, approaching about 10%, but this may be because of study selection. Scoliosis is not a feature.

Because of the mental retardation, the failure of developing speech and paucity of social interactions raise questions about the suitability of these patients for orthopaedic treatment. Braces, physical therapy, and surgery for tight heel cords are justifiable. Upper extremity surgery is not indicated unless improved performance capacity is ensured. Patients with de Lange syndrome do not use upper extremity prostheses. Lower extremity prostheses, however, should be prescribed. Because the gastroesophageal reflux and swallowing disorders may persist well past the first year, there is a higher risk of anesthesia complications.[285]

FAMILIAL DYSAUTONOMIA

The features of familial dysautonomia (i.e., Riley-Day syndrome) are the consequence of absent or defective functioning of the autonomic nervous system and sensory system. This disorder has a unique ethnic distribution, limited to the Ashkenazi Jews of Eastern Europe. Is an autosomal recessive disorder, with a gene carrier frequency of 1 in 30 people. The gene locus has not been found, but attempts to localize it have so far excluded it from 60% of the genome.[289] There is no prenatal diagnosis possible, and a carrier test is yet to be determined. The specific biochemical defects in this disorder remain elusive.[287,295,303] The clinical features are manifestations of a disturbed autonomic and sensory nervous system. Infants have difficulty swallowing, with misdirected fluids going to the lungs, resulting in pneumonia. There is a poor suck response and a curious absence of tears.

During childhood, the autonomic dysfunction becomes more apparent, with wide swings in blood pressure and body temperature. There are cyclic vomiting episodes; these crises often last hours or days. Swallowing remains poor. The skin is blotchy. There is relative insensitivity to pain and poor hot-cold distinction. Intelligence, however, is normal.

Scoliosis affects 100% of patients.[296,298,302,305] It has an early onset, and progression is often rapid. Kyphosis, accentuated by tight anterior pectoralis muscles, appears in about one half of patients. Fractures occur frequently and often go unrecognized because of the insensitivity to pain.[297] Roentgenographic evidence of avascular necrosis is common, but the pathobiology is entirely unknown.[296,299,305] There are Legg-Perthes changes in the hips. Osteochondritis dissecans of the knees is often extensive, involving both femoral condyles (Fig. 8-33). It may be difficult to differentiate the ossification changes in the knee due to osteochondritis dissecans from what may be an early Charcot joint.[290,291] Hip dysplasia may be seen in patients with this syndrome.

Pathologic anatomy reveals a paucity of neurons in cervical sympathetic ganglia, dorsal sensory roots, and abdominal parasympathetic nerves.[300] The number of small axons is depleted from the sensory nerves and the dorsal columns. Because of a primary failure to develop axons, the symptoms are present at birth, and there is a loss of nerve cells and progression of symptoms as the patient ages.

The natural history of familial dysautonomia is characterized by a relatively high mortality rate in infancy attributed to aspiration pneumonia.[287] Sudden death in childhood and adolescence occurs, because the child is unable to respond appropriately to stress

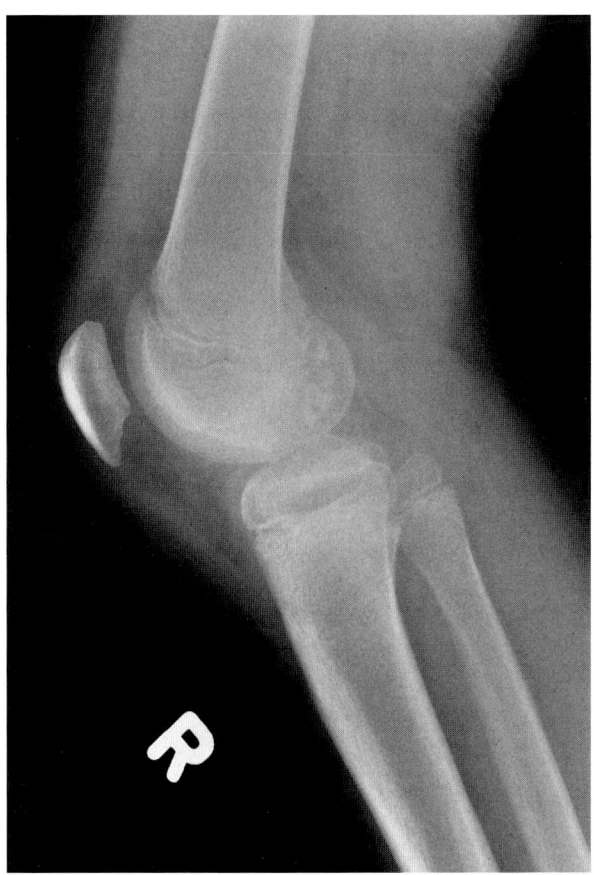

FIGURE 8-33. Familial dysautonomia. Irregular ossifications of the distal femoral epiphysis mimic osteochondritis dissecans.

or hypoxia. Early recognition of this syndrome and appropriate care leads to a life expectancy of many decades. There have been successful pregnancies brought to term in affected mothers.[301]

The scoliosis is poorly suited for management with an orthosis because of pain insensitivity, respiratory difficulty, and easy vomiting with abdominal pressure. Only a few curves have been arrested with braces. Surgery is needed for most patients, and it is best done as soon as scoliosis progression has been confirmed. The inability of these patients to have normal homeostatic responses makes scoliosis fusion an anesthesia nightmare.[292,293] The goal of surgery is to be expeditious and with utmost efficiency insert a spinal fixation system that promotes fusion without the need for postoperative immobilization. Attempts at heroic corrections that prolong operative or anesthesia time or predispose the patient to further homeostatic instability must be avoided. Stretching of the pectoralis muscles may improve the kyphotic posture.[294]

The physician should be suspicious of occult fractures in patients who have had trauma and swelling but experience minimal tenderness. Fractures usually heal quite well, but early diagnosis and avoiding displacement is the goal. It may be difficult to differentiate the ossification changes in the knee due to osteochondritis dissecans from what may be an early Charcot joint.[290,291] Orthostatic hypotension seems to get worse during adolescence, and wearing elastic stockings helps to control the symptoms. Gastrostomy and fundoplications are routine measures to control vomiting and ensure nutrition.[288,304]

RUBINSTEIN-TAYBI SYNDROME

The Rubinstein-Taybi syndrome is defined by its most obvious orthopaedic features: a broad thumb and a broad great toe.[316] It is relatively common in the mentally retarded population; with an incidence of 1 in 500.[310] Most cases are sporadic, although there is the possibility of autosomal dominant inheritance.[312] The gene locus for this syndrome has been assigned to chromosome 16p13.3.[307,308,311]

One of the most characteristic clinical features is the comical face with a Cyrano-like nose and the nasal septum extending below the nostrils (Fig. 8-34). The face may change with time, making this a less reliable finding.[306] Broad terminal phalanges of the thumb are present in 87% of patients, and the great toe is affected in 100%. One half of the patients have radially angulated thumbs, a source of disability. Hallux varus is common, and the physician should consider Rubinstein-Taybi syndrome whenever congenital hallux varus is encountered. Patients have ligamentous laxity and pronated feet, and they have an increased incidence of fractures.[310]

Birth weight and size are normal, but growth retardation is noticed at the end of the first year, and

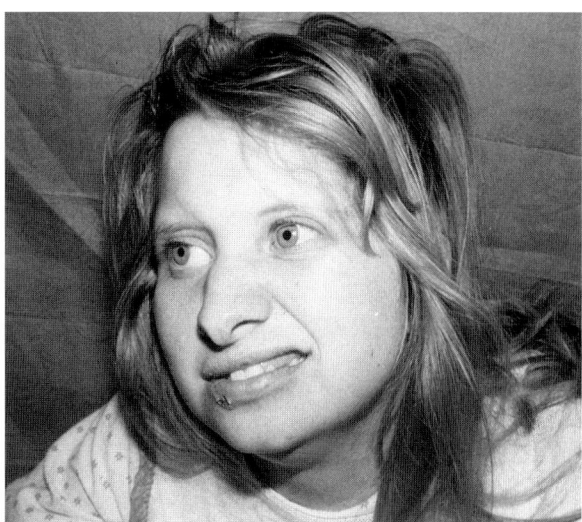

FIGURE 8-34. Rubinstein-Taybi syndrome. In a 10-year-girl, the characteristic Cyrano-like nose has a septum that extends below the nostrils.

there is no true pubertal growth spurt.[318] The patients are mentally retarded, many with microcephaly. IQ can range from 35 to 80, with a delay in acquiring skills. However, these features vary. Associated medical problems include visual disturbances, congenital heart disease, and gastrointestinal abnormalities.

The radiographs are rather characteristic. The thumb shows a wide distal phalanx, with soft tissue hypertrophy and a triangular proximal phalanx (i.e., delta phalanx) that accounts for the radial deviation (Fig. 8-35A) The toe demonstrates duplicated or a broad distal phalanx, but true polydactyly is not part of this syndrome (Fig. 8-35B). There is an assortment of insignificant other skeletal anomalies, many in the axial skeleton.[315] There have been some reports of congenital dislocated patellae, but this may be a coincidental association and not a true part of the syndrome.[313]

Patients with Rubinstein-Taybi syndrome theoretically have normal longevity, with mental retardation the major disability. However, the adults are not healthy. Frequent upper respiratory infections are related to abnormal craniofacial features, severe dental caries are common, and other infections lead to morbidity.[309,314,319]

The thumb is treated if the radial deviation interferes with pinch, in which case, osteotomy of the proximal phalanx should be performed. The deformity is progressive and recurrence is common, as with managing any delta phalanx. The toe rarely requires treatment unless there is a significant congenital hallux varus.

The physician should be aware of the anesthesia complications. About one third of patients have structural or conductive heart defects. Patients are sensitive to many anesthesia drugs, including neuromuscular

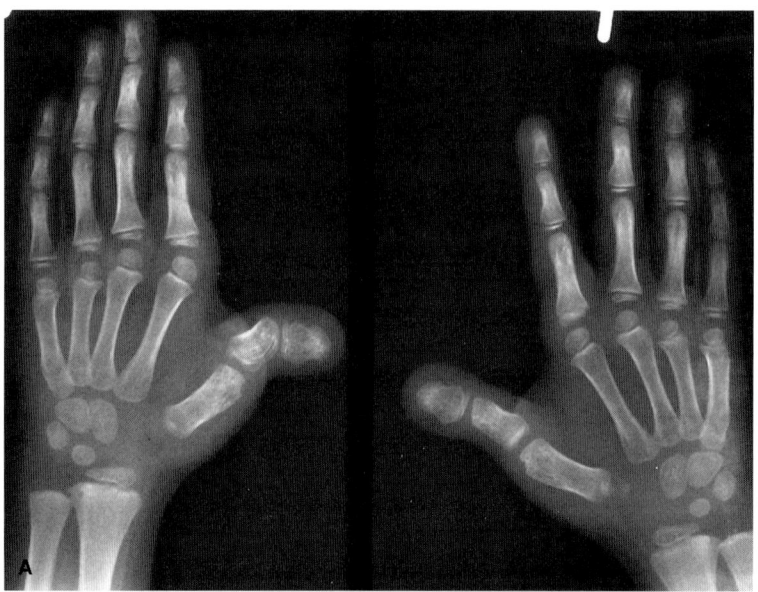
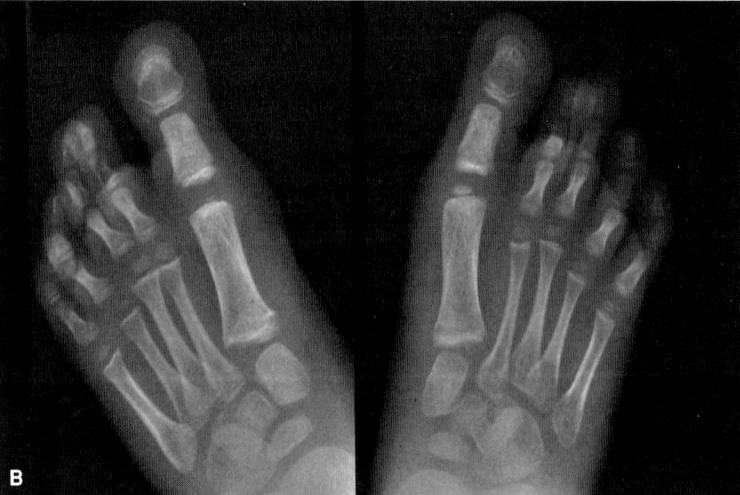

FIGURE 8-35. Rubenstein-Taybi syndrome in a 7-year-old patient. (**A**) The thumbs are malformed, with a trapezoid proximal phalanx. The epiphysis extends around the radial side. (**B**) The feet are more symmetric. Notice the broadening of the distal phalanx of the great toe. (From Goldberg MJ. The dysmorphic child: an orthopaedic perspective. New York: Raven Press, 1987.)

blocking agents, which tend to induce arrhythmias.[320,321] Keloid formation is common.[317]

PROGERIA

Progeria (i.e., Hutchinson-Gilford syndrome) is the best known of many syndromes characterized by premature aging. It is exceedingly rare, with no more than 24 affected children in the United States at any one time. The cause is entirely unknown. Autosomal dominant[333] and autosomal recessive[331] inheritance patterns have been proposed, but a sporadic dominant mutation is more likely.[324] At the cellular level, the fibroblast abnormalities include poor responsiveness to growth factors such as platelet derived growth factor,[326,335] abnormal gene expression of skin fibroblasts,[327] reduced decorin expression leading to formation of abnormal matrix[323], and abnormal glycosylation of fibroblast proteins leading to connective tissue destruction.[325] Abnormally elevated levels of hyaluronic acid excretion have been described.[222,324] How these findings fit into a unified theory remains unclear, but a combination of inactivation of growth factors and a lack of vascular genesis has been suggested.

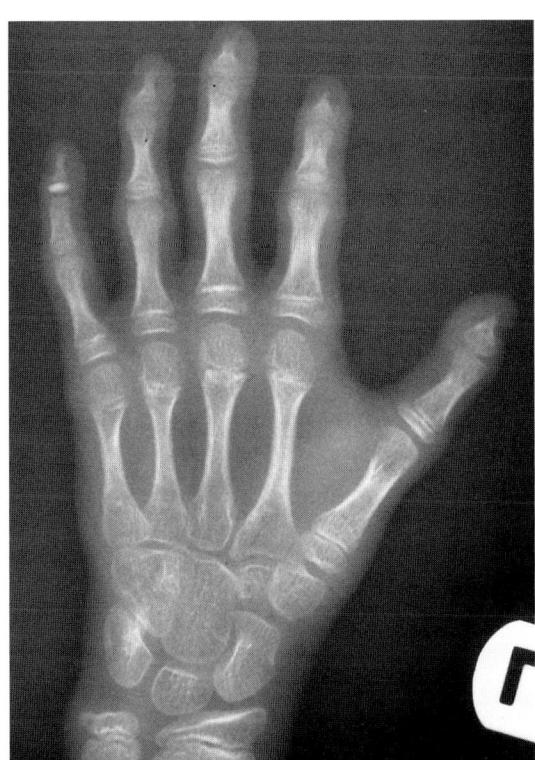

FIGURE 8-36. Progeria. The radiograph shows distal acrolysis with resorption of the distal phalanges. (From Goldberg MJ. The dysmorphic child: an orthopaedic perspective. New York: Raven Press, 1987.)

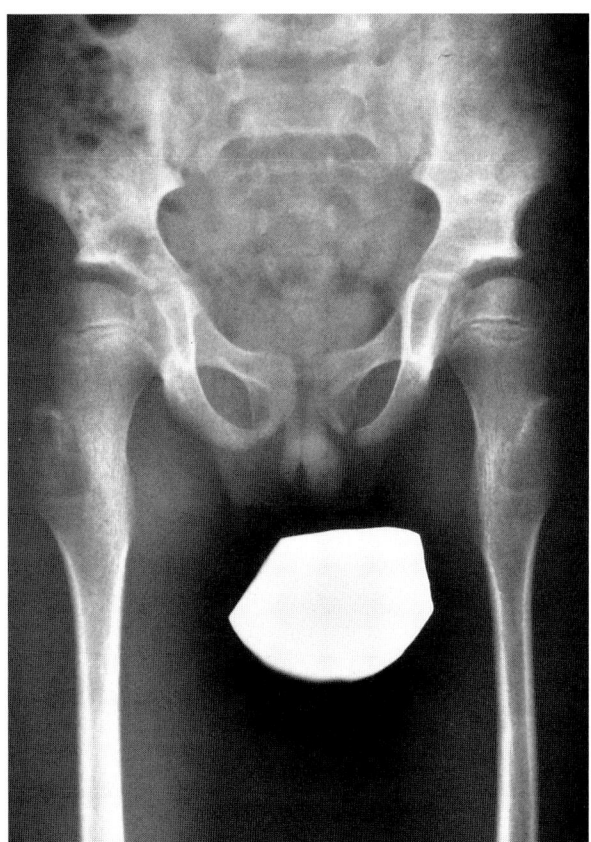

FIGURE 8-37. Progeria in an 11-year-old patient. The radiograph shows a marked degree of coxa valgus and some femoral head uncovering.

Children with progeria are diagnosed between 1 and 2 years of aged according to their clinical features alone. There is severe growth retardation and an inability to gain weight. If there is survival to adolescence, there is no pubertal growth spurt. Alopecia and a loss of subcutaneous fat is dramatic and accounts for the distinctive appearance of a skinny old man or woman.[322,330]

These patients have joint stiffness that is not arthritis; it is a periarticular fibrosis. Osteolysis occurs in the fingertips, clavicle, and proximal humerus (Fig. 8-36).[332,333,334] The vertebrae may become osteopenic, creating fish-mouth vertebral bodies on radiographs.[328,330,333] Fractures are common, often with delayed union. There is late developmental dysplasia of the hip and the onset of a rather significant coxa valga (Fig. 8-37).[328,329] The children do not live long enough to develop arthritis secondary to the acetabular dysplasia. Not all systems age. There are no cataracts; there is no senility. Rather than aging, the normal tissues undergo an atrophic or degenerative change that mimics normal aging. The principal histopathologic atrophic changes occur in the skin, subcutaneous tissue, bone, and cardiovascular system. Atherosclerosis with myocardial infarction by 10 years of age is the rule, and life expectancy rarely exceeds 20 years. There is no senility, and the major complaints of these patients are social.

The children are vital until struck down by myocardial infarction. Despite a short life, it is imperative not to permit any suffering. Hip surgery is indicated only if there is a documented functional impairment. Surgery is not indicated to prevent future arthritis. There is no medical treatment for the basic disease process.

RUSSELL-SILVER DWARFISM

The patient with Russell-Silver syndrome is defined clinically as a short child with body asymmetry and a characteristic face (Fig. 8-38).[336,342,346] The cause is unclear. Some suggest autosomal dominant inheritance and others an abnormal intrauterine environment.[337,343] The associated genitourinary malformations and the variation in the pattern of sexual maturation chemically (increased gonadotropin secretion) or clinically (precocious sexual development) have suggested hypothalamic or other endocrine disturbance contributing to the pathogenesis. Affected children are small at birth and remain below the third percentile throughout growth, with a marked delay in skeletal maturation. Body asymmetry with hemihypertrophy affects 80%. It averages about 2 cm at maturity but can be as much as 6 cm. Regardless of the magnitude of the discrepancy, it is clinically more apparent because the child is small. The face is characteristically triangular and seemingly too small for the cranial vault. There have been several reports of variations in sexual maturation pattern, chemically or clinically. Malformation of the genitourinary systems have been described.

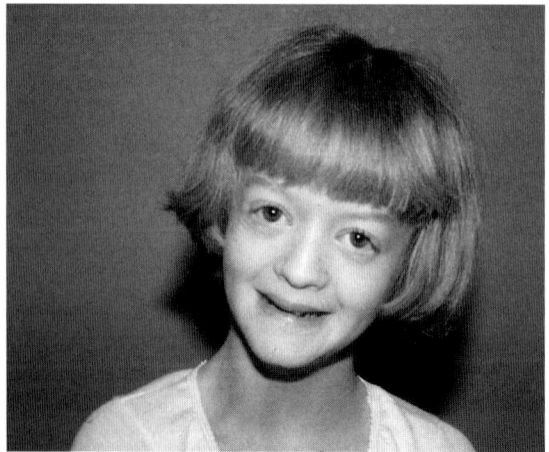

FIGURE 8-38. Russell-Silver syndrome. The triangular face is seemingly small for the size of the skull.

Radiologic analysis discloses a remarkable array of orthopaedic findings, but it is not clear which are part of the syndrome and which are coincidental.[339–341,344] Scoliosis is usually idiopathic. Hand and foot abnormalities include clinodactyly, polydactyly, and hallux varus. Developmental hip dysplasia, avascular necrosis of the femoral head, and slipped capital femoral epiphysis may be present.[331] Many x-ray changes, such as the minor hand abnormalities, suggest a disturbed morphogenesis.[338]

Treatment consists of managing leg length equality. This can be difficult because individual growth curves may vary, the skeletal age is very retarded, and puberty may be very abnormal. It is easy to miss the appropriate timing for epiphyseodesis. Growth hormone has been administered to improve stature. In the short term, it increases velocity, but the final height is not increased.[345]

TURNER SYNDROME

The affected girl has short stature, sexual infantilism, a webbed neck, and cubitus valgus, features associated with a single X chromosome. This chromosome disorder is remarkably common, affecting 1 of 2500 live births, but the rate of intrauterine lethality is 95%. The cause is a single X chromosome. In two thirds of cases, all cells are XO, and parental origin of the single X chromosome is the mother in 70% of the cases.[349] XX/XO mosaicism occurs in about one third of patients, and in 1%, there is deletion of only a part of an X chromosome. The mechanisms that relate an absent X chromosome to the characteristic phenotype are unknown.[348,349]

The identification of particular features at a particular age raises suspicion for this syndrome. At birth, the child has a webbed neck, widely spaced nipples, and edema of the hands and feet. The foot edema may persist for several months. During childhood, the low hairline, webbed neck, cubitus valgus, and short stature become more apparent. The adolescent has short stature and sexual infantilism. The most important features that call for chromosome analysis are edema of the hands and feet at birth, short stature in childhood, and sexual infantilism as an adolescent.

Growth retardation is a cardinal feature, with an ultimate height about 140 cm (56 in).[354] Bone maturation is normal until 8 to 9 years of age, and then, because sex hormone stimulation is absent, there is neither skeletal maturation nor pubertal growth spurt. There is no puberty at all, and the girls remain without secondary sexual characteristics unless exogenous estrogen is administered. The web neck looks like a feature of Klippel-Feil syndrome, but the cervical spine radiographs are normal. It is a cutaneous web only, and the cause may be related to an intrauterine cystic hygroma.[352] It is cosmetically unsightly, and plastic surgery is effective.[364] Idiopathic scoliosis is common, and the curve usually develops in juveniles. The delayed skeletal maturation allows a long period for curve progression. Growth hormone, which is almost always administered to girls with this syndrome, accelerates curve progression. Cubitus valgus is present in 80%, but there is a normal range of elbow motion and no disability.[347] Genu valgum is also apparent, but osteotomy is rarely needed. There is a medial bony protuberance not unlike an osteochondroma, arising off the proximal tibia in some.[350]

Osteoporosis is a significant problem. It is because of the low estrogen and an altered renal vitamin D metabolism, which is correctable with the administration of growth hormone.[351,353,355,360] Even in childhood, there may be the sequelae of osteoporosis, with a high incidence of wrist fractures reported.[358]

Intelligence is normal, but there is a high frequency of learning disabilities.[359,362] The life expectancy is normal, overall medical status is excellent, and social acceptance is good.[363] There are some heart and kidney abnormalities reported at a somewhat higher incidence than for the normal population.[361] Having only one X chromosome enables the patient to have X-linked recessive disorders, such as Duchenne muscular dystrophy.

Children with Turner syndrome are treated with growth hormone through adolescence, which results in a modest increase in growth velocity and final height: from an average of 140 cm (55 in) to just under 149 cm (58.5 in).[356,357] Growth hormone is not continued after skeletal maturity. Cyclic sex hormones (usually oxandrolone) are administered during adolescence and throughout adulthood. Estrogen is necessary for the development of secondary sexual characteristics, and the estrogen and possibly the previously administered growth hormone help to prevent osteoporosis. Many with Turner syndrome marry, and obstetric techniques of hormone supplementation and ovum transplantation can result in pregnancy.

NOONAN SYNDROME

The phenotype of Noonan syndrome is reminiscent of Turner syndrome, with short stature, webbed neck, cubitus valgus, and sexual immaturity.[367,369] However, the chromosomes are normal. This syndrome affects boys and girls. The incidence is 1 in 1000, and it is an autosomal dominant disorder.[370] Many clinical features are shared with the Turner phenotype, but what distinguishes this syndrome are the normal gonads, a high incidence of mental retardation, and right-sided congenital heart defects, often with hypertrophic cardiomyopathy.[365,366] Scoliosis is more common (40%) than in Turner patients and more severe.[371] Minor to major vertebral abnormalities may be seen on radiographs. Skeletal maturation is delayed despite normal puberty and menarche. Noonan syndrome is often misdiagnosed and most frequently confused with King-Denborough syndrome, a myopathic arthrogryposis syndrome characterized by short stature, web neck, spinal deformity, and contractures. Recognizing the difference is important, because malignant hyperthermia is part of the King-Denborough syndrome.[360]

PRADER-WILLI SYNDROME

Prader-Willi is a syndrome of hypotonia, obesity, hypogonadism, short stature, small hands and feet, and mental deficiency.[374,378,381] The incidence is 1 in 5000 births, with a prevalence in the population of 1 in 16,000 to 25,000. A specific genetic defect accounts for this syndrome: a deletion of a small part of chromosome 15 (15q11-13).[375,383] This syndrome also is a product of genomic imprinting.[385] Genomic imprinting suggests that it makes a difference which chromosome comes from which parent and that specific parental chromosomes protect against certain diseases. Angelman syndrome or happy puppet syndrome is phenotypically dissimilar to Prader-Willi. Angelman patients are small and mentally retarded, and they have athetosis and seizures. However, they have the exact chromosome deletion that occurs in Prader-Willi: 15q11-13.[383] Although it is the same chromosome deletion, the difference is which parent donated the chromosome. When the defective chromosome 15 is from the father, the child gets Prader-Willi syndrome, and when the defective chromosome 15 is from the mother, the child has Angelman syndrome.

As a newborn, those with Prader-Willi are floppy babies, having hypotonia, poor feeding, and delayed milestones.[372] They may mimic infants with spinal muscular atrophy. About 10% have developmental dysplasia of the hip. The syndrome may be remembered with an H mnemonic: hypotonia, hypogonadism, hyperphagia, hypomentation, and small hands, all probably based on a hypothalamic disorder.

After 1 or 2 years of age, a different clinical picture appears.[376] A characteristic face of upward-slanting, almond-shaped eyes becomes apparent (Fig. 8-39). Obesity begins, and a Prader-Willi diagnosis is usually suspected because of the onset of a voracious eating disorder. The patient has a preoccupation with food and an insatiable appetite.[373,377] Obesity has a central distribution, sparing the distal limbs. Complex behavioral modification programs are occasionally effective, and a trial using fenfluramine has had limited suc-

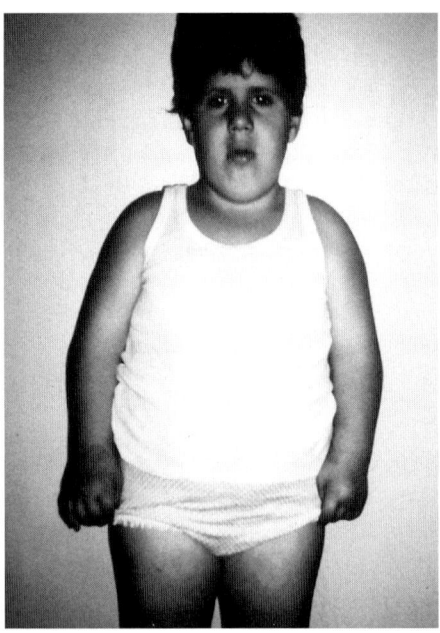

FIGURE 8-39. Prader-Willi syndrome in a 7-year-old patient. The features include truncal obesity and a round face with almond-shaped eyes. (From Goldberg MJ. The dysmorphic child: an orthopaedic perspective. New York: Raven Press, 1987.)

cess.[387] The patient has short stature, below the 10th percentile, with an ultimate height of 150 cm (59 in). There is no adolescent growth spurt. The genitalia are hypoplastic, and the patient has small hands and feet.[382] Mental retardation is present but is extremely variable. Nevertheless, skills for independent living are almost nonexistent, and most reside in sheltered workshop–homes.[373,388]

The most significant orthopaedic problem is juvenile-onset scoliosis, which affects 50% to 90% (Fig. 8-40). It is difficult to control with an orthosis because of the truncal fat.[379,380,386] Those who come to surgery have a significant anesthesia risk because of the morbid obesity.[384] The legs are malaligned, with genu valgum and pes planus, but the condition has limited or no effect on the functional health and physical performance.

BECKWITH-WIEDEMANN SYNDROME

Beckwith-Wiedemann syndrome is a curious triad of organomegaly, omphalocele, and a large tongue.[393]

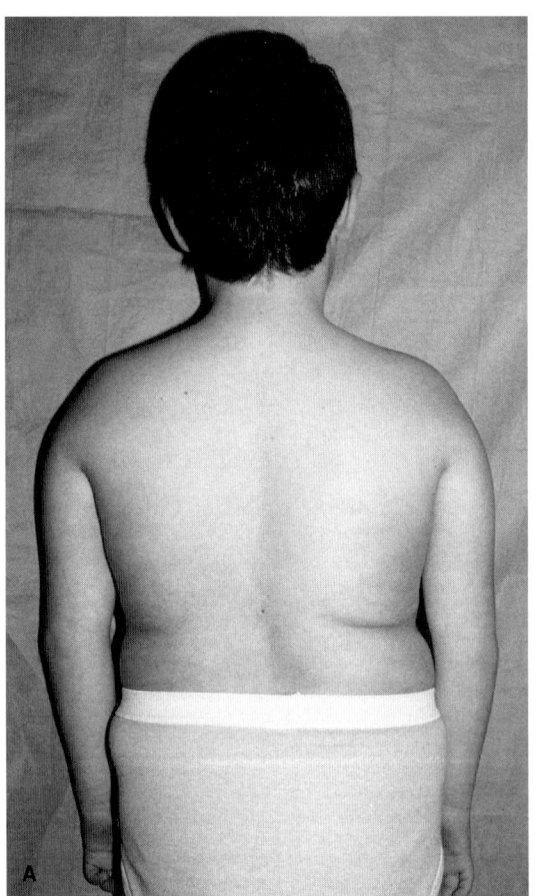
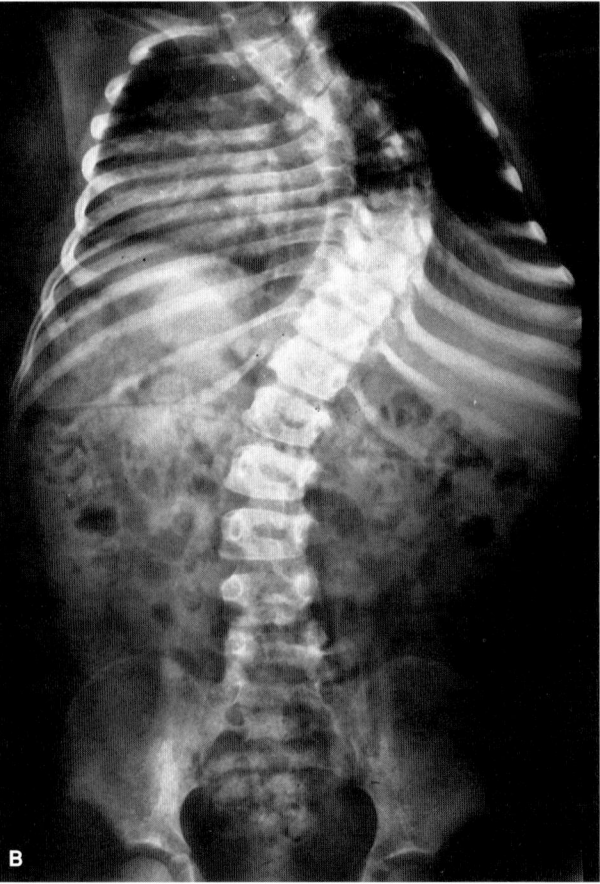

FIGURE 8-40. Prader-Willi syndrome in a 6-year-old patient. (**A**) Scoliosis is difficult to detect because of the truncal obesity. (**B**) The roentgenogram of this patient discloses a 50-degree thoracic curve. (**B** from Goldberg MJ. The dysmorphic child: an orthopaedic perspective. New York: Raven Press, 1987.)

The incidence is 1 in 14,000, and it is probably an autosomal dominant trait of variable expression. It is genetically linked to chromosome 11p15, which is near the Wilms tumor gene (11p13) and the insulin-like growth factor gene (11p15.5).[394] There may be some paternal genomic imprinting (see Prader-Willi section).[389,397] The closeness of the Beckwith-Wiedemann gene locus and the embryonal tumor gene loci accounts for the higher incidence of tumors seen in this syndrome.

The patient is large, although this feature is not always noticed at birth.[390] The child is in the 97th percentile by 1 year of age. The tongue is gigantic at birth, and although it tends to regress, hemiglossectomy is sometimes needed. Omphalocele is common, and 15% of the babies born with omphaloceles have Beckwith-Wiedemann syndrome. The abdominal viscera are enlarged, and a single-cell hypertrophy accounts for the large organs: in the adrenals, giant cortical cells; in the gonads, increased number of interstitial cells; and in the pancreas, islet cell hyperplasia. This underlies the 10% risk of developing benign or malignant tumors. Wilms tumor is the most common.

Pancreatic islet cell hyperplasia causes hypoglycemia in the newborn, a significant cause of future disability. Seizures may occur at day 2 or 3, often contributing later to a cerebral palsy diagnosis. The diagnosis can occasionally be made prenatally by ultrasound.[392,395] It is critical for the neonatologist to diagnose this syndrome early to prevent the consequences of hypoglycemia.

Clinical features that make the orthopaedist suspect this diagnosis is the unusual combination of two otherwise common problems: spastic cerebral palsy and hemihypertrophy (Fig. 8-41). The spasticity is thought to be a result of the neonatal hypoglycemic episodes, especially if accompanied by neonatal seizures, but spastic hemiplegia is most commonly seen. In general, children with cerebral palsy tend to be small; Beckwith-Wiedemann syndrome should be suspected if a large child has spastic cerebral palsy. Asymmetric growth affects about 20%. It is usually true hemihypertrophy, but it can be significant if the spastic hemiplegia affects the smaller side. Those with hemihypertrophy must be followed for tumor formation with regularly scheduled renal ultrasound examinations.[396] There is no consensus regarding periodicity. Because the major concern is about the development of Wilms tumor, several clinics empirically perform ultrasound examinations twice each year until the child is 6 years of age, at which time the incidence of Wilms tumor drops significantly.

Scoliosis is common; it is usually idiopathic, but there may be insignificant morphogenic variations, such as 13 ribs. It is managed as any idiopathic curve. Other orthopaedic findings include cavus feet, dislo-

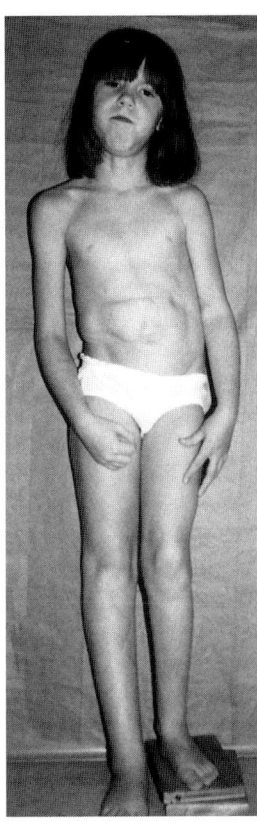

FIGURE 8-41. Beckwith-Wiedemann syndrome in an 8-year-old patient. Hemihypertrophy on right, a part of this syndrome, is combined with hemiatrophy on left due to acquired encephalopathy secondary to hypoglycemic seizures as a newborn, yielding a significant leg length discrepancy of 4.6 cm. Abdominal scars are a consequence of omphalocele repair. (From Goldberg MJ. The dysmorphic child: an orthopaedic perspective. New York: Raven Press, 1987.)

cated radial heads, and occasional cases of polydactyly.[391]

STICKLER SYNDROME

The name hereditary progressive arthroophthalmopathy better describes the important clinical features of the Stickler syndrome: an array of joint complaints and progressive loss of vision in a person with a Marfan habitus.[402] It is relatively common, especially in the Midwest. Its inheritance pattern is autosomal dominant, but variations in expression makes ascertainment difficult.[404,405] Type II collagen abnormalities have been detected, and at least some of the features appear to be caused by a procollagen gene mutation (*COL2A1*).[398,401] Because of the roentgenographic changes in the epiphyses, it may also be considered a primary epiphyseal dysplasia.

Clinically, these patients are tall and marfanoid, with lax ligaments. As children, the symptoms may mimic juvenile rheumatoid arthritis, with morning stiffness, that usually affects the ankles and then involves other joints. Adolescents experience ankle, knee, or hip pain. Despite the joint pain, there are no findings suggesting an inflammatory arthritis. Osteochondritis dissecans is common, and in some patients, loose bodies are found in the knees or ankles.[403]

The radiographs show a broad array of findings suggesting an epiphyseal dysplasia with precocious joint degeneration. The manifestations include irregular ossification centers with hints of avascular necrosis, joint narrowing and loose bodies, protrusio acetabuli, narrow intervertebral discs, and end plate irregularity.[399] The pain, loss of motion, and roentgenographic narrowing at a joint space imply chondrolysis. Abnormalities in the shape of the long bones include a narrow diaphysis with widened epiphyses and metaphyses, coxa valga with occasional subluxation, and a wide femoral neck. The unusual combination of coxa valga and protrusio acetabuli suggests Stickler syndrome.[400]

Variations make the natural history difficult to determine, but the worse cases have progressive joint destruction. Treatment is physical therapy for the stiffness, arthroscopy for the loose bodies, and arthroplasty as a young and middle-aged adult. The face demonstrates midface hypoplasia, and there is a high incidence of cleft lip and cleft palate. The greatest disability arises from a progressive loss of vision. Among these patients, there is a high rate of myopia, often congenital, and then later in life, total retinal detachment leads to blindness.

VACTERLS AND VATER ASSOCIATION

VATER, as the syndrome was previously known, has been expanded to VACTERLS.[409] The letters of VACTERLS in this syndrome's name constitute an acronym for the systems and defects involved: vertebral, anus, cardiac, tracheal, esophageal, renal, limb, and single umbilical artery.

The cause is entirely unknown. It is a nonrandom association, but the simultaneous occurrence of these defects by chance is unlikely.[406] The physician does not need to find examples of all seven categories of anomalies to diagnose the syndrome. The syndrome can be diagnosed prenatally by visualizing several of the malformations on ultrasound. Prenatally and at birth, the radial ray defect is most obvious; the others are more occult. The orthopaedist should be aware that 5% to 10% of radial club hands indicate VACTERLS.

The vertebral defects include disturbed spinal segmentation with vertebral bars and blocks.[408,411] The child may need early surgery for the accompanying congenital scoliosis. Thoracic anomalies are worse in those with tracheoesophageal fistula, and lumbar anomalies are more common with those who have imperforate anus. Occult intraspinal pathology is common,[407,410] and a screening MR study of the entire spine is recommended at some time during the first few years of life.

Congenital heart defects affect in one half of these patients. Ventricular septal defect is the the most common problem. Duodenal atresia may be found in this syndrome. The VACTERLS patient often has a single kidney. Other collecting system anomalies occur frequently among this group.

The limb anomalies range from a hypoplastic thumb to a radial club hand. The defect may be unilateral or bilateral; bilateral defects are always asymmetric.[408] The legs are spared 80% of the time. When the lower extremities are involved, a duplicated hallux is the most common finding.

The normal umbilical cord has two arteries and one vein. The absence of an artery, detectable only at the time of delivery or in the immediate newborn period, reflects the broad range of morphologic defects dating back to placental formation.

Developmental delay may be observed and is thought to be the consequence of skeletal anomalies of the arms, scoliosis, and surgery for gastrointestinal or genitourinary malformations. Nevertheless, several central nervous system malformations (e.g., encephalocele hydrocephalus) may be associated with VACTERLS and must be excluded.[407,410] If the patient survives the gastrointestinal anomalies and correction of the cardiac defects, the prognosis for a normal life is excellent. For treatment, the reader is referred to the sections on congenital scoliosis and radial clubhand. It is imperative to look for each member of the association before undertaking treatment of a radial clubhand.

GOLDENHAR SYNDROME

The name ocular-auricular-vertebral dysplasia points to the areas where anomalies are found: the eye, ear, and vertebrae.[412] The defects vary in severity and frequently are associated with other malformations.[416,419] It is not a rare syndrome, with an incidence of 1 in 3000 to 5000 births. Neither the cause nor the recurrent risks are known. It is sporadic, but marked geographic variation and segregation analysis suggests a genetic disorder.[414]

The typical eye defect is an epibulbar dermoid on the conjunctiva (Fig. 8-42A). Preauricular fleshy skin tags are found in front of the ear, and pits extend from the tragus to the corner of the mouth (Fig. 8-42B). In some patients, the ear may be hypoplastic or absent.

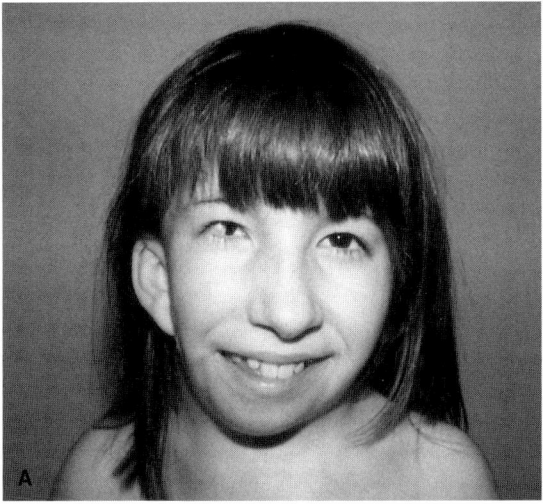
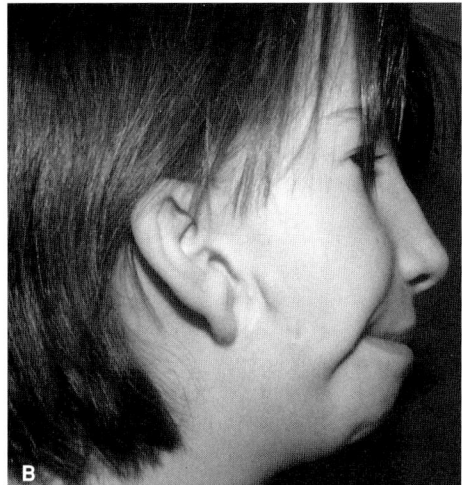
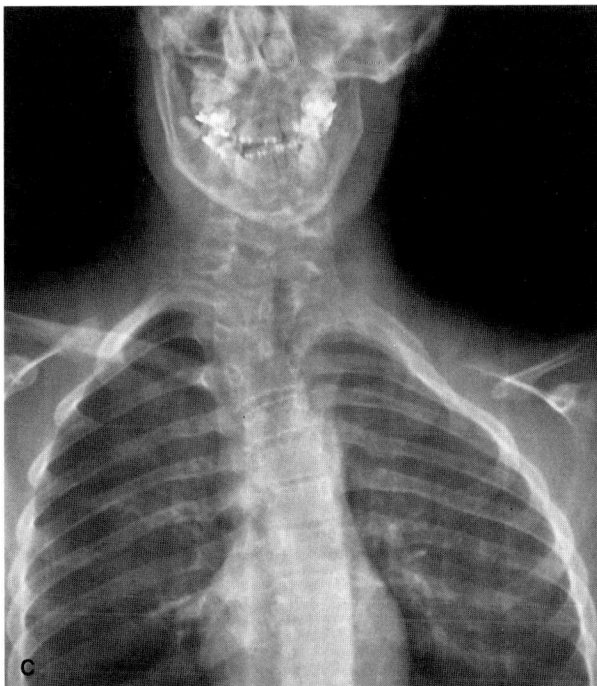

FIGURE 8-42. Goldenhar syndrome. (**A**) Facial asymmetry and epibulbar dermoid of the right eye. (**B**) Malformed ears with preauricular tags and sinuses. (**C**) The x-ray film demonstrates the congenital anomalies of the lower cervical and upper thoracic spine. Hypoplasia of the ascending ramus of the mandible accounts for the facial asymmetry. The clavicle is absent on the same side as the deformed face. (From Goldberg MJ. The dysmorphic child: an orthopaedic perspective. New York: Raven Press, 1987.)

The eye and ear anomalies are unilateral in 85% of these children, and facial asymmetry is the result of a hypoplastic mandibular ramus, invariably on the same side as the ear anomalies (Fig. 8-42C).

The vertebral anomalies may occur anywhere along the spine, although the lower cervical and upper thoracic predominate (Fig. 8-42C). Hemivertebrae are the most common defect, with an occasional block fusion found. Neural tube defect occurs more often than expected in the general population, and it may involve lumbar spine, cervical spine, or the skull (i.e., encephalocele). About one half of patients have clinically detectable scoliosis. The scoliosis initially was thought to be benign, but progression is reported on a regular basis, although the risk factors for progression are unknown.[413] An idiopathic curve below the congenital curve is often more troublesome than the congenital curve itself.

As with any congenital scoliosis involving the cervical-thoracic spine, Sprengel deformity and rib anomalies may be present. Other anomalies include congenital heart disease (e.g., ventricular septal defect),[416] cleft lip, and cleft palate.[418] Mental retardation, affecting 10% to 25% of patients, is usually limited to cases involving microphthalmia or an encephalocele.[417]

Orthotic management of scoliosis is difficult. The curves are often too high for a low-profile thoracolumbar orthosis. A Milwaukee brace adversely affects the facial hypoplasia and is probably ineffective for curves with an apex above T6. Early fusion is recommended if there is progression, but it is important to watch for hidden myelodysplasia. A preoperative CT or MRI is recommended. Intubation for anesthesia may be difficult because of the small jaw, stiff neck, and upper airway dysmorphology.[415]

TRICHORHINOPHALANGEAL SYNDROME

Unfortunately, the name of this syndrome causes confusion, because textbooks describe trichorhinophalangeal syndrome, trichorhinophalangeal syndrome with exostosis, and Langer-Giedion syndrome. It is best to think of two relatively distinct trichorhinophalangeal (TRP) syndromes: types I and II. Despite the clinical overlaps between the two, there are enough features to separate them into distinct syndromes.

Patients with TRP-I have a pear-shaped, bulbous nose, prominent ears, sparse hair, and cone epiphyses. Those with TRP-II have similar facial features and cone epiphyses, but they also have exostoses. TRP-II and Langer-Giedion syndrome are identical. TRP-I is an autosomal dominant disorder. In TRP-II, a defect is found in chromosome 8, a deletion of 8q24.1.[422] Both syndromes can present with signs and symptoms suggesting other orthopaedic conditions, such as Legg-Perthes disease, multiple hereditary exostosis, osteogenesis imperfecta, or Ehlers-Danlos syndrome.

Patients with TRP-I have mild growth retardation and the characteristic face described previously. The thumbs are broad, and the fingers are often angled at the distal interphalangeal and proximal interphalangeal joints. The hips mimic a Perthes-like disease in radiographs and symptoms.[423] There may be lax ligaments.

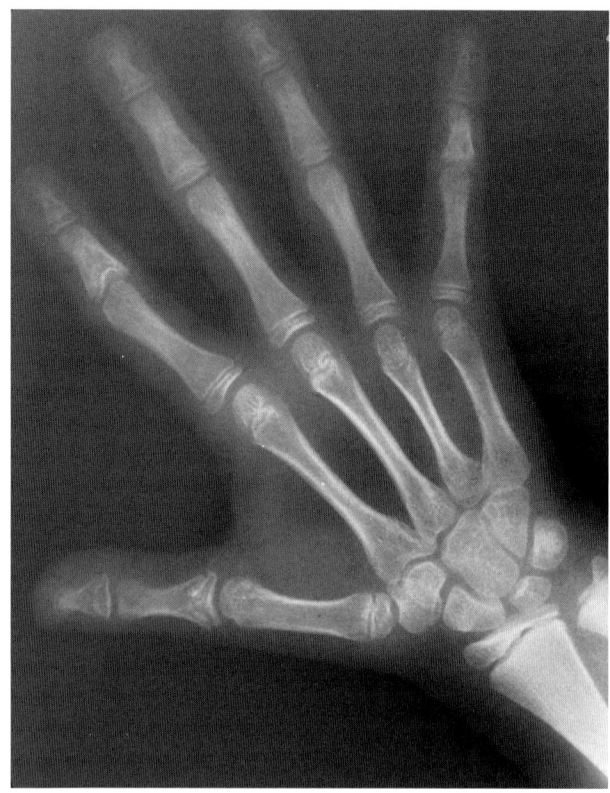

FIGURE 8-43. Trichorhinophalangeal syndrome. This 11-year-old patient has cone or chevron-shaped epiphyses in the hand and a broad thumb and distal phalanx.

Patients with TRP-II have microcephaly, large and protruding ears, a bulbous nose, and sparse scalp hair. In infancy, the skin is redundant and loose, which may be severe enough to mimic Ehlers-Danlos syndrome. Marked ligamentous laxity may further support this error in diagnosis. Multiple exostoses of the

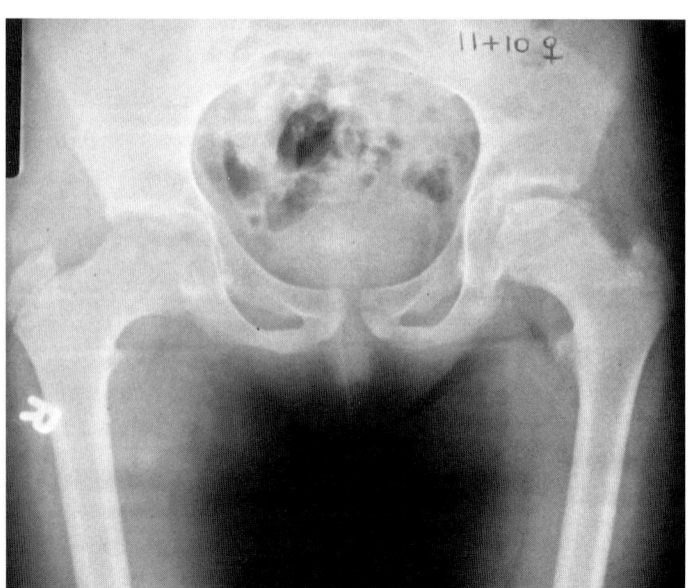

FIGURE 8-44. Trichorhinophalangeal syndrome, type I. The changes mimic Legg-Perthes disease, but by 12 years of age, they did not resolve. On the right is a small but spherical epiphyis. On the left, the changes are similar to those seen in Perthes disease and in multiple epiphyseal dysplasia.

long tubular bones and small bones creates a picture that mimics multiple hereditary exostosis, with a preponderance of exostoses in the lower extremities. There is a tendency toward fractures. Similar to TRP-I, the Perthes-like picture is expressed in TRP-II, as well as all the hand anomalies.[420]

Radiographically, the hand in a patient with TRP-I or TRP-II shows short fourth and fifth metacarpals, cone epiphyses, a short and broad thumb, and finger with angled proximal and distal interphalangeal joints (Fig. 8-43).[421] The cone epiphyses, so characteristic of this syndrome are not seen until after 3 or 4 years of age. The pelvis shows the unilateral or bilateral changes of Perthes in TRP-I and TRP-II, but rather than resolution, the Perthes-like picture persists, evolving into a pattern more like multiple epiphyseal dysplasia with precocious arthritis (Fig. 8-44). Despite the wealth of x-ray abnormalities, the hands rarely have functional disturbances. Osteotomy of the thumb is occasionally needed. The hips need to be managed as in symptomatic Perthes, but there are insufficient data about outcomes. Occasionally, an exostosis may be large or symptomatic enough to require excision.

MUCOPOLYSACCHARIDOSES

This group of genetic disorders is characterized by mucopolysaccharide excretion in the urine.[432] There are at least 12 types (Table 8-1). The mild to severe mucopolysaccharidoses have similar radiographs and various clinical features, but each produces a particular sugar in the urine because of a specific enzyme defect.[432,438] Changes in the naming and numbering of systems over the years have introduced considerable confusion in understanding the mucopolysaccharidoses. The incidence in general is 1 in 10,000.

The patients have somewhat thickened and coarse facial features and short stature, and many develop stiff joints (Fig. 8-45), especially in the hands. Stiffness is postulated to be the result of the deposition of mucopolysaccharide in the capsule and periarticular structures and to reflect the loss of joint congruity. Radiographs reveal oval vertebral bodies that often are beaked anteriorly; a pelvis with wide, flat ilia; capacious acetabulae; unossified femoral head cartilage; and coxa valga. The x-ray and clinical features are usually not apparent at birth but become more apparent as the child gets older. It is difficult to diagnose mucopolysaccharidosis during the first year of life.

All the mucopolysaccharides are autosomal recessive except for mucopolysaccharides type II (Hunter), which is X linked. The most common mucopolysaccharidoses are type I (Hurler) and type IV (Morquio).

The mucopolysaccharidoses can be diagnosed by urine screening, using a toluidine blue spot test. If the initial results are positive, specific blood testing is done for the associated sugar abnormality. Spot tests are

TABLE 8-1 Mucopolysaccharidoses

DESIGNATION	NAME	ENZYME DEFECT	STORED SUBSTANCE	INHERITANCE PATTERN
MPS I	Hurler/Scheie	α-L-iduronidase	HS + DS	Autosomal recessive
MPS II	Hunter	Iduronate-2-sulfatase	HS + DS	X-linked recessive
MPS IIIA	Sanfilippo A	Heparan-sulfate sulfatase (sulfamidase)	HS	Autosomal recessive
MPS IIIB	Sanfilippo B	α-N-acetylglucosaminidase	HS	Autosomal recessive
MPS IIIC	Sanfilippo C	Acetyl-CoA: α-glucosaminide-N-acetyltransferase	HS	Autosomal recessive
MPS IIID	Sanfilippo D	Glucosamine-6-sulfatase	HS	Autosomal recessive
MPS IVA	Morquio A	N-acetyl galactosamine-6-sulfate sulfatase	KS, CS	Autosomal recessive
MPS IVB	Morquio B	β-D-galactosidase	KS	Autosomal recessive
MPS IVC	Morquio C	Enzyme defect uncertain	KS	Autosomal recessive
MPS V	Formerly Scheie disease, no longer used			
MPS VI	Maroteaux-Lamy	Arylsulfatase B, N-acetylgalactosamine-4-sulfatase	DS, CS	Autosomal recessive
MPS VII	Sly	β-D-glucuronidase	CS, HS, DS	Autosomal recessive
MPS VIII		Glucoronate-2-sulpitatase	CS, HS	Autosomal recessive

CS, chondroitan sulfate; DS, dermatan sulfate; HS, heparan sulfate; KS, karatan sulfate; MPS, mucopolysaccharidosis.

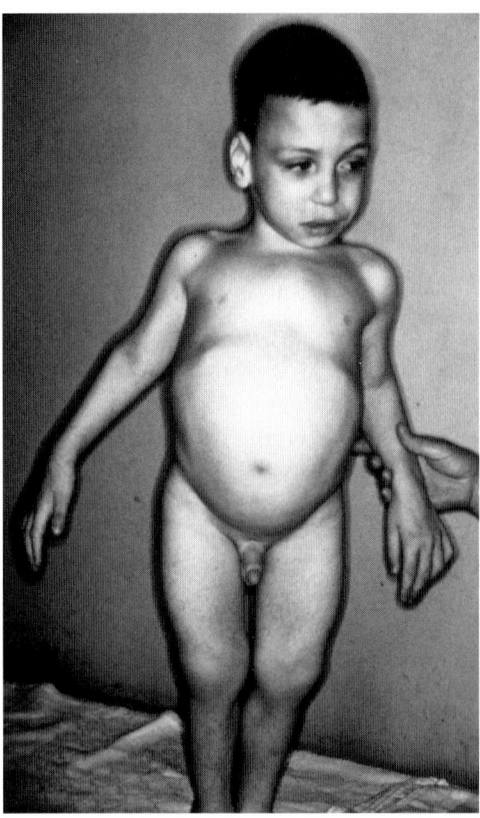

FIGURE 8-45. The classic appearance of a mucopolysaccharidosis in a 3-year-old patient include facial features that are mildly coarsened, an abdominal protuberance from an enlarged spleen and liver, a short trunk, and stiff interphalangeal joints of the fingers.

quick and inexpensive but have high false-positive and high false-negative rates.

The pathobiologic mechanisms are similar for the mucopolysaccharidoses. Each has a deficiency of a specific lysosomal enzyme that degrades the sulfated glycosamine glycans: heparan sulfate, dermatan sulfate, keratan sulfate, and chondroitin sulfate. The incomplete degradation product accumulates in the lysozymes themselves; the mucopolysaccharidoses are part of a larger group of disorders known as the lysosomal storage diseases. The incomplete product accumulates in the tissues, such as the brain, the viscera, and the joints. This unremitting process leads to the clinical progression of the disease. The child is normal at birth, but a problem may be chemically detectable by 6 to 12 months of age, and clinical progression is apparent by 2 years of age.

Mucopolysaccharidosis type I is the clinical prototype. It is characterized by a deficiency of α-L-iduronidase, the enzyme that degrades dermatan sulfate and heparan sulfate. The Hurler and Sheie forms represent the severe and mild ends of the clinical spectrum in mucopolysaccharidosis type I. Children with the Hurler form have progressive mental retardation; severe, multiple skeletal deformities; considerable organ and soft tissue deformities; and death before 10 years of age. The Sheie form is characterized by joint stiffness, corneal clouding, and no mental retardation; the diagnosis is usually made at about 15 years of age, and the patient has a normal life expectancy. Many patients with mucopolysaccharidosis I fall in the middle of this clinical spectrum. The clinical variation is determined by where and what kind of mutation occurs along the gene for α-L-iduronidase. Different mutations of the same gene may produce phenotypic variations that may be mistaken for different diseases rather than a spectrum of the same disorder.[430,433]

There is no specific medical treatment, although gene therapy offers promise. Marrow transplantation is effective in getting the enzyme to all affected sites and offers the best treatment in the long term.[428,429,432,435] Decisions for orthopaedic treatment must balance the severity of the local problem with the overall severity of the patient.

Morquio Syndrome

Between 1929 and 1959, there was a miscellany of skeletal diseases called Morquio syndrome, including several types of spondyloepiphyseal dysplasia. Morquio is an autosomal recessive disorder with an incidence of 3 per 1,000,000 members of the population. Three types of Morquio syndrome are classified as subtypes of mucopolysaccharidosis type IV. All are caused by enzyme defects involved in degradation of keratan sulfate.[430,436]

Patients with severe classic mucopolysaccharidosis type IVA are short-trunked dwarfs, although they appear normal at birth. They develop corneal opacities. The bone dysplasia is radiographically obvious, and the final height is less than 125 cm (50 inches). Patients have abnormal dentition. The deficient enzyme is N-acetyl galactosamine-6-sulfate sulfatase, and the chromosomal defect occurs at 16q24.3.[424]

Patients with intermediate mucopolysaccharidosis type IVB have the same but milder phenotypes as those with type IVA. They are taller, with final heights greater than 125 cm (50 inches), and they have normal dentition. Here the enzyme defect is β-D-galactosidase.

Patients with mild mucopolysaccharidosis type IVC have very mild clinical manifestations. The enzyme involved is unknown.

The three forms of Morquio mucopolysaccharidoses type IV can be separated by the severity of symptoms and the patient's age at detection. All patients are normal at birth. For patients with the severe type IVA, the diagnosis is made between 1 and 3 years of age; those with the mild type IV are diagnosed as teenagers; and those with the intermediate form are diagnosed somewhere in the middle of this age range. The three forms may also be separated by the severity of the radiographic changes.

Intelligence is normal in all of the mucopolysaccharidosis IV types and only rarely are the facial features coarsened. Similarly, all are short-trunked dwarfs with ligamentous laxity; the laxity is rather profound in mucopolysaccharidosis type IVA. The degree of genu valgus is significant, aggravated by the lax ligaments.[425,426,431,434] Management of the knee proves difficult because of the osseous malalignment and the lax ligaments. Despite the observation that the fingers and joints are becoming stiff, the medial and lateral instability of the knee remains. Realignment osteotomies can restore plumb alignment, but braces are often needed to control the instability during ambulation. The prophylactic use of braces to prevent initial valgus or recurrent deformity after surgery has not been effective. The hips and knees develop early arthritis. It is difficult to imagine that the roentgenograms

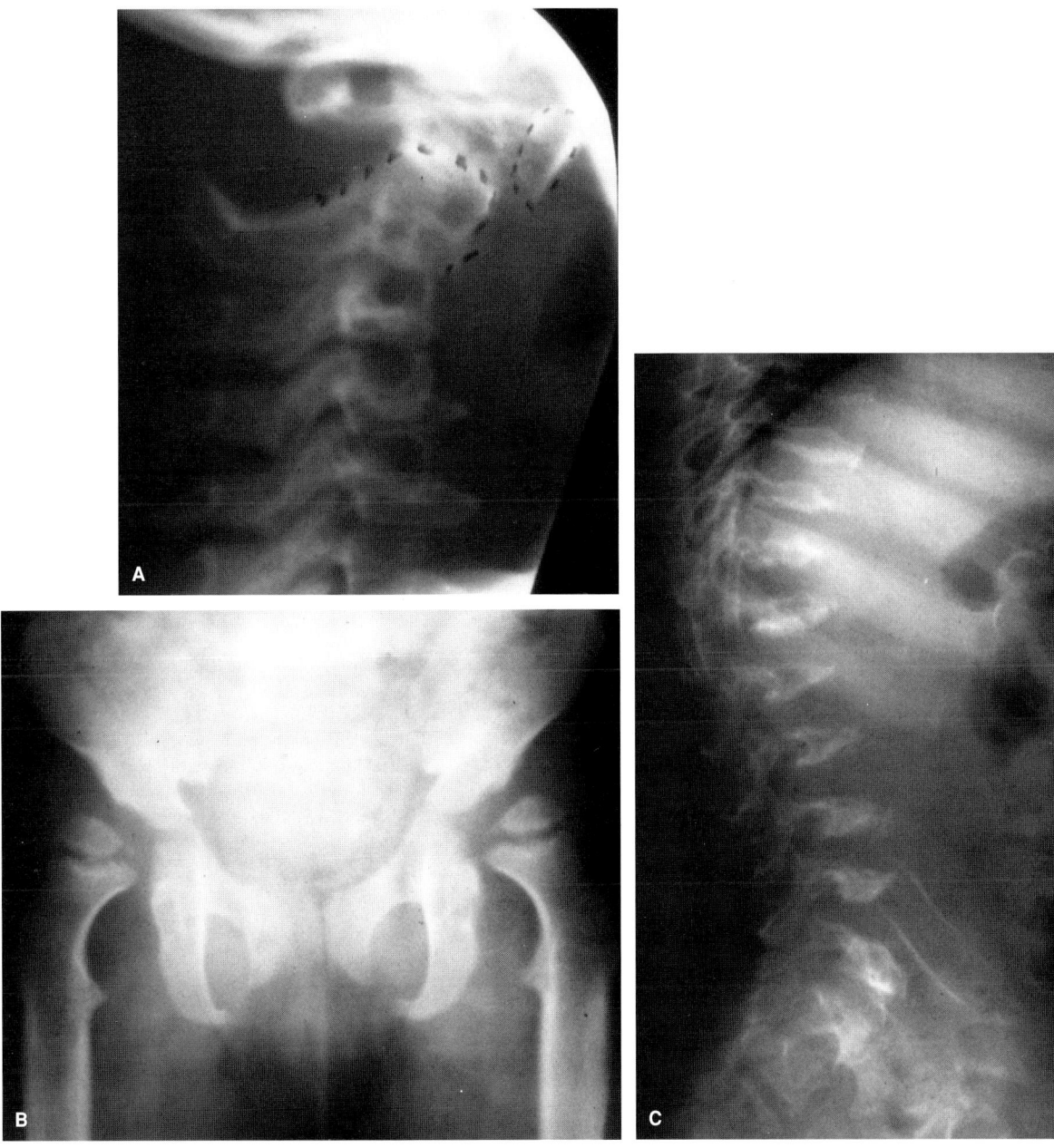

FIGURE 8-46. Morquio syndrome. The roentgenographic features include (**A**) an absent odontoid, (**B**) a pelvis with capacious acetabulae and coxa valga, and (**C**) a marked platyspondyly at 12 years of age. It is difficult to imagine these vertebrae were normal at birth.

of a child with Morquio were almost normal at birth. The hips show a progressive acetabular dysplasia. Early arthrograms may show substantial cartilage modeling within the capacious bony acetabulum, but in time, it disappears. The femoral capital epiphyses are initially advanced for the patient's age, but between 4 and 9 years of age, the femoral heads grow smaller and then disappear altogether (Fig. 8-46B, C).

The progressive hip disease is a consequence of the basic mucopolysaccharide gene defect, and neither medication nor surgery have improved the prognosis. A prominent pectus carinatum is a characteristic feature of Morquio syndrome. Odontoid hypoplasia or aplasia is universal, with resultant C1–C2 instability (Fig. 8-46A).[427,431,434,437] Although radiographs to detect this abnormality are indicated, neurologic monitoring, especially of upper extremity strength, tone, and function, is probably more important than measuring distances.

Sudden deaths of patients with Morquio disease have been reported, and they typically attributed to the C1–C2 subluxation. However, neurologic symptoms are caused by a build up of extra dural soft tissue anterior to the cord rather than to the mechanical atlantoaxial instability itself.[437,439] The onset of the myelopathy can occur early in life, progressing as the soft tissue hypertrophies, with the C1–C2 instabilities only aggravating the situation. C1–C2 fusion before the onset of symptoms is controversial but promoted by some.[437,439] Others think the best surgery is occipital cervical fusion because it reduces the anterior soft tissue mass.[439] Elsewhere in the spine, the vertebrae show a progressive platyspondyly with a thoracic kyphosis. No treatment is effective.

Despite these problems, many patients with Morquio disease live for decades. Cardiorespiratory disease is common, but the problems at the upper cervical spine account for most disability.

References

General

1. Goldberg MJ. The dysmorphic child: an orthopedic perspective. New York: Raven Press, 1987.
2. Hecht JT, Scott CI Jr. Genetic study of an orthopedic referral center. J Pediatr Orthop 1984;4:208.
3. Jones KL. Smith's recognizable patterns of human malformation. 4th ed. Philadelphia: WB Saunders, 1992.
4. Jones KL, Robinson LK. An approach to the child with structural defects. J Pediatr Orthop 1983;3:238.
5. McKusick VA. Mendelian inheritance in man. Catalogs of autosomal dominant, autosomal recessive, and X-linked phenotypes. 10th ed. Baltimore: The Johns Hopkins University Press, 1992.
6. Van Regemorter N, Dodion J, Druart C, et al. Congenital malformations in 10,000 consecutive births in a university hospital: need for genetic counseling and prenatal diagnosis. J Pediatr 1984;104:386.

Neurofibromatosis

7. Akbarnia BA, Gabriel KR, Beckman E, Chalk D. Prevalence of scoliosis in neurofibromatosis. Spine 1992;17:S244.
8. Alldred AJ. Congenital pseudarthrosis of the clavicle. J Bone Joint Surg [Br] 1963;45:312.
9. Anderson DJ, Schoenecker PL, Sheridan JJ, Rich MM. Use of an intramedullary rod for the treatment of congenital pseudarthrosis of the tibia. J Bone Joint Surg [Am] 1992;74:161.
10. Baker JK, Cain TE, Tullos HS. Intramedullary fixation for congenital pseudarthrosis of the tibia. J Bone Joint Surg [Am] 1992;74:169.
11. Bayne LG. Congenital pseudarthrosis of the forearm. Hand Clin 1985;1:457.
12. Bensaid AH, Dietemann JL, Kastler B, et al. Neurofibromatosis with dural ectasia and bilateral symmetrical pedicular clefts: report of two cases. Neuroradiology 1992;34:107.
13. Betz RR, Iorio R, Lombardi AV, et al. Scoliosis surgery in neurofibromatosis. Clin Orthop Rel Res 1989;245:53.
14. Brill CB. Neurofibromatosis: clinical overview. Clin Orthop Rel Res 1989;245:10.
15. Calvert PT, Edgar MA, Webb PJ. Scoliosis in neurofibromatosis. The natural history with and without operation. J Bone Joint Surg [Br] 1989;71:246.
16. Chee CP. Lateral thoracic meningocele associated with neurofibromatosis: total excision by posterolateral extradural approach. A case report. Spine 1989;14:129.
17. Coleman BG, Arger PH, Dalinka MK, et al. CT of sarcomatous degeneration in neurofibromatosis. AJR 1983;140:383.
18. Craig JB, Govender S. Neurofibromatosis of the cervical spine. J Bone Joint Surg [Br] 1992;74:575.
19. Crawford AH Jr, Bagamery N. Osseous manifestations of neurofibromatosis in childhood. J Pediatr Orthop 1986;6:72.
20. Crawford AH. Pitfalls of spinal deformities associated with neurofibromatosis in children. Clin Orthop Rel Res 1989;245:29.
21. Crossett LS, Beaty JH, Betz RR, et al. Congenital pseudarthrosis of the tibia. Long-term follow-up study. Clin Orthop Rel Res 1989;245:16.
22. Dolynchuk KN, Teskey J, West M. Intrathoracic meningocele associated with neurofibromatosis: case report. Neurosurgery 1990;27:485.
23. Egelhoff JC, Bates DJ, Ross JS, et al. Spinal MR findings in neurofibromatosis types 1 and 2. AJNR 1992;13:1071.
24. Elster AD. Radiologic screening in the neurocutaneous syndromes: strategies and controversies. AJNR 1992;13:1078.
25. Ezekowitz RA, Mulliken JB, Folkman J. Interferon alpha-2a therapy for life threatening hemangiomas of infancy. N Engl J Med 1992;326:1456.
26. Folkman J. Successful treatment of an angiogenic disease. N Engl J Med 1989;320:1211.
27. Funasaki H, Winter RB, Lonstein JB, Denis F. Pathophysiology of spinal deformities in neurofibromatosis. An analysis of 71 patients who had curves associated with dystrophic changes. J Bone Joint Surg [Am] 1994;76:692.
28. Graham PW, Oehlschlaeger FH. Articulating the Elephant Man. Joseph Merrick and his interpreters. Baltimore: Johns Hopkins University Press, 1992.
29. Gregg PJ, Price BA, Ellis HA, Stevens J. Pseudarthrosis of the radius associated with neurofibromatosis. A case report. Clin Orthop 1982;171:175.
30. Gutmann DH, Collins FS. Recent progress toward understanding the molecular biology of von Recklinghausen neurofibromatosis. Brief review. Ann Neurol 1992;31:555.
31. Gutmann DH, Collins FS. The neurofibromatosis type 1 gene and its protein product, neurofibromin. Review. Neuron 1993;10:335.

32. Hruban RH, Shiu MH, Senie RT, Woodruff JM. Malignant peripheral nerve sheath tumors of the buttock and lower extremity. A study of 43 cases. Cancer 1990;66:1253.
33. Hsu LCS, Lee PC, Leong JCY. Dystrophic spinal deformities in neurofibromatosis. Treatment by anterior and posterior fusion. J Bone Joint Surg [Br] 1984;66:495.
34. Huson SM, Compston DAS, Harper PS. A genetic study of von Recklinghausen neurofibromatosis in south east Wales. II. Guidelines for genetic counseling. J Med Genet 1989;26:712.
35. Huson SM. Recent developments in the diagnosis and management of neurofibromatosis. Arch Dis Child 1989;64:745.
36. Isu T, Miyasaka K, Abe H, et al. Atlantoaxial dislocation associated with neurofibromatosis. Report of three cases. J Neurosurg 1983;58:451.
37. Joseph KN, Bowen JR, MacEwen GD. Unusual orthopedic manifestations of neurofibromatosis. Clin Orthop Rel Res 1992;278:17.
38. Kaempffe FA, Gillespie R. Pseudarthrosis of the radius after fracture through normal bone in a child who had neurofibromatosis. A case report. J Bone Joint Surg [Am] 1989;71:1419.
39. Kameyama O, Ogawa R. Pseudarthrosis of the radius associated with neurofibromatosis: report of a case and review of the literature. J Pediatr Orthop 1990;10:128.
40. Kaufman A, Sherman FC, Black W, Duban S. Osseous destruction by neurofibroma diagnosed in infancy as "desmoplastic fibroma." J Pediatr Orthop 1984;4:239.
41. Konishi K, Nakamura M, Yamakawa H, et al. Case Report: hypophosphatemic osteomalacia in von Recklinghausen neurofibromatosis. Am J Med Sci 1991;301:322.
42. Kozlowski K, Lipson A. Bony tuberculosis misinterpreted—a cautionary tale. Aust Radiol 1993;37:119.
43. Listernick R, Charrow J, Greenwald M. Emergence of optic pathway gliomas in children with neurofibromatosis type 1 after normal neuroimaging results. J Pediatr 1992; 121:584.
44. Locht RC, Huebert HT, McFarland DF. Subperiosteal hemorrhage and cyst formation in neurofibromatosis: a case report. Clin Orthop 1981;155:141.
45. Lubs ML, Bauer MS, Formas ME, Djokic B. Lisch nodules in neurofibromatosis type 1. N Engl J Med 1991;324:1264.
46. Maffulli N, Fixsen JA. Pseudoarthrosis of the ulna in neurofibromatosis. A report of four cases. Arch Orthop Trauma Surg 1991;110:204.
47. Mandell GA, Harcke T, Scott CI, et al. Protrusio acetabuli in neurofibromatosis: nondysplastic and dysplastic forms. Neurosurgery 1992;30:552.
48. Mapstone TB. Neurofibromatosis and central nervous system tumors in childhood. Neurosurg Clin North Am 1992;3:771.
49. Masihuz-Zaman MB. Pseudarthrosis of the radius associated with neurofibromatosis. A case report. J Bone Joint Surg [Am] 1977;59:977.
50. Meis JM, Enzinger FM, Martz KL, Neal JA. Malignant peripheral nerve sheath tumors (malignant schwannomas) in children. Am J Surg Pathol 1992;16:694.
51. Morrissy RT, Riseborough EJ, Hall JE. Congenital pseudarthrosis of the tibia. J Bone Joint Surg [Br] 1981;63:367.
52. Morrissy RT. Congenital pseudarthrosis of the tibia. A long-term follow-up study. Clin Orthop 1982;166:14.
53. National Institutes of Health. Neurofibromatosis. Consensus development conference statement. Arch Neurol 1988;45:575.
54. Ostrowski DM, Eilert RE, Waldsten G. Congenital pseudarthrosis of the ulna: a report of two cases and a review of the literature. J Pediatr Orthop 1985;5:463.
55. Riccardi VM. Type 1 neurofibromatosis and the pediatric patient. Curr Probl Pediatr 1992;66.
56. Rockower S, McKay D, Nason S. Dislocation of the spine in neurofibromatosis. A report of two cases. J Bone Joint Surg [Am] 1982;64:1240.
57. Samuelsson B, Riccardi VM. Neurofibromatosis in Gothenburg, Sweden. Neurofibromatosis 1989;2:78.
58. Shufflebarger HL. Cotrel-Dubousset instrumentation in neurofibromatosis spinal problems. Clin Orthop Rel Res 1989; 245:24.
59. Sirois JL III, Drennan JC. Dystrophic spinal deformity in neurofibromatosis. J Pediatr Orthop 1990;10:522.
60. So CB, Li DKB. Anterolateral cervical meningocele in association with neurofibromatosis: MR and CT studies. J Comput Assist Tomogr 1989;13:692.
61. Sorensen SA, Mulvihill JJ, Nielsen A. Long-term follow-up of von Recklinghausen neurofibromatosis. Survival and malignant neoplasms. N Engl J Med 1986;314:1010.
62. Viskochil D, White R, Cawthon R. The neurofibromatosis type 1 gene. Annu Rev Neurosci 1993;16:183.
63. Wanebo JE, Malik JM, VandenBerg SR, Wanebo HJ, Driesen N, Persing JA. Malignant peripheral nerve sheath tumors. A clinicopathologic study of 28 cases. Cancer 1993;71:1247.
64. Warrier RP, Kini KR, Ragu U, et al. Neurofibromatosis and malignancy. Clin Pediatr 1985;24:584.
65. Weinstein RS, Harris RL. Hypercalcemic hyperparathyroidism and hypophosphatemic osteomalacia complicating neurofibromatosis. Calcif Tissue Int 1990;46:361.
66. Winter RB, Moe JH, Bradford DS, Lonstein JE, Pedras CV, Weber AH. Spine deformity in neurofibromatosis. A review of one hundred and two patients. J Bone Joint Surg [Am] 1979;61:677.
67. Winter RB. Spontaneous dislocation of a vertebra in a patient who had neurofibromatosis. Report of a case with dural ectasia. J Bone Joint Surg [Am] 1991;73:1402.
68. Wong-Chung J, Gillespie R. Lumbosacral spondyloptosis with neurofibromatosis. Spine 1991;16:986.
69. Zlotogora J. Mutations in von Recklinghausen neurofibromatosis: an hypothesis. Am J Med Genet 1993;46:182.

Proteus Syndrome

70. Aylsworth AS, Friedmann PA, Powers SK, Kahler SG. New observations with genetic implications in two syndromes: (1) father to son transmission of the Nager acrofacial dysostosis syndrome; and (2) parental consanguinity in the Proteus syndrome. Am J Hum Genet 1987;41:A43.
71. Azouz EM, Costa T, Fitch N. Radiologic findings in the Proteus syndrome. Pediatr Radiol 1987;17:481.
72. Barkmakian JT, Posner MA, Silver L, et al. Proteus syndrome. J Hand Surg 1992;17:32.
73. Bobenhouse J, Moeschler JB. Proteus syndrome: case reports and review. Am J Hum Genet 1987;41:A49.
74. Clark RD, Donnai D, Rogers J, et al. Proteus syndrome: an expanded phenotype. Am J Med 1987;25:99.
75. Cohen MM Jr. Understanding Proteus syndrome. Unmasking the elephant man, and stemming elephant fever. Neurofibromatosis 1988;1:260.
76. Cremin BJ, Viljoen DL, Wynchank S, Beighton P. The Proteus syndrome: the magnetic resonance and radiological features. Pediatr Radiol 1987;17:486.
77. Demetriades MD, Hager J, Nikolaides N, et al. Proteus syndrome: musculoskeletal manifestations and management: a report of two cases. J Pediatr Orthop 1992;12:106.
78. Graham PW, Oehlschlaeger FH. Articulating the Elephant Man. Joseph Merrick and his interpreters. Baltimore: Johns Hopkins University Press, 1992.
79. Goodship J, Redfearn A, Milligan D, et al. Transmission of Proteus syndrome from father to son? J Med Genet 1991; 28:781.

80. Hotamisligil GS. Proteus syndrome and hamartoses with overgrowth. Dysmorphol Clin Genet 1990;4:87.
81. Kalen V, Burwell DS, Omer GE. Macrodactyly of the hands and feet. J Pediatr Orthop 1988;8:311.
82. Lacombe D, Taieb A, Vergnes P, et al. Proteus syndrome in 7 patients: clinical and genetic considerations. Genet Couns 1991;2:93.
83. Malamitsi-Puchner A, Dimitriadis D, et al. Proteus syndrome: course of a severe case. Am J Med Genet 1990;35:283.
84. Mayatepek E, Kurczynski TW, Ruppert ES, et al. Expanding the phenotype of the Proteus syndrome: a severely affected patient with new findings. Am J Med Genet 1989;32:402.
85. Stricker S. Musculoskeletal manifestations of Proteus syndrome: report of two cases with literature review. J Pediatr Orthop 1992;12:667.
86. Tibbles SA, Rogers JG. Macrodactyly, hemihypertrophy, and connective tissue nevi: report of a new syndrome and review of the literature. J Pediatr 1976;89:924.
87. Tibbles JA, Cohen MM. The Proteus syndrome: the Elephant Man diagnosed. Br Med J 1986;293:683.
88. Vaughn RY, Selinger AD, Howell CG, et al. Proteus syndrome: diagnosis and surgical management. J Pediatr Surg 1993;28:5.
89. Viljoen DL, Nelson MM, de Jong G, et al. Proteus syndrome in Southern Africa. Natural history and clinical manifestations in six individuals. Am J Med Genet 1987;27:87.
90. Wiedemann HR, Burgio GR, Alenjoff P, et al. The Proteus syndrome: partial gigantism of the hands and/or feet, nevi, hemihypertrophy, subcutaneous tumors, macrocephaly or other skull anomalies and possible accelerated growth and visceral affections. Eur J Pediatr 1983;140:5.

Arthrogryposis

91. Atkins RM, Bell MJ, Sharrard WJW. Pectoralis major transfer for paralysis of elbow flexion in children. J Bone Joint Surg [Br] 1985;67:640.
92. Banker BQ. Neuropathologic aspects of arthrogryposis multiplex congenita. Clin Orthop 1985;194:30.
93. Bayne LG. Hand assessment and management of arthrogryposis multiplex congenita. Clin Orthop 1985;194:68.
94. Bennet JB, Hansen PE, Granberry WM, Cain TE. Surgical management of arthrogryposis in the upper extremity. J Pediatr Orthop 1985;5:281.
95. Brown LM, Robson MJ, Sharrard WJW. The pathology of arthrogryposis multiplex congenita neurologica. J Bone Joint Surg [Br] 1980;62:291.
96. Carlson WO, Speck GJ, Vicari V, Wenger DR. Arthrogryposis multiplex congenita. A long-term follow-up study. Clin Orthop 1985;194:115.
97. Clarren SK, Hall JG. Neuropathologic findings in the spinal cords of 10 infants with arthrogryposis. J Neurol Sci 1983;58:89.
98. Daher YH, Lonstein JE, Winter RB, Moe JH. Spinal deformities in patients with arthrogryposis. A review of 16 patients. Spine 1985;10:608.
99. Davidson J, Beighton P. Whence the arthrogrypotics? J Bone Joint Surgery [Br] 1976;58:492.
100. Diamond LS, Alegado R. Perinatal fractures in arthrogryposis multiplex congenita. J Pediatr Orthop 1981;1:189.
101. Doyle JR, James PM, Larsen W, Asley RK. Restoration of elbow flexion in arthrogryposis multiplex congenita. J Hand Surg 1980;5:149.
102. Fahy MJ, Hall JG. A retrospective study of pregnancy complications among 828 cases of arthrogryposis. Genet Couns 1990;1:3.
103. Goldberg MJ. The dysmorphic child: an orthopedic perspective. New York: Raven Press, 1987:1.
104. Green ADL, Fixsen JA, Lloyd-Roberts GC. Talectomy for arthrogryposis multiplex congenita. J Bone Joint Surg [Br] 1984;66:697.
105. Guidera KJ, Drennan JC. Foot and ankle deformities in arthrogryposis multiplex congenita. Clin Orthop 1985;194:93.
106. Guidera JK, Kortright L, Barber V, Ogden JA. Radiographic changes in arthrogrypotic knees. Skeletal Radiology 1991;20:193.
107. Hahn G. Arthrogryposis. Pediatric review and rehabilitative aspects. Clin Orthop 1985;194:105.
108. Hall JG, Reed SD. Teratogens associated with congenital contractures in humans and animals. Teratology 1982;25:173.
109. Hall JG, Reed SD, Driscoll EP. Part I. Amyoplasia: a common, sporadic condition with congenital contractures. Am J Med Genet 1983;15:571.
110. Hall JG, Reed SD, McGillvray BC, et al. Part II. Amyoplasia: twinning in amyoplasia—a specific type of arthrogryposis with an apparent excess of discordantly affected identical twins. Am J Med Genet 1983;15:591.
111. Hall JG. Genetic aspects of arthrogryposis. Clin Orthop 1985;194:44.
112. Hoffer MM, Swank S, Eastman F, et al. Ambulation in severe arthrogryposis. J Pediatr Orthop 1983;3:293.
113. Hsu LCS, Jaffray D, Leong JCY. Talectomy for club foot in arthrogryposis. J Bone Joint Surg [Br] 1984;66:694.
114. Huurman WW, Jacobsen ST. The hip in arthrogryposis multiplex congenita. Clin Orthop 1985;194:81.
115. Otto AW. A human monster with inwardly curved extremities. Clin Orthop 1985;194:4.
116. Palmer PM, MacEwen GD, Brown JR, Mathews PA. Passive motion therapy for infants with arthrogryposis. Clin Orthop 1985;194:54.
117. Quinn CM, Wigglesworth JS, Heckmatt J. Lethal arthrogryposis multiplex congenita: a pathological study of 21 cases. Histopathology 1991;19:155.
118. Robertson WL, Glinski LP, Kirkpatrick SJ, Pauli RM. Further evidence that arthrogryposis multiplex congenita in the human sometimes is caused by an intrauterine vascular accident. Teratology 1992;45:345.
119. Robinson RO. Arthrogryposis multiplex congenita: feeding, language and other health problems. Neuropediatrics 1990;21:177.
120. St. Clair HS, Zimbler S. A plan of management and treatment results in the arthrogrypotic hip. Clin Orthop 1985;194:74.
121. Sarwark JF, MacEwen GD, Scott CI. Current concepts review. Amyoplasia (a common form of arthrogryposis). J Bone Joint Surg [Am] 1990;72:465.
122. Sodergard J, Ryoppy S. The knee in arthrogryposis multiplex congenita. J Pediatr Orthop 1990;10:177.
123. Staheli LT, Chow DE, Elliott JS, Mosca VS. Management of hip dislocations in children with arthrogryposis. J Pediatr Orthop 1987;7:681.
124. Swinyard CA, Bleck EE. The etiology of arthrogryposis (multiplex congenita contracture). Clin Orthop 1985;194:15.
125. Thomas B, Schopler S, Wood W, Oppenheim WL. The knee in arthrogryposis. Clin Orthop 1985;194:87.
126. Thompson GH, Bilenker RM. Comprehensive management of arthrogryposis multiplex congenita. Clin Orthop 1985;194:6.
127. Weston PJ, Ives EJ, Honore RL. Monochomonic diamniotic minimally conjoined twins. Am J Med Genet 1990;37:558.
128. Williams P. The management of arthrogryposis. Orthop Clin North Am 1978;9:67.
129. Williams PF. Management of upper limb problems in arthrogryposis. Clin Orthop 1985;194:60.

130. Wynne-Davies R, Williams PF, O'Connor JCB. The 1960's epidemic of arthrogryposis multiplex congenita. A survey from the United Kingdom, Australia and the United States of America. J Bone Joint Surg [Br] 1981;63:76.
131. Yonenobu K, Tada K, Swanson B. Arthrogryposis of the hand. J Pediatr Orthop 1984;4:599.
132. Zimbler S, Craig CL. The arthrogrypotic foot. Plan of management and results of treatment. Foot Ankle 1983;3:211.

Larsen Syndrome

133. Bowen JR, Ortega K, Ray S, MacEwen GD. Spinal deformities in Larsen's syndrome. Clin Orthop 1985;197:159.
134. Habermann ET, Sterling A, Dennis RI. Larsen's syndrome: a heritable disorder. J Bone Joint Surg [Am] 1976;58:558.
135. Houston CS, Reed MH, Desautels JEL. Separating Larsen syndrome from the "arthrogryposis basket". J Can Assoc Radiol 1981;32:206.
136. Kiel EA, Frias JL, Victorica BE. Cardiovascular manifestations in the Larsen syndrome. Pediatrics 1983;71:942.
137. Klenn PJ, Iozzo RV. Larsen's syndrome with novel congenital anomalies. Hum Pathol 1991;22:1055.
138. Larsen LJ, Schottstaedt ER, Bost FC. Multiple congenital dislocations associated with characteristic facial abnormality. J Pediatr 1950;37:574.
139. Laville JM, Lakermance P, Limouzy F. Larsen's syndrome: review of the literature and analysis of thirty-eight cases. J Pediatr Orthop 1994;14:63.
140. Marques MdeNT. Larsen's syndrome: clinical and genetic aspects. J Genet Hum 1980;28:83.
141. Micheli LJ, Hall JE, Watts HG. Spinal instability in Larsen's syndrome. Report of three cases. J Bone Joint Surg [Am] 1976;58:562.
142. Munk S. Early operation of the dislocated knee in Larsen's syndrome. A report of two cases. Acta Orthop Scand 1988;59:582.
143. Oki T, Terashima Y, Murachi S, Nogami H. Clinical features and treatment of joint dislocations in Larsen's syndrome. Report of three cases in one family. Clin Orthop 1976;119:206.
144. Stanley D, Seymour N. The Larsen syndrome occurring in four generations of one family. Int Orthop 1985;8:267.
145. Steel HH, Koh EJ. Multiple dislocations associated with other skeletal anomalies (Larsen's syndrome) in three siblings. J Bone Joint Surg [Am] 1972;54:75.
146. Stevenson GW, Hall SC, Palmieri J. Anesthetic considerations for patients with Larsen's syndrome. Anaesthesia 1991;75:142.

Distal Arthrogryposis

147. Bui TH, Lindholm H, Demir N, Thomasin P. Prenatal diagnosis of distal arthrogryposis type I by ultrasonography. Prenat Diagn 1992;12:1047.
148. Dhaliwal AS, Myers TL. Digitotalar dysmorphism. Orthop Rev 1985;14:90.
149. Hageman G, Jenekens FGI, Vette JK, Willemse J. The heterogeneity of distal arthrogryposis. Brain Dev 1984;6:273.
150. Hall JG, Reed SD, Greene G. The distal arthrogryposes: delineation of new entities-review and nosologic discussion. Am J Med Genet 1982;11:185.
151. Kasai T, Oki T, Nogami H. Familial arthrogryposis with distal involvement of the limbs. Clin Orthop 1982;166:182.
152. McCormack MK, Coppola-McCormack P, Lee M. Autosomal-dominant inheritance of distal arthrogryposis. Am J Med Genet 1980;6:163.
153. Robinow M, Johnson GF. The Gordon syndrome: autosomal dominant cleft palate, camptodactyly, and club feet. Am J Med Genet 1981;9:139.
154. Rozin MM, Hertz M, Goodman RM. A new syndrome with camptodactyly, joint contractures, facial anomalies, and skeletal defects: a case report and review of syndromes with camptodactyly. Clin Genet 1984;26:342.
155. Salis JG, Beighton P. Dominantly inherited digito-talar dysmorphism. J Bone Joint Surg [Br] 1972;54:509.
156. Zancolli E, Zancolli E Jr. Congenital ulnar drift of the fingers. Pathogenesis, classification, and surgical management. Hand Clinics 1985;1:443.

Freeman Sheldon Syndrome

157. Dallapiccola B, Giannotti A, Lembo A, Sagni L. Autosomal recessive form of whistling face syndrome in sibs. Am J Med Genet 1989;33:542.
158. Duggar RG, DeMars PD, Bolton VE. Whistling face syndrome: general anesthesia and early postoperative caudal analgesia. Anesthesiology 1989;70:545.
159. Estrada R, Rosenfeld W, Salazar JD, Jhaveri R. Freeman-Sheldon syndrome with unusual hand and foot anomalies. J Natl Med Assoc 1981;73:664.
160. Freeman EA, Sheldon JH. Cranio-carpo-tarsal dystrophy. An undescribed congenital malformation. Arch Dis Child 1938;13:277.
161. Galaini CA, Matt BH. Laryngomalacia and intraneural striated muscle in an infant with Freeman-Sheldon syndrome. Int J Pediatr Otolaryngology 1993;25:243.
162. Jones R, Dolcourt JL. Muscle rigidity following halothane in two patients with Freeman-Sheldon. Anesthesiology 1992;77:599.
163. Malkawi H, Tarawneh M. The whistling face syndrome, or craniocarpaltarsal dysplasia. Report of two cases in a father and son and review of the literature. J Pediatr Orthop 1983;3:364.
164. Marasovich WA, Mazaheri M, Stool SE. Otolaryngologic findings in whistling face syndrome. Arch Otolaryngol Head Neck Surgery. 1989;115:1373.
165. O'Connell DJ, Hall CM. Cranio-carpo-tarsal dysplasia. A report of seven cases. Radiology 1977;123:719.
166. Rinsky LA, Bleck EE. Freeman-Sheldon ("whistling face") syndrome. J Bone Joint Surg [Am] 1976;58:148.
167. Sauk JJ, Delaney JR, Reaume C, et al. Electromyography of oral-facial musculature in craniocarpotarsal dysplasia (Freeman-Sheldon syndrome). Clin Genet 1974;6:132.
168. Walker BA. Whistling face—windmill vane syndrome (craniocarpotarsal dystrophy; Freeman-Sheldon syndrome). Birth Defects 1969;5:228.
169. Wenner SM, Shalvoy RM. Two stage correction of thumb adductor contracture in Freeman-Sheldon syndrome. J Hand Surg 1989;14:937.
170. Wettstein A, Buchinger G, Braun A, Bazan UB. A family with whistling face syndrome. Hum Genet 1980;55:177.

Pterygia Syndromes

171. Addison A, Webb PJ. Flexion contractures of the knee associated with popliteal webbing. J Pediatr Orthop 1983;3:376.
172. Crawford A. Treatment of popliteal pterygium syndrome. J Pediatr Orthop 1982;2:443.
173. Cunningham LN, Keating MA, Snyder HM, Duckett JW. Urologic manifestations of the popliteal pterygium syndrome. J Urology 1989;141:910.
174. De Die-Smulders CE, Schrander-Stompel CT, Fryns JP. The

lethal multiple pterygium syndrome: a nosological approach. Genet Couns 1990;1:13.
175. De Die-Smulders CE, Vonsee MJ, Zandvoort JA, Fryns JP. The lethal multiple pterygium syndrome: prenatal ultrasonographic and postmortem findings. Eur J Obstet Gynecol Reprod Biol 1990;35:283.
176. Escobar V, Weaver D. Popliteal pterygium syndrome. A phenotypic and genetic analysis. J Med Genet 1978;15:35.
177. Froster-Iskenns VG. Popliteal pterygium syndrome. J Med Genet 1990;27:320.
178. Hall JG, Reed SD, Rosenbaum KN, et al. Limb pterygium syndromes: a review and report of 11 patients. Am J Med Genet 1982;12:377.
179. Hall JG. Genetic aspects of arthrogryposis. Clin Orthop 1985;194:44.
180. Hansson LI, Hansson V, Jonsson K. Popliteal pterygium syndrome in a 74-year old woman. Acta Orthop Scand 1976;47:525.
181. Hartwig NG, Vermeij-Keers C, Bruijn JA, van Groningen K. Case of lethal multiple pterygium syndrome with special references to the origin of pterygia. Am J Med Genet 1989;33:537.
182. Herold HZ. Popliteal pterygium syndrome. Clin Orthop 1986;299:194.
183. Hunter A. The popliteal pterygium syndrome: report of a new family and review of literature. Am J Med Genet 1990;36:196.
184. Koch H, Grzonka M, Koch J. Popliteal pterygium syndrome with special consideration of the cleft malformation. Cleft palate. Craniofac J 1992;29:80.
185. McCall RE, Buddon J. Treatment of multiple pterygium syndrome. Orthopedics 1992;15:1417.
186. Moerman P, Fryns JP, Corneilis A, et al. Pathogenesis of the lethal multiple pterygium syndrome. Am J Med Genet 1990;35:415.
187. Oppenheim WL, Larson KR, McNabb MB, et al. Popliteal pterygium syndrome: an orthopaedic perspective. J Pediatr Orthop 1990;10:58.
188. Penchaszadeh VB, Salszberg B. Multiple pterygium syndrome. J Med Genet 1981;18:451.
189. Saleh M, Gibson MF, Sharrard WJ. Femoral shortening in correction of congenital knee flexion deformity with popliteal webbing. J Pediatr Orthop 1989;9:609.
190. Winter RB. Scoliosis and the multiple pterygium syndrome. J Pediatr Orthop 1983;3:125.
191. Wynne JM, Fraser AG, Herman R. Massive oral membrane in the popliteal web syndrome. J Pediatr Surg 1982;17:59.

Down Syndrome

192. Aprin H, Zink WP, Hall JE. Management of dislocation of the hip in Down syndrome. J Pediatr Orthop 1985;5:428.
193. Barden HS. Growth and development of selected hard tissues in Down syndrome: a review. Hum Biol 1983;55:539.
194. Bennet GC, Rang M, Roye DP, Aprin H. Dislocation of the hip in trisomy 21. J Bone Joint Surg [Br] 1982;64:289.
195. Brock DJH. Molecular genetics for the clinician. Cambridge, UK: Cambridge University Press, 1993.
196. Caffey J, Ross S. Pelvic bones in infantile mongoloidism: roentgenographic features. AJR 1958;80:458.
197. Cremers MJ, Beijer HJ. No relation between general laxity and atlantoaxial instability in children with Down syndrome. J Pediatr Orthop 1993;13:318.
198. Cronk C, Crocker AC, Pueschel SM, et al. Growth charts for children with Down syndrome: 1 month to 18 years of age. Pediatrics 1988;81:102.
199. Diamond LS, Lynne D, Sigman B. Orthopedic disorders in patients with Down's syndrome. Orthop Clin North Am 1981;12:57.
200. Dugdale TW, Renshaw TS. Instability of the patellofemoral joint in Down syndrome. J Bone Joint Surg [Am] 1986;68:405.
201. Fidone GS. Degenerative cervical arthritis and Down's syndrome. N Engl J Med 1986;314:320.
202. Gabriel KR, Mason DE, Carango P. Occipito-atlantal translation in Down's syndrome. Spine 1990;15:997.
203. Gath A. Parental reactions to loss and disappointment: the diagnosis of Down's syndrome. Dev Med Child Neurol 1985;27:392.
204. Gore DR. Recurrent dislocation of the hip in a child with Down's syndrome. J Bone Joint Surg [Am] 1981;63:823.
205. Herring JA, Fielding JW. Cervical instability in Down's syndrome and juvenile rheumatoid arthritis. J Pediatr Orthop 1982;2:205.
206. Hresko MT, McCarthy JC, Goldberg MJ. Hip disease in adults with Down syndrome. J Bone Joint Surg [Br] 1993;75:604.
207. Kolata G. Down syndrome—Alzheimer's linked. Science 1985;230:1152.
208. Levack B, Roper BA. Dislocation in Down's syndrome. Dev Med Child Neurol 1984;26:122.
209. MacLachlan RA, Fidler KE, Yeh H, et al. Cervical spine abnormalities in institutionalized adults with Down's syndrome. J Intellect Disabil Res 1993;37:277.
210. Martich V, Ben-Ami T, Yousefzadeh DK, Roizen NJ. Hypoplastic posterior arch of C-1 in children with Down syndrome: a double jeopardy. Radiology 1992;183:125.
211. Menezes AH, Ryken TC. Craniovertebral abnormalities in Down's syndrome. Pediatr Neurosurg 1992;18:24.
212. Miele JF, Piasio MA, Goldberg MJ. Orthopedic deformity occurring in Down syndrome patients with juvenile rheumatoid arthritis. Orthop Trans 1986;10:130.
213. Nogi J. Hip disorders in children with Down's syndrome. Dev Med Child Neurol 1985;27:86.
214. Nyberg DA, Resta RG, Luthy DA, et al. Humerus and femur length shortening in the detection of Down's syndrome. Am J Obstet Gynecol 1993;168:534.
215. Ohsawa T, Izawa T, Kuroki Y, Ohnari K. Follow-up study of atlanto-axial instability in Down's syndrome without separate odontoid process. Spine 1989;14:1149.
216. Parker AW, Bronks R. Gait of children with Down syndrome. Arch Physiol Med Rehabil 1980;61:345.
217. Pueschel SM, Herndon JH, Gelch MM, et al. Symptomatic atlanto-axial subluxation in persons with Down syndrome. J Pediatr Orthop 1984;4:682.
218. Pueschel SM, Scola FH, Tupper TB, Pezzullo JC. Skeletal anomalies of the upper cervical spine in children with Down syndrome. J Pediatr Orthop 1990;10:607.
219. Pueschel SM, Moon AC, Scola FH. Computerized tomography in persons with Down syndrome and atlantoaxial instability. Spine 1992;17:735.
220. Pueschel SM, Scola FH, Pezzullo JC. A longitudinal study of atlanto-dens relationships in asymptomatic individuals with Down syndrome. Pediatrics 1992;89:1194.
221. Rast MM, Harris SR. Motor control in infants with Down syndrome. Dev Med Child Neurol 1985;27:682.
222. Roberts GM, Starey N, Harper P, Nuki G. Radiology of the pelvis and hips in adults with Down's syndrome. Clin Radiol 1980;31:475.
223. Rotmensch S, Luo JS, Liberati M, et al. Fetal humeral length to detect Down syndrome. Am J Obstet Gynecol 1992;166:1330.
224. Selby KA, Newton RW, Gupta S, Hunt L. Clinical predictors and radiological reliability in atlantoaxial subluxation in Down's syndrome. Arch Dis in Childhood 1991;66:876.
225. Shaw ED, Beals RK. The hip joint in Down's syndrome. A

study of its structure and associated disease. Clin Orthop Rel Res 1992;278:101.
226. Sherk HH, Pasquariello PS, Watters WC. Multiple dislocations of the cervical spine in a patient with juvenile rheumatoid arthritis and Down's syndrome. Clin Orthop 1982;162:37.
227. Stein SM, Kirchner SG, Horev G, Hernanz-Schulman M. Atlanto-occipital subluxation in Down syndrome. Pediatr Radiol 1991;21:121.
228. Tangerud A, Hestnes A, Sand T, Sunndalsfoll S. Degenerative changes in the cervical spine in Down's syndrome. J Ment Defic Res 1990;34:179.
229. Tredwell SJ, Newman DE, Lockitch G. Instability of the upper cervical spine in Down syndrome. J Pediatr Orthop 1990;10:602.
230. Twining P, Whalley DR, Lewin E, Foulkes K. Is a short femur length a useful ultrasound marker for Down's syndrome? Br J Radiol 1991;64:990.
231. White KS, Ball WS, Prenger EC, et al. Evaluation of the craniocervical junction in Down syndrome: correlation of measurements obtained with radiography and MR imaging. Radiology 1993;186:377.

Fetal Alcohol Syndrome

232. Abel EL, Sokol RJ. A revised conservative estimate of the incidence of FAS and its economic impact. Alcoholism 1991;15:514.
233. Autti-Ramo I, Gaily E, Granstrom ML. Dysmorphic features in offspring of alcoholic mothers. Arch Dis Child 1992;67:712.
234. Clarren SK. Neural tube defects and fetal alcohol syndrome. J Pediatr 1979;95:328.
235. Crain LS, Fitzmaurice NE, Mondry C. Nail dysplasia and fetal alcohol syndrome. Am J Dis Child 1983;137:1069.
236. Cremin BJ, Jaffer Z. Radiological aspects of the fetal alcohol syndrome. Pediatr Radiol 1981;11:151.
237. Day NL, Richardson GA. Prenatal alcohol exposure: a continuum of effects. Semin Perinatol 1991;4:271.
238. Ernhart CB. Clinical correlations between ethanol intake and fetal alcohol syndrome. Recent Dev Alcohol 1991;9:127.
239. Goldstein G, Arulanantham K. Neural tube defect and renal anomalies in a child with fetal alcohol syndrome. J Pediatr 1978;93:636.
240. Halmesmaki E, Raivio K, Ylikorkala O. A possible association between maternal drinking and fetal clubfoot. N Engl J Med 1985;312:790.
241. Jaffer Z, Nelson M, Beighton P. Bone fusion in the foetal alcohol syndrome. J Bone Joint Surg [Br] 1981;63:569.
242. Knupfer G. Abstaining for foetal health: the fiction that even light drinking is dangerous. Br J Addiction 1991;86:1057.
243. Leicher-Duber A, Schumacher R, Spranger J. Stippled epiphyses in fetal alcohol syndrome. Pediatr Radiol 1990;20:369.
244. Little RE, Wendt JK. The effects of maternal drinking in the reproductive period: an epidemiologic review. J Subst Abuse 1991;3:187.
245. Lowry RB. The Klippel-Feil anomalad as part of the fetal alcohol syndrome. Teratology 1977;16:53.
246. Neidengard L, Carter TE, Smith DW. Klippel-Feil malformation complex in fetal alcohol syndrome. Am J Dis Child 1978;132:929.
247. Rosett HL, Weiner L. Prevention of fetal alcohol effects. Pediatrics 1982;69:813.
248. Rosett HL, Weiner L, Lee A, et al. Patterns of alcohol consumption and fetal development. Obstet Gynecol 1983;61:539.
249. Rostand A, Kaminski M, Lelong N, et al. Alcohol use in pregnancy, craniofacial features, and fetal growth. J Epidemiol Commun Health 1990;44:302.
250. Smith DF, Sandor GG, MacLeod PM, et al. Intrinsic defects in the fetal alcohol syndrome: studies on 76 cases from British Columbia and the Yukon Territory. Neurobehav Toxicol Teratol 1981;3:145.
251. Spiegel PG, Pekman WM, Rich BH, et al. The orthopedic aspects of the fetal alcohol syndrome. Clin Orthop 1979;139:58.
252. Streissguth AP, Clarren SK, Jones KL. Natural history of the fetal alcohol syndrome: a 10-year follow-up of eleven patients. Lancet 1985;2:85.
253. Tredwell SJ, Smith DF, MacLeod PJ, Wood BJ. Cervical spine anomalies in fetal alcohol sydrome. Spine 1982;7:331.
254. Van Rensburg LJ. Major skeletal defects in the fetal alcohol syndrome. J Afr Med J 1981;59:687.
255. West JR, Black AC Jr, Reimann PC, Alkana RL. Polydactyly and polysyndactyly induced by prenatal exposure to ethanol. Teratology 1981;24:13.

Nail-Patella Syndrome

256. Beals RK, Eckhardt AL. Hereditary onycho-osteodysplasia (nail-patella syndrome). A report of nine kindreds. J Bone Joint Surg [Am] 1969;51;505.
257. Daniel CR, III., Osment LS, Noojin RL. Triangular lunulae. A clue to nail-patella syndrome. Arch Dermatol 1980;116:448.
258. Darlington D, Hawkins CF. Nail-patella syndrome with iliac horns and hereditary nephropathy. Necropsy report and anatomical dissection. J Bone Joint Surg [Br] 1967;49-B;164.
259. Drut RM, Chandra S, Latorraca R, Gilbert-Barness E. Nail-patella syndrome in a spontaneously aborted 18-week fetus: ultrastructural and immunofluorescent study of the kidneys. Am J Med Genet 1992;43:693.
260. Guidera KJ, Satterwhite Y, Ogden JA, et al. Nail patella syndrome: a review of 44 orthopaedic patients. J Pediatr Orthop 1991;11:737.
261. Hogh J, Macnical MF. Foot deformities associated with onycho-osteodysplasia. A familial study and a review of associated features. Int Orthop 1985;9:135.
262. Ioan DM, Maximilian C, Fryns JP. Madelung deformity as a pathognomonic feature of the onycho-osteodysplasia syndrome. Genet Couns 1992;3:25.
263. Letts M. Hereditary onycho-osteodysplasia (nail-patella syndrome). A three generation familial study. Orthop Rev 1991;20:267.
264. Lommen EJ, Hamel BC, te Slaa RL. Nephropathy in hereditary osteo-onycho dysplasia (HOOD): variable expression or genetic heterogeneity? Prog Clin Biol Res 1989;305:157.
265. Loomer RL. Shoulder girdle dysplasia associated with nail patella syndrome. A case report and literature review. Clin Orthop Rel Res 1989;238:112.
266. Papadakos VT, Swan A, Bhalla AK. Nail-patella syndrome associated with mixed crystal deposition arthropathy. Clin Rheumatol 1992;11:413.
267. Yakish SD, Fu FH. Long-term follow-up of the treatment of a family with nail-patella syndrome. J Pediatr Orthop 1983;3:360.

De Lange Syndrome

268. Bruner JP, Hsia YE. Prenatal findings in Brachmann-de Lange syndrome. Obstet Gynecol 1990;76:966.
269. Cates M, Billmire DF, Bull MJ, Grosfeld JL. Gastroesophageal dysfunction in Cornelia de Lange syndrome. J Pediatr Surg 1989;24:248.
270. Condron CJ. Limb anomalies in Cornelia de Lange syndrome—infant patient. Birth Defects 1969;5:226.

271. Curtis JA, O'Hara AE, Carpenter GG. Spurs of the mandible and supracondylar process of the humerus in Cornelia de Lange syndrome. AJR 1977;129:156.
272. De Die-Smulders C, Theunissen P, Schranger-Stumpel C, Frijns JP. On the variable expression of the Brachmann–de Lange syndrome. Clin Genet 1992;41:42.
273. Dossetor DR, Couryer S, Nicol AR. Massage for very severe self-injurious behaviour in a girl with Cornelia de Lange syndrome. Dev Med Child Neurol 1991;33:636.
274. Drolshagen LF, Durmon G, Berumen M, Burks DD. Prenatal ultrasonographic appearance of "Cornelia de Lange" syndrome. J Clin Ultrasound 199;220:470.
275. Filippi G. The de Lange syndrome. Report of 15 cases. Clin Genet 1989;35:343.
276. Filippi G, Renuart AW. Limb anomalies in the Cornelia de Lange syndrome—adult patient. Birth Defects 1969;5:228.
277. Fraser WI, Campbell BM. A study of six cases of de Lange Amsterdam dwarf syndrome, with special attention to voice, speech and language characteristics. Dev Med Child Neurol 1978;20:189.
278. Greenberg F, Robinson LK. Mild Brachmann–de Lange syndrome: changes of phenotype with age. Am J Med Genet 1989;32:90.
279. Halal F, Preus M. The hand profile in de Lange syndrome: diagnostic criteria. Am J Med Genet 1979;3:317.
280. Ireland M, English C, Cross I, et al. A de novo translocation t (3;17)(q26.a3;q23.1) in a child with Cornelia de Lange syndrome. J Med Genet 1991;28:639.
281. Joubin J, Pettrone CF, Pettrone FA. Cornelia de Lange's syndrome. A review article (with emphasis on orthopedic significance). Clin Orthop 1982;171:180.
282. Lakshminarayana P, Nallasivam P. Cornelia de Lange syndrome with ring chromosomes 3. J Med Genet 1990;27:405.
283. Pashayan HM, Fraser FC, Pruzansky S. Variable limb malformations in the Brachmann-Cornelia de Lange syndrome. Birth Defects 1975;11:147.
284. Rosenbach Y, Zahavi I, Dinari G. Gastroesophageal dysfunction in Brachmann-de Lange syndrome. Am J Med Genet 1992;42:379.
285. Sargent WW. Anesthetic management of a patient with Cornelia de Lange syndrome. Anesthesiology 1991;74:1162.
286. Shear CS, Nyhan WL, Kirman BH, Stern J. Self-mutilative behavior as a feature of the de Lange syndrome. J Pediatr 1971;78:506.

Familial Dysautonomia (Riley-Day Syndrome)

287. Axelrod FB, Abularrage JJ. Familial dysautonomia: a prospective study of survival. J Pediatr 1982;101:234.
288. Axelrod FB, Gouge TH, Ginsburg HB, et al. Fundoplication and gastrostomy in familial dysautonomia. J Pediatr 1991;118:388.
289. Blumenfeld A, Axelrod FB, Trofatter JA, et al. Exclusion of familial dysautonomia from more than 60% of the genome. J Med Genet 1993;30:47.
290. Brunt PW. Unusual cause of Charcot joints in early adolescence (Riley-Day syndrome). Br Med J 1967;4:277.
291. Chillag KJ, Stevens DB. Idiopathic neurogenic arthropathy. J Pediatr Orthop 1985;5:597.
292. Cox RG, Sumner R. Familial dysautonomia. Anaesthesia 1983;38:293.
293. Foster JMG. Anaesthesia for a patient with familial dysautonomia. Anaesthesia 1983;38:391.
294. Ganz SB, Levine DB, Axelrod FB, Kahanovitz N. Physical therapy management of familial dysautonomia. Phys Ther 1983;63:1121.
295. Goto S, Hirano A, Pearson J. Calcineurin and synaptophysin in the human spinal cord of normal individuals and patients with familial dysautonomia. Acta Neuropathol 1990;79:647.
296. Grunebaum M. Radiological manifestations in familial dysautonomia. Am J Dis Child 1974;128:176.
297. Guidera KJ, Multhopp H, Ganey T, Ogden JA. Orthopaedic manifestations in congenitally insensate patients. J Pediatr Orthop 1990;10:514.
298. Hensinger RN, MacEwen GD. Spinal deformity associated with heritable neurological conditions: spinal muscular atrophy, Friedreich's ataxia, familial dysautonomia, and Charcot-Marie-Tooth disease. J Bone Joint Surg [Am] 1976;58:13.
299. Mitnick JS, Axelrod FB, Genieser NB, Becker M. Aseptic necrosis in familial dysautonomia. Radiology 1982;142:89.
300. Pearson J, Pytel BA, Grover-Johnson N, et al. Quantitative studies of dorsal root ganglia and neuropathologic observations on spinal cords in familial dysautonomia. J Neurol Sci 1978;35:77.
301. Porges RF, Axelrod FB, Richards M. Pregnancy in familial dysautonomia. Am J Obstet Gynecol 1978;132:485.
302. Robin GC. Scoliosis in familial dysautonomia. Bull Hosp Joint Dis Orthop Inst 1984;44:16.
303. Strasberg P, Yeger H, Warren I. Increased globotriaosylceralmide in familial dysautonomia. Lipids 1992;27:978.
304. Udassin R, Seror D, Vinograd I, et al. Nissen fundoplication in the treatment of children with familial dysautonomia. Am J Surg 1992;164:332.
305. Yoslow W, Becker MH, Bartels J, Thompson WAL. Orthopaedic defects in familial dysautonomia. A review of sixty-five cases. J Bone Joint Surg [Am] 1971;53:1541.

Rubinstein Taybi

306. Allanson JE. Rubinstein-Taybi syndrome: the changing face. Am J Med Genet Suppl 1990;6:38.
307. Breuning MH, Dauwerse HG, Fugazza G, et al. Rubinstein-Taybi syndrome caused by submicroscopic deletions within 16p13.3. Am J Hum Genet 1993;52:249.
308. Hennekam RC, Tilanus M, Hamel BC, et al. Deletion at chromosome 16p13.3 as a cause of Rubinstein-Taybi syndrome: clinical aspects. Am J Hum Genet 1993;52:255.
309. Hennekam RC, Van Doorne JM. Oral aspects of Rubinstein-Taybi syndrome. Am J Med Genet Suppl 1990;6:42.
310. Hennekam RC, Van Den Boogaard MJ, Sibbles BJ, Van Spijker HG. Rubinstein-Taybi syndrome in The Netherlands. Am J Med Genet Suppl 1990;6:17.
311. Lacombe D, Saura R, Taine L, Battin J. Confirmation of assignment of a locus for Rubinstein-Taybi syndrome gene to 16p13.3. Am J Med Genet 1992;44:126.
312. Marion RW, Garcia DM, Karasik JB. Apparent dominant transmission of the Rubinstein-Taybi syndrome. Am J Med Genet 1993;46:284.
313. Moran M, Calthorpe D, McGoldrick F, Fogarty E, Dowling F. Congenital dislocation of the patella in Rubinstein Taybi syndrome. Ir Med J 1993; 86:34.
314. Partington MW. Rubinstein-Taybi syndrome: a follow-up study. Am J Med Genet Suppl 1990;6:65.
315. Robson MJ, Brown LM, Sharrad WJW. Cervical spondylolisthesis and other skeletal abnormalities in Rubinstein-Taybi syndrome. J Bone Joint Surg [Br] 1980;62:297.
316. Rubinstein JH. Broad thumb-hallux (Rubinstein-Taybi) syndrome 1957-1988. Am J Med Genet Suppl 1990;6:3.
317. Selmanowitz VJ, Stiller MJ. Rubinstein-Taybi syndrome. Cutaneous manifestations and colossal keloids. Arch Dermatol 1981;117:504.
318. Stevens CA, Hennekam RC, Blackburn BL. Growth in the Rubinstein-Taybi syndrome. Am J Med Genet Suppl 1990;6:51.

319. Stevens CA, Carey JC, Blackburn BL. Rubinstein-Taybi syndrome: a natural history study. Am J Med Genet Suppl 1990;6:30.
320. Stirt JA. Anesthetic problems in Rubinstein-Taybi syndrome. Anesth Analg 1981;60:534.
321. Stirt JA. Succinylcholine in Rubinstein-Taybi syndrome. Anesthesiology 1982;57:429.

Progeria (Hutchinson Gilford) Syndrome

322. Badame AJ. Progeria. Arch Dermatol 1989;125:540.
323. Beavan LA, Quentin-Hoffmann E, Schonherr E, et al. Deficient expression of decorin in infantile progeroid patients. J Biol Chem 1993;268:9856.
324. Brown WT. Progeria: a human-disease model of accelerated aging. Am J Clin Nutr 1992;55(Suppl 6):1222S.
325. Clark MA, Weiss AS. Elevated levels of glycoprotein gp200 in progeria fibroblasts. Mol Cell Biochem 1993;120:51.
326. Colige A, Nusgens B, Lapiere CM. Altered response of progeria fibroblasts to epidermal growth factor. J Cell Sci 1991;100:649.
327. Colige A, Roujeau JC, De la Rocque F, Nusgens B, Lapiere CM. Abnormal gene expression in skin fibroblasts from a Hutchinson-Gilford patient. Lab Invest 1991;64:799.
328. Fernandez-Palazzi F, McLaren AT, Slowie DF. Report on a case of Hutchinson-Gilford progeria, with special reference to orthopedic problems. Eur J Pediatr Surg 1992;2:378.
329. Gamble JG. Hip disease in Hutchinson-Gilford progeria syndrome. J Pediatr Orthop 1984;4:585.
330. Gillar PJ, Kaye CI, McCourt JW. Progressive early dermatologic changes in Hutchinson-Gilford progeria syndrome. Pediatr Dermatol 1991;8:199.
331. Khalifa MM. Hutchinson-Gilford progeria syndrome: report of a Libyan family and evidence of autosomal recessive inheritance. Clin Genet 1989;35:125.
332. Moen C. Orthopaedic aspects of progeria. J Bone Joint Surg [Am] 1982;64:542.
333. Monu JU, Benka-Coker LB, Fatunde Y. Hutchinson-Gilford progeria syndrome in siblings. Report of three new cases. Skeletal Radiol 1990;19:585.
334. Reichel W, Bailey JA II, Zigel S, et al. Radiological findings in progeria. J Am Geriatr Soc 1971;19:657.
335. Winkles JA, O'Connor ML, Friesel R. Altered regulation of platelet-derived growth factor A-chain and c-fos gene expression in senescent progeria fibroblasts. J Cell Physiol 1990;144:313.

Russell-Silver Dwarfism

336. Angehrn V, Zachmann M, Prader A. Silver-Russell syndrome. Observations in 20 patients. Helv Paediatr Acta 1979;34:297.
337. Escobar V, Gleiser S, Weaver DD. Phenotypic and genetic analysis of the Silver-Russell syndrome. Clin Genet 1978;13:278.
338. Herman TE, Crawford JD, Cleveland RH, Kushner DC. Hand radiographs in Russell-Silver syndrome. Pediatrics 1987;79:743.
339. Limbird TJ. Slipped capital femoral epiphysis associated with Russell-Silver syndrome. South Med J 1989;82:902.
340. Moseley JE, Moloshok RE, Freiberger RH. The Silver syndrome: congenital asymmetry, short stature and variations in sexual development. Roentgen features. AJR 1966;97:74.
341. Moss SH, Switzer HE. Congenital hypoplastic thumb in the Silver syndrome—a case report and review of upper extremity anomalies in the world literature. J Hand Surg 1983;8:480.
342. Saal HM, Pagon RA, Pepin MG. Reevaluation of Russell-Silver syndrome. J Pediatr 1985;107:733.
343. Samn M, Lewis K, Blumberg B. Monozygotic twins discordant for the Russell-Silver syndrome. Am J Med Genet 1990;37:543.
344. Spect EE, Hazelrig PE. Orthopaedic considerations of Silver's syndrome. J Bone Joint Surg [Am] 1973;55:1502.
345. Stanhope R, Ackland F, Hamill G, et al. Physiological growth hormone secretion and response to growth hormone treatment in children with short stature and intrauterine growth retardation. Acta Paediatr Scand Suppl 1989;349:47.
346. Tanner JM, Lejarraga H, Cameron N. The natural history of the Silver-Russell syndrome: a longitudinal study of thirty-nine cases. Pediatr Res 1975;9:611.

Turner Syndrome

347. Beals RK. Orthopedic aspects of the XO (Turner's) syndrome. Clin Orthop 1973;97:19.
348. Gicquel C, Cabrol S, Schneid H, et al. Molecular diagnosis of Turner's syndrome. J Med Genet 1992;29:547.
349. Jacobs PA, Betts PR, Cockwell AE, et al. A cytogenetic and molecular reappraisal of a series of patients with Turner's syndrome. Ann Hum Genet 1990;54:209.
350. Kosowicz J. The deformity of the medial tibial condyle in nineteen cases of gonadal dysgenesis. J Bone Joint Surg [Am] 1960;42:600.
351. Mora S, Weber G, Guarneri MP, et al. Effect of estrogen replacement therapy on bone mineral content in girls with Turner syndrome. Obstet Gynecol 1992;79:747.
352. Mostello DJ, Bofinger MK, Siddigi TA. Spontaneous resolution of fetal cystic hygroma and hydrops in Turner syndrome. Obstet Gynecol 1989;73:862.
353. Naeraa RW, Brixen K, Hansen RM, et al. Skeletal size and bone mineral content in Turner's syndrome: relation to karyotype, estrogen treatment, physical fitness, and bone turnover. Calcif Tissue Int 1991;49:77.
354. Naeraa RW, Nielsen J. Standards for growth and final height in Turner's syndrome. Acta Paediatr Scand 1990;79:182.
355. Neely EK, Marcus R, Rosenfeld RG, Bachrach LK. Turner syndrome adolescents receiving growth hormone are not osteopenic. J Clin Endocrinol Metab 1993;76:861.
356. Rosenfeld RG. Growth hormone therapy in Turner's syndrome: an update on final height. Acta Paediatr Suppl 1992;383:3.
357. Rosenfeld RG, Frane J, Attie KM, et al. Six year results of a randomized, prospective trial of human growth hormone and oxandrolone in Turner syndrome. J Pediatr 1992;121:49.
358. Ross JL, Long LM, Feuillan P, et al. Normal bone density of the wrist and spine and increased wrist fractures in girls with Turner's syndrome. J Clin Endocrinol Metab 1991;73:355.
359. Rovet JF. The psychoeducational characteristics of children with Turner syndrome. J Learn Disabil 1993;26:333.
360. Saggese G, Federico G, Bertelloni S, Baroncelli GI. Mineral metabolism in Turner's syndrome: evidence for impaired renal vitamin D metabolism and normal osteoblast function. J Clin Endocrinol Metab 1992;75:998.
361. Subramaniam PN. Turner's syndrome and cardiovascular anomalies: a case report and review of the literature. Am J Med Sci 1989;297:260.
362. Swillen A, Fryns JP, Kleczkowska A, et al. Intelligence, behaviour and psychosocial development in Turner syndrome. A cross-sectional study of 50 pre-adolescent and adolescent girls (4–20 years). Genet Couns 1993;4:7.
363. Sylven L, Hagenfeldt K, Brondum-Neilsen K, von Schoultz B. Middle-aged women with Turner's syndrome. Medical status, hormonal treatment and social life. Acta Endocrinol 1991;125:359.
364. Thomson SJ, Tanne NS, Mercer DM. Web neck deformity;

anatomical considerations and options in surgical management. Br J Plast Surg 1990;43:94.

Noonan Syndrome

365. Burch M, Mann JM, Sharland M, et al. Myocardial disarray in Noonan syndrome. Br Heart J 1992;68:586.
366. Campbell AM, Bousfield JD. Anaesthesia in a patient with Noonan's syndrome and cardiomyopathy. Anaesthesia 1992;47:131.
367. Collins E, Turner G. The Noonan syndrome—a review of the clinical and genetic features of 27 cases. J Pediatr 1973;83:941.
368. Hunter A, Pinsky L. An evaluation of the possible association of malignant hyperpyrexia with the Noonan syndrome using serum creatine phosphokinase levels. J Pediatr 1975;86:412.
369. Sharland M, Burch M, McKenna WM, Paton MA. A clinical study of Noonan syndrome. Arch Dis Child 1992;67:178.
370. Sharland M, Morgan M, Smith G, et al. Genetic counselling in Noonan syndrome. Am J Med Genet 1993;45:437.
371. Wedge JH, Khalifa MM, Shokeir MHK. Skeletal anomalies in 40 patients with Noonan's syndrome. Orthop Trans 1987;11:40.

Prader-Willi Syndrome

372. Aughton DJ, Cassidy SB. Physical features of Prader-Willi syndrome in neonates. Am J Dis Child 1990;144:1251.
373. Borghgraef M, Fryns JP, Van den Berghe H. Psychological profile and behavioral characteristics in 12 patients with Prader-Willi syndrome. Genet Couns 1990;1:141.
374. Cassidy SB. Prader-Willi syndrome. Curr Probl Pediatr 1984;14:1.
375. Cassidy SB, ed. Prader-Willi syndrome and other chromosome 15q deletion disorders. NATO ASI series—series H: cell biology, vol 61. Heidelberg: Springer, 1992:265.
376. Char F. A photographic study: the natural history of Prader-Willi syndrome. J Clin Dysmorphol 1984;2:2.
377. Curfs LM, Verhulst FC, Fryns JP. Behavioral and emotional problems in youngsters with Prader-Willi syndrome. Genet Couns 1991;2:33.
378. Gavranich J, Selikowitz M. A survey of 22 individuals with Prader-Willi syndrome in New South Wales. Aust Paediatr J 1989;25:43.
379. Gurd AR, Thompson TR. Scoliosis in Prader-Willi syndrome. J Pediatr Orthop 1981;1:317.
380. Holm VA, Laurnen EL. Prader-Willi syndrome and scoliosis. Dev Med Child Neurol 1981;23:192.
381. Holm VA, Cassidy SB, Butler MG, et al. Prader-Willi syndrome: consensus diagnostic criteria. Pediatrics 1993;91:398.
382. Hudgins L, Cassidy SB. Hand and foot length in Prader-Willi syndrome. Am J Med Genet 1991;41:5.
383. Knoll JH, Wagstaff J, Lalande M. Cytogenetic and molecular studies in the Prader-Willi and Angelman syndromes: an overview. Am J Med Genet 1993;46:2.
384. Mayhew JF, Taylor B. Anaesthetic considerations in the Prader-Willi syndrome. Can Anaesth Soc J 1983;30:565.
385. Nicholls RD. Genomic imprinting and uniparental disomy in Angelman and Prader-Willi syndromes: a review. Am J Med Genet 1993;46:16.
386. Rees D, Jones MW, Owen R, Dorgan JC. Scoliosis surgery in the Prader-Willi syndrome. J Bone Joint Surg [Br] 1989;71:685.
387. Selikowitz M, Sunman J, Pendergast A, Wright S. Fenfluramine in Prader-Willi syndrome: a double blind, placebo controlled trial. Arch Dis Child 1990;65:112.
388. Waters J, Clarke DJ, Corbett JA. Educational and occupational outcome in Prader-Willi syndrome. Child Care Health Dev 1990;16:271.

Beckwith-Wiedemann Syndrome

389. Brown KW, Gardner A, Williams JC, et al. Paternal origin of 11p15 duplications in the Beckwith-Wiedemann syndrome. A new case and review of the literature. Cancer Genet Cytogenet 1992;58:66.
390. Goldberg MJ. Beckwith-Wiedemann syndrome. In: Goldberg MJ, ed. The dysmorphic child. An orthopedic perspective. New York: Raven Press, 1987:175.
391. Lee FA. Radiology of the Beckwith-Wiedemann syndrome. Radiol Clin North Am 1972;10:261.
392. Lodeiro JG, Byers JW III, Chuipek S, Feinstein SJ. Prenatal diagnosis and perinatal management of the Beckwith-Wiedemann syndrome: a case and review. Am J Perinatol 1989;6:446.
393. Martinez y Martinez R, Martinez-Carboney R, Ocampo-Campos R, et al. Wiedemann-Beckwith syndrome: clinical, cytogenetical and radiological observations in 39 new cases. Genet Couns 1992;3:67.
394. Ping AJ, Reeve AE, Law DJ, et al. Genetic linkage of Beckwith-Wiedemann syndrome to 11p15. Am J Hum Genet 1989;44:720.
395. Shah YG, Metlay L. Prenatal ultrasound diagnosis of Beckwith-Wiedemann syndrome. J Clin Ultrasound 1990;18:597.
396. Shah KJ. Beckwith-Wiedemann syndrome: role of ultrasound in its management. Clin Radiol 1983;34:313.
397. Viljoen D, Ramesar R. Evidence for paternal imprinting in familial Beckwith-Wiedemann syndrome. J Med Genet 1992;29:221.

Stickler Syndrome

398. Ahmad NN, McDonald-McGinn DM, Zackai EH, et al. A second mutation in the type II procollagen gene (COL2A1) causing Stickler syndrome (arthro-ophthalmopathy) is also a premature termination codon. Am J Hum Genet 1993;52:39.
399. Beals RK. Hereditary arthro-ophthalmopathy (the Stickler syndrome): report of a kindred with protrusio acetabuli. Clin Orthop 1977;125:32.
400. Bennett JT, McMurray SW, Stickler syndrome. J Pediatr Orthop 1990;10:760.
401. Brown DM, Nichols BE, Weingeist TA, et al. Procollagen II gene mutation in Stickler syndrome. Arch Ophthalmol 1992;110:1589.
402. Liberfarb RM, Hirose T, Holmes LB. The Wagner-Stickler syndrome—a study of 22 families. J Pediatr 1981;99:394.
403. Trepman E. Osteochondritis dissecans of the knee in an adult with Stickler syndrome. Orthop Rev 1993;22:371.
404. Vintiner GM, Temple IK, Middleton-Price HR, Baraitser M, Malcolm S. Genetic and clinical heterogeneity of Stickler syndrome. Am J Med Genet 1991;41:44.
405. Zlotogora J, Sagi M, Schuper A, Leiba H, Merin S. Variability of Stickler syndrome. Am J Med Genet 1992;42:337.

VATER Association

406. Beals RK, Rolfe B. VATER association. A unifying concept of multiple anomalies. J Bone Joint Surg [Am] 1989;71:948.
407. Chestnut R, James HE, Jones KL. The VATER association and spinal dysraphia. Pediatr Neurosurg 1992;18:144.
408. Lawhorn SM, MacEwen GD, Bunnell WP. Orthopaedic aspects of the VATER association. J Bone Joint Surg [Am] 1986;68:424.
409. Quan L, Smith DW. The VATER association: *V*ertebral defects,

Anal atresia, T-E fistula with esophageal atresia, Radial and Renal dysplasia: a spectrum of associated defects. J Pediatr 1973;82:104.
410. Raffel C, Litofsky S, McComb JG. Central nervous system malformations and the VATER association. Pediatr Neurosurg 1990–91;16:170.
411. Wulfsberg EA, Phillips-Dawkins TL, Thomas RL. Vertebral hypersegmentation in a case of the VATER association. Am J Med Genet 1992;42:766.

Goldenhar Syndrome

412. Cohen MM JR, Rollnick BR, Kaye CI. Oculoauriculovertebral spectrum: an updated critique. Cleft Palate J 1989;26:276.
413. Darling DB, Feingold M, Berkman M. The roentgenological aspects of Goldenhar's syndrome (oculoauriculovertebral dysplasia). Radiology 1968;91:254.
414. Kaye CI, Martin AO, Rollnick BR, et al. Oculoauriculovertebral anomaly: segregation analysis. Am J Med Genet 1992;43:913.
415. Madan R, Trikha A, Venkataraman RK, Barra R, Kalia P. Goldenhar's syndrome: an analysis of anaesthetic management. A retrospective study of seventeen cases. Anaesthesia 1990;45:49.
416. Morrison PJ, Mulholland HC, Craig BG, Nevin NC. Cardiovascular abnormalities in the oculo-auriculo-vertebral spectrum (Goldenhar syndrome). Am J Med Genet 1992;44:425.
417. Schrander-Stumpel CT, de Die-Smulders CE, Hennekam RC, et al. Oculoauriculovertebral spectrum and cerebral anomalies. J Med Genet 1992;29:326.
418. Sherk HH, Whitaker LA, Pasquariello PS. Facial malformations and spinal anomalies. A predictable relationship. Spine 1982;7:526.
419. Van Bever Y, van den Ende JJ, Richieri-Costa A. Oculo-auriculo-vertebral complex and uncommon associated anomalies: report on 9 unrelated Brazilian patients. Am J Med Genet 1992;44:683.

Trichorhinophalangeal Syndrome

420. Bauermeister S, Letts M. The orthopaedic manifestations of the Langer-Giedion syndrome. Orthop Rev 1992;21:31.
421. Burgess RC. Trichorhinophalangeal syndrome. South Med J 1991;84:1268.
422. Ludecke HJ, Johnson C, Wagner MJ, et al. Molecular definition of the shortest region of deletion overlap in the Langer-Giedion syndrome. Am J Hum Genet 1991;49:1197.
423. Minguella I, Ubierna M, Escola J, Roca A, Prats J, Pintos-Morell G. Trichorhinophalangeal syndrome, type I, with avascular necrosis of the femoral head. Acta Paediatr 1993;82:329.

Morquio Syndrome and the Mucopolysaccharidoses

424. Baker E, Guo XH, Orsborn AM, et al. The Morquio A syndrome (mucopolysaccharidosis IVA) gene maps to 16q24.3. Am J Hum Genet 1993;52:96.
425. Bassett GS. Orthopaedic aspects of skeletal dysplasias. Instruct Course Lect 1990;39:381.
426. Bassett GS. Lower-extremity abnormalities in dwarfing conditions. Instruct Course Lect 1990;39:389.
427. Bethem D, Winter RB, Luther L, et al. Spinal disorders of dwarfism: review of the literature and report of eighty cases. J Bone Joint Surg [Am] 1981;63:1412.
428. Breider MA, Shull RM, Constantopoulos G. Long-term effects of bone marrow transplantation in dogs with mucopolysaccharidosis I. Am J Pathol 1989;134:677.
429. Field RE, Buchanan JAF, Copplemans MGJ, Aichroth PM. Bone marrow transplantation in Hurler's syndrome. J Bone Joint Surg [Br] 1994;76:975.
430. Fukada S, Tomatsu S, Masue M, et al. Mucopolysaccharidosis type IVA. N-acetyl galactosamine-6-sulfate sulfatase exonic point mutations in classical Morquio and mild cases. J Clin Invest 1992;90:1049.
431. Goldberg MJ. Orthopedic aspects of bone dysplasia. Orthop Clin North Am 1976;7:445.
432. Hopwood JJ, Morris CP. The mucopolysaccharidoses. Diagnosis, molecular genetics and treatment. Mol Biol Med 1990;7:381.
433. Jin WD, Jackson CE, Desnick RJ. Mucopolysaccharidosis type VI: identification of three mutations in the arylsulfatarase B gene of patients with severe and mild phenotypes provides molecular evidence for genetic heterogeneity. Am J Hum Genet 1992;50:795.
434. Kopits SE. Orthopaedic complications of dwarfism. Clin Orthop 1976;114:153.
435. Lenarsky C, Kohn DB, Weinberg KI, Parkman R. Bone marrow transplantation for genetic diseases. Hematol Oncol Clin North Am 1990;4:589.
436. Nelson J, Broadhead D, Mossman J. Clinical findings in 12 patients with MPS IVA (Morquio's disease): further evidence for heterogeneity. Part 1: clinical and biochemical findings. Clin Genet 1988;33:111.
437. Nelson J, Thomas PS. Clinical findings in 12 patients with MPS IVA (Morquio's disease): further evidence for heterogeneity. Part III: odontoid dysplasia. Clin Genet 1988;33:126.
438. Scriver CR, Beaudet AL, Sly WS, Valle D, eds. The metabolic basis of inherited disease. 6th ed. New York: McGraw-Hill, 1989.
439. Stevens JM, Kendall BE, Crockard HA. The odontoid process in Morquio-Brailsford disease. The effects of occipitocervical fusion. J Bone Joint Surg [Br] 1991;73:851.

Chapter 9

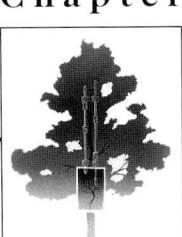

Localized Disorders of Bone and Soft Tissue

Paul D. Sponseller

Congenital and Developmental Disorders
Soft Tissue or Generalized Disorders
Disorders Involving Bone or Joint

Acquired Disorders
Myositis Ossificans
The Osteochondroses
Congenital Quadriceps Fibrosis
Reflex Sympathetic Dystrophy

Many disease processes affect the pediatric skeleton in a local or regional manner, but they are not unique to one area of the body and are not part of a systemic abnormality. The pathologic process itself is the unifying feature. The condition may be congenital or developmental and may involve bone or soft tissue. Klippel-Trenaunay syndrome is an example of this; the same gross and microscopic vascular pathology may occur in any area of the skeleton, and the associated anomalies are highly variable. This chapter was designed to unify such disorders and make recommendations for evaluation and treatment. The conditions discussed are grouped according to whether they are congenital or acquired and whether they involve multiple tissues in a region or bone alone.

CONGENITAL AND DEVELOPMENTAL DISORDERS

Soft Tissue or Generalized Disorders

Klippel-Trenaunay Syndrome

In 1900, Klippel and Trenaunay described their eponymous disorder, which has three essential features: a cutaneous hemangioma or vascular nevus, varicose veins, and hypertrophy of the involved limbs in length, girth, or both dimensions. The hemangioma usually is revealed first. It usually does not cross the midline of the body.[3,4,5,7] The entire limb is not uniformly affected. The severity of the varicose veins varies, but they tend to get larger with age. The hypertrophy usually involves bone and soft tissue.

The condition is probably related to a mesodermal defect that causes microscopic arteriovenous malformations from the embryonic state to persist.[2,6] It is presumed that this vascular malformation induces the hypertrophy of other tissues (e.g., adipose, muscle, bone), but there also may be primary mesodermal abnormalities in these cases.[12] The absence of deep venous drainage is not likely to be a causative factor, because deep veins are missing in only 14% of patients.[3]

CLINICAL FEATURES. Although most cases are evident from the time of birth or infancy, a few cases have been reported in which features appeared as late as 6 years of age. There is no recognized pattern of inheritance. The lower extremities are affected at least ten times more often as the upper extremities. The affected limb is longer than normal in 90% of patients.[10,14] Usually, all bones and soft tissues are involved in the hypertrophy (Fig. 9-1).

The growth patterns of the involved limbs have not been rigorously studied over time, but there are enough reported cases of nonuniform overgrowth to caution the physician that prediction of an eventual

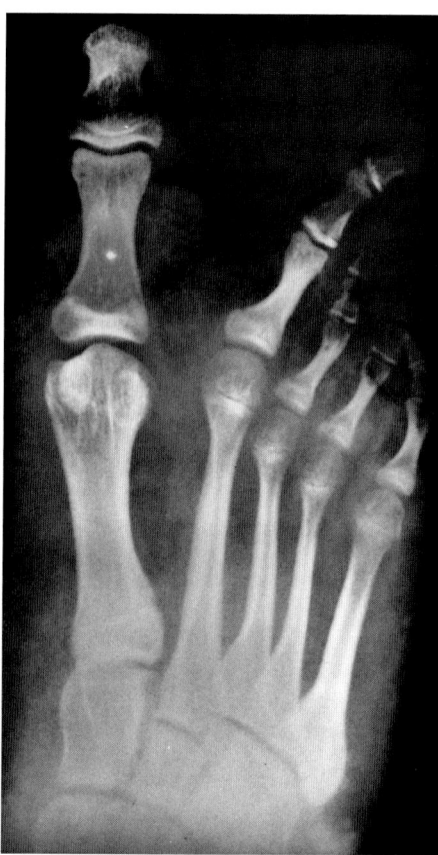

FIGURE 9-1. Standing radiograph of the foot of a 14-year-old boy with Klippel-Trenaunay syndrome. Although cutaneous hemangioma extended from the buttocks to the foot and the circumference of the involved limb was increased, limb lengths were equal. The foot malformation caused difficulty with fitting and wearing shoes. Notice the soft tissue radiodensities.

discrepancy should be done only as a rough estimate. In addition to the extremity hypertrophy, there is evidence of fundamental embryologic regulatory defects, especially distally, with 25% of patients having anomalies of fingers or toes, such as macrodactyly, syndactyly, polydactyly, and clinodactyly.[10] Scoliosis affects at least 5% of patients, although it rarely requires surgery. Systemic involvement may occur. In the central nervous system, arteriovenous malformations and cerebral and cerebellar hypertrophy have been described.[1,11] The gastrointestinal and genitourinary system may be involved, resulting in bleeding in some cases. Kasabach-Merritt syndrome may occur in severely involved patients; this is a coagulopathy caused by fibrinogen consumption and platelet sequestration. Surface bleeding from the hemangioma occurs in 25% of patients, and 15% have clinical pulmonary emboli, spontaneously or after operation.[3] Congestive heart failure may occur in patients with massive hypertrophy. Despite these complications, the life expectancy is not markedly decreased.

PATHOLOGY. Most notably, venous fibromuscular dysplasia, consisting of hypertrophied, irregular, or absent medial layers of the veins, allows dilatation. Valves are anomalous; they are absent or obstructed. Deep venous channels are usually present, and gross arteriovenous malformations are rare.[6] If fistulas are prominent, the designation of Parkes-Webber syndrome is preferred. Other tissues, such as nerve and subcutaneous tissue, may be hypertrophied.

DIFFERENTIAL DIAGNOSIS. Neurofibromatosis may produce massive hypertrophy without prominent nevi. Maffucci syndrome often includes limb length inequality with hemangiomas, but it is differentiated by the presence of intraosseous enchondromas. Beckwith-Wiedemann syndrome involves localized overgrowth but also includes aniridia, macroglossia, and Wilms tumor. Proteus syndrome is a more severe disorder involving virtually all the features of Klippel-Trenaunay, but it also includes soft tissue tumors, pigmented skin lesions, and thickened palms and soles.[4] The term congenital soft tissue dysplasia has been applied to a group of disorders, including this syndrome, neurofibromatosis, and Klippel-Trenaunay syndrome.[12] Parkes-Webber syndrome includes hemangioma with significant arteriovenous fistula.

IMAGING. Venography should be done if major limb surgery is planned to detect any significant venous anomalies. Arteriography may be helpful in planning for hemipelvectomy or hip disarticulation to map major vessels and anticipate significant bleeding.[14]

TREATMENT. Surgery has a limited role in this condition and should be done only for disabling problems and when the benefit is fairly predictable.[8] Instead, initial therapy should consist of compression. Intermittent pneumatic compression should be applied at night, using a custom-fitted garment and a home pump, inflated every 90 seconds to a pressure midway between diastolic and systolic.[13] Just before arising, a Jobst compression garment is applied and worn throughout the day. If this regimen is used properly, rather dramatic improvement has resulted in some cases, including resolution of lymphedema and a marked decrease in limb girth, resolution of cardiac overload and dependent syncope, and marked improvement in function. Consultation with a vascular surgeon may be beneficial for most of these patients.

Surgery is beneficial in selected situations, including cardiac failure from shunting, not responding to compressive therapy, rapid enlargement in limb size, encroachment of internal hemangiomas on vital structures, coagulopathy, reconstruction of selected cases of syndactyly or polydactyly, and for severely disfiguring, dysfunctional limbs for which reconstruction is not an option and amputation may provide a more functional limb. If amputation is indicated, it may be possible in some cases to amputate more distally than the soft tissues would predict, because the vascular hypertrophy in the residual limb may partially involute after removal of the abnormal segment. Occasionally, a proximal limb disarticulation is needed in neonates as a lifesaving procedure. For patients in this age group, hypothermia and total circulatory arrest for up to 60 minutes has been successful as an adjunct to minimize blood loss.[9]

Certain procedures have low success rates. Surgery to debulk the extremities has usually resulted in recurrence or minimal improvement. Varicose vein ligation may provide relief of local symptoms, but the varicosities often recur, and ligation should be avoided if the deep venous system is not patent. Epiphyseodesis usually does not have a role because growth patterns are unpredictable, and the procedure does not decrease width of involved extremities.

If surgery is planned, the involved skin should be protected, and the increased risk of deep thrombosis borne in mind.

Other Conditions Associated With Hemangiomas

Hemangiomas occur in different forms, corresponding to different abnormalities in the embryologic stages of vascular development.[16,18] They may be solitary or may be the organizing features of various syndromes.[17]

Capillary or strawberry hemangiomas are the most common variety. They are dermal-epidermal malformations. They have small capillary lumens lined by large endothelial cells. Although red, they blanch poorly. These hemangiomas occur in 1 of 200 children; 95% of the lesions involute spontaneously by 5 years of age.[21] If enlargement occurs, compression therapy may be started, and prednisone has been used successfully in resistant cases.

Port wine stains are intradermal hemangiomas. They are usually bluish and do not blanch well. Sturge-Weber, painful neuronevus, and Klippel-Trenaunay syndromes are characterized by these stains.

Verrucous hemangiomas are raised, large hemangiomas of unknown origin. They are treated by excision if bothersome.

Cavernous hemangiomas usually involve the deep subcutaneous or muscle layers and represent the most common hemangiomas presenting as masses. These are large, bluish, arteriovenous lakes with slow blood flow. They do not involute spontaneously. Often, their presence is signaled radiographically by phleboliths: large, round stones that form in the vessel lumen. Some venogram results may be negative for cavernous hemangiomas if the flow in them is slow.[19] Solitary lesions are discussed in Chapter 13. Surgery should be limited to patient conditions with severe pain or deformity caused by the hemangioma; the lesion tends to recur after surgery because the involvement of the muscle is extensive and difficult to discern. The wider the resection, the less likely is recurrence.

The options for imaging vascular lesions include plain films, which show abnormalities in most cases of deep hemangiomas, including phleboliths and enlargement or distortion of soft tissue planes.[14,17] Ultrasound and computed tomography (CT) scans demonstrate similar findings but do not add significant new information to the plain films. They may be used to direct aspiration or needle biopsy if a limited specimen is useful. Magnetic resonance imaging (MRI) adds significant anatomic detail. Hemangiomas produce a very high T2 signal, presumably because of the pooling of blood with low flow. The signal is nonuniform because of the fibrous and fatty septae within the hemangioma. Angiography or venography are recommended only if surgery is planned and an arteriovenous fistula is suspected. MRI is proving to be a noninvasive way to determine the extent of deep hemangiomas and differentiate the vascular elements from surrounding tissues. However, MRI cannot differentiate feeding arteries from veins, and angiography is the only way to obtain this information.

Other syndromes are highlighted by hemangiomas (Table 9-1).[15] The blue rubber bleb nevus syndrome has a sporadic inheritance pattern.[17,20] Multiple cavernous hemangiomas, or the nevi, are usually present at birth and appear as bluish, raised, compressible, blanching nodules on the skin. They may also appear on other viscera, especially the gastrointestinal tract. The main orthopaedic implications are interference with grip if the nevi occur on the hands and leg length inequality, which is usually not severe enough to require surgical treatment, unlike some other hemangioma syndromes. Hemangiomas sometimes occur in joints and cause decreased range of motion or bleeds. There is also a slightly increased risk of malignant transformation in multiple organ systems.

Sturge-Weber syndrome is a nonhereditary condition characterized by a port wine stain located in the distribution of the trigeminal nerve.[17] There may be other hemangiomas in other areas of the body, but they are inconstant. The hemangiomas are nonprogressive. The most important feature of this condition is the possibility of unseen hemangiomas of the arachnoid and pial coverings of the brain. These may lead to seizures, cerebrovascular accidents, and paresis. This diagnosis should be kept in mind for patients

TABLE 9-1   Associations of Hemangiomas in Children

SYNDROME	TYPE AND LOCATION	CLINICAL PROBLEMS	ORTHOPAEDIC CONCERNS	MODE OF INHERITANCE
Hemangiomas on Limbs				
Klippel-Trenaunay	Port wine stain anywhere, arteriovenous malformations in the extremities	Varicose veins, cardiac overload	Limb hypertrophy	
Blue rubber bleb nevus	Cavernous, scattered over skin, in gastrointestinal and musculoskeletal systems	Gastrointestinal bleeding	Limb hypertrophy, internal derangement of joints	Autosomal dominant
Maffucci	Cavernous; in the subcutaneous tissues	Malignant tumors	Enchondroma with skeletal deformity, overgrowth, and sarcoma	
Sturge-Weber	Port wine stain on face, hemangioma on brain	Seizures, mental retardation, glaucoma	Hemiplegia, hemiatrophy (neurogenic)	
Central Hemangiomas With Indirect Effects on Skeleton				
Osler-Weber-Rendu (hereditary hemorrhagic telangiectasia)	Telangiectasia on the lips, tongue, mucous membranes, gastrointestinal and genitourinary systems, and the skin	Bleeding from all sites, anemia, pulmonary arteriovenous malformations	Skeletal hemangioma (hands, wrist, axial skeleton)	Autosomal dominant
Kasabach-Merritt	Solitary or multiple cavernous hemangiomas on trunk or extremities	Thrombocytopenia and consumption coagulopathy	Usually none	
Ataxia-telangiectasia (Louis-Bar)	Telangiectasia on conjunctivae, face, neck, and arms	Progressive ataxia, sinus and pulmonary infections, lymphomas	Mimics Friedreich ataxia	Autosomal dominant

Adapted from Goldberg MJ. The dysmorphic child. New York: Raven Press, 1989:63. Permission requested.

suspected of having cerebral palsy, because the hemangiomas may cause a hemiplegia.

Von Hippel-Lindau disease may involve central nervous system dysfunction. It is heralded by hemangiomas in the retina and the cerebellum; visual loss may ensue.

Osler-Weber-Rendu is an eponym describing multiple hereditary telangiectasias of the mucous membranes, especially the mouth, nose, and lips. Arteriovenous fistulas may occur in the gastrointestinal tract or lungs. All of these lesions have a risk of ulceration and bleeding.

Ataxia-telangiectasia is an autosomal recessive condition in which the telangiectasias are primarily on the upper part of the body: the face, neck, arms, and conjunctivae. Ataxia increases with time, and contractures, especially for the foot, may develop.

Maffuci syndrome is characterized by cavernous hemangiomas in the subcutaneous tissues, along with multiple enchondromas. There is no consistent genetic basis.[17] The hemangiomas are present at birth in only 25% of patients; in the remainder, the lesions become evident by 5 years of age. The clinical appearance is of a blue discoloration on the skin. X-ray films may show calcified thrombi in addition to the enchondromas. The skeletal manifestations include short stature, limb length inequality, angular deformities, and scoliosis. The patient's risk potential for malignant transformation is 30%; this may include the vascular lesions undergoing transformations to angiosarcoma or fibrosarcoma.

Lymphangioma

Lymphangiomas may affect any area of the body, although they are most commonly seen in central areas. Although usually falling within the province of the general pediatric surgeon, a lymphangioma may first be noticed as a mass of unknown origin in a limb or as a cause of osteolysis or nerve compression. Most are problems of youth.

The four types are capillary lymphangiomas, cavernous lymphangiomas, cystic lymphangiomas, and lymphangiohemangiomas.[31] They are thought to arise from anomalies in development of the lymphatic system. Capillary lymphangiomas present as superficial, vesicular structures. Cavernous lymphangiomas have superficial and deep components. The treatment of these two types is complete excision if clinically indicated. Cystic lymphangiomas include the well-known cystic hygromas. Although three quarters of these cases involve the neck, other sites of orthopaedic importance include the retroperitoneum, pelvis, groin and axilla.[22,24] Although they are benign, they are locally aggressive and may compress or invade adjacent structures (Fig. 9-2).

Diagnosis may be aided by transillumination, ultrasound, CT, or MRI. Lymphangiomas tend to have a characteristic MRI appearance, with a heterogenous low signal on T1-weighted images, similar to that of muscle, but a very high T2-weighted signal, greater than that of fat.[30] Other congenital anomalies may affect the patient with lymphangioma.

A small percentage of lymphangiomas may regress spontaneously. In the others, if clinically troublesome, meticulous excision should be done. Radical procedures, with removal of important adjacent structures, are not indicated to alter the course of the disease.

Lymphedema may occur at various ages. If present in childhood, it is called Milroy disease, a congenital lymphedema, which is autosomal dominant. Cases with onset slightly later in the first or in the second decade are called Meige disease and have the same inheritance pattern. Lymphedema is also seen as part of Turner syndrome and Noonan syndrome (i.e., Turner phenotype with normal appearing chromosomes and mental retardation). Treatment in all of these cases is conservative: elevation when possible and compression with a Jobst stocking or intermittent pneumatic compression.[31]

Osseous lymphangiomas may include solitary intraosseous or more extensive forms. Solitary intraosseous lymphangiomas are rare. They are lytic and well demarcated but variably circumscribed. The appearance resembles a simple cyst, but involvement within bone is more extensive. Curettage and bone graft has been reported with success.[27]

Gorham disease (i.e., massive osteolysis) has also been called disappearing bone disease.[26] This is a lymphohemangiomatous dysplasia with a wide spectrum that may include significant morbidity. The onset is usually between the ages 10 and 30 years. Inheritance is uncertain. It may involve any area of the skeleton but prefers the shoulder and pelvic girdles, especially the clavicles, ribs, ilia, and spine.[28] It may present as dull, aching weakness in involved segments, with increasing deformity, or with pathologic fracture. Soft tissue fibrosis may be detected. Patients with lesions extending outside of bone have a high mortality rate, approaching 50% from chylothorax, chylopericardium, chyloperitoneum, and cachexia.[22,25]

RADIOGRAPHIC FINDINGS. The radiographic findings of lymphangioma include an expanding lytic area in the cortex or the medulla, progressing to frank distortion and dissolution of bone (Fig. 9-3); there is no sclerosis. If a pathologic fracture occurs, the bony lesion may be overlooked initially if the lysis is minimal. Unlike normal fracture healing, the bone ends eventually become tapered, and there is no evidence of new callus forming. The differential diagnosis includes other rare causes of idiopathic osteolysis, including hereditary multicentric osteolysis (i.e., carpotarsal type), nonhereditary multicentric osteolysis with nephropathy, and others.

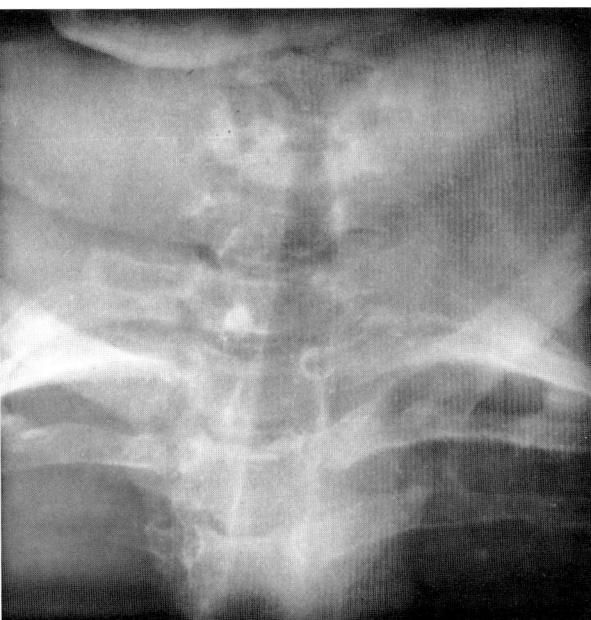

FIGURE 9-2. Lymphangioma of the neck in a 15-year-old boy led to cervical osteolysis and eventual death from respiratory obstruction. Diffuse resorption of the lower four cervical vertebrae and loss of the cortical margins cause blurred appearance. The overlying neck soft tissue folds are prominent because of enlargement by lymphangioma.

HISTOPATHOLOGY. Histologic studies show elements of lymphangioma and hemangioma in most cases. There are capillary and sinusoidal vessels, but lymphangioma elements prevail. The bone shows extensive osteoclastic activity. The cause is unclear, but

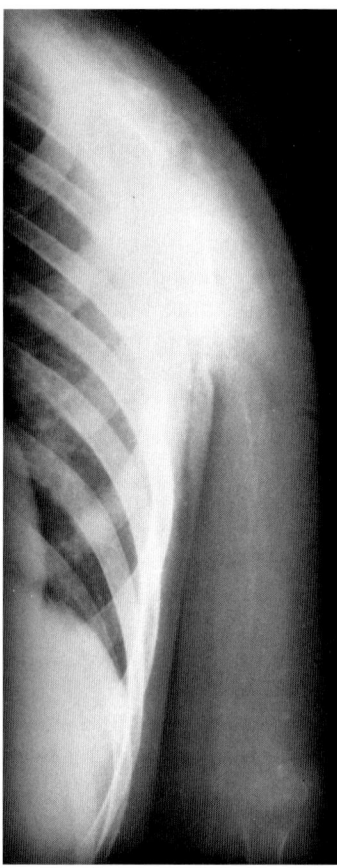

FIGURE 9-3. Gorham disease, with osteolysis of the entire humerus of a 16-year-old patient. No other areas of the skeleton were involved.

perivascular cells of the lesion show the characteristics of osteoclast precursors.[23]

TREATMENT. No treatment is consistently successful. Chemotherapy and irradiation are not recommended. Some cases, especially those without significant involvement of chest or abdominal cavities, stabilize spontaneously, although return of the "vanished" bone does not occur. Amputation may be effective in limiting spread and improving function in selected cases.[28] Success has also been reported with resection and bone grafting for limited lesions, and in one extensive case of proximal femoral involvement, a free vascularized fibular graft from distal femur to pelvis was successful.[29] Resection and limb salvage by prosthetic reconstruction may also be successful.

Hemihypertrophy and Hemihypotrophy

Orthopaedic surgeons frequently are called on to assess persons with differences in limb size. This may be a localized disorder of growth, or it may be part of a broader syndrome. This section discusses the diagnostic and therapeutic considerations. Further elaboration of certain syndromes may be found in Chapter 8, and an advanced discussion of prediction and treatment of lower limb length inequality is contained in Chapter 27.

DIFFERENTIAL DIAGNOSIS. Studies have shown that 95% of the population have a limb length discrepancy of less than 1.1 cm between sides.[38] Hemihypertrophy or hemihypotrophy has been arbitrarily defined to consist of a growth discrepancy of more than 5%.[44] This may include differences in the circumference and length. In many of the conditions discussed subsequently, there are variable patterns of involvement; just one limb, an upper and lower limb on opposite sides of the body, or an entire half of the body may be affected. A basic determination must be made about whether the limb inequality represents overgrowth of the long side or undergrowth of the short side.[40] Overgrowth may be seen with normal limb tissue development, as in idiopathic hemihypertrophy (Table 9-2) and Beckwith-Wiedemann syndrome, or it may involve hemartomatous disorders, as in Klippel-Trenaunay syndrome, lymphangiomas, neurofibromatosis, or Proteus syndrome. Undergrowth may be seen with idiopathic hypotrophy, mosaicism for Turner syndrome, Russell-Silver syndrome, neurologic asymmetry (e.g., cerebral palsy, polio), or skeletal dysplasias such as multiple exostoses, enchondromas, or polyostotic fibrous dysplasia.

CLINICAL FEATURES. Differentiation of overgrowth from undergrowth is based on comparison of the limb with its expected length in proportion to the rest of the body. This may be visually obvious and straightforward for full-blown cases, or it may be difficult to discern in milder cases. The examiner may search for anomalies that herald the "abnormal" limb. Vascular malformations and associated digital malformations or macrodactyly usually signify overgrowth conditions; obvious muscle hypotrophy, focal neurologic abnormality, mental retardation, or cruciate laxity may accompany undergrowth. If no such clues are found, a graph of normative sitting heights can be used to determine the patient's trunk height percentile, and a graph of normal lengths of the tibia and femur can be used to see which side falls on a percentile that most closely matches it.[42] This exercise is usually largely academic, because it usually does not affect treatment decisions.

Idiopathic hemihypertrophy is a condition of unknown cause affecting approximately 1 per 50,000 members of the population.[32,44,48] There is no clear inheritance pattern. Although often primarily evident in just one limb, it may also affect upper and lower limbs, the trunk, the face (Fig. 9-4), and internal organs. Growth is largely proportional and linear until maturity, with physeal closure at the same time on both sides.[47] There are cases of resolution of inequality

TABLE 9-2 Differential Diagnosis of Hemihypertrophy and Hemihypotrophy

CONDITION	FEATURES	GROWTH PATTERN	TREATMENT IMPLICATION
Hypertrophy of Normal Tissues			
Idiopathic Hemihypertrophy	Increase in length and breadth of one extremity or one half of body ± renal malformation	Proportionate, linear	Monitor for increased risk of Wilms or other neoplasm
Beckwith-Weidemann syndrome	Large body size, hemihypertrophy of whole body, macroglossia, omphalocele, pancreatic hyperplasia	Irregular	Risk of Wilms or adrenal tumor
Hemartomatous Disorders			
Klippel-Trenaunay syndrome	Limb length discrepancies, hemangioma (may be on long or short side) varicosities	Often irregular, does not affect all segments equally	Prediction for epiphyseodesis inaccurate, operate for function, amputation sometimes needed, compression therapy
Lymphangioma	Limb length discrepancies, pitting edema		
Neurofibromatosis	Café-au-lait spots (>5) plus family history of subcutaneous neurofibroma, dystrophic bone changes	Irregular	
Proteus syndrome	Epidermal nevi, skin thickening, macrodactyly, subcutaneous masses	Irregular	Valgus often coexists, skeletal age delayed or disassociated
Hemi-3 syndrome	Hemihypertrophy, hemihypasthesia, hemiarexia	Hypertrophy of girth, not length	
Undergrowth of Limb			
Idiopathic hemihypotrophy	Greater dysmorphism than hemihypertrophy, congenital scoliosis, genitourinary malformation	Proportionate	Discrepancy rarely exceeds 2 cm by maturity, treatment rarely indicated
Turner/mosaic (XO/XX)	Short stature, low hairline, peripheral edema, valgus of knees or elbows	Discrepancy accelerated near puberty	Keloids common
Russell-Silver syndrome	Very short stature (<3%), small, triangular face, one limb or whole side short, developmental dysplasia of the hip, scoliosis, genitourinary anomalies common	Eventual limb length discrepancy of 1–6 cm	Skeletal age is delayed
Neurogenic (e.g., hemiplegic, polio)	Undergrowth is proportional to weakness	Proportionate, affects weakest limb segments	Lengthening rarely indicated in weak limb
Skeletal dysplasia or dyostoses	Polyostotic fibrous dysplasia, multiple exostoses, multiple enchondromas		

in early childhood or disproportionate exaggeration of the discrepancy during puberty, but these are unusual.[45] The total lower extremity discrepancy rarely exceeds 5 cm by maturity.[41,44] Two thirds of patients in most series have some type of surgery for limb length equalization.[35] The tibia is overgrown as much as or slightly more than the femur.[44] Limb girth is also increased, but it is usually not as strikingly as in the hamartomatous disorders.

Mental capacities are usually normal, unlike those

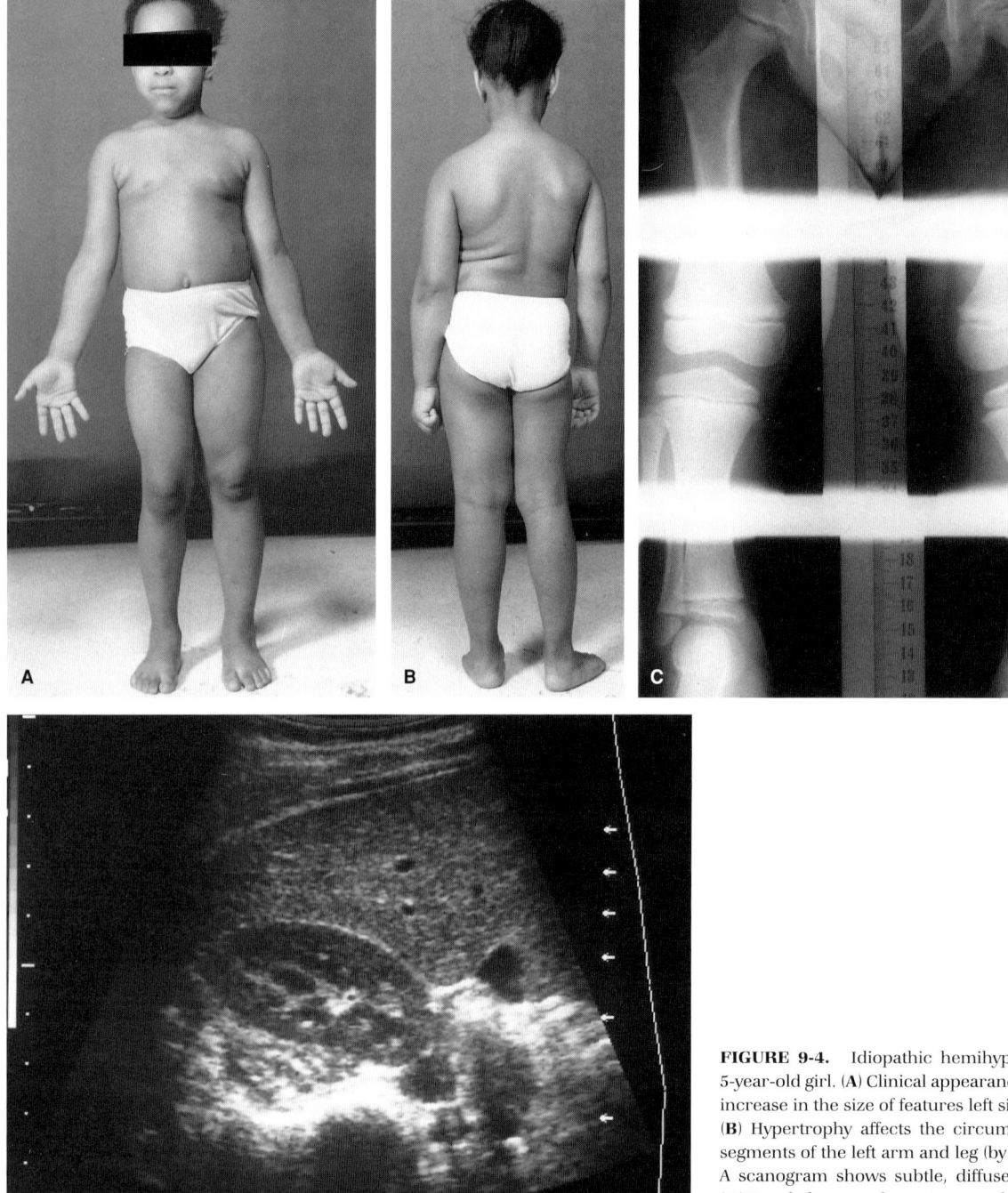

FIGURE 9-4. Idiopathic hemihypertrophy in a 5-year-old girl. (**A**) Clinical appearance, with a mild increase in the size of features left side of the face. (**B**) Hypertrophy affects the circumference of all segments of the left arm and leg (by 1 to 2 cm). (**C**) A scanogram shows subtle, diffuse hypertrophy. (**D**) Renal ultrasound scan is normal. It was recommended for surveillance for Wilms tumor.

of patients with idiopathic hemihypotrophy and contrary to earlier reports.[32] However, there is an increased frequency of renal malformations, such as medullary sponge kidney. The most important feature of this syndrome is its association with intraabdominal neoplasms, such as Wilms tumor, which occurs in about 2% of these patients. These renal abnormalities may be ipsilateral or contralateral to the hemihypertrophied limb, and the relative timing of the findings varies. One case report described hemihypertrophy developing 4 years after successful treatment of Wilms tumor.[39] Because of this variability in timing and the rather low frequency of Wilms tumor, there is controversy about whether and when to perform routine tumor screening.[37] The National Wilms Tumor Study Group suggests that there is no evidence that routine diagnostic imaging is better than physical examinations. Nevertheless, until this issue is better studied, it is common orthopaedic practice to obtain an ultrasound scan of the abdomen at the diagnosis of hemihypertrophy and every 6 to 12 months thereafter until the patient is 5 years of age; more than 90% of associated Wilms tumors occur before this age. Cutaneous birthmarks may be seen in these patients.[38] The chance of scoliosis also is increased,[34] even after leg length equalization, and may be the result of vertebral body asymmetry. Uncommon skeletal anomalies are syndactyly, lobster-claw hand, developmental dysplasia of the hip, and clubfoot.[45]

Beckwith-Wiedemann syndrome is slightly more common than idiopathic hemihypertrophy. This is a syndrome of total body overgrowth with superimposed hemihypertrophy. It usually is discovered at birth with omphalocele, macroglossia, and pancreatic islet cell hyperplasia. The risk of Wilms tumor in this condition is slightly higher than in idiopathic hemihypertrophy, raising the possibility of fundamental similarities between the two. This is even more intriguing, because there have been cases of Beckwith-Wiedemann syndrome, aniridia, and Wilms tumor with abnormalities of chromosome 11. Nevertheless, a genetic basis for most cases has not been established.

Hamartomatous disorders with limb length inequality include neurofibromatosis, Proteus syndrome, Klippel-Trenaunay syndrome, and lymphangiomas.[36,96]

A rare disorder, known as the hemi-3 syndrome, may be associated with hemihypertrophy, mostly of limb width.[43] Its other features include hemihypesthesia, hemiareflexia, and scoliosis. It appears to be a neural crest disorder.

Hemihypotrophy is more likely to be associated with diffuse skeletal abnormalities than is hemihypertrophy.[32] The term hypotrophy is preferred to atrophy, because there is decreased development instead of a loss of previous normal tissue bulk.

Idiopathic hemihypotrophy appears to be about one half as frequent as idiopathic hemihypertrophy.[32] These patients, however, have a higher incidence of other dysmorphic features, including cleft palate and facial malformations, congenital scoliosis, and genitourinary malformations. Mental retardation is common, but Wilms tumor is not associated with the condition.[38] Rarely does this syndrome require orthopaedic treatment, because in most cases, the discrepancy is less than 2.5 cm.

Russell-Silver syndrome has some features in common with idiopathic hemihypotrophy, but it is characterized by overall short stature, with most patients never exceeding a height of 152 cm (5 ft). These patients have a characteristic small, triangular face and renal and genital malformations.[38] Scoliosis is common and may be congenital or idiopathic-like. The limb hypotrophy is usually minimal, but as much as 5 cm has been reported.

Patients who are mosaic for the Turner syndrome (XO/XX) may have hemihypotrophy, as may patients who have multiple enchondromas or osteochondromas, with mean discrepancies of 9 and 4 cm, respectively, for those with patients with limb length inequality. Neurogenic inequalities vary in proportion to the asymmetry of the neurologic involvement, rarely exceeding 2.5 cm in the lower extremities in cerebral palsy or 6 cm in polio patients.[47] In assessing patients with localized overgrowth or undergrowth, it should not be assumed that the growth alteration is proportional. Shapiro[47] described five patterns of limb length discrepancy, and even within a given diagnosis, multiple patterns may be seen. Periodic assessment should be done, if possible, during growth to determine the pattern being followed. Predictions are then more accurate. If significant joint contractures are present, plain radiographs or scans may not measure limb length accurately, and CT scans may be needed. For treatment of significant upper extremity inequalities, normative growth data is also available.[33]

Macrodactyly

Also known as localized gigantism, macrodactyly involves primary hyperplasia of all tissue elements of a single or several adjacent rays or digits of the hand or foot. Two types exist: the more common static type, in which the proportion of enlargement remains the same, and the progressive type, in which this proportion or ratio increases with time.[48]

Macrodactyly most commonly occurs as an isolated condition, but it may also occur in patients with neurofibromatosis, lymphedema, hemangiomas, or Proteus syndrome.[50] It may not be possible in infancy to completely rule out these conditions, because cafe-au-lait spots and hemangiomas may appear later.

CLINICAL FEATURES. Most cases of macrodactyly are evident from birth, although occasionally the dynamic type may not become apparent until later in infancy, when relentless enlargement occurs (Fig. 9-5). The upper extremities are more commonly affected than lower extremities. Unilateral involvement occurs in 95% of cases, although in 67% of patients, more than one digit on the involved side is affected. The second ray is the most commonly enlarged, followed in descending frequency by the third, first, fourth, and fifth rays. Syndactyly may coexist. Usually, the palmar or plantar surface is more hypertrophied than the dorsal, causing a hyperextended posture to develop.[54] If two adjacent digits are affected, they grow apart from each other. In static macrodactyly, the involved digits are about one and one-half times the normal length and width. In the dynamic type, even more striking enlargement may occur. The bone age is advanced in the involved phalanges in either type. To a lesser degree, the metacarpals or metatarsals are also enlarged, widening the hand or foot. The width

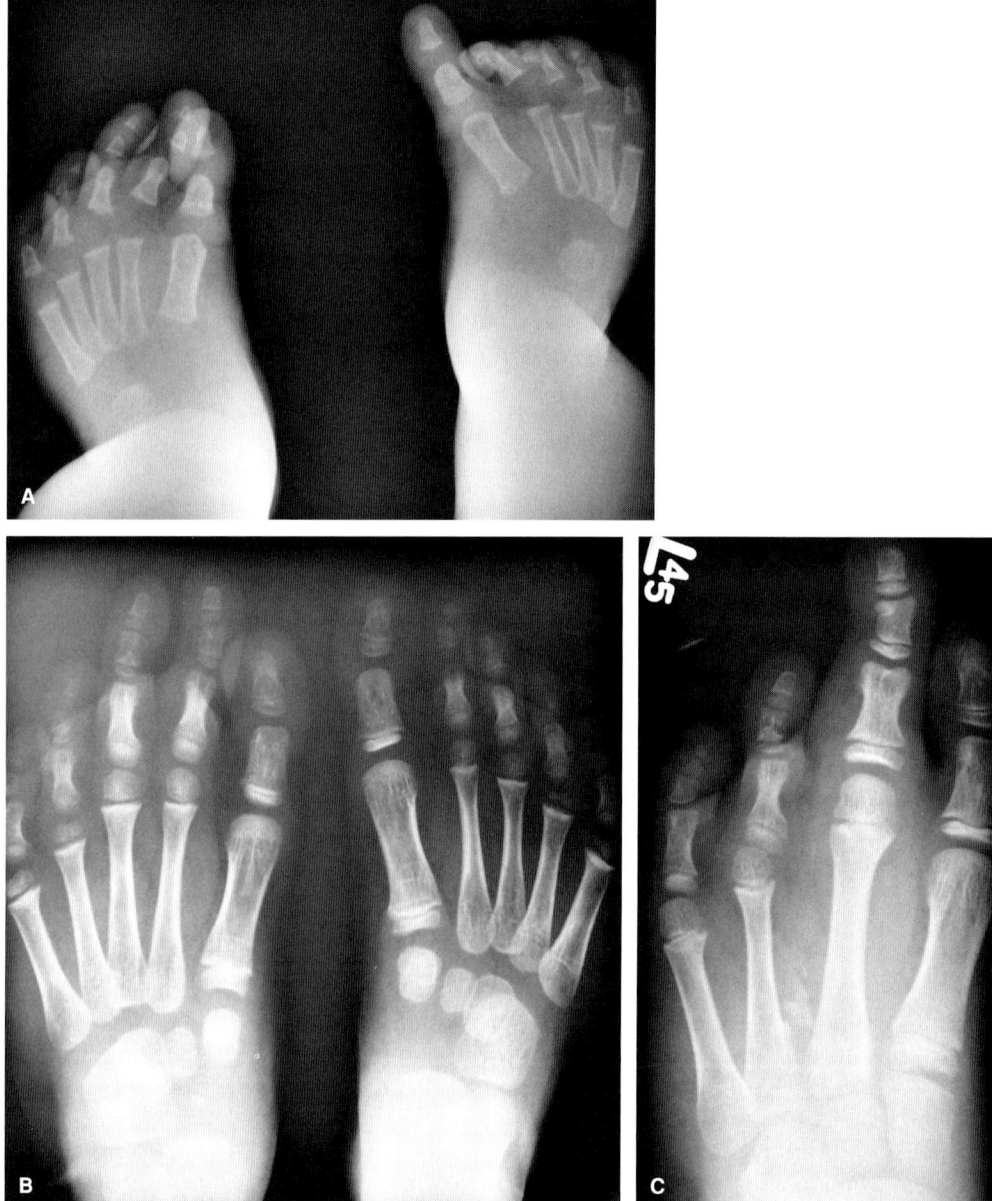

FIGURE 9-5. Progressive macrodactyly of the left foot. (**A**) At 1 year of age, the typical mild enlargement of the second and third rays is greatest distally. (**B**) More noticeable overgrowth is present at 3 years of age; notice the increased foot width. (**C**) Third ray amputation was performed at 5 years of age and the foot narrowed to match the contralateral side. Epiphyseodesis of all phalanges was later performed to equalize their lengths.

of the same-side forearm, leg, thigh, or arm may also be subtly increased.[51] Not long after skeletal maturity, interphalangeal joint stiffness and degenerative changes may supervene prematurely, even in untreated cases.

PATHOLOGY. All tissue types are enlarged in the involved digit. Fibrofatty proliferation accounts for the greatest bulk.[51] Vessels, bone, and dermis are also enlarged, and the changes are greatest distally. In one case, marked proliferation of the basal layer of the periosteum was seen.[46] Pathologic changes are greatest in the digital nerves, with thick epineurium, fatty infiltration, and hypertrophied endoneurial tissue.[52] This has led some experts to speculate that neural abnormalities are primary in this condition, but the theory remains unproven. The cause is still unknown. Occult neurofibromatosis was once thought to be the cause, but long-term follow-up studies, including one of 26 years, have failed to reveal development of other features of neurofibromatosis besides the macrodactyly itself.[49] Because the problem is acral and central in the limb, it may be related to abnormalities in growth factors found in the apical ridge.

TREATMENT. Treatment varies with the degree of enlargement. Treatment should always be aimed toward creating a functional foot or hand, because a perfect cosmetic result is almost never possible. In moderate cases, if length is not a problem, soft tissue wedge-debulking procedures may be done, first on one side and then on the other at least 3 months later. Epiphyseodesis may effectively stop the growth in length, especially if done before 8 years of age, and it must be done on all of the involved segments.[52] If the patient is seen at an older age, bone-shortening procedures may be needed. Neither of these procedures, however, addresses or prevents the increase in width, which occurs at the metacarpal-tarsal level and the digital level. This is one disorder in which the hand is less of a problem than the foot, because accommodating even a small excess of width into a shoe may be difficult. Soft tissue debulking must be combined with bone procedures and often must be repeated. Amputation at the metatarsophalangeal or metacarpophalangeal joint may be done if the problem is one of length more than width. Close observation for hallux valgus should follow, although this may not develop.[49] An interesting question is whether early, ablative procedures decrease the tendency toward more proximal enlargement, which is sometimes noticed later. There is no evidence that this is the case.

Ray resection is a more definitive solution to the multiple dimensions of enlargement often encountered. One or two rays may be taken, although the first ray of the foot should not be amputated in isolation because of its unique function in balance and weight bearing. Ray resection prevents crossover of the adjacent digits and eliminates "gap" formation and soft tissue enlargement. A three-ray foot is the minimum that is functionally serviceable. In the foot, more extensive involvement would necessitate midfoot or Syme disarticulation, depending on the extent of overgrowth.

As the patient matures, a subtle increase in width may be seen in all levels of the limb. Herring reported a case of macrodactyly with width increase in the absence of any overall limb length discrepancy.[53] The family should be counseled from the first visit that this condition is complex and involves multiple tissues and levels. They need to know that multiple procedures may be necessary and that early appropriate "aggressive" resections involving all affected dimensions may decrease the total number of surgeries required. For example, as soon as it becomes apparent that length and width may be excessive, resection of one or several rays, with shortening or epiphyseodesis of an adjacent ray, may be appropriate. Often, several consultations with one or different surgeons may be necessary to help families achieve this realization.

Congenital Constriction Band Syndrome

This condition is known by several different names: Streeter dysplasia, amniotic band syndrome, and pseudoainhum. It has not been conclusively proven that the condition is caused by amniotic bands; the term "congenital constriction band syndrome" is preferred because it refers only to the physical findings of bands. The three major components of this syndrome are circumferential transverse bands, acrosyndactyly, and terminal amputations (Fig. 9-6), although all three are not required for the diagnosis.[56,62,66] The other, more varied components that may also occur are discussed subsequently.

Congenital constriction band syndrome is the most common cause of terminal congenital malformation of a limb. Its incidence is approximately 1 per 10,0000 live births.[64] There is no gender difference in incidence, and no evidence of hereditary transmission. In two reported sets of involved twins, there were marked variations in the extent and locations of involvement.[67,68]

CLINICAL FEATURES. Patterson[64] reported four types of involvement in his classification: simple constriction ring, constriction ring with vascular-lymphatic obstruction, constriction ring with syndactyly, and intrauterine amputation.[63] In all types, involvement of the upper limbs is twice as common as that of the lower limbs. The greatest involvement is seen in the most distal (acral) parts of the limbs, especially distal to the metacarpophalangeal joints. The longest fingers (digits 2–4) are most often affected, perhaps because the added length increases the chance of entanglement in a band. An average of three limbs per patient are involved. In the infant, circulatory compromise may be seen at birth if the bands are deep (Fig. 9-7). Alternatively, compromise may develop with time and growth if the band does not accommodate limb growth.

Associated anomalies are seen in one half of the cases overall. Amputations are the most common component of the syndrome. These tend to be transverse terminal amputations at various levels in different digits. Syndactyly is seen in 50% of patients and has a characteristic appearance known as fenestrated syndactyly. This refers to the clefts between the digits proximal and distal to the syndactyly. Polydactyly is also seen in some patients with constriction bands and must be related to abnormalities early in limb development.[60] Nail deformities are often seen and usually signal an underlying bony syndactyly. The in-

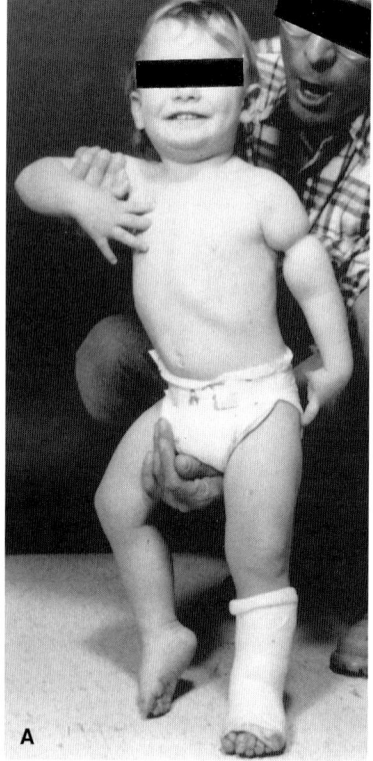
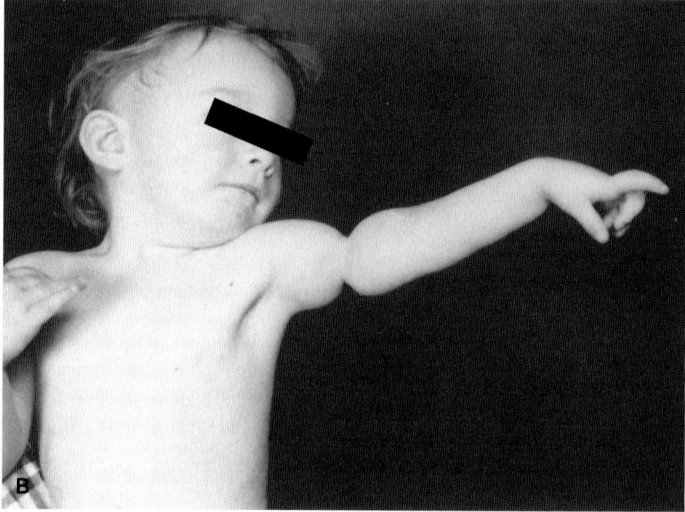

FIGURE 9-6. An infant with congenital constriction band syndrome illustrates the four features of his condition: a deep band in the left proximal humerus, partial amputation of the right long finger distal phalanx, distal paresis of the radial and median nerves, and an idiopathic clubfoot.

volved digits are usually shorter than normal (i.e., brachydactyly or brachysyndactyly).

Clubfoot is seen in 23% of patients. The clubfoot cases are about evenly split between paralytic and nonparalytic types. The paralytic type occurs because of deep compression of the peroneal nerve below the fibular head, with or without vascular involvement. Several of these cases have had surgical confirmation

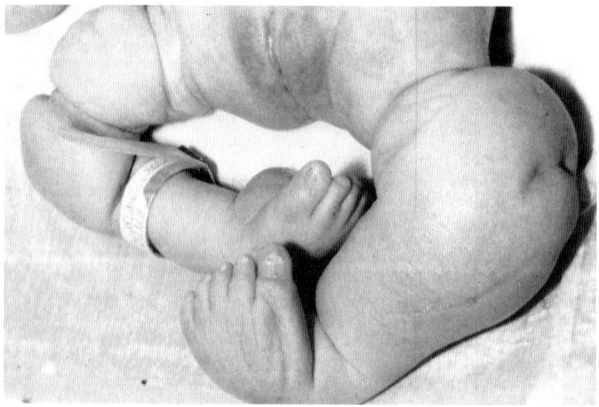

FIGURE 9-7. Multiple constriction bands caused paralytic clubfeet and distal venous obstruction on one side.

and release of the nerve lesion, usually an axonotmesis or neurotmesis under the band. These patients eventually require tendon transfers to restore muscle balance. Other patients with clubfeet have no constriction bands proximally in the limb.[56] In these patients, the clubfoot is presumed to result from temporary oligohydramnios, leakage of fluid leading to uterine crowding and pressure and possible stretching of the peroneal nerve. Because disorders in this group respond to normal treatment methods, they are classified as idiopathic-like clubfeet.

Cranial and facial malformations, especially cleft palate, may coexist with constriction bands in approximately 5% of patients. These include some obvious band-induced clefts and more embryologically fundamental malformations. Leg length inequality of more than 2.5 cm has been found in one quarter of patients who have constriction bands and therefore should be searched for in the ongoing evaluation of these patients, even after their deformities and bands have been dealt with.[58] Long bone diaphyseal malformations include anterolateral tibial bowing and pseudarthrosis of tibia and of the forearm. The pseudoarthroses usually heal after simple fixation and bone grafting, unlike the problems usually seen in neurofibromatosis or isolated congenital pseudarthrosis. No natural history is available regarding the cases of anterolateral bowing; these have been treated satisfactorily with osteotomy.

ETIOLOGIC THEORIES. There are two basic theories about the cause of this syndrome: band formation as a result of factors intrinsic to the embryo or fetus (i.e., developmental aberration or infarcts) or constriction from factors external to the embryo, such as amniotic bands.

The first point of view had been held by Streeter in his 1930 paper.[65] He thought that the features of the syndrome were a result of a germ plasm defect, an abnormality of the apical ectodermal ridge. Focal necrosis may result in the formation of annular scars in a limb. The thumb and index finger, which are least frequently involved with this syndrome, have separate digital vessels and theoretically would be least susceptible to necrosis from emboli. Several cases of constriction syndrome have been documented by ultrasound to have occurred in the absence of amniotic bands in fetuses which were at risk for embolic events.[67] One of these was a neonate who developed constriction bands after in utero death of a co-twin, which may have produced emboli through placental anastomoses. Another was in a neonate who had other evidence of placental emboli transmitted through the umbilical vein.

The second point of view, causation by external constriction, is supported by the finding of actual bands in some patients at the time of delivery and by the experimental production of limb defects and clubfoot after amniocentesis in animals. Because of the variability of the syndrome, it is possible that intrinsic and extrinsic factors may play a role in causation.

The differential diagnosis is limited, but there are some interesting conditions to consider. The "Michelin tire baby syndrome" consists of multiple benign circumferential skin creases. This is an autosomal dominant condition that has been traced through as many as four generations in one family. These creases are present from birth, disappear by 5 years of age, and predominantly involve the extremities.[57] Hair thread constriction may occur in infants, usually younger than 2 years of age, and cause circulatory compromise.[55] Strands of hair may become wrapped around fingers and toes and become wrapped tightly enough that distal swelling occurs. At that time, it may be difficult to see the hair causing the problem to differentiate it from congenital constriction bands. General anesthetic is often needed to identify and remove the offending strands.

Ainhum is a disorder characterized by ulceration at the base of the fifth toe on the plantar surface, which progresses to a circumferential constriction ring with autoamputation. It is mainly seen in Africa.[60]

TREATMENT. Constriction bands may be released by excision and multiple Z-plasties.[61] This may be done urgently, in the newborn period, if there is significant swelling and circulatory compromise. Alternatively, it may be done electively at an older age, as appearance and function dictate. In the acute phase, the surgeon should check for compartment syndrome before and after ring release. Fasciotomies should be done if compartmental pressures are elevated. A small margin of normal skin (1–2 mm) should be resected on either side of the scar to prevent recurrence. Extreme care should be taken to identify major nerves and vessels, because they may be directly under the band. These are best identified at a distance from the band. Neurolysis of underlying nerves is not recommended. The flaps of the Z-plasty should be at approximately 60-degree angles. The entire constriction ring may be revised by Z-plasty at one session, rather than staging release as two isolated procedures.[59] This is possible because the blood flow to the flaps of the Z-plasty comes from segmental myocutaneous vessels perpendicular to the skin, not crossing the constriction band itself.

Disorders Involving Bone or Joint

Progressive Diaphyseal Dysplasia

This disorder is one of the sclerosing bone dysplasias. It was first described by Camurati in 1922[69] and Engelman in 1929 and often is called by their eponyms jointly. However, it was renamed by Neuhauser in 1949, and his term, progressive diaphyseal dysplasia, is more descriptive. It is characterized by symmetrically widened, sclerotic diaphyses, with epiphyseal sparing, muscle weakness, and muscle wasting. Although it affects multiple bones throughout the skeleton, it does not usually involve all, and the extraskeletal features are limited. It is considered here under regional disorders instead of dysplasias.

CLINICAL FEATURES. This disorder is rare, with an incidence of less than 1 per 1,000,000. It is transmitted as an autosomal dominant trait, but penetrance and expressivity are variable, and there are many sporadic cases.[73] Boys are slightly more often affected than girls (3:2 ratio). Clinical presentation is usually in the first decade, with weakness, pain in the limbs, a waddling gait, an inability to run, and fatigue.[70] Stenzler[75] reported two patients who were initially diagnosed as having muscular dystrophy because of the weakness, until incidental radiographs showed diaphyseal sclerosis. On the other end of the spectrum, the diagnoses of several cases have been delayed until middle age. The best tabulation of clinical features of these rare cases reported in the literature is given by Hundley.[71] Limb musculature is asthenic to atrophic. Valgus may develop at the knees, and osteoarthrosis may be present by middle adulthood. Some enlargement of the cranial vault and frontal bossing may occur. Puberty is usually delayed, and there may be hypogonadism. The clinical severity of the disease does not correlate well with radiographic extent.[73] The progression of symptoms in a given patient varies, and in some cases, progression is spontaneously halted. Life expectancy is normal.

Laboratory studies are not very helpful. The alkaline phosphatase level may be mildly elevated in 20% of patients. There have been some reports of elevated urinary hydroxyproline excretion.[72] Electromyographic results are normal. Muscle biopsy, when performed (usually for presumptive diagnosis of myopathy), is nonspecific.

RADIOGRAPHIC FEATURES. The main feature of this disorder is diaphyseal widening and cortical thickening (Fig. 9-8).[76] The tibia is most frequently involved (approximately 90% of cases), followed by the femur and the humerus. Symmetry of involvement is the rule. Usually, the earliest radiographic abnormality is middiaphyseal sclerosis, followed by diaphyseal widening and cortical thickening (see Fig. 9-8). The medullary canal becomes narrow. The cortex may become irregular. In two-bone limb segments, such as the forearm and leg, valgus angular deformity may occur because of an overgrowth of the radius and tibia. Eventually, the skull and pelvis may display widening and sclerosis. In the spine, sclerosis affects mainly the posterior elements and posterior cortex of vertebral body. CT scans have shown that the sclerosing process may be rather focal; in some cases, it is all posterior, confined to the region of the linea aspera. Technetium 99m bone scans illustrate bone modelling activity. The scan is "hot" in multiple long bones early in the disease, when plain films show minimal to no characteristic changes. It later shows less isotope uptake or no increased uptake in the more mature or quiescent phases, when plain film changes are more established.[73,74] It may be helpful in confirming the diagnosis in the early stages, if such confirmation is needed.

PATHOLOGY. Histologic examination reveals the expected changes but is not pathognomonic. The cortex and the periosteum of the involved bones is thickened. There is evidence of increased osteoblastic and osteoclastic activity, although presumably the balance is in favor of the former. The epiphyses appear

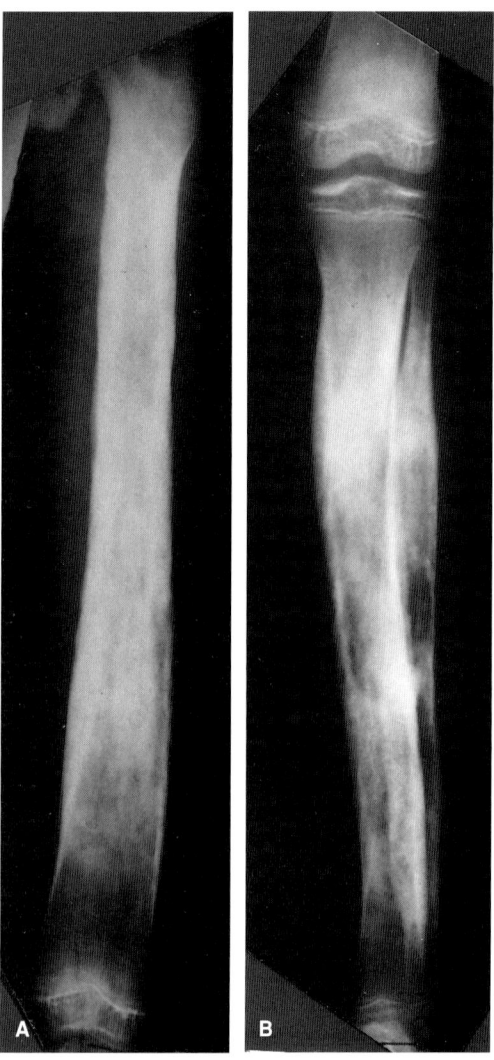

FIGURE 9-8. Progressive diaphyseal dysplasia involving (**A**) the femur and (**B**) the tibia. The physes and epiphyses are relatively normal. Contralateral involvement was similar.

relatively normal because they are products of endochondral bone formation. The marrow of the diaphyses later becomes replaced by loose mesenchymal and fibrous tissue.

ETIOLOGY. No elucidation of the basic cause of this syndrome is available. A hormonal or growth factor abnormality may account for the relative osteoblastic stimulation and the somatic abnormalities.

DIFFERENTIAL DIAGNOSIS. There are several sclerosing bone dysplasias that must be considered in the differential diagnosis. The classification of Greenspan[88] is organized according to whether the abnormality involves enchondronal bone formation as does osteopetrosis, intramembranous bone formation (as in progressive diaphyseal dysplasia), or both. Ribbing disease is a sclerosing dysplasia that has a similar radiographic appearance but affects only the lower extremities. These patients have normal muscles. The presentation is in adulthood, and it is nonprogressive. Osteopetrosis may be differentiated by its epiphyseal and diaphyseal involvement, and tendency to pathologic fracture.

A patient with Caffey disease (i.e., infantile cortical hyperostosis) presents at a much earlier age (0–8 weeks) than a progressive diaphyseal dysplasia patient, and the disease involves different bones: mandible, ribs, and clavicle. It is less symmetric and regresses after infancy.

Polyostotic fibrous dysplasia has some similarities, including widening of the diaphysis and loss of distinction between the cortex and the medullary canal but is usually less sclerotic and highly asymmetrical.

Juvenile Paget disease, sclerosing osteomyelitis, and heavy metal poisoning should also be considered. Progressive diaphyseal dysplasia should be included in the differential diagnosis of the child with a clinical picture of muscle weakness.[73]

TREATMENT. There is no specific treatment for this disease. Nonsteroidal antiinflammatory agents may alleviate symptoms. Physical therapy may provide assistive devices and streamline the activities of daily living, but it should not be expected to reverse the myopathy. Attention should be given to an appropriate and common reactive depression.

Some experience has been reported with the use of steroids, which may produce clinical and radiographic improvement. They should be reserved for the more incapacitating cases in the spectrum of progressive diaphyseal dysplasia. A loading dose of 20 mg/kg/day of prednisone, followed by a maintenance dose of 5 to 10 mg/kg/day is recommended.[75] Other researchers dispute the effectiveness of steroids for this condition.[73] Surgery is rarely needed. Clawson, however, reported the use of distal femoral extension and proximal tibial varus osteotomies to correct flexion-valgus knee deformities in one case, resulting in uneventful healing and improved function.[70]

Melorheostosis

Melorheostosis, first described in 1922, is characterized by asymmetric longitudinal hyperostotic streaks, limb pain, and soft tissue contractures.[81] Its name is derived from the Greek description of the appearances, "melos" (limb) and "rhein" (flowing, as in wax).

CLINICAL FEATURES. There is no genetic pattern of inheritance. The limbs are affected asymmetrically, with the lower extremities much more frequently involved than the upper extremities. One or multiple bones in a limb may become involved, and the process is usually progressive in proportion to the growth velocity. The usual presentation in childhood is a painless contracture before 6 years of age that is usually misdiagnosed.[79] The difference in the clinical pictures of children and adults was pointed out in 1979 by Younge and colleagues,[82] who collected the experience of the North American Shriners Hospitals to report the largest pediatric series. Significant pain does not develop until late adolescence, which is when the characteristic radiographic features become better developed. Knee flexion contracture with or without valgus is the most common joint deformity, followed by ankle, hip, and finger flexion contractures. Further flexion is also limited. The overlying skin is usually tight and shiny, and underlying tissues are fibrotic. Limb length inequality is common, with the affected limb usually but not always being the shorter, by a mean of 4 cm. Closure of the affected physis often occurs early. Shoe fitting is difficult. A slightly increased frequency of soft tissue tumors, such as lipoma and desmoid and even osteosarcoma has been reported.[80] All laboratory studies are unremarkable. Life expectancy is normal.

RADIOGRAPHIC FEATURES. The classic appearance of melorheostosis is that of flowing streaks of bone, which seem to follow dermatomes and may involve the epiphyses and even cross joints (Fig. 9-9). This appearance is somewhat different in children; the streaking is endosteal and not as well demarcated or mature as in adults. However, the same patient, at maturity, develops extraosseous changes in the same regions. The epiphysis may also develop small, dense patches resembling osteopoikilosis.

PATHOLOGY. Pathologic analysis reveals nonspecific dense areas of otherwise normal bone with normal-appearing haversian systems and thickened trabeculae. Soft tissues show dense fibrosis.

The cause of this condition has not been determined. Because the sclerosis appears to follow roughly a dermatomal distribution, it has been postulated that there may be a neurogenic origin.

The differential diagnosis includes osteomyelitis, osteopetrosis, and osteopathia striata for radiographically obvious reasons. The asymmetry, internal irregularities, and length discrepancies create a resemblance to enchondromatosis, although the latter does not have soft tissue fibrosis. Focal scleroderma may

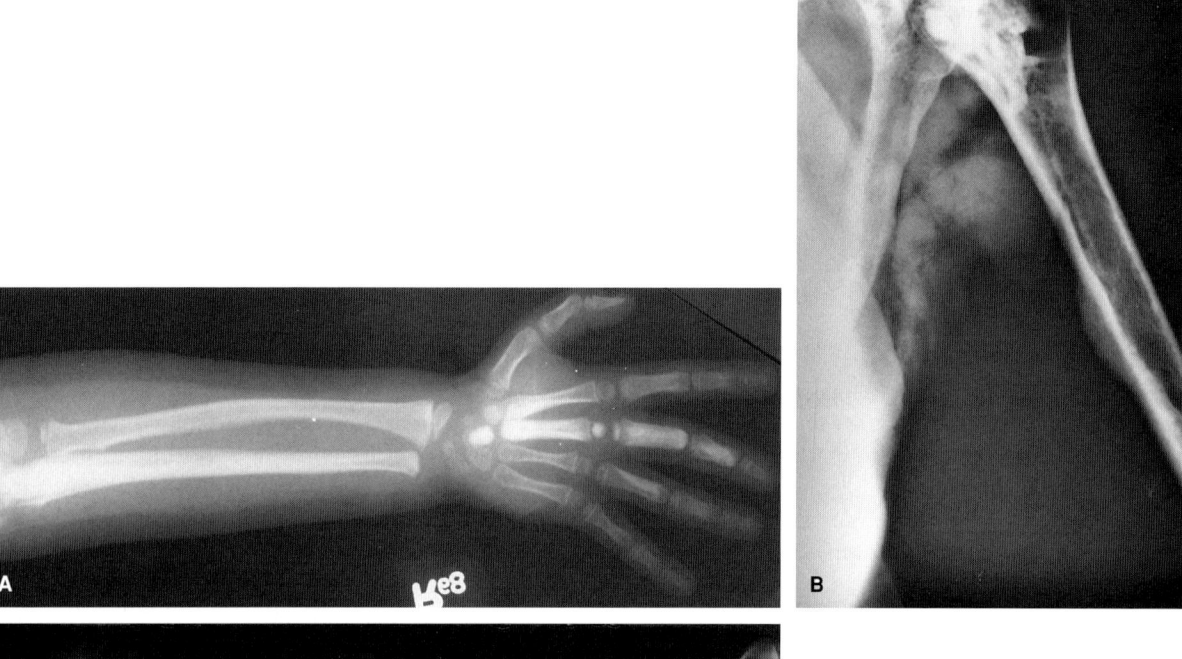

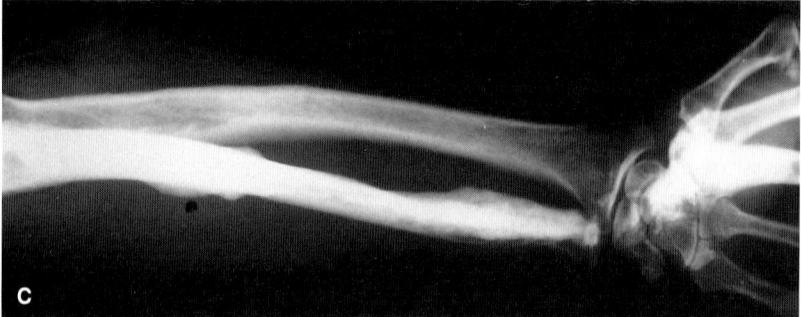

FIGURE 9-9. Melorheostosis. Longitudinal hyperostolic streaks impart the flowing-wax appearance and linear involvement in the upper extremity of (**A**) a child, and (**B, C**) an adult. The cortical thickening appears to be more endosteal in the child and more appositional and pronounced in the adult.

produce soft tissue fibrosis and contractures in children, but the bones are radiographically normal.[78]

TREATMENT. Analgesia is offered for moderate cases. Bracing may be used on affected limbs during periods of rapid growth to prevent progressive contractures. The patient should be counseled about the progressive nature of the limb deformities. Surgery does not have a high success rate for correcting contractures or length inequality, but it may be offered in extreme cases, particularly if amputation is the alternative. Contracture releases should include radical capsulotomies and tenotomies, accompanied by bony shortening if rapid intraoperative correction is desired. Traditional osteotomies and angular correction are limited by the tightness of soft tissues, nerves, and vessels. Complications such as pseudarthrosis, recurrence, or stretch-induced ischemia requiring amputation have been reported after osteotomies.[82] There is a report of successful use of Ilizarov gradual distraction methods for correction of an angular knee deformity with shortening, although the follow-up period was short.[77]

Osteopoikilosis

Osteopoikilosis, also known by the straightforward description osteopithia condensans disseminata (i.e., spotted bones), is characterized by multiple dense ovoid spots in cancellous bone.

CLINICAL FEATURES. Osteopoikilosis is a rare autosomal dominant condition, with a prevalence of approximately 1 in 10,000,000.[83] Most cases are discovered incidentally on radiographs taken for other reasons. There are no symptoms associated with the skeletal involvement. Several reports exist of concurrence of osteopoikilosis with multiple cutaneous dermatofibromas, an association called Buschke-Ollendorff syndrome, but still having few clinical implications unless the dermatofibromas are large.[86] Although there is one case report each of osteosarcoma and of chondrosarcoma developing in patients with osteopoikilosis, reliably estimating the risk of malignancy in this condition is difficult because many patients probably go undetected.

RADIOGRAPHIC FEATURES. The radiodense nodules are round to oval and 2 to 10 mm. They are located primarily in the epiphyses and metaphyses of long tubular bones, especially the carpals and tarsals; much less commonly, they develop in the diaphyses (Fig. 9-10). The ribs, clavicles, and skull rarely demonstrate lesions. The pelvis is often involved. The bones most involved are those derived from the C6–C7 and L3–L4 sclerotomes, as determined by Chigira and colleagues.[84] This finding led them to speculate about an etiologic factor in utero that expressed itself during limb and bud formation at the end of the fourth week. As the patient grows, the lesions may increase or decrease in number.

PATHOLOGIC FEATURES. The lesions consist of condensations of compact lamellar bone within the spongiosa.[85] The pathology of the dermatofibromas in Buschke-Ollendorff syndrome reveals intradermal bundles of collagen, which may be pathologically related to the bony lesions.

TREATMENT. No recommendations exist for routine surveillance of these patients. If osteopoikilosis is found incidentally, the patients can be reassured that the spots have no known clinical implications.

Osteopathia Striata

Osteopathia striata is another of the sclerosing bone dysplasias, characterized by linear striations in the cancellous bone of the metaphyseal region and sclerosis of the skull base.[87,88]

CLINICAL FEATURES. Osteopathia striata is about as rare as osteopoikilosis; its frequency is well under 1 per 1,000,000, although in view of the benign nature, many cases may not be recognized. The inheritance pattern is autosomal dominant. No clinical symptoms are associated with the disorder. Several

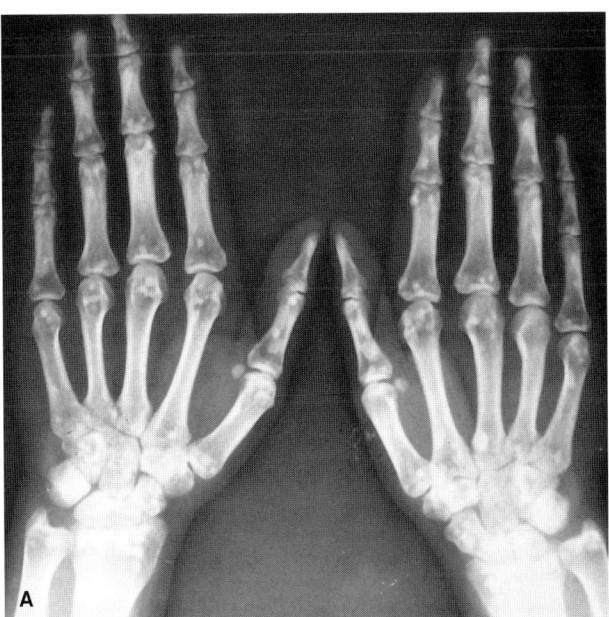
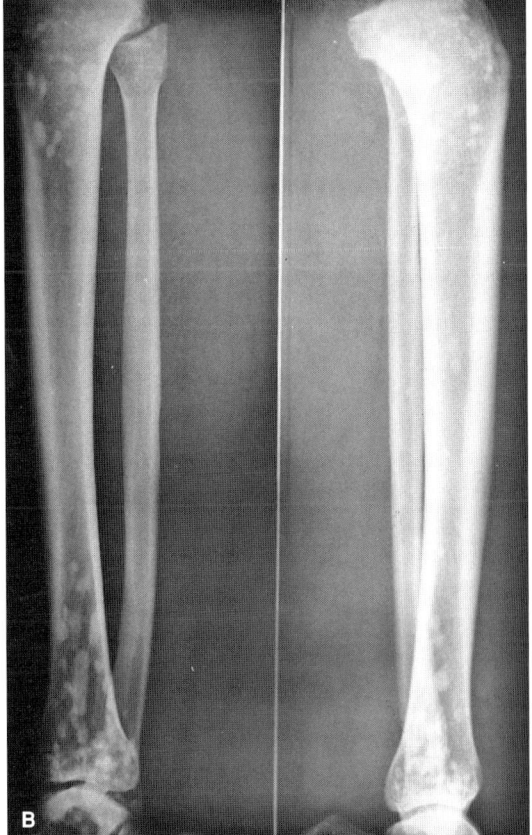

FIGURE 9-10. Osteopoikilosis. This asymptomatic patient demonstrates symmetric involvement of the ends of all tubular bones and the pelvis. (Courtesy of Edward McCarthy, Jr., M.D.)

cases have coexisted with focal dermal hypoplasia consisting of skin atrophy and pigmentation.

RADIOGRAPHIC FEATURES. Striations may involve few or many long bones and are usually bilaterally symmetric. They are dense and may extend into the epiphysis (Fig. 9-11). In the ilia, they radiate laterally from the center of each iliac wing, giving a sunburst appearance. They do not change with time. Coexistence of cranial sclerosis is necessary for diagnosis of this condition. The differential diagnosis involves the other sclerosing bone dysplasias.[88] Osteopathia striata may be differentiated from melorheostosis by the fine intraosseous nature of the streaks, like thickening of normal trabeculae, and by the bilateral symmetry.

TREATMENT. Treatment is not needed for this asymptomatic condition.

Congenital Pseudarthrosis of the Tibia

This rare disorder poses one of the greatest challenges of orthopaedic practice and has stimulated development of treatment methods and literature far out of proportion to its incidence of 1 per 190,000 members of the population.[100] In this condition, the affected tibia displays sclerosis, cyst formation, tapering, and anterolateral bowing in early childhood and usually progresses to develop pathologic fracture. This bone displays virtually no tendency toward union after fracture occurs. Because only a few cases display fracture from birth, the term congenital should be applied loosely; it refers more to the fact that the bone is abnormal from birth.

CLINICAL FEATURES. There is no predominance of the right or left leg, as there is in clavicle pseudarthrosis. Bilateral cases are rare. Most series report a preponderance of affected male patients. Anterolateral bowing is usually discovered in the first or second year of life. It may be differentiated from physiologic genu varum by noticing that the apex of bowing is in the distal part of the tibia and by the unilateral involvement. Fracture usually occurs by 2 to 3 years of age, usually with minimal or no trauma. Those cases fracturing after 5 years of age are called late onset and have several different features. The latest fracture reported occurred in a patient 11 years of age.[107] Slight leg length inequality is evident from the start.

Several conditions may be associated with congen-

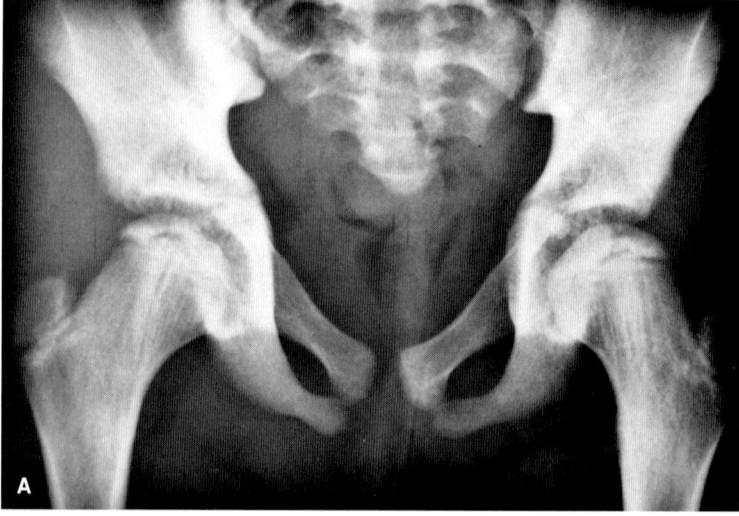
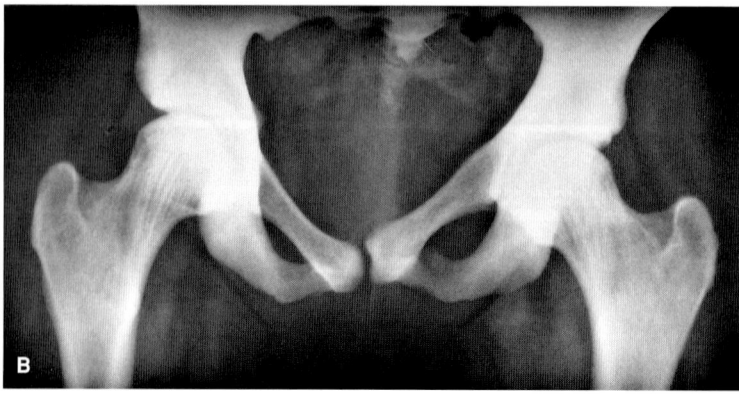

FIGURE 9-11. Osteopathia striata. The streaking of the proximal femurs did not change much in this patient between the ages of (**A**) 12 years and (**B**) 25 years. Notice the flattened femoral epiphysis.

ital pseudarthrosis. The most common is neurofibromatosis, which occurs in approximately 55% of cases.[89,110] This diagnosis is made by finding of two or more of Crowe's criteria: café-au-lait spots (i.e., five or more spots greater than 0.5 cm in diameter), characteristic dystrophic bone changes, positive family history, subcutaneous neurofibromas, or positive lesion biopsy. Because not all findings of neurofibromatosis are expressed from birth, it cannot be ruled out in early childhood. There is no evidence that pseudarthrosis in neurofibromatosis has a lower rate of successful treatment.

Other conditions are more rarely associated. Fibrous dysplasia has been reported in several series[109] and Ehlers-Danlos syndrome in at least one. Constriction band syndrome has been associated with pseudarthrosis and vascular compromise. Rarely, pseudarthrosis may be associated with the orofaciodigital syndrome.[104] Approximately 45% patients with tibial pseudarthrosis have no underlying disorder. Patients with late-onset pseudarthrosis are less likely to have any underlying disorder and rarely have dystrophic changes. They seem to respond more readily to treatment methods than younger patients.[107]

RADIOGRAPHIC FEATURES. The level of bowing or pseudarthrosis is at the junction of the middle and distal thirds of the tibia. A fibular pseudarthrosis is usually present.[95] There are at least three different classification methods for congenital pseudarthrosis.[92,109,111] The two most widely used are those of Boyd[92] and of Anderson[89] (Table 9-3; Fig. 9-12). The basic point of the classifications is to define the appearance of the involved segment of tibia as constricted, cystic, or sclerotic and to differentiate those who have a pseudarthrosis from birth. Those with an hourglass constriction are more likely to have neurofibromatosis. The radiographic type is only moderately correlated with response to treatment. Those tibiae pres-

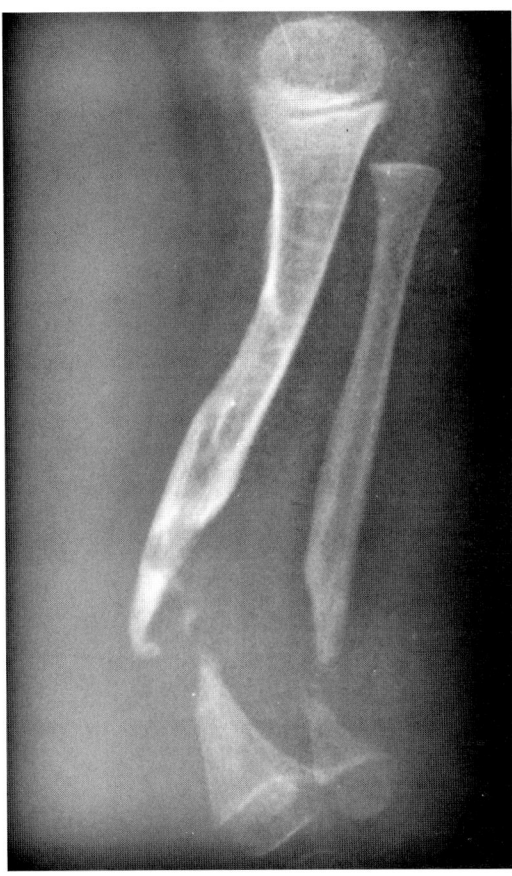

FIGURE 9-12. Early (Boyd type I) congenital pseudoarthrosis of the tibia and fibula in a patient with neurofibromatosis.

enting as cystic have a better prognosis than those which are dysplastic or fractured at birth.

Differential diagnoses also includes focal fibrocartilaginous dysplasia, a rare cause of anterolateral bow of proximal tibia.[93] The tibia in this condition has a focal bow at the site of a medial cortical indentation (Fig. 9-13); the anterior bow is less. Spontaneous correction is the rule. Posteromedial bow of the tibia produces a striking radiographic and clinical appearance, but usually the bowing spontaneously resolves, although leaving the involved limb as much as 4 cm short.[108]

Scanograms should be used to follow limb length inequality after the congenital pseudarthrosis is healed. In some cases, the femur on the affected side is longer than its opposite side. Usually, by maturity, the limb with pseudarthrosis is short by 2 to 6 cm if no equalization treatment is performed. Arteriography is recommended preoperatively for patients undergoing vascularized fibular grafting, especially in a previously operated limb.[111]

PATHOLOGY. The most cited gross pathologic observation is a thick hamartomatous cuff of tissue surrounding the pseudarthrotic lesion.[94] Theoreti-

TABLE 9-3   Classification of Treatment of Congenital Pseudarthrosis of the Tibia

BOYD SYSTEM	ANDERSON SYSTEM
I Fracture present at birth	
II Hourglass constriction of tibia often associated with neurofibromatosis	Dysplastic type
III Bone cysts	Cystic type
IV Sclerotic segment of tibia without constriction, stress frature results	Sclerotic type
V Dysplastic fibula	Fibular type
VI Intraosseous neurofibroma	Clubfoot or congenital band type

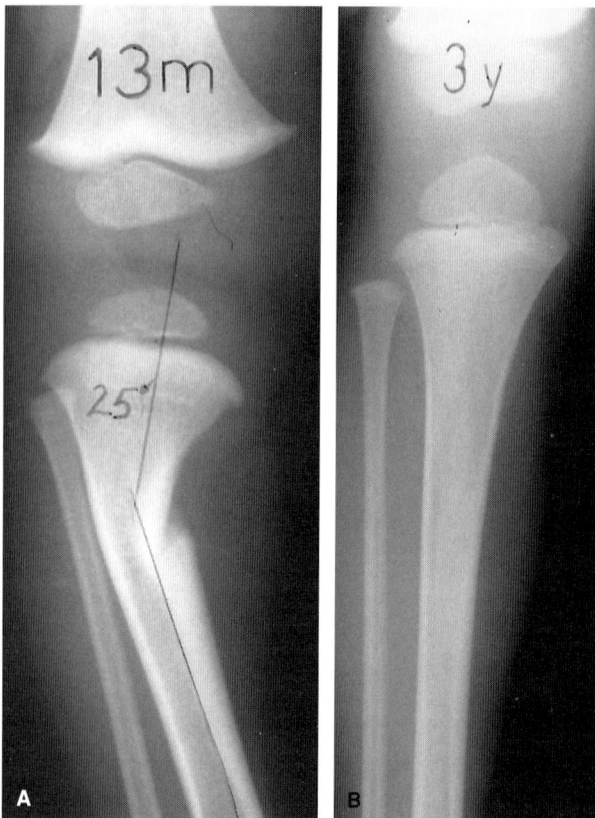

FIGURE 9-13. Focal fibrocartilaginous dysplasia. (**A**) Initial radiograph of the patient at 6 months of age shows anterior and lateral bowing of the tibia, but it is more proximal than in congenital pseudarthrosis. (**B**) The deformity resolved spontaneously, as seen in a radiograph made at 3 years of age.

cally, this may function as an internal constriction band. The tissue from the pseudarthrosis itself does not resemble a neurofibroma. The usual findings are inactive fibroblasts without basement membranes.[92] There are no Schwann cells, axons, or perineural cells. There is a predominance of subperiosteal osteoclasts. The pseudarthrosis is microscopically indistinguishable by standard and electron microscopy from pseudarthrosis due to other causes.

ETIOLOGY. The cause of congenital pseudarthrosis of the tibia remains speculative. It may represent a defect in the cartilaginous anlage of the tibia or in the formation of the primary ossification center, which begins at the area of the tibia, typically the site of pseudarthrosis.[108]

NATURAL HISTORY. If left untreated, there is no tendency for the pseudarthrosis lesion to heal spontaneously.[110] However, the response to treatment and the tendency toward recurrent deformity seem to improve near puberty. The treatment of this condition involves achieving union, preventing refracture, correcting angulation, and equalizing leg lengths. Within the past two decades, there have been several major treatment advances with reasonable rates of union. However, initial union is not an endpoint; more often than not, the previously mentioned problems recur and may be dealt with successfully. Crossett[95] showed that only at skeletal maturity can the result be considered final. Occasionally, patients may come to amputation even as adults. Patients with neurofibromatosis have a significant risk of central nervous system gliomas and sarcomas in childhood or adulthood.[109]

PREVENTION OF FRACTURE. If dysplastic changes are diagnosed before fracture, most researchers recommend prophylactic treatment of some type, despite the lack of clear proof of efficacy. Two centers each braced four patients and successfully prevented fracture in most of them.[110] A long-leg brace or a floor-reaction clamshell brace may have benefit.[106] However, the benefit of prophylactic bracing is not definitively established because of the small numbers of patients and short follow-up periods in these reports.

Prophylactic bypass grafting has been advocated. Strong[110] collected nine such cases and found that fracture was prevented in six. The bypass graft of rib or contralateral tibia is placed posterior and medial to the bow slotted into the tibia along the axis of weight bearing. Allograft bone should not be used, because it is uniformly resorbed. This prophylactic procedure has not gained wide acceptance. It should probably only be used if definite worsening of the bow has been documented. The surgeon should not perform a corrective osteotomy before fracture. Because of the poor healing rate, it is likely to precipitate problems. It is better to let nature take its course.

TREATMENT OF ESTABLISHED FRACTURE. Methods of simple bone grafting and plating have a discouraging success rate of well under 50%.[103] Several other methods have been developed (Table 9-4; Fig 9-14).

ELECTRICAL STIMULATION. Electrical stimulation has several beneficial effects on a nonunion.[91] It increases the calcification of fibrocartilage found in the gap, decreases bone resorption, and promotes angiogenesis. The stimulation may be delivered by external coils, percutaneous electrodes, or an implanted system. In the implanted technique, this is usually combined with bone grafting and intramedullary rods, correcting the deformity.[105] All techniques employ prolonged cast immobilization for 3 to 6 months, and stimulation is continued even after healing has occurred. Success rates of 57% to 75% have been reported in terms of achieving union, but the criteria

TABLE 9-4 *Options for Treatment of Congenital Pseudarthrosis of the Tibia*

METHOD	RATE OF UNION	ADVANTAGES	DISADVANTAGES
Electrical stimulation	55%–80%	Noninvasive, may be combined with other techniques	Limited ability to correct deformity, long time in cast
Intramedullary rod with bone graft (Williams, Coleman)	90%–100%	Corrects deformity, provides long-term internal splint	May cause slight ankle stiffness, does not correct severe, established shortening
Free vascularized bone graft	90%–95% eventual	Provides excellent bone stock, may add slight length	Requires specialized skill, relatively long operation, distal angulation hard to correct
External fixator (circular or monolateral frame)	90%–100%	Corrects nonunion length, angulation	High risk of refracture, bowing, long-term follow-up not available

for definition of union are not firm, and there is a 30% refracture rate.[91,106] For the implanted-stimulator regimen, it is impossible to determine which is the key step: rod, bone graft, or stimulator. Nevertheless, this is the most widely used of the electrical stimulation methods, because all three steps may be combined to achieve mechanical and biologic stimulation.

The role for preventive electrical stimulation (before fracture) is unproven. Electrical stimulation by itself is becoming less widely used, because more effective surgical techniques are evolving. It is probably best used in conjunction with other techniques.

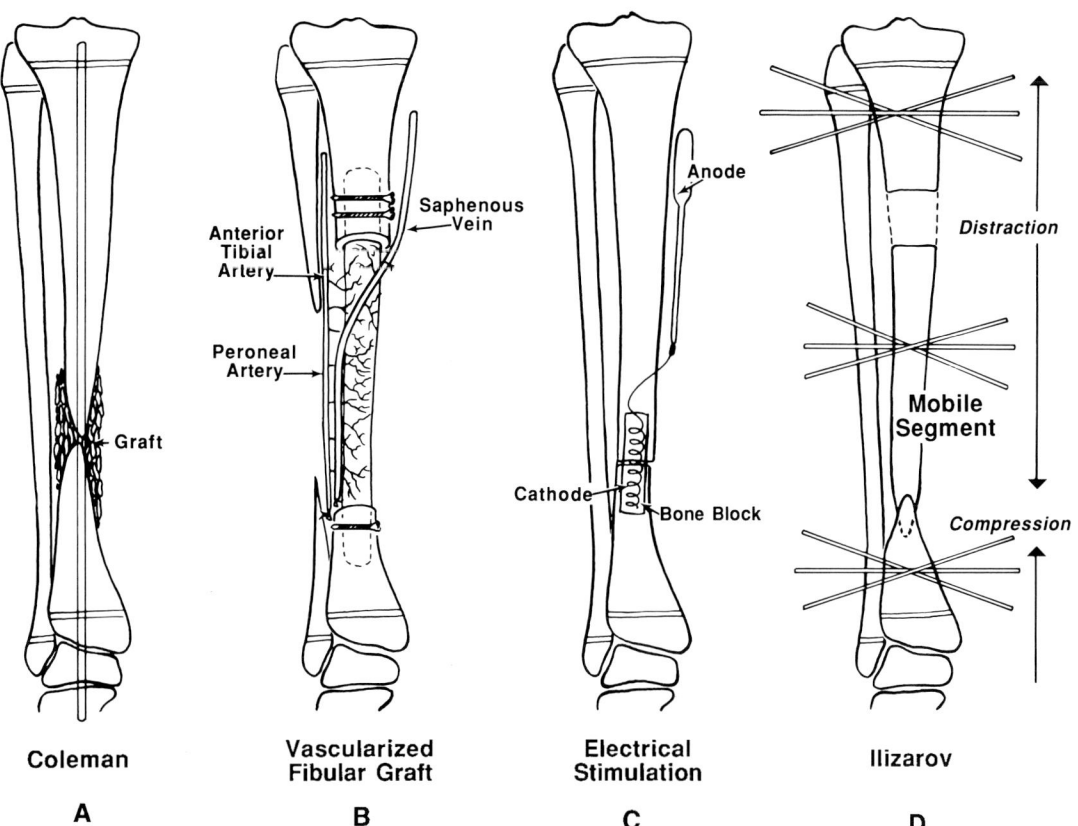

FIGURE 9-14. Operative options for pseudarthrosis of the tibia. (**A**) Coleman osteosynthesis. (**B**) Vascularized fibular graft from the opposite leg. (**C**) Electrical stimulation. (**D**) Ilizarov technique of lengthening above and compression of the pseudarthrosis to achieve union.

INTRAMEDULLARY ROD. In treating congenital pseudarthrosis, the surgeon must achieve union and prevent repeat bowing and refracture and must do this despite poor bone density. These are similar principles to the treatment of osteogenesis imperfecta. It is only fitting that techniques developed for osteogenesis imperfecta have been successfully adapted to congenital pseudarthrosis of the tibia. The best known of these are the Williams rod technique[90] and the Sheffield technique.[98] They employ an intramedullary rod long enough to stabilize virtually the entire tibia and allow graft healing, while realigning it and allowing growth to occur with the rod in place.

The technique of rodding involves resecting the dysplastic segment of the tibia back to normal bone, usually 1 to 3 cm. A medullary canal is created. A rod is inserted next.[90] In the Williams technique, a rod as large as the canal allows is passed from the fracture antegrade through the foot and then retrograde up across the fracture to a level across the center of the proximal tibial physis. The rod remains across the ankle into the calcaneus to buttress the small distal tibial fragment and allow growth. The Williams rod has a threaded inserter and may be custom made by the hospital equipment department. In estimating rod length, the surgeon should add the amount of length to be gained by correcting the angulation but subtract that lost during resection of pseudarthrosis. The largest possible rod should be used and electrical stimulation employed, if desired. The valgus of the distal fragment should be corrected during initial rod passage.

Bone graft is placed around the fracture. The fibula, if involved, may be rodded to lend additional stability. The fascia of the leg should not be closed. Postoperatively, bracing is continued indefinitely. As the tibia grows, the foot and ankle grow beyond the fixed rod. At that point, ankle motion may be allowed in a hinged orthosis, but bracing should be continued until skeletal maturity. The rod should be left in place until skeletal maturity and then removed only if problematic. Anderson's review of this technique shows a 100% (10 of 10) initial union rate, but five refractured and required repeat rod insertion and graft; all eventually healed.[90] Three patients in whom ankle valgus became excessive required corrective osteotomy or medial stapling of the distal tibial physis. Forty percent of patients had more than 2 cm of leg length inequality. Only one fifth of patients had less than 25 degrees of ankle motion.

As an alternative to the solid, single-piece Williams rod, the surgeon may use an extensible rod such as the Bailey-Dubow rod or the Sheffield rod. The wide, hollow rod should be placed distally and the narrow rod proximally, because the pseudarthrosis is distal and represents the site of maximal stress. Because the ends of these rods are anchored in the epiphysis, they do not need to cross the ankle joint and theoretically may minimize some of the loss of motion that is seen in some ankles.[90] The Sheffield experience of five reported patients was that union occurred in all cases, and there was 19% elongation of the rod.[98]

The procedures using intramedullary rods are attractive because they do not require long operative times or unusual surgical skills. They do, however, require attention to details such as rod size and length, tibial alignment, and follow-up. This is the most widely preferred technique for established pseudarthroses. The rod provides long-term support for the tibia until a biologically more favorable age is reached. Valgus of the distal fragment should be corrected. If a refracture occurs in the meantime, it may heal with the rod in place if it is still an appropriate size.

The following techniques are usually reserved for cases with multiple failed surgeries or because of surgeon's technical preference (see Table 9-4).

VASCULARIZED BONE GRAFT. The use of living, normal bone graft seems to circumvent the abnormal biologic factors present at the pseudarthrosis site and has yielded a much higher success rate than nonvascularized bone grafts (Fig. 9-15). The forerunner of this technique was the Farmer operation, a cross-leg delayed pedicle flap that transferred a portion of the opposite, normal tibia. With the advent of microvascular techniques, the ease and the success rate of viable bone transfer has improved. The vascularized donor bone is usually the contralateral fibula, but it may be the ipsilateral fibula, if it is not involved and can be moved on a vascular pedicle to bridge the gap.

Vascularized bone grafting is most commonly done if prior treatment by bone graft and intramedullary rod has failed to produce a union. Preoperative arteriography is recommended to plan the anastomosis and rule out anomalies. If available, two operative teams may be used, one to obtain the graft and one to prepare the bed depending on surgeon's preference.[111] The pseudarthrosis is resected back to more normal bone in which a medullary canal may be created, and the artery for anastomosis identified (usually the anterior tibial). The fibula with a length of 6 to 8 cm is transferred with its peroneal vascular pedicle, anastomosed, and anchored into the proximal and distal medullary canal. Distal anchorage is usually poor because of the small, osteopenic distal fragment. Unfortunately, an intramedullary rod cannot be used at the time of initial surgery because it may impair graft vascularity. The ipsilateral fibula should be rodded or synostosed distally to the tibia. The distal remnant of the donor fibula should also be synostosed to the tibia to prevent later ankle valgus deformity developing with growth.

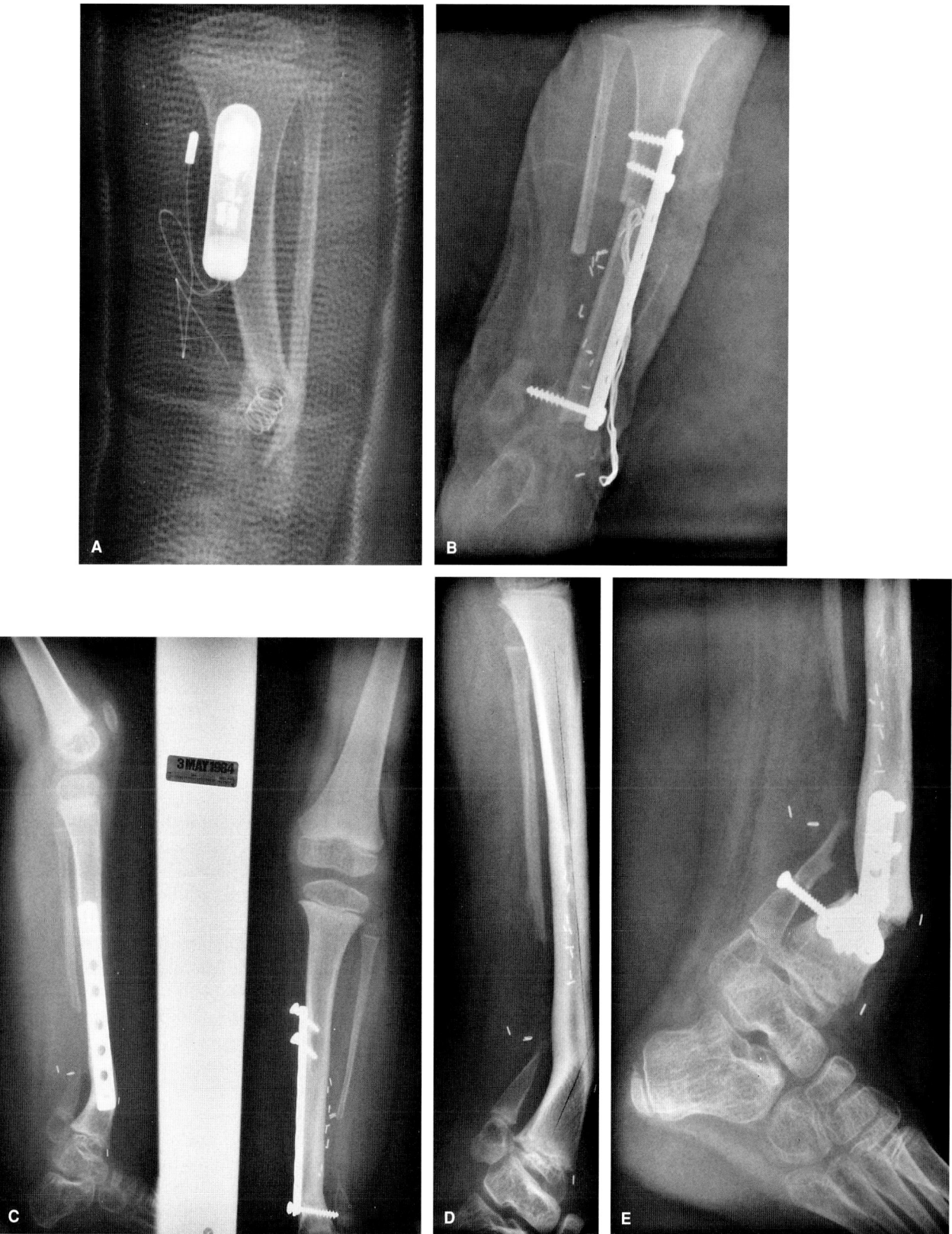

FIGURE 9-15. One patient's treatment for congenital pseudarthrosis of the tibia. (**A**) A fracture developed in infancy; 6 months of treatment with electrical stimulation were unsuccessful. (**B**) A vascularized graft from the contralateral fibula was performed at 2 years of age. Notice the small, osteopenic, valgus distal fragment. (**C**) Union and hypertrophy of the fibula has occurred, but the anterolateral bow persists. (**D**) The increasing bow was treated with an osteotomy, (**E**) which failed to unite. (**F**) Osteotomy and intramedullary rod led to a union persisting to maturity, but a constant 4-cm shortening of the involved limb remained. (**G**) After treatment with contralateral epiphyseodesis of the proximal and distal tibia and ipsilateral hemiepiphyseodesis of the distal-medial tibia, the limb lengths are equal, and alignment is acceptable.

(continued)

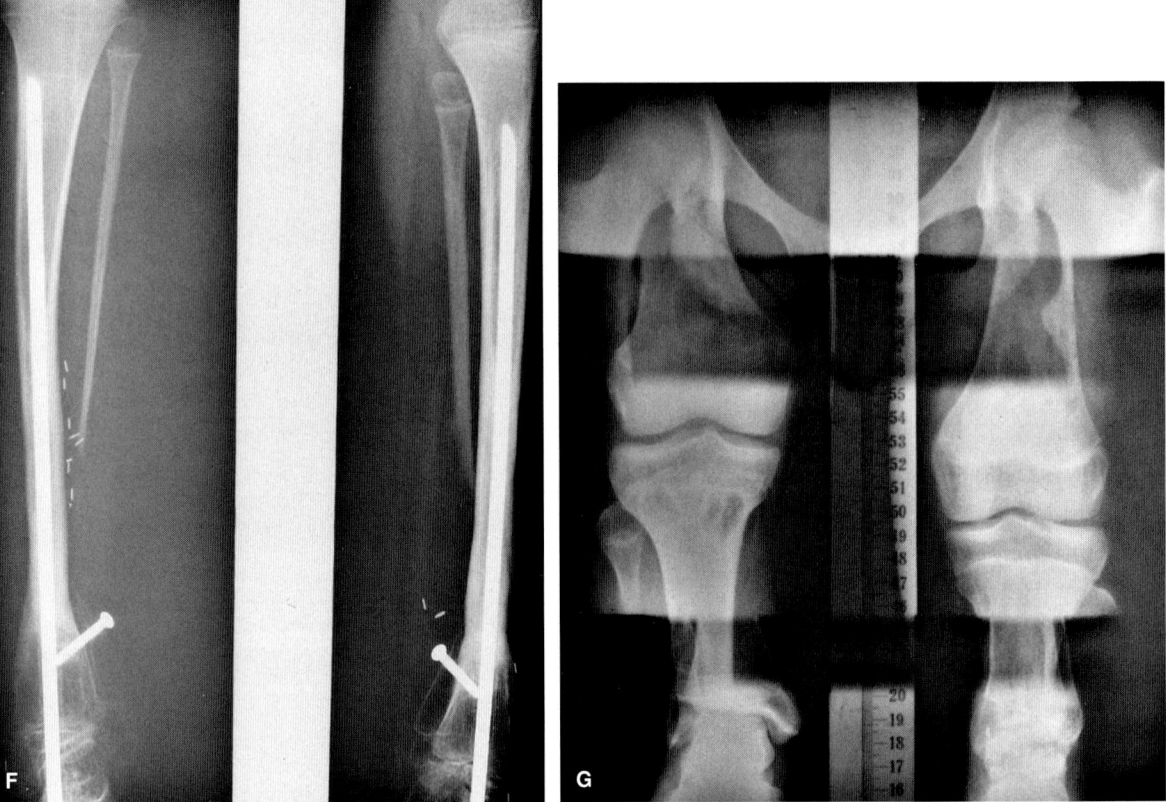

FIGURE 9-15. (Continued).

The success rate of this procedure is 92%[99] to 95%[102] in terms of viability of the graft. However, nonunion can occur, especially distally, and may require revision osteosynthesis. Weiland reported five nonunions of proximal or distal ends in 19 patients after the index operation, and two refractures. His 19 patients eventually required 25 additional operations.[111] These were mostly bone grafts or correction of residual anterolateral angulation. Hypertrophy of the fibula was impressive after union occurred. Reports have shown that osteotomy and distraction can later be carried out through the vascularized fibula site with a success rate similar to normal bone.[101]

EXTERNAL COMPRESSION-DISTRACTION TREATMENT. External fixator-lengthening devices have been used successfully to unite the pseudarthrosis. This may be accomplished by compression followed by distraction at the pseudarthrosis site or by two-level correction, with proximal corticotomy and internal bone transport to promote compression at the pseudarthrosis. The pseudarthrosis itself may need to be grafted. If bone quality is adequate, the problems of nonunion, angulation, and length may all be addressed with this device. Fabry[97] and Plowecky[106] each report three of three cases successfully treated all were over age five. Because follow-up is short, and numbers are small, it is not yet certain if these results may be generalized to all cases. It is also unknown what the lower age limit for successful treatment is and whether there are frequent problems with angulation and refracture in longer follow-up until maturity. At one large U.S. center, the initial union is followed by a recurrence of bowing or fracture in nearly one half of cases.* The advantages of the external fixator in preserving local blood supply may be offset by the lack of long-term mechanical support.

Amputation is necessary in at least 5% of cases in almost all series. This should not necessarily be regarded as a failure, because the biology seems to vary between cases, and these are likely to be the most severely involved. Some patients may require multiple operations to obtain union if it is achieved at all, with resultant severe angulation, shortening, and ankle stiffness. In these patients, the limb and the patient may be less functional than if an earlier amputation and prosthetic fitting had been performed. The decision must be individualized, but if there have been repeated failures of technically well-done, definitive

---

* Herzenberg J, personal communication, 1994.

procedures (e.g., intramedullary rod, free vascularized graft, external fixator), or there is severe ankle stiffness, pain or excessive residual deformity (i.e., shortening or angulation), amputation may be elected (Fig. 9-16).

Perhaps counterintuitively, an ankle disarticulation of the Syme or Boyd type rather than an amputation through the lesion is the preferred method.[100] This prevents spike formation in the end of the stump with growth, maximizes length of the limb residual, and gives good end-bearing skin. The pseudarthrotic tibia and fibula may be rodded and bone grafted to correct angulation. Although fewer than one half of the pseudarthroses healed before maturity in Jacobsen's series, the function was still good, and the technique was recommended.[100] An exception may be in the older adolescent with a distal pseudarthrosis, in which case length and growth may not be problems, and a below-knee amputation would be satisfactory.

After union is achieved, the tibia should be protected with a brace and sports restricted until maturity. Limb length inequality should be treated if more

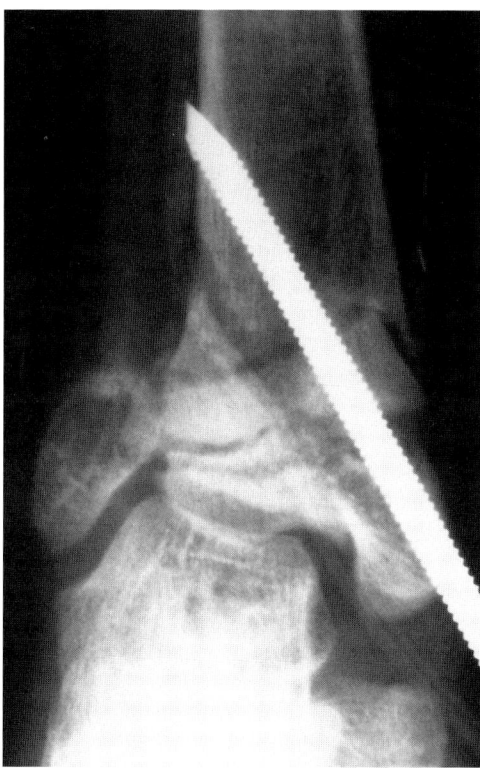

FIGURE 9-17. Residual ankle valgus from a tilt of the distal tibia is often a problem in congenital pseudarthrosis patients.

than 2 cm, and valgus of the ankle should be corrected by medial tibial hemiepiphyseodesis in the young patient or a Wiltse osteotomy for older patients (Fig. 9-17).[112] The family should be counseled from the outset that multiple procedures are the rule to achieve a long-term success, so they do not despair at short-term complications.

Congenital pseudarthrosis infrequently may involve the radius, ulna, or humerus. The principles of treatment are similar.

Congenital Pseudarthrosis of the Fibula

Pseudarthrosis of the fibula may occur in the absence of tibial pseudarthrosis. The tibia, however, is abnormal and shows anterolateral bowing, although it may not go on to fracture. The clinical picture is one of ankle varus initially, changing to valgus after the fibula fractures and shortens.[111] Only 15 cases are reported in the literature.[113-115] Neurofibromatosis seems to be more frequently associated with this entity than with congenital pseudarthrosis of the tibia. Radiographically, the tibia demonstrates cortical thickening and only moderate bow, with no constriction; this corresponds to Boyd type IV (Fig. 9-18) or type V. There is significant overlap with the various categories of tibial pseudarthrosis.

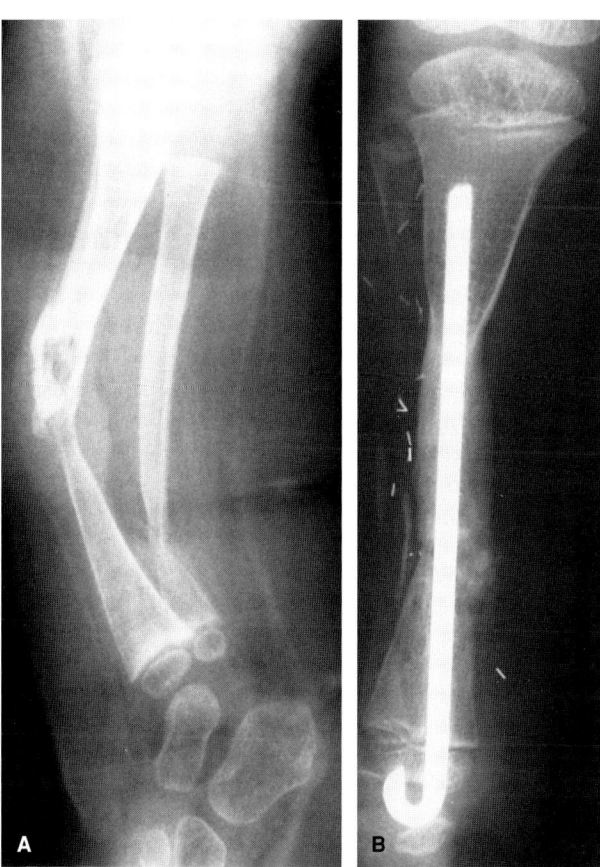

FIGURE 9-16. (A) Congenital pseudarthrosis of the tibia before treatment in a patient with neurofibromatosis. (B) Vascularized grafts from the contralateral and then from the ipsilateral fibulas were rapidly resorbed. Eventually, Boyd disarticulation was performed. This took several years to unite solidly but allowed early function in a prosthesis.

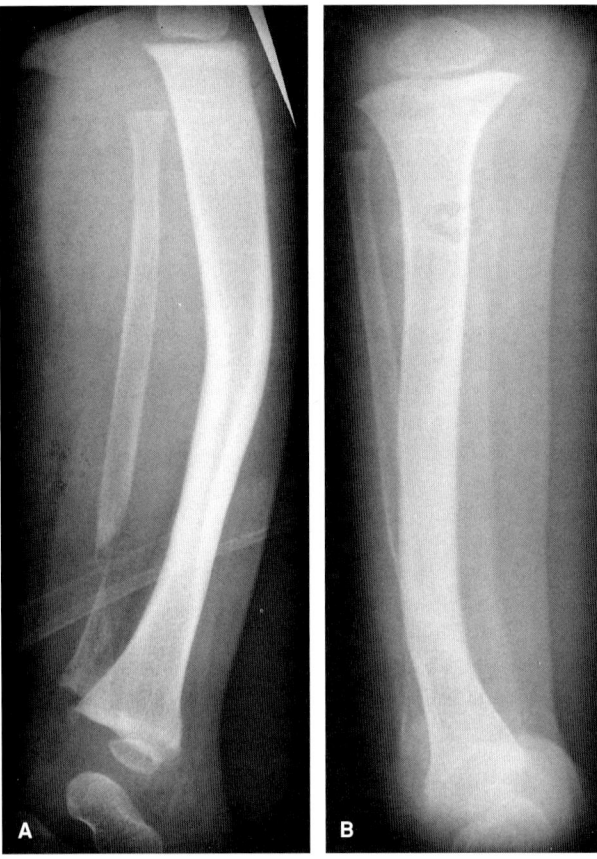

FIGURE 9-18. Congenital pseudarthrosis of the fibula. The tibia has an anterolateral bow but never fractured.

Treatment depends on the degree of clinical deformity. For cases with anterolateral bow but no significant ankle valgus, an ankle-foot orthosis may be used for prevention of ankle deformity. If there is ankle valgus, it may be minimized by repair or synostosis of the fibula, although no controlled studies exist. The fibula may be repaired by an intramedullary rod and onlay bone graft. The peroneal and Achilles tendons may need to be lengthened. If union is not achieved, the fibular pseudarthrosis should be excised and distal tibiofibular fusion performed as described by Langenskiold.[115] This is done to prevent further fibular migration and valgus. Iliac crest bone is used to create synostosis of the distal fibular fragment to the tibial metaphysis. In no case should a varus osteotomy of an intact tibia be performed until puberty, because there is a high risk of a persistent tibial pseudarthrosis developing.[113]

Congenital Pseudarthrosis of the Clavicle

The clavicle can be fractured at birth and usually heals with abundant callus. Congenital pseudarthrosis of the clavicle is an interesting condition characterized by the absence of any of the typical signs or symptoms of a fracture.[117]

CLINICAL FEATURES. The patient presents with a visible and palpable prominence in which the two ends may be thought to be separately mobile. There is no prior history of tenderness or pseudoparalysis suggesting fracture and no history of trauma. The physical effects of the shortened clavicle are evident; the shoulder appears dropped and the arm slightly closer to the midline. The cosmetic defect is thought by some researchers to progress over time.[124] The medial segment is above the lateral segment and is generally larger. There is no association with neurofibromatosis, as there is with other long bone pseudarthroses. Most cases involve the right clavicle, 10% are bilateral, and only a few cases involve just the left clavicle. Cases that do affect only the left side have been reported to have dextrocardia.[119] Bilateral cases are often associated with cervical ribs.

In some cases, there is a complaint by the patient of pain or weakness with activity, especially sports or overhead lifting. In other cases, with a greater degree of displacement, the "bump" itself may be the presenting complaint. There have been a few cases of thoracic outlet syndrome due to what appears to be congenital pseudarthrosis.[116] In some cases, symptoms are minimal enough that patients only come to medical attention incidentally.

RADIOGRAPHIC FEATURES. The pseudarthrosis is in the central one third of the clavicle (Fig. 9-19). The bone ends are usually enlarged, as in hyper-

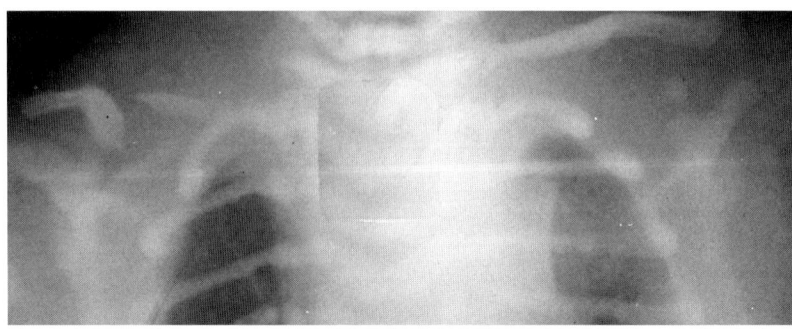

FIGURE 9-19. Congenital pseudarthrosis of the right clavicle. There are no signs of healing.

trophic type of pseudarthrosis, unlike the wispy, atrophic appearance of congenital pseudarthrosis of the tibia. There is, however, no attempt at healing or periosteal reaction.

DIFFERENTIAL DIAGNOSIS. Cleidocranial dysostosis is an autosomal dominant condition that involves partial or total absence of the clavicle. The missing portion, however, is more than just the central one third. These patients also have frontal bossing and diastasis of the symphysis pubis. Birth fracture should be differentiated by the clinical picture, with pseudoparalysis and swelling or hypertrophic callus.[120] Neurofibromatosis has occasionally been reported to occur with pseudarthrosis of the clavicle, but most patients presenting with clavicle pseudarthrosis do not have neurofibromatosis.[121]

ETIOLOGY. The two major etiologic theories about the formation of congenital pseudoarthrosis involve intrinsic failure of development and extrinsic pressure on the clavicle. In support of the former, it has been observed that the clavicle develops from two centers of ossification, a sternal and an acromial nucleus, which fuse in the seventh week of gestation.[120] It is possible that failure of these to coalesce may be a cause of the problem. Alternatively, Lloyd-Roberts observed that the right-sided predominance may be the result of the higher subclavian artery on the right side of normal individuals.[119] He theorized that constant arterial pulsations may contribute to the pseudarthrosis. This view is neatly supported by the finding of left-sided congenital pseudarthrosis in persons with dextrocardia. Cervical ribs may cause localized pressure leading to pseudarthrosis, because the pseudarthrosis is usually located where the artery crosses the rib. Cervical ribs have been seen in cases of bilateral congenital pseudarthrosis.[123]

TREATMENT. Most cases described in the literature were symptomatic and were surgically repaired, and it is not known whether asymptomatic cases are common. Patients may present because of the "bump" and the associated cosmetic concerns. Tachdjian[108] thinks that the clavicular shortening is progressive and recommends repair within the first year of life. Most researchers, however, operate on the basis of symptoms and recommend waiting until 3 to 6 years of age.[118,122,123] Tachdjian recommends using a threaded pin and cast as well as iliac bone graft.[124] This should be viewed with caution because of the tendency of even threaded clavicular pins to migrate. Other techniques involve a plate and intercalary bone graft.[118,123] Ogden presents a unique point of view and regards the problem as one of failure of ossification centers to meet.[118] He opens and sutures the periosteum of the two bone ends, without bone grafting or fixation. He reports union in each of his eight cases. The high union rate with each of the procedures mentioned is in marked contrast to the dismal results in tibial pseudarthrosis. Cosmetically, treatment changes the bump to a scar.

Dysplasia Epiphysealis Hemimelica

This localized disorder is also known as Trevor disease, after the researcher who reported eight cases in 1950, calling it tarsoepiphyseal aclasia.[132] The association with the tarsus has been deemphasized, because many cases do not involve the foot. The most sensible name is epiphyseal osteochondroma, because it describes the pathology well. The customary name, dysplasia epiphysealis hemimelica, alludes to the occasional involvement of multiple joints, usually on one side of the limb.

CLINICAL FEATURES. The incidence is approximately 1 per 1,000,000. It is more common in boys than in girls for unknown reasons.[130] Patients usually present before 14 years of age with complaints of a mass, decreased range of motion,[127] or of joint locking, rather than pain.[128] The involved limb may overgrow or develop angulation. Degenerative joint disease in the involved joints may supervene in adulthood, but this is not uniform. There is no consistent familial inheritance pattern. Growth of the involved area proceeds proportionately to the patient's overall growth. The medial side is affected more frequently than the lateral side.

Azouz[125] described three types: localized (i.e., one epiphysis involved), classic (i.e., more than one bone involved in single limb) and generalized. Classic involvement is the most common.[128]

Unusual presentations are the rule: progressive angulation of the joint due to growth of an intraarticular lesion or progressive limp and widening of the joint due to the cartilaginous mass. Cases of carpal and hip involvement have also been described.[129,131] A case of rigid flatfoot has been described due to a late-recognized lesion in the medial subtalar joint.[129]

RADIOGRAPHIC FEATURES. Sites most often involved include the knee (especially distal femur), ankle (distal tibia), talus, and tarsal navicular. The radiographic appearance varies with age. First, the joint enlarges in response to the space-occupying unossified cartilage. The epiphysis may appear early. Multicentric ossification takes place in the mass, which then coalesces with the main epiphysis itself (Fig. 9-20). There is some streaking of the metaphysis in the in-

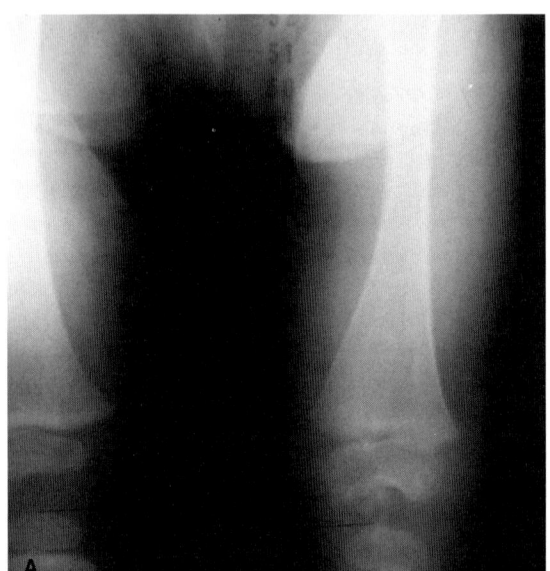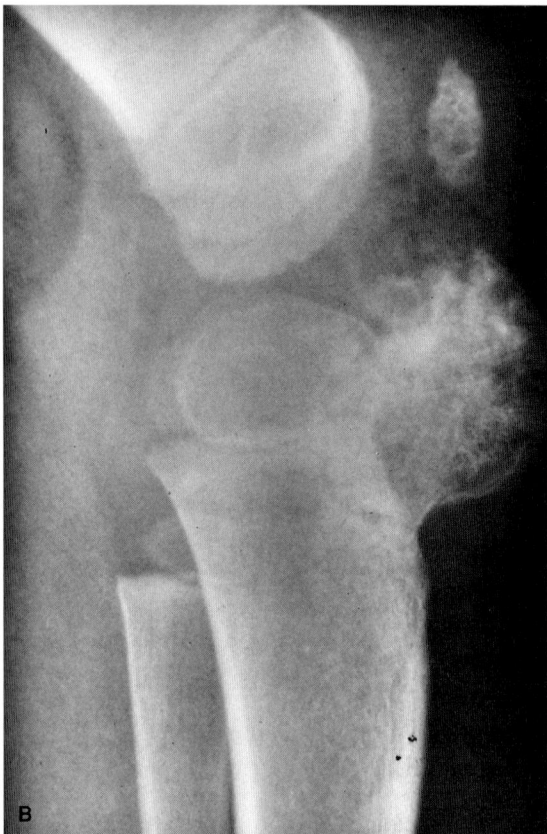

FIGURE 9-20. Dysplasia epiphysealis hemimelica of the distal femur in a 3-year-old patient. There are only scattered calcifications in the lesion at this young age. (**B**) Dysplasia epiphysealis hemimelica caused a mass and limitation of extension in a 10-year-old boy. No other joints were involved.

volved region, similar to osteopathia striata. The limb length may overgrow.

MRI may be helpful, especially before skeletal maturity, to define the plane between lesion and normal epiphysis and thereby allow more anatomic surgical resection.[128]

PATHOLOGY. Grossly, the lesion resembles an osteochondroma. It may be sessile or somewhat pedunculated, but never with a stalk as well developed as seen in metaphyseal osteochondromas. Microscopically, there is a cartilage boundary between the lesion and the normal epiphysis. The arrangement of chondrocytes is like that in osteochondromas, producing endochondral ossification through germinal, hypertrophic, and calcifying zones.[129]

ETIOLOGY. The cause is unknown. Trevor postulated an abnormality of maturation of cells of the epiphyseal growth plate.[132] The frequent involvement of both sides of a joint points to a problem occurring before joint cavitation, when a common fibrocartilaginous anlage is present representing both adjacent epiphyses. The longitudinal lateralization of some cases (e.g., medial side of several successive joints) mimics a tendency seen in melorheostosis.

TREATMENT. The treatment should address the presenting problem but not damage the joint unnecessarily. The prominent masses should be removed, but the surgeon should limit resection of as much true articular cartilage as possible. Maylock et al[125] described the technique of an intraepiphyseal wedge resection for angular overgrowth, preserving a flap of the articular surface and suturing it to the base of the resected wedge. This may be useful if defining and preserving normal articular surface apart from the lesion is difficult.

Recurrence of the overgrowth is common, especially before skeletal maturity.[128] Malignant degeneration has not been reported.

Fibrodysplasia Ossificans Progressiva

Fibrodysplasia ossificans progressiva involves progressive development of multiple foci of heterotopic ossification with progressive, disabling ankylosis and characteristic shortening or valgus deformity of the great toe and other malformations. Excellent clinical studies of the genetic transmission, clinical course, and histology have been done by Kaplan, Zaslof, and their colleagues.[134,138,139] Although it is not purely a localized disorder, it is included here because it initially appears so and resembles myositis ossificans.

CLINICAL FEATURES. The incidence of this disorder is low, less than 1 per 1,000,000 members of the population.[133,136] Most affected patients appear to have had spontaneous mutations. However, two families with parent-child transmission suggest autosomal dominant transmission, including one well-documented family with a father and all three offspring affected.[138] Some parents of fully affected children have only the great toe deformity.[133] Affected patients do not usually have offspring. The sexes are affected equally.

The children are born without restricted range of motion or heterotopic nodules; only the great toe deformities are present at birth. Heterotopic ossification begins at a mean age of 5 years, often after blunt trauma, and progresses steadily, although the diagnosis is often delayed because of the rarity of the condition. The initial painful, erythematous nodule in tendon, ligament, or fascia gradually becomes hard. Nodules may also form in the absence of any trauma. Progressive involvement follows a relatively predictable pattern, proceeding from the posterior neck and shoulder girdle region in a proximal-to-distal, axial-to-appendicular, and posterior-to-anterior sequence (Fig. 9-21).[132] The upper extremities are affected before the lower extremities. If the clinical picture is characteristic, a confirmatory biopsy is contraindicated, because it may accelerate the process and is not likely to be definitive.[138] The shoulder and hips and other major joints are stiffened by extraarticular ankylosis, and the patient may have difficulty sitting. The progression seems to be less rapid after skeletal maturity. The process does not involve the diaphragm, extraocular muscles, heart, or smooth muscle.

The characteristic great toe morphology is seen in more than 90% of patients and involves some or all of these elements: shortening of the entire ray, malformed (i.e., short, delta-shaped) proximal phalanx, interphalangeal joint fusion, and valgus alignment from various causes.[133,136] There may be reduction defects in the other toes or clinodactyly. The thumb is affected in a smaller percentage of patients.

Conductive hearing loss occurs in 25% of patients, deafness in 25%, and mental retardation in 5%; premature generalized thinning of the hair affects many patients. Laboratory study results are normal, except for mild elevation of serum alkaline phosphatase levels during early periods of heterotopic ossification. Patients often develop decubiti because of an unfortunate combination of the bony prominences, poor nutrition, and decreased mobility. Most patients survive well into adulthood. Life expectancy is variably foreshortened, with death caused by restrictive lung disease from ankylosis of the ribs or poor nutrition due to stiffness of the jaw.

RADIOGRAPHIC FEATURES. The abnormal ossification evolves in a sequence similar to myositis ossificans, with diffuse calcification developing into peripheral maturation and sometimes well-developed linear extraosseous bridges, such as from the scapula to humerus, pelvis to femur, or spine to occiput (see Fig. 9-21).[123] The toe deformities are characteristic. The femoral necks are short and broad. Cervical vertebrae have diminutive bodies and large spinous processes.[134]

PATHOLOGY. Specimens are available from several biopsies done in cases for which the diagnosis was not suspected. If fibrodysplasia is the leading entity in the differential diagnosis, it is not recommended to biopsy nodules.

Three phases are seen in the process of endochondral ossification.[134] In the earliest phase, there is loose myxoid fibrous tissue infiltrating and replacing normal fibrous tissue and muscle. The stains for S100 protein are positive, which in connective tissue indicates presence of chondroblastic cells. Later, there is fairly well-organized endochondral ossification. In the third or mature stage, there is mature lamellar bone with fatty marrow. The ossification process appears to be endochondral rather than intramembranous. Late sarcomatous transformation has not been reported.

ETIOLOGY. The cause of this debilitating condition remains speculative but will probably be elucidated by insights into bone-regulating proteins. Kaplan has observed that the progressive sequence of ectopic ossification recapitulates normal embryologic skeletal development.[139] Because of the abnormal development of the toes and femurs and the sometime occurrence of osteochondromas, he postulates that there is defective regulation of the induction of endochondral ossification as the predominant pathogenetic mechanism of this disorder.[137]

TREATMENT. The physician should aim first to do no harm. Skeletal surgery has no role in treating this condition. Diphosphonates have been tried to decrease the ossification process. A slight benefit has

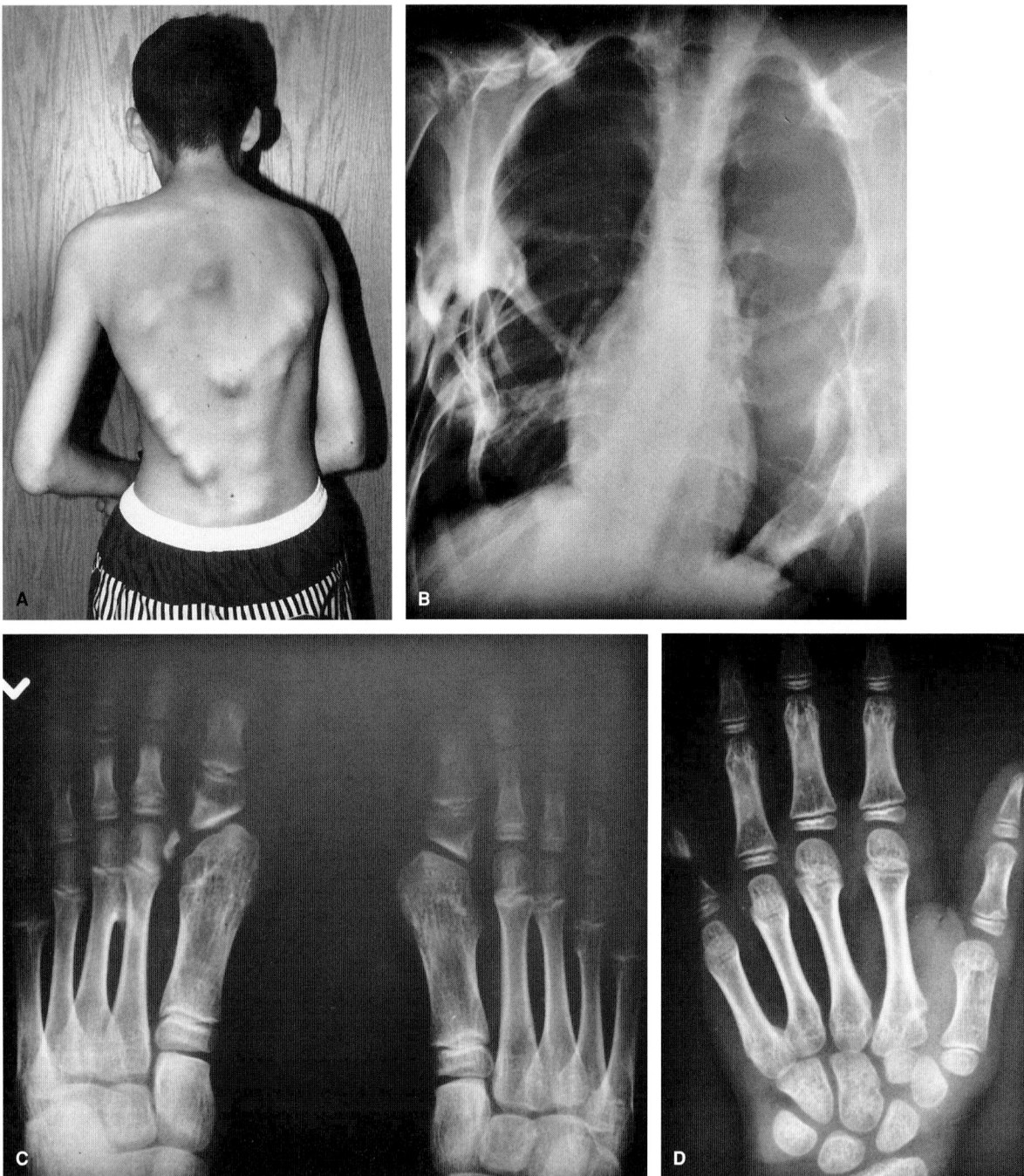

FIGURE 9-21. Fibrodysplasia ossificans progressiva. (A) Clinical appearance. The proximal and posterior areas are most involved. (B) Radiograph of the same region. (C) One of the several types of characteristic deformity of the great toe and proximal phalanx. Notice the small osteochondromas on the lesser metatarsals. (D) The thumb is also foreshortened. (E) Bridging ossification in the cervical extensors. (F) Osteochondromas of the proximal tibias. (G) Clinical appearance of the feet.

been observed in a few patients, but it has been temporary, and the medication is not widely used.[133,140] Education and padding to prevent pressure sores are helpful. Sophisticated motorized transport devices have been developed to accommodate difficulty in arising and walking.[137] Nutrition should be monitored and supplemented if indicated.

ACQUIRED DISORDERS

Myositis Ossificans

The term myositis ossificans refers to a benign, solitary mass in soft tissue, usually in skeletal muscle. There may or may not be a history of prior trauma. Other,

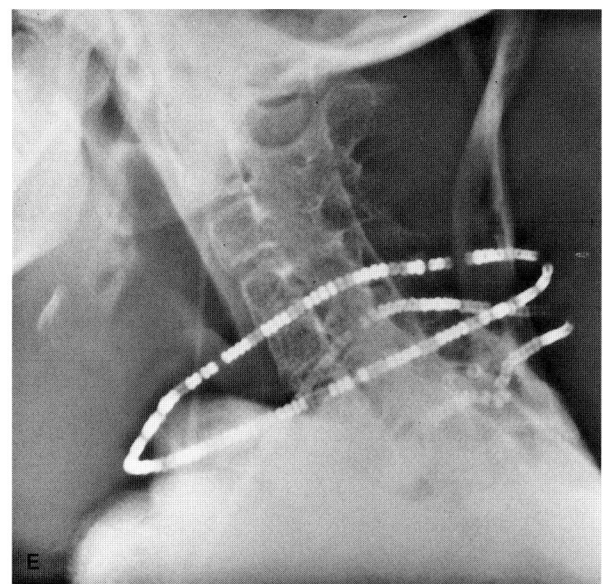
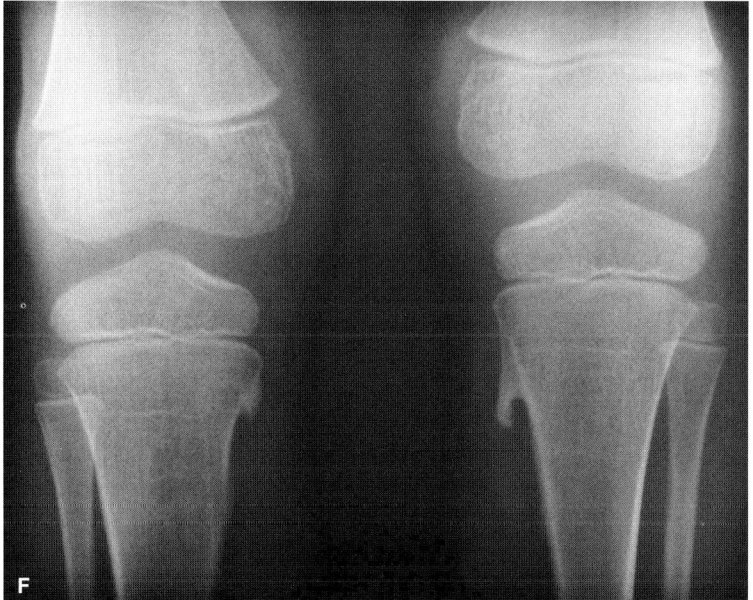
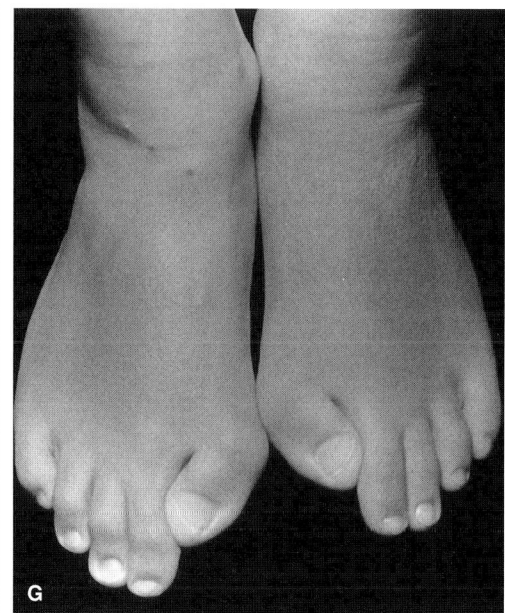

FIGURE 9-21. *(Continued).*

less common names include pseudomalignant myositis ossificans or myositis ossificans circumscripta.[150,152] It is part of a broader spectrum of ectopic ossification in various tissues from various causes, which possibly share pathogenetic mechanisms.

Clinical Features

This entity merits description in a pediatric orthopaedic context, because although it is primarily thought of as a disorder of young adults, as many as 25% of patients may be diagnosed before skeletal maturity, usually in teens and preteens.[142,147] Onset before 10 years of age is rare, although there are case reports of a 5-month-old and a 2-year-old child.[146]

More than one half of cases follow recognized trauma, usually blunt but occasionally repetitive. Any cause of hematoma, such as injection, may precede the process.[148] There are several cases in which no trauma was recalled; it is uncertain whether they were truly spontaneous or occurred after an unrecognized minor injury.[152]

Symptoms include a tender, progressively expanding mass that is often most symptomatic 1 to 3 weeks after an injury. Fever and a mildly elevated erythrocyte sedimentation rate may be seen. Serum calcium and phosphorous are normal. If the lesion is observed, it becomes harder and nontender by 2 to 3 months after injury. The lower extremities are more frequently affected than the upper extremities, and the trunk is involved in 20% of cases. Quadriceps and brachialis muscles are the most commonly affected, although involvement of virtually all regions of the skeleton have been reported.

Radiographic Features

Most lesions are located in the diaphyseal region of an extremity. Calcification begins at about 2 weeks after onset of the lesion. It is usually peripherally located about the lesion. Serial x-ray films at short intervals should show progressive zonal maturation to confirm the diagnosis. CT is especially good for demonstrating the zones, with the periphery being most mature.[149] MRI is relatively nonspecific. Early in the course, it shows surrounding edema and hemorrhage, gradually changing over 2 months to a well-defined inhomogeneous mass with a well-defined rim of low signal intensity (Fig. 9-22).[146,147,148]

The differential diagnosis includes child abuse (an overlapping diagnosis) and fibrodysplasia ossificans progressiva. This entity is characterized by onset of multiple foci of ossification before 5 years of age and by characteristic great toe malformations. The physician should also consider an extraosseous osteosarcoma or rhabdomyosarcoma and interstitial calcinosis.[143] If possible, observation of the natural history usually provides the diagnosis.

Pathologic Features

The lesion usually occurs in skeletal muscle but may instead involve tendon or subcutaneous fat. It is typically 3 to 6 cm in diameter. The histologic patterns

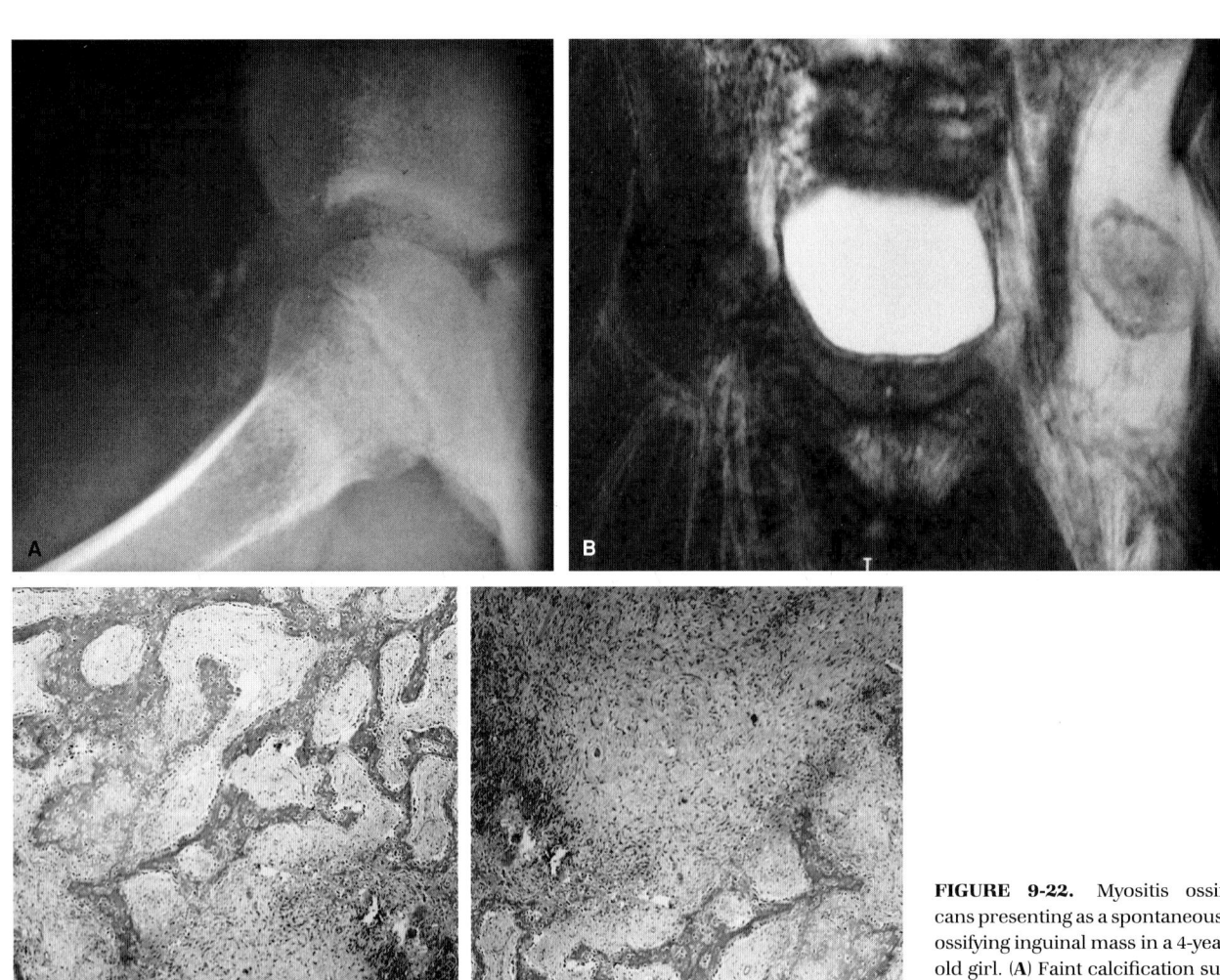

FIGURE 9-22. Myositis ossificans presenting as a spontaneously ossifying inguinal mass in a 4-year-old girl. (**A**) Faint calcification suggests the possibility of a tumor, but it is greatest peripherally. (**B**) The magnetic resonance image shows demarcation. (**C**) Histologic examination reveals a typical zonal maturation, which is greatest peripherally. (Courtesy of J. David Thompson, M.D.)

of traumatic and atraumatic cases are identical. Although called myositis, the lesion does not have the histology of inflammation. Four zones have been described by Ackerman[139]: a central, undifferentiated zone; just peripheral to this, a well-oriented zone of cellular osteoid; outside of this, new bone formation; and an outer zone of well-organized bone in the maturing lesion by 6 to 8 weeks. If a subtotal excision is done, the pathologist needs to know the precise site the sample was taken from to interpret it. Fine needle aspirates have been reported to be adequate by one researcher, but this is not universally accepted, and biopsy technique should be discussed with the pathologist.[148] The zonation described is different from that of osteosarcoma, which usually has the reverse zonal arrangement. The reason for this may be that the tumor is growing centripetally, but the lesion of myositis matures by revascularization from the periphery.

Etiology and Pathogenesis

The origin of the cells producing the lesion is only beginning to be understood.[151-153] Illes, using lectins to probe the cells in lesions of different ages, suggests that they are bone marrow–derived myofibroblast cells responsible for bone formation within damaged muscle.[147]

Treatment

Rest is important in the early stages, because an overly aggressive range of motion may exaggerate the myositis.[144,148] Activity should be to tolerance as pain and spasm subside. The clinical and radiographic appearance of early myositis ossificans may at times resemble malignancy. The discrete nature of the mass or a history of trauma suggests myositis ossificans. If this is in the differential diagnosis, it is best confirmed by observing radiographs at 7- to 10-day intervals to demonstrate the characteristic zonal maturation. If this can be demonstrated, biopsy is rarely needed. Nonsteroidal inflammatory agents alleviate symptoms, and a good response may confirm the diagnosis. The lesion tends to involute partially or totally with time. Excision is therefore unnecessary unless the tissue is interfering with function.[142] If so, it should be deferred until the new bone is radiographically mature, usually about 1 year after onset.

The Osteochondroses

The term osteochondrosis refers to a disturbance of endochondral ossification, including chondrogenesis and osteogenesis, in a previously normal endochondral growth region. This process has been observed sporadically in nearly every growth center of the skeleton.[155,158] This includes epiphyses, apophyses, and physes. Many of these disorders have specific features related to their region of occurrence, and most have eponyms. Discussions of major entities are covered in sections of this text approximate for the anatomic location. This section delineates the common features and highlights the universal vulnerability of the growth regions to vascular and mechanical stress. Eponyms for some of the more common osteochondroses are given in Table 9-5.

Clinical Features

The growth disturbance itself is only minimally symptomatic. Symptoms occur when significant osseous weakening occurs, such as of the tibial tubercle in Osgood-Schlatter disease or the femoral head in Perthes, or when mechanical alteration causes ligamentous strain, such as in adolescent tibia vara. Symptoms generally include local tenderness, effusion, restriction of motion, and visible alteration in growth. Acute pain occurs mainly if there is articular irregularity, such as a free osteochondrotic defect or a subchondral fracture in Perthes.

Etiology

It is important to study normal endochondral growth at various sites to understand how they may be affected. The major longitudinal growth plates are similar in structure. The epiphyses are also surrounded on all other sides by an epiphyseal growth plate, which grows at a much slower rate. On the

---

TABLE 9-5 Examples of Osteochondroses by Region

Upper Extremity
Capitellum, (Panner)
Carpal
Navicular, (Kienboch)
Phalangeal epiphysis (Theemann)
Distal radial epiphysis (Madelung)

Vertebral End Plates
Schuermann

Lower Extremity
Capital femoral epiphysis (Legg-Perthes)
Proximal tibial physis (Blount)
Tibial tubercle (Osgood-Schlatter)
Calcaneal apophysis (Severe)
Tarsal navicular (Kohler)
Metatarsal heads, 2, 3, or 4 (Freiberg)

General
Osteochondritis dissecans, especially knee, ankle, elbow

articular regions of an epiphysis, there is another zone peripheral to the epiphyseal growth cartilage, the articular cartilage. These two layers are not readily differentiated on gross sections. Articular cartilage is nourished solely by synovial fluid, but epiphyseal cartilage and the major physis are nourished by vessels from within the epiphysis. Apophyses such as the trochanter and tibial tubercle often develop from a common cartilage anlage with the adjacent epiphyses and grow in a similar manner. Epiphysioid bones of the hands and feet also develop in a manner like epiphyses, with greatest growth in regions under an articular surface.

Endochondral growth disturbance occurs through mechanical or vascular mechanisms. Excessive load results in disordered growth through direct cellular or a local microvascular overload. Carlson,[154] for example, has shown a high incidence of spontaneous osteochondrosis in the femoral condyles of swine, which is directly related to weight gain, because they gain almost 70 kg within the first 4 months of life. It appears that necrosis occurs first in the epiphyseal cartilage and affects subchondral bone only secondarily. In a separate step, they were then able to produce osteochondrotic lesions by interrupting only the epiphyseal cartilage blood supply through its cartilage canals, leaving the epiphyseal bone vascularized. Whether this is a valid model for human osteochondritis dissecans is unknown.

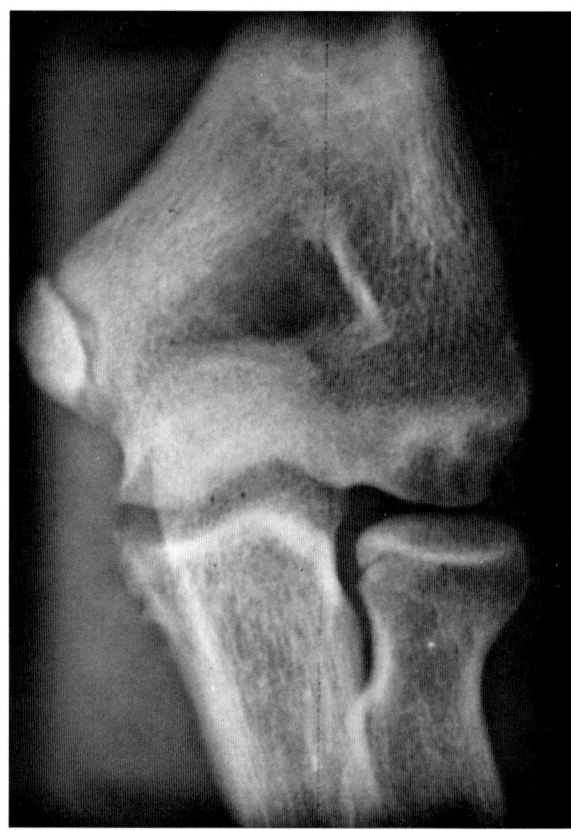

FIGURE 9-23. One example of osteochondrosis, Panner disease of the capitelum, is a primary articular type.

Radiographic Features

Certain stages are common to all osteochondroses.[157] First, there is an arrest in ossification of the affected region, making it appear radiographically smaller. Second, during revascularization, there is bony resorption (Fig. 9-23). Third, reossification occurs and may reveal an alteration in shape of the region. Much later, degenerative changes sometimes occur.

A bone scan may tell if the lesion is early or late. Disruption of cartilage surface can be inferred from an arthrogram or MRI scan.

Treatment

For all locations, the prognosis and treatment are determined by the growth potential of the involved area, and a younger age is a significant positive prognostic factor. General treatment principles include rest from loading until symptoms subside, usually while maintaining range of motion. If a significant but intact osteochondral fragment persists, drilling may stimulate revascularization.[156] If it is unstable, internal fixation with bone grafting as needed is recom-

mended. In some cases, bony realignment can help to minimize causative stress, as in Blount disease.

Congenital Quadriceps Fibrosis

Quadriceps muscle contracture in early childhood is caused by fibrosis of one or more of its four components. It presents with limitation of flexion and may be associated with patellar dislocation.

Clinical Features

Presentation may occur in one of four patterns: a stiff, hyperextended knee at birth; progressive loss of normal knee motion after birth; habitual dislocation of the patella in later childhood; and a painful knee in young adulthood due to the above factors.[161] Girls seem to be more commonly affected. A history of multiple injections into the quadriceps may be elicited, especially in countries where the medical facilities make intravenous access difficult to maintain.[159,161] Patella alta is usually present. If patellar dislocation coexists, the knee flexes a little while the patella is held in the groove but then permits almost full flexion after the point of patellar dislocation.[159] There is an increased reported incidence of congenital anomalies. Some patients, however, are otherwise normal children who present with an acquired contracture and no known history of injections.

Etiology

Trauma, as caused by injections, is the most commonly recognized associated factor related to quadriceps contracture. The reason that this affects primarily children may be that the volume of their quadriceps muscle is smaller in relation to the volume of drugs given.[159] A quadriceps contusion or stretch injury may also cause fibrosis. The physician should rule out mild forms of arthrogryposis or spinal dysraphism.

Pathology

Of the four components of the quadriceps, the vastus intermedius is the most consistently involved. The vastus lateralis is the next most frequently affected, in which case patellar dislocation and valgus deformity may occur. A few reports of rectus femoris involvement exist. The histologic appearance is that of straightforward fibrosis, distally greater than proximally. In longstanding cases in which flexion remains limited (usually those without patellar dislocation), secondary changes may occur, consisting of flattening of the femoral condyles and tightness of the capsule, which further impair the patient's potential for regaining flexion.

Treatment

An organized stretching program is the start of conservative management, followed by serial casting if this fails.[160] These methods have a low yield in the severe cases.

Surgical release is indicated if flexion beyond 60 degrees cannot be achieved. It is done through a midline or anterolateral incision, exploring the fibrotic components and releasing what is tight, typically the vastus intermedius with or without the lateralis and iliotibial band.[159,160] A quadricepsplasty may be necessary in severe cases. The knee is immobilized at 90 degrees of flexion for 3 weeks, followed by work on strength and range of motion. In most reported cases, flexion of at least 135 degrees was obtained, with quadriceps strength of grade 4+ to 5 on a scale of 0 to 5.[159,160] Best results were obtained in patients operated on at a young age, before femoral flattening occurred.

Reflex Sympathetic Dystrophy

Reflex sympathetic dystrophy is a localized disorder characterized by unexplained or exaggerated pain in an extremity and by evidence of autonomic dysfunction.[163] The diagnosis may be substantiated by response to sympathetic-modulating treatments. Synonyms include sympathetically maintained pain, Sudeck atrophy, and causalgia. The latter term refers to the syndrome when it results from direct trauma to a major nerve trunk.[170]

Clinical Features

The manifestations of this disorder vary among individuals and with the stage of the process. These include edema, increased or decreased sweating, erythema, cyanosis, atrophy, or dystrophic skin changes. Dietz described a very high frequency of the sign *tache cerebrale*.[164] This is a sign of autonomic dysfunction elicited by stroking the skin with a blunt object (e.g., head of a safety pin), which is followed in 15 to 30 seconds by a red line. This response should be absent in the contralateral limb.

Criteria for diagnosis of reflex sympathetic dystrophy vary. The criteria which are most established are those of Wilder and colleagues (Table 9-6).[170]

In childhood reflex sympathetic dystrophy, girls are five times more frequently affected than boys, although there is a much more narrow female preponderance among adults.[164] Affected individuals are described as emotionally labile or psychologically predisposed. This theme appears in virtually all reports, but it is not scientifically proven.[169] Signs of de-

TABLE 9-6 Reflex Sympathetic Dystrophy in Children: Criteria for Diagnosis and Stages

NEUROPATHIC PAIN DESCRIPTORS*	SIGNAL AUTONOMIC DYSFUNCTION*
Burning	Cyanosis
Dyesthesia	Mottling of skin
Paresthesia	Hyperhidrosis
Mechanical allodynia	Edema
Hyperalgesia to cold	Coolness of extremity

Stages of Reflex Sympathetic Dystrophy

Acute stage:	Intense pain, hyperesthesia, vasodilation
Dystrophic stage:	Lessened pain, generalized woody edema, early atrophy
Atrophic stage:	Coolness, cyanosis, diminished subcutaneous tissue, stiffness, atrophy, osteoporosis

* At least two from each category are needed for the diagnosis.
From Wilder RT, Berde CB, Wolohan M, et al. Reflex sympathetic dystrophy in children. J Bone Joint Surg [Am] 1992; 74:910.

pression, including decreased appetite, decreased energy, and anhedonia, should be searched for. The lower extremities are five times more frequently involved than the upper extremities in children; the reverse trend is seen in adults. For most children, the onset occurs after some type of trauma, but usually it is vague, and for some, no clear injury can be identified; it may also begin after surgery. A very high percentage of children with this diagnosis participate in organized sports; this has been suggested as a predisposing factor.[170]

In most cases of reflex sympathetic dystrophy, the diagnosis is delayed for almost 1 year.[167] A form of dystrophy localized to the knee region exists and may be frequently misclassified as anterior knee pain syndrome.

Reflex sympathetic dystrophy typically evolves through characteristic stages.[166,167,170] The acute stage is characterized by intense pain, vasodilation, and early edema. The dystrophic stage demonstrates disuse, woody edema, and muscle wasting. The atrophic stage includes smooth, glossy, atrophic skin; pallor; decreased subcutaneous tissue; stiffness; and osteoporosis.

The differential diagnosis includes two basic groups of disorders: any skeletal condition which by itself can explain the symptoms and any recognized psychiatric abnormality. Examples of the former include osteoid osteoma and stress fracture; examples of the latter include conversion reaction, depression, and Munchausen syndrome. The evaluation team should include specialists able to assess the patient for these types of problems.

Radiographic Features

Usually, there is progressive osteopenia with time, but it is not the typical mottling seen in the adult case of reflex sympathetic dystrophy. The bone scan yields variable results, with nearly equal percentages of patients showing increased, decreased, or equal but delayed isotope uptake compared with the normal side.[165] If increased and decreased uptake are considered positive, the sensitivity of bone scans is only 60%, and specificity is 86%.[165] The main value of the scan is to rule out occult skeletal disorders such as stress fracture, neoplasm, and other conditions.[170]

Etiology

Most theories invoke a disturbance of autonomic (sympathetic) function, but all are still speculative. Leading theories include abnormal firing by damaged peripheral nerves, triggering sympathetic response; resetting of the central reticular "bias" because of loss of sensory input from the damaged extremity; and artificial synapses between injured peripheral nerve endings. It is not known whether some of the personality traits of the typical patient are related to the cause or are the result of chronic pain.

Treatment

Treatment involves a stepwise approach, trying different therapies while returning the patient to function.[169,170] There is no single treatment with a distinctively high success rate nor a universal algorithm. However, one approach that has been widely tested is given in Figure 9-24.[165] This proceeds from least to

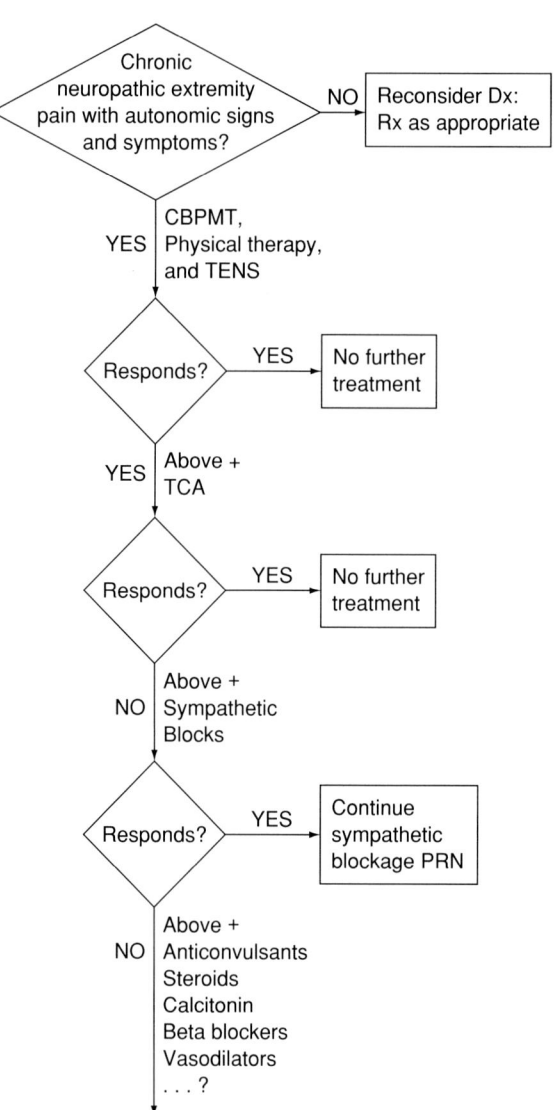

FIGURE 9-24. Algorithm for the treatment of reflex sympathetic dystrophy. (CBPMT, cognitive-behavioral pain-management techniques; Dx, diagnosis, PRN, Rx, therapy; TCA, tricyclic antidepressants; TENS, transcutaneous electrical nerve stimulation; from Wilder RT, Berde CB, Wolohan M, et al. Reflex sympathetic dystrophy in children. J Bone Joint Surg 1992; 74A:910.)

greater degrees of invasiveness and risk, and involves the basic steps of physical and behavior therapy, tricyclic antidepressants, sympathetic block, and miscellaneous agents such as anticonvulsants, steroids, and β-blockers. Sympathetic blocks are used on a continuous basis, using a catheter for 7 to 10 days, as part of a structured behavioral program. Long-term sympatholysis can be done if the blocks yield adequate but only temporary relief.[168] Tricyclic agents are used if depressive features are present in addition to the sympathetic findings. The most effective treatments are sympathetic blocks followed by physical therapy and antidepressants.

Treatment of this disorder is best carried out by a team including specialists in pain management, rehabilitation, and orthopaedics. In general, the surgeon should avoid immobilization (i.e., cast), opioids, and steroids in children because of the risks and lack of efficacy.

The long-term outlook is one of improvement but often not complete relief of symptoms. In Wilder's study, although most patients were improved at a mean follow-up of 3 years, 55% still had some residual pain and dysfunction.[170] Early treatment yields the best results. Predictors of better outcome were age younger than 13 years and minimal time out of school.

Reflex sympathetic dystrophy in children is characterized by predominant involvement of the lower extremities, much higher incidence in girls, stress such as organized sports or family disorder, and delayed diagnosis. A stepwise, team approach can lead to improvement for most patients.

References

Klippel-Trenaunay Syndrome

1. Anlar B, Yalaz R, Erzen C. Klippel-Trenaunay-Weber syndrome: a case with cerebral and cerebellar hemihypertrophy. Neuroradiology 1988;30:360.
2. Baskerville PA, Ackroyd JS, Browse NL. The etiology of the Klippel-Trenaunay syndrome. Ann Surg 1985;292:624.
3. Baskerville PA, Ackroyd JS, Lea Thomas M, et al. The Klippel-Trenaunay syndrome. Clinical, radiological and hemodynamic features and management. Br J Surg 1985;72:232.
4. Guidera KJ, Brinker MR, Koussoff BG, et al. Overgrowth management in Klippel-Trenaunay and Proteus syndromes. J Pediatr Orthop 1993;13:459.
5. Klippel M, Trenaunay P. Du naevus variquex ostephypertrophique. Arch Gen Med (Paris) 1900;185:641.
6. Lie JT. Pathology of angiodysplasia in Klippel-Trenaunay syndrome. Pathol Res Pract 1988;183:747.
7. Lindenauer SM. The Klippel-Trenaunay syndrome. Ann Surg 1965;162:303.
8. Moor JJ, Warren FH, Arensman RM. Klippel-Trenaunay syndrome: rarely a surgical disease. South Med J 1988;81:83.
9. McCarthy RE, Lytle JD, VanDevanter S. The use of total circulatory arrest in the surgery of giant hemangioma and Klippel-Trenaunay syndromes in neonates. Clin Orthop 1983;289:237.
10. McGrory BJ, Amadio PC, Dobyns JH, et al. Anomalies of the fingers and toes associated with Klippel-Trenaunay syndrome. J Bone Joint Surg [Am] 1991;73:1537.
11. Oyesiku NM, Gahm NJ, Goldman RL. Cerebral arteriovenous fistula in Klippel-Trenaunay-Weber syndrome. Dev Med Child Neurol 1988;30:245.
12. Pelleren D, Martelli H, Lutoiche X, et al. Congenital soft tissue dysplasia: a new malformation entity and concept. Prog Pediatr Surg 1989;22:1.
13. Stringel G, D'Astous J. Klippel-Trenaunay syndrome and other cases of lower limb hypertrophy: pediatric surgical implications. J Pediatr Surg 1987;22:645.
14. Yousem DM, Scott WW Jr, Fishman EK. Case report 440: Klippel-Trenaunay syndrome of right lower extremity. Skeletal Radiol 1987;16:652.

Hemangioma

15. Beninson J, Hurley JP. Hemolymphangioma in a neonate. Angiology 1988;39:1043.
16. Greenspan A, McGahan JP, Vogelsang P, et al. Imaging strategies in the evaluation of soft tissue hemangiomas of the extremities. Skeletal Radiol 1992;21:11.
17. Goldberg M. Hemangioma syndromes. In: Goldberg M, ed. The dysmorphic child. New York: Raven Press, 1987.
18. Kaplan EN. Vascular malformations of the extremities. In: Williams HB, ed. Symposium in vascular malformations and melanotic lesions. St. Louis: CV Mosby, 1983:144.
19. Levine C. Imaging of body asymmetry and hemihypertrophy. Crit Rev Diagn Imaging 1990;31:1.
20. McCarthy JE, Goldberg MJ, Zimbler S. Orthopaedic dysfunction in the blue rubber-bleb nevus syndrome. J Bone Joint Surg [Am] 1982;64:280.
21. Moroz B. Long term follow-up of hemangioma in children. In: Williams HB, ed. Symposium in vascular malformations and melanotic lesions. St. Louis: CV Mosby, 1983:162.

Lymphangioma

22. Gupta AK, et al. Mediastinal and skeletal lymphangiomas in a child. Pediatr Radiol 1991;21:129.
23. Heyden G, Knidblom LG, Nielson M. Disappearing bone disease. J Bone Joint Surg [Am] 1971;79:57.
24. Hoeffel JG, Marchal AC, Pierre E, Derelle J. Cystic lymphangioma of the pelvis in childhood. Br Radiol 1990;63:813.
25. Joseph J, Bartal EG. Disappearing bone disease. J Pediatr Orthop 1987;7:584.
26. Gorham LW, Stout AP. Massive osteolysis. J Bone Joint Surg [Am] 1955;37:985.
27. Jumbelic M, Fuerstien M, Dorfman HD. Solitary intraosseous lymphangioma. J Bone Joint Surg [Am] 1984;66:75.
28. Mendez AA, Keret D, Robertson W, MacEwen GD. Massive osteolysis of the femur. J Pediatr Orthop 1989;9:604.
29. Picault C, Comtet JJ, Imbert JC, Boyer JM. Surgical repair of extensive idiopathic osteolysis of the pelvic girdle. J Bone Joint Surg [Br] 1984;66:148.
30. Siegel MJ, Glazer HS, St. Amour TF, Rosenthal DD. Lymphgiomas in children: MRI imaging. Radiology 1989;170:467.
31. Stringel G. Hemangiomas and lymphangiomas. In: Ashcroft KW, Haldor TM, eds. Pediatric surgery. Philadelphia: WB Saunders, 1993.

Hemihypertrophy

32. Beals RK. Hemihypertrophy and hemihypotrophy. Clin Orthop 1992;166:200.

33. Bortel DT, Pritchett JW. Straight-line graphs for prediction of growth of the upper extremity. J Bone Joint Surg [Am] 1993;75:885.
34. Carvell JE, Chopin D. Infantile idiopathic scoliosis in hemihypertrophy with hemangiomatosis. J R Coll Surg Edinb 1984;29:321.
35. Cavaliere RG, McElgun TM. Macrodactyly and hemihypertrophy: a new surgical procedure. J Foot Surg 1988;27:226.
36. Cremin BJ, Viljoen DL, Wynchank S, Beighton P. The Proteus syndrome: MR and radiological features. Pediatr Radiol 1987;17:486.
37. Green DM, Breslow NE, Beckwith JB, Norkool P. Screening of children with hemihypertrophy, aniridia and Beckwith-Wiedemann syndrome in patients with Wilms tumor. Med Pediatr Oncol 1993;21:188.
38. Goldberg MJ. Syndromes of overgrowth. In: Goldberg M, ed. The dysmorphic child. New York: Raven Press, 1987.
39. Janik JS, Steeler RA. Delayed onset of hemihypertrophy in Wilms' tumor. J Pediatr Surg 1976;11:581.
40. Levine CL. The imaging of body asymmetry and hemihypertrophy. Crit Rev Diagn Imaging 1990;31:1.
41. MacEwen GD, Case JL. Congenital hemihypertrophy. Clin Orthop 1967;50:147.
42. McCullough CJ, Kenwright J. The prognosis in congenital lower limb hypertrophy. Acta Orthop Scand 1979;50:307.
43. Nudleman K, Andermann E. Hemi-3 syndrome. Brain 1984;107:533.
44. Pappas AM, Nehme AM. Leg length discrepancy associated with hypertrophy. Clin Orthop 1979;144:198.
45. Phelan EM, Carty HM, Kalos S. Generalized enchondromatosis associated with hemangiomas, soft tissue calcifications and hemihypertrophy. Br J Radiol 1986;59:69.
46. Samlaska CP, Levin SW, James WD, et al. Proteus syndrome. Arch Dermatol 1989;125:1109.
47. Shapiro F. Developmental patterns in lower extremity length discrepancies. J Bone Joint Surg [Am] 1992;64:639.
48. Viljoen D, Pearn J, Beighton P. Manifestations and natural history of idiopathic hemihypertrophy. Clin Genet 1984;26:81.

Localized Gigantism and Macrodactyly

49. Ackland MK, Uthoff HK. Idiopathic localized gigantism: a 26-year follow-up. J Pediatr Orthop 1988;8:618.
50. Barsky AJ. Macrodactyly. J Bone Joint Surg [Am] 1967;49:1255.
51. Ben-Bassat M, Casper J, Laron Z. Congenital macrodactyly. J Bone Joint Surg [Br] 1966;48:359.
52. Dennyson WG, Bear JN, Bhoola KD. Macrodactyly in the foot. J Bone Joint Surg [Br] 1977;59:355.
53. Herring JA, Tolo VT. Instructional case: macrodactyly. J Pediatr Orthop 1984;4:503.
54. Stevens PM. Toe deformities. In: Drennan JC, ed. The child's foot and ankle. New York: Raven Press, 1984.

Congenital Constriction Band Syndrome

55. Abel M, McFarland R. Hair and thread constriction in infants. J Bone Joint Surg [Am] 1993;75:915.
56. Askins G, Ger E. Congenital constriction band syndrome. J Pediatr Orthop 1988;8:461.
57. Bass HN, Caldwell S, Brooks BS. Michelin tire baby syndrome. Am J Med Genet 1993;45:370.
58. Bourne MH, Klassen RA. Congenital annular constricting bands. J Bone Joint Surg 1987;7:218.
59. Greene WB. One-stage release of congenital circumferential constriction bands. J Bone Joint Surg [Am] 1993;75:650.
60. Keane BH, Tucker HA. Etiologic concepts and pathologic aspects of ainhum. Arch Pathol 1986;41:639.
61. Masada K, Tsuyuguchhi Y, Kawabata H, et al. Terminal limb congenital malformation: analysis of 523 cases. J Pediatr Orthop 1986;6:340.
62. Morrissy RT. Release of congenital constriction band. In: Morrissy RT, ed. Atlas of pediatric orthopaedic surgery. Philadelphia: JB Lippincott, 1990.
63. Moses JM, Flatt AE, Cooper RR. Annular constricting bands. J Bone Joint Surg [Am] 1979;61:562.
64. Patterson TJS. Congenital ring constrictions. Br J Plast Surg 1961:14:1.
65. Streeter GL. Focal deficiencies in fetal tissues and their relationship to intrauterine amputation. Contrib Embryol 1930;22:1.
66. Tada K, Yonenobu K, Swanson AB. Congenital constriction band syndrome. J Pediatr Orthop 1984;4:726.
67. VanAllen MI, Siegel-Bartelt J, Dixon J, et al. Constriction bands and limb reduction defects in two newborns. Am J Med Genet 1992;44:598.
68. Zionts LE, Osterkamp JA, Crawford TO, Harvey JP. Congenital annular bands in identical twins. J Bone Joint Surg [Am] 1984;56:450.

Camurati-Engelman Syndrome

69. Camurati M. Dilulraro caso di osteite simmetrica ereditaria degli arti inferriori. Chir Organi Mov 1992;6:662.
70. Clawson DK, Loop JW. Progressive diaphyseal dysplasia (Engelman's disease). J Bone Joint Surg [Am] 1964;46:143.
71. Hundley JD, Wilson FC. Progressive diaphyseal dysplasia: review of the literature and report of seven cases in one family. J Bone Joint Surg [Am] 1973;55:461.
72. Johnston CE. Progressive diaphyseal dysplasia. Orthopaedics 1984;7:133.
73. Kaftori JK, Kleinhaus A, Naveh Y. Progressive diaphyseal dysplasia: radiographic follow-up and CT findings. Radiology 1987;164:772.
74. Naveh Y, Kaftori JK. Progressive diaphyseal dysplasia: genetics and clinical and radiologic manifestations. Pediatrics 1984;74:399.
75. Stenzler S, Grogan DP, Frenchman SM, et al. Progressive diaphyseal dysplasia presenting as neuromuscular disease. J Pediatr Orthop 1989;9:463.
76. Tachdjian MO. Progressive diaphyseal dysplasia. In: Tachdjian MO, ed. Pediatric orthopaedics. Philadelphia: WB Saunders, 1990:804.

Melorheostosis

77. Atar D, Lehmann WB, Grant AD, Strongwater AM. The Ilizarov apparatus for treatment of melorheostosis. Clin Orthop 1992;281:163.
78. Buckley SL, Skinner S, James P, Ashley RK. Focal scleroderma in children. J Pediatr Orthop 1993;13:784.
79. Fryns JP, et al. Melorheostosis in a 3-year old girl. Acta Pediatr Belg 1980;33:185.
80. Ippolito V, Mirra JM, Motta C, et al. Case report 771: melorheostosis in association with desmoid tumor. Skeletal Radiol 1993;22:284.
81. Leri A. Une nouvelle observation de melorheostose: etude clinique, anatomique et experimentale. Bull Mem Soc Med Hosp Paris 1930;54:1210.
82. Younge D, Drummond D, Herring J, Cruess RL. Melorheostosis in children. Clinical features and natural history. J Bone Joint Surg [Br] 1979;61:415.

Osteopoikilosis

83. Benli IT, Akalin S, Boysan E, et al. Epidemiological, clinical and radiological aspects of osteopoikilosis. J Bone Joint Surg [Br] 1992;74:504.
84. Chigira M, Kati K, Mishio K, Shinozaki T. Symmetry of bone lesions in osteopoikilosis. Acta Orthop Scand 1991;62:495.
85. Walker GF. Mixed sclerosing bone dystrophies. J Bone Joint Surg [Br] 1964;46:546.
86. Walpole IR, Manners PJ. Clinical considerations in Buschke-Ollendorf syndrome. Clin Genet 1990;37:59.

Osteopathia Striata

87. Fairbanks HAT. Osteopathia striata. J Bone Joint Surg [Br] 1950;32:117.
88. Greenspan A. Sclerosing bone dysplasias. A target-site approach. Skeletal Radiol 1991;20:561.

Congenital Pseudarthrosis of the Tibia

89. Anderson KS. Congenital pseudarthrosis of the leg. J Bone Joint Surg [Am] 1976;58:657.
90. Anderson DJ, Schoenecker PL, Sheridan JJ, et al. Use of an intramedullary rod for the treatment of congenital pseudarthrosis of the tibia. J Bone Joint Surg [Am] 1992;74:161.
91. Bassett CAL, Schink-Ascani M. Long term pulsed-electromagnetic field results in congenital pseudarthrosis. Calcif Tissue Int 1991;49:216.
92. Boyd HB. Pathology and natural history of congenital pseudarthrosis of the tibia. Clin Orthop 1982;166:5.
93. Bradish CF, Davies SJM, Malone M. Tibia vara due to focal fibrocartilagonous dysplasia. J Bone Joint Surg [Br] 1988;70:106.
94. Briner J, Yunis E. Ultrastructure of congenital pseudarthrosis of the tibia. Arch Pathol 1973;95:97.
95. Crossett LS, Beaty JH, Betz RR, et al. Congenital pseudarthrosis of the tibia: long term follow-up study. Clin Orthop 1989;245:16.
96. Dormans JP, Krajbich JI, Zuker R, Demuynk M. Congenital pseudarthrosis of the tibia: treatment with free vascularized fibula grafts. J Pediatr Orthop 1990;10:623.
97. Fabry G, Lammens J, van Melkebeek J, Stuyck J. Treatment of congenital pseudarthrosis of the fibula with the Ilizarov technique. J Pediatr Orthop 1988;8:67.
98. Fern ED, Stockley I, Bell MJ. Extending intramedullary rods in congenital pseudarthrosis of the tibia. J Bone Joint Surg [Br] 1990;72:1073.
99. Goldberg I, Maor P, Yosipovitch Z. Congenital pseudarthrosis of the tibia treated by a pedicled vascularized graft of the ipsilateral fibula. J Bone Joint Surg [Am] 1988;70:1396.
100. Jacobson ST, Crawford AH, Millar EA, Steel HH. The Symes amputation in patients with congenital pseudarthrosis of the tibia. J Bone Joint Surg [Am] 1983;65:533.
101. Jupiter JB, Palumbo M, Nunley J, et al. Secondary reconstruction after vascularized fibula transfer. J Bone Joint Surg [Am] 1993;75:1442.
102. Manoylovic R, Cheng JC, Levinsohn DG, Gordon L. Free vascularized fibular transfer in the management of congenital pseudarthrosis of the tibia. Microsurgery 1991;12:170.
103. Morrissy RT, Riseborough EJ, Hall JE. Congenital pseudarthrosis of the tibia. J Bone Joint Surg [Br] 1981;63:367.
104. Orstavik RH, Tangsrud SE, Nordshus T, et al. Orofaciodigital syndrome type I in a girl with unilateral tibial pseudarthrosis. J Med Genet 1992;29:827.
105. Paterson DC, Simonis RB. Electrical stimulation in the treatment of congenital pseudarthrosis of the tibia. J Bone Joint Surg [Br] 1985;67:454.
106. Plawecki S, Carpentier E, Lascombes P, et al. Treatment of congenital pseudarthrosis of the tibia by the Ilizarov method. J Pediatr Orthop 1990;19:788.
107. Roach JW, Shindell R, Green NE. Late-onset pseudarthrosis of the dysplastic tibia. J Bone Joint Surg [Am] 1993;75:1593.
108. Sofield HA. Congenital pseudarthrosis of the tibia. Clin Orthop 1971;76:33.
109. Tachdjian MO. Congenital pseudarthrosis of the tibia. In: Tachdjian MO, ed. Pediatric orthopaedics. Philadelphia: WB Saunders, 1990:656.
110. Strong ML, Wong-Chung J. Prophylactic bypass graft of the prepseudarthrotic tibia in neurofibromatosis. J Pediatr Orthop 1991;11:757.
111. Weiland AJ, Weiss AP, Moore JR, Tolo VT. Vascularized fibular grafts in the treatment of congenital pseudarthrosis of the tibia. J Bone Joint Surg [Am] 1990;72:654.
112. Wiltse LL. Valgus deformity of the ankle: a sequelae to acquired or congenital anomalies of the fibula. J Bone Joint Surg [Am] 1972;54:595.

Congenital Pseudarthrosis of the Fibula

113. DalMonte A, Danzelli O, Sudanese A. Congenital pseudarthrosis of the fibula. J Pediatr Orthop 1987;7:14.
114. Dooley BJ, Menelaus MB, Paterson DC. Congenital pseudarthrosis and bowing of the fibula. J Bone Joint Surg [Br] 1974;56:739.
115. Langenshkiold A. Pseudarthrosis of the fibula and progressive valgus deformity of the ankle in children. J Bone Joint Surg [Am] 1967;49:463.

Congenital Pseudarthrosis of the Clavicle

116. Bargar WL, Marcus RF, Ittleman FP. Late thoracic outlet syndrome secondary to pseudarthrosis of the clavicle. J Trauma 1984;24:857.
117. Gardner IE. The embryology of the clavicle. Clin Orthop 1968;58:9.
118. Grogan DP, Love SM, Guidera KJ, Ogden JA. Operative treatment of congenital pseudarthrosis of the clavicle. J Pediatr Orthop 1991;11:176.
119. Lloyd-Roberts GC, Apley AG, Pyrford OR. Reflections on the etiology of congenital pseudarthrosis of the clavicle. J Bone Joint Surg [Br] 1975;57:24.
120. Morin LR, Fossey FP, Besselievre A, et al. Congenital pseudarthrosis of the clavicle. Acta Obstet Gynecol Scand 1993;72:120.
121. Laws JL, Pallis C. Spinal deformities in neurofibromatosis. J Bone Joint Surg [Br] 1963;45:674.
122. Schoenecker PL, John GE, Howard B, Capelli AM. Congenital pseudarthrosis of the clavicle. Orthop Rev 1992;21:855.
123. Schnall SB, King JD, Marrero G. Congenital pseudarthrosis of the clavicle: a review of the literature and surgical results of six cases. J Pediatr Orthop 1988;8:316.
124. Tachdjian MO. Congenital pseudarthrosis of the clavicle. In: Tachdjian MO, ed. Pediatric orthopaedics. Philadelphia: WB Saunders, 1991.

Dysplasia Epiphysealis Hemimelica (Trevor Disease)

125. Azouz RM, Slomic AM, Marton D. The variable manifestations of dysplasia epiphysealis hemimelia. J Pediatr Radiol 1985;15:44.

126. Fairbank TJ. Dysplasia epiphysealis hemimelia (tarso-epiphysial aclasis). J Bone Joint Surg [Br] 1956;38:237.
127. Graves SC, Kuester DJ, Richardson EG. Dysplasia epiphysealis hemimelica presenting in peroneal spastic flatfoot. Foot Ankle 1991;12:55.
128. Keret D, Spatz D, Caro P, Mason DE. Dysplasia epiphysealis hemimelica: diagnosis and treatment. J Pediatr Orthop 1992;12:365.
129. Kettelkamp DB, Campbell CJ, Bonfiglio M. Dysplasia epiphysealis hemimelica. A report of fifteen cases and a review of the literature. J Bone Joint Surg [Am] 1966;48:746.
130. Maylack FH, Manske PR, Strecker WB. Dysplasia epiphysealis hemimelica at the metacarpophalangeal joint. J Hand Surg [Am] 1988;13:916.
131. Mendez AA, Keret D, MacEwan GD. Isolated dysplasia epiphysealis hemimelica of the hip joint. J Bone Joint Surg [Am] 1988;70:921.
132. Trevor D. Tarso-epiphysial aclasis: a congenital error of epiphyseal development. J Bone Joint Surg [Br] 1950;32:204.

Fibrodysplasia Ossificans Progressiva

133. Bruni L, Giammaria P, Tozzi MC, et al. Fibrodysplasia ossificans progressiva. Acta Paediatr Scand 1990;79:994.
134. Cohen RB, Hahn GV, Tabas JA, et al. Natural history of heterotopic ossification in patients who have fibrodysplasia ossificans progressiva. J Bone Joint Surg [Am] 1993;75:215.
135. Connor JM, Evans DAP. Fibrodysplasia ossificans progressiva: clinical features and natural history of 34 patients. J Bone Joint Surg [Br] 1982;64:76.
136. Fairbanks HAT. Myositis ossificans progressiva. J Bone Joint Surg [Br] 1950;32:108.
137. Hoeksema AF, Postuma A. A remarkable transport device for a fibrodysplasia ossificans progressive patient. Prosthet Orthot Int 1992;16:64.
138. Kaplan FS, McClusky W, Hahn G, et al. Genetic transmission of fibrodysplasia ossificans progressiva: report of a family. J Bone Joint Surg [Am] 1993;75:1214.
139. Kaplan FS, Tabas JA, Gannon FH, et al. The histopathology of fibrodysplasia ossificans progressiva. J Bone Joint Surg [Am] 1993;75:220.
140. Rogers JG, Geho WB. Fibrodysplasia ossificans progressiva. J Bone Joint Surg [Am] 1979;61:909.

Myositis Ossificans

141. Ackerman LV. Extraosseous localized non-neoplastic bone and cartilage formation. J Bone Joint Surg [Am] 1958;40:279.
142. Carlson WO, Klassen RA. Myositis ossificans of the upper extremity: a long-term follow-up. J Pediatr Orthop 1984;4:693.
143. Clapton WK, James CL, Morris LL, et al. Myositis ossificans in childhood. Pathology 1992;24:311.
144. Cushner FD, Morwessel RM. Myositis ossificans traumatica. Orthop Rev 1992;21:1319.
145. DeSmet AA, Norris MA, Fisher DR. Magnetic resonance imaging of myositis ossificans. Skeletal Radiol 1992;21:503.
146. Heifetz SA, Galliana CA, DeRosa GP. Myositis (fasciitis) ossificans in an infant. Pediatr Pathol 1992;12:223.
147. Illes T, Dubousset J, Szendroi M, Fischer J. Characterization of bone-forming cells in post-traumatic myositis ossificans by lectins. Pathol Res Pract 1992;188:172.
148. Jackson DW, Feagin JA. Quadriceps contusion in young athletes: relationship of severity of injury to treatment and prognosis. J Bone Joint Surg [Am] 1973;55:95.
149. Krandorf MJ, Meis JM, Jelinek JS. Myositis ossificans: MR appearance with radiologic pathologic correlation. AJR 1991;157:1243.
150. Merkow SJ, St. Clair HS, Goldberg MJ. Myositis ossificans masquerading as sepsis. J Pediatr Orthop 1985;5:601.
151. Michelsson JE, Granroth G, Andersson LC. Myositis ossificans following forcible manipulation of the leg. A rabbit model for the study of heterotopic bone formation. J Bone Joint Surg [Am] 1980;62:811.
152. Ogilvie-Harris DJ, Fornasier VL. Pseudomalignant myositis ossificans. Heterotopic new bone formation without a history of trauma. J Bone Joint Surg [Am] 1980;62:1274.
153. Roser B, Herrlin K, Rydholm A, et al. Pseudomalignant myositis ossificans. Acta Orthop Scand 1989;60:457.

The Osteochondroses

154. Carlson CS, Neuten DJ, Richardson DC. Ischemic necrosis of cartilage in spontaneous and experimental lesions of osteochondrosis. J Orthop Res 1991;9:317.
155. Mubarak SJ. Osteochondrosis of the lateral cuneiform. J Bone Joint Surg 1992; 74:285.
156. Ruch DS, Poehling GG. Arthroscopic treatment of Panner's disease. Clin Sports Med 1992;10:629.
157. Siffert RS. Classification of the osteochondrosis. Clin Orthop 1981;158:10.
158. Tallroth K, Schlenzka D. Spinal stenosis subsequent to juvenile lumbar osteochondrosis. Skeletal Radiol 1986:19:203.

Quadriceps Fibrosis

159. Gunn DR. Contracture of the quadriceps muscle. A discussion on the etiology and relationship to recurrent dislocation of the patella. J Bone Joint Surg [Br] 1964;46:492.
160. Karlen A. Congenital fibrosis of the vastus intermedius muscle. J Bone Joint Surg [Br] 1984;46:488.
161. Williams PF. Quadriceps contractures. J Bone Joint Surg [Br] 1968;49:389.

Reflex Sympathetic Dystrophy

162. Berde CB, Sethna NF, Micheli LJ. A technique for continuous lumbar sympathetic blockade for severe reflex sympathetic dystrophy in children and adolescents. Anesth Analg 1988;67(Suppl):514.
163. Bernstein BH, Singsen BH, Kent TJ, et al. Reflex sympathetic dystrophy in children. J Pediatr 1978;43:211.
164. Dietz FR, Matthews KD, Montgomery WJ. Reflex sympathetic dystrophy in children. Clin Orthop 1990;258:225.
165. Intenzo C, Kim S, Mellin J, et al. Scantigraphic patterns of the reflex sympathetic dystrophy syndrome of the lower extremities. Clin Nucl Med 1989;14:657.
166. Lynch ME. Psychological aspects of reflex sympathetic dystrophy. Pain 1992;49:337.
167. Pillemer FG, Micheli LJ. Psychological considerations in youth sports. Clin Sports Med 1988;7:679.
168. Schutzer SF, Gossling HR. Current concepts review: the treatment of reflex sympathetic dystrophy. J Bone Joint Surg [Am] 1984;66:625.
169. Silber JJ, Magid M. Reflex sympathetic dystrophy in children and adolescents. Am J Dev Child 1988;142:1325.
170. Wilder RT, Berde CB, Wolohan M, et al. Reflex sympathetic dystrophy in children. J Bone Joint Surg [Am] 1992;74:910.

Chapter 10

Diseases Related to the Hematopoietic System

Walter B. Greene

Disorders of Erythrocytes
  Iron Deficiency Anemia
  Diamond-Blackfan Anemia
  Fanconi Anemia
  Sickle Cell Disorders
  Thalassemia
Disorders of Granulocytes
  Schwachman-Diamond Syndrome
  Chronic Granulomatous Disease
Disorders of Lymphocytes and the Immune System
  X-Linked Agammaglobulinemia
  Cartilage-Hair Hypoplasia
  Acquired Immunodeficiency Syndrome

Disorders of the Monocyte-Macrophage System
  Gaucher Disease
  Neimann-Pick Disease
  Langerhans Cell Histiocytosis
Disorders of Hemostasis
  Thrombocytopenia With Absent Radius Syndrome
  Hemophilia
Leukemia

The hematopoietic system includes the circulating blood, the bone marrow, the spleen, the lymph nodes, and the reticuloendothelial cells scattered throughout the body. The multiple cells that compose the hematopoietic system lead to a large number and variety of disorders.[1,2] This chapter focuses on pediatric disorders of the hematopoietic system that alter the function and development of the spine and the extremities (Table 10-1).

DISORDERS OF ERYTHROCYTES

The erythrocyte, with its unique hemoglobin molecule, delivers oxygen from the lungs to the tissue and transports carbon dioxide in the reverse direction. The intravascular journey of an erythrocyte is approximately 175 miles in its normal life span of 120 days. Any process that impairs production of the erythrocyte, alters the structure of the erythrocyte, or disrupts the function of the hemoglobin molecule causes a reduced number or a reduced life span of the erythrocyte, or both. Anemia is the common resultant.

Iron Deficiency Anemia

Iron deficiency anemia is the most common nutritional deficiency in the western world and the most common cause of anemia worldwide.[5,8,10] The peak incidence characteristically is between 6 months and 3 years of age and during adolescence, age groups that are characterized by rapid growth and an expanding erythrocyte mass. With a mild anemia the child is asymptomatic, but lethargy, easy fatigability, irritability, and growth retardation of weight are observed with a severe hemoglobin deficiency.[8] Skeletal changes reflect the severity of the anemia and the degree of marrow hyperplasia.[7] The skull, in particular, may

TABLE 10-1   Diseases of the Hematopoietic System Associated with Skeletal Changes in Children

Disorders of erythrocytes
  Impaired production
    Iron deficiency anemia
    Congenital hypoplastic anemia (Diamond-Blackfan syndrome)
    Fanconi aplastic anemia
  Hemoglobinopathy
    Sickle cell disease
      SS disease
      SC disease
      Sβ disease
    β-Thalassemia
Disorders of granulocytes
  Hereditary neutropenia
    Schwachman-Diamond syndrome
  Disorders of granulocyte function
    Chronic granulomatous disease
Disorders of lymphocytes and the immune system
  Dysfunction of B cells
    X-Linked agammaglobulinemia
  Dysfunction of T cells
    Cartilage-hair hypoplasia
    Acquired immunodeficiency syndrome
Disorders of the monocyte-macrophage system
  Lysosomal storage disease
    Gaucher disease
    Niemann-Pick disease
  Langherhans cell histiocytosis and eosinophilic granuloma
Disorders of hemostasis
  Disorders of platelets
    Thrombocytopenia with absent radius syndrome
  Disorders of coagulation factors
    Hemophilia
Leukemia

show widening of the diploic space with striations. Skeletal abnormalities and the low body weight will resolve following iron supplement therapy, but developmental deficiencies secondary to chronic anemia in young children are not fully reversible.[6,10,13]

Risk factors for iron deficiency anemia in young children include prematurity, low socioeconomic status, introduction of cow's milk before age 6 months, and unfortified formulas.[6,8,10] Recognition of these risk factors and the Supplemental Food Program for Women, Infants and Children (WIC) has greatly reduced the incidence of anemia in young children in the United States.[3,9,13,14–16] Some authors now question routine screening of all infants for anemia.[4]

Girls are the group at risk during adolescence. The prevalence of iron deficiency in this group is 6% to 8% and has not changed during the past 10 to 15 years.[3,5] Risk factors for this group include poor nutrition, increased duration or frequency of menstrual flow, chronic use of certain analgesic medications, and prolonged training for long distance running.[11]

The orthopaedic surgeon most likely will encounter iron deficiency anemia during the preoperative evaluation of another problem; however, obtaining preoperative hemoglobin levels on all pediatric patients is not necessary.[12] I obtain this test on adolescent girls who have started menstruating or who have other risk factors, on infants at risk who did not receive adequate supplementation, and on any patient whose history or physical examination suggests anemia. Hemoglobin levels of less than 11 g/dL in infants and less than 12 g/dL in adolescents should be referred for further evaluation and treatment. Patients who have mild anemia during infancy and adolescence can be evaluated by simple laboratory screening studies and a 4-week therapeutic trial of iron. An increase of 1 g/dL in the hemoglobin concentration is considered diagnostic of iron deficiency anemia.[8,10] Severe anemia, or anemia occurring during the middle period of growth, will require more extensive laboratory studies to exclude other causes of hemoglobin deficiency.

Diamond-Blackfan Anemia

The hematologic manifestations of Diamond-Blackfan anemia (i.e., congenital hypoplastic anemia) are not apparent at birth. Associated malformations, however, may be obvious. Anomalies of the thumb are the most common skeletal abnormality.[17,18,22,24,26] Alter[19] reviewed 270 patients reported in the literature and noted a 9% incidence of thumb anomalies, including 12 cases of triphalangeal, 7 duplicated or bifid, 2 subluxed, and 3 hypoplastic thumbs. Incomplete radial hemimelia has been reported,[23,24] but forearm deficits are uncommon in Diamond-Blackfan anemia. Klippel-Feil syndrome also is seen, and in Alter's review,[19] 6% of the patients had a short or webbed neck. Cervical spine and hand abnormalities may be present in the same patient, and Greenspan and colleagues[22] described a patient with Klippel-Feil syndrome, Sprengel deformity, an omovertebral bone, and hypoplasia of the first ray of the hand. Other abnormalities seen in patients with Diamond-Blackfan anemia include low birth weight (11%), small jaw and cleft palate (6%), congenital heart disease (4%), and renal anomalies (3%).

Infants with Diamond-Blackfan syndrome, although apparently healthy at birth, develop the insidious onset of listlessness, irritability, and pallor, usually by the age of 2 to 3 months or later in the first year of life.[19–21,23,25] Sometimes, a patient will not develop anemia until the age of 6 years. Laboratory studies demonstrate a striking normocytic anemia with hemoglobin levels of 3 to 4 g/dL. Platelet and white blood counts are usually normal. Marrow aspiration reveals virtual absence of nucleated erythroid cells but no depression of granulocyte or platelet precursors. The etiology and genetics of Diamond-Blackfan anemia are uncertain.

The first line of therapy is corticosteroids,[19,21,23,25] and the overall response rate is approximately 67%. The most common pattern of the responders is a long-term dependence on steroid medications but at a reduced dosage. Supportive transfusions are necessary for patients who do not respond to steroids or who develop side effects from the medications. With repeated transfusions, chelation therapy minimizes the complications associated with hemosiderosis. Experience with bone marrow transplantation is limited, but the initial results are not promising. In a series of four patients, two died and one developed chronic problems with graft-versus-host disease.[27]

Fanconi Anemia

Fanconi anemia is an autosomal recessive disorder that ultimately causes pancytopenia.[19,29,30,32] Congenital anomalies as well as breakages, gaps, and constrictions in chromosomes are common. The chromosomal aberrations do not correlate with the presence of congenital anomalies or the severity of the anemia, but they may permit prenatal diagnosis.[28]

Onset of the pancytopenia is delayed and averages 6 to 7 years of age for boys and 8 to 9 years of age for girls (range, birth–35 years).[19,29,31] Thrombocytopenia is usually the first manifestation. Granulocytopenia and anemia follow in that order. If treatment is limited to blood transfusions, 80% of patients die within 2 years. Steroids and androgens may result in long-term remissions. Leukemia may develop and rarely may occur before the onset of the pancytopenia. Bone marrow transplantation is an option but should be used with caution because these patients have a greater risk of developing a second malignancy, particularly leukemia.[19]

Many of the anomalies observed in patients with Fanconi anemia, similar to those with Diamond-Blackfan syndrome, are obvious at birth. Approximately half of the patients have low birth weight and growth retardation with short stature, and a relatively short trunk is observed in 50% to 75%.[19,30,32] Café-au-lait spots are a common skin abnormality, occurring in approximately 80% of patients. The most common skeletal anomaly is a radial deficiency of the hand or forearm.[30,31] In a review of 68 patients with Fanconi anemia, Minagi and Steinbach[32] recorded 9 with radial hemimelia and 25 with deficiencies limited to the hand, either hypoplasia or absence of the thumb. Other skeletal abnormalities are less frequent and include Klippel-Feil syndrome, Sprengel deformity, hip dislocation, and syndactyly of the second and third toes. Renal abnormalities, mental retardation, and malformation of the ears also are seen in Fanconi anemia.

Sickle Cell Disorders

Sickle cell disorders include patients homozygous for hemoglobin S (SS), patients with sickle cell–C (SC) disease, those with sickle cell β-thalassemia, and those who have other rarer conditions in which hemoglobin S is combined with another abnormal β-globulin chain. People who are heterozygous for hemoglobin S and a normal β-globulin chain have no clinical problems under physiologic conditions and may participate in athletic events without restriction.

Hemoglobin S results from an abnormality of the β-globulin gene on chromosome 11 that causes substitution of valine for glutamic acid at the 6th codon from the amino-terminus.[70,74] The gene for hemoglobin S is common in the black race, occurring in about 8% of African-American people living in the United States.[69,78] In central Africa, 40% of some ethnic groups carry this gene.[70] The frequency of patients who are homozygous SS (i.e., those with sickle cell anemia) is much less and was 1.4 per thousand in a study of 249,000 African-American people.[78]

Hemoglobin C occurs when lysine is substituted for the same glutamic acid affected in hemoglobin S.[70,74] Patients heterozygous for one HbS gene and one HbC gene have SC disease. This disorder is the second most common type of sickle cell disease in the United States.[78] Patients with SC disease have similar but less frequent complications compared with patients with SS disease.

The β-thalassemia gene results in reduced synthesis of the β-globulin polypeptide. Patients heterozygous for hemoglobin S and β-thalassemia have clinical manifestations of sickle cell disease that depend on the output of the β-thalassemia gene.[74] If no HbA is produced, these patients are listed as Sβ^0 and have a clinical course comparable to patients with SS disease. If there is some production of HbA from the β-thalassemia gene, the patients are classified as Sβ^+ and have a milder clinical course similar to that of SC disease.

Sickle cell disorders cause hemolytic anemia and vasoocclusion.[58,61,71,73,74] Under conditions of low oxygen tension or reduced blood flow, HgbS polymerizes and soluble HbS is changed to a gel of intertwined fibers. As a result, the erythrocyte becomes distorted, fragile, and rapidly destroyed. The paradox is that sickle cells are not only more fragile but are relatively rigid and more viscous. Therefore, in addition to increased hemolysis, these erythrocytes clog small blood vessels and infarct tissues. Other factors, such as cellular dehydration and erythrocyte adhesion to the endothelium, also may be important factors in the vasoocclusion.

Musculoskeletal problems in sickle cell disorders result directly or indirectly from vasoocclusion and include dactylitis, osteomyelitis, avascular necrosis, septic arthritis, and reactive arthritis. The hemolytic anemia in these patients causes erythroid hyperplasia of the bone marrow with resultant increased size of the medullary spaces, osteoporosis, thinning of the long bone cortices, and biconcavity of the vertebra (Fig. 10-1). Fortunately, this aspect of sickle cell disorders usually has limited clinical significance.

Considerable heterogeneity is observed in patients with sickle cell disease. For example, painful crises occur every few days in some patients, whereas others have less than 1 painful crisis per year. The basis of this heterogeneity is not well understood but probably involves a variety of genetic and environmental factors. Patients who inherit a gene for hereditary persistence of fetal hemoglobin clearly have a mild disease, and for that reason hydroxyurea, a drug that elevates hemoglobin F levels, is under investigation.[71] The concomitant presence of α-thalassemia genes in patients with HgbSS causes the erythrocytes to be smaller and lighter. These patients have improved hematologic parameters (i.e., higher hemoglobin levels and fewer reticulocytes) but may be at greater risk for vasoocclusive disorders.[70]

Dactylitis, or hand-foot syndrome, is secondary to infarction of a bone in the hand or foot and frequently is the first clinical manifestation seen after hemoglobin F has been replaced by hemoglobin S. The typical case is of a child younger than 2 years of age who presents with an acutely swollen and tender hand or foot.[47,55,83,89] In a prospective study, Stevens and colleagues[83] reported a 45% incidence of dactylitis, with 41% of the affected patients demonstrating recurrent episodes until 4 years of age. This problem ceases with the disappearance of hematopoietic marrow in the hands and feet, and no series has reported dactylitis in patients older than 6 years of age.

Dactylitis may be difficult to differentiate from osteomyelitis and, therefore, appropriate treatment of osteomyelitis may be delayed (Fig. 10-2).[36,50,52] The temperature in patients with dactylitis may be normal, but it is frequently greater than 38°C and rarely, greater than 39°C.[80,89] The leukocyte count may be normal or elevated. Radiographic findings are similar in dactylitis and osteomyelitis, with initial x-ray films demonstrating soft tissue swelling and subsequent examinations characterized by periosteal elevation, subperiosteal bone reaction, bone lysis, and ultimately bone reformation.[47] Technetium bone scans have not proven as effective in differentiating osteomyelitis from dactylitis.[77] A temperature greater than 39°C and an unusual degree of pain should raise questions of osteomyelitis

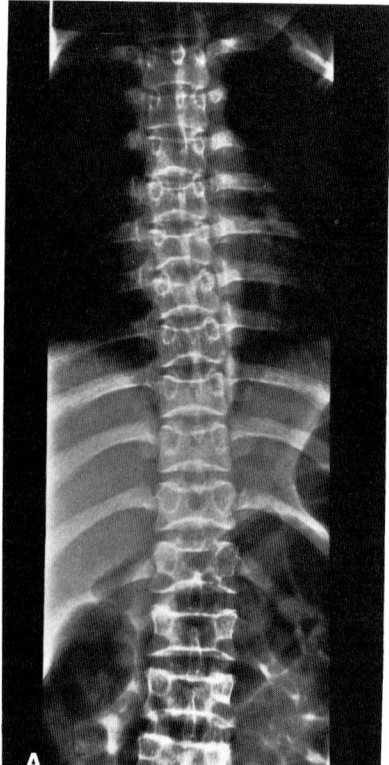
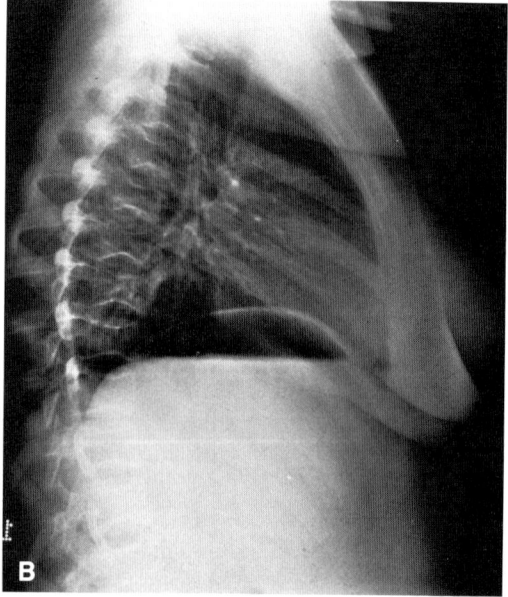

FIGURE 10-1. Sixteen-year-old girl with sickle cell anemia. Anteroposterior and lateral radiographs of the spine show the typical biconcavity of multiple vertebrae.

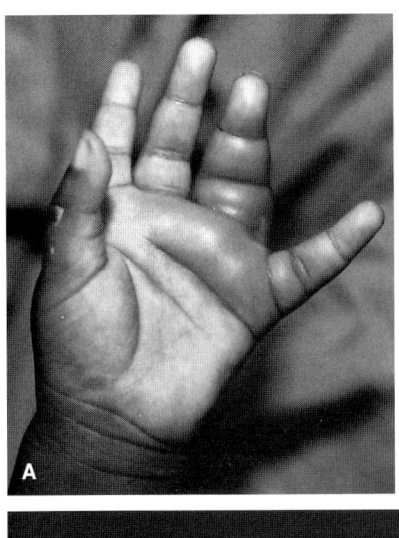
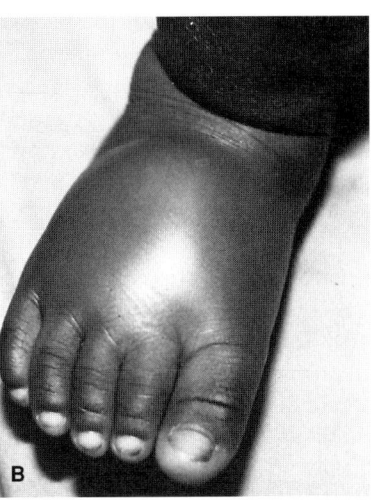
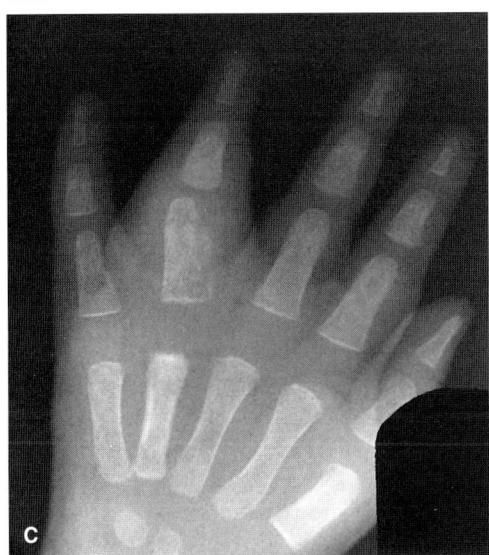
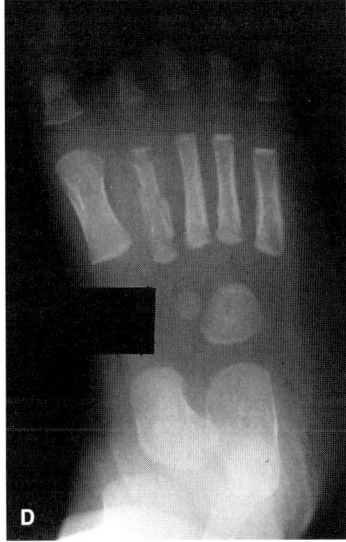

FIGURE 10-2. Osteomyelitis in a 7-month-old boy with sickle cell anemia. Patient presented with swelling of the hand and foot. Initial diagnosis was dactylitis. Because of persistent swelling and elevated temperature, aspiration was performed 48 hours after admission. Purulent material was obtained, and cultures demonstrated *Salmonella* organisms. Antibiotic therapy and surgical drainage of the hand and foot successfully resolved the infection. (**A**) Forty-eight hours after admission, the hand shows marked swelling in the region of the ring finger. (**B**) Forty-eight hours after admission, there is swelling on the dorsum of the foot. (**C**) Anteroposterior radiograph of the hand on the 15th hospital day. (**D**) Anteroposterior radiograph of the foot on the 15th hospital day. Osteolysis and periosteal elevation is noted in the proximal phalanx of the ring finger and second metatarsal. Although this patient had osteomyelitis, the radiographic appearance also is consistent with a healing dactylitis. (From Greene WB, MacMillian CW. Salmonella osteomyelitis and hand/foot syndrome in a child with sickle cell anemia. J Pediatr Orthop 1987;7:716.)

in a child who presents with apparent dactylitis.[52] Aspiration of the affected bone usually will differentiate these two clinical problems.

Sickle cell crises are the most common cause of extremity pain in patients with sickle cell disease. These episodes typically begin after a child is 3 to 4 years of age. In a study of 3578 patients, the average rate of crisis requiring medical treatment was 0.8/year in SS disease, 1.0/year in Sβ^0, and 0.4/year in SC and Sβ^+.[75] An elevated fetal hemoglobin level was associated with a lower rate of crises. Considerable variation, however, occurs within groups, and 39% of the SS patients recorded no crisis.

A sickle cell crisis results from a localized area of bone marrow infarction, and the subsequent excruciating pain is probably secondary to the subsequent inflammatory response.[62,66] In children, the humerus, the tibia, and the femur, in that order, are the most common sites of long bone infarction.[62] Swelling of the extremity and limitation of motion typically is mild.

Temperature elevation is usually low grade, but 21% of the episodes in the study by Keeley and Buchanan[62] had a temperature greater than 39°C. A sickle cell crisis typically lasts 3 to 5 days. Supportive measures have been the mainstay of therapy,[70,74] but Griffin and colleagues,[53] reported that a high dose of intravenous methylprednisolone significantly reduced the duration of severe pain in children and adolescents with sickle cell anemia.

Infection is more common in patients with sickle cell disease because of hypersplenism, defective opsonization mechanisms, and other ill-defined factors; however, compared with the number of sickle cell crises, the rate of osteomyelitis is low. Osteomyelitis in patients with sickle cell anemia has some unique features. *Salmonella* is the most common bacterial agent recorded in most[34,37,48,51,65,72,84] but not all series.[50] In a review of 68 well-documented and culture-proven cases of osteomyelitis, Givner and colleagues[51] found that *Salmonella* organisms accounted for 74% of the cases, whereas *Staphylococcus aureus* was noted in only 10%. Microscopic bowel infarctions provide an avenue for hematogenous spread of *Salmonella* organisms to bone marrow that also may be infarcted. Diaphyseal involvement of the humerus, the tibia, or the femur also is characteristic[34,50,65] Multiple sites of involvement may occur, with the rate of polyostotic cases ranging from 12% to 47% (Fig. 10-3).[34,50,72]

Differentiating bone infarction from osteomyelitis may be difficult. The degree of fever and leukocytosis overlap and the initial radiographs do not show abnormalities in either disorder. Owing to the shape of the erythrocyte and other factors, the erythrocyte sedimentation rate is unreliable in sickle cell disorders.[41] Furthermore, the usual radionuclide studies frequently are inconclusive.[54,65] A paired bone scan and bone marrow scan may be helpful if performed shortly after the onset of pain; however, 7 days after the onset of symptoms, the patterns of infarction may not differ from that of advanced osteomyelitis.[63] Kahn and colleagues[60] found that the sequential use of technetium bone marrow and gallium scans was helpful in distinguishing osteomyelitis from infarction in patients with sickle cell disorders. Sequential gallium scans, however, result in significant exposure to radiation.

The key to avoiding or minimizing complications associated with osteomyelitis in patients with sickle cell anemia is early recognition (see Fig. 10-3). Identifying an organism will provide the diagnosis. Blood cultures and aspiration of the affected area should be performed in patients who have temperatures above 39°C and in those who appear ill or who have persistent pain that does not resolve with the usual supportive therapy for sickle cell crisis.

If osteomyelitis is a possibility, antibiotic therapy is instituted with chloramphenicol or ampicillin to cover *Salmonella* and oxacillin to provide protection against *S aureus*. The emergence of resistant *Salmonella* species has caused some authors to suggest that a third generation cephalosporin should be used as the initial antibiotic.[40,42] With a delay in diagnosis, surgical drainage and prolonged parenteral antibiotic therapy is needed. Epps and colleagues[50] recommend making a cortical window in all patients and leaving the wound open. I make a small drill hole in the bone and enlarge it to a cortical window only if pus exuded from the drill hole. The wound should be left open when a large subperiosteal abscess is present.

Pathologic fractures complicating long bone osteomyelitis are more common in patients with sickle cell anemia[48,50] and occurred in 10% of patients in one large series.[48] In this study, fractures were more common in the first decade of life, in acute rather than chronic osteomyelitis, and in patients whose treatment was delayed. Approximately 10% to 15% of the fractures were complicated by delayed union, malunion, or joint stiffness.

Compared with osteomyelitis, septic arthritis is relatively uncommon in sickle cell disease.[35,47,49,84] Most reported cases of septic arthritis are caused by organisms other than *Salmonella* unless the joint infection is secondary to direct penetration from an adjacent osteomyelitis.[84] Because of the delay in diagnosis, septic arthritis of the hip is more likely to be complicated by avascular necrosis or dislocation in patients with sickle cell disease.[49]

Reactive arthritis causing a sterile joint effusion also may occur in children with sickle cell anemia.[56,79] The knees and elbows are most frequently involved, but symptoms may occur in other joints. The onset of pain is acute in one or more joints. Fever is commonly present and may range from low grade to greater

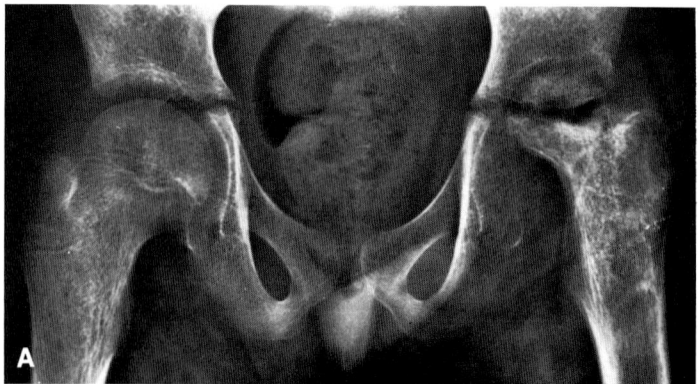
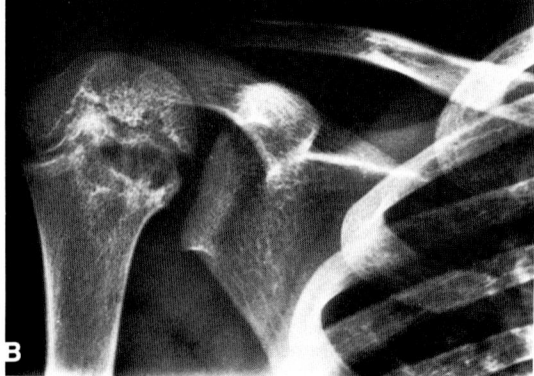

FIGURE 10-3. Eight-year-old boy with sickle cell anemia who presented with high fever and bilateral shoulder and left hip pain. Cultures from the left hip and right shoulder demonstrated *Salmonella* organisms. (**A**) Pelvic radiograph 4 months after diagnosis demonstrates progressive destruction of the left femoral head due to osteonecrosis from the concomitant septic arthritis and osteomyelitis. (**B**) Anteroposterior radiograph of the right shoulder demonstrates osteolytic changes in the humeral head and the metaphysis. Similar changes were observed on the contralateral side.

than 39°C. Synovial fluid analysis typically reveals a leukocyte count of less than 20,000/mm³. Joint effusions usually last 1 to 2 weeks, and joint arthralgia lasts for a few days to 2 months. Because reactive arthritis associated with *Salmonella* gastroenteritis has been reported in patients with hemoglobinopathy,[85] it is possible that reactive arthritis in patients with sickle cell disease is associated with minor episodes of *Salmonella* enteritis. Another possible mechanism is microvascular thrombosis in the synovial tissue. Treatment for reactive arthritis is splinting and analgesic medication.

Osteonecrosis of the femoral head is common in sickle cell disease. In a radiographic study of 2890 patients older than 5 years of age[67] the overall prevalence was 9.7%, with the rate dependent on the patient's age and the type of sickle cell disease (Table 10-2). Patients with SC or Sβ^+ genotype tended to develop osteonecrosis at a later age. Within the SS group, those who were also homozygous for the α-thalassemia gene were 2.4 times more likely to have osteonecrosis (21.2% when homozygous for α-thalassemia, 11.5% when heterozygous for α-thalassemia, and 8.7% in SS patients without an α-thalassemia gene). This provides further evidence that the association of the α-thalassemia gene increases the risk of vasoocclusion. Bilateral disease occurred in 54% of the patients, but this factor was not affected by genotype.

Sickle cell patients with osteonecrosis of the femoral head may be asymptomatic for several years. In a large radiographic study, almost half were asymptomatic at the time of diagnosis, but 21% of this group became symptomatic in the follow-up period, which averaged 5.6 years.[67] Children with sickle cell anemia have a better prognosis, but disability and symptoms frequently are observed in studies having long periods of observation.[59,81] With an average follow-up of 19 years, Hernigou and colleagues[59] found that only 5 of 14 hips had a Harris hip score lower than 80 points when the osteonecrosis occurred before 10 years of age. By comparison, 51 of 81 hips had a low hip rating when the osteonecrosis developed between 10 and 14 years of age. Therefore, although repetitive vascular insults may occur, young children with sickle cell disease have a reasonable potential for healing avascular necrosis of the femoral head.[43] The prognosis, however, is guarded when osteonecrosis develops in older children.

Magnetic resonance imaging (MRI) is not helpful in early detection of avascular necrosis in sickle cell disease.[87] MRI, however, is helpful in defining the extent of the osteonecrosis (Fig. 10-4). Furthermore, MRI frequently shows that segments of the femoral head are involved to varying degrees, suggesting a different pathophysiology of avascular necrosis in patients with sickle cell disease, that is, different segments of the femoral head were infarcted at different times.[76]

Several series have documented poor results after total joint arthroplasty in patients with sickle cell disease.[33,39,45,57] Both acute and late complications are increased with the incidence of infection and early revision being alarmingly high. The results of reconstructive procedures for osteonecrosis in patients with sickle cell disease are unknown, but the poor results after total joint arthroplasty and the poor long-term results for children 10 years of age or older necessitates consideration of realignment osteotomy for this group. The extent of the avascular necrosis should be defined by radiographs and MRI. If the lateral pillar is maintained, nonoperative treatment may be satisfactory,[88] but with total head involvement or deficiency of the lateral pillar a femoral or pelvic osteotomy should be considered. Severe involvement may require a combined femoral and pelvic osteotomy. Crutch ambulation or abduction bracing is a better alternative for children younger than 10 years of age (see Fig. 10-4), but loss of motion and total head involvement require further evaluation and consideration of other therapeutic alternatives.

Osteonecrosis of the humeral head also occurs in sickle cell disorders. The prevalence rate was 5.6% in a study of 2524 patients 5 years of age or older.[68] Similar to that of osteonecrosis of the femoral head, the prevalence of osteonecrosis of the humeral head was dependent on age and type of sickle cell disease (Table 10-3). Patients with SS disease and concomitant α-thalassemia also had a higher rate of osteonecrosis: 10% when homozygous for α-thalassemia, 7.1% when heterozygous, and 4.7% in SS patients without an α-thalassemia gene. The incidence of osteonecrosis before age 25 was extremely low in Sβ^+ and SC disease. Compared with the femur, bilateral disease of the humerus was more common and occurred in 67%. Con-

TABLE 10-2 Prevalence of Femoral Head Osteonecrosis in Sickle Cell Disease

AGE (Y)	PERCENT WITH FEMORAL HEAD OSTEONECROSIS	TYPE OF SICKLE CELL DISORDER	
		Genotype	Percent*
5–9	1.3	Sβ^0	13.1
10–14	4.6	SS	10.2
15–24	8.2	SC	8.8
25–34	18.8	Sβ^+	5.8
35–44	21.9		
≥45	32.5		

* Age-adjusted rate.
Adapted from Milner PF, Kraus AP, Sebes JI, et al. Sickle cell disease as a cause of osteonecrosis of the femoral head. N Engl J Med 1991;325:1476.

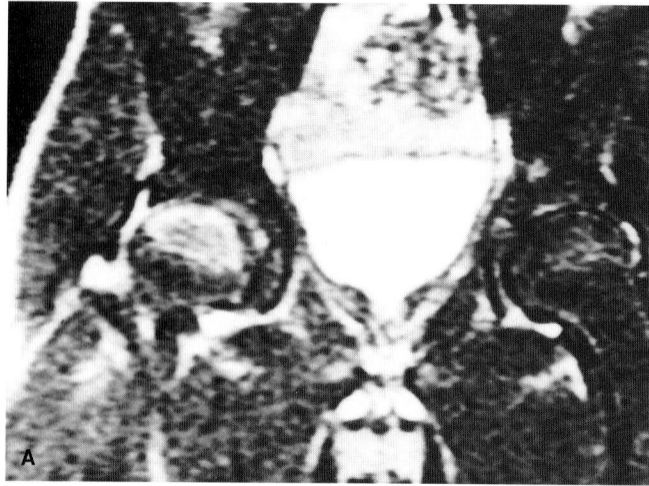
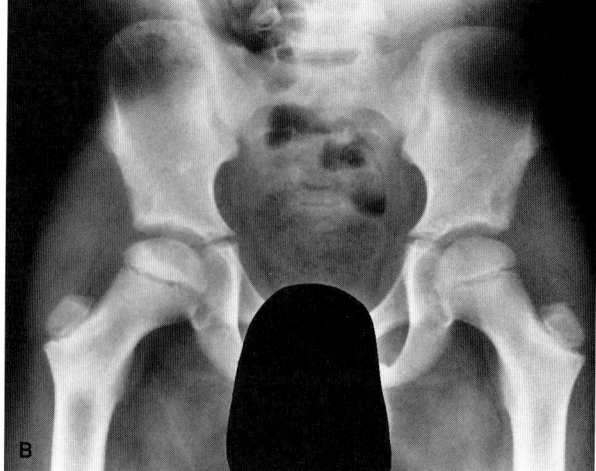

FIGURE 10-4. (A) Magnetic resonance image of a 7-year, 4-month-old boy with sickle cell anemia. Patient complained of pain in the right hip. The T2-weighted image is consistent with avascular necrosis of the right femoral head. On other views, abnormal signals also were present in the left femoral head, although not to the degree seen in the right femur. (B) Anteroposterior radiograph of the pelvis 5 months later demonstrates sclerosis of the lateral and inferior margin of the epiphysis, consistent with the creeping substitution healing of osteonecrosis. Patient had been maintained in an abduction brace. (Adapted from Greene WB. Disease of the hematopoietic system and chronic inflammatory arthritides: musculoskeletal complications in children. In: Bowen JR, Epps CE, eds. Complications in pediatric orthopaedic surgery. Philadelphia: JB Lippincott, 1995.)

comitant humeral and femoral head osteonecrosis was common, and occurred in 76% of SS and 75% of SC patients.

Compared with the femoral head, disability and pain are less frequent with osteonecrosis of the humeral head.[44,68] In a large radiographic survey,[68] 79% of the patients were asymptomatic at diagnosis. The disease process, however, may progress. The crescent sign and collapse of the humeral head typically begin in the superior medial quadrant. Further fragmentation and joint incongruity will cause symptoms and restricted motion, but the need for prosthetic replacement is uncommon. This is fortunate, because David and colleagues[46] observed that both of their patients with shoulder arthroplasty had prosthetic loosening. The prognosis for healing is better in children, and Chung and Ralston[44] recorded remarkable resolution of humeral head osteonecrosis in an 11-year-old boy.

Cerebral infarction occurs in approximately 8% of patients with sickle cell anemia. These strokes may occur in young children and result in a permanent spastic hemiplegia.[64] The risk of recurrent strokes can be reduced significantly by a program of chronic hypertransfusion.

Bone marrow transplantation also has been described in patients with sickle cell disease.[38,86] Results are preliminary and still under investigation. Complications are significantly less if the patient is young, without major chronic organ damage, and with a healthy HLA-identical relative. Using these criteria, Vermylen and colleagues[86] reported that 25 of 27 patients were free of vasoocclusive-related manifestations at follow-up ranging from 4 to 78 months.

The desirable level of hemoglobin and the need for packed erythrocytes or exchange transfusion prior to elective surgery remains controversial and is under investigation by a multicenter study. Special intraoperative considerations for patients with sickle cell disease include adequate hydration, avoidance of hypothermia and deoxygenation, and maintenance of blood volume.[43] The use of a tourniquet does not seem to

TABLE 10-3 Prevalence of Humeral Head Osteonecrosis in Sickle Cell Disease

AGE (Y)	PERCENT WITH HUMERAL HEAD OSTEONECROSIS	TYPE OF SICKLE CELL DISEASE	
		Genotype	Percent*
5–9	1.2	SS	6.0
10–14	2.6	Sβ^0	5.7
15–24	3.8	SC	4.6
25–34	9.7	Sβ^+	3.6
35–44	18.7		
≥45	22.0		

* Age-adjusted rate.
Adapted from Milner PF, Kraus AP, Sebes JI, et al. Osteonecrosis of the humeral head in sickle cell disease. Clin Orthop 1993;289:136.

cause increased sickling,[82] but I make an effort to exsanguinate the limb in these patients before inflating the pneumatic tourniquet. In the postoperative period, intravascular volume should be maintained and supplemental oxygen prescribed when appropriate.

Thalassemia

Normal hemoglobin is composed of two α- and two non–α-globulin (usually β-globulin) polypeptide chains that combine with heme to form a hemoglobin tetramer. Normally, two α- and two β-globulin chains pair to form hemoglobin A, a molecule that is both highly soluble and stable.

The thalassemia group is heterogeneous and characterized by absent or deficient synthesis of either the α- or β-globulin chains.[91,103] The consequence ranges from a severe anemia to laboratory abnormalities of no clinical significance. Thalassemia major, also known as Cooley anemia or β-thalassemia, is secondary to homozygous mutations of the β-globulin gene that result in absent or severely deficient synthesis of the β-polypeptide chain. Therefore, in β-thalassemia many of the hemoglobin molecules are composed of unpaired α chains. This molecule is extremely insoluble and causes intracellular precipitates. The circulating erythrocytes are distorted, extremely small, and have a markedly reduced amount of hemoglobin. In addition, increased hemolysis occurs as these damaged erythrocytes are removed at an accelerated rate. The clinical consequences are severe anemia, growth retardation, hepatosplenomegaly, and bone marrow expansion with its associated complications.

Chains of α-globulin are duplicated on each number 16 chromosome and, therefore, each human cell contains four copies of the α-globulin gene. If all four α-globulin genes are affected, the result is hydrops fetalis and death in utero. Otherwise, patients with α-thalassemia have significantly less problems than patients with β-thalassemia.[103] This is because unpaired β-globulin chains can form a relatively stable tetramer (HbH). Even with three mutant α-globulin genes, only a moderately severe hemolytic anemia occurs.

Untreated, patients with homozygous β-thalassemia major present with severe anemia during the first months of life, and most will die before the first 5 years of life.[105] Transfusion programs to maintain hemoglobin levels greater than 9 to 10 g/dL and chelation therapy to prevent hemosiderosis have markedly altered life expectancy and other problems seen in thalassemia[91,92,101,103,104]; however, even when patients begin serial transfusions at an early age they still may develop growth retardation, endocrine abnormalities, and die of cardiac dysfunction in middle age.[92,101,103]

Owing to the long-term problems of chronic transfusion therapy and the risk of blood-borne diseases, bone marrow transplantation increasingly is being used for patients with thalassemia major.[90,95,97,100,104] The best results are seen in young patients who have not received a large number of transfusions, who have not developed hepatomegaly or portal fibrosis, and who receive a bone marrow transplant from an HLA identical donor after undergoing a preoperative conditioning regimen. In this group, Baronciani and colleagues[90] reported a 97% survival rate, a 93% disease-free survival rate, and a 4% rejection rate at a follow-up of more than 6 years. The growth rate also is improved in children with thalassemia who undergo bone marrow transplantation before 8 years of age.[100] Bone marrow transplantation should prevent cardiac and other long-term complications associated with iron overload, but it is still too early to tell if the long-term outcome will be better than a diligent program of transfusion and chelation therapy.

Skeletal abnormalities seen in sporadically treated thalassemia result from extreme erythroid hyperplasia that causes widening of the marrow space, thinning of the cortex, and striking osteoporosis.[93] The earliest changes are noted in the hands and feet. The metacarpals, metatarsals, and phalanges are expanded to a rectangular and then a convex shape. The changes observed in these peripheral areas diminish in older children as the distal red marrow is replaced by fatty marrow; however, the skull, the spine, and the pelvis in these patients may show progressive radiologic changes (Figs. 10-5 and 10-6).

Earlier studies noted that fractures following minimal trauma occurred in 40% to 50% of patients with thalassemia at an average age of 10 to 16 years.[96,98,99] Transfusion therapy has decreased the incidence and nature of this complication. For example, Michaelson and Cohen[102] recorded a fracture incidence of 21% at an average age of 25 years when a transfusion program was started during early childhood. Furthermore, fractures in these patients occurred after a more appropriate level of trauma and healed within an expected time, and without the deformity commonly seen in earlier studies. To enhance fracture healing, the level of vitamin C, which is lowered by chelation therapy, may need to be increased by supplementation.[102] This should be done with caution, however, because too much vitamin C can cause cardiac arrhythmias.

Premature fusion of the physis also was observed in earlier studies of thalassemia patients.[94,96] This problem was noted in 15% to 20% of the patients and was particularly common in the proximal humeral physis. The etiology of the premature physeal fusion was unclear, but the problem was observed more frequently

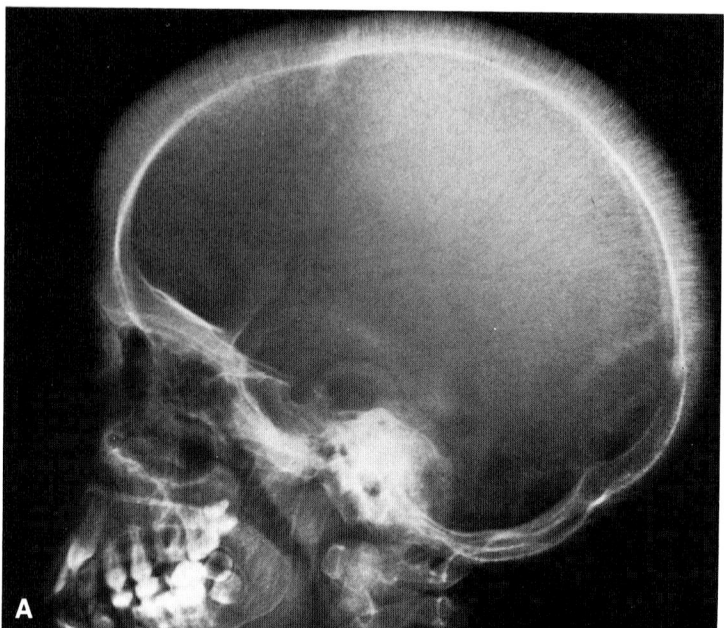
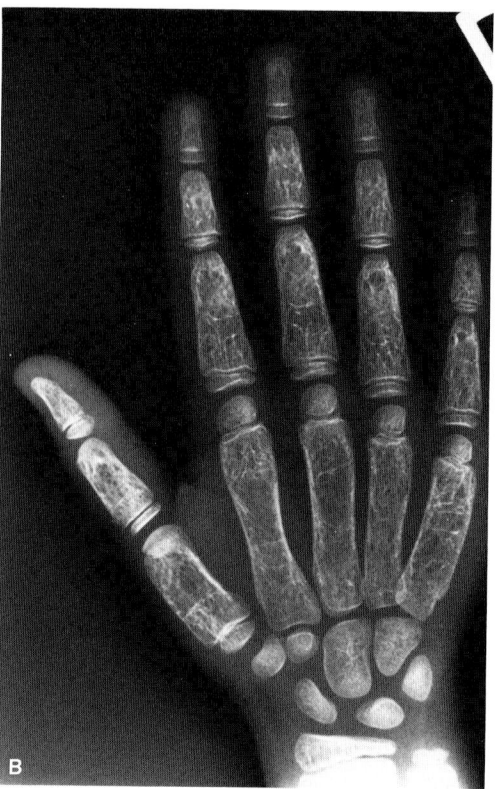

FIGURE 10-5. (A) Lateral radiograph of the skull showing the radial striations of the calvarium in an 11-year-old boy with thalassemia major. (B) Note the widened marrow cavities of the metacarpals and phalanges and the marked osteoporosis.

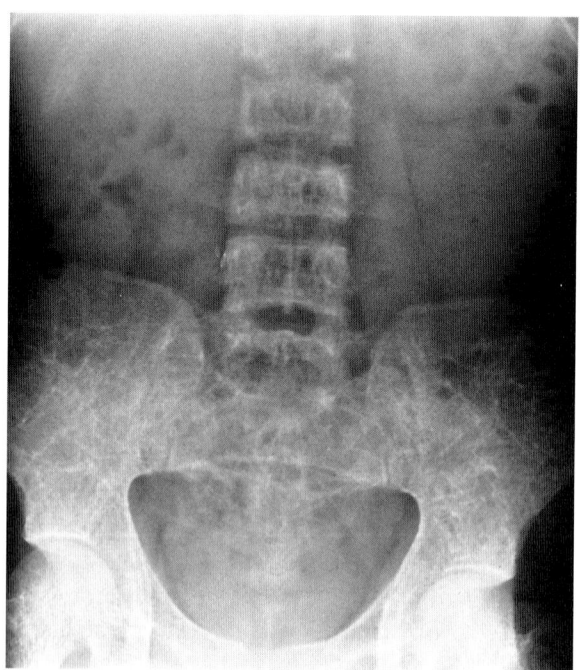

FIGURE 10-6. Anteroposterior radiograph of the lumbar spine and pelvis in a 26-year-old man with homozygous β-thalassemia. Radiographs show marked osteoporosis and lacy trabeculae secondary to marrow hypoplasia. (From Green WB. Disease of the hematopoietic system and chronic inflammatory arthritides: musculoskeletal complications in children. In: Bowen JR, Epps CE, eds. Complications in pediatric orthopaedic surgery. Philadelphia: JB Lippincott, 1995.)

in the group with a delay in beginning transfusion therapy.[94]

DISORDERS OF GRANULOCYTES

Granulocytes primarily act to clear bacterial infections. Included in the granulocyte family are neutrophils, eosinophils, and basophils, of which the neutrophils are by far the most numerous. A variety of humeral factors elaborated by a bacterial invasion or tissue necrosis mobilize neutrophils to the area of inflammation (i.e., chemotaxis). Opsonized bacteria (i.e., those coated with a specific antibody in the complement system) are phagocytized by neutrophils. Through a process called degranulation, granules of the neutrophil are discharged into the phagocytic vacuole, and the bacteria are killed and digested.

Childhood disorders of neutrophils are uncommon and are characterized by recurrent infections, particularly involving the skin and respiratory system. By comparison, bone and joint infections are relatively uncommon. Two representative disorders are discussed in this chapter. The Schwachman-Diamond syndrome is characterized by a chronic, cyclical neutropenia and skeletal dysplasia. In chronic granulomatous disease the neutrophils are dysfunctional. Osteomyelitis is more common and has some unique features in this disorder.

Schwachman-Diamond Syndrome

Except for cystic fibrosis, the Schwachman-Diamond syndrome[111] is the most common cause of exocrine pancreatic insufficiency in children.[107] These children present during the first year of life with failure to thrive, malabsorption with diarrhea and steatorrhea, and frequent respiratory and cutaneous infections.[19,106,107] Laboratory studies show normal sweat chloride tests but excessive fecal fat and deficient pancreatic trypsin, lipase, and amylase in the stool and duodenal secretions. Biopsy specimens of the pancreas demonstrate preservation of the islets of Langerhans but fatty tissue replacement of the remainder of the organ. Cyclical neutropenia with the neutrophil count periodically being less than 1500/mm^3 is seen in approximately 95% of these children.[106] Intermittent thrombocytopenia (i.e., platelet count <100,000/mm^3) occurs in approximately 50%, and pancytopenia also may develop.[19,106,107] Metaphyseal chondrodysplasia and other skeletal abnormalities may be seen in patients with Schwachman-Diamond syndrome.[106,108,110] In a review of 21 patients, Agett and colleagues[106] observed that short stature and delayed bone age was always present. The short stature was proportionate and was initially noted between the first and second year of life. Radiographic changes of metaphyseal chondrodysplasia were recorded in 13 of the 21 patients; however, this may be an underestimation because the radiographic features of this skeletal dysplasia may not be obvious in older adolescents or adults. Marked coxa vara was noted in 4 of 13 patients. Osteonecrosis, misdiagnosed as Legg-Calvé-Perthes disease, has been observed in one patient who also exhibited progressive coxa vara.[110] Clinodactyly (48%), genu varum (33%), and abnormally short ribs with flared anterior ends (47%) were also observed in the study by Agett and colleagues.[106] Two often-quoted case reports describing the bony histopathology in Schwachman-Diamond syndrome[109,112] are of questionable value because one patient did not have pancreatic tests performed, and the other case involved normal pancreatic exocrine laboratory studies.

Treatment for patients with Schwachman-Diamond syndrome includes high doses of pancreatic extract and medium chain triglyceride supplementation.[19,106,107] Although this will significantly improve the malabsorption, it does not affect either the limb growth or neutropenia. Respiratory and sinus tract infections are frequent, but respond to prompt treatment with antibiotics. Although the malabsorption seems to improve with age, infections continue to be a problem. The mortality rate is between 15% and 25% and is secondary to infections and an increased risk of leukemia.[19,107]

Chronic Granulomatous Disease

Chronic granulomatous disease is a group of inherited disorders characterized by deficiency in the nicotinamide-adenine dinucleotide phosphate (NADPH) oxidase system.[114–117,123,124] Phagocytosis is normal, but granulocytes have decreased ability to kill microbes that are catalase negative, organisms unable to destroy their endogenously produced hydrogen peroxide. In normal phagocytosis, neutrophils rapidly activate the membrane and cytosolic components of the NADPH system. As a result, oxygen is reduced by one electron to superoxide, which combines with hydrogen to produce hydrogen peroxide, a necessary metabolite for killing the ingested microbes.

Four subgroups of chronic granulomatous disease have been identified. Two mutations affect cytochrome B (i.e., the membrane components of NADPH oxidase), and two mutations affect cytosol proteins that are necessary for functional reconstitution of the NADPH oxidase system. Patients with cytochrome B defects are more severely involved than those with cytosol protein deficiency. The most common subgroup, transmitted by sex-linked recessive inheritance, accounts for approximately 60% of the patients and affects the glycosylated subunit of cytochrome B. The other subgroups are transmitted by autosomal-recessive inheritance. Within each group, different mutations may produce identical enzymatic defects.[113]

Patients with chronic granulomatous disease typically develop symptoms of recurrent infections in the first or second year of life, although some patients do not have problems until later childhood or adulthood.[118,122] A history of recurrent infections associated with persistent lymphadenopathy suggests the possibility of chronic granulomatous disease. The diagnosis can be confirmed by measuring neutrophil superoxide generation using the nitroblue tetrazolium test or related assays.[116]

Sites of recurrent infection include superficial abscesses with lymphadenitis (96%), chest infections (61%–80%), liver abscess (25%–38%), gastrointestinal tract (34%), and osteomyelitis (31%–36%; Fig. 10-7).[115,118,122,125] The organisms commonly cultured are those which are catalase negative, including *Staphylococcus*; certain Gram negative bacteria, such as *Serratia*, *Escherichia*, and *Klebsiella*; and fungi, such as *Aspergillus*, *Nocardia*, and *Candida albicans*.[114] The severity of chronic granulomatous disease is not uniform. An adverse prognostic indicator is development of symptoms before 1 year of age,[118] a factor that may reflect the site of mutation.

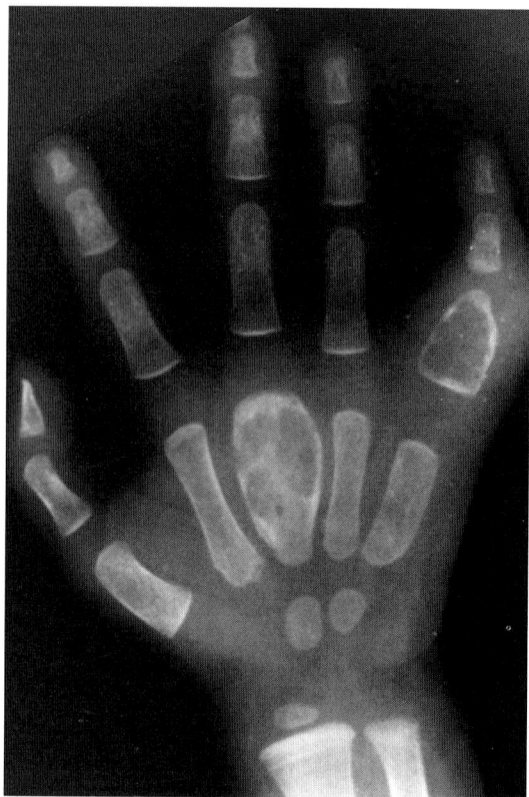

FIGURE 10-7. Fifteen-month-old boy with a 2-month history of progressive swelling of the right hand. Anteroposterior radiograph of the hand demonstrates fusiform swelling and osteolysis of the third metacarpal and proximal phalanx of the little finger. The patient had a past history of tuberculosis meningitis. Because the chest radiograph demonstrated infiltrates the preoperative diagnosis was tuberculosis dactylitis. A drainage procedure was performed. Cultures demonstrated *Serratia marcescens*; subsequent tests confirmed diagnosis of chronic granulomatous disease.

Earlier reports of bone infections in children with chronic granulomatous disease indicated that the hands and feet were most commonly involved and that operative procedures should be performed with reluctance.[126] A recent comprehensive review questioned these earlier recommendations. In 13 children who developed 20 episodes of osteomyelitis, Sponseller and colleagues[125] observed that the spine, the ribs, the hands, and the feet were the most common sites of infection. The causative organism was *Aspergillus* in 7 cases, *Serratia marcescens* in 5, and *Nocardia* in 4 cases. The route of the infection was direct spread from a lung abscess in 9 patients. The diagnosis often was delayed and, in contrast to other reports, Sponseller and colleagues[125] did not find that bone infection in these patients responded to antibiotics alone. Best results were obtained with preoperative imaging to define the extent of the bony infection, temporary withholding of antibiotics to obtain reliable intraoperative cultures, thorough debridement of the infected tissue, and leaving the wound open to allow healing by secondary intention.

Long-term prophylactic antibiotics and aggressive early treatment of infections are important.[114,115,117] A large multicenter double-blind study demonstrated that recombinant interferon resulted in a 72% reduction in the rate of serious infection.[121] Interferon was more beneficial in patients younger than 10 years of age, but the use of prophylactic antibiotics, as well as the type of chronic granulomatous disease, did not affect the risk of infection.[119,121] The clinical benefit of interferon therapy apparently is not secondary to enhanced neutrophil NADPH oxidase activity.[127] Heinrich and colleagues[120] also reported the benefits of interferon in controlling a well-established *Aspergillus* osteomyelitis.

DISORDERS OF LYMPHOCYTES AND THE IMMUNE SYSTEM

Lymphocytes can be divided into two main categories. Bone marrow–derived lymphocytes, the B cells, are precursors for humoral immunity cells (i.e., plasma cells that secrete antibodies). Thymus-derived lymphocytes, or T cells, control cell-mediated immunity and have both effector and regulatory functions. Effector functions include delayed hypersensitivity and graft-versus-host reactivity. Regulatory function includes enhancement and suppression of both cell-mediated and humoral immunity.

Three disorders of lymphocytes affect the musculoskeletal system. X-linked agammaglobulinemia affects the β cells, whereas cartilage hair hypoplasia and acquired immunodeficiency syndrome (AIDS) belong to the group of T-cell disorders.

X-Linked Agammaglobulinemia

X-Linked agammaglobulinemia is a disease manifested by recurrent bacterial infections.[128] It typically begins after 6 months of age, when maternal immunoglobulins have been largely metabolized. Physical findings, even lymphadenopathy, are absent, but a history of recurrent dermatitis, otitis media, pneumonia, and meningitis, will initiate appropriate laboratory studies. The disease is confirmed by IgG of less than 100 mg/mL and IgM, IgA, and IgE of less than 1% normal values. Circulating B cells are absent because of a block in maturation at the pre–B-cell level.[129] Cell-mediated immunity and response to viral disorders is normal.

The unique musculoskeletal problem seen in these affected boys, and in other disorders causing hypogammaglobulinemia, is aseptic arthritis. In a review of 69 patients with X-linked agammaglobulinemia, 15% had aseptic arthritis at presentation and 4% subsequently developed the complication.[131] The arthritis is usually nonerosive and either oligoarticular or polyarticular, and it most commonly affects the knees, the wrists, the ankles, and the fingers.[132] The etiology of the arthritis is unclear, but it involves the T-cell system and is therefore different from rheumatoid arthritis.[130] Typically the arthritis responds to the institution of immunoglobulin therapy; however, some patients develop a chronic arthritis.[132,134,135]

Untreated, patients with agammaglobulinemia usually develop bronchiectasis and die of pulmonary complications. The prognosis is significantly improved with immunoglobulin therapy and prompt institution of antibiotics for infections. Liese and colleagues[133] reported a significant reduction in infections when using higher doses of immunoglobulin (>400 mg/Kg every 3 weeks).

Cartilage-Hair Hypoplasia

Cartilage-hair hypoplasia is an autosomal recessive, short-limbed skeletal dysplasia associated with fine, sparse hair and defective cell-mediated immunity. In 1965, McCusick and colleagues[138] described the clinical and genetic characteristics of this disorder in 77 patients belonging to the Old Amish sect. Cartilage-hair hypoplasia has subsequently been described in the non-Amish population.[136,141] A recent review of 63 such patients observed that their clinical and laboratory manifestations were similar to those of the Amish population.[141]

Short stature (<3rd percentile) is a consistent finding.[138,141] The limbs are disproportionately short, and these patients superficially resemble people with achondroplasia; however, the sparse head hair and normal-sized skull permit ready differentiation. Furthermore, narrowing of the interpedicular distance is absent, and overgrowth occurs at the distal fibula in patients with cartilage hair hypoplasia. Immunodeficiency in cartilage-hair hypoplasia was first suspected because of atypical response to varicella infection. McCusick and colleagues[138] observed that two patients died of this disease, and three others had such virulent attacks that small pox was seriously considered. Subsequent studies have documented mild to moderate lymphopenia in approximately 75%.[141] Pierce and Polmar[139] observed an intrinsic proliferative defect in most lymphocytic subtypes. Chronic neutropenia also has been described in a small number of patients with cartilage-hair hypoplasia.[136,137,141] Recurrent viral respiratory tract infections are common during childhood, but the impaired cellular immunity is mild enough that adults with cartilage-hair hypoplasia typically have no health problems. Vaccination against polio should only be performed with attenuated virus, because vaccinia-related paralytic poliomyelitis has been reported.[140]

Acquired Immunodeficiency Syndrome

AIDS is secondary to infection by the human immunodeficiency virus (HIV). Children who develop AIDS most likely belong to one of the following population groups: hemophiliac children who received clotting factor concentrates prior to 1985, those who received blood products from HIV seropositive donors, and those born to HIV-infected mothers. With purification of clotting concentrates it is now rare to see a child with hemophilia who is HIV seropositive. Likewise, improved screening of blood donors and the expanding practice of autologous donation makes it unlikely that a child will be infected by a blood transfusion. At present, the majority of children with AIDS are born to HIV-infected mothers.[151]

The World Health Organization estimates that 10 to 12 million men and women and over 1 million children have been infected with HIV since the middle of 1992.[147] Approximately 7 million infections have occurred in sub-Saharan Africa, and more than 1 million have occurred in both Asia and Latin America. The increasing rate of HIV infection in women parallels the increased incidence of AIDS in children, and the vertical transmission of HIV from mother to child accounts for 80% of the pediatric AIDS cases in the United States.[156] In the United States, approximately 1800 infants per year are born with HIV infection,[151] and the number of pediatric AIDS cases will continue to increase, particularly in inner city areas.[142]

HIV is a retrovirus that infects the CD4 helper lymphocyte. Once inside the lymphocyte, the viral RNA is transcribed into DNA by a reverse transcriptase enzyme that is unique to this viral group.[144] Viral DNA is then integrated into the host cell chromosome and, when activated, the proviral DNA is transcribed to RNA, which is then translated to produce multiple HIV viruses that are released into the bloodstream. The infected CD4 lymphocyte becomes dysfunctional and sustains an early demise. Because the CD4 lymphocyte plays a key role in many segments of the immune system, an HIV-infected child ultimately will develop an immune-compromised infection and be classified as having AIDS.

Approximately 25% to 30% of the children born to HIV-infected women will become HIV seropositive.[149,151,154] Diagnosing an infected infant can be difficult because maternal IgG crosses the placenta and causes a false-positive reaction on standard tests.[156] Development of additional assays, such as the immune complex–dissociated HIVp24 antigen[150] and the IgG-Fc capture enzyme,[153] may allow earlier identification of infected neonates. Children who are congenitally infected typically develop the criteria for AIDS at an earlier age, with 20% to 50% having symptoms in the first year of life.[144,151] Exceptions occur, and experienced observers note that some children with perinatally acquired infection still are not symptomatic at 7 to 10 years of age. Perhaps because immunoglobulins are not well developed, HIV-infected children are more likely to develop recurrent bacterial infections, but certain opportunistic infections seen in seropositive adults, such as toxoplasmosis and cryptococcal meningitis, are infrequent.[144] Kaposi sarcoma and lymphomas also are relatively uncommon in HIV-infected children. On the other hand, lymphocytic interstitial pneumonitis, a diffuse and progressive reticulonodular pulmonary infiltrate, is frequently seen in children with AIDS.

Growth retardation and developmental delay are unique features of HIV-infected children. The growth retardation is proportional, with both weight and height being low for the child's age.[149] Early recognition of retarded growth and failure to thrive may be signs that identify the infected infant of an HIV seropositive mother.[145,149]

Developmental delays are common in children with perinatally acquired HIV infection.[143,152,155] In a study from central Africa (thereby excluding the effect of cocaine abuse), Msellati and colleagues[152] demonstrated frequent developmental delays in HIV-infected children compared with unaffected children born to seropositive mothers and unaffected children born to seronegative mothers. Developmental delays primarily involved gross motor function and were observed as early as 6 months of age. A static encephalopathy also may occur, and the orthopaedic surgeon may be consulted concerning management of the child's cerebral palsy–like problems. Occasionally a child may develop a profound and rapidly progressive encephalopathy.

The etiology of the developmental delay and encephalopathy has not been proven, but this problem is probably caused by direct effect of the HIV virus on the brain.[144] Monocytes also are invaded by the HIV virus and, although not particularly cytopathic to the monocytes, this cell may be the vehicle that spreads HIV to the central nervous system.

The orthopaedic surgeon primarily interacts with HIV-infected children who have musculoskeletal infections, static encephalopathy, or hemophilia. Musculoskeletal infections do occur but are surprisingly uncommon in HIV-infected children.[144] As with any immunocompromised patient, antibiotic therapy should be prolonged. Similarly, drainage of a soft tissue or bony abscess and debridement of necrotic tissue will facilitate the eradication of the infection. In hemophiliacs, septic arthritis occurs most frequently in joints that have an associated arthropathy. In these patients, the diagnosis is frequently delayed because the swelling and pain initially is thought to be a hemarthrosis. Owing to the delay in diagnosis and immune compromise, I have observed better results in these patients when they have been treated with arthroscopic drainage in addition to vigorous antibiotic therapy.

Because it may be difficult to predict whether an HIV-infected child has a stable or slowly progressive encephalopathy, and because children with perinatally acquired HIV infection have a limited life expectancy, it would seem appropriate to treat muscle and joint contractures in these children by nonoperative means whenever possible. As therapeutic modalities improve, operative intervention should be considered for the atypical older child who remains asymptomatic with satisfactory CD4 lymphocyte counts.

HIV-infected children with hemophilia progress to AIDS at a slower rate than either adults with hemophilia or children with perinatally acquired infection.[148] Therefore, if these patients are disabled by recurrent hemarthroses a synovectomy should be considered. The decision to do surgery should be individualized, but the risk of postoperative infection seems to be relatively small, and even patients with CD4 lymphocyte counts lower than 200/mm^3 have good results.[146]

DISORDERS OF THE MONOCYTE-MACROPHAGE SYSTEM

Cells of the monocyte-macrophage system arise from a common stem cell in the bone marrow. After differentiation into monocytes these cells circulate in the peripheral blood and migrate to different tissues, where they may change and develop highly specialized functions. One class of monocyte-macrophage cells is antigen-processing and phagocytic. Osteoclasts, Kupffer cells of the liver, pulmonary macrophages, and sinusoidal histiocytes of the lymph nodes are in this group of specialized tissue macrophages. The other class of monocyte-macrophage cells are the antigen-presenting, nonphagocytic dendritic cells. Included in this group are the Langerhans cells of the skin and reticulum cells of the lymph node.

Accumulation or proliferation of cells is characteristic of monocyte-macrophage system disorders. In lysosomal storage disorders catabolic enzymes are deficient and certain cellular products cannot be excreted. Abnormal accumulation of macrophages subsequently occur. Langerhans cell histiocytosis, another disorder affecting the monocyte-macrophage system, includes solitary and multifocal eosinophilic granuloma of bone and is probably an aberrant response to an unknown stimulus.

Gaucher Disease

Gaucher disease, initially described in 1882 by Philippe Charles-Ernest Gaucher, is the most common lysosomal storage disease, with an overall incidence of 1 per 40,000.[192] A sentinel study by Brady and colleagues[166] proved that Gaucher disease was caused by a deficiency of glucocerebrosidase, the lysosomal enzyme that hydrolizes glucocerebroside. Glucocerebroside, an important component of cell wall membranes, cannot be metabolized in Gaucher disease. Therefore, normal necrosis of cells, especially leukocytes, causes a gradual accumulation of glucocerebroside in macrophages. The resultant Gaucher cell is a large, lipid-laden cell that mostly accumulates in the red pulp of the spleen, the liver sinusoids, and the bone marrow. Clinical manifestations of Gaucher disease are directly attributable either to accumulation of these abnormal macrophages or a secondary consequence of the resultant organ dysfunction. For example, the clotting deficiency that results from splenomegaly and hepatomegaly may precipitate leg or back pain in a Gaucher crisis.

Three forms of the Gaucher disease are recognized.[184] All are characterized by autosomal recessive inheritance. Type I, mostly confined to the spleen, the liver, and the bones, is by far the most common type and is particularly prevalent among Ashkenazi Jews (i.e., those of eastern European descent). The frequency of the gene for Gaucher disease in this population has been calculated as 0.04, which is equivalent to a carrier frequency of 8.9% and a birth incidence of 1:450.[164] Type II Gaucher disease, also known as the acute neuronopathic or infantile type, is rare, has no ethnic predilection, involves the central nervous system, and causes death before age 2 years. Type III Gaucher disease, also called the chronic neuronopathic type, has the heterogenic features of type I disease and demonstrates slowly progressive neurologic dysfunction. Most patients with type III Gaucher disease live in Norbotten, a northern district of Sweden.

The gene for glucocerebrosidase has been mapped, and mutation analysis has been performed on several patients with type I Gaucher disease.[194,196] As expected, the specific mutation, the genotype, causes variable deficiency of the enzyme and provides the best correlation for clinical severity and age at presentation. Zimran and colleagues[196] studied 53 patients: 39 Ashkenazi Jews, 13 non-Jewish people, and 1 person with one Jewish parent. The most common mutation, 1226G, creates a restriction site that allows some production of the enzyme. Mutation 1226G was identified in 65 alleles (77% frequency in Jewish and 24% frequency in non-Jewish patients). Other common mutations, 84GG and 1448C, had severely deficient or no production of glucocerebrosidase. The most common genotype was 1226G/1226G. These patients had relatively mild disease and later onset of symptoms. Other common genotypes, such as 1226G/1448C and 1226G/84GG, were associated with more severe clinical manifestations and an earlier onset of symptoms.

Clinical heterogeneity also is noted among Gaucher patients with the same genotype.[196] Possible explanations for this phenomenon include the existence of other mutations in the same allele, unknown modifying genes that link with the cerebroside enzyme, and nongenetic events, such as the effect of viral infections on splenomegaly and the effect of a traumatic event on the skeletal manifestations of the disease.

The age at onset of symptoms reflects the clinical heterogeneity of Gaucher disease[189] and ranges from early childhood to the older adult years. In the study by Zimran and colleagues[196] the age at diagnosis averaged 25 years (range, 8 months–70 years). The most common symptom at presentation is an abnormality of coagulation, such as epistaxis, ease of bruising, or prolonged bleeding after superficial wounds. An incidental finding of splenomegaly or thrombocytopenia also may prompt diagnosis before symptoms occur. Bone pain or fracture may herald the disease, but this is uncommon, noted in only 13% of patients.[196] Skeletal involvement, however, is a major cause of the morbidity and disability recorded in long-term follow-up studies.[158,184,191,196]

Splenomegaly is a cardinal feature of Gaucher disease.[184,191,196] Splenic enlargement may be enormous, occupying half of the abdomen, and may cause aching pain, protuberant abdomen, and altered posture. The resultant hypersplenism most often causes thrombocytopenia and a mild anemia, but pancytopenia also may be present. Total splenectomy is followed by accelerated deposition of glucocerebroside in the liver and bones.[186,193] Therefore, subtotal splenectomy is indicated for hypersplenism in Gaucher disease.[159,170,193] Subtotal splenectomy also protects the patient against complications associated with postsplenectomy sepsis. The splenic remnant, however, may regenerate.[170,193] To minimize the risk of recurrent hypersplenism, Zer and Freud[193] recommend leaving a small amount of spleen, approximately the size of the operated child's fist.

Hepatomegaly also occurs as glucocerebroside accumulates in Kupffer cells, the specialized macrophage cells lining the walls of the sinusoids of the liver. Compared with the spleen, the degree of hepatomegaly is not as severe or as frequent.[184,191] Abnormal liver function tests often occur, but they usually are of limited consequence. An exception is the effect of liver dysfunction on clotting factors. The resultant coagulopathy may complicate treatment of fractures or operations for arthritic conditions. On occasion, severe liver disease does occur and may be associated with pulmonary dysfunction, portal hypertension, and esophageal varices.[184]

The skeletal changes seen in Gaucher disease include abnormal widening of the metaphysis, osteopenia, Gaucher crisis or pseudoosteomyelitis, osteomyelitis, pathologic fractures, hemorrhagic cysts, avascular necrosis, and subsequent arthritis.[157,158,162,169,177,184,189–191] Infiltration of the bone marrow by the Gaucher cells is the primary cause of the skeletal problems. Quantitative MRI demonstrates that the degree of marrow infiltration, as measured by the percentage reduction of marrow fractions, correlates with the disease severity as measured by splenic enlargement and musculoskeletal complications.[173,176,187,188]

Approximately 70% of patients with Gaucher disease have abnormal flaring of the metaphysis, or the Erlenmeyer-flask deformity (Fig. 10-8).[196] The distal femur is most often involved, but the proximal tibia and proximal humerus also may exhibit a widened metaphysis.[158] In Gaucher disease, this bony deformity most likely results from expansion of a relatively weak metaphyseal cortex by the abundant Gaucher cells.

Osteopenia in Gaucher disease is most obvious in the vertebra and proximal portion of the appendicular skeleton, where the hematopoietic marrow is concentrated. Osteoporosis, however, is diffuse as indicated by Mankin and colleagues'[184] report of decreased bone mass on densitometry studies of the distal radius in 15 adult patients. Accumulation of Gaucher cells in the marrow may be the sole explanation for the osteopenia, although metabolic studies suggest a possible role of altered vitamin D metabolism and abnormal absorption of vitamin D and calcium.[184] Patients with significant osteopenia may complain of aching in the bones or loss of height secondary to vertebral wedging. The primary significance of the osteopenia, however, is its predisposition to pathologic fractures.

A Gaucher crisis is characterized by intense pain that is acute in onset and relatively well localized.[179,184,191] Common sites of involvement include the distal femur, the proximal tibia, and the proximal femur. Mild swelling, localized tenderness, and fever are often present. The leukocyte count is elevated and ranged from 13,100 to 19,800 in one series.[178] Likewise, the erythrocyte sedimentation rate is elevated, typically in the range of 40 to 120 mm/h. These symptoms mimic osteomyelitis, and hence the alternative nomenclature for Gaucher crisis is pseudoosteomyelitis. A crisis may be the first clinical manifestation of Gaucher disease. The finding of concomitant splenomegaly will suggest the correct diagnosis.

The etiology of a Gaucher crisis is hemorrhage in the intramedullary canal and, on occasion, the subperiosteal space.[173,175] Damage to the vascular endothelium with sudden leakage of blood into the intramedullary cavity is probably caused by thrombocytopenia and clotting deficiencies in the environment of a crowded bone marrow. Blood under pressure explains the intense pain of Gaucher crisis and why the acute symptoms mimic osteomyelitis.

Intramedullary hemorrhage during a Gaucher crisis also causes localized ischemia and explains the findings on x-ray film and bone scan. Radiographs are normal at the onset of a Gaucher crisis, whereas a technetium bone scan will show decreased uptake.[165,179,184] Consistent with the subsequent inflammatory and remodeling response, a few weeks after a Gaucher crisis radiographs demonstrate periosteal elevation and lytic areas within the medullary canal (Fig. 10-9).[158] Bone scans at this time show increased uptake surrounding a central photopenic area.[179] Several months after the crisis, the bone scans return to normal but radiographs show areas of sclerosis in the intramedullary canal or areas of osteonecrosis in the femoral head, the tibial plateau, the femoral condyles, or the humeral head (Figs. 10-10 and 10-11; see Fig. 10-9).

Treatment during the acute phase of a Gaucher crisis is supportive. The pain typically is severe for 1 to 3 days, and during this time intravenous narcotics are required. The pain then gradually subsides over 2 to 4 weeks. Continued observation is warranted to

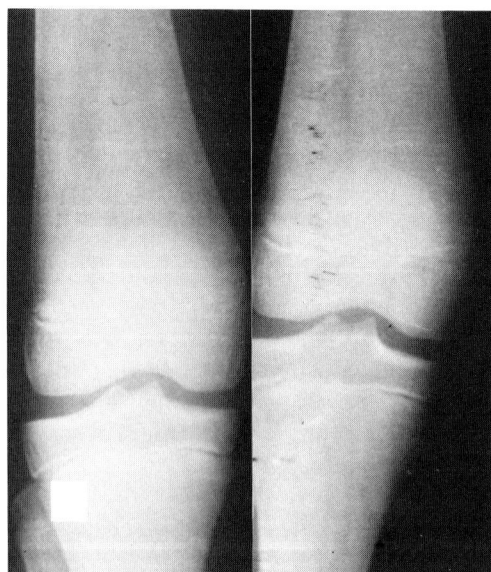

FIGURE 10-8. Flaring of the distal femoral metaphysis, known as Erlenmeyer-flask deformity, in a child with Gaucher disease. (Courtesy of Henry J. Mankin, M.D.)

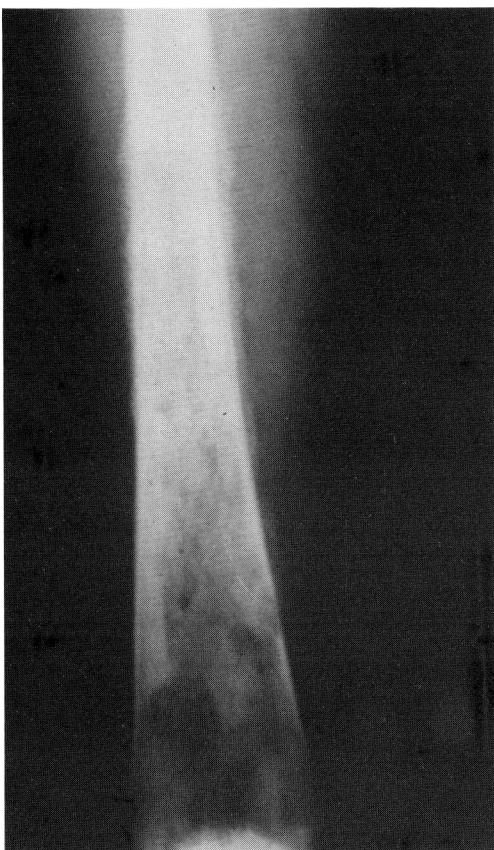

FIGURE 10-9. Bone destruction, sclerosis, and periosteal new bone formation in the femoral shaft following a Gaucher crisis. (Courtesy of Henry J. Mankin, M.D.)

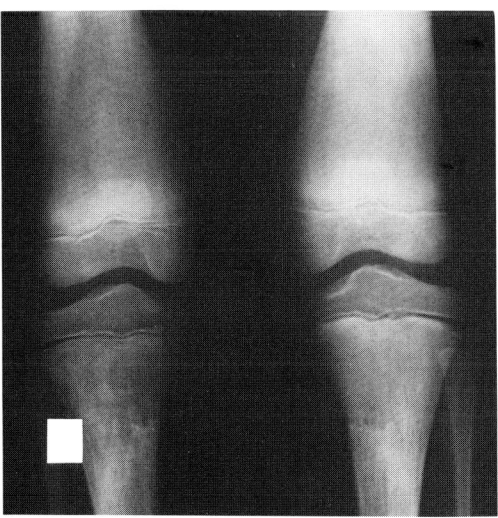

FIGURE 10-10. Radiolucency and osteosclerosis in the proximal tibial metaphysis are a result of Gaucher crisis. Note the Erlenmeyer-flask appearance of the distal femur. (Courtesy of Henry J. Mankin, M.D.)

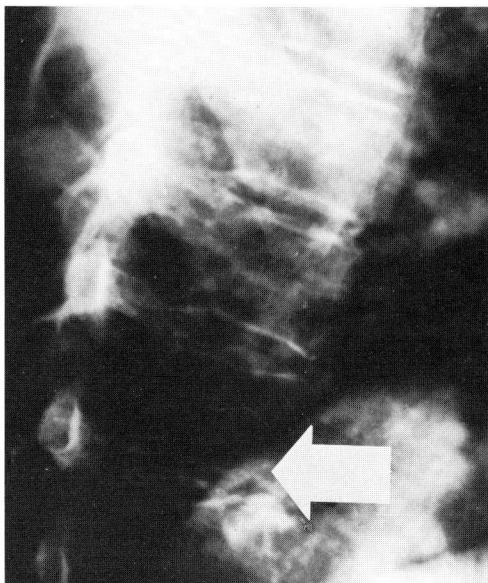

FIGURE 10-11. Compression fracture of a vertebra in Gaucher disease. (Courtesy of Henry J. Mankin, M.D.)

see whether a complication such as osteonecrosis of the femoral head develops after a crisis.

Similar to sickle cell anemia, osteomyelitis in Gaucher is uncommon.[169] In Gaucher disease, osteomyelitis often follows a crisis and is characterized by delay in diagnosis and an increased prevalence of anaerobic organisms. No doubt, regions of ischemic bone marrow predispose to infection by these organisms. Laboratory and imaging studies may not differentiate a crisis from osteomyelitis. A bone biopsy should be performed with caution and strict aseptic technique, as Bell and colleagues[162] recorded several cases with Gaucher crisis who developed osteomyelitis after aspiration or surgical drainage.

Pathologic fractures also may occur in children with Gaucher disease. Katz and colleagues[177] reported 23 fractures occurring in 9 children at an average age of 12 years (range, 6–18 years old). Fifteen fractures (65%) occurred at a site that had been affected by a crisis 2 to 12 months previously. Therefore, the common location for fracture included the distal femur, the proximal tibia, and the base of the femoral neck. Delayed union and nonunion are common in patients with Gaucher disease, but nonoperative therapy is usually necessitated by associated medical problems.[184] Fractures of the femoral neck occur more often in children younger than 10 years of age and are frequently complicated by coxa vara, pseudoarthrosis, and avascular necrosis.[158,172]

Back pain in patients with Gaucher disease may be severe and secondary to either a crisis or pathologic fracture (see Fig. 10-11), or the pain may be mild and presumably secondary to osteopenia. In a series of 19 involved children and adolescents, Katz and colleagues[180] noted 9 episodes of nonspecific mild pain in the thoracic spine that lasted 2 to 5 days. Three patients had severe pain that was typical for Gaucher crisis. One of these patients progressed to thoracic kyphosis, but the other two did not develop altered spinal alignment. Pathologic fractures presented with an insidious onset of pain 1 to 2 months prior to diagnosis. The most common fracture pattern was rectangular compression and a "bone-within-a-bone" appearance of 2 to 3 adjacent vertebra. In these patients, the vertebra healed with a central depression, but kyphosis or scoliosis was an infrequent complication. Anterior wedge compression fracture of one or more vertebra also may occur, and these patients may develop severe kyphosis, which causes spinal cord compression.[174,180]

Osteonecrosis involving the femoral head, the femoral condyles, the tibial plateau, and the humeral head can cause severe disability in patients with Gaucher disease.[157,158,184,191] In 53 patients evaluated at an average age of 33 years (range, 1–72 years old), Zimran and colleagues[196] observed avascular necrosis of the femoral head in 11 patients. Two patients had undergone total hip arthroplasty, and two patients had undergone total knee replacement. The prognosis for children who develop avascular necrosis of the femoral head is guarded (Fig. 10-12). In 8 patients (13 hips) who developed osteonecrosis of the femoral head at an average age of 9 years (range, 6–12 years old) Katz and colleagues[178] observed that all but 3 hips had poor Mose ratings at an average follow-up of 26 years. These patients, however, were asymptomatic with daily activities. Osteonecrosis of the humeral head in patients with Gaucher disease is similar to sickle cell anemia in that joint incongruity may cause limitation of motion, but the disability usually is not severe enough to limit routine activities or require total joint arthroplasty.

Operative intervention for osteomyelitis, fractures, or arthritis should be carefully considered in patients with Gaucher disease. Thrombocytopenia secondary to hypersplenism and other clotting deficiencies secondary to hepatic dysfunction may cause excessive bleeding, and osteoporosis limits fixation of implants.[157,158,181,182,184] Total joint arthroplasty in these patients has been complicated by excessive perioperative hemorrhage and an accelerated rate of symptomatic loosening.

Recent developments in medical therapy are exciting.[183] Previous attempts to administer glucocerebrosidase had been a failure because the deficient enzyme could not be transported intracellularly. Barton and colleagues[160] discovered that by exposing a mannose residue, the resultant enzyme, aglucerase (Ceredase), could be transported across the cell membrane and was functional. Subsequent studies of patients treated for 6 to 24 months with aglucerase have consistently observed decreased splenic volume and increased hemoglobin concentration.[160,163,167,168,185] In addition, most patients showed increased platelet count and decreased hepatic volume and serum acid phosphatase activity. Changes in the skeleton were not obvious in early studies that had administered aglucerase for less than 24 months. The slow response of the skeleton may be caused by limited delivery of the enzyme to the bone marrow and the large reservoir of accumulated glucocerebroside within the marrow compartment. The skeleton may eventually respond to long term enzyme replacement, as indicated by a case report of a child treated for 3.5 years who showed definite improvement on both radiographs and MRI studies.[161]

The present cost of enzyme replacement therapy for Gaucher disease is often prohibitive.[171] The initial study transfused 60 U/kg of body weight every 2 weeks. This amount of enzyme administered to a 70 kg patient costs 382,000 U.S. dollars per year. Other studies[163,168,185] have administered only 30 U/kg of aglucerase each month in fractionated doses, one fourth as much enzyme. On this regimen, I noted an equivalent effect on blood counts and liver and spleen size. Home transfusion therapy of this reduced dosage also has been successful.[195] Whether the reduced dosage will be as effective in altering the skeletal changes is still unanswered. That, and many other questions, are under study. The cost and need for repeated intravenous administration make therapy unwarranted in patients

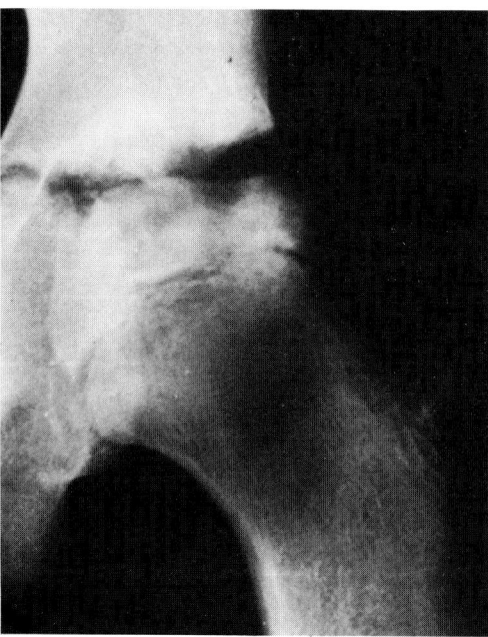

FIGURE 10-12. Late phases of osteonecrosis of the femoral head demonstrate flattening and incongruity. (Courtesy of Henry J. Mankin, M.D.)

with mild disease; however, there is little doubt that the crippling effects of Gaucher disease on patients with moderate and severe enzyme deficiency will be radically ameliorated in the years to come. Even if the skeletal abnormalities cannot be eliminated, the improved hematologic manifestations should make operative intervention more feasible.

Niemann-Pick Disease

Our understanding of the Niemann-Pick group of diseases is evolving. It is now clear that there are two main subgroups with different enzymatic effects. Both groups are lysosomal storage diseases characterized by accumulation of foam cells in the bone marrow and varying degrees of hepatosplenomegaly.[206] In addition, both types of Niemann-Pick disease are transmitted by autosomal recessive inheritance.

Type I disease, also described as type A or B, is secondary to deficiency of acid sphingomyelinase.[199,206] This enzyme is necessary for normal degradation of sphingomyelin, a phospholipid found in relatively high concentration in normal liver, spleen, and brain tissue. Patients with severe type I Niemann-Pick disease (type A) have mutations that cause the enzyme to be nonfunctional, whereas in the less severe type B disease, the enzyme is defective but has residual catabolic activity.[198,202,203,207]

The diagnosis of type A Niemann-Pick disease is made shortly after birth. Progressive and massive enlargement of the liver and spleen is accompanied by progressive pulmonary infiltration and progressive deterioration of the central nervous system.[198,199,206] Cherry red spots in the macula, similar to Tay-Sachs disease, are seen in 50% of the patients.[206] Spasticity, blindness, and deafness eventually occur. At present there is no effective treatment for type A Niemann-Pick disease, and attempts at bone marrow transplantation have not been successful.[197] These patients usually die by age 1 to 2 years in an emaciated state.

Radiographs in type A Niemann-Pick disease show delayed bone age, osteoporosis, and metaphyseal splaying.[201] The altered shape of the metaphysis is consistent with bone marrow infiltration. Flaring of the metaphyseal contour is not striking, and this may reflect the deficient nutritional status of these patients. The vertebrae, particularly in the lumbar region, have relatively long pedicles. This, perhaps, is secondary to accumulation of sphingomyelin in the spinal cord tissue.

Patients with type B Niemann-Pick disease present during childhood with enlargement of the spleen and the liver.[198,199,206] The onset of pulmonary infiltrates and neurologic dysfunction is variable, and patients often survive into adulthood. Bone changes have not been well categorized, but osteoporosis, delayed bone age, and widening of the diaphysis and metaphysis have been reported.[198,205] In contrast to Gaucher disease, these patients do not have a classic Erlenmeyer flask deformity, crisis, or osteonecrosis.

One case of pseudoosteomyelitis has been reported in a 9-year-old girl with type B Niemann-Pick disease.[204] Her clinical picture and the operative findings, however, were different from Gaucher disease, because this patient had a 3-day history of apparently mild-to-moderate right shoulder pain, radiographs that showed periosteal elevation, and a bone biopsy specimen that demonstrated foam cells and necrotic tissue. Cultures were negative, and the patient's pain resolved following the operative decompression and intravenous antibiotics.

Type II Niemann-Pick disease, commonly called type C, is caused by an abnormality in the intracellular translocation of exogenous cholesterol. Unesterified cholesterol accumulates in the lysosomes.[199,206,208] The diagnosis can be confirmed by measuring the rate of esterification after challenging a culture of the patient's skin fibroblasts with low-density lipoproteins. Considerable variability in disease onset and progression is seen in patients with type C Niemann-Pick disease. Patients generally are classified into three groups.[200,206] In the infantile group, psychomotor delay and severe hepatic dysfunction become evident before 18 months of age. These patients typically die between the ages of 3 to 5 years, with progressive spasticity and dementia. In the juvenile form of type C Niemann-Pick disease, the most common presentation is an ataxic gait that develops during early childhood. Mild hepatosplenomegaly is common but not invariably found. Progressive central nervous system involvement results in death, typically during the second decade. The late onset form of type C Niemann Pick disease presents during adolescence or adulthood with apparent psychiatric dysfunction.

The foam cells seen in the bone marrow of patients with type C Niemann-Pick disease are fewer in number and are not as mulberry-like in appearance.[206] No apparent clinical problems occur from the bone marrow infiltration in type C Niemann-Pick disease. Orthopaedic surgeons, however, may see these patients at the onset of their disease, when they are being evaluated for a possible cerebral palsy.

Langerhans Cell Histiocytosis

Eosinophilic granuloma of bone was first described in 1940 by Lichenstein and Jaffe[251] and Otani and Ehrlich.[258] Green and Faber,[236] in 1942, observed that the histopathology of eosinophilic granuloma was similar to that seen in Hand-Schüller-Christian disease and the more severe Letterer-Siwe disease. Because proliferating histiocytes are common to all three disorders, Lichstein[249,250] designated this group of diseases as histiocytosis X. Because the Langerhans cell histiocyte is unique to these disorders the Histiocyte Society, in 1985, recommended the term Langerhans cell histiocytosis,[228] and that nomenclature is preferred. Eosinophilic granuloma, however, is still commonly used when describing a patient with solitary bone involvement.

Ordinary histiocytes are components of the mononuclear phagocyte system, whose stem cells may undergo metamorphosis to mononuclear cells, foam cells, macrophages, multinucleated giant cells, osteoclasts, and so forth.[245] A Langerhans cell histiocyte is a dendritic cell found in normal tissues. Its origin is debatable, and it may arise as a specialized cell of the mononuclear phagocyte system or as a cell of separate bone marrow lineage.[232] Compared with other histiocytes, the unique structural aspect of the Langerhans cell is tubular or racket-shaped granules seen in electron microscopy and first described by Birbeck and colleagues.[215] These granules, or organelles, apparently result from internalization of antigen complexes formed at the cell membrane.[232] Cambazard and colleagues[219] produced a monoclonal antibody from an eosinophilic granuloma lesion of one patient that specifically recognized normal Langerhans cells as well as proliferating cells from bone and skin lesions of other patients with Langerhans cell histiocytosis.

The pathogenesis of Langerhans cell histiocytosis is still speculative. The disease is not a neoplasm, at least not in the classic sense; there is no evidence of aneuploidy and no prognostic significance based on cellular atypia.[229,259] A reactive immunologic process causing bone and soft tissue destruction is the probable cause.[232] Some stimulus, perhaps a virus, causes a poorly regulated activation of histiocytes with some of the histiocytes becoming Langerhans cells. Proliferation of Langerhans cells and related histiocytes, the effects of cytokines released by these cells, or some combination of these mechanisms could explain the subsequent tissue destruction. Eosinophil degranulation and subsequent binding of eosinophil peroxidase may be impressive in these lesions and most likely plays a role in the inflammatory and destructive process.[271]

Histopathologic features vary depending on the stage of the disease, the tissue involved, and unknown factors.[245,253] The classic lesion of bone contains groups of lipid-laden histiocytes and a variable number of acute and chronic inflammatory cells. The granulocytes predominantly are eosinophils, although these cells may be sparse or virtually absent. Not all of the histiocytes in these lesions are Langerhans cells, the typical granules being found in 2% to 79% of the histiocytes.[255] Early in the disease process the lesions tend to be dominated by histiocytes. More mature lesions may be difficult to differentiate from a subacute or chronic osteomyelitis, but foci of necrosis, granulomatous changes with variable amounts of fibrosis, multinucleated giant cells with a histiocytoid nuclei, and the presence of Langerhans histiocytes usually distinguishes the lesion as Langerhans histiocytosis. Immunochemical markers, such as CD1, LN3, peanut lectin, S100 neuroprotein, mannosidase, and α_1-antichymotrypsin, may be helpful in distinguishing an ordinary histiocyte from the Langerhans cell.[229,232] Definitive diagnosis requires electron microscopy demonstration of Birbeck granules in lesional histiocytes or the presence of a certain antigen in a typical histopathologic setting.[225]

The clinical manifestations of Langerhans cell histiocytosis are protean, and it is now recognized that the previous categories of Letterer-Siwe disease and Hand-Schüller-Christian are too restrictive; however, it is necessary to evaluate the patient for multisystem involvement and to classify the disorder. Classification defines prognosis, clarifies appropriate treatment options, and identifies possible future complications. Furthermore, ongoing evaluation is needed because the extent of the disease and its classification may change. A patient with Langerhans cell histiocytosis should be classified as having solitary bone involvement, multiple bone involvement without soft tissue involvement, bone and soft tissue involvement, or soft tissue involvement alone. Furthermore, the presence of organ dysfunction also should be determined[246] (Table 10-4).

TABLE 10-4 Criteria of Organ Dysfunction in Langerhans Cell Histiocytosis

Liver
Albumin < 2.5 gm/dL
Bilirubin > 1.5 mg/dL
Edema
Ascites

Pulmonary System[*]
Cough
Cyanosis
Dyspnea
Pleural effusion
Pneumothorax

Hematopoietic System
Anemia < 10 mg/dL[†]
Leukopenia < 4000/dL
Neutropenia < 1500/dL
Thrombocytopenia < 100,000/dL

---

[*] Not secondary to pulmonary infection.
[†] Not attributable to iron deficiency anemia.

Adapted from Lahey ME. Histiocytosis X—an analysis of prognostic factors. J Pediatr 1975;87:184.

Common sites of soft tissue involvement include the skin, the pituitary stalk, the lungs, the liver, the spleen, and the bone marrow. Skin involvement may vary from a few discrete pinhead lesions to a generalized pustular eczematous eruption. Although it is not the cause of death, generalized skin disease is a poor prognostic factor[217,245,247] and is a typical presenting feature in children younger than 2 years of age. Involvement of other organs, such as the lungs, the liver, the spleen, and the bone marrow, is the usual cause of death.[213,214,217,246,247,254,261] Fatal dissemination occurs more often in children 2 years of age and younger at onset, but it also may occur when the disease is diagnosed in later childhood or even in the adult years.[257]

Diabetes insipidus occurs in 12% to 50% of children with multiple system involvement.[214,231,247] It may be the only abnormality at the onset of the disease,[266] but more often it occurs after Langerhans cell histiocytosis already has been diagnosed. Diabetes insipidus is the most frequent soft tissue abnormality that subsequently develops in patients who only have bone involvement at the onset of disease. More generalized involvement of the brain occurs in adults and in children with disseminated disease.[240]

Skeletal lesions are common, occurring in 80% to 97% of patients with Langerhans cell histiocytosis.[216,217,230,247,261] The skull, the spine, the pelvis, the ribs, and the femur are the common sites of bony lesions.[239] Involvement of other long bones also occurs, but lesions in the hands and the feet are rare. Skull lesions have a well-defined, punched-out appearance[227,264] (Fig. 10-13B). Vertebra plana, first described by Compere and colleagues,[226] is the typical spinal lesion. The vertebral body is markedly collapsed, but in contrast to infection the adjacent disc space is preserved. Posterior elements usually are spared. In the series by Ruppert and colleagues[264] a thoracic vertebra

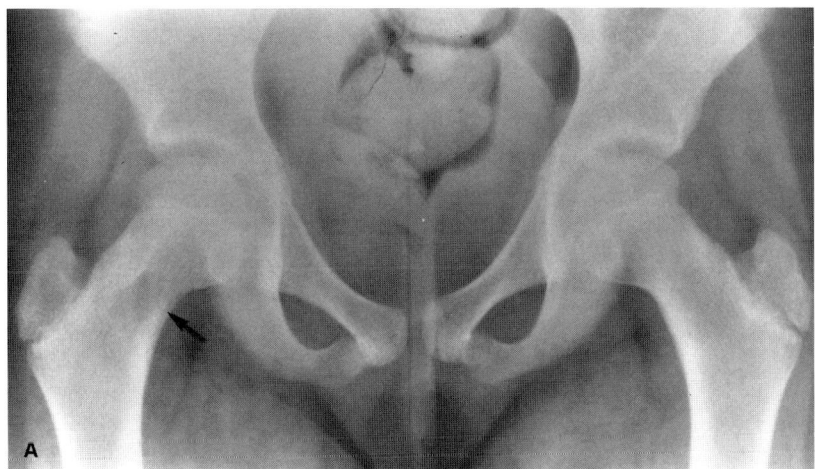

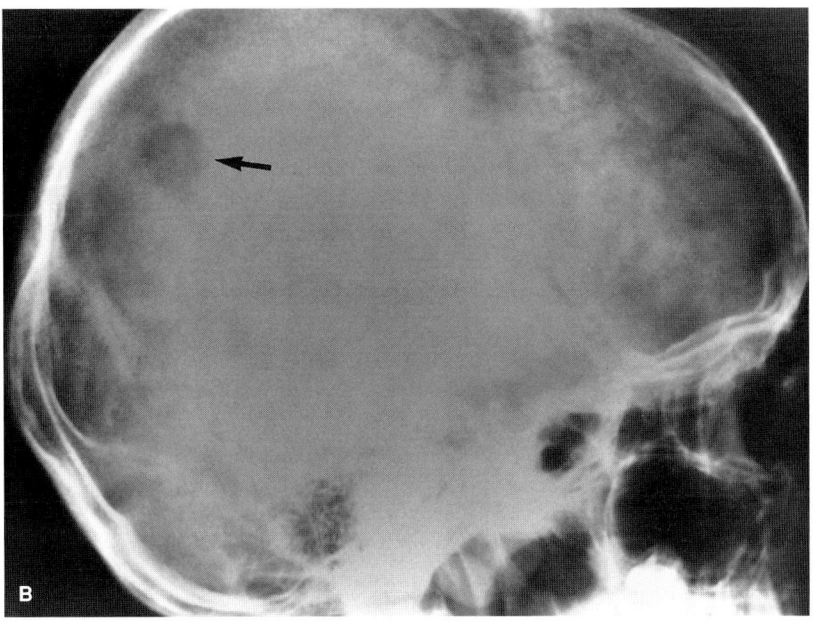

FIGURE 10-13. Eosinophilic granuloma with multiple bone involvement in a 9-year-old girl who had progressive symptoms of pain and limp involving the right hip. (**A**) Anteroposterior radiograph of the pelvis demonstrates a lytic lesion in the right femoral neck. Biopsy defined the diagnosis. Follow-up radiographs taken 5 months later show complete resolution of the lesion. (**B**) Lateral radiograph of the skull 5 months after biopsy of the femur. At that time, the patient had a sore spot on the back of the head. Radiographs show the typical "punched-out" appearance of eosinophilic granuloma. Three months later, the patient developed a third bony lesion in the left proximal femur. Subsequent follow-up showed a full resolution of symptoms without therapy.

was most often affected (54%) and a cervical vertebra was least often involved (11%).

A typical long bone lesion is lytic and is located in the diaphysis or metaphysis[227] (see Fig. 10-13). Other radiographic features include endosteal scalloping, cortical thinning, and widening of the medullary cavity.[264] Lamellated periosteal elevation simulating Ewing sarcoma or osteomyelitis may occur (Fig. 10-14) and accounts for approximately 5% of the solitary eosinophilic granulomas. In a series of 25 children presenting with unilateral midfemoral periosteal new bone formation, 10 cases were secondary to Ewing sarcoma, and 7 were diagnosed as eosinophilic granuloma.[243] Patients with Ewing sarcoma are more likely to show definite Codman triangles as well as intramedullary and cortical destruction. Epiphyseal or transphyseal involvement is uncommon but has been reported.[234,248,264] In a series of 15 solitary lucent epiphyseal lesions, only one case was secondary to eosinophilic granuloma.[234]

Although bone scans may identify lesions that are not seen on radiographs, these imaging studies are not routinely obtained because the false-negative rate is high.[216] MRI changes also are nonspecific because the low signal intensity on T1-weighted images and the high signal intensity on T2-weighted images does not differentiate eosinophilic granuloma from osteomyelitis or Ewing sarcoma.[212] On the other hand, bone scans, computed tomography, and MRI may be useful in localizing a site of unexplained pain or in finding spinal cord compression.

A bony lesion without soft tissue involvement is the most common presentation of Langerhans cell histiocytosis, accounting for 50% to 77% of the pediatric cases.[216,230,247,261] Patients with solitary bone involvement at disease onset have the best prognosis, and in this group of patients no deaths have been reported.[213,214,216,217,224,233,247,261] By comparison, patients with organ dysfunction at disease onset have a mortality rate of 30% to 70%.[214,247,254,261] Evolution to multiple bone lesions or soft tissue involvement, or both, is also uncommon in patients with solitary bone involvement at disease onset. Bollini and colleagues[216] reviewed 216 patients from 8 series who had solitary bone involvement. Evolution to multiple bone lesions occurred in 7%, mostly during the first year after diagnosis, and only 1% developed soft tissue involvement. Dimentberg and Brown[230] found a 30% incidence of new bony lesions in patients with initial solitary involvement. Their protocol, however, included periodic skeletal surveys, and 55% of their new lesions were asymptomatic.

Multiple bone involvement without soft tissue involvement has a good prognosis; however, the incidence of additional bone lesions and subsequent soft tissue involvement is higher in this group compared with patients who have solitary bony lesions at disease onset.[230] The mortality rate is low in this group and was observed in only 1 of 22 patients reported by Raney and D'Angio.[261] Diabetes insipidus is the most common soft tissue problem that occurs in this group.

The presenting complaint of patients with a solitary bone lesion is localized swelling, pain, or limp (Fig. 10-15). The child also may be asymptomatic, and the diagnosis may be made on radiographs obtained for unrelated circumstances. These patients should be evaluated for possible soft tissue and additional bone lesion involvement. The parents should be questioned specifically for symptoms of lethargy, polyuria or polydypsia, chronic cough, dyspnea, and feeding difficulties. Physical examination should assess the possibility of skin rash; otitis media; exophthalmos; tachypnea; sinusitis; hepatomegaly; jaundice; splenomegaly; growth retardation; and swelling over the skull, the facial bones, the spine, and the extremities. A lateral skull radiograph is a good screening study for a child with a solitary bone lesion of unknown etiology. Additional laboratory studies that should be considered for a child with known Langerhans cell histiocytosis include a complete blood count and smear, liver function tests, serum and urine osmolarity, and radiographic survey of the chest and skeleton.[230] Unless clinically indicated, hand and feet radio-

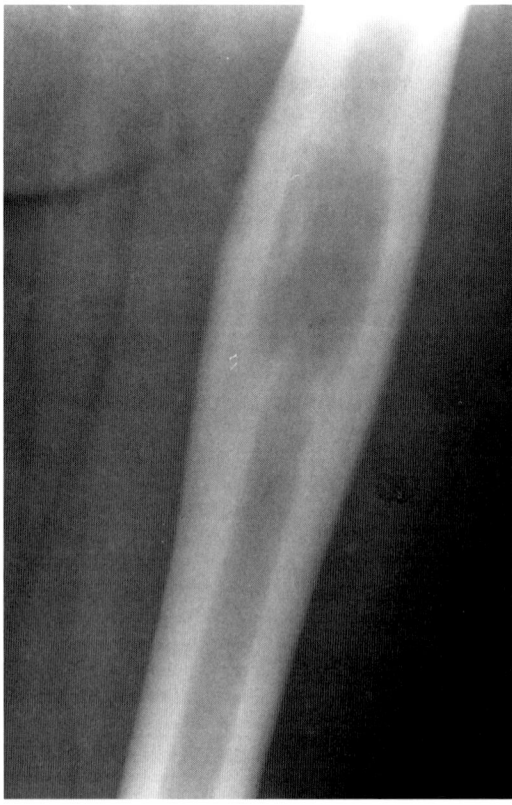

FIGURE 10-14. Eosinophilic granuloma in a 12-year-old girl who had pain in the thigh for 3 to 4 months. Radiograph of the femur shows an expansile lesion with periosteal reaction.

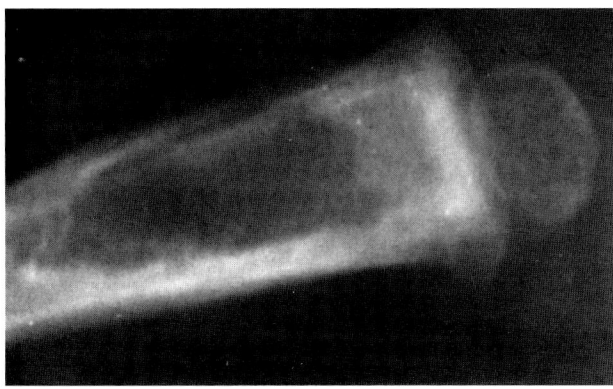

FIGURE 10-15. Eosinophilic granuloma in a 9-month-old boy who had a 2-week history of a mass in the thigh. Prior to transfer, the patient had received several days of antibiotic therapy. Lateral radiograph of the distal femur shows a large lytic lesion with periosteal elevation. After biopsy and curettage, the femur was protected with a spica cast. No other lesions developed, and follow-up 10 years later demonstrated no abnormalities.

graphs are not necessary because these regions are rarely involved. For patients with significant risk of organ dysfunction, such as those with obvious soft tissue involvement or those younger than 3 years of age who have multiple bone lesions, Dimentberg and Brown[230] recommend additional studies to include arterial blood gas, bone marrow aspirate, computed tomography scan of the chest, abdominal ultrasound, audiology assessment, dental assessment, and immunologic profile.

A tissue biopsy specimen is necessary to confirm the suspected diagnosis. The exception is patients with classic multifocal radiographic findings. When involved, skin lesions are the preferred site of biopsy. A typical lytic lesion of bone can be biopsied by a transcutaneous needle aspiration.[210,216,242] Open biopsy is preferred when curettage is indicated or for middiaphyseal lesions characterized by periosteal elevation.

Treatment of bone lesions in patients without soft tissue involvement should be limited to either observation, curettage, or steroid injection. In a study evaluating treated and untreated bone lesions in Langerhans cell histiocytosis, the mode of treatment did not influence the rate of healing.[270] Solitary eosinophilic granuloma, in particular, may be a self-limiting disease requiring no treatment.[252] Low-dose radiotherapy should not be used because there are two reports documenting secondary malignancy after this treatment modality was used for solitary bone involvement.[230,237] Curettage is an adjunct to an open biopsy. In addition, this mode of therapy, with or without supplemental bone graft, may be selected for lesions associated with intense pain or significant risk of fracture. Capanna and colleagues[221] and other authors[210,218,265] have reported favorable results after in-

jecting steroids by a technique similar to that used for unicameral bone cysts. Owing to the variable rate of healing and self-limited nature of eosinophilic granuloma, it is difficult to know whether this treatment influences the natural history. Steroid injections, however, may be preferred for vertebral body lesions[210] or for lesions with persistent pain and slow healing following curettage.

Solitary spinal lesions in patients typically cause pain and may be associated with postural adaptations, such as torticollis or scoliosis. On the other hand, multiple sites of asymptomatic spinal involvement may be present in patients with disseminated soft tissue involvement. Vertebra plana without posterior arch involvement is the most common pattern, but cases have been reported of lesions limited to the posterior arch and those involving the vertebral body without causing collapse and the spinal cord without bony involvement.[211,263,264,269] Most patients do not have neurologic deficit and can be treated symptomatically by short-term immobilization after the diagnosis has been confirmed. Reconstitution of vertebral height to a variable but effective amount is the natural history,[256] and long-term follow-up studies have not observed back or neck dysfunction.[220,256,263]

Although uncommon, eosinophilic granuloma of the spine may cause neurologic deficit.[210,224,235,244,263] In these patients, clinical and MRI examinations should be able to differentiate nerve root involvement from spinal cord compression. With nerve root impingement, treatment should include bed rest, immobilization, and perhaps steroid injection. For patients with spinal cord compression, surgical decompression and stabilization should be considered unless there is disseminated disease and an unfavorable prognosis. Radiotherapy may be indicated with this degree of involvement.

Chemotherapy, like radiotherapy, has a more limited role in patients with Langerhans cell histiocytosis.[254,260] Patients with solitary bone involvement are no longer treated with chemotherapy. Treatment remains controversial for the patients with multiple bone site involvement. In a study of 92 patients with multiple bone lesion, Berry and colleagues[214] noted no progression of the disease in 25 patients, continuous progression in 53, and intermittent recurrence in 13. A favorable prognostic factor, however, was involvement limited to bone. Therefore, most authors now agree that systemic chemotherapy generally is reserved for patients who have constitutional symptoms, such as fever and weight loss, and those who have severe skin involvement and organ dysfunction, as defined by Lahey.[260,267] Even in this group, a short course of prednisolone may be the best initial treatment.[254] Monochemotherapy with etoposide or vinblastine[222,223,241,268] as opposed to combination chemotherapy with agents

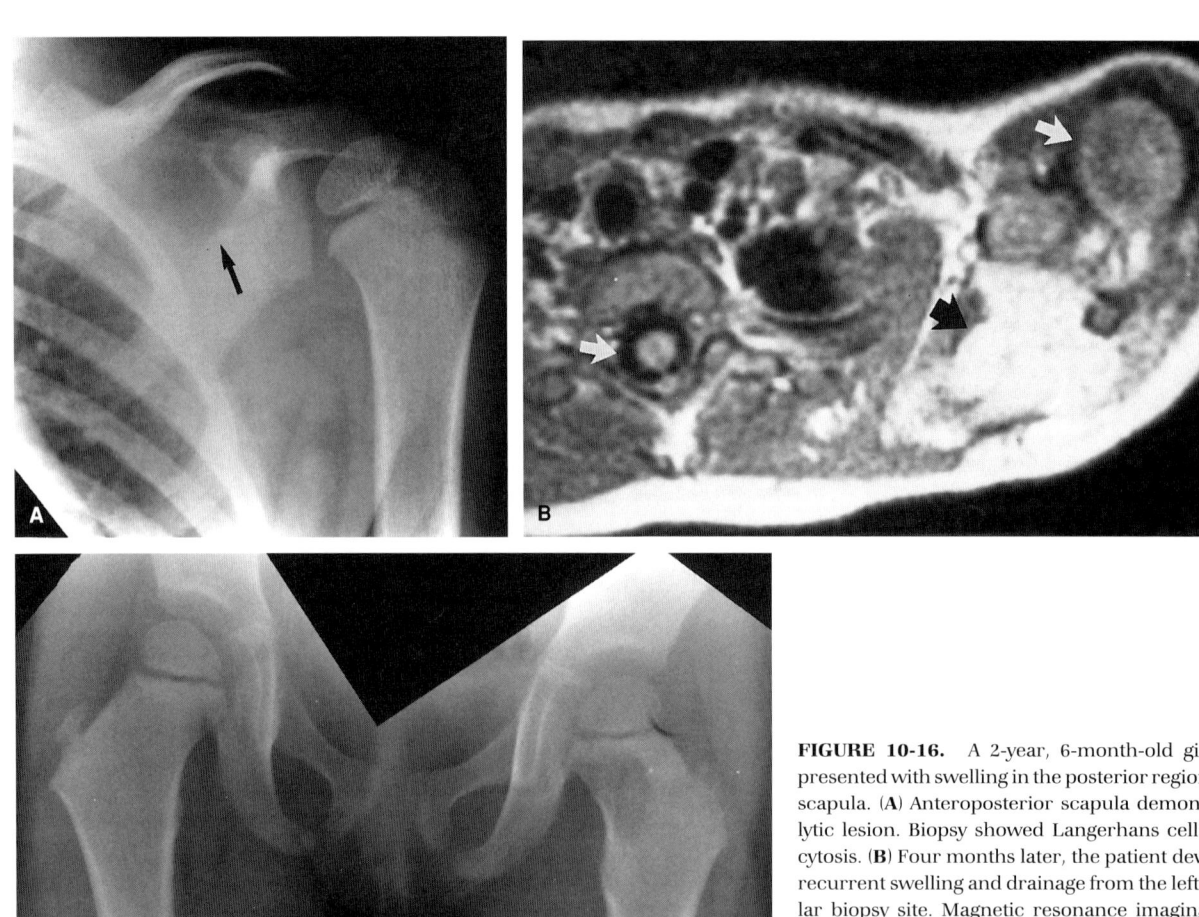

FIGURE 10-16. A 2-year, 6-month-old girl who presented with swelling in the posterior region of the scapula. (A) Anteroposterior scapula demonstrated lytic lesion. Biopsy showed Langerhans cell histiocytosis. (B) Four months later, the patient developed recurrent swelling and drainage from the left scapular biopsy site. Magnetic resonance imaging prior to the second biopsy of the scapula shows increased signal intensity with spread into soft tissues anterior and posterior to the scapula. *White arrow* points to humeral head and spinal cord. *Black arrow* points to the mass invading the scapula. Repeat biopsy also demonstrated Langerhans cell histiocytosis. The scapular lesion subsequently resolved without problems. (C) Anteroposterior radiograph of the pelvis at age 3 years, 4 months. At that time, the patient had developed a limp and pain in the left leg. Radiographs show a lytic lesion in the proximal femur. Spica cast immobilization was used for 7 weeks. (D) Frog-leg lateral radiograph of the left hip at age 3 years, 4 months. (E) Anteroposterior radiograph of the pelvis at age 3 years, 6 months. (F) Frog-leg lateral radiograph of the pelvis at age 3 years, 6 months. Trabecular pattern indicates progressive healing of the Langerhans cell histiocytosis. (Courtesy of Gary D. Bos, M.D.)

such as adriamycin, methotrexate, vinblastine, and 6-mercaptopurine may be a better alternative. Bone marrow transplantation also has been reported in isolated cases that did not respond to multiple regimen chemotherapy.[238,262]

The earliest radiographic finding seen with healing of appendicular skeletal lesions is change to a trabecular pattern (Fig. 10-16). In the study by Alexander and colleagues[209] the trabecular pattern occurred at 6 to 10 weeks following diagnosis in patients who had uneventful healing. Complete healing then occurred within the next 36 to 40 weeks. Therefore, it is reasonable to repeat radiographs of the involved lesion approximately 2 months after diagnosis. If a trabecular pattern has developed, the next radiologic examination can be scheduled at the 6-month interval. However, if no evidence of trabeculation has occurred, repeat radiographs are warranted in another 2 months. If there is no evidence of healing at 4 months following diagnosis, additional therapy may be indi-

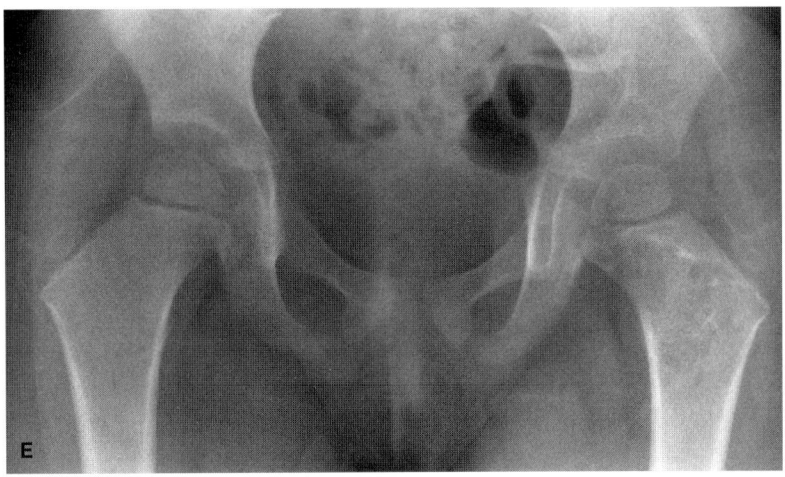
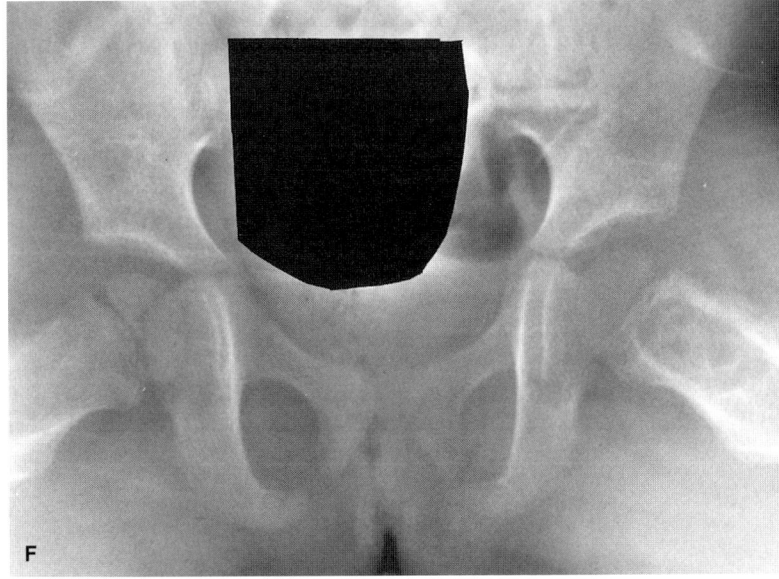

FIGURE 10-16. (*Continued*)

cated. Routine skeletal surveys as well as a complete physical examination are performed every 6 months for at least 2 years.[230] These surveys will diagnose new bony and soft tissue lesions in a timely fashion.

In summary, Langerhans cell histiocytosis is a fascinating disorder that is probably secondary to an aberrant reactive immunologic process that causes tissue destruction. Solitary bony involvement is most common. In these patients, treatment probably does not influence healing, and making a diagnosis and classifying the extent of involvement is more important. Periodic reexamination is needed because the disease classification may change. Patients with organ dysfunction have a guarded prognosis, and systemic chemotherapy is indicated.

DISORDERS OF HEMOSTASIS

Hemostasis not only permits safe surgery but also protects us from the many bumps of everyday activity. Injury to a blood vessel initiates a highly integrated set of reactions to restore hemostasis. Although the reactions overlap, it is helpful to divide the clotting process into vascular, platelet, and plasma phases.

The vascular phase includes the grossly evident vasoconstriction and exposure of tissue elements that promote adhesion and aggregation of platelets, release tissue thromboplastin to activate the extrinsic coagulation pathway, and activate factor XII to initiate the intrinsic coagulation pathway. The platelet phase of coagulation includes adhesion of platelets to vascular tissues (assisted by factor VIII–related von Willebrand factor), aggregation of platelets to each other, and consolidation of the platelet plug by deposition of fibrin within it.

The plasma phase of restoring hemostasis has an intrinsic and extrinsic pathway. Both sets of reactions produce thrombin (Fig. 10-17), which is the key to formation and stabilization of the fibrin clot. In the extrinsic pathway, tissue thromboplastin activates factor VII, which in the presence of ionic calcium activates factor X. The intrinsic coagulation cascade is more important and begins with sequential activation

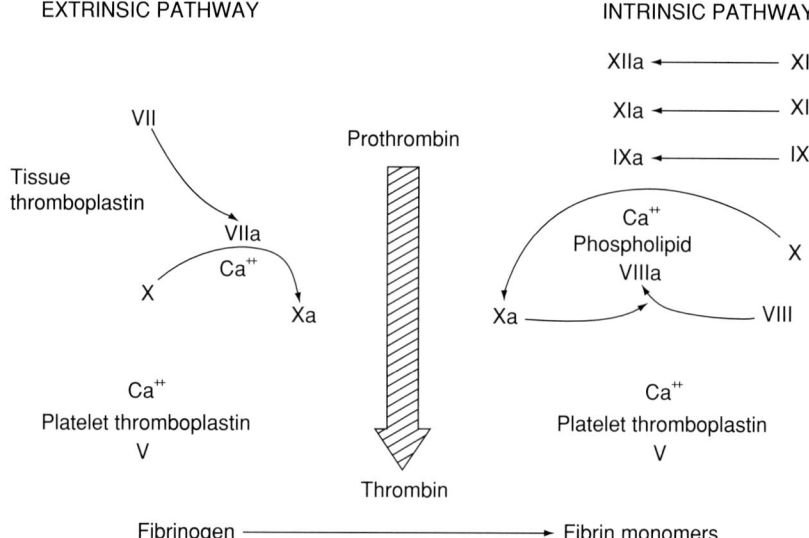

FIGURE 10-17. Formation of thrombin.

of factors XII, XI, and IX. Factor VIII, when activated by thrombin and activated factor X, markedly accelerates the activation of factor X by activated factor IX. Activated factor X, whether derived from the intrinsic or the extrinsic pathway, combines with factor V, ionic calcium, and platelet thromboplastin to convert prothrombin to thrombin. Thrombin acts to cleave peptides from fibrinogen, creating fibrin monomers that consolidate the platelet plug.

Thrombocytopenia With Absent Radius Syndrome

Thrombocytopenia with absent radius (TAR) syndrome is a unique autosomal recessive condition that always has upper extremity skeletal deficiencies and frequently demonstrates congenital abnormalities of the lower extremity. In 1969, Hall and colleagues[276] reviewed 40 patients and clearly defined the association of thrombocytopenia with absence of the radius. A more recent review of 100 cases with adequate documentation has further clarified the clinical spectrum of this disorder.[277] The juxtaposition of skeletal abnormalities and thrombocytopenia is intriguing. It is likely that the genes responsible for each defect are located at similar geographic positions on the same chromosome.[277]

Upper extremity deficiencies in TAR are characterized by an intercalary radial hemimelia with the thumb always being present.[273,276,277] Hypoplasia of the thumb, however, does occur. By contrast, in Diamond-Blackfan anemia and Fanconi anemia, the upper extremity abnormalities are mostly at the thumb, and radial deficiencies of the forearm are either absent or mild. Furthermore, in TAR the remainder of the upper extremity is frequently involved (Table 10-5). Hypopla-

TABLE 10-5 **Skeletal Deficiency in Thrombocytopenia with Absent Radius Syndrome**

DEFICIENCY	PRESENCE/NUMBER PATIENTS WITH ADEQUATE DOCUMENTATION
Upper Extremity	
Bilateral absent radius	99/100
Unilateral absent radius	1/100
Thumbs present	100/100
Thumbs hypoplastic	48/92
Ulnar involvement	50/68
Short and bowed	35
Unilaterally absent	3
Bilaterally absent	12
Humerus involvement	36/87
Hypoplastic	22
Absent	14
Shoulder girdle involvement (hypoplastic or absent scapular and clavicle)	10/49
Middle phalanx little finger (hypoplastic and absent)	35/41
Lower Extremity	
Hip dislocation	6/79
Lower extremity phocomelia	5/100
Stiff knee	9/100
Genu varum	29/92
Patella abnormalities	13/92
Clubfoot	4/100
Face	
Mandibular hypoplasia	11/79

Adapted from Hedberg VA, Lipton JM. Thrombocytopenia with absent radii. Am J Pediatr Hematol Oncol 1988;10:51.

sia, or absence of the middle phalanx of the little finger, also has been noted in 85% of the cases with adequate documentation.

Thrombocytopenia may necessitate a delay in centralization of the hand and wrist (Fig. 10-18). Early and prolonged splinting and frequent stretching exercises will prevent the resultant soft tissue contractures.[272] With shortening of the humerus and the ulna, centralization may be contraindicated.

Lower extremity abnormalities in TAR are mostly at the knee. Genu varum associated with flexion contracture and internal tibial torsion was the most common abnormality recorded by Schoenecker and colleagues[278] in their detailed description of 21 patients. Absence or hypoplasia of the patella also was observed and in some patients was accompanied by either lateral or medial dislocation. Hypoplasia of the medial femoral condyle was a primary factor in the genu varum caused by joint malalignment. Recurrent varus was a frequent finding following osteotomies and patella realignment procedures. Gounder and colleagues[274] reported on soft tissue release of the knee followed by postoperative bracing but did not provide adequate information concerning long-term follow-up to determine whether soft tissue releases performed at an early age were better than osteotomy for the knee deformities in TAR.

Micrognathia, secondary to mandibular hypoplasia, also may be present (see Table 10-5). Cardiac anomalies have been reported in 22% of patients with TAR with tetralogy of Fallot, atrial septal defect, and ventricular septal defect being the most common lesions.[277]

Hematologic manifestations, in contrast to Fanconi anemia, typically begin during the neonatal period. The onset of the thrombocytopenia was noted by the first week of life in 58% of subjects, between 1 and 6 weeks of age in 19%, and before 1 year of age in 11%. Delayed onset of the thrombocytopenia, however, does occur and was noted after 2 years of age in 6 of 75 cases.[277]

Thrombocytopenia in patients with TAR syndrome tends to be episodic and precipitated by nonspecific stresses, such as upper respiratory tract infections and gastrointestinal disturbances.[275] The platelet count is typically in the range of 15,000 to 30,000/mm^3 but may be more depressed.[275] Platelet function is normal and, therefore, bleeding tendencies correlate with platelet counts. Anemia may occur as a consequence of the bleeding. Periodic leukemoid reactions may be observed and temporally correlate with the thrombocytopenic episodes.

Supportive therapy with platelet transfusions has significantly altered the mortality risk.[277] Appropriate transfusions are prescribed for bleeding episodes, but to minimize the risk of multiple platelet transfusions, prophylactic therapy is only prescribed when the platelet count approaches 5000/mm^3. The thrombocytopenia typically resolves by early childhood, and steroids or splenectomy are not necessary. The timing of operations for the skeletal deformities has to be individualized but is usually feasible between 6 months and 6 years of age.[274,277]

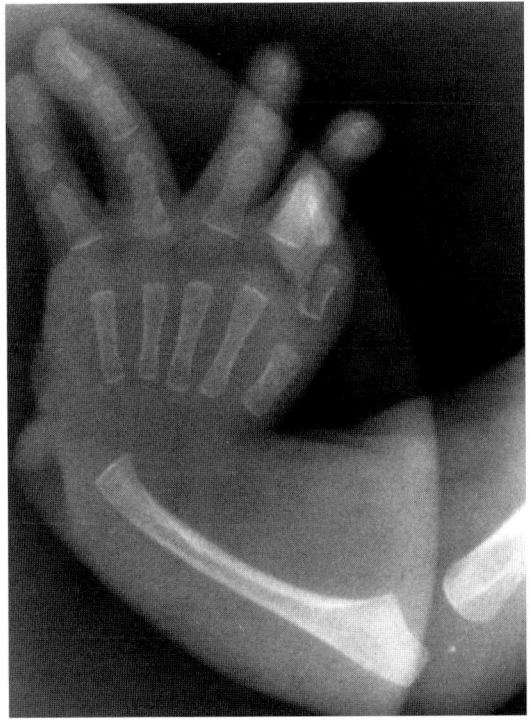

FIGURE 10-18. Anteroposterior radiograph of the left hand of a 1-month-old infant with bilateral radial hemimelia and essentially normal thumbs. Patient was started on a program of progressive casting and splinting, with anticipation of centralization at 6 months of age. At age 2 months, laboratory studies obtained for evaluation of gastroenteritis revealed thrombocytopenia with a platelet count of 17,000/mm^3. Low platelet count continued, and centralization of the wrist had not been performed as of the age of 1-year, 9-months.

Hemophilia

Any of the thirteen coagulation factors may be deficient, but musculoskeletal problems are primarily seen in patients with deficits of either factor VIII or factor IX coagulant activity. Factor VIII deficiency, also known as classic hemophilia or hemophilia A, constitutes about 75% of all inherited clotting disorders and affects 60 to 80 per 1 million people in the general population.[324] Factor IX deficiency, also known as Christmas disease or hemophilia B, is the second most common inherited clotting disorder and affects about 12% of people affected by a clotting disorder. The other inherited coagulation disorders are not only less common but, more importantly, are characterized by mucosal hemorrhages, such as epistaxis and menorrhagia, and rarely demonstrate hemorrhage into a joint except after major trauma.

The diagnosis of hemophilia usually has been made before joint bleeds develop. Bleeding at the time of circumcision, atypical bruising with neonatal immunizations, and lip lacerations in toddlers learning to walk arouse clinical suspicion and investigation of a possible coagulation disorder. Both factor VIII and factor IX deficiencies are transmitted by a sex-linked recessive gene and, therefore, both disorders are largely restricted to the male population. A history of affected males on the maternal side of the family combined with a history of hemorrhage should lead to the appropriate laboratory test. The partial thromboplastin time (PTT) is abnormal in both factor VIII and factor IX deficiency. Specific factor assays are used to establish the deficiency and its degree of severity.

Coagulation factors are quantitated in units; 1 unit is equal to the activity of the clotting factor in 1 mL of pooled, normal plasma. The concentration of factors VIII and IX is commonly designated as percent activity, representing units per deciliter. Therefore, factor VIII and IX activity in a normal person should be 100%, but a range from 50% to 200% is within normal limits. Deficiencies of either factor VIII or factor IX are commonly graded as severe, less than 1% activity; moderate, 1% to 5% activity; and mild, greater than 5% activity.[302] In patients who have a severe clotting deficiency, hemorrhage may occur with minimal trauma or spontaneously during normal daily activities. A hemarthrosis rarely develops in a patient with mild deficiency unless significant trauma occurs. Patients with moderate deficiency have intermediate symptoms but typically develop significantly less joint arthropathy than those with severe disorders.

Neither acute bleeding episodes nor surgery can be managed effectively in hemophiliacs without appropriate replacement of the missing clotting factor. When only whole blood or plasma was available, the volume requirements for even a single transfusion were so great that transfusions were only administered in limb-threatening and life-threatening situations. The discovery of cryoprecipitates, in 1965,[338] made the effective treatment of acute hemorrhages possible. The subsequent development of concentrates[285,353] made it possible to deliver a total blood volume of clotting factor in a 50 mL solution. Starting in the 1970s, these concentrates also made elective operations and home transfusion therapy feasible.

Both factor VIII and factor IX concentrates were initially prepared from plasma that was pooled from many donors. This process allowed transmission of blood-borne diseases. In the 1970s, hepatitis was a recognized complication of transfusion therapy, and most hemophiliacs at that time had hepatitis-associated antibodies, although few developed chronic hepatitis.[309] In the early 1980s, AIDS clearly was identified in hemophiliacs. Heat treatment of the concentrates, however, virtually eliminated the HIV virus so that hemophiliacs who received their initial transfusion after 1984 did not get infected by the HIV virus.[302] Both factor VIII and factor IX can now be manufactured using recombinant DNA techniques that produce a purified product. Therefore, at this time, most pediatric patients with hemophilia are seronegative for both HIV and hepatitis viruses.[148]

Inhibitors, antibodies that inhibit the infused product, develop in about 15% of patients with severe factor VIII deficiencies.[344] The prevalence in patients with factor IX deficiency is much less.[326] Patients with an inhibitor do not bleed more frequently but have limited options for transfusion. The potency of a patient's inhibitor status is defined in Bethesda units per milliliter of plasma. Inhibitor titers greater than 10 to 20 Bethesda units/mL plasma cannot be overwhelmed with high doses of factor VIII, and therefore elective surgery is not feasible.[302] The exception is the selective situation in which a patient has undergone multiple, sequential transfusions to induce immune tolerance.[283,293] Emergency lifesaving or limb-saving surgery in patients with high titer inhibitors may be accomplished with agents such as activated factor VII or porcine factor VIII. The possibility of uncontrolled bleeding with these agents demands that their use be selective. The likelihood of developing a high-titer inhibitor is remote if a patient has received 100 transfusions,[350] and elective surgery may proceed in these people without apprehension that this complication will develop in the postoperative period.

With development of effective concentrates, administering the clotting factor at home became a reality.[312] Home transfusion therapy has minimized bleeding complications. Active encouragement by physicians and training by nurse specialists make it feasible to institute home replacement therapy in approximately 80% of hemophilia patients before 5 years of age. For routine treatment of muscle or joint hemorrhages, the patient or the patient's parents transfuse 20 to 25 units of factor per kilogram of body weight. This amount of transfusion typically keeps the clotting factor greater than 1% for at least 48 hours (Fig. 10-19). Home transfusion therapy has reduced the severity and incidence of hemophilic arthropathy but has not eliminated this problem.

Arthropathy in a hemophiliac person begins with a hemarthrosis, particularly when 2 or 3 bleeding episodes occur in a joint within a short period. As the blood inside the joint is catabolized, the breakdown products must be absorbed by the synovium. Iron seems to be the most damaging element.[279,302,321,347] Synovial cells can absorb a limited amount of iron, but when that quantity is exceeded the cell disintegrates

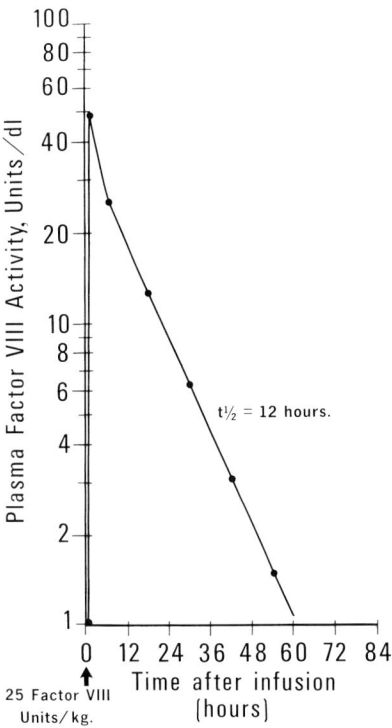

FIGURE 10-19. Typical fall-off curve after infusion of 25 U/kg body weight of factor VIII in a patient with severe hemophilia. (From Green WB. Disease of the hematopoietic system and chronic inflammatory arthritides: musculoskeletal complications in children. In: Bowen JR, Epps CE, eds. Complications in pediatric orthopaedic surgery. Philadelphia: JB Lippincott, 1995.)

and releases lysosomes that not only destroy articular cartilage but inflame the synovial tissue. The result is a hypertrophic and hypervascular synovium that, in a person with a clotting deficiency, is friable and tends to bleed easily (Fig. 10-20). Thus begins a vicious cycle of recurrent hemarthrosis followed by more synovitis and joint destruction.

Blood breakdown products also affect the chondrocytes. Even in the early stage of joint disease the chondrocytes contain siderosomes (secondary lysosomes containing iron ferritin granules) and show intracellular evidence of cell disruption.[302,342] With disintegration of the chondrocyte, not only are lysosomes released to destroy the matrix of the cartilage, but the factory, or the chondrocyte, also is destroyed (Fig. 10-21). The result of this is an arthropathy that may progress rapidly (Figs. 10-22 and 10-23).

With advanced hemophilic arthropathy, the synovium loses its marked villous formation, is largely replaced by fibrous tissue, and therefore is not as hypertrophic.[347,351] This, in combination with erosion of the articular surfaces, causes loss of joint motion.[316] The result may be a progressive arthropathy that causes a disabling arthritis at an early age (see Fig. 10-21).

Radiographic changes in the early stages of hemophilic arthropathy are similar to those observed in rheumatoid arthritis. With initiation of synovitis, the radiographic findings include soft tissue swelling, osteopenia, and overgrowth of the epiphysis.[279] As the disease progresses, marginal erosions, subchondral cysts, subchondral irregularity, widening of the intercondylar notch of the femur, squaring of the patella, enlargement of the radial head, and widening of the trochlear notch of the olecranon are characteristic changes. With end-stage arthropathy, narrowing of the articular cartilage is obvious, but the subchondral bone is more sclerotic in hemophiliacs compared with that in patients with rheumatoid arthritis.

Hemophilic arthropathy may be staged by radiographic classification. Using range of motion and muscle torque, Greene and colleagues[305] compared the classification system developed by Arnold and Hilgartner[279] with the one described by Pettersson and col-

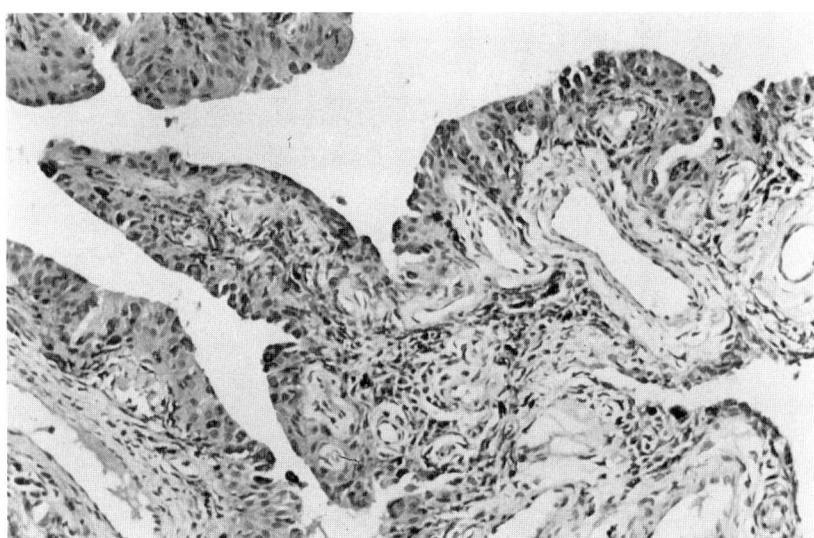

FIGURE 10-20. Synovium from an 8-year-old boy with hemophilia who had an 18-month history of hypertrophic synovitis and recurrent hemarthrosis in the knee. Note villous formation, markedly increased vascularity, and chronic inflammatory cell infiltrates. (From Greene WB, McMillan CW. Nonsurgical management of hemophilic arthropathy. Instr Course Lect. 1989;38:367.)

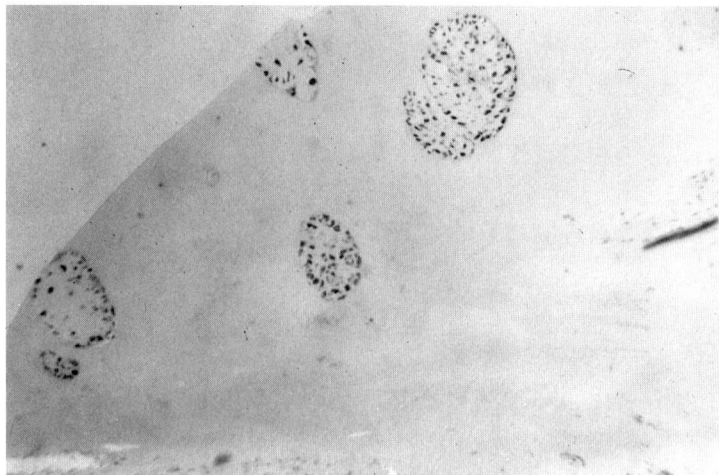

FIGURE 10-21. Cartilage shaving from patellar erosions in an 11-year-old boy with factor IX hemophilia. The patient had had only a 9-month history of difficulty with this knee. Chondrocytes demonstrate disintegration with iron deposition around the periphery (Perls stain). (From Greene WB, McMillan CW. Nonsurgical management of hemophilic arthropathy. Instr Course Lect. 1989;38:367.)

leagues.[335] The Pettersson classification was more difficult to use but was better for staging advanced arthropathy. Greene and colleagues[305] found that the Pettersson classification could be simplified without losing accuracy if it was reduced to a four-part, seven-point classification system (Table 10-6).

MRI demonstrates soft tissue abnormalities and articular cartilage erosion better than plain radiographs.[336,358] Nuss and colleagues[330] reported that MRI was helpful in making the decision for synovectomy in children with hemophilic arthropathy.

The knee, the ankle, and the elbow are the joints most commonly affected in hemophiliacs.[279,280,296,297,315] In small children, the ankle is frequently the target joint because it is vulnerable to jumping, an activity that is prominent in the play of this age group. After the age of 5 years, the knee joint assumes a more prominent role. In adolescents, Aronstam and colleagues[280] observed that the elbow was the most common site of bleeding, but other series[296,297,315] have noted that the knee or the ankle is most frequently affected at that age. The shoulder, the hip, and the wrist joints

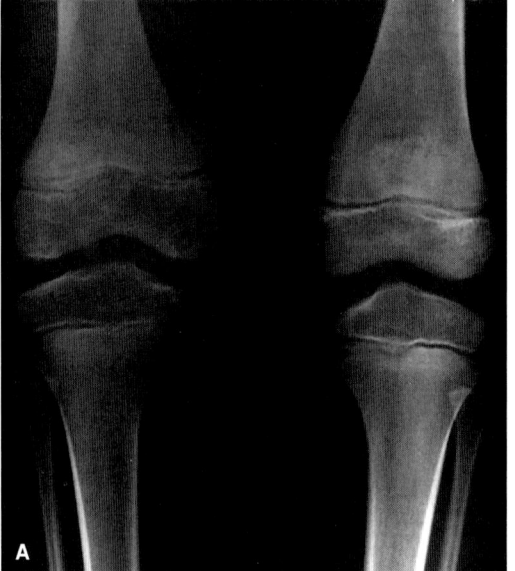
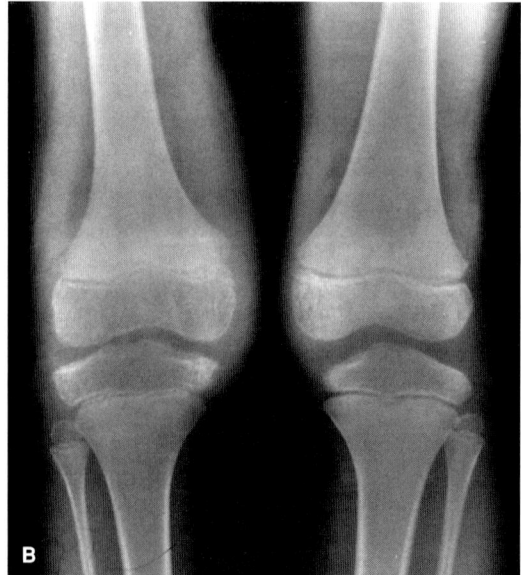

FIGURE 10-22. (A) Anteroposterior standing radiograph of the knee in a 7-year 2-month-old male with factor VIII deficiency. Early changes of hypertrophic synovitis and hemophilic arthropathy are present in the right knee. Note the widening of the intercondylar notch. (B) Anteroposterior standing radiograph of both knees 8 months later. The arthropathy has progressed despite good compliance with home transfusion therapy and 6 months of prophylactic transfusions. Significant joint narrowing and cartilage erosions are observed in the right knee. (From Greene WB. Diseases of the hematopoietic system and chronic inflammatory arthritides: Musculoskeletal complications in children. In: Bowen JR, Epps CE, eds. Complications in pediatric orthopaedic surgery. Philadelphia: JB Lippincott, 1995.)

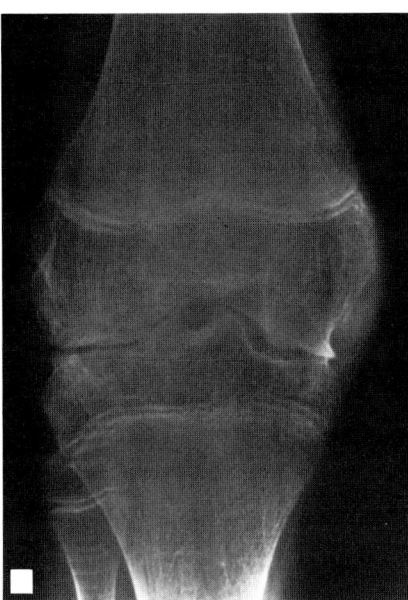

FIGURE 10-23. Radiograph of the knee of a 14-year-old boy with advanced hemophilic arthropathy.

rarely are affected by a hemarthrosis and, in this era of home therapy, they rarely progress to significant arthropathy.

The physical signs of a minor hemarthrosis include increased warmth, swelling, and some limitation of motion. A prodrome of pain or discomfort frequently is perceived by the older child before joint swelling is obvious. A minor hemarthrosis can be treated at home by transfusing the appropriate concentrate as soon as possible. Ice packs and mild analgesics are useful adjuncts in controlling pain and swelling. For a bleed into a weight-bearing joint, crutches are used until the pain has fully subsided and until 90 degrees of knee motion or full ankle dorsiflexion has been achieved.

A major hemarthrosis is different. This type of bleed usually occurs after significant trauma or as a recurrent hemarthrosis in a joint that already is affected by synovitis. A major hemarthrosis is painful. Furthermore, with a large amount of blood in the joint recurrent hemarthrosis and hypertrophic synovitis are likely sequelae. In addition to transfusion therapy, a major hemarthrosis should be treated by aspiration, short-term splinting, a defined rehabilitation program, and most importantly, repeated transfusions to minimize the risk of developing hypertrophic synovitis.

Aspiration is critical in treating a major hemarthrosis.[302,306] Removing the bulk of blood within the joint greatly reduces the amount of iron that is absorbed by the synoviocytes and chondrocytes and reduces the risk of synovitis and recurrent hemorrhage. Aspiration also dramatically reduces the severe pain associated with a major hemarthrosis. The procedure is performed in the outpatient clinic. Routine sterile precautions should virtually eliminate iatrogenic sepsis. In fact, the risk of infection may be reduced by aspirating this pool of blood because septic arthritis in hemophiliacs with normal immune function typically has occurred in joints affected by a large hemarthrosis that was not treated or was treated only by transfusion on a delayed basis.[313,314,355]

A short period of prophylactic transfusions is needed to protect the joint while it is recovering from a major hemarthrosis. Transfusions are repeated every 48 hours. This schedule keeps factor VIII or factor IX at more than 1%, a level that prevents a recurrent hemorrhage caused by minimal trauma. Typically, the prophylactic transfusions are continued for 5 to 14 days after the major hemarthrosis. By that time, joint motion and muscle strength have been regained, the macrophages and synoviocytes have sequestered any iron remaining in the joint without synovitis developing.

With advanced arthropathy, a hemarthrosis only can distend the fibrotic synovium a limited amount, and treatment usually is limited to transfusion and symptomatic splinting. Aspiration in this situation is not only more difficult but also typically yields only 5 to 10 mL of bloody fluid.

When synovitis develops, the affected joint is swollen by the hypertrophic, boggy synovium. Joint mo-

TABLE 10-6 Radiographic Grading of Hemophilic Arthropathy

CLASSIFICATION	SCORE
Subchondral Irregularity	
Absent	0
Mild (≤ 50% of joint surface)	1
Pronounced	2
Joint Space Narrowing	
Absent	0
≤50%	1
>50%	2
Joint Margin Erosion	
Absent	0
Present	1
Joint Surface Incongruity	
Absent	0
Mild	1
Pronounced	2

Adapted from Greene WB, Yankaskas BC, Guilford WB. Comparison of radiologic classification of hemophilic arthropathy with clinical parameters. J Bone Joint Surg 1989;71A:237.

tion, however, is not particularly painful or restricted at this early stage unless a hemarthrosis recently has occurred. Recurrent hemarthroses, however, are typical. Furthermore, between episodes of obvious joint bleeds, some patients have constant oozing of blood from the hypervascular friable synovium. This not only perpetuates the synovitis but creates an ongoing serosanguineous synovial effusion.

The standard therapy used for most patients with synovitis, antiinflammatory drugs, is not feasible in a child with hemophilia. Prophylactic transfusions may prevent joint bleeds and allow resolution of the synovitis.[333] At our center, a protocol of prophylactic transfusions is instituted when 3 bleeding episodes occur in a joint within 6 weeks or when persistent synovial hypertrophy is noted 6 weeks after the last apparent hemarthrosis. Transfusions (25 U/kg of body weight) are given 3 times per week for the first 3 weeks and then 2 times per week for the next 3 weeks. Transfusions 3 times per week essentially maintain clotting factor levels greater than 1%. When transfusions are given 2 times per week, there are instances when the factor level falls to less than 1%, but this regimen has the advantages of decreased costs and decreased venue punctures.

At the end of 6 weeks, the patient's joint is reevaluated. If synovial hypertrophy is still present, the patient continues the prophylactic transfusions for a minimum of 4 additional months. Transfusions are given 2 times per week unless breakthrough bleeding is occurring routinely. In this case the transfusions are administered 3 times per week. In a previous evaluation of this protocol in 20 children with 34 affected joints, the rate of hemarthrosis in the affected joint averaged 3.6 per month before therapy and 1.7 per month after treatment.[302] Results, graded 1 year after completing treatment, were good in 17 joints, fair in 7, and poor in 10. Good results demonstrated greater than 50% reduction in the hypertrophic synovium and less than 1.5 transfusions per month in the affected joint.

Synovectomy in hemophiliacs initially was reported by Storti and colleagues[349] in 1969. Since then, many centers[287,289,291,300,318–320,325,328,329,331,337,339,343,346,348,352,354,356] have reported the results of this operation in hemophiliacs.

Reduction in the rate of hemarthrosis is a consistent result and is the only noncontroversial aspect of this procedure. This, however, is important because reducing the incidence of hemarthrosis has both functional and economic benefits. An acute hemarthrosis is painful and will limit ambulation and function for 1 to 10 days, even when transfusions are promptly administered.[280] Therefore, when hemarthroses are occurring 3 to 6 times a month, the child is severely disabled. In addition, by 1 year after synovectomy, the reduction in transfusion requirements actually offsets the cost of transfusion required to do the operation.[356]

Whether a synovectomy stops progression of hemophilic arthropathy is more difficult to answer. Although the data is not conclusive, the reports of knee synovectomy with long term follow-up,[318,325,328,331,339,343,348,352] and my personal observations, support the concept that the procedure delays but does not eliminate the progression of the arthropathy. Joints with less advanced changes at the time of synovectomy have demonstrated less progression.[318,325,328,339,352] Although recurrent synovitis is uncommon after a synovectomy, it is not surprising that the arthropathy continues to progress because articular cartilage erosions already are present in many hemophiliac people at the time of synovectomy.

Most synovectomies have been performed on the knee. The initial technique was an open procedure managed with conventional postoperative therapy. In these cases, loss of motion was common and significant, even with prolonged inpatient therapy.[287,289,322,328,332,352] For example, in a series of 13 cases Montane and colleagues[328] observed that 11 patients lost an average of 43 degrees of motion. Continuous passive motion and performing the operation by arthroscopic technique has improved the results of knee synovectomy in hemophiliac patients.[288,299,318,320,329,337,352,354] Most authors who advocate arthroscopic knee synovectomy also recommend postoperative continuous passive motion.[288,318,320,329,354] By using these techniques the range of knee motion can be maintained. Arthroscopic synovectomy of the knee in a hemophiliac person is a demanding and time-consuming procedure. The hypertrophic, fibrotic synovium can be difficult to remove, and thorough removal is necessary to prevent recurrent hemarthroses. In addition, arteriovenous fistula has been reported after performing this procedure in hemophiliac patients.[286,290]

I prefer open synovectomy of the knee, because it permits more effective and less traumatic removal of the synovium, where it inserts at the margin of the articular cartilage. Joint motion is maintained by preserving the joint capsule in the suprapatellar region and instituting continuous passive motion immediately after the operation. Preserving the suprapatellar capsule provides an interface for movement of the quadriceps tendon over the distal femur. This tissue, however, has become attenuated by the hypertrophic synovium and must be dissected carefully from the underlying synovium. Because articular changes typically are present in these patients at the time of synovectomy, it is mandatory that an arc of motion be established immediately. Otherwise, adhesions develop, and it is difficult to rehabilitate the joint.

Elbow synovectomy usually is accompanied by radial head excision in the older adolescent or adult.[319,339,346] The enlarged and incongruent radial head is probably secondary to the hypervascular synovium stimulating aberrant growth. After the radial head has been removed, it is easy to excise the remainder of the synovium. For a younger child, excision of the radial head is contraindicated. In this situation it is difficult to perform an open synovectomy without taking down the collateral ligaments. Arthroscopic synovectomy would seem to be a better approach in younger children, and Busch and Kurczynski[286] have reported good results in 3 patients treated by arthroscopic synovectomy of the elbow.

The results of ankle synovectomy in children with hemophilia only recently have been reported. Greene[300] described a three-incision technique that allowed a complete synovectomy. Continuous passive motion was not required in these patients, and rehabilitation was easy and effective, even though three of the five children were younger than 5 years of age. The rate of hemarthrosis in the involved ankle averaged 3.4 per month prior to synovectomy, compared with 0.1 per month after the operation. In addition, the range of ankle motion increased by an average of 10 degrees. Busch and Kurczynski[286] have presented similar results following arthroscopic synovectomy of the ankle. One of their 17 ankle synovectomies developed a pseudoaneurysm of the anterior tibial artery.

Radioactive synovectomy is an alternative and may be the only option for a patient with an inhibitor. Radioactive isotopes cause fibrosis of synovial tissue; however, articular cartilage is relatively resistant to the effects of radiation, and joint function is maintained. Among the advantages of radioactive synovectomy is the low cost of the procedure. It can be performed on an outpatient basis, and more importantly, transfusion of the expensive clotting factor is only necessary for 1 to 3 days. The disadvantage is the theoretical concern of causing a malignancy or chromosomal damage. For that reason, most of the experience with radioactive synovectomy in children with hemophilia has been in European centers; however, radioactive synovectomy is now being performed under investigational protocols in this country.

Gold (^{198}Au), yttrium (^{90}Y), rhenium (^{186}Rh), chromic phosphate (^{32}P), and dysprosium (^{165}Dy) are the radioisotopes that have been used in hemophiliac patients. ^{165}Dy has a short half-life (2.3 hours) and therefore can only be used in centers that are adjacent to nuclear reactors. For that reason, it only has been reported in a few patients with hemophilia.[359] ^{198}Au and ^{186}Rh have a relatively short half-life (2.7 and 3.7 days respectively) and have been used successfully in patients with hemophilia.[294,327,332] These agents, however, have the disadvantage of a relatively shallow depth of penetration, and therefore they may not be optimal for large joints, such as the knee. Furthermore, leakage outside the joint may be higher with these agents.

Good results in patients with hemophilia have been reported with ^{90}Y,[292,310] an agent that has a relatively short half-life of 2.7 days but a greater depth of penetration (mean, 3.6 mm versus 1.2 mm for ^{198}Au and ^{186}Rh). Heim and colleagues[310] used ^{90}Y in 50 joints of 43 hemophilia patients of whom 4 had inhibitors. The rate of hemarthrosis of the affected joint decreased from 1 bleed per month to 1 bleed per week. Eight joints required a second injection. Erken and colleagues[292] reported on 58 joints in 35 hemophiliacs ranging in age from 5 to 20 years. Factor levels were raised to 80% at the time of injection and were maintained at more than 50% for 3 days. An estimated dose of 5 mCi ^{90}Y was injected into the knee joint and less into smaller joints. The joints were immobilized for 48 to 60 hours to minimize leakage of their radioisotope from the joint.[292,308,357] The frequency of hemorrhage decreased from 4 per month prior to the injection to 0.2 per month at a mean follow-up of 7 years. Eight patients required a repeat injection. After the second injection, the rate of hemarthrosis was decreased in 4 and unchanged in 4.

Some authors favor ^{32}P, a radioactive agent that has a half-life of 14 days. The theoretical advantage of a prolonged half-life is that an acute inflammatory reaction and subsequent hemorrhage would not occur. Therefore, ^{32}P could be safer for patients with an inhibitor. The long half-life also means that only a single transfusion prior to the injection is necessary. The theoretical disadvantage is the greater risk of this agent accumulating in tissues outside the joint. Two centers have reported good results with ^{32}P in people with hemophilia.[340,341,345] In a recent report, Siegel and colleagues[345] observed no significant leakage of the radioisotope, improved range of motion in 67%, and moderate to marked decrease in the frequency of hemarthrosis in 80%.

The role of radioactive synovectomy in hemophilia is evolving. The percentage of patients with recurrent hemarthrosis is higher than observed after surgical synovectomy, but the results are acceptable. The expense of transfusion therapy for a surgical synovectomy and the low morbidity of the procedure are obvious advantages that are particularly germane in developing countries. In centers performing these procedures, careful monitoring is needed to document the possible side effects of radiotherapy on children.

Muscle hemorrhages are common in patients with severe factor VIII or IX deficiency and may occur after minimal trauma. Characteristic sites include the volar compartment of the forearm, the iliopsoas, the quadriceps, and the anterior and posterior calf muscles. Clinical symptoms progress from stiffness to pain on movement to pain at rest. In a study of lower-extremity muscle bleeds in children, the quadriceps muscle was involved in 44%, the posterior calf muscles in 35%, the adductors in 7%, and the anterior calf muscles in 7%.[281] Most bleeding episodes in this study were transfused within 3 hours, and the time for complete restoration of joint motion averaged 3.5 days.

Home transfusion therapy is effective for minor muscle bleeds. A single infusion usually is adequate if administered shortly after the onset of the hemorrhage. For lower extremity bleeds, crutches are used until normal range of motion has been regained. Patients and parents are instructed to call their physicians if they have symptoms of severe pain or neurologic dysfunction. With symptoms suggestive of a compartment syndrome in a hemophiliac who does not have an inhibitor, the factor levels are raised to 100%, and then evaluation and management should be routine. This means that compartment pressures are measured, and fasciotomy is performed when indicated.

Patients with a high-titer inhibitor are at increased risk for complications from a muscle hemorrhage (Fig. 10-24). These patients should seek medical attention early so that alternative transfusions can be started. To minimize the risk of a compartment syndrome and contractures, nonoperative modalities, such as protective dressings, elevation, and splinting, should be aggressively pursued.

Hemorrhage into the iliopsoas muscle sometimes is misclassified as a retroperitoneal hemorrhage. Goodfellow and colleagues[298] demonstrated that hemorrhage into the iliacus muscle was the cause of the associated femoral nerve paralysis. Because the iliacus muscle is confined between the pelvic wall and the overlying fascia, a relatively small hemorrhage in this muscle also will cause marked pain. The patient holds the hip in a flexed position, and pain is markedly increased by attempts at hip extension. Hemarthrosis into the hip joint can be differentiated by flexing the hip to 90 degrees. With this degree of flexion, rotation of the hip will be relatively normal with a muscle hemorrhage, but rotation will remain limited when the bleed is into the joint. If the location of the hemorrhage is unclear on clinical examination, an ultrasonography or a computed tomography scan may be used to define the site of bleeding. In the 1970s, femoral nerve palsies were found in approximately 60% of the iliacus bleeds.[315] The increased use of home therapy has reduced the incidence of this complication.

The standard treatment for femoral nerve palsy associated with an iliopsoas bleed is bed rest and continuous transfusion to maintain factor levels at 50% or higher for 7 to 14 days. With this therapy the femoral nerve paralysis resolves, but several months may elapse before the quadriceps muscle regains sufficient strength to extend the knee against gravity. Growe and Meek[307] reported a case that was treated by open decompression of the iliopsoas muscle. This patient had symptoms for 5 days, a severe flexion contracture, paralysis of the femoral nerve, and a compartment pressure measurement of 166 mm Hg with the hip in extension and 60 mm Hg with the hip flexed. At operation, a large organized clot was evacuated from the interval between the psoas and iliacus muscle. The patient's hip flexion contracture resolved within 1 week, and the quadriceps muscle function was normal within 1 month.

An equinus contracture may develop following hemorrhage into the gastrocnemius soleus muscle,[282] particularly when there is a delay in transfusion for more than 6 to 12 hours (Fig. 10-25). Aggressive use of sequential splints and casts prevents this problem, even in patients with inhibitors. After a single transfusion the leg should be immobilized in a compressive dressing and posterior splint. If an equinus contracture is present after 48 hours, a short-leg walking cast is applied with the ankle held in maximum dorsiflexion. The cast aids ambulation but more importantly minimizes the establishment of an equinus contracture as the hematoma organizes. The cast is changed every few days until the ankle can be positioned in neutral dorsiflexion with the knee extended. Stretching exercises then are used to gain further dorsiflexion.

Fixed knee flexion contractures rarely develop in patients on home transfusion therapy. The exception is a patient with an inhibitor. In these patients, the alternatives for transfusion are not always effective, and an acute hemarthrosis may evolve into a fixed knee flexion contracture. Traction, if instituted in an

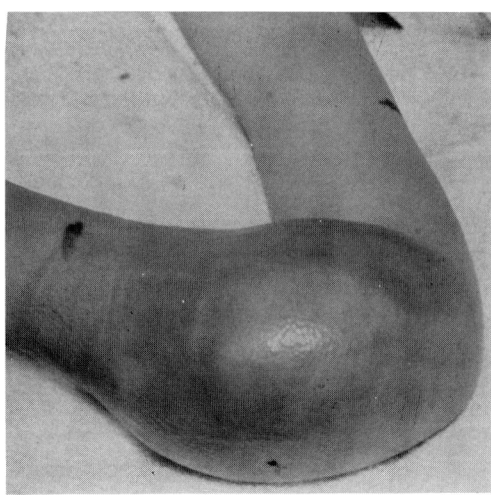

FIGURE 10-24. Massive soft tissue hemorrhage in the forearm of a 5-year-old patient with hemophilia can lead to Volkmann contractures.

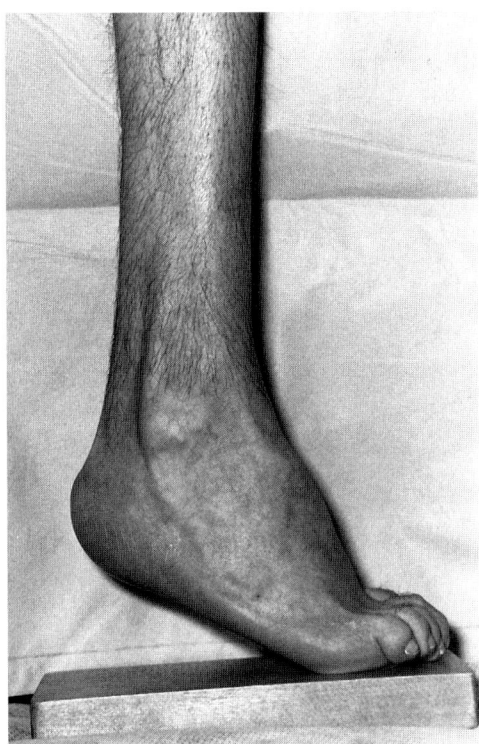

FIGURE 10-25. A 29-year-old man with hemophilia and high titer inhibitor sustained multiple calf hemorrhages during childhood that resulted in a fixed equinus contracture. Consistent and persistent treatment with serial casts could have greatly minimized the deformity and enhanced the patient's lower extremity function. (From Green WB. Chronic inflammatory arthritides and diseases related to the hematopoietic system. In: Drennan JC. The child's foot and ankle. New York: Raven Press, 1992.)

early and timely fashion, will regain full knee extension in 3 to 7 days.

Severe knee flexion contractures that are chronic may be complicated by posterior subluxation of the tibia.[279,301,302,317] If the patient also has an inhibitor that precludes elective surgery, the flexion contracture and subluxation of the tibia may be corrected by a Quengel cast (Fig. 10-26).[302,317] The offset subluxation hinges pull the proximal tibia forward, and the toggle stick allows windlass correction of the flexion deformity.[304] The Quengel cast usually can correct the contracture to approximately 15 degrees. Further extension is attained with standard cast-wedging techniques.

Whether using traction or casting, the goal is to correct the knee flexion contracture to 5 to 10 degrees. If less correction is attained, recurrent contractures are more likely. Furthermore, a typical patient will subsequently lose a few degrees correction, but if the knee flexion contracture remains less than 15 degrees, knee function is maximized and stress across the joint is minimized.[333] Therefore, after the contracture is corrected, a period of bracing is necessary. Over several months the patient gradually is weaned from the brace while a program of muscle strengthening and range of motion is instituted.

The necessity of Quengel casting and bracing for a chronic contracture does not mean that the knee will be stuck in extension. Approximately half of the patients who I treated ultimately regained more than 100 degrees of knee motion, despite having a flexion contracture of more than 40 degrees at initiation of treatment.[299] Factors associated with good results included no significant joint erosions at initiation of therapy, no breakthrough bleeding during treatment, and a good compliance during the period of bracing.

A pseudotumor, or hemophiliac cyst, starts as a hemorrhage that is intramuscular, subperiosteal, or intraosseous.[295] A fibrous capsule eventually surrounds and sequestrates the large mass of blood, which ultimately is transformed to necrotic erythrocytes and reactive tissues. Pseudotumors continue to enlarge, probably secondary to small and asymptomatic hemorrhages from blood vessels lining the capsular wall. Although the lining of the capsule of the pseudotumor has a relatively sparse vasculature, the coagulation defects in these patients allow ongoing bleeding. This may be secondary to altered pressure gradients that develop when the extravasated blood is catabolized. As the pseudotumor expands, the surrounding soft tissue is displaced and erosion of adjacent bones occurs (Fig. 10-27). Eventually, a clinically apparent mass or pathologic fracture causes the patient to seek evaluation.

The radiographs of a pseudotumor typically demonstrate a soft tissue mass, areas of soft tissue calcification, varying degrees of osseous destruction, and reactive new bone formation.[284] The differential diagnosis includes aneurysmal bone cysts, osteomyelitis, and some types of sarcoma.

Pseudotumors were more common prior to the development of effective concentrates. At that time, pseudotumors in young children were more likely in the bones of the hands and feet. In a series of 19 pseudotumors, Martinson[323] observed that 9 occurred in the carpometacarpal or tarsometatarsal bones of skeletally immature people. In my experience, which is during the era of concentrates and home transfusion therapy, most pseudotumors have been located in the pelvis and probably originated from a bleed in the iliacus muscle. Other sites, however, may be involved. Since the mid-1980s, I have treated patients with pseudotumors of the proximal humerus, the olecranon, and the proximal femur.

The pseudotumor should be excised if at all possible. Delay in operation will only allow further expansion of the pseudotumor and destruction of surrounding structures. A computed tomography scan is adequate to demonstrate the extent of the mass.[311] In most situations, a lesional excision is indicated, but in

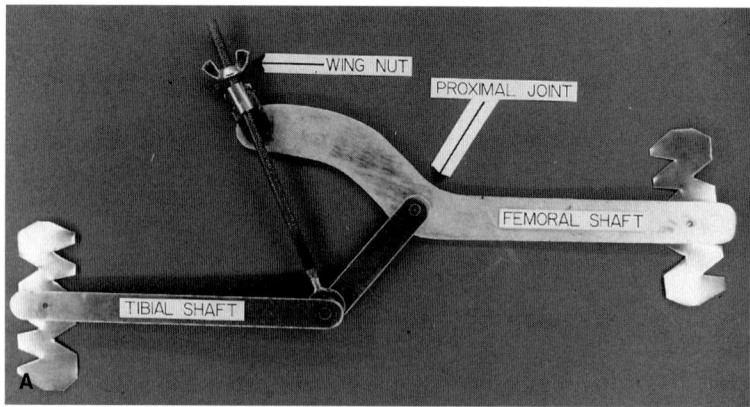

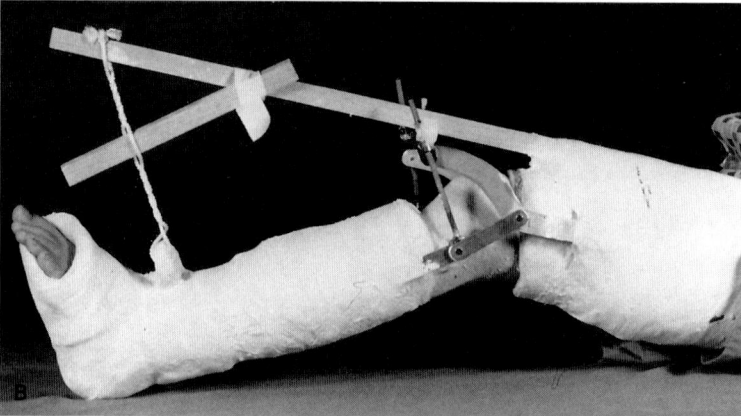

FIGURE 10-26. (A) Quengel cast antisubluxation hinge. (B) Completed Quengel cast applied to a patient. (From Greene WB, Wilson FC. Nonoperative management of hemophilic arthropathy and muscle hemorrhage. Instr Course Lect. 1983;32:223.)

large pseudotumors of the pelvis portions of the inner wall of the pseudotumor capsule may be left. This minimizes the risk of massive hemorrhage from adherent internal iliac vessels.

In a hemophiliac person with normal joint mobility, fracture patterns are similar to injuries observed in other children, but differences are noted in patients who have significant arthropathy of the lower extremities. Limited mobility of the lower extremities coupled with disuse osteoporosis makes supracondylar fracture of the femur and fractures of the femoral neck more likely.

Fracture in these patients, even if nondisplaced, will cause more bleeding, swelling, and risk of compartment syndrome. Transfusion therapy should be instituted immediately and most of these patients will need to be admitted, at least overnight, for observation. For fractures that can be treated by nonoperative means, the amount and duration of transfusion is individualized, depending on the location of the fracture, the amount of apparent hemorrhage, and the social situation. Some patients receive continuous transfusion to maintain a factor level of 50% or more for 2 to 7 days. Other patients, after the initial period of observation, can be treated as outpatients with daily, or every other day, transfusions for 3 to 7 days. Patients who require open reduction will be transfused using standard protocols for surgical procedures.

LEUKEMIA

Leukemia is the most common neoplasm in children. In one survey of the United States, leukemia accounted for 34% of the malignancies in white children and 24%

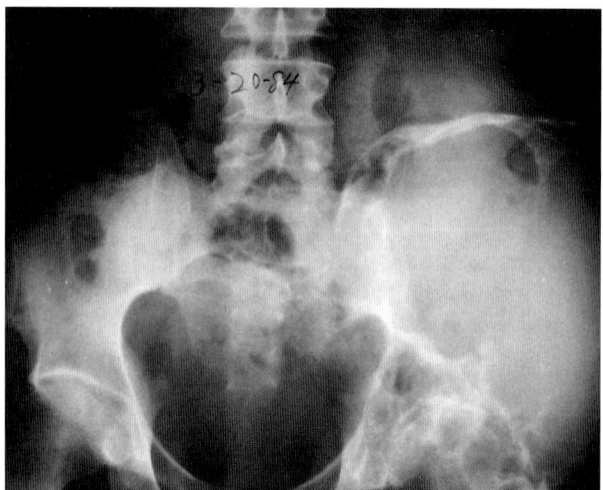

FIGURE 10-27. Pseudotumor of the ilium in a 39-year-old man with severe factor VIII deficiency and low titer inhibitor. There is marked destruction of the left illium.

in African-American children.[366] Acute lymphoblastic leukemia (ALL), characterized by a predominance of immature lymphoid precursors, is the most common type and accounts for approximately 80% of the leukemias seen in children.[371] The peak incidence of ALL is between the ages of 1 and 5 years, and the frequency progressively declines in the older childhood age groups. With intensive combination chemotherapy and CNS prophylaxis the survival rate of ALL has significantly improved so that the 5-year survival rate is now approximately 80%. Adverse risk factors include certain T-cell phenotypes and chromosomal abnormalities, a leukocyte count greater than 25,000/mm^3, and a delay in diagnosis.

Leukemia is primarily a disease of the bone marrow and the peripheral blood, but any organ may be infiltrated by the malignant cells. For that reason, the signs and symptoms at diagnosis can vary (Table 10-7). Pain in the extremities or a limp may be the initial complaint, and the first physician evaluating these children may be an orthopaedic surgeon. The incidence of extremity pain at diagnosis typically ranges from 15% to 32%,[367,370,371,373,374] although one study observed a 56% incidence of this problem at disease onset.[365] Extremity pain is most frequently localized to the metaphyseal portion of bone in the region of the knee, the ankle, and the wrist.[370,371] Painful swelling of a joint is less frequent but may also herald the onset of leukemia.[368,371,372] Multiple joints and migratory joint pain may occur.[372] Back pain secondary to infiltration of the marrow also may be noted at the time of diagnosis. In addition, pathologic fracture of the vertebral body is the initial complaint in 2% to 7% of children with ALL[365,369,370] (Fig. 10-28).

Radiographic changes at the onset of disease are approximately twice as frequent as musculoskeletal symptoms, with the incidence of radiographic abnor-

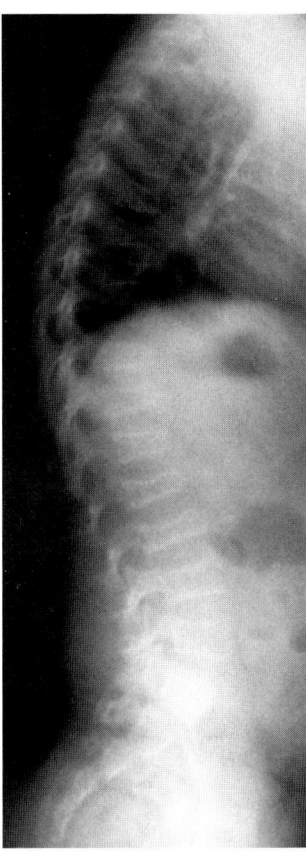

FIGURE 10-28. A 6-year-old girl presented with acute pain and an inability to walk. Radiographic examination revealed diffuse osteopenia and multiple compression fractures. Diagnostic evaluation revealed acute leukemia. (From Greene WB. Idiopathic juvenile osteoporosis. In: Weinstein SL, ed. The pediatric spine. New York: Raven Press, 1994.)

TABLE 10-7 *Signs and Symptoms of Diagnosis of Acute Lymphoblastic Leukemia in 137 Children*

SIGNS AND SYMPTOMS	PATIENTS* (%)
Lethargy or malaise	36
Fever or infection	31
Extremity or Joint pain	23
Bleeding manifestation	18
Anorexia	12
Abdominal pain	7
Central nervous system manifestation	2

* Some patients presented with more than one sign or symptom.
Adapted from Sallan SE, Weinstein HJ. Childhood acute leukemia. In: Nathan DG, Oski FA, eds. Hematology of infancy and childhood. 3rd ed. Philadelphia: WB Saunders; 1987:1028.

malities ranging from 44% to 57%.[360,365,367,370,373] Characteristic findings include localized and generalized osteoporosis, radiolucent metaphyseal bands, osteolytic defects, cortical defects, osteosclerosis, and periosteal reactions (Figs. 10-29 and 10-30). Osteopenia is the most common radiologic abnormality in some studies,[360,373] whereas other reports observe metaphyseal lucent bands as being most frequent.[361,365] The metaphysis is the most common site of involvement, although diaphyseal radiolucency as a presenting sign also has been reported.[362]

Children who present with leukemic skeletal pain may be misdiagnosed as having osteomyelitis, septic arthritis, or juvenile rheumatoid arthritis.[368,370-372] Laboratory studies do not always differentiate these disorders because children with leukemia may have a fever, an elevated erythrocyte sedimentation rate, and a nondiagnostic leukocyte count that is elevated, depressed, or normal. The correct diagnosis is suggested by a greater degree of osteopenia than one would expect with an acute infectious process. Radiographs also should be carefully examined for the presence of more

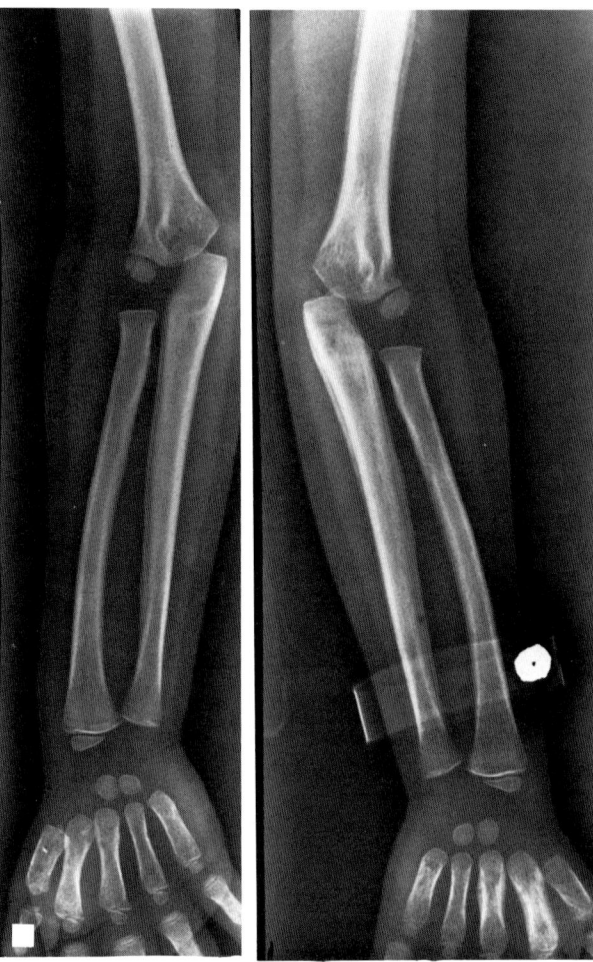

FIGURE 10-29. A 3-year-old boy with acute lymphocytic leukemia shows periosteal new bone formation involving large segments of the radius, the ulna, and the humerus. A metaphyseal band is present at the distal radius.

morning stiffness was common in patients with juvenile rheumatoid arthritis but was not observed in the leukemia patients. Nonarticular bone pain was found in all of the leukemia patients but was not seen in the arthritis patients. Thrombocytosis was seen in 80% of the children with rheumatoid arthritis but in only 20% of the patients with leukemia. Neutrophilia was present in arthritis patients, but lymphocytosis predominated in leukemia patients. Finally, abnormalities on radiographs were limited to joint effusions in arthritis patients, whereas the leukemia patients frequently had other abnormalities.

Leukemic bone and joint pain typically resolves with institution of chemotherapy; however, during the early phase of chemotherapy, osteoporosis may increase and pathologic fractures may occur.[371] Whether bone involvement at the onset of disease is a prognostic factor remains controversial. Ribeiro and colleagues[369] demonstrated that the presence of a vertebral compression fracture did not affect the treatment outcome. Other studies have observed that skeletal involvement at the onset of ALL does not affect prognosis[360,361,367]; however, Heinrich and colleagues[365] noted that children with ALL who presented with 5 or more skeletal lesions had a reduced survival rate, presumably caused by a longer duration of symptoms prior

characteristic lesions, such as metaphyseal lucent bands. Other findings that suggest leukemia instead of a septic process include a depressed hemoglobin level, a normal leukocyte count, and an inconsistent technetium bone scan. Bone scans in children with leukemia may show increased uptake in an asymptomatic region or normal or decreased uptake in areas that have obvious lysis on plane radiographs.[363,364] With any combination of these findings, a diagnostic bone marrow aspiration should be considered.

Making the correct diagnosis in children with leukemia who present with multiple joint pain may be challenging. In a study that compared children with systemic juvenile rheumatoid arthritis with children who were referred initially for rheumatologic evaluation but in whom leukemia was ultimately diagnosed, Ostrov and colleagues[368] observed that lymphadenopathy, splenomegaly, and hepatomegaly were equivalent in both groups. Musculoskeletal night pain, however, frequently was seen in the children with leukemia but was not reported in arthritis patients. In addition,

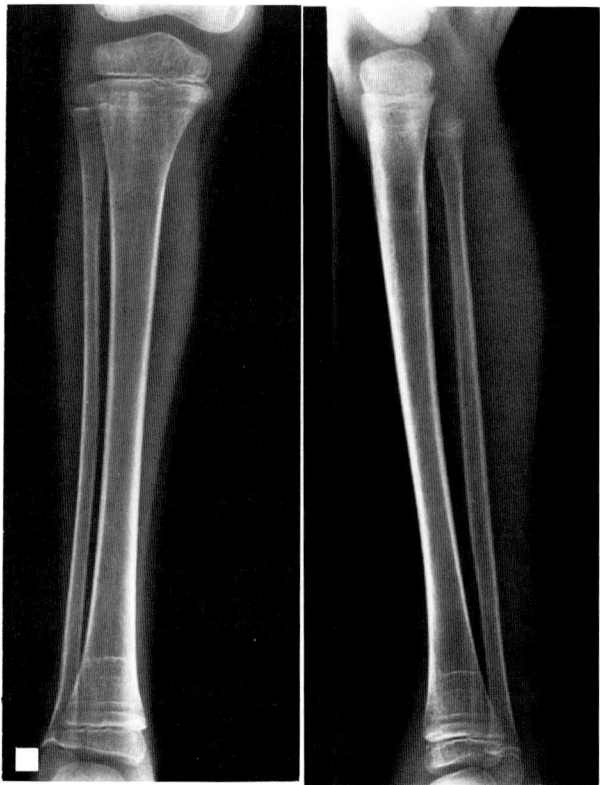

FIGURE 10-30. A 6-year-old girl with acute myelogenous leukemia shows multiple growth rest lines, generalized osteopenia, and a metaphyseal band.

to diagnosis. In this study, children with 1 to 4 radiographic lesions had an indolent form of leukemia and the best prognosis, whereas children without radiographic skeletal abnormalities had an aggressive form of leukemia. The survival rate of the group without skeletal abnormalities and the group with 5 or more skeletal lesions was similar. Appell and colleagues,[360] however, used similar classifications and found no significant correlation in the survival rate of children with no skeletal involvement, those with skeletal involvement of less than 3 bones, and those with skeletal involvement of 3 or more bones.

ACKNOWLEDGMENT

I gratefully acknowledge the assistance of Gail M. Darden in the writing of this chapter.

References

1. Miller DR, Baehner RL, Miller LP. Blood diseases of infancy and childhood. 6th ed. St. Louis: CV Mosby, 1989.
2. Nathan DG, Oski FA, eds. Hematology of infancy and childhood. 3rd ed. Philadelphia: WB Saunders, 1987.

Iron Deficiency Anemia

3. Ballin A, Berar M, Rubinstein U, Kleter Y, Hershkovitz A, Meytes D. Iron state in female adolescents. Am J Dis Child 1992;146:803.
4. Dallman PR. Has routine screening of infants for anemia become obsolete in the United States? Pediatrics 1987;80:439.
5. Dallman PR, Yip R, Johnson C. Prevalence and causes of anemia in the United States, 1976 to 1980. Am J Clin Nutr 1984;39:437.
6. Filer LJ. Iron needs during rapid growth and mental development. J Pediatr 1990;117:S143.
7. Lanzkowsky P. Radiological features of iron-deficiency anemia. Am J Dis Child 1968;116:16.
8. Lukens JN. Iron metabolism and iron deficiency. In: Miller DR, Baehner RL, Miller LP, eds. Blood diseases of infancy and childhood. 6th ed. St. Louis: CV Mosby, 1989:170.
9. Miller V, Swaney S, Deinard A. Impact of the WIC program on the iron status of infants. Pediatrics 1985;75:100.
10. Oski FA. Iron deficiency in infancy and childhood. N Engl J Med 1993;329:190.
11. Raunikar RA, Sabio H. Anemia in the adolescent athlete. Am J Dis Child 1992;146:1201.
12. Roy WL, Lerman J, McIntyre BG. Is preoperative haemoglobin testing justified in children undergoing minor elective surgery? Can J Anaesth 1991;38:700.
13. Stockman JA. Iron deficiency anemia: have we come far enough? JAMA 1987;258:1645.
14. Vazquez-Seoane P, Windom R, Pearson HA. Disappearance of iron-deficiency anemia in a high-risk infant population given supplemental iron. N Engl J Med 1985;313:1239.
15. Yip R, Binkin NJ, Fleshood L, Trowbridge FL. Declining prevalence of anemia among low-income children in the United States. JAMA 1987;258:1619.
16. Yip R, Walsh KM, Goldfarb MG, Binkin NJ. Declining prevalence of anemia in childhood in a middle-class setting: a pediatric success story? Pediatrics 1987;80:330.

Diamond-Blackfan Anemia

17. Aase JM, Smith DW. Congenital anemia and triphalangeal thumbs: a new syndrome. J Pediatr 1969;74:471.
18. Alter BP. Thumbs and anemia. Pediatrics 1978;62:613.
19. Alter BP. The bone marrow failure syndromes. In: Nathan DG, Oski FA, eds. Hematology of infancy and childhood. 3rd ed. Philadelphia: WB Saunders Company, 1987:159.
20. Diamond LK, Blackfan KD. Hypoplastic anemia. Am J Dis Child 1938;56:464.
21. Glader BE. Diagnosis and management of red cell aplasia in children. Hematol Oncol Clin North Am 1987;1:431.
22. Greenspan A, Cohen J, Szabo RM. Klippel-Feil syndrome: an unusual association with Sprengel deformity, omovertebral bone, and other skeletal, hematologic, and respiratory disorders. Bull Hosp Joint Dis Orthop Inst 1991;51:54.
23. Halperin DS, Freedman MH. Diamond-Blackfan anemia: etiology, pathophysiology, and treatment. Am J Pediatr Hematol Oncol 1989;11:380.
24. Hurst JA, Baraitser M, Wonke B. Autosomal dominant transmission of congenital erythroid hypoplastic anemia with radial abnormalities. Am J Med Genet 1991;40:482.
25. Miller DR. Erythropoiesis, hypoplastic anemias, and disorders of heme synthesis. In: Miller DR, Baehner RL, Miller LP, eds. Blood diseases of infancy and childhood. 6th ed. St. Louis: CV Mosby, 1989:124.
26. Murphy S, Lubin B. Triphalangeal thumbs and congenital erythroid hypoplasia: report of a case with unusual features. J Pediatr 1972;81:987.
27. Saunders EF, Olivieri N, Freedman MH. Unexpected complications after bone marrow transplantation in transfusion-dependent children. Bone Marrow Transp 1993;12(S2):88.

Fanconi Anemia

28. Auerbach AD, Sagi M, Adler B. Fanconi anemia: prenatal diagnosis in 30 fetuses at risk. Pediatrics 1985;76:794.
29. Fanconi G. Familial constitutional panmyelocytopathy, Fanconi's anemia (F.A.). Semin Hematol 1967;4:233.
30. Gmyrek D, Syllm-Rapoport I. Zur Fanconi-Anamie (FA). Eur J Pediatr 1964;91:297.
31. Miller DR, O'Reilly RJ. Aplastic anemia. In: Miller DR, Baehner RL, Miller LP, eds. Blood diseases of infancy and childhood. 6th ed. St. Louis: CV Mosby, 1989:464.
32. Minagi H, Steinbach HL. Roentgen appearance of anomalies associated with hypoplastic anemias of childhood: Fanconi's anemia and congenital hypoplastic anemia (erythrogenesis imperfecta). AJR 1966;97:100.

Sickle Cell Disorders

33. Acurio MT, Friedman RJ. Hip arthroplasty in patients with sickle-cell haemoglobinopathy. J Bone Joint Surg [Br] 1992;74:367.
34. Al-Salem AH, Ahmed HA, Qaisaruddin S, Al-Jam'a A, Elbashier AM, Al-Dabbous I. Osteomyelitis and septic arthritis in sickle cell disease in the eastern province of Saudi Arabia. Int Orthop 1992;16:398.
35. Barrett-Connor E. Bacterial infection and sickle cell anemia. An analysis of 250 infections in 166 patients and a review of the literature. Medicine 1971;50:97.
36. Bennett OM. Salmonella osteomyelitis and the hand-foot syndrome in sickle cell disease. J Pediatr Orthop 1992;12:534.
37. Bennett OM, Namnyak SS. Bone and joint manifestations of sickle cell anemia. J Bone Joint Surg [Br] 1990;72:494.
38. Bernaudin F, Souillet G, Vannier JP, et al. Bone marrow transplantation (BMT) in 14 children with severe sickle cell disease

(SCD): the French experience. Bone Marrow Transp 1993;12(S1):118.
39. Bishop AR, Roberson JR, Eckman JR, Fleming LL. Total hip arthroplasty in patients who have sickle cell hemoglobinopathy. J Bone Joint Surg [Am] 1988;70:853.
40. Bryan JP, Rocha H, Scheld WM. Problems in salmonellosis: rationale for clinical trials with lower b-lactam agents and quinolones. Rev Infect Dis 1986;8:189.
41. Cardiello P, Starr DS. Salmonella osteomyelitis in a hemoglobin SC patient. Clin Pediatr (Phila) 1990;29:98.
42. Chadwick EG, Connor EM, Shulman ST, Yogev R. Efficacy of ceftriaxone in treatment of serious childhood infections. J Pediatr 1983;103:141.
43. Chung SMK, Alavi A, Russell MO. Management of osteonecrosis in sickle-cell anemia and its genetic variants. Clin Orthop 1978;130:158.
44. Chung SMK, Ralston EL. Necrosis of the humeral head associated with sickle cell anemia and its genetic variants. Clin Orthop 1971;80:105.
45. Clarke HJ, Jinnah RH, Brooker AF, Michaelson JD. Total replacement of the hip for avascular necrosis in sickle cell disease. J Bone Joint Surg [Br] 1989;71:465.
46. David HG, Bridgman SA, Davies SC, Hine AL, Emery RJH. The shoulder in sickle-cell disease. J Bone Joint Surg [Br] 1993;75:538.
47. Diggs LW. Bone and joint lesions in sickle-cell disease. Clin Orthop 1967;52:119.
48. Ebong WW. Pathological fracture complicating long bone osteomyelitis in patients with sickle cell disease. J Pediatr Orthop 1986;6:177.
49. Ebong WW. Septic arthritis in patients with sickle-cell disease. Br J Rheumatol 1987;26:90.
50. Epps CH, D'Orsay DB, Coles MJM, Castro O. Osteomyelitis in patients who have sickle-cell disease. J Bone Joint Surg [Am] 1991;73:1281.
51. Givner LB, Luddy RE, Schwartz AD. Etiology of osteomyelitis in patients with major sickle cell hemoglobinopathies. J Pediatr 1981;99:411.
52. Greene WB, McMillan CW. Salmonella osteomyelitis and hand-foot syndrome in a child with sickle cell anemia. J Pediatr Orthop 1987;7:716.
53. Griffin TC, McIntire D, Buchanan GR. High-dose intravenous methylprednisolone therapy for pain in children and adolescents with sickle cell disease. N Engl J Med 1994;330:733.
54. Guze BH, Hawkins RA, Marcus CS. Technetium-99m white blood cell imaging: false-negative result in salmonella osteomyelitis associated with sickle cell disease. Clin Nucl Med 1989;14:104.
55. Haggard ME, Schneider RG. Sickle cell anemia in the first two years of life. J Pediatr 1961;58:785.
56. Hanisssian AS, Silverman A. Arthritis of sickle cell anemia. South Med J 1974;67:28.
57. Hanker GJ, Amstutz HC. Osteonecrosis of the hip in the sickle-cell diseases. J Bone Joint Surg [Am] 1988;70:499.
58. Hebbel RP. Beyond hemoglobin polymerization: the red blood cell membrane and sickle cell disease pathophysiology. Blood 1991;77:214.
59. Hernigou P, Galacteros F, Bachir D, Goutallier D. Deformities of the hip in adults who have sickle-cell disease and had avascular necrosis in childhood. J Bone Joint Surg [Am] 1991;73:81.
60. Kahn CE, Ryan JW, Hatfield MK, Martin WB. Combined bone marrow and gallium imaging. Differentiation of osteomyelitis and infarction in sickle hemoglobinopathy. Clin Nucl Med 1988;13:443.
61. Kaul DK, Nagel RL. Sickle cell vasoocclusion: many issues and some answers. Experientia 1993;49:5.
62. Keeley K, Buchanan GR. Acute infarction of long bones in children with sickle cell anemia. J Pediatr 1982;101:170.
63. Kim HC, Alavi A, Russell MO, Schwartz E. Differentiation of bone and bone marrow infarcts from osteomyelitis in sickle cell disorders. Clin Nucl Med 1988;14:249.
64. Lane PA. Sickle hemoglobinopathies. Curr Opin Pediatr 1993;5:74.
65. Mallouh A, Talab Y. Bone and joint infection in patients with sickle cell disease. J Pediatr Orthop 1985;5:158.
66. Mankad VN, Williams JP, Harpen MD, et al. Magnetic resonance imaging of bone marrow in sickle cell disease: clinical, hematologic, and pathologic correlations. Blood 1990;75:274.
67. Milner PF, Kraus AP, Sebes JI, et al. Sickle cell disease as a cause of osteonecrosis of the femoral head. N Engl J Med 1991;325:1476.
68. Milner PF, Kraus AP, Sebes JI, et al. Osteonecrosis of the humeral head in sickle cell disease. Clin Orthop 1993;289:136.
69. Motulsky AG. Frequency of sickling disorders in US Blacks. N Engl J Med 1973;288:31.
70. Ohene-Frempong K, Schwartz E. Sickle cell disease and other disorders of abnormal hemoglobin. In: Miller DR, Baehner RL, Miller LP, eds. Blood diseases of infancy and childhood. 6th ed. St. Louis: CV Mosby, 1989:387.
71. Orringer EP, Parker JC. Hydroxyurea and sickle cell disease. Hematol Pathol 1992;6:171.
72. Piehl FC, Davis RJ, Prugh SI. Osteomyelitis in sickle cell disease. J Pediatr Orthop 1993;13:225.
73. Platt OS. Easing the suffering caused by sickle cell disease. N Engl J Med 1994;330:783.
74. Platt OS, Nathan DG. Sickle cell disease. In: Nathan DG, Oski FA, eds. Hematology of infancy and childhood. 3rd ed. Philadelphia: WB Saunders, 1987:655.
75. Platt OS, Thorington BD, Brambilla DJ, et al. Pain in sickle cell disease: rates and risk factors. N Engl J Med 1991;325:11.
76. Rao VM, Mitchell DG, Steiner RM, et al. Femoral head avascular necrosis in sickle cell anemia: MR characteristics. Magn Reson Imaging 1988;6:661.
77. Rao S, Solomon N, Miller S. Scintigraphic differentiation of bone infarction from osteomyelitis in children with sickle cell disease. J Pediatr 1985;107:685.
78. Schneider RG, Hightower B, Hosty TS, et al. Abnormal hemoglobins in a quarter million people. Blood 1976;48:629.
79. Schumacher HR, Andrews R, McLaughlin G. Arthropathy in sickle-cell disease. Ann Intern Med 1973;78:203.
80. Sebes JI. Diagnostic imaging of bone and joint abnormalities associated with sickle cell hemoglobinopathies. AJR 1989;152:1153.
81. Sebes JI, Kraus AP. Avascular necrosis of the hip in the sickle cell hemoglobinopathies. J Can Assoc Radiol 1983;34:136.
82. Stein RE, Urbaniak J. Use of the tourniquet during surgery in patients with sickle cell hemoglobinopathies. Clin Orthop 1980;151:231.
83. Stevens MCG, Padwick M, Serjeant GR. Observations on the natural history of dactylitis in homozygous sickle cell disease. Clin Pediatr (Phila) 1981;20:311.
84. Syrogiannopoulos GA, McCracken GH, Nelson JD. Osteoarticular infections in children with sickle cell disease. Pediatrics 1986;78:1090.
85. Trull AK, Eastmond CJ, Panayi GS, Reid TM. Salmonella reactive arthritis: serum and secretory antibodies in eight patients identified after a large outbreak. Br J Rheum 1986;25:13.
86. Vermylen C, Cornu G, Ferster A, Ninane J, Sariban E. Bone marrow transplantation in sickle cell disease: the Belgian experience. Bone Marrow Transp 1993;12(S1):116.
87. Ware HE, Brooks AP, Toye R, Berney SI. Sickle cell disease and silent avascular necrosis of the hip. J Bone Joint Surg [Br] 1991;73:947.

88. Washington ER, Root L. Conservative treatment of sickle cell avascular necrosis of the femoral head. J Pediatr Orthop 1985;5:192.
89. Watson RJ, Burko H, Megas H, Robinson M. The hand-foot syndrome in sickle-cell disease in young children. Pediatrics 1963;31:975.

Thalassemia

90. Baronciani D, Galimberti M, Lucarelli G, et al. Bone marrow transplantation in class 1 thalassemia patients. Bone Marrow Transp 1993;12(S1):56.
91. Benz EI, Schwartz E. Thalassemia syndromes. In: Miller DR, Baehner RL, Miller LP, eds. Blood diseases of infancy and childhood. 6th ed. St. Louis: CV Mosby, 1989:428.
92. Borgna-Pignatti C, Zurlo MG, DeStefano P, et al. Outcome of thalassemia treated with conventional therapy. Bone Marrow Transp 1993;12(S1):2.
93. Caffey J. Cooley's anemia: a review of the roentgenographic findings in the skeleton. AJR 1957;78:381.
94. Colavita N, Orazi C, Danza SM, et al. Premature epiphyseal fusion and extramedullary hematopoiesis in thalassemia. Skeletal Radiol 1987;16:533.
95. Di Bartolomeo P, Di Girolamo G, Angrilli F. Treatment of thalassemia by allogeneic bone marrow transplantation. Bone Marrow Transp 1993;12(S1):37.
96. Dines DM, Canale VC, Arnold WD. Fractures in thalassemia. J Bone Joint Surg [Am] 1976;58:662.
97. Evans DIK. Bone marrow transplantation for thalassemia major. J Clin Pathol 1992;45:553.
98. Exarchou E, Politou C, Vretou E, et al. Fractures and epiphyseal deformities in beta-thalassemia. Clin Orthop 1984; 189:229.
99. Finsterbush A, Farber I, Mogle P, et al. Fracture patterns in thalassemia. Clin Orthop 1985;192:132.
100. Gaziev J, Galimberti M, Giardini C, Baronciani D, Lucarelli G. Growth in children after bone marrow transplantation for thalassemia. Bone Marrow Transp 1993;12(S1):100.
101. Kattamis C, Liakopoulou T, Kattamis A. Growth and development in children with thalassemia major. Acta Paediatr Suppl 1990;366:111.
102. Michelson J, Cohen A. Incidence and treatment of fractures in thalassemia. J Orthop Trauma 1988;2:29.
103. Nienhuis AW, Wolfe L. Disorders of hemoglobin: the thalassemias. In: Nathan DG, Oski FA, eds. Hematology of infancy and childhood. 3rd ed. Philadelphia: WB Saunders, 1987:699.
104. Piomelli S, Loew T. Management of thalassemia major (Cooley's anemia). Hematol Oncol Clin North Am 1991;5:557.
105. Silvestroni E, Bianco I. Screening for microcytemia in Italy: analysis of data collected in the past 30 years. Am J Hum Genet 1975;27:198.

Schwachman-Diamond Syndrome

106. Aggett PJ, Cavanagh NPC, Matthew DJ, Pincott JR, Sutcliffe J, Harries JT. Schwachman's syndrome. Arch Dis Child 1980;55:331.
107. Baehner RL. Disorders of granulopoiesis. In: Miller DR, Baehner RL, Miller LP, eds. Blood diseases of infancy and childhood. 6th ed. St. Louis: CV Mosby, 1989:515.
108. Burke V, Colebatch JH, Anderson CM, Simons MJ. Association of pancreatic insufficiency and chronic neutropenia in childhood. Arch Dis Child 1967;42:147.
109. Danks DM, Haslam R, Mayne V, Kaufmann HJ, Holtzapple PG. Metaphyseal chondrodysplasia, neutropenia, and pancreatic insufficiency presenting with respiratory distress in the neonatal period. Arch Dis Child 1976;51:697.
110. Dhar S, Anderton JM. Orthopaedic features of Schwachman syndrome. J Bone Joint Surg [Am] 1994;76:278.
111. Schwachman H, Diamond LK, Oski FA, Khaw KT. The syndrome of pancreatic insufficiency and bone marrow dysfunction. J Pediatr 1964;65:645.
112. Spycher MA, Giedion A, Shmerling DH, Rüttner JR. Electron microscopic examination of cartilage in the syndrome of exocrine pancreatic insufficiency, neutropenia, metaphyseal dysostosis and dwarfism. Helv Paediatr Acta 1974;29:471.

Chronic Granulomatous Disease

113. Ariga T, Nakanishi M, Tomizawa K, et al. Genetic heterogeneity in patients with X-linked recessive chronic granulomatous disease. Pediatr Res 1992;31:516.
114. Baehner RL. Disorders of granulocyte function. In: Miller DR, Baehner RL, Miller LP, eds. Blood diseases of infancy and childhood. 6th ed. St. Louis: CV Mosby, 1989:549.
115. Curnutte JT, Boxer LA. Disorders of granulopoiesis and granulocyte function. In: Nathan DG, Oski FA, eds. Hematology of infancy and childhood. 3rd ed. Philadelphia: WB Saunders, 1987:797.
116. Dinauer MC. Leukocyte function and nonmalignant leukocyte disorders. Curr Opin Pediatr 1993;5:80.
117. Dinauer MC, Orkin SH. Chronic granulomatous disease. Annu Rev Med 1992;43:117.
118. Finn A, Hadžić N, Morgan G, Strobel S, Levinsky RJ. Prognosis of chronic granulomatous disease. Arch Dis Child 1990;65:942.
119. Gallin JI. Interferon in the management of chronic granulomatous disease. Rev Infect Dis 1991;13:973.
120. Heinrich SD, Finney T, Craver R, Yin L, Zembo MM. Aspergillus osteomyelitis in patients who have chronic granulomatous disease. J Bone Joint Surg [Am] 1991;73:456.
121. The International Chronic Granulomatous Disease Cooperative Study Group. Controlled trial of interferon gamma to prevent infection in chronic granulomatous disease. N Engl J Med 1991;324:504.
122. Johnston RB Jr, Newman SL, Struth AG. Chronic granulomatous disease. Pediatr Clin North Am 1977;24:365.
123. Quie PG, White JG, Holmes B, Good RA. In vitro bactericidal capacity of human polymorphonuclear leukocytes: diminished activity in chronic granulomatous disease in childhood. J Clin Invest 1967;46:668.
124. Segal AW. Biochemistry and molecular biology of chronic granulomatous disease. J Inherit Metab Dis 1992;15:683.
125. Sponseller PD, Malech HL, McCarthy EF, Horowitz SF, Jaffe G, Gallin JI. Skeletal involvement in children who have chronic granulomatous disease. J Bone Joint Surg [Am] 1991;73:37.
126. Wolfson JJ, Kane WJ, Laxdal, SD, Good, RA, Quic PG. Bone findings in chronic granulomatous disease of childhood: a genetic abnormality of leukocyte function. J Bone Joint Surg [Am] 1969;51:1573.
127. Woodman RC, Erickson RW, Rae J, Jaffe HS, Curnutte JT. Prolonged recombinant interferon-γ therapy in chronic granulomatous disease: evidence against enhanced neutrophil oxidase activity. Blood 1992;79:1558.

X-Linked Agammaglobulinemia

128. Baehner RL. Lymphocytes. In: Miller DR, Baehner RL, Miller LP, eds. Blood diseases of infancy and childhood. 6th ed. St. Louis: CV Mosby, 1989:578.
129. Campana M, Farrant J, Inamdar N, Webster ADB, Janossy G. Phenotypic features and proliferative activity of B cell pro-

genitors in X-linked agammaglobulinemia. J Immunol 1990;145:1675.
130. Chattopadhyay C, Nativg JB, Chattopadhyay H. Excessive suppressor T-cell activity of the rheumatoid synovial tissue in X-linked hypogammaglobulinaemia. Scand J Immunol 1980;11:455.
131. Hansel TT, Haeney MR, Thompson RA. Primary hypogammaglobulinaemia and arthritis. Br Med J 1987;295:174.
132. Lee AH, Levinson AI, Schumacher HR. Hypogammaglobulinemia and rheumatic disease. Semin Arthritis Rheum 1993;22:252.
133. Liese JG, Wintergerst U, Tympner KD, Belohradsky BH. High vs low-dose immunoglobin therapy in the long-term treatment of X-linked agammaglobulinemia. Am J Dis Child 1992;146:335.
134. McLaughlin JF, Schaller J, Wedgwood RJ. Arthritis and immunodeficiency. J Pediatr 1972;81:801.
135. Taborn JD. Rice bodies in hypogammaglobulinemic arthritis. J Rheum 1981;8:165.

Cartilage-Hair Hypoplasia

136. Beals RK. Cartilage-hair hypoplasia. J Bone Joint Surg [Am] 1968;50:1245.
137. Lux SE, Johnston RB, August CS, et al. Chronic neutropenia and abnormal cellular immunity in cartilage-hair hypoplasia. N Engl J Med 1970;282:231.
138. McKusick VA, Eldridge R, Hostetler JA, Ruangwit U, Egeland JA. Dwarfism in the Amish. Bull Johns Hopkins Hosp 1965;116:285.
139. Pierce GF, Polmar SH. Lymphocyte dysfunction in cartilage-hair hypoplasia: evidence for an intrinsic defect in cellular proliferation. J Immunol 1982;129:570.
140. Saulsbury FT, Winklestein JA, Davis LE, et al. Combined immunodeficiency in vaccine-related poliomyelitis in a child with cartilage-hair hypoplasia. J Pediatr 1975;86:862.
141. Van der Burgt I, Haraldsson A, Oosterwijk JC, van Essen AJ, Weemaes C, Hamel B. Cartilage hair hypoplasia, metaphyseal chondrodysplasia type McKusick: description of seven patients and review of the literature. Am J Med Genet 1991;41:371.

Acquired Immunodeficiency Syndrome

142. Cartelli N, Stanton B, Feigelman S, et al. Prevalence of human immunodeficiency virus among pediatric patients attending a Baltimore inner city primary health care center. Pediatr AIDS HIV Infect 1991;2:68.
143. Diamond GW, Gurdin P, Wiznia AA, Belman AL, Rubinstein A, Cohen HJ. Effects of congenital HIV infection on neurodevelopmental status of babies in foster care. Dev Med Child Neurol 1990;32:999.
144. Falloon J, Eddy J, Wiener L, Pizzo PA. Human immunodeficiency virus infection in children. J Pediatr 1989;114:1.
145. Fein JA, Friedland LR, Rutstein R, Bell LM. Children with unrecognized human immunodeficiency virus infection. Am J Dis Child 1993;147:1104.
146. Greene WB, DeGnore LT, White GC. Orthopaedic procedures and prognosis in hemophilic patients who are seropositive for human immunodeficiency virus. J Bone Joint Surg [Am] 1990;72:2.
147. Heymann D. HIV/AIDS: the global epidemic. AIDS Res Hum Retroviruses 1993;9:S13S.
148. Hilgartner MW. AIDS in children with hemophilia. Pediatr AIDS HIV Infect 1991;2:275.
149. McKinney RE, Robertson WR, Duke Pediatric AIDS Clinical Trial Unit. Effect of human immunodeficiency virus infection on the growth of young children. J Pediatr 1993;123:579.
150. Miles SA, Balden E, Magpantay L, et al. Rapid serologic testing with immune-complex–dissociated HIV p24 antigen for early detection of HIV infection in neonates. N Engl J Med 1993;328:297.
151. Mofenson LM, Wright PF, Fast PE. Summary of the working group on perinatal intervention. AIDS Res Hum Retroviruses 1992;8:1435.
152. Msellati P, Lepage P, Hitimana DG, Van Goethem C, Van De Perre P, Dabis F. Neurodevelopmental testing of children born to human immunodeficiency virus type 1 seropositive and seronegative mothers: a prospective cohort study in Kigali, Rwanda. Pediatrics 1993;92:843.
153. Parekh BS, Shaffer N, Coughlin R, et al. Dynamics of maternal IgG antibody decay and HIV-specific antibody synthesis in infants born to seropositive mothers. AIDS Res Hum Retroviruses 1993;9:907.
154. Pizzo PA. Pediatric AIDS: problems within problems. J Infect Dis 1990;161:316.
155. Wachtel RC, Tepper VJ, Houck DL, Nair P, Thompson C, Johnson JP. Neurodevelopment in pediatric HIV-1 infection: a prospective study. Pediatr AIDS HIV Infect 1993;4:198.
156. Yogev R. Pediatric acquired immunodeficiency virus syndrome. Pediatr Infect Dis 1990;9:767.

Gaucher Disease

157. Amstutz HC. The hip in Gaucher's disease. Clin Orthop 1973;90:83.
158. Amstutz HC, Carey EJ. Skeletal manifestations and treatment of Gaucher's disease. J Bone Joint Surg [Am] 1966;48:670.
159. Bar-Maor JA and Govrin-Yehudain J. Partial splenectomy in children with Gaucher's disease. Pediatrics 1985;76:398.
160. Barton NW, Brady RO, Dambrosia JM, et al. Replacement therapy for inherited enzyme deficiency—Macrophage-targeted glucocerebrosidase for Gaucher's disease. N Engl J Med 1991;324:1464.
161. Barton NW, Brady RO, Dambrosia JM, et al. Dose-dependent responses to macrophage-targeted glucocerebrosidase in a child with Gaucher disease. J Pediatr 1992;120:277.
162. Bell RS, Mankin HJ, Doppelt SH. Osteomyelitis in Gaucher's disease. J Bone Joint Surg [Am] 1986;68:1380.
163. Beutler E, Kay A, Saven A, et al. Enzyme replacement therapy for Gaucher disease. Blood 1991;78:1183.
164. Beutler E, Nguyen NJ, Henneberger MW, et al. Gaucher disease: gene frequencies in the Ashkenazi Jewish population. Am J Hum Genet 1993;52:85.
165. Bilchik TR, Heyman S. Skeletal scintigraphy of pseudo-osteomyelitis in Gaucher's disease: two case reports and a review of the literature. Clin Nucl Med 1992;17:279.
166. Brady RO, Kanfer JN, Shapiro D. Metabolism of glucocerebrosides. II. Evidence of an enzymatic deficiency in Gaucher's disease. Biochem Biophys Res Commun 1965;18:221.
167. Fallet S, Grace ME, Sibille A, et al. Enzyme augmentation in moderate to life-threatening Gaucher disease. Pediatr Res 1992;31:496.
168. Figueroa ML, Rosenbloom BE, Kay AC, et al. A less costly regimen of alglucerase to treat Gaucher's disease. N Engl J Med 1992;327:1632.
169. Finkelstein R, Nachum Z, Reissman P, et al. Anaerobic osteomyelitis in patients with Gaucher's disease. Clin Infect Dis 1992;15:771.
170. Fleshner PR, Astion DJ, Ludman MD, Aufses AH, Grabowski

GA, Dolgin SE. Gaucher disease: fate of the splenic remnant after partial splenectomy—a case of rapid enlargement. J Pediatr Surg 1989;24:610.
171. Garber AM. No price too high? N Engl J Med 1992;327:1676.
172. Goldman AB, Jacobs B. Femoral neck fractures complicating Gaucher disease in children. Skeletal Radiol 1984;12:162.
173. Hermann G, Shapiro RS, Abdelwahab IF, Grabowski G. MR imaging in adults with Gaucher disease type I: evaluation of marrow involvement and disease activity. Skeletal Radiol 1993;22:247.
174. Hermann G, Wagner LD, Gendal ES, Ragland RL, Ulin RI. Spinal cord compression in type I Gaucher disease. Radiology 1989;170:147.
175. Horev G, Kornreich L, Hadar H, Katz K. Hemorrhage associated with "bone crisis" in Gaucher's disease identified by magnetic resonance imaging. Skeletal Radiol 1991;20:479.
176. Johnson LA, Hoppel BE, Gerard EL, et al. Quantitative chemical shift imaging of vertebral bone marrow in patients with Gaucher's disease. Radiology 1992;182:451.
177. Katz K, Cohen IJ, Ziv N, Grunebaum M, Zaizov R, Yosipovitch Z. Fractures in children who have Gaucher disease. J Bone Joint Surg [Am] 1987;69:1361.
178. Katz K, Horev G, Grunebaum M, Yosipovitch Z. The natural history of osteonecrosis of the femoral head in children and adolescents with Gaucher disease. Unpublished data.
179. Katz K, Mechlis-Frish S, Cohen IJ, Horev G, Zaizov R, Lubin E. Bone scans in the diagnosis of bone crisis in patients who have Gaucher disease. J Bone Joint Surg [Am] 1991;73:513.
180. Katz K, Sabato S, Horev G, Cohen IJ, Yosipovitch Z. Spinal involvement in children and adolescents with Gaucher disease. Spine 1993;18:332.
181. Lachiewicz PF, Lane JM, Wilson PD. Total hip replacement in Gaucher's disease. J Bone Joint Surg [Am] 1981;63:602.
182. Lau MM, Lichtman DM, Hamati YI, Bierbaum BE. Hip arthroplasties in Gaucher's disease. J Bone Joint Surg [Am] 1981;63:591.
183. Mankin HJ. Gaucher's disease: a novel treatment and an important breakthrough. J Bone Joint Surg [Br] 1993;75:2.
184. Mankin HJ, Doppelt SH, Rosenberg AE, Barrenger JA. Metabolic bone disease in patients with Gaucher's disease. In: Avioli LA, Krane SM, eds. Metabolic bone disease and clinically related disorders. 2nd ed. Philadelphia: WB Saunders, 1990:730.
185. Pastores GM, Sibille AR, Grabowski GA. Enzyme therapy in Gaucher disease type I: dosage efficacy and adverse effects in 33 patients treated for 6 to 24 months. Blood 1993;82:408.
186. Rose JS, Grabowski GA, Barnett SH, Desnick RJ. Accelerated skeletal deterioration after splenectomy in Gaucher type 1 disease. Am J Radiol 1982;139:1202.
187. Rosenthal DI, Barton NW, McKusick KA, et al. Quantitative imaging of Gaucher disease. Radiology 1992;185:841.
188. Rosenthal DI, Scott JA, Barrenger J, et al. Evaluation of Gaucher disease using magnetic resonance imaging. J Bone Joint Surg [Am] 1986;68:802.
189. Sidrasky E, Ginns EI. Clinical heterogeneity among patients with Gaucher's disease. JAMA 1993;269:1154.
190. Springfield DS, Landfried M, Mankin HJ. Gaucher hemorrhagic cyst of bone. J Bone Joint Surg [Am] 1989;71:141.
191. Stowens DW, Teitelbaum ST, Kahn AJ, Barranger JA. Skeletal complications of Gaucher disease. Medicine 1985;64:310.
192. Whittington R, Goa KL. Aglucerase. Drugs 1992;44:72.
193. Zer M, Freud E. Subtotal splenectomy in Gaucher's disease: towards a definition of critical splenic mass. Br J Surg 1992;79:742.
194. Zimran A, Gelbart T, Westewood B, Grabowski GA, Beutler E. High frequency of the Gaucher disease mutation at nucleotide 1226 among Ashkenazi Jews. Am J Hum Genet 1991;49:855.
195. Zimran A, Hollak CEM, Abrahamov A, van Oers MHJ, Kelly M, Beutler E. Home treatment with intravenous enzyme replacement therapy for Gaucher disease: an international collaborative study of 33 patients. Blood 1993;82:1107.
196. Zimran A, Kay A, Gelbart T, et al. Gaucher disease: clinical, laboratory, radiologic, and genetic features of 53 patients. Medicine 1992;71:337.

Niemann-Pick Disease

197. Bayever E, Kamani N, Ferreira P, et al. Bone marrow transplantation for Niemann-Pick type 1A disease. J Inherit Metab Dis 1992;15:919.
198. Crocker AC, Farber S. Niemann-Pick disease: a review of eighteen patients. Medicine 1958;37:1.
199. Elleder M. Niemann-Pick disease. Pathol Res Pract 1989;185:293.
200. Fink JK, Filling-Katz MR, Sokol J, et al. Clinical spectrum of Niemann-Pick disease type C. Neurology 1989;39:1040.
201. Grünebaum M. The röntgenographic findings in the acute neuronopathic form of Niemann-Pick disease. Br J Radiol 1976;49:1018.
202. Levran O, Desnick RJ, Schuchman EH. Niemann-Pick type B disease: identification of a single codon deletion in the acid sphingomyelinase gene and genotype/phenotype correlations in type A and B patients. J Clin Invest 1991;88:806.
203. Levran O, Desnick RJ, Schuchman EH. Identification and expression of a common missense mutation (L302P) in the acid sphingomyelinase gene of Ashkenazi Jewish type A Niemann-Pick disease patients. Blood 1992;80:2081.
204. Özsoylu S, Koçak N, Aksoy A. Pseudo-osteomyelitis in Niemann-Pick disease. Clin Pediatr (Phil) 1988;27:394.
205. Pavone L, Fiumara A, LaRosa M. Niemann-Pick disease type B: clinical signs and follow-up of a new case. J Inherit Metab Dis 1986;9:73.
206. Spence MW, Callahan JW. Sphingomyelin-cholesterol lipidoses: the Niemann-Pick group of diseases. In: Scriver CR, Beaudet AL, Sly WS, Valle D, eds. The metabolic basis of inherited disease. 6th ed. New York: McGraw Hill, 1989:1655.
207. Takahashi T, Suchi M, Desnick RJ, Takada G, Schuchman EH. Identification and expression of five mutations in the human acid sphingomyelinase gene causing types A and B Niemann-Pick disease. J Biol Chem 1992;267:12552.
208. Vanier MT, Pentchev P, Rodriguez-LaFrasse C, Rousson R. Niemann-Pick disease type C: an update. J Inherit Metab Dis 1991;14:580.

Langerhans Cell Histiocytosis

209. Alexander JE, Seibert JJ, Berry DH, Glasier CM, Williamson SL, Murphy J. Prognostic factors for healing of bone lesions in histiocytosis X. Pediatr Radiol 1988;18:326.
210. Alley RM, Sussman MD. Rapidly progressive eosinophilic granuloma. Spine 1992;17:1517.
211. Baber WW, Numaguchi Y, Nadell JM, Culicchia F, Robinson AE. Eosinophilic granuloma of the cervical spine without vertebrae plana. J Comput Tomogr 1987;11:346.
212. Beltran J, Aparisi F, Bonmati LM, Rosenberg ZS, Present D, Steiner GS. Eosinophilic granuloma: MRI manifestations. Skeletal Radiol 1993;22:157.
213. Berry DH, Becton DL. Natural history of histiocytosis-X. Hematol Oncol Clin North Am 1987;1:23.
214. Berry DH, Gresik MV, Humphrey GB, et al. Natural history of

histiocytosis X: a pediatric oncology group study. Med Pediatr Oncol 1986;14:1.
215. Birbeck MD, Breathnach AJ, Everall JD. An electron microscope study of basal melanocytes and high-level clear cells (Langerhans cells) in vitiligo. J Invest Dermatol 1961;37:51.
216. Bollini G, Jouve JL, Gentet JC, Jacquemier M, Bouyala JM. Bone lesions in histiocytosis X. J Pediatr Orthop 1991; 11:469.
217. Broadbent V. Favourable prognostic features in histiocytosis X: bone involvement and absence of skin disease. Arch Dis Child 1986;61:1219.
218. Camargo OP, De Oliveira NRB, Andrade JS, Filho RC, Croci AT, Filho TEPDB. Eosinophilic granuloma of the ischium: long-term evaluation of a patient treated with steroids. J Bone Joint Surg [Am] 1992;74:445.
219. Cambazard F, Dezutter-Dambuyant C, Staquet MJ, Schmitt D, Thivolt J. Eosinophilic granuloma of bone and biochemical demonstration of 49-kDa CD1a molecule expression by Langerhans cell histiocytosis. Clin Exp Dermatol 1991;16:377.
220. Canadall J, Villa C, Martinez-Denegri J, Azcarate J, Imizcoz A. Vertebral eosinophilic granuloma. Spine 1986;11:767.
221. Capanna R, Springfield DS, Ruggieri P, et al. Direct cortisone injection in eosinophilic granuloma of bone: a preliminary report on 11 patients. J Pediatr Orthop 1985;5:339.
222. Ceci A, Terlizzi M, Colella R, et al. Etoposide in recurrent childhood Langerhans' cell histiocytosis: an Italian cooperative study. Cancer 1988;62:2528.
223. Ceci A, Terlizzi M, Colella R, et al. Langerhans cell histiocytosis in childhood: results from the Italian cooperative. Med Pediatr Oncol 1993;21:259.
224. Cheyne C. Histiocytosis X. J Bone Joint Surg [Br] 1971;53:366.
225. Chu T, D'Angio GJ, Favara B, Ladisch S, Nesbit M, Pritchard J. Histiocytosis syndromes in children. Lancet 1987;1:208.
226. Compere EL, Johnson WE, Coventry MB. Vertebra plana (Calve's disease) due to eosinophilic granuloma. J Bone Joint Surg [Am] 1954;36:969.
227. Conway WF, Hayes CW. Miscellaneous lesions of bone. Radiol Clin North Am 1993;31:339.
228. D'Angio GJ, Favara BE, Ladisch S. Workshop on the childhood histiocytosis: concepts and controversies. Med Pediatr Oncol 1986;14:104.
229. Dehner LP. Morphologic findings in the histiocytic syndromes. Semin Oncol 1991;18:8.
230. Dimentberg RA, Brown KLB. Diagnostic evaluation of patients with histiocytosis X. J Pediatr Orthop 1990;10:733.
231. Dunger DB, Broadbent V, Yeoman E, et al. The frequency and natural history of diabetes insipidus in children with Langerhans-cell histiocytosis. N Engl J Med 1989;321:1157.
232. Favara BE. Langerhans' cell histiocytosis pathobiology and pathogenesis. Semin Oncol 1991;18:3.
233. Fiorillo A, Sadile F, DeChiara C, et al. Bone lesions in Langerhans cell histiocytosis. Clin Pediatr (Phil) 1993;32:118.
234. Gardner DJ, Azouz EM. Solitary lucent epiphyseal lesions in children. Skeletal Radiol 1988;17:497.
235. Green NE, Robertson WW, Kilroy AW. Eosinophilic granuloma of the spine with associated neural deficit. J Bone Joint Surg [Am] 1980;62:1198.
236. Green WT, Farber S. Eosinophilic or solitary granuloma of bone. J Bone Joint Surg [Am] 1942;24:499.
237. Greenberger JS, Crocker AC, Vawter G, Jaffe N, Cassidy JR. Results of treatment of 127 patients with systemic histiocytosis (Letterer-Siwe disease, Schüller-Christian syndrome and multifocal eosinophilic granuloma). Medicine 1981;60:311.
238. Greinix HT, Storb R, Sanders JE, Petersen FB. Marrow transplantation for treatment of multisystem progressive Langerhans cell histiocytosis. Bone Marrow Transplant 1992;10:39.
239. Greis PE, Hankin FM. Eosinophilic granuloma: the management of solitary lesions of bone. Clin Orthop 1990;257:204.
240. Grois N, Barkovich AJ, Rosenau W, Ablin AR. Central nervous system disease associated with Langerhans' cell histiocytosis. Am J Pediatr Hematol Oncol 1993;15:245.
241. Ishii E, Matsuzaki A, Okamura J, et al. Treatment of Langerhans cell histiocytosis in children with etoposide. Am J Clin Oncol 1992;15:515.
242. Katz RL, Silva EG, DeSantos LA, Lukeman JM. Diagnosis of eosinophilic granuloma of bone by cytology, histology, and electron microscopy of transcutaneous bone-aspiration biopsy. J Bone Joint Surg [Am] 1980;62:1284.
243. Kozlowski K, Diard F, Padovani J, Sprague P, Pietron K. Unilateral mid-femoral periosteal new bone of varying aetiology in children. Pediatr Radiol 1986;16:475.
244. Kumar A. Eosinophilic granuloma of the spine with neurological deficit. Orthopedics 1990;12:1310.
245. Ladisch S, Miller DR. The spleen and disorders involving the monocyte-macrophage system. In: Miller DR, Baehner RL, Miller LP, eds. Blood diseases of infancy and childhood. 6th ed. St. Louis: CV Mosby, 1989:722.
246. Lahey ME. Histiocytosis X–an analysis of prognostic factors. J Pediatr 1975;87:184.
247. Leavey P, Varughese M, Breatnach F, O'Meara A. Langerhans cell histiocytosis—a 31-year review. Irish J Med Sci 1991;160:271.
248. Leeson MC, Smith A, Carter JR, Makley JT. Eosinophilic granuloma of bone in the growing epiphysis. J Pediatr Orthop 1985;5:147.
249. Lichtenstein L. Histiocytosis X: integration of eosinophilic granuloma of bone, "Letterer-Siwe disease," and "Schüller-Christian disease" as related manifestations of a single nosologic entity. Arch Pathol 1953;56:84.
250. Lichtenstein L. Histiocytosis X (eosinophilic granuloma of bone, Letterer-Siwe disease, and Schüller-Christian disease). J Bone Joint Surg [Am] 1964;46:76.
251. Lichenstein L, Jaffe H. Eosinophilic granuloma of bone with report of a case. Am J Pathol 1940;16:595.
252. Mackenzie WG, Morton KS. Eosinophilic granuloma of bone. Can J Surg 1988;31:264.
253. Makley JT, Carter JR. Eosinophilic granuloma of bone. Clin Orthop 1986;204:37.
254. McLelland J, Broadbent V, Yeomans E, Malone M, Pritchard J. Langerhans cell histiocytosis: the case for conservative treatment. Arch Dis Child 1990;65:301.
255. Mierau GW, Favara BE, Brenman JM. Electron microscopy in histiocytosis X. Ultrastruct Pathol 1982;3:137.
256. Nesbit ME, Kieffer S, D'Angio GJ. Reconstitution of vertebral height in histiocytosis X: a long-term follow-up. J Bone Joint Surg [Am] 1968;51:1360.
257. Novice FM, Collison DW, Kleinsmith DM, Osband ME, Burdakin JH, Coskey RJ. Letterer-Siwe disease in adults. Cancer 1989;63:166.
258. Otani S, Ehrlich J. Solitary granuloma of bone simulating primary neoplasm. Am J Pathol 1940;16:479.
259. Rabakin MS, Wittwer CT, Kjeldsberg CR, et al. Flow-cytometric DNA content of histiocytosis X (Langerhans cell histiocytosis). Am J Pathol 1988;131:283.
260. Raney RB. Chemotherapy for children with aggressive fibromatosis and Langerhans' cell histiocytosis. Clin Orthop 1991;262:58.
261. Raney RB, D'Angio GJ. Langerhans' cell histiocytosis (histiocytosis X): experience at the Children's Hospital of Philadelphia, 1970–1984. Med Pediatr Oncol 1989;17:20.
262. Ringdén O, Åhström L, Lönnqvist B, Båryd I, Svedmyr E, Gahrton G. Allogeneic bone marrow transplantation in a patient with chemotherapy-resistant progressive histiocytosis X. N Engl J Med 1987;316:733.

263. Robert H, Dubousset J, Miladi L. Histiocytosis X in the juvenile spine. Spine 1987;12:167.
264. Ruppert D, Oria RA, Kumar R, et al. Radiologic features of eosinophilic granuloma of bone. AJR 1989;153:1021.
265. Scaglietti O, Marchetti PG, Bartolozzi P. Final results obtained in the treatment of bone cysts with methylprednisolone acetate (Depo-Medrol) and a discussion of results achieved in other bone lesions. Clin Orthop 1982;165:33.
266. Schmitt S, Martin E, Zachmann M, Schoenle EJ. Pituitary stalk thickening with diabetes insipidus preceding typical manifestations of Langerhans cell histiocytosis in children. Eur J Pediatr 1993;152:399.
267. Starling KA. Chemotherapy of histiocytosis-X. Hematol Oncol Clin North Am 1987;1:119.
268. Viana MB, Oliveira BM, Silva CM, Leite VHR. Etoposide in the treatment of six children with Langerhans cell histiocytosis (histiocytosis X). Med Pediatr Oncol 1991;19:289.
269. Whelan HT, Clinton ME, Fogo A, Smith H. Histiocytosis-X isolated to the cervical spinal cord. Am J Pediatr Hematol Oncol 1987;9:228.
270. Womer RB, Raney RB, D'Angio GJ. Healing rates of treated and untreated bone lesions in histiocytosis X. Pediatrics 1985;76:286.
271. Zabucchi G, Soranzo MR, Menegazzi R, et al. Eosinophilic granuloma of the bone in Hand-Schüller-Christian disease: extensive in vivo eosinophil degranulation and subsequent binding of released eosinophil peroxidase (EPO) to other inflammatory cells. J Pathol 1991;163:225.

TAR Syndrome

272. Dell PC, Sheppard JE. Thrombocytopenia, absent radius syndrome. Clin Orthop 1982;162:129.
273. Fromm B, Niethard FU, Marquardt E. Thrombocytopenia and absent radius (TAR) syndrome. Int Orthop 1991;15:95.
274. Gounder DS, Pullon HW, Ockelford PA, Nicol RO. Clinical manifestations of the thrombocytopenia and absent radii (TAR) syndrome. Aust NZ J Med 1989;19:479.
275. Hall, JG. Thrombocytopenia and absent radius (TAR) syndrome. J Med Genet 1987;24:79.
276. Hall JG, Levin J, Kuhn JP, Ottenheimer EJ, van Berkum KAP, McKusick VA. Thrombocytopenia with absent radius (TAR). Medicine 1969;48:411.
277. Hedberg VA, Lipton JM. Thrombocytopenia with absent radii. Am J Pediatr Hematol Oncol 1988;10:51.
278. Schoenecker PL, Cohn AK, Sedgwick WG, Manske PR, Salafsky I, Millar EA. Dysplasia of the knee associated with the syndrome of thrombocytopenia and absent radius. J Bone Joint Surg [Am] 1984;66:421.

Hemophilia

279. Arnold WD, Hilgartner MW. Hemophilic arthropathy: current concepts of pathogenesis and management. J Bone Joint Surg [Am] 1977;59:287.
280. Aronstam A, Browne RS, Wassef M, Hamad Z. Clinical features of early haemarthroses in severely affected adolescent haemophiliacs. Clin Lab Haematol 1984;6:9.
281. Aronstam A, Rainsford SG, Painter MJ. Patterns of bleeding in adolescents with severe haemophilia A. Br Med J 1979;1:469.
282. Atkins RM, Henderson NJ, Duthie RB. Joint contractures in the hemophilias. Clin Orthop 1987;219:97.
283. Brackmann HH, Gormsen J. Massive factor-VIII infusion in hemophiliac with factor-VIII inhibitor, high responder. Lancet 1977;2:933.
284. Brant EE, Jordan HH. Radiologic aspects of hemophilic pseudotumors in bone. AJR 1972;115:525.
285. Brinkhous KM, Shanbrom E, Roberts HR, Webster WP, Fekete L, Wagner RH. A new high-potency glycine-precipitated antihemophilic factor (AHF) concentrate. JAMA 1968;205:613.
286. Busch M, Kurczynski E. The role of arthroscopic synovectomy in the treatment of children with hemophilia. Presented at Pediatric Orthopaedic Society of North America Meeting, White Sulpher Springs, WV, May 4, 1993.
287. Canale ST, Dugdale M, Howard BC. Synovectomy of the knee in young patients with hemophilia. South Med J 1988;81:1480.
288. Casscells CD. Commentary: the argument for early arthroscopic synovectomy in patients with severe hemophilia. Arthroscopy 1987;3:78.
289. Clark MW. Knee synovectomy in hemophilia. Orthopedics 1978;1:285.
290. Cohen B, Griffiths L, Dandy DJ. Arteriovenous fistula after arthroscopic synovectomy in a patient with haemophilia. Arthroscopy 1992;8:373.
291. DeGnore LT, Wilson FC. Surgical management of hemophilic arthropathy. Instr Course Lect 1989;38:383.
292. Erken EHW. Radiocolloids in the management of hemophilic arthropathy in children and adolescents. Clin Orthop 1991;264:129.
293. Ewing NP, Sanders NL, Dietrich SL, Kasper CK. Induction of immune tolerance to factor VIII in hemophiliacs with inhibitors. JAMA 1988;259:65.
294. Fernandez-Palazzi F, de Bosch NB, de Vargas AF. Radioactive synovectomy in haemophilic haemarthrosis. Follow-up of fifty cases. Scand J Haematol 1984;33(Suppl 40):291.
295. Fernandez de Valderrama JA, Matthews JM. The haemophilic pseudotumor or haemophilic subperiosteal haematoma. J Bone Joint Surg [Br] 1965;47:256.
296. Gamble JG, Bellah J, Rinsky LA, Glader B. Arthropathy of the ankle in hemophilia. J Bone Joint Surg [Am] 1991;73:1008.
297. Gilbert MS. Musculoskeletal manifestations of hemophilia. Mt Sinai J Med 1977;44:339.
298. Goodfellow J, Fearn CB, Matthews JM. Iliacus haematoma: a common complication of haemophilia. J Bone Joint Surg [Br] 1967;49:748.
299. Greene WB. Use of continuous passive slow motion in the postoperative rehabilitation of difficult pediatric knee and elbow problems. J Pediatr Orthop 1983;3:419.
300. Greene WB. Synovectomy of the ankle for hemophilic arthropathy. J Bone Joint Surg [Am] 1994;76:812.
301. Greene WB, Howes CL, Mathewson AB. Treatment of knee flexion contractures in hemophiliacs with inhibitors and preexistent arthropathy. In: Gilbert MS, Greene WB, eds. Musculoskeletal problems in hemophilia. New York: The National Hemophilia Foundation, 1990:74.
302. Greene WB, McMillan CW. Nonsurgical management of hemophilic arthropathy. Instr Course Lect 1989;38:367.
303. Greene WB, McMillan CW, Dykstra W, Warren M. Treatment of hypertrophic synovitis and recurrent hemarthrosis in children with severe hemophilia. Dev Med Child Neurol 1983;25:112.
304. Greene WB, Wilson FC. Nonoperative management of hemophilic arthropathy and muscle hemorrhage. Instr Course Lect 1983;32:223.
305. Greene WB, Yankaskas BC, Guilford WB. Comparison of radiologic classification of hemophilic arthropathy with clinical parameters. J Bone Joint Surg [Am] 1989;71:237.
306. Gregosiewicz A, Wosko I, Kandzierski G. Intraarticular bleeding in children with hemophilia: the prevention of arthropathy. J Pediatr Orthop 1989;9:182.
307. Growe GH, Meek R. Decompression of the iliopsoas muscle. In: Gilbert MS, Greene WB, eds. Musculoskeletal problems in hemophilia. New York: The National Hemophilia Foundation, 1990:45.

308. Gumpel JM, Williams ED, Glass HI. Use of yttrium 90 in persistent synovitis of the knee. Ann Rheum Dis 1973;32:223.
309. Hasiba U, Eyster ME, Gill FM, et al. Liver dysfunction in Pennsylvania's multitransfused hemophiliacs. Dig Dis Sci 1980;25:776.
310. Heim M, Horoszowski H, Lieberman L, Varon D, Martinowitz U. Methods and results of radionucleotide synovectomies. In: Gilbert MS, Greene WB, eds. Musculoskeletal problems in hemophilia. New York: The National Hemophilia Foundation 1990:98.
311. Hermann G, Yeh HC, Gilbert MS. Computed tomography and ultrasonography of the hemophilic pseudotumor and their use in surgical planning. Skeletal Radiol 1986;15:123.
312. Hilgartner MW. Home care for hemophilia: current state of the art. Scand J Haematol 1977;30(Suppl):58.
313. Hofmann A, Wyatt R, Bybee B. Septic arthritis of the knee in a 12-year-old hemophiliac. J Pediatr Orthop 1984;4:498.
314. Houghton GR. Septic arthritis of the hip in a hemophiliac: report of a case. Clin Orthop 1977;129:223.
315. Houghton GR, Duthie RB. Orthopaedic problems in hemophilia. Clin Orthop 1979;138:197.
316. Johnson RP, Babbitt DP. Five stages of joint disintegration compared with range of motion in hemophilia. Clin Orthop 1985;201:36.
317. Jordan HH. Orthopedic appliances. Springfield: Charles C Thomas, 1963:21.
318. Klein KS, Aland CM, Him HC, Eisele J, Saidi P. Long-term follow-up of arthroscopic synovectomy for chronic hemophilic synovitis. Arthroscopy 1987;3:231.
319. Le Balc'h T, Ebelin M, Laurin Y, Lambert T, Verroust F, Larrieu M. Synovectomy of the elbow in young hemophilic patients. J Bone Joint Surg [Am] 1987;69:264.
320. Limbird TJ, Dennis SC. Synovectomy and continuous passive motion (cpm) in hemophilic patients. Arthroscopy 1987;3:74.
321. Mainardi CL, Levine PH, Werb Z, Harris, Jr. Proliferative synovitis in hemophilia: biochemical and morphologic observations. Arthritis Rheum 1978;21:137.
322. Mannucci PM, de Franchis R, Torri G, Pietrogrande V. Role of synovectomy in hemophilic arthropathy. Israel J Med Sci 1977;13:983.
323. Martinson, A. Hemophilic pseudotumors. In: Boone DC, ed. Comprehensive management of hemophilia. Philadelphia: FA Davis, 1976:94.
324. May RB, McMillan CW. Bleeding disorders in the newborn. In: Conn HF, Conn RB, eds. Current diagnosis. Philadelphia: WB Saunders 1977:1045.
325. Matsuda Y, Duthie DB. Surgical synovectomy for haemophilic arthropathy of the knee joint: long-term follow-up. Scand J Haematol 1984;33(Suppl 40):237.
326. McMillan CW, Greene WB, Blatt PM, White GC II, Roberts HR. The management of musculoskeletal problems in hemophilia. Instr Course Lect 1983;33:210.
327. Merchan ECR, Magallon M, Martin-Villar J, Galindo E, Ortega F, Pardo JA. Long-term follow-up of haemophilic arthropathy treated by AU-198 radiation synovectomy. Int Orthop 1993;17:120.
328. Montane I, McCollough NC, Lian EC. Synovectomy of the knee for hemophilic arthropathy. J Bone Joint Surg [Am] 1986;68:210.
329. Nicol RO, Menelaus MB. Synovectomy of the knee in hemophilia. J Pediatr Orthop 1986;6:330.
330. Nuss R, Kilcoyne RF, Geraghty S, Wiedel J, Manco-Johnson M. Utility of magnetic resonance imaging for management of hemophilic arthropathy in children. J Pediatr 1993;123:388.
331. O'Connell FD. Open surgical synovectomy of the knee in hemophilia: long-term follow-up. In: Gilbert MS, Greene WB, eds. Musculoskeletal problems in hemophilia. New York: The National Hemophilia Foundation, 1989:91.
332. Ortonowski G, Ziemski JM, Kucharski W, Woy-Wojciechowski J. Synoviorthesis with ^{198}Au colloid gold in haemophilia patients. A preliminary report. Folia Haematol 1990;117:505.
333. Perry J, Antonelli D, Ford W. Analysis of knee-joint forces during flexed-knee stance. J Bone Joint Surg [Am] 1975;57:961.
334. Petrini P, Lindvall N, Egberg N, Blombäck M. Prophylaxis with factor concentrates in preventing hemophilic arthropathy. Am J Pediatr Hematol 1991;13:280.
335. Pettersson H, Ahlberg A, Nilsson IM. A radiologic classification of hemophilic arthropathy. Clin Orthop 1980;149:153.
336. Pettersson H, Gillespy T, Kitchens C, Kentro T, Scott KN. Magnetic resonance imaging in hemophilic arthropathy of the knee. Acta Radiologica 1987;28:621.
337. Poggini L, Chistolini A, Mariani G, Mariani PP. Arthroscopic synovectomy in the treatment of haemophilic arthropathy: preliminary results in eight patients. Ital J Orthop Traumatol 1989;15:457.
338. Pool JG, Shannon AE. Production of high-potency concentrates in antihemophilic globulin in a closed-bag system: assay in vitro and in vivo. N Engl J Med 1965;273:1443.
339. Post M, Watts G, Telfer M. Synovectomy in hemophilic arthropathy: a retrospective review of 17 cases. Clin Orthop 1986;202:139.
340. Rivard GE. Synoviorthesis with radioactive colloids in hemophiliacs. Prog Clin Biol Res 1990;324:215.
341. Rivard GE, Girard M, Lamarre C, et al. Synoviorthesis with colloidal ^{32}P chromic phosphate for hemophilic arthropathy: clinical follow-up. Arch Phys Med Rehabil 1985;66:753.
342. Roy S. Ultrastructure of articular cartilage in experimental hemarthrosis. Arch Pathol 1968;86:69.
343. Scarponi R, Silvello L, Landonio G, Baudo F, DeCataldo F. Long-term evaluation of knee-joint function after synovectomy in haemophilia. Br J Haematol 1982;52:337.
344. Shapiro SS. Antibodies to blood coagulation factors. Clin Haematol 1979;8:207.
345. Siegel HJ, Luck JV, Siegel ME, Llinas A, Kasper CK. P-32 chromic phosphate colloid radiosynovectomy for hemarthrosis and synovitis in hemophilia (abstract). XXI International Congress of the World Federation of Hemophilia, Mexico City, Mexico, 1994.
346. Sneppen O, Beck H, Holsteen V. Synovectomy as a prophylactic measure in recurrent haemophilic haemarthrosis. Acta Paediatr Scand 1978;67:491.
347. Stein H, Duthie RB. The pathogenesis of chronic haemophilic arthropathy. J Bone Joint Surg [Br] 1981;63:601.
348. Storti E, Ascari E, Gamba G. Postoperative complications and joint function after knee synovectomy in haemophiliacs. Br J Haematol 1982;50:544.
349. Storti E, Traldi A, Tosatti E, Davol PG. Synovectomy, a new approach to haemophilic arthropathy. Acta Haematol 1969;41:193.
350. Strauss HS. Acquired circulating anticoagulants in hemophilia A. N Engl J Med 1969;281:866.
351. Swanton MC. Hemophilic arthropathy in dogs. Lab Invest 1959;8:1269.
352. Triantafyllou SJ, Hanks GA, Handal JA, Greer RB. Open and arthroscopic synovectomy in hemophilic arthropathy of the knee. Clin Orthop 1992;283:196.
353. Wagner RH, McLester WD, Smith M, Brinkhous KM. Purification of antihemophilic factor (factor VIII) by amino acid precipitation. Thromb Diath Haemorrh 1964;11:64.
354. Wiedel JD. Arthroscopic synovectomy for chronic hemophilic synovitis of the knee. Arthroscopy 1985;3:205.
355. Wilkins RM, Wiedel JD. Septic arthritis of the knee in a hemophiliac: a case report. J Bone Joint Surg [Am] 1983;65:267.
356. Wilson FC, Mayhew DE, McMillan CW. Surgical management of musculoskeletal problems in hemophilia. Instr Course Lect 1983;32:233.

357. Winfield J, Crawley JCW, Hudson EA, Fisher M, Gumpel JM. Evaluation of two regimens to immobilise the knee after injections of yttrium-90. Br Med J 1979;1:986.
358. Yulish BS, Lieberman JM, Strandjord SE, Bryan PJ, Mulopulos GP, Modic MT. Hemophilic arthropathy: assessment with MR imaging. Radiology 1987;164:759.
359. Zuckerman JD, Solomon GE, Shortkroff S, Sledge CB. Principles of radiation synovectomy. In: Gilbert MS, Greene WB, eds. Musculoskeletal problems in hemophilia. New York: The National Hemophilia Foundation 1990:93.

Leukemia

360. Appell RG, Buhler T, Willich E, Brandeis WE. Absence of prognostic significance of skeletal involvement in acute lymphocytic leukemia and non-Hodgkin lymphoma in children. Pediatr Radiol 1985;15:245.
361. Aur RJA, Westbrook HW, Riggs W. Childhood acute lymphocytic leukemia: initial radiologic bone involvement and prognosis. Am J Dis Child 1972;124:653.
362. Bos GD, Simon MA, Spiegel PG, Moohr JW. Childhood leukemia presenting as a diaphyseal radiolucency. Clin Orthop 1978;135:66.
363. Caudle RJ, Crawford AH, Gelfand MJ, Gruppo RA. Childhood acute lymphoblastic leukemia presenting as "cold" lesions on bone scan: a report of two cases. J Pediatr Orthop 1987;7:293.
364. Clausen N, Gøtze H, Pedersen A, Riis-Petersen J, Tjalve E. Skeletal scintigraphy and radiography at onset of acute lymphocytic leukemia in children. Med Pediatr Oncol 1983;11:291.
365. Heinrich SD, Gallagher D, Warrior R, Phelan K, George VT, MacEwen GD. The prognostic significance of the skeletal manifestations of acute lymphoblastic leukemia of childhood. J Pediatr Orthop 1994;14:105.
366. Li FP, Bader JL. Epidemiology of cancer in childhood. In: Nathan DG, Oski FA, eds. Hematology of infancy and childhood. 3rd ed. Philadelphia: WB Saunders, 1987:918.
367. Masera G, Carnelli V, Ferrari M, Recchia M, Bellini F. Prognostic significance of radiological bone involvement in childhood acute lymphoblastic leukaemia. Arch Dis Child 1977;52:530.
368. Ostrov BE, Goldsmith DP, Athreya BH. Differentiation of systemic juvenile rheumatoid arthritis from acute leukemia near the onset of disease. J Pediatr 1993;122:595.
369. Ribeiro RC, Pui CH, Schell MJ. Vertebral compression fracture as a presenting feature of acute lymphoblastic leukemia in children. Cancer 1988;61:589.
370. Rogalsky RJ, Black GB, Reed MH. Orthopaedic manifestations of leukemia in children. J Bone Joint Surg [Am] 1986;68:494.
371. Sallan SE, Weinstein HJ. Childhood acute leukemia. In: Nathan DG, Oski FA, eds. Hematology of infancy and childhood. 3rd ed. Philadelphia: WB Saunders, 1987:1028.
372. Schaller J. Arthritis as a presenting manifestation of malignancy in children. J Pediatr 1972;81:793.
373. Silverman FN. The skeletal lesions in leukemia: clinical roentgenographic observations in 103 infants and children, with a review of the literature. Am J Radiol 1948;59:819.
374. Thomas LB, Forkner CE Jr, Frei E, Besse BE Sr, Stabenau JR. The skeletal lesions of acute leukemia. Cancer 1961;14:608.

Chapter 11

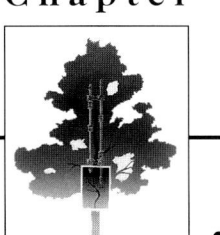

Juvenile Rheumatoid Arthritis and Seronegative Spondyloarthropathies

David D. Sherry
Vincent S. Mosca

Juvenile Rheumatoid Arthritis
   Pauciarticular Onset
   Polyarticular Onset
   Systemic Onset
Seronegative Spondyloarthropathies
   Ankylosing Spondylitis
   Other Seronegative
      Spondyloarthropathies
Etiology
Pathology and Radiology
Differential Diagnosis of Childhood
   Arthritis and Arthralgia
   Septic Arthritis
   Leukemia
   Systemic Lupus Erythematosus
   Acute Rheumatic Fever
   Henoch-Schönlein Purpura
   Toxic Synovitis of the Hip
   Reflex Neurovascular Dystrophy
   Pigmented Villonodular Synovitis
   Sarcoidosis
   Lyme Disease
   Foreign Body Synovitis
   Hypermobility Syndrome
   Miscellaneous Conditions
Approach to the Child With Joint Swelling,
   Limited Motion, and Pain
   History
   Physical Examination
   Laboratory Tests
   Radiography
   Arthrocentesis and Synovial Biopsy

Management of Arthritis Syndromes in
   Children
   Medical Therapy
   Intraarticular Steroid Injections
   Physical and Occupational Therapy
   Other Issues
Orthopaedic Surgical Treatment
   Special Considerations
   Synovectomy
   Soft Tissue Release
   Osteotomy
   Arthrodesis
   Total Joint Arthroplasty
   Epiphyseodesis
Joint-Specific Orthopaedic Treatment
   Hip
   Knee
   Foot and Ankle
   Cervical Spine
   Hand and Wrist
   Elbow
   Shoulder
Orthopaedic Surgery in Seronegative
   Spondyloarthropathies

In 1897, nearly a century after the first description of rheumatoid arthritis in adults, George F. Still published the first English-language description of chronic joint disease in children.[84] He observed significant clinical and pathologic differences between adult and childhood chronic arthritis and also recognized several kinds of arthritis in children. Both observations have withstood the test of time.

Still's report concentrated on the description of the form of chronic childhood arthritis characterized by severe systemic symptoms associated with multiple joint involvement. In the United States, this systemic-onset form of chronic arthritis in children is known as Still disease; in Great Britain, all forms of chronic childhood arthritis are referred to as Still disease. In 1977, because of problems with nomenclature, the European League Against Rheumatism (EULAR) suggested the term *juvenile chronic arthritis* to define this entire group of disorders.[92] Unfortunately, neither this nor any other term has been universally accepted.

Both the American Rheumatism Association (ARA) and EULAR agree that there are several subgroups of chronic arthritis in children. The ARA defines JRA as that group of diseases in which

- chronic synovial inflammation of unknown cause is present
- onset is in children younger than 16 years of age
- objective evidence of arthritis is present in one or more joints for 6 consecutive weeks
- other diseases are excluded from the diagnosis.[12]

Arthritis is defined as swelling of a joint or limitation of motion with heat, pain, or tenderness. This is in contrast to arthralgia, which is merely joint pain. The EULAR definition of juvenile chronic arthritis differs from JRA because the arthritis must be present for a minimum of 12 weeks, and the seronegative spondyloarthropathies are included.[1,92] There has been interest in eliminating both terms and replacing them with the term juvenile arthritis but the nomenclature controversy continues.[34] We will use the ARA definition of JRA in this chapter and discuss the seronegative spondyloarthropathies separately.

The seronegative spondyloarthropathies comprise a group of diseases for which ankylosing spondylitis is the prototype. They are characterized by axial skeleton arthritis, peripheral arthritis that is often asymmetric in distribution, eye or mucocutaneous involvement, urethritis or dysentery, enthesitis, absence of rheumatoid factor (RF) and antinuclear antibodies in the blood, a tendency to be familial, and a high association with the human lymphocyte antigen B27 (HLA-B27).[62,71]

The purpose of this chapter is to describe the clinical spectrum of JRA and the seronegative spondyloarthropathies; to present a practical approach to the diagnosis of swollen, painful joints in children; and to discuss the medical and surgical treatment modalities for these conditions.

JUVENILE RHEUMATOID ARTHRITIS

Juvenile rheumatoid arthritis is the most common chronic childhood rheumatic disease, affecting about 200,000 children in North America.[18] There are three generally recognized patterns or subgroups of JRA (Table 11-1).[1,36,72,85] Pauciarticular-onset JRA is defined by the involvement of four or fewer joints after the first 6 months of arthritis, whereas in polyarticular-onset JRA, five or more joints are involved. Regardless of the number of joints involved, when the illness begins with high, spiking fevers greater than 39.3°C (103°F), the term systemic-onset JRA is used. Children within each subgroup also share other characteristics.

Pauciarticular Onset

Pauciarticular-onset JRA is the most frequently encountered subgroup, comprising 40% to 60% of children with JRA. The peak age of onset is 2 years. Girls are affected four times more frequently than boys. The arthritis is usually insidious in onset and can be painless. Swelling, warmth, and restriction of motion are prominent features. The knee, ankle, and fingers are the most frequently involved joints, although the elbow and wrist also may be affected.[79] Hip involvement is unusual and creates a diagnostic dilemma when it is the first joint involved. Cervical spine involvement is rare.

The erythrocyte sedimentation rate (ESR), C-reactive protein (CRP), and leukocyte count are frequently normal in pauciarticular JRA. The RF test is rarely positive in these children. When it is positive, it portends eventual conversion to a polyarticular clinical course.[67] As many as 50% of children have a positive result in an antinuclear antibody (ANA) test.[36,60] Titers are usually low, rarely exceeding 1 : 320. These titers can change over time; therefore, when initially negative, the test should be repeated in 1 year.

The ANA test result is positive in 64% to 88% of JRA patients with chronic iridocyclitis,[60,74] a disease of unknown etiology that can insidiously lead to visual impairment and blindness.[19,68] Chronic iridocyclitis, or iritis, occurs in 20% of patients with pauciarticular disease, is asymptomatic in its early stages, and can either precede the arthritis or develop many years later. Onset is usually within 7 years after onset of

TABLE 11-1 Chronic Inflammatory Arthritis in Childhood

	PAUCIARTICULAR JRA (40%–60%)	POLYARTICULAR JRA (30%–40%)	SYSTEMIC JRA (20%)	SERONEGATIVE SPONDYLOARTHROPATHY
Age (y)	1–3	1–3 or adolescence	Any	>8
Gender predominance	4 : 1 female	3 : 1 female	Equal	4 : 1 males
Joint (n)	<5	>4	Any	Any
Joints	Large	Large and small	Any	Lower extremity
Enthesitis	Negative	Negative	Negative	Positive
Iritis				
Chronic	20%	10%	5%	Negative
Acute	Negative	Negative	Negative	Positive
ESR	Normal–low	Normal–moderate	Moderate–high	Normal–Moderate
CRP	Normal	Normal–low	High	Normal–High
ANA-positive	30%–50%	30%	15%	Negative
RF-positive	<5%	15%–50%	5%	Negative
Systemic signs	none	Low fever Nodules Felty vasculitis	High fever Rash Hepatosplenomegaly Anemia Lymphadenopathy Leukocytosis Pericarditis Myocarditis	None
HLA association	DR5, DR8	DR4 (if RF-positive)		B27
Prognosis	Very good; iritis can blind	Good; fair in adolescents	Variable	Good in childhood
Destructive arthritis	Uncommon	10%–15% RF-negative; 25%–50% RF-positive	25%–50%	Uncommon

ANA, antinuclear antibodies; CRP, C-reactive protein; ESR, erythrocyte sedimentation rate; HLA, human lymphocyte antigen; JRA, juvenile rheumatoid arthritis; RF, rheumatoid factor.

arthritis. Untreated, chronic inflammation in the anterior chamber of the eye leads to the formation of adhesions between the iris and lens. These adhesions, called posterior synechiae, cause the pupil to deform (Fig. 11-1). Cataract formation with band keratopathy may follow, further obscuring vision. Children with iritis early in the course of their JRA are at the highest risk for losing their vision. Therefore, when a child presents for evaluation with arthritis and an irregular pupil, immediate referral to an ophthalmologist is indicated. Otherwise, the schedule of routine ophthalmologic surveillance is shown in Table 11-2.[78]

Prognosis for the child with pauciarticular JRA is generally excellent; more than 70% of those affected are in remission, with little or no functional impairment, 15 years after onset.[15,35] Although mild to moderate joint space narrowing and erosions may be seen in long-term follow-up, fewer than 15% of children have severe joint destruction and disability.

*TABLE 11-2 Routine Schedule of Iritis Surveillance**

ANA-positive pauciarticular and polyarticular onset—younger than 7 years of age at onset: every 3 to 4 months for 4 years, then every 6 months for 3 years, then yearly

ANA-negative pauciarticular and polyarticular onset—younger than 7 years of age at onset: every 6 months for 7 years, then yearly

ANA-positive or ANA-negative pauciarticular and polyarticular onset—7 years of age or older at onset: every 6 months for 4 years, then yearly

Systemic onset: yearly

* ANA, antinuclear antibody.

These are surveillance recommendations for those children who do not have iritis. If iritis develops, more frequent care by the ophthalmologist is required.

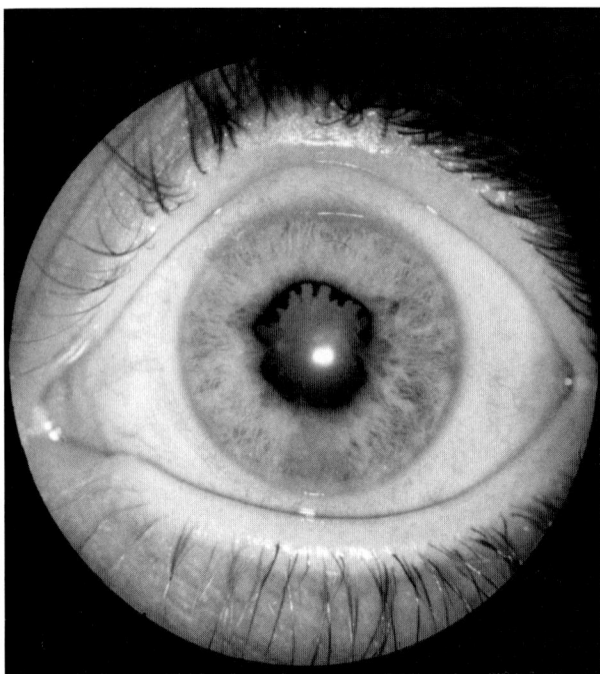

FIGURE 11-1. Iritis in pauciarticular juvenile rheumatoid arthritis. Posterior synechiae are finger-like adhesions between the iris and lens and as seen well during pupil dilation.

Subluxation, especially at the knee, can occur in children with large flexion contractures and aggressive disease. Leg length inequality is common in children with pauciarticular disease with unilateral knee involvement.[81] Hyperemia associated with the inflammatory process stimulates overgrowth of the adjacent growth plates, causing the involved leg to grow longer. Premature closure of the growth plates may eventually lead to ipsilateral shortness, however.

The pauciarticular disease course usually takes several years but can be as short as several months. Occasionally, pauciarticular-onset JRA later develops a polyarticular course that can lead to widespread joint destruction and disability. A final note on prognosis is that the iritis may be more devastating than the arthritis.

Polyarticular Onset

The next most common form of JRA is polyarticular onset, which is found in 30% to 40% of children with JRA. As with pauciarticular JRA, girls predominate. There are two peak ages of onset: 1 to 3 years of age and early adolescence. By definition, these patients have at least five involved joints; many exceed that number. Both large and small joints are affected, frequently in a symmetric pattern. In the first year, however, there may be an asymmetric involvement of joints. Symmetric involvement of the knees, wrists, and ankles is most characteristic. The proximal interphalangeal and metacarpophalangeal joints are involved in more than 20% of patients. Involvement of the cervical spine, hips, shoulders, and temporomandibular joints is not uncommon. In most patients, onset of polyarticular JRA is insidious, although in a few, the disease begins with low-grade fever and acute polyarthritis.

About 30% of patients have positive ANA test results.[36,60] Patients with polyarticular JRA are at risk for developing asymptomatic chronic iritis but at less risk than children in the pauciarticular group.[19,68]

Rheumatoid factor is rarely present in the younger patient but is common in the adolescent.[36] In the latter group, polyarticular disease closely resembles adult rheumatoid arthritis; affected children are more likely to have rheumatoid nodules, joint erosions, and Felty syndrome (i.e., rheumatoid arthritis, splenomegaly, and leukopenia).

Prognosis for children with active polyarticular JRA is generally good, with 60% of patients in remission 15 years after onset.[15,35] Ten percent to 15% of the younger-onset subgroup and 25% to 50% of the adolescent-onset subgroup develop severe destructive arthritis.[70] Severe hip disease is a major cause of late disability.[41,44]

Systemic Onset

The least common form of JRA is systemic-onset, affecting about 20% of children with JRA, girls and boys about equally. Typically, systemic-onset JRA begins between ages 5 and 10 years but it can occur from infancy through adulthood. Fever is the key finding, although patients may have a plethora of other systemic manifestations. Frequently, the fever precedes the arthritis. This makes diagnosis more difficult and necessitates extensive diagnostic evaluation.

Initially, fever may be erratic, but usually there is a quotidian (daily) or double quotidian (twice daily) pattern. The peak of the fever curve is usually in the evening and by definition must exceed 39.3°C (103°F). By morning, the child feels better and has a normal or subnormal temperature. At onset, these fevers can be associated with intense arthralgia and myalgia, occasionally inhibiting the child's movements. Cervical spine stiffness is common and can mimic meningismus, although severe neck pain and torticollis are rare. It is best to look for the characteristic rash of systemic-onset JRA when the child is febrile.[16] This rash is usually nonpruritic, pink to salmon in color, macular or maculopapular, evanescent, and forms small discrete spots with central clearing. It is seen most frequently on the trunk and especially in the axillae. Rash may be induced by mild trauma, such as scratching the skin (i.e., Kobner phenomenon) and occasionally may be widespread (Fig. 11-2). The child without arthritis but with the typical fever and rash, with or without other manifestations, may be considered to have probable systemic-onset JRA once other causes are excluded.[12]

Other systemic manifestations include pericarditis or myocarditis, generalized lymphadenopathy especially in the axillary nodes, hepatosplenomegaly, abdominal pain, growth retardation, vasculitis including the central nervous system, and asymptomatic iritis. Children with systemic-onset JRA are the most anemic and may have leukocytosis exceeding 40,000 leukocytes/μL. Leukopenia and thrombocytopenia are rarely seen in this subgroup and make the diagnosis suspect. The CRP measurement is quite high, as is that of the ESR, which frequently exceeds 100 mm/hour. Rheumatoid factor and ANA are rarely positive in these children.[36]

With time, the child with systemic-onset JRA may develop a few or many inflamed joints. The arthritis tends to be more painful than that found in the other subgroups of JRA, although occasionally a child has painless arthritis.

The prognosis for children with systemic-onset JRA is highly variable.[15,35] The systemic manifestations of the disease usually last from a few to many months. If the arthritis remits when the systemic signs subside, permanent joint destruction or functional limitation is rare. The 25% to 50% of children who develop persistent moderate to severe arthritis can have destructive disease,[39] which can quickly (i.e., within 1 or 2 years) lead to marked disability. As with polyarticular JRA, severe hip disease is a major cause of late disability.[41,44]

SERONEGATIVE SPONDYLOARTHROPATHIES

Seronegative spondyloarthropathies include those types of arthritis associated with sacroiliitis, spinal arthritis, and enthesitis.[62,71] Seronegativity is defined as the absence of RF in the blood. ANA are usually absent but exist in as many as 10% of normal children. Patients are frequently HLA-B27–positive, however. Ankylosing spondylitis, Reiter syndrome, reactive arthritis, and the spondyloarthropathies associated with both psoriasis and inflammatory bowel disease make up this group. All these diseases are more common in adults than in children. In the childhood forms, boys are four times more likely than girls to be affected, and their symptoms are usually more severe than those of girls.[59]

The iritis associated with seronegative spondyloarthropathies is an acute inflammatory process causing redness, pain, and photophobia.[6] It is self-limited and rarely leads to visual impairment. This is in sharp contrast to the chronic iritis of JRA.

Other systemic manifestations of these conditions are low-grade fevers, malaise, weight loss, and aortitis, which can develop silently and lead to aortic insufficiency.[66]

Ankylosing Spondylitis

Ankylosing spondylitis is a painful and progressive arthritis of the sacroiliac joints and spine, which most typically occurs in 20- to 40-year-old Caucasian men. It can develop in childhood, however, with presenting features indistinguishable from pauciarticular JRA.[62,71] These patients are usually boys older than age 8 years, having an asymmetric pattern of peripheral arthritis or arthralgia of the lower extremities. Involvement of the hips, knees, ankles, toes, and rarely, upper extremity joints may be seen and may precede onset of low back pain by several years. Radiographic changes in the axial skeleton are usually a late finding. The peripheral arthritis is often acutely painful but rarely chronic and destructive.

Ankylosing spondylitis may also be seen in children with the more classic adult pattern of low back

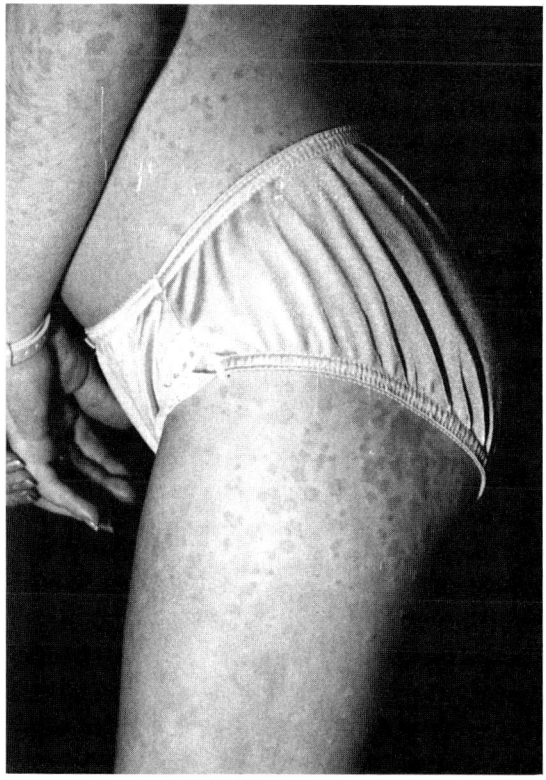

FIGURE 11-2. Maculopapular rash of systemic-onset juvenile rheumatoid arthritis. Central clearing is seen in some spots on the lateral thigh.

and hip girdle pain and stiffness.[71] Symptoms are typically worse in the morning or in the middle of the night. Back motion is limited and there is loss of lumbar lordosis. Involvement of the costovertebral joints causes restriction of chest expansion.

The ESR is often elevated during active disease and a mild anemia may be present. The ANA and RF are negative. HLA-B27 is present in the blood of 8% of normal Caucasians and 4% of normal blacks but it is present in more than 90% of Caucasians and 60% of blacks with ankylosing spondylitis.[75,76] A positive test is also found in 50% to 90% of patients with other seronegative spondyloarthropathies.[59] Therefore, the presence of HLA-B27 is sensitive but not specific for ankylosing spondylitis.

Prognosis for patients with ankylosing spondylitis is good for pain relief by a combination of medical treatment and natural history. Chronic peripheral arthritis and chronic iritis are rare.[62]

Other Seronegative Spondyloarthropathies

Arthritis, conjunctivitis, and urethritis are the three cardinal manifestations of Reiter syndrome, a disease with a strong genetic basis that is triggered by dysentery or sexually transmitted diseases.[46,71] All three features are not necessarily present at the same time. Urethritis is usually associated with dysuria, although it may be painless and manifest by sterile pyuria. Conjunctivitis is usually mild. The arthritis of Reiter syndrome is generally in the lower extremities and is more painful than that in JRA. Sacroiliitis and spondylitis may occur, with radiographic changes somewhat dissimilar to those in ankylosing spondylitis (see Pathology and Radiology).

Postenteric Reiter syndrome is a sequela of infections with *Salmonella*, *Shigella*, *Yersinia*, or *Campylobacter* species in young children.[71,89] In older children and adolescents, a similar disease is seen after sexually transmitted infections caused by *Chlamydia* or *Ureaplasma* organisms. The patient may be asymptomatic, and a history of sexual activity is frequently denied. The arthritis lasts fewer than 6 weeks, and recurrences are rare. A reactive arthritis identical to Reiter syndrome but without urethral or eye involvement also may follow these infections.

Between 7% and 21% of children with inflammatory bowel disease develop a transient peripheral arthritis or a spondylitis similar to ankylosing spondylitis.[52] Arthritis usually follows the onset of gastrointestinal symptoms.

Psoriatic arthritis, occurring in as many as 7% of patients with psoriasis, may assume several patterns in childhood, including a spondylitis form.[71,80] Other forms are predominant distal interphalangeal joint involvement, symmetric polyarticular or oligoarticular arthritis, and asymmetric arthritis. Psoriasis may not be manifest for years after onset of arthritis. Usually, there is a family history of psoriasis; however, 1% of the population has psoriasis, so this is not specific.

Enthesopathy (i.e., pain at ligament and tendon insertions) is found frequently in children with seronegative spondyloarthropathies.[62,69] It can be present with arthritis or arthralgia and may occur long before any low back symptoms. Enthesitis is usually asymmetric and occurs in the lower extremities. The most frequent sites are the metatarsal heads, plantar fascia origin, and Achilles tendon insertion. The tibial tubercle, patella (especially at the 2-, 6-, and 10-o'clock positions), greater trochanter, iliac crest, sacroiliac joints, and clavicle are other frequently involved sites.

The prognosis for most children with enthesopathies or seronegative spondyloarthropathies is good.[71] They respond well to medical therapy; as in adults, indomethacin is particularly effective.[82] Most patients have symptoms sporadically for years but they remain functional and have little disability. Rarely in childhood does severe spondylitis develop. Those who are HLA-B27–positive and have early-onset hip disease are at highest risk.

ETIOLOGY

The etiologies of JRA and the seronegative spondyloarthropathies are unknown. Investigations into the cause of the various forms of JRA fall into two general areas: infectious (especially chronic viral and other nonbacterial organisms) and immunologic (with investigations including immunoregulation mechanisms, cytokine production, and immunogenetics).[49] JRA may be caused by a combination of both. The clustering of disease within some families and the HLA associations suggest that genetic influences play a role. That role may be either in the development of these diseases or in a predisposition to manifest an arthritic response to an antigenic stimulus such as an infection. This is well-demonstrated in individuals who possess the HLA-B27 antigen, because they are likely to have postinfectious Reiter syndrome.[89] Children with either subtle or overt immunodeficiency (e.g., IgA deficiency, agammaglobulinemia, heterozygous C2 deficiency) have an increased incidence of arthritides, some of which are indistinguishable from JRA.

The etiology of systemic-onset JRA is most likely infectious. Its abrupt onset, with high spiking fever, rash, pericarditis, hepatosplenomegaly, and arthritis, is typical for various infections. Furthermore, in Kansas and the Canadian prairie provinces, but not the coastal provinces, it has been reported that the onset of the systemic subgroup of JRA is more common in autumn. Another Canadian study noted a coincidence of a 3-year peak incidence onset of both pauciarticular and polyarticular JRA with that of *Mycoplasma pneumoniae*. Rubella has been cultured from peripheral and synovial leukocytes in a few children within each of the three subgroups of JRA. Data suggesting chronic persistent antigenic material from influenza A have been reported from a single cohort of children with JRA in England. The clinical observation that intercurrent viral infections may cause an exacerbation of JRA supports the idea of persistent viral antigens within the synovium. Direct infection has not been demonstrated in JRA, although infection by previously unknown or difficult to culture organisms (e.g., demonstrated in Lyme disease)[83] is always a possibility. Short-lived arthritis can be caused by a host of viruses, including adenovirus, coxsackievirus, cytomegalovirus, echovirus, Epstein-Barr virus, hepatitis B, parvovirus, rubella, varicella, and others.[63] Some of these are occasionally implicated in chronic arthritis. Chronic arthritis in animals has been caused by various mycoplasma species, *Chlamydia*, reovirus, and retrovirus.

Immunologic abnormalities observed in these patients have involved both the humeral and cellular systems. The most commonly encountered and studied autoantibodies are ANA and RF. The prevalence of each in the various subsets of JRA is shown in Table 11-1. Children with pauciarticular disease with ANA are at the highest risk for asymptomatic iritis, although the titer is not correlated with the severity of eye or joint disease. Erosive changes and prolonged polyarticular disease, much like adult rheumatoid arthritis, are associated with the presence of classic IgM RF (i.e., IgM directed against the Fc portion of IgG). Specialized research laboratories have reported hidden IgM RF (IgM molecules complexed to serum IgG, which are therefore not detected by standard methods), IgG RF, and IgA RF in children with JRA. The clinical significance of these remains to be determined, although one study found that hidden IgM RF correlated with disease activity better than did ESR. Another study found hidden IgA RF in those patients with severe polyarticular JRA. Immune complex formation has been proposed as one mechanism of perpetuating synovitis but an etiologic role for ANA, RF, or circulating immune complexes remains speculative. Interestingly, several patients have been noted to become ANA-negative after the disease goes into remission. Other autoantibodies such as anticollagen antibodies are of interest but incomplete and inconsistent data preclude any conclusions.[61]

Studies of the cellular immune system have not been etiologically enlightening. Generally, the absolute number of peripheral T and B lymphocytes is normal. T-lymphocyte proliferative responses to some antigens are normal and to others are variable, decreased, or delayed, which at times correlates with disease activity. Natural killer cell activity is decreased in peripheral blood, synovial fluid, and synovial tissue, although the number of natural killer surface markers is normal. Inconsistent results regarding production of various cytokines have been reported.

Immunologic studies have been hampered by incomplete knowledge of pathogenic versus nonspecific inflammatory responses, differences between subgroups of JRA, varying disease activity in the subjects, and imperfect assay techniques. Energy is being directed at isolating these confounding factors and establishing pathogenic mechanisms.

PATHOLOGY AND RADIOLOGY

Although the cause of inflammatory arthritis is unknown, the underlying pathology is that of inflammation.[14] The histology is the same for all three subgroups of JRA and adult rheumatoid arthritis. Synovial biopsy is not specific for the diagnosis of JRA but may help to eliminate other conditions, such as sarcoidosis or tuberculosis.

The synovial lining of joints is comprised of a thin (1–3 cells thick) layer of synovial cells overlying fibroadipose tissue, which is comprised of type I collagen, fat, blood vessels, and unmyelinated nerves, without a discrete basement membrane. Of the two endothelial cell types, synovial A cells predominate and are phagocytic, whereas synovial B cells are more similar to fibroblasts.

The hallmarks of inflammation are lymphocytic infiltration (mostly helper T cells) and increased vascularity. On a molecular level, one of the first steps is getting the neutrophils to the inflammatory site. This is regulated by a variety of adhesion molecules produced by the endothelial cells and neutrophils. A variety of substances then more firmly adhere the neutrophils to the endothelium, cause migration into the tissue, and produce chemotaxis (both early and late chemotactic molecules). Angiogenesis is closely related to cellular proliferation. This is associated with hyperemia and edema, with secretion of large amounts of protein-rich synovial fluid into the joint. Numerous leukocytes migrate to the joint, undoubtedly because of the chemotactic substances produced; most potent of the early chemotactic molecules are C5a, leukotriene B4, and platelet-activating factor. Synovial-fluid cell counts in JRA usually range from 4000 to 30,000/μL but counts exceeding 50,000/μL and even 100,000/μL can be seen, especially in systemic-onset JRA.

At this stage, histologic study demonstrates lymphocytic infiltration and villi that protrude into the joint cavity and are composed of hypervascular hypertrophic synovium. Continued synovial inflammation leads to expansion of the hypertrophic synovium over the articular cartilage, called pannus. This pannus invades the cartilage using lysosomal hydrolases, which break down the proteoglycans and collagen. Eventually, this process reaches the subchondral bone, causing erosions and cyst formation. At the margins of the cartilage and the synovium, the lining is discontinuous, which exposes bare bone. This area is especially vulnerable to pannus, which then leads to the marginal erosions seen on radiographs. It is only after significant amounts of cartilage have been destroyed that joint space narrowing is manifest radiographically. In the late stages, subchondral bone cysts may collapse, leading to marked joint irregularity and avascular necrosis. Fibrous ankylosis and even bony fusion may finally occur.

The periarticular structures are also involved in the inflammatory process. Capsular hypertrophy and thickening, periosteal new bone formation, and osteoporosis are seen. Synovial cysts are not uncommon, although most are small and do not present a problem. Adjacent tendons and muscles can become inflamed. Synovial inflammation leads to pain and muscle spasm, with involuntary, then fixed, loss of joint movement. Ligaments are stretched or destroyed, and periarticular contractures ensue. Normal alignment of the bones is lost, with deformities noted both clinically and radiographically. Articular cartilage requires movement and physiologic pressures for its nourishment and health. When these are lost, the destructive process begun by pannus is compounded.

Children are uniquely affected by the inflammatory process because their bones are not fully grown. Inflammatory hyperemia may cause stimulation of adjacent growth plates, with overgrowth of bones or in some cases, early physeal closure with shortening. The effect on any growth plate may be symmetric or asymmetric. Leg length discrepancy is a recognized complication of monoarticular and pauciarticular JRA, with predominant involvement of the knee. This problem been quantitated and analyzed.[81] The findings suggest that overgrowth of the involved extremity occurs when disease onset is earlier than age 9 years. The major discrepancy develops within the first 3 to 4 years, then increases slowly, decreases, or remains the same. Overgrowth rarely exceeds 3 cm and premature closure of the growth plates, with shortening of the involved extremity, does not occur. In patients with disease onset after age 9 years, premature closure of the growth plates, with shortening of the involved extremity, may occur and the discrepancies can be substantial, occasionally reaching 6 cm. This is in sharp contrast to the hip, in which disease onset in young patients is associated with premature growth arrest of the acetabulum and the femoral head.[41,44]

Radiographic changes in the cervical spine of patients with JRA have been reclassified into seven types:[38]

1. Anterior erosion of the odontoid process
2. Anteroposterior erosion of the odontoid process, the apple-core odontoid (Fig. 11-3)
3. Subluxation of C1 on C2
4. Focal soft tissue calcification anterior to the ring of C1
5. Ankylosis of the apophyseal joints, often eventually leading to ankylosis and fusion of the vertebral bodies (Fig. 11-4)
6. Longitudinal and circumferential growth abnormalities of adjacent vertebral bodies after spontaneous posterior fusions (see Fig. 11-4)
7. Subaxial subluxations between C2 and C7, often associated with ankylosis of facet joints above and below the area of subluxation (Fig. 11-5).

In ankylosing spondylitis, there is an ascending ankylosis of the axial skeleton that is detectable clinically and radiographically.[14,62] Inflammation of the zygoapophyseal joints causes pain, muscle spasm, restriction of motion, and eventually joint destruction, with bony ankylosis. Radiographically, the earliest findings are symmetric, bilateral subchondral erosions of the sacroiliac joints, which make the joints appear widened and fuzzy. Subchondral sclerosis follows, first on the

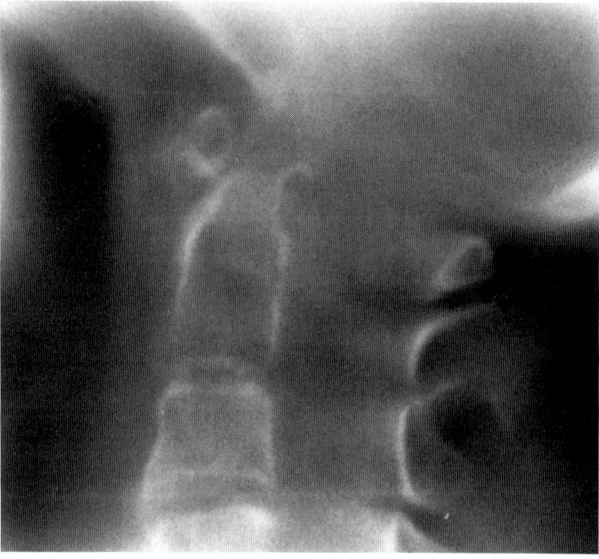

FIGURE 11-3. Apple-core odontoid in polyarticular juvenile rheumatoid arthritis. Tomogram shows anterior and posterior erosion.

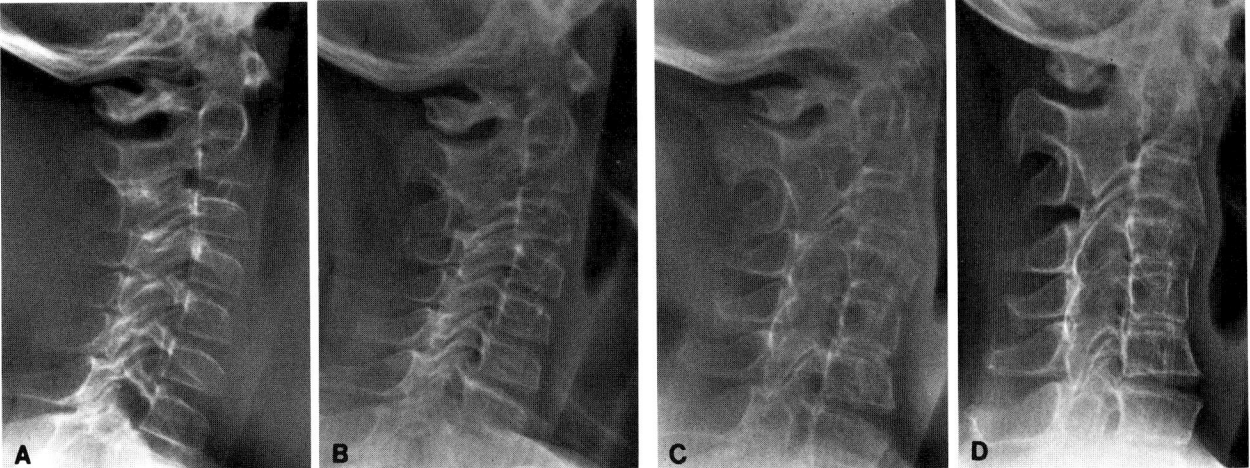

FIGURE 11-4. The cervical spine in systemic-onset juvenile rheumatoid arthritis. (A) Age 9 years; early C2–C3 apophyseal ankylosis. (B) Age 10 years; solid C2–C3 apophyseal fusion and early C4–C6 apophyseal ankylosis. (C) Age 14 years; solid C2–C3 and C4–C6 apophyseal fusions, with ankylosis and growth abnormalities of corresponding vertebral bodies. (D) Age 15 years; more advanced deformity.

iliac side and then on both sides of the joints. As the disease ascends, the lumbar and then thoracic spine straighten. The vertebrae appear squared-off on the lateral radiograph. The longitudinal ligaments and annulus fibrosis ossify, creating marginal syndesmophytes and giving the classic bamboo spine–appearance from sacrum to occiput. Facet joints are simultaneously obliterated. In Reiter syndrome and psoriatic arthritis, beak-like nonmarginal syndesmophytes may be seen.

DIFFERENTIAL DIAGNOSIS OF CHILDHOOD ARTHRITIS AND ARTHRALGIA

Many medical conditions share certain clinical features with JRA and the seronegative spondyloarthropathies. Because JRA is a diagnosis of exclusion, the orthopaedist should have a working knowledge of the full differential diagnosis. One way to organize these diseases is by mode of onset and the general

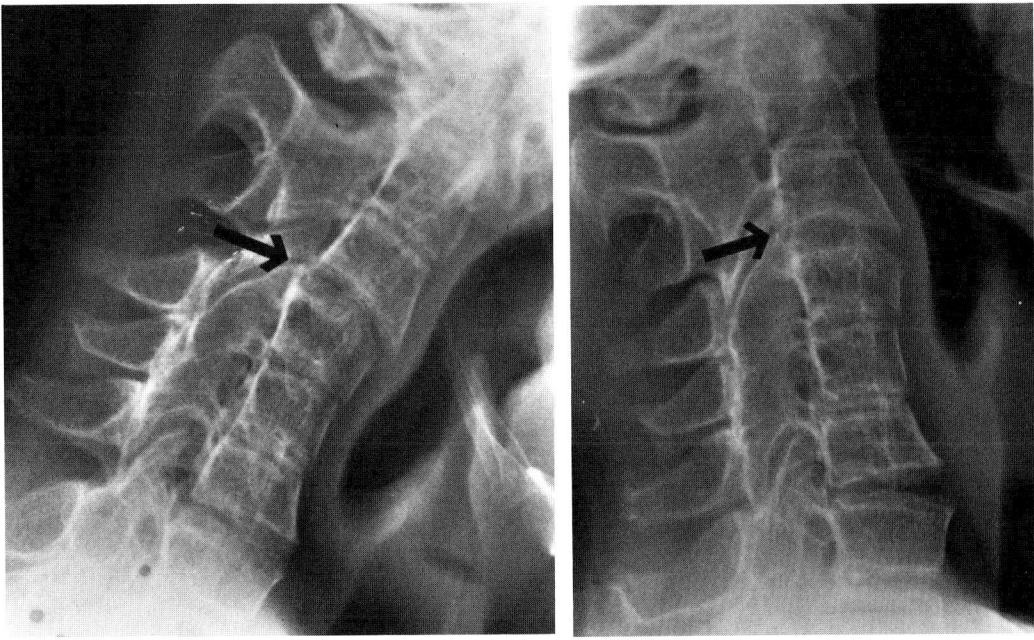

FIGURE 11-5. Systemic-onset juvenile rheumatoid arthritis. Subaxial subluxation at C3–C4, associated with fusions at levels above and below.

TABLE 11-3 Differential Diagnosis

ACUTE ONSET	INSIDIOUS ONSET
Toxic Child	
Systemic JRA	Systemic JRA
Infection (bacterial, viral)	Infection (tuberculosis, fungal)
Leukemia	Sarcoidosis
Systemic lupus erythematosis	Neuroblastoma
Reiter syndrome	Other neoplasia
Reactive arthritis	
Sickle cell disease	
Serum sickness	
Acute rheumatic fever	
Vasculitities (Henoch-Schönlein purpura, Kawasaki syndrome)	
Inflammatory bowel disease	
Well Child	
Trauma	Pauciarticular JRA
Toxic synovitis	Polyarticular JRA
Reflex neurovascular dystrophy	Seronegative spondyloarthropathies
Hemophilia	Osteochondroses (Legg-Calvé-Perthes, Osgood-Schlatter)
SCFE (acute)	SCFE (chronic)
Pigmented villonodular synovitis	Lyme disease
	Mechanical
	Discitis
	Osteoid osteoma
	Foreign body synovitis
	Hypermobility
	Patellofemoral joint disease
	Synovial hemangioma

JRA, juvenile rheumatoid arthritis; SCFE, slipped capital femoral epiphysis.

well-being or toxicity of the child (Table 11-3). Several of these diseases are highlighted here.

Septic Arthritis

Septic arthritis is discussed in Chapter 16. Monoarticular septic arthritis and JRA should rarely be confused. Among the 30% of children treated for culture-negative septic arthritis, however, a few children later prove to have had a chronic inflammatory or reactive arthritis.[42] Joint fluid with a leukocyte count exceeding 100,000/μL is suggestive of but not pathognomonic for septic arthritis and may be seen in inflammatory joints.

Infection of multiple joints can be mistaken for JRA. Outside of the neonatal period, wherein multiple different organisms may be responsible, the two most likely etiologic agents are *Haemophilus influenzae* and *Neisseria gonorrhea*. The former is becoming less common with the advent of an effective immunization program. History of sexual exposure in those with gonorrhea, even with a positive culture result, can be impossible to elicit in many children and adolescents. Appropriate child abuse authorities need to be contacted. Children with multiple joints infected with *Staphylococcus* organisms are extremely ill and not easily confused with patients having JRA.

Children with long-standing arthritis are at an increased risk of developing septic arthritis (usually as a result of *Staphylococcus*), and treatment should not be delayed if clinically suspected.

Leukemia

Leukemia usually affects young children. Most appear systemically ill. This disease can mimic systemic-onset JRA by its skeletal and extraskeletal manifestations. The joint disease is usually monarticular (frequently a hip), although it may be polyarticular and is painful. Bone pain is common. Symptoms can be present for months before the child is seen but a few weeks is more typical. A complete blood count (CBC) without blast forms does not exclude leukemia; therefore, bone marrow examination is required to make the diagnosis of leukemia or to rule it out.[73]

Systemic Lupus Erythematosus

Systemic lupus erythematosus typically affects teen-aged girls and is marked by constitutional symptoms, malar rash (i.e., butterfly pattern); major organ disease (especially renal, bone marrow, central nervous system, and cardiopulmonary); and a painful, debilitating, red, hot arthritis. The arthritis responds quickly to steroids and rarely leads to deformity.[25]

Acute Rheumatic Fever

Acute rheumatic fever is an autoimmune reactive process, occurring 2 to 4 weeks after a streptococcal infection. Children 5 to 15 years of age are most susceptible; younger children are rarely affected. Criteria for its diagnosis are shown in Table 11-4. The arthritis of rheumatic fever is unlike that of JRA because joints are exquisitely tender, red, and hot and the arthritis migrates from joint to joint over a period of hours. Its rapid response to aspirin therapy is almost diagnostic. Rheumatic fever lasts fewer than 6 weeks.[86]

Henoch-Schönlein Purpura

Henoch-Schönlein purpura is a small vessel vasculitis, usually involving the skin, joints, gut, and kidneys. Boys

TABLE 11-4	Modified Jones Criteria* for the Diagnosis of Rheumatic Fever
MAJOR	MINOR
Carditis Polyarthritis Chorea Erythema marginatum Subcutaneous nodules	Clinical: fever to 39°C, arthralgia Laboratory: acute-phase reaction (elevated ESR, elevated CRP); prolonged PR interval
PLUS	
Supporting evidence of preceding streptococcal infection (elevated or rising streptococcal antibody titers, positive throat culture for group A streptococci, or positive rapid streptococcal antigen test).	

CRP, C-reactive protein; ESR, erythrocyte sedimentation rate.
* The presence of two major critera or one major and two minor critera indicates a high probability of the presence of rheumatic fever.

are more frequently affected. The mean age of onset is 6 years. The rash is typically from the waist down but it can involve the arms and face. It begins as urticaria but quickly turns into petechiae, then purpura. Severe episodic abdominal pain and hematochezia denote gut involvement. Occasionally, intussusception occurs. Microscopic hematuria is the most common manifestation of kidney disease but rarely, chronic renal failure can develop. The arthritis is usually quite painful but can be relieved by nonsteroidal medication. The entire course usually lasts fewer than 6 weeks but recurrences are common.[26]

Toxic Synovitis of the Hip

Toxic synovitis of the hip is a relative short-lived acute inflammatory process, usually seen in boys aged 2 to 10 years. It frequently follows an upper respiratory tract infection. Findings include pain in the hip area, muscle spasm, restriction of motion, refusal to walk, and occasionally, low-grade fever. This condition is more typically confused with septic arthritis than with JRA. The ESR and leukocyte count are elevated but to a lesser extent than in septic arthritis. The pain and dysfunction are also less severe.[37]

Reflex Neurovascular Dystrophy

Reflex neurovascular dystrophy (reflex sympathetic dystrophy) usually occurs in 8- to 16-year-old children, in girls more often than boys. Pain is the primary symptom. Patients show marked dysfunction and signs of sympathetic overdrive, such as cyanosis, coldness, edema, and hyperhydrosis. Hyperesthesia with an incongruent affect is typical. Children with RND are usually compliant and pseudomature. Underlying psychosocial stress from school, family, or both is almost always present. Aggressive physical therapy is curative but psychologic evaluation is imperative.[8]

Pigmented Villonodular Synovitis

Pigmented villonodular synovitis is a slow-growing, benign, and locally invasive tumor of the synovium. It is usually monoarticular and most frequently involves the knee. It can also occur in the hip, ankle, elbow, and any other joint. Acute episodic attacks of pain and swelling may occur. Most have hemorrhagic, dark brown synovial fluid. Biopsy is diagnostic.[24]

Sarcoidosis

Children with sarcoidosis have nontender boggy synovium that does not limit range of motion significantly. They may have fevers, rash, and iritis, which can resemble JRA. Pulmonary disease, erythema nodosum, abdominal pain, liver enlargement, and perihilar adenopathy may also be present.[57]

Lyme Disease

Lyme disease is a tick-borne spirochetal infection leading to widespread symptoms including rash (i.e., erythema chronicum migrans), constitutional symptoms, neurologic symptoms, carditis, and either acute episodic or chronic arthritis. It is most prevalent in the northeastern part of the country, in Wisconsin, and in northern California, although it has been reported in most states. Antibody response to the organism helps with the diagnosis. Tetracycline, penicillin, and erythromycin therapy each have been successful.[83]

Foreign Body Synovitis

Occasionally, a piercing injury may leave a splinter or thorn embedded in a joint. This leads to chronic inflammation indistinguishable from JRA, although it is almost always monoarticular. Diagnosis is made by observing organic matter in the biopsy specimen under polarized light. Synovectomy is curative.

Hypermobility Syndrome

Hypermobility is usually seen in younger children and is defined as the presence of four of the five following signs:

1. Thumb abduction to touch the forearm
2. Finger hyperextension to parallel the forearm

3. More than 10 degrees of hyperextension of the elbow
4. More than 10 degrees of hyperextension of the knee
5. Ability to touch palms to floor with knees extended.[10]

If pain occurs, it is usually nocturnal and involves the lower extremities symmetrically and nonfocally. Pain may be worse after a particularly active day. Physical findings are lacking. Leg aches or growing pains are other terms used to describe these symptoms, whether or not hypermobility coexists. Reassurance and discontinuing secondary gain are usually sufficient treatment.

Miscellaneous Conditions

A host of other rheumatologic conditions can initially mimic JRA. Other associated physical findings, the course of the disease over time, and the response to therapy clear up any diagnostic dilemma in most cases. For example, skin changes are notable in scleroderma. Some children with linear scleroderma present with a flexion contracture of a joint but no arthritis is apparent. Oral and genital ulcers are present in children with Behçet syndrome. Fever and rash are seen in polyarteritis nodosa; multiple other systemic signs are present when major organs are involved. Most children with familial Mediterranean fever have discrete, relatively short-lived episodes of arthritis, fever, and abdominal pains. Many do not have a positive family history and, in North America, are not of Mediterranean extraction. A description of many of the other conditions listed in Table 11-3 can be found elsewhere in this text.

APPROACH TO THE CHILD WITH JOINT SWELLING, LIMITED MOTION, AND PAIN

The old adage holds true that if you do not think of it, you will not diagnose it. The corollary is that if you think of it, you ought to know how to evaluate it or where to refer it. For the orthopaedic surgeon faced with a child with one or more swollen, stiff, painful, warm, or tender joints, the differential diagnosis is broad but the diagnoses that must be immediately ruled out are few and familiar. The conditions requiring immediate diagnosis and treatment are pyogenic infection, fracture, tumor, and slipped capital femoral epiphysis.

The orthopaedist may not be as familiar with the rheumatologic conditions in the differential diagnosis as with other conditions. Unfortunately, there is no single laboratory test that can be used to make a definitive diagnosis of JRA or many of the other conditions mentioned in this chapter. Juvenile rheumatoid arthritis is a diagnosis of exclusion. The orthopaedist should therefore familiarize himself with this group of diseases. The key to any diagnosis, and particularly to JRA, is a complete and accurate history and physical examination, supplemented by appropriate laboratory tests and radiographs.

It is not our purpose here to discuss the entire evaluation of joint swelling, stiffness, and pain in children. It is to point out the special features of the history and physical examination that should lead the physician to entertain the possibility of JRA or the spondyloarthropathies and to discuss the evaluation process for these diagnoses.

History

A detailed history should ascertain the nature of onset, the duration of symptoms, the pattern of joint involvement, and the child's general state of health. Was there obvious antecedent trauma or infection or was the onset insidious? How long have the signs or symptoms been present? How many joints are involved? Which joints are involved? Is the involvement migratory or stationary? Has the child been ill? Are there any underlying illnesses? Are diarrhea, dysuria, eye irritation, psoriasis, or rash either current or remote problems? Additionally, the quality of the pain is determined. If a lower extremity joint is involved, does the child bear weight? When the answers to these questions are considered in the context of the patient's age and gender, the differential diagnosis quickly narrows. Family history should be explored, particularly in children with long-standing symptoms.

The quality of pain is important. The affected joints in septic arthritis, acute rheumatic fever, SLE, Reiter syndrome, leukemia, and the vasculitis syndromes are extremely painful. The child generally does not bear weight on the involved lower extremity and does not tolerate even slow and gentle movement of the joint. The joints in JRA are less painful; the child generally walks on the affected extremity and allows some manipulation. The pain in JRA typically improves with use of the affected joint.

Morning stiffness is commonly reported. As previously stated, diagnosis of JRA requires the presence of objective arthritis for a minimum of 6 weeks; therefore, JRA should not be high in the differential for joint symptoms of shorter duration.

Single joint symptoms of short duration are usually seen with a history of antecedent trauma or infection. Trauma is obvious. Infection may not be so obvious but acute onset of single joint systems in a child who looks sick usually leads to the appropriate evaluation and diagnosis. Leukemia is another possibility.

If the single affected painful joint is the hip and the symptoms are mild, consider toxic synovitis in the young child, Legg-Calvé-Perthes disease in the 4- to 10-year-old boy, and slipped capital femoral epiphysis in the 10- to 15-year-old adolescent. Monoarticular JRA of the hip is rare. Pauciarticular or polyarticular JRA presenting first with hip involvement is also rare. The exception may be the boy older than 8 years with the peripheral arthritis presentation of ankylosing spondylitis. Sacroiliac and low back symptoms should then be explored.

Based on the history alone, when the single affected joint is the knee and the symptoms are mild or moderate, consider patellofemoral joint disease in the adolescent girl or a periarticular tumor in any age group. The knee is the most common site of musculoskeletal tumors in children. In evaluating the knee, a history of tick bite or rash in an area endemic for Lyme disease should be sought. Hemophilia as the cause of joint swelling and pain is suggested by the history of present or previous joint symptoms, the family history, and the gender of the child. Orthopaedic surgeons are generally sophisticated in the evaluation of internal derangements of the adult knee. The adult forms of internal derangement are less common in children, however, and other considerations should include a discoid meniscus, osteochondritis dissecans, and a painless noncommunicating popliteal cyst.

The knee is the most frequently affected joint in monoarticular and pauciarticular JRA. In otherwise healthy girls younger than age 5 years, a history of several weeks of swelling, warmth, and mild pain or tenderness of a knee, ankle, or elbow should raise suspicions of pauciarticular JRA. Although it is in this female age group that the frequency and morbidity of chronic iritis is high, rarely is the eye symptomatic at the time of presentation. Therefore, the absence of a history of eye symptoms does not rule out diagnosis of JRA. It is necessary to inquire about eye symptoms in the older boy with arthritis, in whom acute iritis may suggest a diagnosis of ankylosing spondylitis. A history of enthesitis or a family history of spondyloarthropathy should be sought in these boys.

Two to four swollen, warm, and moderately painful or tender joints in an asymmetric pattern in a child suggest JRA, trauma, leukemia, tuberculous or fungal infections, hemophilia, and Lyme disease. The distinctive diagnostic features have already been mentioned. When the child is febrile or appears ill and has polyarticular symptoms of short duration, consider acute rheumatic fever, leukemia, child abuse, rheumatoid disease, and infectious, reactive, or gonococcal arthritis. The longer the duration of symptoms the greater the likelihood of rheumatologic disease. Any history of rash should be considered. Knowledge of the fever pattern can help differentiate acute rheumatic fever (sustained pattern) from JRA (spiking pattern). Migratory polyarthritis suggests acute rheumatic fever or gonococcal disease. Symmetric polyarthritis in this setting strongly suggests JRA. Although it is unlikely that a child with systemic-onset JRA with spiking fevers, rash, hepatosplenomegaly, and arthritis will present to the orthopaedist for diagnosis, the possibility exists and should not be discounted.

Rheumatic disease should be high on the list of possible diagnoses for children who are afebrile, presenting with symmetric polyarthritis of long duration. A history of neck stiffness or pain should be ascertained when considering this subgroup of JRA. A positive family history of rheumatic disease in a teenaged girl is helpful with the clinical diagnosis of seropositive polyarticular disease.

A detailed history and a thorough knowledge of the diagnostic possibilities can lead the orthopaedist to arrive at a reasonable differential diagnosis of joint swelling, stiffness, and pain in children even before the physical examination.

Physical Examination

Some of the characteristic features of JRA joints have already been mentioned. The arthritic joint often looks worse than it feels; in fact, the only finding may be swelling. As a rule, children walk on these joints despite the presence of fusiform swelling, warmth, discomfort, and limitation of motion. There is generally greater active and passive motion and less pain than usually found in a similar-appearing joint caused by trauma or infection. Tenderness is diffuse and nonfocal. Atrophy and weakness of the adjacent muscles, suggesting chronicity, may already be present at the time of diagnosis. Measurement of limb circumference can be helpful in this case. In contrast, children with septic arthritis, acute rheumatic fever, SLE, Reiter syndrome, leukemia, and vasculitis do not tolerate even slow and gentle movement of the affected joint: move the joint and move the child. Warmth and tenderness are common to all of these diagnoses but are more intense in the more painful joints. Severe and disabling pain with la belle indifference, and an incongruent affect, should raise the suspicion of RND.

Knowledge of the pattern of joint involvement can be helpful. Symmetric involvement of many joints usually means polyarticular JRA. Asymmetric involvement of a few joints may mean pauciarticular JRA, early polyarticular JRA, or seronegative spondyloarthropathy. Examine other large joints in children with monoarticular symptoms for possible painless or nontender swelling and warmth.

Measurement of leg lengths may be revealing in a young girl presenting with a swollen knee. In older boys, the low back and sacroiliac joints should be examined and chest expansion measured (<2.5 cm is abnormal).[7] Range of motion of the cervical spine is tested in all children suspected of having JRA. Limitation of extension is the initial finding. Normally, neck extension pinches the examiner's finger when it is placed at the seventh cervical vertebra.[38] A careful neurologic examination is performed, especially to look for long tract signs.

In adolescents with arthritis, enthesopathy may be found, unknown to the child, at sites distant from the initial complaint, such as plantar fascia insertion tenderness in a patient with hip pain.[62]

Extending the physical examination beyond the extremities and spine, the orthopaedist should examine the skin for rashes, the fingernails for pitting (psoriatic arthritis), the eyes for conjunctivitis or pupil irregularity, the abdomen for hepatosplenomegaly, and the lymph nodes for enlargement or tenderness. Although not performed by the orthopaedist, the most important part of the examination of the child suspected of having pauciarticular or polyarticular JRA is the slit-lamp eye examination. It may be the only positive diagnostic finding.

Laboratory Tests

Assuming that JRA is a strong consideration for a diagnosis based on the history and physical examination, the initial laboratory evaluation should include an ESR, CRP, CBC, ANA, RF, and urinalysis. These tests try to pinpoint JRA. Other tests should be performed to rule out other disease possibilities. It cannot be overemphasized that JRA is a diagnosis of exclusion.

The ESR assesses evidence of inflammation and can be used to monitor the degree of disease activity. The CRP is an acute phase–reactant molecule that rises and falls in response to disease activity more rapidly than the ESR.[47] It is not influenced by the hematocrit, which makes it particularly useful for the many patients with arthritis who are anemic. The CRP is usually normal in pauciarticular and polyarticular disease, high in systemic-onset JRA, and may be high in reactive arthritis. It is normal in SLE, even when the ESR is high, unless there is a concurrent infection. The CBC is important to screen for neoplasia or collagen vascular disease. The platelet count may be elevated as an acute-phase reactant or it may be normal in children with chronic arthritis. The leukocyte count should be normal or elevated; it can be elevated in systemic-onset JRA. Low platelet or leukocyte measurements may indicate leukemia, SLE, or sarcoidosis. The hematocrit is usually normal or slightly low in chronic arthritis. A significantly low hematocrit can be indicative of any chronic disease, inflammatory bowel disease, neoplasia, SLE, or an underlying hematopoietic disease such as sickle cell or thalassemia.

Urinalysis is a useful screen for many collagen vascular diseases such as SLE, and it can pick up sterile pyuria in Reiter syndrome. Only rarely does JRA cause renal problems.

Rheumatoid factor is an IgM anti-IgG antibody. It is not specific for JRA and may be seen in conditions such as subacute bacterial endocarditis. The RF is negative in the seronegative spondyloarthropathies and only rarely positive in JRA. It is suggestive but not diagnostic of JRA when positive, especially in the older girl with polyarticular involvement. Those with RF are at greater risk of developing erosive disease. When RF is present in pauciarticular disease, a polyarticular course is likely.

As many as 10% of normal children have a low-titer positive ANA test using HEp-2 cells as substrate. This may be a nonspecific cross-reaction from a recent infection. A low-titer ANA (<1 : 640) in a young girl with pauciarticular involvement is highly suggestive of JRA; its presence is a marker for those children at high risk for developing asymptomatic iritis. A high-titer ANA (1 : 640 or higher) may require further evaluation to rule out SLE or mixed connective tissue disease.[25] This should include measuring complement (CH50) and antibodies to DNA and extractable nuclear antigens.

Depending on the particular circumstances, other tests may be helpful. The HLA-B27 antigen is normal in 8% of the Caucasian population, so its presence is not necessarily abnormal. In an older boy with pauciarticular symptoms or in one whose signs and symptoms fall between pauciarticular JRA and spondyloarthropathy, the presence of HLA-B27 would tend to support the latter. Thus, the child would be at an increased risk for acute iritis, enthesitis, and involvement of the sacroiliac and hip joints. The presence of HLA-B27 portends a more severe course, especially regarding the low back.

Radiography

Early radiographs in JRA and the spondyloarthropathies are not diagnostic, often showing only soft tissue swelling or osteopenia (Fig. 11-6). They are helpful, however, in ruling out other diagnoses and in establishing a baseline for later joint changes. Computed tomography or magnetic resonance imaging of some joints, such as the sacroiliac or the hip, may be helpful in selected patients because they show abnormalities (e.g., edema, effusions, bony changes) before plain radiographs. Radionuclide bone scans may help differentiate synovitis, leukemia, osteoid osteoma, aseptic necrosis, osteomyelitis, and RND.[23] As a baseline and before any anesthetic, a child with suspected or known JRA should have lateral flexion and extension cervical spine radiographs to assess atlantoaxial instability and subaxial ankylosis.

Arthrocentesis and Synovial Biopsy

Arthrocentesis is not routinely performed. It should be performed in the acute setting to evaluate possible

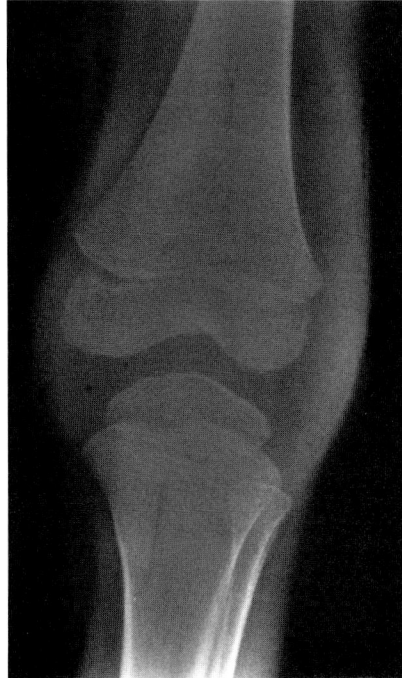 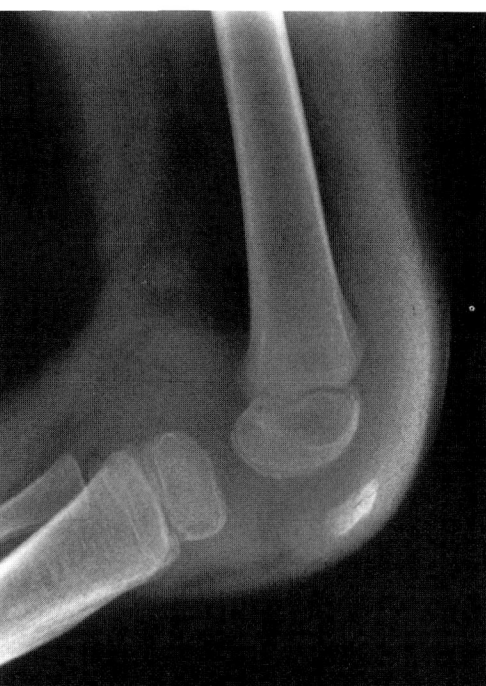

FIGURE 11-6. Knee effusion and osteopenia several months after onset of pauciarticular disease in a 4-year-old girl.

septic arthritis. In the chronic setting, it should be performed only when the history, physical examination, and laboratory studies fail to point to a clear diagnosis. The pain and cost are not justified otherwise.

Juvenile rheumatoid arthritis usually produces an inflammatory fluid, with leukocytes in the 2000 to 50,000/μL range, although counts can exceed 100,000/μL. In JRA, polymorphs predominate, glucose is not significantly depressed, and protein is elevated. The broad overlap in test results between inflammatory and infectious cases makes the interpretation of joint fluid analysis difficult. Additionally, children with septic arthritis may have sterile joint fluid in as many as 30% of cases.[42]

A synovial biopsy specimen should be obtained in the presence of otherwise undiagnosable, continuous, monoarticular arthritis. This may help to rule out pigmented villonodular synovitis, foreign body synovitis, synovial hemangioma, or neoplasia. Although tuberculosis is rare in North America, it may require biopsy for diagnosis. A biopsy specimen is necessary to diagnose sarcoidosis.

MANAGEMENT OF ARTHRITIS SYNDROMES IN CHILDREN

Juvenile rheumatoid arthritis and the seronegative spondyloarthropathies are painful chronic diseases for which there are no known cures. Although about 70% of patients with JRA and even more patients with spondylitis eventually enter long remissions without significant joint damage, these diseases take a toll on the physical, emotional, social, and educational growth of affected children. The goals of medical management are pain relief, prevention of deformity, and maintenance of function—all in the context of the total care of the child and his or her family. These children require the services of many health and education professionals of varying degrees of intensity during the course of disease. A team, including a pediatric rheumatologist, physical therapist, occupational therapist, nurse specialist, social worker, and orthopaedic surgeon, is desirable for optimal communication and coordination of health services. An anesthesiologist familiar with the special problems of airway management in these children is important. The educator, psychologist, and nutritionist should be considered to be part of the extended-care team.

Management of JRA and seronegative spondyloarthropathies in children consists of drug therapy for control of pain and inflammation, selective intraarticular steroid injections, physical and occupational therapy and splinting to prevent deformity and maintain function, and selective orthopaedic surgery to control pain, reduce deformity, and maintain or improve function. Bed rest and joint immobilization should be kept to a minimum, especially during the acute phase of disease.

Medical Therapy

The aim of medical therapy is remission. Aggressive disease should be met with aggressive therapy. Those children at the highest risk for long-term disability can often be identified in the first 6 months of the disease. Early treatment of these children is mandatory to significantly affect their futures. Most centers have seen a dramatic decrease in the number of severely involved children by treating earlier and more intensely. Because of the unknown etiology of these diseases and the incomplete ability to modify the pathogenic process, uniform success is not possible.

The first line of therapy is the nonsteroidal antiinflammatory drugs (NSAIDs), for which aspirin has traditionally been the gold standard.[11,13] These drugs interfere with several steps in the inflammatory process, the major effect being inhibition of cyclooxygenase.[30] Each nonsteroidal agent has varying effects on this and other steps, such as the lipoxygenase pathway, oxygen radical generation, and chemotaxis. Therefore, in any given child, one NSAID may have a vastly different effect or side effect than another NSAID.

Published pediatric doses for most of these drugs are shown in Table 11-5. Only aspirin, tolmetin sodium, and naproxen, however, are approved for use in children younger than 14 years of age. Aspirin is usually effective, well tolerated, and inexpensive; however, it is one of the more hepatotoxic NSAIDs. Therapeutic blood levels are between 20 to 30 mg/dL. The physician needs to wait a minimum of 5 days before checking a salicylate level to allow a steady state to occur. There is an increased risk for Reye syndrome in young children taking aspirin during exposure to chickenpox or influenza.[90] For that reason, nonaspirin NSAIDs are being used more frequently.

Although NSAIDs rarely cause gastrointestinal upset in children, the dose should always be given after eating. Tinnitus is a common side effect that is difficult to diagnose in a young child. Frequently, poor hearing is noted by the parents, or the child complains of a bug in his or her ear. Central nervous system effects are less common but can be seen with all the NSAIDs. These include hyperactivity, lethargy, headache, depression, and other personality changes. Some atopic children may have a bronchospastic reaction to NSAIDs. Prolonged bleeding time is an effect of all NSAIDs because of interference with platelet function. Bruising is the main consequence. For safety, however, aspirin should be discontinued 1 week before elective surgery. For the other NSAIDs, 2 days is sufficient. Spontaneous resolution of most untoward effects occurs quickly after the offending drug is stopped.

Nonsteroidal antiinflammatory drugs should be instituted in the early stages of joint inflammation. They do not cause all signs of inflammation to disappear when JRA is the underlying diagnosis. Therefore, if in 6 weeks all signs of arthritis are gone, it is most likely that the child had a reactive or viral arthritis, and medication should be discontinued.

In JRA, an NSAID is usually given for a minimum of 6 weeks before changing to a different NSAID for lack of effectiveness.[11] There is little to recommend one NSAID over another. Individual variation may result in better response to a different NSAID if one fails.[11,30] Medications with daily or twice-daily dosage schedules may increase compliance. Liquids are frequently more suitable for small children, in whom ease of swallowing and titration of dosage are important considerations.

Use of aspirin and the other NSAIDs in similar doses is generally effective in the spondyloarthropathies also. If these fail, especially in the management of severe back pain in children older than age 14 years, indomethacin in doses of 50 to 150 mg/day (2–3 mg/kg/day) is often helpful. Headaches, gastrointestinal irritation, and psychologic changes are common side effects.

Second-line drugs, or slow-acting remittive drugs (SARDs), are indicated when NSAIDs fail to control marked or prolonged synovitis.[13] They should be used as soon as indicated, which may be well before there is evidence of joint destruction. The least toxic of these drugs include sulfasalizine, hydroxychloroquine (an antimalarial), and auranofin (oral gold). Injectable gold (gold sodium thiomalate or aurothioglucose) and D-penicillamine are relatively more toxic and require more frequent laboratory monitoring. All SARDs require several months to evaluate their effectiveness in an individual child. Nonsteroidal antiinflammatory drugs may be used simultaneously because SARDs lack analgesic and antiinflammatory properties.

Third-line therapy consists of the cytotoxic agents,

TABLE 11-5 Nonsteroidal Antiinflammatory Drug Dosages

DRUG	DAILY DOSAGE Total (mg/kg)	Maximum (mg)
Aspirin	80–130	4500
Choline magnesium trisalicylate*‡	50	3000
Indomethacin,‡ indomethacin-SR*	2–3	200
Ibuprofen‡	40	3200
Tolmetin sodium	20–30	2000
Fenoprofen calcium	40	3200
Naproxen‡	10–20	1000
Sulindac*	4.5–6	400
Meclofenemate sodium	4.5–6	400
Piroxicam†	0.3–0.6	20

* Twice daily.
† Every day.
‡ Liquid.

with methotrexate the most widely used. About 70% of children respond to methotrexate.[91] The toxicity of other cytotoxic drugs that have been used for JRA limits their usefulness. Methotrexate does not cause sterility or malignancy.

Steroid drugs have multiple uses in the chronic inflammatory arthritides, although rarely as daily oral therapy because of the associated side effects.[13] Most children do well on doses as low as 2 to 7.5 mg/day. Severe systemic manifestations such as pericarditis may warrant high-dose therapy. Pulse intravenous steroid therapy can be less toxic while useful in treating systemic flares. Ophthalmologic steroids are frequently used along with mydriatics in controlling iritis.

Intraarticular Steroid Injections

Intraarticular steroid injections are useful for a child with a limited number of affected joints that have failed medical treatment, are inappropriate for surgical treatment, and are causing major disability. Synovial cysts, especially popliteal cysts, usually respond nicely to joint injection. Triamcinolone hexacetonide is used in large joints, whereas triamcinolone acetonide is used in medium and smaller joints. The former has more of a tendency to cause skin atrophy and hypopigmentation, although it has a longer-lasting effect. Up to 1 mg/kg is used. Repeat injections may be beneficial even if the first injection was not. If more than three injections per joint per year or if more than five or six total injections are required, more aggressive medical or surgical management is in order.

Physical and Occupational Therapy

Most children with chronic inflammatory arthritis require physical and occupational therapy. This therapy is aimed at improving and maintaining strength and range of motion while protecting joints. Children with arthritis can and should work hard to maintain their functional skills in everyday activities. Pain is less of an issue when medical therapy adequately controls the synovitis; however, some children unavoidably experience pain with their therapy program. It is paramount that they maintain as much function as possible because, with loss of function, loss of age-appropriate developmental skills inevitably follows. Therefore, therapy needs to include more than passive and active range of motion and progressive resistive exercises. Functional skills need to be monitored and appropriately acquired.

Nighttime splinting of the wrist and hand, knee, and ankle may decrease morning stiffness and help prevent flexion contractures. Serial casting of knees, ankles, wrists, fingers, and even elbows can restore mild loss of extension. This needs to be gentle to avoid iatrogenic fractures and physeal injuries.

Children with unequal leg lengths require shoe lifts, not only to improve gait but to decrease the tendency to develop a flexion contracture on the long (involved) side. Enthesitis at the metatarsal heads can be greatly relieved by redistributing the weight posteriorly with a shoe insert. Ice, heat, ultrasound, or a combination of these can be helpful in restoring motion and relieving pain in joints wherein muscle spasm is the main cause of disability.

Other Issues

School can present a problem for these children. Medication with a thrice-daily dosage schedule may have to be administered by a nurse or office personnel. This may draw unwanted attention to the child's arthritis. Those patients with gelling (i.e., excessive stiffness from prolonged immobilization) should be allowed to get up occasionally to keep their joints loose. A double set of books, one for school and one for home, is helpful to many patients. Rarely, a child needs an altered school day to allow time to work out marked morning stiffness. Home tutoring is almost never indicated.

Physical education and sports present a difficult problem. Most children do well when allowed to participate in the sport they desire. Many need to be allowed to pace themselves, especially for endurance-training activities. Extra attention to preactivity and postactivity stretching and sport-specific safety precautions need to be emphasized. A child's desires and disease activity, however, need to be balanced. There are no hard and fast rules, and we rarely restrict our patients after informing them of the risks involved. The risks relate to osteopenia, delayed reflexive protective mobility, and increased stress on already stressed joints.

Remission can be difficult to recognize in an individual child, especially when permanent joint damage has occurred. It is defined as absence of signs of inflammation, minimal to no joint tenderness, and morning stiffness not exceeding 15 minutes. Laboratory evidence of inflammation, such as the ESR and CBC measurements, should likewise be normal. Children on NSAIDs at the time of remission should be continued on their medication for about 6 months before discontinuation. When an SARD or third-line drug induces the remission, it should be continued, along with any NSAID, for a prolonged period. The exception is injectable gold, which can be progressively spaced out to every 2 to 3 weeks. Discontinuation of these medications is always a matter of trial and error. Children at risk for iritis require continued eye surveillance regardless of arthritic remission because these conditions are not concordant.

ORTHOPAEDIC SURGICAL TREATMENT

Although about 70% of children with JRA eventually enter long remissions without significant permanent joint damage, orthopaedic surgery can play an important role in maximizing the outcome for many. The orthopaedic surgeon should be a regular member of the health care team to help assure the use of effective procedures in both early and late stages of disease.

The chief disabilities addressed by orthopaedic surgery are the same ones that medical treatment and physical therapy try to prevent—namely, joint deformity, loss of movement, and pain. Problems related to asymmetric acceleration or deceleration of growth may also need surgical intervention. The chief surgical modalities are synovectomy, soft tissue release, osteotomy, arthroplasty, arthrodesis, and joint excision. Based on the known pathology of JRA, orthopaedic intervention can be divided into early and late treatment. Synovectomy and soft tissue releases are considered in the early stages, before significant joint destruction is evident. Once the joint is destroyed, osteotomy, joint replacement, excision, or fusion is considered. Angular osteotomy for asymmetric growth at a physis and epiphyseodesis for limb length discrepancy are other late-treatment modalities.

Special Considerations

Children with JRA bring to the orthopaedic surgeon a special set of problems that must be appreciated before proceeding with treatment. Hyperemia and disuse lead to osteoporosis, which is compounded when steroids have been used in the medical management.[13] These patients are fragile, and fractures have occurred with intentional and unintentional manipulation under anesthesia. With long-standing disease, cortical bone becomes eggshell thin, often permitting osteotomy with a scalpel, even in the major long bones. Additionally, screws and other orthopaedic hardware may have no hold on these bones.[3]

Hyperemia may lead to significant blood loss in surgical areas in which a tourniquet is impractical or impossible to use, such as the hip. Where a tourniquet is used, special care must be exercised to protect the delicate skin.

Children with JRA are small and their bones are small, especially when systemic steroid drugs have been used. This is of particular significance when considering total joint replacement. Standard components often do not fit.[20,22,48,54,77] Custom-made prostheses cannot be ordered part of the way through the procedure. Although bone stock might be better for prosthetic replacement in younger children, component sizing is an even greater problem, some growth potential may be lost, and subsequent revisions are moved up in time.

It is mandatory to have an anesthesiologist who is aware of the special problems of intubation and airway management in JRA.[3,77] Atlantoaxial instability makes intubation potentially hazardous. Children with seronegative JRA tend to have stiff necks secondary to spontaneous fusion of the posterior facets. This can lead to dangerous instability at the remaining mobile levels.[29,38] Failure of jaw development and stiffness of the temporomandibular joints may compound the problem. Preoperative clinical examination of the cervical spine and lateral flexion and extension radiographs are mandatory. Fiberoptic malleable laryngoscopes have made intubation less of a problem. Alternatively, intravenous ketamine hydrochloride can be used without intubation, although it may cause unpleasant dreams and cause increased bleeding due to its hypertensive action.

It is important to consider the activity of disease at the time of planned surgery because this certainly affects the outcome. It would perhaps seem desirable to perform surgery at a stable point during remission but this is not always possible. The present and potential future condition of adjacent joints must also be considered.

Finally, the success of the extensive and often painful rehabilitation program after surgery requires a fairly mature and cooperative patient. For that reason, age 6 years is considered the earliest age for procedures such as synovectomy.[28,45] Regardless of age, short-term rehabilitation in the hospital may be required.

Synovectomy

The role of synovectomy in JRA is controversial. In 1900, Mignon first reported a synovectomy in chronic arthritis but it was not until 1923 that Swett reported and analyzed a series of 15 synovectomies performed for "chronic infectious arthritis."[87] He reported marked pain relief, increase in joint motion, and no recurrences in his patients. The rationale for the procedure was to remove the diseased synovial tissue to slow down or stop the destructive process and allow regeneration of normal synovium. Studies, however, have clearly shown that the regenerated synovial tissue has many of the same pathologic features as the original tissue, although the amount of regenerated synovium is usually less.[31,43,53,58,65]

Since 1923, there have been many reports on synovectomy for rheumatoid arthritis in children and adults. The difficulty in analyzing the results of these studies is that the indications, timing, and evaluation criteria have been variable, the length of follow-up short, and only three studies used controls (in a disease with a generally good prognosis).[4,5,88] Despite these problems, most authors (except those conducting the controlled studies) have reported favorable short-term clinical results from synovectomy in JRA.[27,28,32,43,45,50,53,55] The most consistent improvements are in joint swelling and pain, whereas range of motion is generally unchanged or diminished. Results tend to be better in large joints than in small joints.[32] Recurrences are reported in all series. Synovectomy does not seem to stop radiographic deterioration of joints, except perhaps in pauciarticular disease, in which there may be less erosion after early synovectomy, but no difference in joint-space narrowing or osteoporosis.[43] Early synovectomy is the term used for surgery in joints with a good preoperative range of motion, minimal radiographic destruction, and little more than proliferative synovium seen at surgery.[45] Late synovectomy is the term used for surgery in joints not meeting these criteria. Surgical results for late synovectomy are not as good as for early synovectomy. A theoretic advantage of synovectomy is the decrease in local blood flow, which may decrease stimulation of adjacent growth plates.[53]

The best discussion and perspective on synovectomy is in the study by the Arthritis Foundation Committee on Evaluation of Synovectomy, sponsored by the ARA and the Arthritis Foundation.[4] This is an ongoing prospective, controlled, relatively long-term multicenter evaluation of synovectomy in adult rheumatoid arthritis. Their 5-year results found surgical synovectomy to have little long-term value in the general treatment of rheumatoid arthritis, in the prevention of recurrence of disease activity, or in the prevention of progressive articular damage. Although their results cannot legitimately and without qualification be applied to JRA, the discussion section in this chapter pertains equally well to both diseases and to the literature on both diseases.

From the foregoing, a set of relative indications and contraindications emerges. Because the results of synovectomy in JRA may not be as favorable as initially suggested, it is particularly important that the patient has an adequate trial of medical treatment first. An adequate trial for most patients includes 6 months of therapeutic NSAIDs and SARDs, along with adequate splinting, physical therapy, and intraarticular steroid injections. If this treatment fails, evidenced by persistent swelling, pain, difficulty controlling spasm, early loss of motion, and the development of contractures, a certain group of children may be considered for synovectomy. This group is generally older than age 6 years, with monoarticular or pauciarticular (and rarely polyarticular) JRA of large joints, without significant radiographic joint destruction, and with the ability to cooperate with a difficult rehabilitation program.

Pain is not always a significant finding in JRA, as it is in adult-onset disease. Synovectomy may also be indicated for children with persistent swelling from relatively painless synovitis if they also meet the other criteria. Anatomic constraints prevent complete synovectomy in most joints. Arthroscopic surgery may improve the ability to perform more complete synovectomy in certain large joints but the advantages of complete versus partial synovectomy in JRA have not been critically evaluated. Nevertheless, most authors recommend as complete a synovectomy as possible, whether an open or arthroscopic technique is used. For open synovectomy, this means more than one incision per joint. For arthroscopy, it means more than one portal. In both techniques, a pneumatic tourniquet is essential and early mobilization is critical.

An advantage of arthroscopic synovectomy is in reducing the morbidity of open synovectomy. Postoperative pain is significant after open procedures and requires a cooperative, mature patient to achieve the maximum outcome from the difficult rehabilitation program. Continuous passive motion after synovectomy in JRA would seem to be beneficial but there are no large controlled series addressing this issue.

Finally, range of motion does *not* improve after synovectomy. Therefore, other procedures must be considered, either simultaneously or sequentially, if loss of motion is significant. More important than the incision is the decision to perform synovectomy, with the limited goals fully appreciated by the surgeon, patient, and family.

Soft Tissue Release

Loss of joint motion in JRA can occur early or late (i.e., before or after radiographic changes are seen). Lower extremity joint contractures, with or without accompanying pain, can impair the child's ability to walk. The energy required to walk with a crouched gait may exceed the child's strength and endurance. The decreased arc of joint motion puts persistent and excessive nonphysiologic pressure on the articular cartilage surfaces, which are in direct contact, whereas the remainder of the articular cartilage loses its normal mechanisms of nourishment (motion and intermittent pressure). This leads to exacerbation of the joint destruction and fibrosis started by pannus. As noted previously, synovectomy does not improve motion in a joint that has become contracted by JRA. Other procedures, alone or in combination with synovectomy, must be performed to improve range of motion.

The goals of soft tissue release are to release contractures to put the joint in a more functional position, to increase range of motion to improve function and articular cartilage nourishment, and to relieve pain. Improved strength from reestablishing the child's activity level is an added benefit.

The literature on soft tissue release operations is

limited but encouraging.[2,3] In most cases, contracture and pain are relieved and range of motion is increased. Unexpectedly, radiographic appearance is often improved with widening of the articular space (Fig. 11-7). The assumption is that this represents healing by fibrocartilage as motion and nourishment are reestablished. It is believed that the release also acts to decompress the joint, thereby relieving vascular congestion. In cases wherein the disease undergoes lasting remission, later radical procedures are unnecessary. If the disease persists or recurs, the joint is in better alignment for subsequent prosthetic replacement.

Surgical release is appropriate for contractures of at least moderate severity that have failed to respond to conservative treatment. In most joints, except the hip, a prerequisite for soft tissue release is radiographic evidence of a good joint space. Releases at the hip and knee seem to be the most beneficial, although the technique has been used with some success in other joints. Postoperative aggressive physical therapy and splinting are important adjuncts to maximize the surgical outcome.

Osteotomy

When a young child presents with a painless, severe contracture in a nonfunctional position and with moderate to severe radiographic evidence of joint incongruity or subluxation, neither soft tissue release nor prosthetic replacement is appropriate. Periarticular extention osteotomy, especially at the knee, may be used in this situation to correct the overall extremity alignment without changing the intraarticular relations. Unfortunately, intertrochanteric hip osteotomy has not been successful because postoperative immobilization in a spica cast is unacceptable and internal fixation is not secure enough in these bones to obviate the cast.

Angular deformity at joints may occur due to epiphyseal compression fractures or to asymmetric growth of physes. There is no effective conservative treatment, and the mechanical stresses of weight bearing may perpetuate or increase the problem. Corrective osteotomy can be used also. Hemiepiphyseal stapling has been recommended by some authors but has the disadvantages of unpredictability and ugly scars.

Rotational deformities may also develop in the lower extremities of children with JRA.[2] Excessive femoral anteversion and lateral tibial torsion can exist separately or together for reasons that are not entirely clear. If they coexist as compensatory deformities, an acceptable foot-progression angle can be maintained without treatment. Patella problems may result when genu valgum is also present, however. Rotational deformity may also cause problems with prosthetic replacement at the knee. Rotational osteotomy can be helpful in these situations. It is rarely performed alone but is more commonly combined with angular osteotomy.

Arthrodesis

For isolated severe joint destruction in children with deformity and pain caused by other diseases (e.g., in-

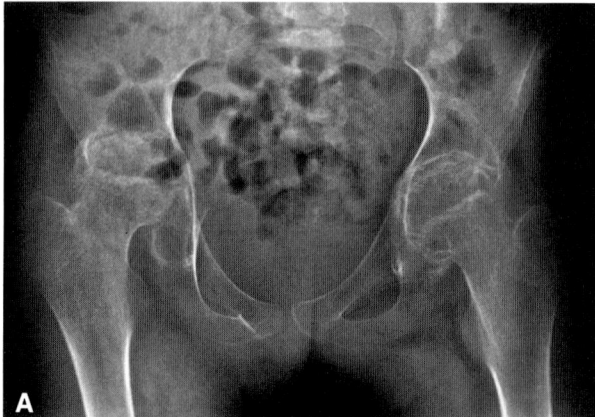
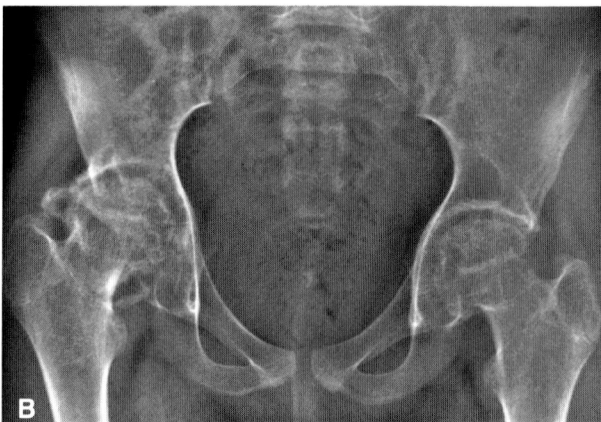
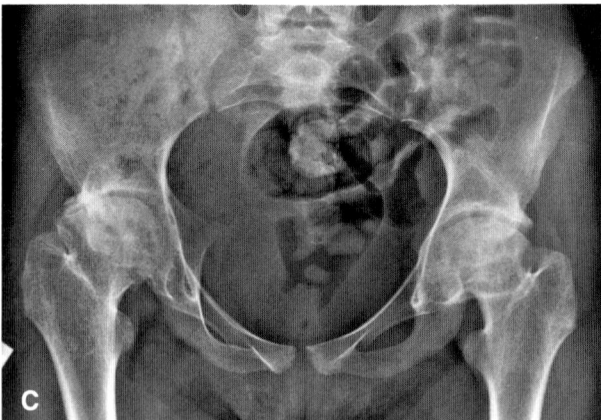

FIGURE 11-7. Polyarticular juvenile rheumatoid arthritis in a girl with bilateral hip ankylosis and pain. (**A**) At age 13 years, 8 months, there is marked joint space narrowing and protrusio acetabulum. The right side is worse than the left. (**B**) Age 14 years 6 months; 10 months after bilateral adductor and psoas tenotomies and right hip capsulectomy. Improved joint space, motion, and pain bilaterally. (**C**) Age 16 years 5 months. Improvements persist despite development of osteophytes.

fection) or trauma, arthrodesis is the treatment of choice. This is not appropriate for the hip or knee in JRA because it does not sufficiently relieve functional disability in the patient with multiple joint involvement. Arthrodesis puts added stress on adjacent joints and increases the risk of fracture by creating long, fragile, rigid lever arms.

Fusion of joints in JRA, therefore, has limited indications. The usual goal of treatment is maintenance or improvement of joint motion. Rare exceptions to this rule, when fusion may be indicated, are in painful, severe wrist or hindfoot destruction and with cervical instability, with pain and neurologic impairment.

Total Joint Arthroplasty

Despite optimal medical management, a small group of children with JRA develop severe hip and knee destruction, causing marked functional impairment or disabling pain. Pain in these end-stage joints is not always as significant a problem as is deformity. The resultant loss of ambulation ability and even transfer skills can be devastating. Therefore, TJA is recommended for these end-stage joints. Joints other than the hip and knee may be replaced but the indications are not as clear and the results have not been as critically analyzed.

Results of cup arthroplasty in patients with JRA have been poor and inconsistent. Surface arthroplasty is contraindicated because of severe osteoporosis, frequent avascular necrosis of the femoral head and neck, small acetabulum with protrusio, and torsional deformity of the proximal femur. Replacement therefore should be total. The issue of cemented versus uncemented is unsettled but cement was used in the reported series.

Because of the known problems and complications of joint replacement surgery generally and in young people in particular,[20] all earlier treatment is aimed at delaying or preventing the need for TJA. Medical treatment, physical therapy, serial casting, traction, synovectomy, soft tissue release, and osteotomy are all used when indicated. As noted previously, none of these treatment modalities cures JRA. They are all used to relieve pain and maintain function while the disease runs its course. In most cases they are successful. When they are not successful in eliminating the need for TJA, they can at least help relieve pain and maintain more functional joint position, muscle strength, and ambulation while delaying arthroplasty. Neither the number nor types of previous surgeries has been shown to adversely affect the outcome of TJA in these patients.[77]

The complications of total joint replacements, specifically loosening and infection, are well known to orthopaedic surgeons. In addition to those sobering facts, the special concerns for joint replacement in JRA are the age of the patient, growth remaining, size of the bones, other joint involvement, ability to use walking aids based on upper extremity involvement, and the great discrepancy between the life expectancy of the patient and the prosthesis.

The clinical results of total joint replacement in adult rheumatoid arthritis patients have been quite good despite radiographic evidence of loosening in some patients. This is presumably because of the decreased demands placed on these joints. Unfortunately, infection has been a greater than average problem in these patients.

With that information and with the important goals of improved function and pain relief and with no other options available, cautious and skilled arthroplasty surgeons have applied their expertise to these patients, with generally good short-term results.[17,20,22,48,54,77]

Age at time of replacement is a major issue because it relates directly to growth remaining, size and quality of the bone, size of the components, health of the periarticular soft tissues, and ability to cooperate with the rehabilitation program. The recommendation is to delay TJA until skeletal maturity if possible. This delay must be weighed against the adverse effects on bones, soft tissues, and motivation that prolonged non–weight bearing and severe ankylosis can create. The surgical procedure is also made more difficult by waiting too long. Even with waiting, as many as 50% of cases require custom-made prosthetic components.[22,54,77] Careful preoperative planning with measured radiographs is mandatory.

When ipsilateral hip and knee replacement are indicated, the hip is operated on first. If all four joints need replacement, both hips are treated before the knees.[77] There are several reasons for this. It is possible to rehabilitate a hip joint in the presence of a flexed, contracted knee joint but not the reverse. During hip surgery, a contracted knee can be manipulated or casted to gain some extension in anticipation of later surgery on that joint. Although hip pain is relieved by the procedure at that joint, the component of knee pain that is referred from the hip is also relieved.

For the specifics of surgical techniques, the references by Carmichael and Chaplin, Chandler and colleagues, Colville and Raunio, Lachiewicz and associates, Mogensen and colleagues, and Scott and associates are recommended.[17,20,22,48,54,77]

It will be many more years before we know the long-term results and problems of TJA in JRA but the early results and the advances in the technology and biology of TJA are encouraging.

Epiphyseodesis

For leg length discrepancies in monarticular and pauciarticular JRA, the predicted discrepancy at maturity can be determined using the Green-Anderson data and the Moseley straight line graph once a stable growth pattern has been established.[56] Appropriately timed Phemister-type epiphyseodesis can then be performed if the predicted discrepancy at maturity is more than 2 cm.[64]

JOINT-SPECIFIC ORTHOPAEDIC TREATMENT

Hip

Hip involvement is uncommon in pauciarticular disease but is a major cause of late disability in systemic-onset and polyarticular JRA. Flexion contracture develops early in the course of disease, followed later by internal rotation and adduction deformity. Children with the onset of hip involvement after age 10 years usually follow the adult pattern of fibrous ankylosis and loss of joint space, with progression to protrusio acetabulum and osteophytosis (see Fig. 11-7A). In younger children with hip involvement, the inflammatory process accelerates arrest of growth cartilage in the acetabulum and the femoral head. Premature fusion of the triradiate cartilage creates acetabular dysplasia. Circumferential undergrowth of the femoral head can occur. Coxa breva, coxa valga, or coxa vara may be seen, depending on the pattern of growth arrest in the capital femoral physis. Hip subluxation results from a combination of these effects (Fig. 11-8).[41,44]

Soft tissue release is indicated in young patients who develop fixed hip flexion contractures despite adequate medical treatment, physical therapy, hydrotherapy, prone lying, and intraarticular steroids, regardless of the radiographic appearance of the joint. Limited open adductor and psoas tenotomy followed by immediate physical therapy and mobilization have been shown to reduce flexion contracture, increase range of motion, relieve pain, and improve the radiologic appearance of the joint. Arthroscopy has been recommended by some authors as a diagnostic tool to identify candidates for synovectomy.[40] These are the same authors who believe that synovectomy has a role in the management of hip disease in JRA.[55] Their critics believe that the beneficial effects of hip synovectomy are actually due to the mandatory soft tissue release that accompanies the procedure.[2,3] Intertrochanteric osteotomy does not play a role in these patients because it tends to increase stiffness. The internal fixation is rarely secure enough to obviate the need for spica immobilization. Long immobilization and non–weight bearing are devastating to the child's motivation, bone stock, and muscle strength.

With care and attention, most hips can make it

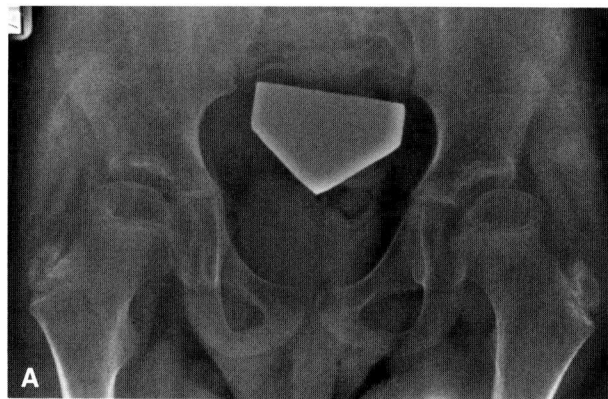
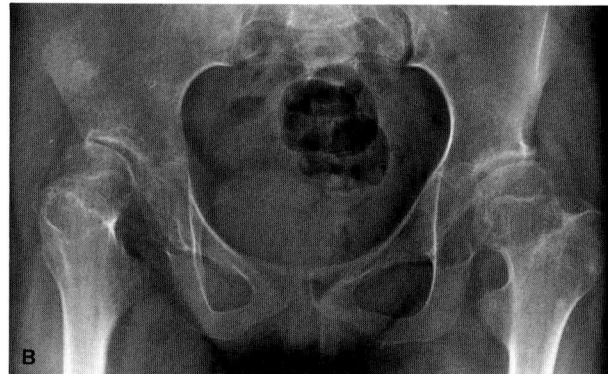

FIGURE 11-8. Progressive hip subluxation in polyarticular juvenile rheumatoid arthritis. (**A**) At age 9 years, there is early subluxation, acetabular dysplasia, and osteopenia. (**B**) At age 15 years, there is marked subluxation, acetabular dysplasia, and osteopenia; marginal joint space narrowing; and coxa breva caused by early physeal closure.

through without need for arthroplasty but when severe functional disability with deformity or pain occur, TJA is indicated. Because it is most common for such severe hip disease to be found in patients with multiple joint involvement, arthrodesis is not a consideration. Ideally, TJA should be performed at or after skeletal maturity. The special considerations have been discussed previously. The orthopaedist can expect good short-term clinical results with careful preoperative planning and meticulous attention to detail but the long-term results are unknown.

Knee

The knee is one of the most frequently involved joints in JRA. Pain and swelling lead to flexion contracture and restricted range of motion, sometimes with valgus deformity and often with posterior subluxation of the tibia. Intraarticular destruction occurs at variable rates and to different degrees. In unilateral disease with onset younger than age 9 years, overgrowth of the adjacent physes occurs. With older onset of unilateral disease, early growth arrest may be anticipated.

As the middle of the three joints in the lower extremity, the knee must be considered in relation to the hip and ankle/foot. When planning correction of a flexed, valgus knee, the orthopaedic surgeon must consider the effect that it would have on the flexed, adducted, internally rotated hip and the externally rotated tibia and varus foot.

Unlike the hip joint, the knee is accessible. Intraarticular steroid injections can often help control swelling and pain in an isolated joint that has failed medical management. Physical therapy, positioning, and splinting should be used early to prevent or treat mild flexion deformities of up to 15 degrees. For contractures of 15 to 25 degrees with no posterior subluxation, serial casting can be carried out. This should be performed with great care and without undue force, which might otherwise cause anterior compression of the tibial plateau and femoral condyles or posterior subluxation of the tibia (Fig. 11-9). Walking should continue during this treatment. If early subluxation is already present with the mild flexion contracture, traction can be employed as described by Bianco and Peterson.[9] For this, the patient is in the 90-degree/90-degree position, with a proximal tibial pin pulled vertically and skin traction on the leg pulled horizontally. The extremity is gradually extended as joint reduction occurs. Return to regular activities should be as rapid as possible.

As discussed at some length previously in the section by the same name, synovectomy has a limited role in JRA. It may be useful to control persistent swelling and pain in children with pauciarticular disease who do not have significant radiographic joint destruction, who are older than age 6 years and who have failed an intensive 6-month trial of medical treatment. Synovectomy cannot be expected to increase range of motion.

Soft tissue release has a definite role in knee flexion contractures greater than 25 degrees at the outset or in smaller contractures with subluxation that have not responded to other measures. A prerequisite is that a good joint space is preserved radiographically. Posteromedial and posterolateral incisions are used to lengthen the hamstring muscles, release the origins of the gastrocnemius muscle, and divide the iliotibial band and posterior joint capsule. If posterior subluxation is present, the posterior cruciate ligament is also divided. Three weeks of casting with early postoperative weight bearing is used when pure flexion deformity is corrected. The casts may be changed during that interval to gradually gain more extension than the neurovascular bundle originally allowed. If subluxation is also corrected, traction is used postoperatively. Intensive physical therapy and prolonged nighttime splinting are essential to maintain correction.

If fixed knee flexion in a skeletally immature patient is associated with joint incongruity, irregularity, or significant subluxation, supracondylar extension osteotomy is indicated. In a patient with good bone density, an anteriorly based wedge of bone can be removed and the fragments internally fixed after usual orthopaedic principles. In patients with significant osteopenia, a short medial incision is made just proximal to the growth plate. A hand-held osteotome is pushed

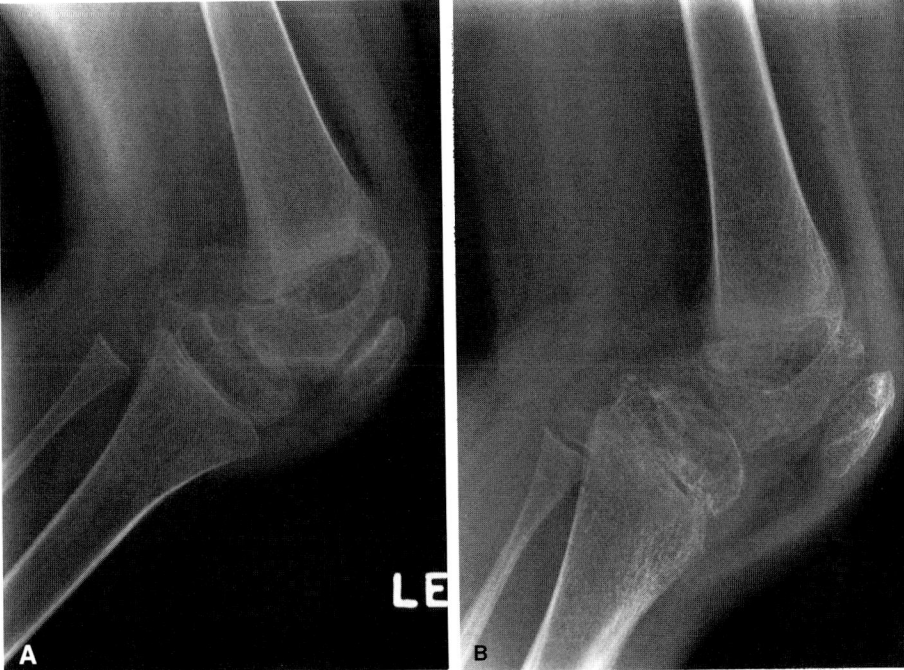

FIGURE 11-9. Eight-year-old boy with polyarticular juvenile rheumatoid arthritis. (**A**) Knee ankylosis and flexion contracture, with mild posterior subluxation of tibia. (**B**) Anterior compression of proximal tibia, caused by serial casting, attempts to forcibly extend the knee.

through the bone, leaving a posterior osteoperiosteal hinge. If significant valgus is also present, a small posterolateral hinge is left instead.

The deformity is corrected by impaction of fragments, and a straight leg cast is applied. Early weight bearing is enforced and immobilization is kept to a minimum. When the cast is removed, aggressive but controlled range of motion and strengthening exercises are instituted.

Valgus deformity may occur as an isolated deformity or in association with flexion or rotation. Preoperative standing radiographs are obtained to assess the weight bearing mechanical axis and the degree of instability. The goal is a straight leg with a horizontal joint line during standing. Supracondylar osteotomy is usually the ideal site to correct the deformity or deformities with the least risk. Occasionally, proximal tibial osteotomy is more appropriate for the deformity but the added neurovascular risk of osteotomy at this level must be carefully considered (Fig. 11-10). Postoperative management is as described above.

For end-stage destructive arthritis of the knee in a child at or near skeletal maturity and in whom deformity or pain cause significant functional impairment, TJA is recommended. The special considerations have previously been discussed in this chapter. Soft tissue

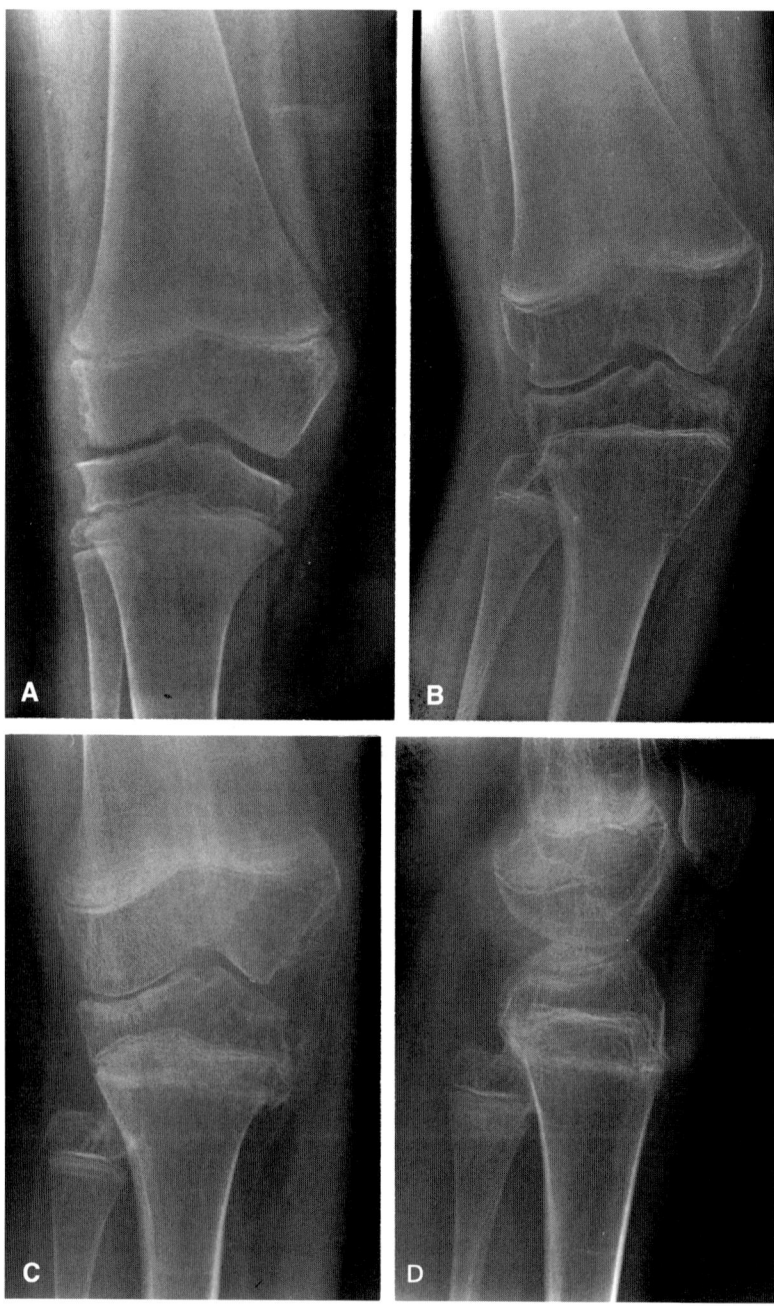

FIGURE 11-10. Genu valgum in polyarticular juvenile rheumatoid arthritis. (**A**) At age 9 years, there is osteopenia and marginal epiphyseal erosions. Good axial alignment is seen on standing radiograph. (**B**) At age 15 years, marked valgus caused by asymmetric growth of proximal tibial physis is seen in a standing radiograph. (**C** and **D**) Six weeks after varus, impaction osteotomy of proximal tibia.

release and osteotomy should be used early in the course of the disease in an attempt to maintain the best position and motion in anticipation of later TJA.

Finally, the surgical management of leg length discrepancy by epiphyseodesis at the knee is the same in JRA as in other conditions. The changing rate of growth and the expected growth pattern must, however, be taken into consideration in preoperative planning.

Foot And Ankle

The foot and ankle are frequently involved in JRA, although surgery is infrequently necessary. Many of the problems are managed by special shoe wear, orthotics, or braces to accommodate the deformity and relieve pain. Prevention of deformity when possible by splinting and exercising is important at this anatomic area, as it is elsewhere. The goal is a plantigrade, mobile, and painless foot.[2]

Involvement of the ankle or subtalar joint is frequently seen in patients with pauciarticular disease. In polyarticular JRA, simultaneous involvement of both of these joints and the remainder of the foot is common. The ankle contracts in equinus. The subtalar joint may develop a varus or valgus deformity. In the early stages of deformity, if conservative treatment is not effective, manipulation under anesthesia and casting in a plantigrade position often relieves pain and corrects deformity. A walking cast is used for 4 weeks, followed by night splinting. If deformity or pain quickly recur, the procedure is repeated but then followed by a daytime orthosis. Only rarely is hindfoot arthrodesis performed because of the stress it puts on the other joints of the foot and the ankle. Corrective osteotomies are preferred over arthrodeses to achieve a plantigrade position in a stiff foot. Occasionally, however, spontaneous fusions of the tarsals occur (Fig. 11-11).

Claw toes, hallux valgus, and metatarsalgia are common forefoot problems in JRA, as they are in the adult disease. The inflammatory process in the metatarsophalangeal joints causes the proximal phalanges to subluxate dorsally and the interphalangeal joints to claw. The metatarsal heads are pushed down, thereby leading to the development of painful plantar callouses. Soft prefabricated arch supports or metatarsal bars may be used initially. Soft tissue surgical procedures are performed before significant joint destruction occurs. The role of synovectomy is unclear.[32] Resection of the metatarsal heads is reserved for painful deformity with severe joint destruction. The treatment of hallux valgus should be individualized but basically reduces to a choice between osteotomy or excision.

Soft accommodative shoeware is vital both before and after surgery. For severe deformity and pain, extradepth shoes with molded polyethylene closed-cell foam liners can improve the quality of life for these patients.

Cervical Spine

The cervical spine is frequently involved in polyarticular and systemic-onset JRA. The exact incidence is unknown but may approach 60%.[29,38] The cervical

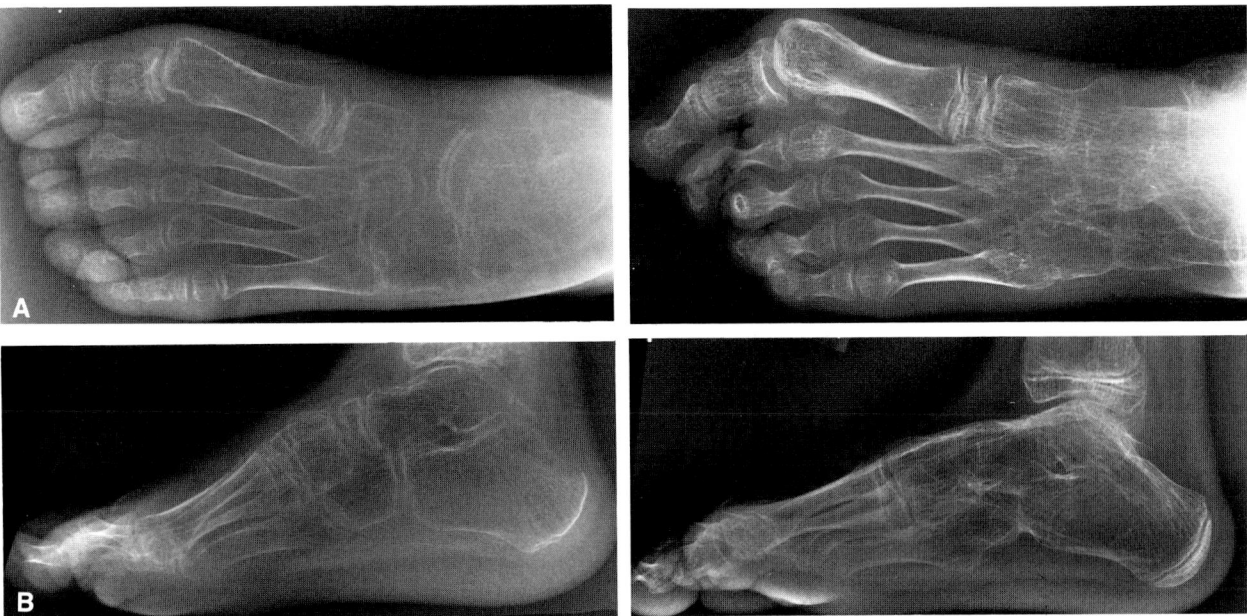

FIGURE 11-11. Polyarticular juvenile rheumatoid arthritis in a girl with foot involvement. (A) At age 8 years, there is osteopenia and joint space narrowing. (B) At age 13 years, there is spontaneous tarsal and tarsometatarsal fusions.

spine is rarely involved in pauciarticular disease. Stiffness is the most common early finding. Pain and torticollis are rare findings early but can occur later. Radiographic abnormalities include atlantoaxial destruction and instability, which is more common in seropositive or polyarticular disease, and posterior facet fusions, which are more common in seronegative or systemic-onset disease. Neurologic involvement is less commonly seen than in adult rheumatoid arthritis, probably because basilar invagination is so rare in JRA.[38] This means that the same amount of atlantoaxial instability causes less spinal cord impingement. Nevertheless, the potential risk of documented instability is hard to ignore. Not only may instability exist without neurologic symptoms but it may exist without pain. All children with JRA should have flexion and extension lateral radiographs of the cervical spine and these should be repeated before anesthetics. There is no consensus on the amount of instability which mandates C1–C2 fusion in the asymptomatic child. Activity restriction is difficult in children, even in those with JRA, and soft cervical collars do not immobilize the atlantoaxial joint. All agree that posterior C1–C2 fusion is indicated for instability with progressive neurologic signs.[29,38]

There is no way to prevent posterior facet fusions and there is little neurologic risk associated but controlling the position of fusion may be beneficial. To this end, well-molded collars have been used with some success. Neurologic risk is small but theoretically possible because the nonfused segments are subjected to more than their usual stresses, and instability can occur.

Hand And Wrist

Stiffness and deformity are the hallmarks of JRA involving the hand and wrist. Pain and instability are less frequently seen than in adults with rheumatoid arthritis.[21,33] The wrist assumes a position of flexion and ulnar deviation, whereas the metacarpophalangeal and interphalangeal joints lose flexion without developing ulnar drift. Synovial joints and synovial tendon sheaths are so prevalent that most patients experience some involvement in this area in the course of their disease. Occupational therapy and splinting can perhaps make their greatest contribution to the management of JRA at these joints. Surgical procedures are rarely indicated.[2,21,33]

Despite sometimes extensive tenosynovitis, tendon rupture is uncommon. Swelling, with restriction of movement, followed by resolution with adhesions is common. Functional splinting at night and occasionally during the day, along with gentle active and passive exercises can help maintain joint position and motion. When flexor tenosynovitis persists, intrathecal injection of steroids can be helpful. Synovectomy during the acute synovitic phase leads to adhesions and stiffness and should be avoided. Later persistent thickening from proliferative synovitis in one or two flexor tendon sheaths may be an indication for synovectomy.[2]

The wrist develops a flexion deformity early in the course of disease. Subluxation of the distal ulna and carpal collapse are seen radiographically (Fig. 11-12).[2,21,33] Spontaneous carpal fusion may occur (Fig. 11-13). Splinting of the wrist in a functional position may obviate the need for surgical procedures. When intractable pain or deformity exist, manipulation under anesthesia and immobilization can be tried, with the hope of achieving a painless ankylosis in a functional position. The other choices are formal arthrodesis or arthroplasty, best performed after skeletal maturity. The former is preferred if there is adequate motion in the ipsilateral elbow and shoulder. Wrist arthroplasty in JRA is still a new technique, without long-term follow-up.

The successful management of JRA involvement of the finger joints also depends on aggressive nonoperative techniques. Synovectomy may have a role in the early treatment of metacarpophalangeal joints that have failed medical treatment. With similar indications, however, results have not even equalled the marginal results achieved in the knee.[4,5,32,88] Additionally,

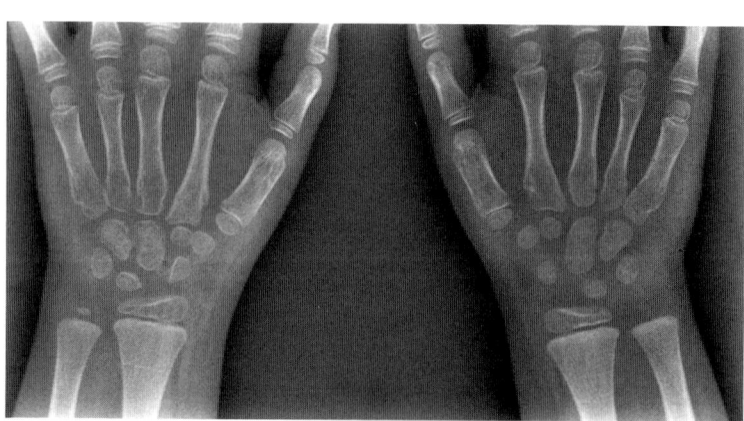

FIGURE 11-12. A 5-year-old girl with systemic-onset juvenile rheumatoid arthritis shows early decreased carpal height of the left wrist.

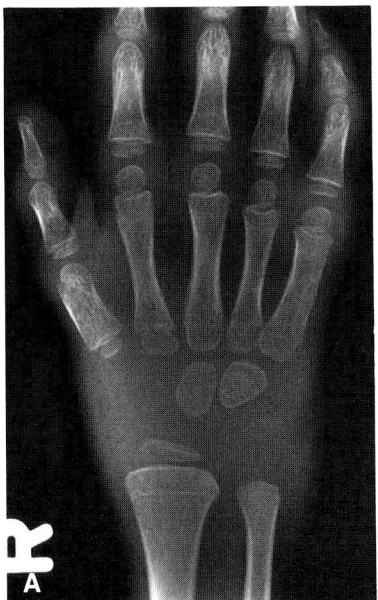 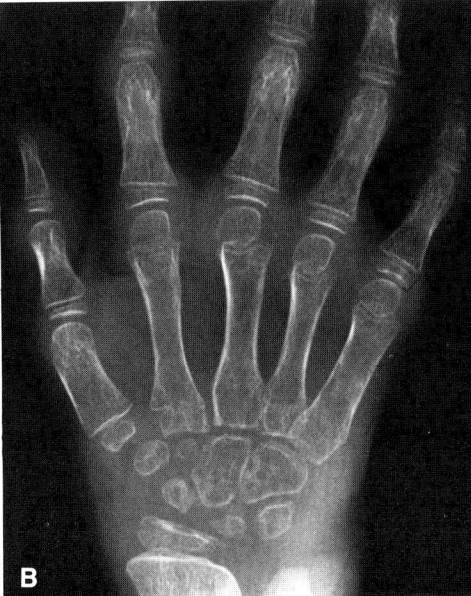 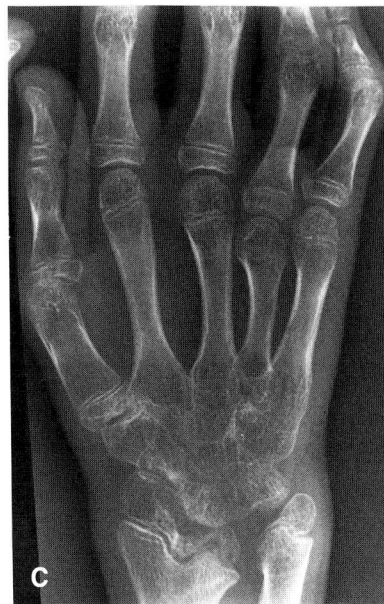

FIGURE 11-13. Polyarticular juvenile rheumatoid arthritis in a girl with wrist involvement. (**A**) At age 4 years, there is fusiform swelling and osteopenia of wrist. (**B**) At age 6 years, there is carpal erosion and collapse, with ulnar drift. (**C**) At age 13 years, spotaneous carpal and carpometacarpal fusions, with subluxation of distal ulna.

the good results may be due to the concurrent soft tissue release.[32] Synovectomy of the interphalangeal joints is not indicated. Soft tissue release of metacarphophalangeal and interphalangeal joints can be used to improve position and relieve pain. Total joint arthroplasty of the fingers is technically demanding for the same reasons noted in other joints, and the prognosis for the prostheses is unknown.

Elbow

Although not frequently involved, JRA of the elbow can lead to disability, with pain, swelling, stiffness, and locking, as in the other synovial joints. There may be instability, overgrowth and subluxation of the radial head, or erosion and obliteration of the joint. The status of the ipsilateral shoulder and wrist are important considerations in the management of the elbow.

Intraarticular steroids and manipulation are used in early disease to relieve pain and improve position and motion. Synovectomy performed early or late can be rewarding in terms of pain relief.[2] Improvement in motion is not as predictable. Resection of a deformed and subluxated radial head that is restricting movement in a skeletally mature patient can sometimes be beneficial. Arthrodesis is disabling and should be avoided.[2] Arthroplasty may be appropriate for the older adolescent if deformity is marked and function is severely impaired. Little has been written on elbow arthroplasty in JRA.

Shoulder

Shoulder involvement in JRA is rarely disabling. All the same principles of conservative early management apply to this joint.[2] The status of the ipsilateral elbow and wrist are important. Subacromial steroids can relieve pain early in the disease. Manipulation and casting in a functional position to achieve painless ankylosis has met with good results. Total joint arthroplasty is an option for the skeletally mature patient with severe joint destruction, pain, and poor joint position. As with all arthroplasties in JRA, the early benefits may be great but the technical difficulties may be greater and the long-term sequelae are unknown.

ORTHOPAEDIC SURGERY IN SERONEGATIVE SPONDYLOARTHROPATHIES

As the prototype disease in this group of disorders, ankylosing spondylitis rarely requires orthopaedic surgical intervention during childhood.[59,62,71,82] The arthralgia is usually transient and nondestructive. Disability comes from spinal ankylosis in flexion. This can be prevented by a regular program of postural and extension exercises, sleeping on a firm mattress prone or supine without a pillow, and occasionally by the use of a brace. Adults with severe flexion deformity can benefit from extension osteotomy of the spine, which, as it sounds, is a formidable procedure.[51] Fracture of the rigid unsegmented spine may occur, with or without accompanying neurologic injury and may require surgical stabilization.

References

1. Ansell BM. Juvenile chronic polyarthritis. ser. 3. Arthritis Rheum 1977;20(Suppl):176.
2. Ansell BM, Swann M. Juvenile chronic arthritis. In: Harris NH, ed. Postgraduate textbook of clinical orthopedics. Bristol: Wright-PSG, 1983.
3. Ansell BM, Swann M. The management of chronic arthritis of children. J Bone Joint Surg [Br] 1983;65:536.
4. Arthritis Foundation Committee on Evaluation of Synovectomy. Multicenter Evaluation of Synovectomy in the Treatment of Rheumatoid Arthritis. Report of results at the end of five years. J Rheumatol 1988;15:764.
5. Arthritis and Rheumatism Council and British Orthopaedic Association. Controlled trial of synovectomy of knee and mcp joints in rheumatoid arthritis. Ann Rheum Dis 1976;35:437.
6. Beckingsale AB, Davies J, Gibson JM, et al. Acute anterior uveitis, ankylosing spondylitis, back pain, and HLA-B27. Br J Ophthalmol 1984;68:741.
7. Bennet PH, Wood PHN. Population studies of the rheumatic diseases. New York: Excerpta Medica, 1968:456.
8. Bernstein BH, Singsen BH, Kent JT, et al. Reflex neurovascular dystrophy in childhood. J Pediatr 1978;93:211.
9. Bianco AJ Jr, Peterson HA. Juvenile rheumatoid arthritis. Orthop Clin North Am 1971;2:745.
10. Biro F, Gewanter HL, Baum J. The hypermobility syndrome. Pediatrics 1983;72:701.
11. Brewer EJ, Arroys I. Use of nonsteroidal antiinflammatory drugs in children. Pediatr Ann 1986;15:575.
12. Brewer EJ, Bass J, Baum J, et al. Current proposed revision of JRA criteria. Arthritis Rheum 1977;20(Suppl):195.
13. Brewer EJ, Giannini EH, Person DA. Juvenile rheumatoid arthritis. Philadelphia: WB Saunders, 1982.
14. Bullough PG, Vigorita VJ. Atlas of orthopaedic pathology with clinical and radiologic correlations. New York: Gower Medical Publishing, 1984:6.14.
15. Calabro JJ, Holgerson WB, Sonpal GM, et al. Juvenile rheumatoid arthritis. A general review and report of 100 patients observed for 15 years. Semin Arthritis Rheum 1976;5:257.
16. Calabro JJ, Marchesano JM. Rash associated with juvenile rheumatoid arthritis. J Pediatr 1968;72:611.
17. Carmichael E, Chaplin DM. Total knee arthroplasty in juvenile rheumatoid arthritis. Clin Orthop 1986;210:192.
18. Cassidy JT, Nelson AM. The frequency of juvenile arthritis. J Rheumatol 1988;15:535.
19. Cassidy JT, Sullivan DB, Petty RE. Clinical patterns of chronic iridocyclitis in children with juvenile rheumatoid arthritis. Arthritis Rheum 1977;20(Suppl):224.
20. Chandler HP, Reineck FT, Wixson RL, et al. Total hip replacement in patients younger than thirty years old. J Bone Joint Surg [Am] 1981;63:1426.
21. Chaplin D, Pulkki T, Saarimaa A, et al. Wrist and finger deformities in juvenile rheumatoid arthritis. Acta Rheumatol Scand 1969;15:206.
22. Colville J, Raunio P. Total hip replacement in juvenile rheumatoid arthritis. Acta Orthop Scand 1979;50:197.
23. Conway JJ. Radionuclide bone scintigraphy in pediatric orthopedics. Pediatr Clin North Am 1986;33:1313.
24. Docken WP. Pigmented villonodular synovitis: a review with illustrative cases. Semin Arthritis Rheum 1979;9:1.
25. Emery H. Clinical aspects of systemic lupus erythematosis in childhood. Pediatr Clin North Am 1986;33:1177.
26. Emery H. Henoch-Schonlein purpura. In: Hicks RV, ed. Vasculopathies of childhood. Littleton, MA: PSG, 1988.
27. Eyring EJ, Longert A, Bass J. Synovectomy in juvenile rheumatoid arthritis. J Bone Joint Surg [Am] 1971;53:638.
28. Fink CW, Baum J, Paradies LH, et al. Synovectomy in juvenile rheumatoid arthritis. Ann Rheum Dis 1969;28:612.
29. Fried JA, Athreya B, Gregg JR, et al. The cervical spine in juvenile rheumatoid arthritis. Clin Orthop 1983;179:102.
30. Furst DE. Are there differences among nonsteroidal antiinflammatory drugs? Arthritis Rheum 1994;37:1.
31. Goldie I. Pathomorphologic features in original and regenerated synovial tissues after synovectomy in rheumatoid arthritis. Clin Orthop 1971;77:295.
32. Granberry WM, Brewer EJ Jr. Results of synovectomy in children with rheumatoid arthritis. Clin Orthop 1974;101:120.
33. Granberry WM, Magnum GL. The hand in the child with juvenile rheumatoid arthritis. J Hand Surg 1980;5:105.
34. Hanson V. From Still's disease and JRA to JCPA, JCA, and JA: medical progress or biased ascertainment? J Rheumatol 1982;9:819.
35. Hanson V, Kornreich HK, Bernstein B, et al. Prognosis of juvenile rheumatoid arthritis. Arthritis Rheum 1977;20(Suppl):279.
36. Hanson V, Kornreich HK, Bernstein B, et al. Three subtypes of juvenile rheumatoid arthritis (correlations of age at onset, sex, and serologic factors). Arthritis Rheum 1977;20(Suppl):184.
37. Haueisen DC, Weiner DS, Weiner SD. The characterization of ''transient synovitis of the hip'' in children. J Pediatr Orthop 1986;6:11.
38. Hensinger RN, DeVito PD, Ragsdale CG. Changes in the cervical spine in juvenile rheumatoid arthritis. J Bone Joint Surg [Am] 1986;68A:189.
39. Hill RH, Herstein A, Walters K. Juvenile rheumatoid arthritis: follow-up into adulthood-medical, sexual, and social status. Can Med Assoc J 1976;76:790.
40. Holgersson S, Brattstrom H, Mogensen B, Lidgren L. Arthroscopy of the hip in juvenile chronic arthritis. J Pediatr Orthop 1981;1:273.
41. Isdale IC. Hip disease in juvenile rheumatoid arthritis. Ann Rheum Dis 1970;29:603.
42. Jackson MA, Nelson JD. Etiology and medical management of acute suppurative bone and joint infections in pediatric patients. J Pediatr Orthop 1982;2:313.
43. Jacobsen ST, Levinson JE, Crawford AH. Late results of synovectomy in juvenile rheumatoid arthritis. J Bone Joint Surg [Am] 1985;67:8.
44. Jacqueline F, Buojot A, Canet L. Involvement of the hips in juvenile rheumatoid arthritis. Arthritis Rheum 1961;4:500.
45. Kampner SL, Ferguson AB Jr. Efficacy of synovectomy in juvenile rheumatoid arthritis. Clin Orthop 1972;88:94.
46. Keat A. Reiter's syndrome and reactive arthritis in perspective. N Engl J Med 1983;309:1606.
47. Kushner I. C-reactive protein in rheumatology. Arthritis Rheum 1991;34:1065.
48. Lachiewicz PF, McCaskill B, Inglis A, et al. Total hip arthroplasty in juvenile rheumatoid arthritis-two to eleven-year results. J Bone Joint Surg [Am] 1986;68:502.
49. Lang BA, Shore A. A review of current concepts on the pathogenesis of juvenile rheumatoid arthritis. J Rheumatol 1990;17(Suppl 21):1.
50. Larsen EH, Reiman I, Revig O. Synovectomy in infantile arthritis. Proceedings of the British Orthopaedic Association. J Bone Joint Surg [Br] 1968;50:221.
51. Law WA. Ankylosing spondylitis and spinal osteotomy. Proc Royal Soc Med 1976;69:715.

52. Lindsley C, Schaller JG. Arthritis associated with inflammatory bowel disease in children. J Pediatr 1974;84:16.
53. McMaster M. Synovectomy of the knee in juvenile rheumatoid arthritis. J Bone Joint Surg [Br] 1972;54:263.
54. Mogensen B, Brattstrom H, Ekelund L, et al. Total hip replacement in juvenile chronic arthritis. Acta Orthop Scand 1983;54:422.
55. Mogensen B, Brattstrom H, Ekelund L, et al. Synovectomy of the hip in juvenile chronic arthritis. J Bone Joint Surg [Br] 1982;64:295.
56. Moseley CF. A straight line graph for leg length discrepancies. J Bone Joint Surg [Am] 1977;59:174.
57. Pattishall EN, Strope GL, Spinola SM, et al. Childhood sarcoidosis. J Pediatr 1986;108:169.
58. Patzakis MJ, Mills DM, Bartholomew BA, et al. A visual, histological, and enzymatic study of regenerating rheumatoid synovium in the synovectomized knee. J Bone Joint Surg [Am] 1973;55:287.
59. Petty RE. Spondyloarthropathies. In: Cassidy JT, ed. Textbook of pediatric rheumatology. New York: John Wiley & Sons, 1982:283.
60. Petty RE, Cassidy JT, Sullivan DB. Clinical correlates of antinuclear antibodies in juvenile rheumatoid arthritis. J Pediatr 1973;83:386.
61. Petty RE, Hunt DWC, Rosenberg AM. Antibodies to type iv collagen in rheumatic diseases. J Rheumatol 1986;13:246.
62. Petty RE, Malleson P. Spondyloarthropathies of childhood. Pediatr Clin North Am 1986;33:1079.
63. Petty RE, Tingle AJ. Arthritis and viral infection. J Pediatr 1988;113:948.
64. Phemister DB. Operative arrestment of longitudinal growth of bones in the treatment of deformities. J Bone Joint Surg 1933;15:1.
65. Ranawat CS, Straub LR, Freyberg R, et al. A study of regenerated synovium after synovectomy of the knee in rheumatoid arthritis. Arthritis Rheum 1971;14:117.
66. Reid GD, Patterson MWH, Patterson AC, et al. Aortic insufficiency in association with juvenile ankylosing spondylitis. J Pediatr 1979;95:78.
67. Rennebohm R, Correll JK. Comprehensive management of juvenile rheumatoid arthritis. Nurs Clin North Am 1984;19:647.
68. Rosenberg AM. Uveitis associated with juvenile rheumatoid arthritis. Semin Arthritis Rheum 1987;16:158.
69. Rosenberg AM, Petty RE. A syndrome of seronegative enthesopathy and arthropathy in children. Arthritis Rheum 1982;25:1041.
70. Schaller JG. Chronic arthritis in children-juvenile rheumatoid arthritis. Clin Orthop 1984;182:79.
71. Schaller JG. The seronegative spondyloarthropathies of childhood. Clin Orthop 1979;143:76.
72. Schaller JG. Juvenile rheumatoid arthritis. Series 1. Arthritis Rheum 1977;20(Suppl):165.
73. Schaller JG. Arthritis as a presenting manifestation of malignancy in children. J Pediatr 1972;81:793.
74. Schaller JG, Johnson GD, Holborow EJ, et al. The association of antinuclear antibodies with the chronic iridocyclitis of juvenile rheumatoid arthritis (Still's disease). Arthritis Rheum 1974;17:409.
75. Schaller JG, Ochs HD, Thomas ED, et al. Histocompatibility antigens in childhood-onset arthritis. J Pediatr 1976;88:926.
76. Schlosstein L, Terasaki PI, Bluestone R, et al. High association of the HLA antigen W27 with ankylosing spondylitis. N Engl J Med 1973;288:704.
77. Scott RD, Sarokhan AJ, Dalziel R. Total hip arthroplasty in juvenile rheumatoid arthritis. Clin Orthop 1984;182:90.
78. Section on Rheumatology and Section of Ophthalmology, American Academy of Pediatrics. Guidelines for ophthalmologic examination in children with juvenile rheumatoid arthritis. Pediatrics 1993;92:295.
79. Sherry DD, Mellins ED, Nepom BS. Pauciarticular-onset juvenile chronic (rheumatoid) arthritis. In: Maddison PJ, Isenberg DA, Woo P, Glass DN, eds. Oxford textbook of rheumatology. Oxford: Oxford University Press, 1993:711.
80. Shore A, Ansell BM. Juvenile psoriatic arthritis—an analysis of 60 cases. J Pediatr 1982;100:529.
81. Simon S, Whiffen J, Shapiro F. Leg-length discrepancies in monarticular and pauciarticular juvenile rheumatoid arthritis. J Bone Joint Surg [Am] 1981;63:209.
82. Smythe H. Therapy of the spondyloarthropathies. Clin Orthop 1979;143:84.
83. Steere AC, Schoen RT, Taylor E. The Clinical Evaluation of Lyme arthritis. Ann Intern Med 1987;107:725.
84. Still GF. On a form of chronic joint disease in children. Med Chir Trans 1897;80:47. (Reprinted in Arch Dis Child 1941;16:156.)
85. Stillman JS, Barry PE. Juvenile rheumatoid arthritis. ser. 2. Arthritis Rheum 1977;20(Suppl):171.
86. Stollerman GH. Rheumatic fever and streptococcal infection. New York: Grune & Stratton, 1975.
87. Swett PP. Synovectomy in chronic infectious arthritis. J Bone Joint Surg 1923;5:110.
88. Thompson M, Douglas G, Davison EP. Synovectomy of the metacarpophalangeal joints in rheumatoid arthritis. Proc R Soc Med 1973;66:197.
89. Valtonen VV, Leirisalo M, Pentikainen PJ, et al. Triggering infections in reactive arthritis. Ann Rheum Dis 1985;44:399.
90. Waldman RJ, Hall WN, McGee H, et al. Aspirin as a risk factor in Reye's syndrome. JAMA 1982;247:3089.
91. Willkens RF, Watson MA, Paxson CS. Low dose pulse methotrexate therapy in rheumatoid arthritis. J Rheumatol 1980;7:501.
92. Wood P. Nomenclature and classification of arthritis methotrexate in children. European League Against Rheumatism Bulletin 1977;6:101.

Chapter 12

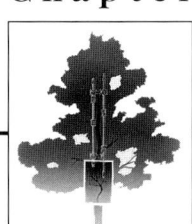

Bone and Soft Tissue Tumors

Dempsey S. Springfield

Origins
Classification
Evaluation
   Chief Complaint
   Medical History
   Review of Systems
   Physical Examination
   Plain Radiograph Examination
   Additional Diagnostic Studies
   Staging
   Biopsy

Specific Bone Tumors
   Bone-Forming Tumors
   Cartilaginous Tumors
   Lesions of Fibrous Origin
   Miscellaneous Lesions
   Soft Tissue Tumors
Chemotherapy for Musculoskeletal Tumors

Primary bone and soft tissue tumors in the pediatric age group are uncommon and, when they occur, usually are benign. There are two primary malignant tumors of bone, osteosarcoma and Ewing sarcoma, and one soft tissue sarcoma, rhabdomyosarcoma, that occur predominantly in the pediatric patient. The orthopaedist must remain alert because the malignant tumor is an unexpected event, and its infrequency can result in improper or delayed initial management. The orthopaedist who sees pediatric patients but is not prepared to manage a malignant or aggressive benign musculoskeletal tumor must be comfortable with evaluating patients with musculoskeletal tumors and know who to refer and who to manage. This chapter reviews the common bone and soft tissue tumors of childhood; it discusses how the patients present, what physical findings to expect, and how the plain radiographs should look; and it suggests additional diagnostic and staging evaluations and treatment. This chapter is not intended to be a definitive text of musculoskeletal pathology and includes only the more common tumors of childhood.

ORIGINS

The first change that must occur for the production of a tumor is for a cell to lose its normal reproductive restraints. Normal cells reproduce by going through the cell cycle but do so under strict control from a variety of cell cycle controlling proteins.[12] When the cell cycle–controlling proteins are not functioning correctly the cell may continue to cycle through the dividing process, making identical daughter cells. These daughter cells will not have lost their normal cell cycle–controlling proteins, and cell production continues unabated.[17]

Although a complete understanding of the mechanisms of origins for musculoskeletal tumors has yet to be developed, the causes are better understood than they were a few years ago, and it may not be much longer before the mystery is fully solved. The key is in understanding nuclear DNA and how alterations in DNA are manifest and corrected. It is believed that genetic alterations are the basis of all tumors.[15] Nuclear DNA controls all of the functions of cells. It directs the cell's functions by controlling the proteins made by the cell, and the proteins are the messenger of the information. An alteration in the DNA may result in overproduction, underproduction, or altered production of a protein that alters the cell's function.

The initial search for altered genetic information was through examining the chromosomes.[13] This lead to the realization that in some tumors there are recognizable alterations in chromosomes characteristic for a specific tumor type. Ewing sarcoma and peripheral neuroectodermal tumor both have a translocation between chromosomes 11 and 22 [t(11:22)(q22:q12)], which is found in all of these tumors. Some pathologists believe that the diagnosis of Ewing sarcoma or peripheral neuroectodermal tumor should not be made unless this chromosomal translocation is documented. Myxoid liposarcomas have a translocation between chromosomes 12 and 16 [t(12:16)(q13:q11)], and alveolar rhabdomyosarcoma has a translocation between chromosomes 2 and 13 [t(2:13)(q35:q14)]. Osteosarcoma, on the other hand, has multiple chromosomal abnormalities but no characteristic alterations. The chromosomal changes are gross alterations of the genetic information, but genetic defects can occur without chromosomal alterations. Point mutations are alterations of genes without changes in chromosomal structure, and those that lead to tumor formation are called oncogenes.

Initially it was believed that oncogenes were only additions to the genetic material (e.g., *MYC*, *MYCN*, *FOS*, *RAS*) whose presence produced the alterations that lead to a tumor, but recently, genes whose normal function is to suppress the production of tumors have been found. They suppress tumor production by controlling the cell cycle. When these genes are missing, or when they malfunction, a tumor is produced. The genes that produce tumors by their presence are called dominant genes, and those that suppress genes are called recessive or tumor suppressor genes.[14] They are recessive because both alleles of the gene have to be missing or malfunctioning before the gene product (i.e., a protein) is changed. Only one allele of a dominant oncogene is necessary for the production of an altered protein. Both the retinoblastoma (*RB*) and the *P53* genes are recessive genes, or tumor suppressor genes. Potential oncogenes are being evaluated, and a complete understanding of the process will not be available for some time.

The *RB* and the *P53* genes are both cell cycle regulatory on genes[16]; the proteins produced under the direction of these genes participate in the regulation of the cell cycle. When these genes malfunction their proteins are either not produced or produced incorrectly, and regulation of the cell cycle malfunctions. As more is learned about cell cycle regulation, is it clear that its control is a complex process with numerous interrelated controlling mechanisms and additional genes and their products need to be found and examined before the entire process is understood.

All of the gene abnormalities that lead to tumor formation do so through the production of abnormal proteins. The place of action of the proteins varies depending on the genetic information. As mentioned, the proteins produced by the *RB* and the *P53* genes are cell cycle regulators. There are probably other genes that produce proteins that participate in cell cycle regulation. Most likely, all tumors, especially malignant tumors, have other gene alterations that produce proteins that increase a cell's response to a growth factor, allow a cell to infiltrate normal tissues, alter the cell's membrane, increase the production of growth factors, or alter functions of the normal cell.

The future of medical science in musculoskeletal oncology is in molecular biology. Through advances in this area, it is probable that these genetic alterations will be understood, and our ability to diagnose and treat musculoskeletal tumors will be greatly improved.

CLASSIFICATION

It is convenient to separate primary tumors of the bone into those that are of bone origin, such as osteoid osteoma, osteoblastoma, osteosarcoma, and its variants; cartilaginous origin, such as enchondroma, osteochondroma, chondromyxofibroma, periosteal chondroma, chondroblastoma, and chondrosarcoma; fibrous origin, such as fibrous dysplasia, nonossifying fibroma, and ossifying fibroma; and a miscellaneous group, including unicameral bone cyst, aneurysmal bone cyst, giant cell tumor of bone, and Ewing sarcoma. This simple grouping separates primary tumors of the bone into similar radiographic and histologic groups. Usually the tissue of origin can be suspected based on the clinical data and a plain radiograph. Recognizing the characteristics of each group helps the physician formulate a reasonable differential diagnosis and, with a reasonable differential diagnosis, design an appropriate evaluation.

Soft tissue tumors also may be classified based on their tissue of origin. These groups include tumors of vascular origin (e.g., hemangioma and its variants), muscular origin (e.g., rhabdomyosarcoma), nerve origin (e.g., neurofibroma, neurolemmoma, neurofibrosarcoma), fibrous tissue origin (e.g., fibromatosis, fibrosarcoma), fat origin (e.g., lipoma, liposarcoma), synovial origin (e.g., pigmented villonodular synovitis [PVNS], synovial chondromatosis), and a miscellaneous group (e.g., malignant fibrous histiocytoma, synovial cell sarcoma). Synovial cell sarcoma may or may not arise from primitive synovial cells, but it does not occur in joints and should not be grouped with the synovial tumors.

EVALUATION

The differential diagnosis for patients who present with a bone or soft tissue mass includes neoplasia, infection, and trauma. Infection and trauma are more common than neoplasia, and one of these is usually the explanation of a mass or abnormality seen on a radiograph. Nonetheless, neoplasia, although less common, should not be forgotten, and as mentioned previously, because neoplasia is less common they should be considered. The consequences of the mismanagement of a patient with a musculoskeletal tumor can be grave. The orthopaedist must remember to include neoplasia in the differential diagnosis and not overlook or mismanage a tumor because its presence was not considered (Fig. 12-1).

Chief Complaint

Pain is the most common presenting complaint of a patient with a musculoskeletal tumor. The characteristics of the pain can help determine the diagnosis. Ask the patient: Where is the pain? How did it begin? Is it sharp, dull, radiating, or constant? Is it associated with activity? Is there a particular activity that makes the pain worse? What makes the pain better? Does it wake you at night? Is the intensity of the pain increasing, staying the same, or diminishing?

Patients who have active benign tumors (e.g., aneurysmal bone cysts, chondromyxofibroma, giant cell tumor) usually have a mild, dull, slowly progressive pain, worse at night and aggravated by activity. Patients with malignant musculoskeletal tumors complain of a more rapidly progressive symptom complex, not specifically related to activity and which often awakens them at night. Occasionally, the pain pattern is diagnostic. The pain of an osteoid osteoma is so typical that the diagnosis should be strongly suspected from the history. The pain of an osteoid osteoma is a constant intense pain, worse at night, and it almost always is relieved by aspirin. The pain caused by a Brodie abscess is similar to that of an osteoid osteoma, but the Brodie abscess pain is rarely relieved by aspirin.

Most children and parents date the onset of symptoms to a traumatic event. The specific nature of the trauma and the relation of the trauma to the current symptoms must be evaluated thoroughly. Trauma without a definitive fracture can be the explanation for an abnormal radiograph but should not be used as the explanation of an abnormal radiograph, not even for a periosteal reaction, unless the history is perfectly consistent. Be cautious about ascribing a lesion to trauma. With the increased level of organized sports for children there has been an increased incidence of fatigue fractures, and these fractures can be confused with a neoplasia. The child presenting with a fracture should be questioned about the specifics of the injury that produced the fracture. Most lesions that lead to a pathologic fracture easily are recognized on a plain radiograph, but occasionally it may not be obvious. When the traumatic event seems insignificant, a pathologic fracture should be suspected. The patient should be asked if they had symptoms, no matter how minimal, before the fracture. Most aggressive benign tumors and malignant tumors produce pain before the bone is weakened enough to fracture. Inactive benign tumors are almost always asymptomatic until the bone breaks.

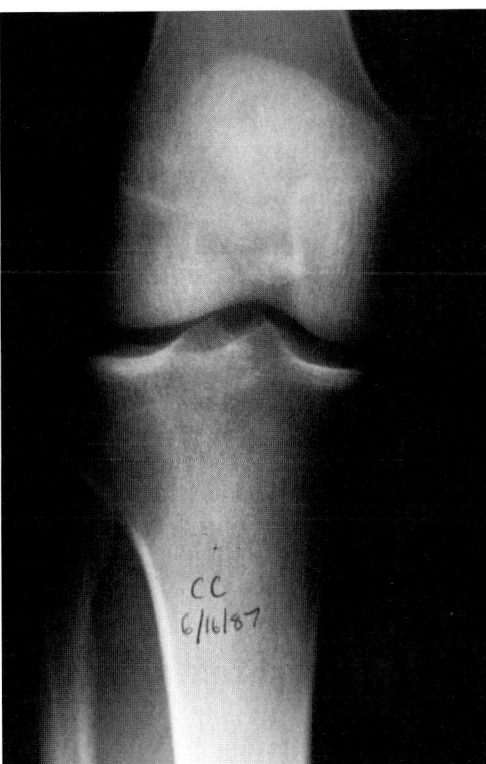

FIGURE 12-1. Anteroposterior radiograph of the knee of a young man who complained of it "giving way." The orthopaedist who saw the patient suspected the derangement, and the patient eventually had arthroscopic surgery. A radiolucent lesion can be seen easily in the lateral aspect of the proximal tibial metaphysis and epiphysis. This giant cell tumor of bone was missed because the physician did not consider this diagnosis when he was examining the patient or the radiograph. By the time the tumor was recognized, it had grown so large that resection and allograft reconstruction were required. Had it been treated when this radiograph was taken, a curettage and bone graft packing or polymethyl methacrylate packing probably would have been done.

Medical History

Most children have no significant past medical history, but inquiries should be made. Has the child had a previous fracture? Has the child had other illnesses? Have previous radiographs been taken? Do not assume that the patient or the family will volunteer significant past medical history. Ask specific questions.

Review of Systems

Ask specifically about systemic symptoms of fever, decreased appetite, irritability, and decreased activity.

Most patients with musculoskeletal tumors do not have systemic symptoms, and the presence of a systemic illness should alert the physician to the possibility of an underlying generalized disorder or osteomyelitis. Patients with Ewing sarcoma may have an elevated temperature, weight loss, and malaise, but this is the exception not the rule. Even children with large primary malignant musculoskeletal tumors usually appear healthy. Patients with cancer do not always present with obvious signs of the underlying malignancy.

Most children with a soft tissue mass do not have symptoms. If the patient is less than 5 years of age, the mass usually is noted first by a parent. The parent is convinced that the mass appeared overnight, but this is rarely the case. Teenagers may report the presence of a mass but often only after a few weeks or months of waiting for it to resolve spontaneously. Painful soft tissue masses are, for the most part, rapidly growing tumors and usually are malignant. The majority of even malignant soft tissue tumors do not produce significant symptoms until they are large. Although most of the soft tissue masses seen in children prove to be benign, all soft tissue masses, even those in children should be considered malignant tumors until proven otherwise. The consequence of mistaking a malignant soft tissue tumor for a benign one can be devastating; the consequences of approaching a benign tumor as if it were a malignancy are minimal.

Physical Examination

All patients with musculoskeletal complaints, especially those in the pediatric age group, should have a complete physical examination. Not only can important information be gained about the specific disorder being evaluated, but other significant abnormalities may be found. Café-au-lait lesions of the skin are a clue that the patient has fibrous dysplasia or neurofibromatosis. Numerous hard, nontender, fixed masses near the ends of long bones are diagnostic of multiple osteochondroma. Exophthalmos and otitis media indicate that the patient has Hand-Schüller-Christian disease.

The affected extremity should be examined carefully. The gait pattern should be recorded, muscular atrophy examined, and abnormalities in the vascular supply and motor and sensory innervation noted. The range of motion of the adjacent joint should be measured. If there is a mass present, it should be measured and the presence of erythema, tenderness, pulsations, bruit, or increased temperature noted.

Soft, movable, nontender masses, especially those in the subcutaneous tissues, usually are benign. These can be felt best when lubricant is applied on the overlying skin. Firm to hard, fixed or tethered, tender masses, especially those deep to the superficial fascia, are more likely to be malignant, but deep lipoma and a cyst usually are firm to the touch. Transilluminate the mass; if light is transmitted more easily through the mass compared with the surrounding tissue, the mass is a fluid-filled cyst.

Plain Radiograph Examination

Patients with musculoskeletal complaints should have at least anteroposterior and lateral plain radiographs. Good quality plain radiographs (at least two views, preferably at 90 degrees) are necessary. The entire lesion must be observed. The radiograph should be reviewed systematically. Look at the bone, all of it and every bone on the radiograph. Ask yourself these questions: Is there an area of increased or decreased density? Is there endosteal or periosteal reaction, and if there is, what are the characteristics of the reaction? Is there cortical destruction? Is it localized or are there multiple defects? Is the margin in the tumor well or poorly defined? Is there a reactive rim of bone surrounding the lesion? Are there densities within a radiolucent lesion? Is the bone of normal, increased, or decreased overall density? Is the joint normal? Is there loss of articular cartilage? Is the subchondral bone normal, thick, or thin? Are there abnormalities in the bone on both sides of the joint? Are there intraarticular densities? Is there a soft tissue mass? Are there calcifications or ossifications in the soft tissue? By looking specifically for abnormalities, it is unlikely that an abnormality will be missed, but a radiograph simply stared at will be poorly interpreted. The pelvis and the scapula are exceptions to this rule. Large tumors of involving the pelvis or the scapula, even those with marked destruction of bone, can be extremely difficult or impossible to see on a plain radiograph. If there is a suggestion that the patient has a pelvic or scapula tumor, bone scan and computed tomography (CT) scan or magnetic resonance imaging (MRI) are recommended.

Enneking[3] teaches that four questions should be asked when looking at plain radiographs of a possible bone tumor:

1. Where is the tumor? This refers to the lesion's anatomic location: long bone or flat bone; epiphyseal, metaphyseal, or diaphyseal; and medullary canal, intracortical or surface.
2. What is the tumor doing to the bone? Is there erosion of the bone, and if so what is the pattern?
3. What is the bone doing to the tumor? Is there periosteal or endosteal reaction? Is it well developed? Is it sharply defined?
4. Are there intrinsic characteristics within the tumor that indicate its histology? Is there bone

formation by the tumor? Is there calcification? Is the lesion completely radiolucent?

The examination of a radiograph should not be a casual glance but a detailed study of all tissue present. Do not forget to specifically examine the soft tissues visible on the radiograph.

Most bone tumors can be diagnosed correctly after obtaining the history, performing a physical examination, and examining the plain radiograph. When the specific diagnosis is made from these examinations, additional studies are requested only if they are necessary for treatment. Specific treatment often can be planned from only the history, physical examination and plain radiographs. For example, a 16-year-old boy with a hard fixed mass in the distal femur that has not increased in size for more than 1 year and has been present for 9 years complains of pain after direct trauma to this mass. Plain anteroposterior and lateral radiographs confirm the clinically suspected diagnosis of osteochondroma. Further evaluation to make the diagnosis is not necessary, but if surgical resection is elected as the treatment a CT scan may be useful in planning the operative procedure.

When the specific diagnosis cannot be made, it should be possible to limit the differential diagnoses to three or four lesions, and appropriate additional evaluations can be requested. Linear tomograms, angiograms, CT, MRI, and nuclear bone scan may reveal findings that are diagnostic or provide needed information from which to plan a subsequent biopsy. For example, a 10-year-old boy complains of mild knee pain that has been present for 3 months, has loss of knee flexion, and on the lateral radiograph of the distal femur there is a bone density lesion attached to the posterior femoral cortex. From this information, the lesion is recognized either as a parosteal osteosarcoma or an osteocartilaginous exostosis. A technetium bone scan with increased activity in the area of the lesion does not distinguish between these two, but both a CT scan and an MRI allow one to distinguish between a parosteal osteosarcoma and an osteocartilaginous exostosis. A parosteal osteosarcoma is attached to the cortex of the bone while an osteocartilaginous exostosis arises from the cortex and has a medullary canal continuous with the medullary canal of the bone. The CT scan or MRI is critical in the evaluation of a patient in this clinical setting.

Additional Diagnostic Studies

Laboratory Examinations

Urine and serum laboratory values in musculoskeletal neoplasia are usually normal. Only a few musculoskeletal disorders are associated with abnormal laboratory values. The erythrocyte sedimentation rate (ESR), or sedimentation rate, is nonspecific but sensitive. Patients with infections or malignant tumors usually have an elevated sedimentation, but patients with benign disease ordinarily have a normal value. A normal ESR value can be used to increase the physician's confidence that a suspected benign, inactive lesion is just that. A markedly elevated value (>80 mm/hour) supports a diagnosis of infection and may be just what is needed to justify an early aspiration of a bone or soft tissue lesion. Patients with active benign or malignant musculoskeletal tumors often have an elevated ESR, but rarely over 80 mm/hour. Patients with Ewing sarcoma are the most likely to have an elevated ESR, but even their ESR rate is not as high as that of a patient with an infection.

Serum alkaline phosphatase is present in most tissues in the body, but the bone and the hepatobiliary system are the predominant sources. In the pediatric age group, conventional high-grade osteosarcoma is associated with an elevated serum alkaline phosphatase. Not all patients with an osteosarcoma have an elevated serum alkaline phosphatase, and therefore a normal value does not exclude osteosarcoma from the diagnosis. A minimal elevation can be observed with numerous processes, even a healing fracture. Adults with an elevated serum alkaline phosphatase secondary to bone disease are most likely to have Paget disease of bone or diffuse metastatic carcinoma. Patients with a primary liver disorder also have an elevated serum alkaline phosphatase, but they also have an elevated serum 5-nucleotidase, leucine aminopeptidase, and a γ-glutamyl transpeptidase deficiency. These are not elevated in primary bone tumors.

Serum and urine calcium and phosphorus should be measured, especially if a metabolic bone disorder is suspected. Other laboratory determinations are not helpful and are not recommended.

Radionuclide Scans

Technetium bone scans are readily available, safe, and an excellent method to evaluate the activity of the primary lesion. In addition, the bone scan is the most practical method to survey the entire skeleton. Technetium 99 attached to a polyphosphate is injected intravenously, and after a delay of 2 to 4 hours the polyphosphate with its attached technetium concentrates in the skeleton proportional to the production of new bone. A disorder that is associated with an increase in bone production increases the local concentration of technetium 99 and produce a "hot spot" on the scan. The technetium bone scan can be used to evaluate the activity of a primary lesion, determine its local extent, and search for other bone lesions. The polyphosphate-technetium 99 compound also concentrates in areas of increased blood flow, and soft tissue tumors usually have increased activity compared with the normal soft tissues. The technetium scan can be used to evaluate blood flow if images are obtained during the early phases, immediately after injection of the technetium. The polyphosphate-technetium 99 is cleared and excreted by the kidneys so the kidneys and the bladder have more activity than other organs.

Gallium 67 imaging is another radionuclide study to evaluate both bone and soft tissue tumors.[27] This examination takes longer to perform (24–72 hours) than a technetium 99 scan (2 hours) but is believed to be useful in the evaluation of musculoskeletal tumors[30] because it can help differentiate a musculoskeletal infection from a neoplasia. I have not found gallium scans useful except when evaluating a patient suspected of having an occult infection. The scan should be performed prior to a surgical procedure because the operative site has increased uptake on the radionuclide scan.

The technetium scan is sensitive but nonspecific. The principle value of a radionuclide scan is as a means of surveying the entire skeleton for clinically unsuspected lesions. Occasionally the bone scan reveals intramedullary extension beyond what is seen on the plain radiograph, but both CT scan and MRI are more accurate. Radionuclide scans, both technetium and gallium, can be useful in evaluating a soft tissue mass. A malignant soft tissue tumor has increased activity, but some benign lesions do not. If a bone or a soft tissue lesion has no increased activity on a radionuclide scan it can be assumed to be benign, but the reverse is not true. In approximately 25% of cases of eosinophilic granuloma and plasmocytoma (an exception to the rule that a normal bone scan means a benign tumor) the bone scan is normal, or there is decreased activity at the site of the lesion.

Linear Tomography

The principal value of linear tomography is its ease and availability, but the quality of its images compared with CT scans is poor. The border between a bone lesion and the normal host bone, the pattern of cortical destruction, and the parosteal reaction are seen on the linear tomography better than on the plain radiograph, but these are seen even better on a CT scan. Linear tomography is more accurate in evaluating the subchondral bone than a plain radiograph or CT scan. An arthrotomogram (i.e., linear tomography after injection of dye into the joint) can help determine if there is intraarticular extension, but MRI is the best method with which to look for intraarticular extension. Although linear tomography is often useful in evaluating fractures, CT scan and MRI have made linear tomography obsolete in the evaluation of musculoskeletal neoplasias. Whole lung linear tomography was once the standard method of locating occult pulmonary metastasis, but whole lung CT scan is the accepted screening technique.

Angiography

Prior to the development of CT and MRI, angiography was the best nonoperative method to determine the extraosseous anatomic extent of a musculoskeletal tumor. The vascular pattern (tortuous small vessels, arteriovenous shunting) was used to predict whether the lesion was malignant or benign, but it proved to be of limited value in determining a specific diagnosis.[37] At present, CT and MRI are used to determine the anatomic extent of a musculoskeletal tumor and have replaced angiography in the evaluation of musculoskeletal neoplasia. Angiography is indicated when the relation of the major vessels and the tumor cannot be determined from the CT or MRI, the tumor appears to encase the major vessel, the patient has had previous surgery adjacent to or including the major vessels, and preoperative embolization is performed or intraarterial chemotherapy is infused.

Computed Axial Tomography

Computed axial tomography has dramatically improved our ability to evaluate bone and soft tissue tumors. The exact anatomic extent of a tumor can be determined. The relation of a cortical lesion to the cortex, the intraosseous extent of a bone tumor, and the involved soft tissue can be determined by CT. Often a specific diagnosis can be made or a suspected diagnosis confirmed after seeing the CT scan. Smaller nodules can be seen on a whole lung CT scans than can be seen with plain chest radiographs or whole lung linear tomography. With a CT scan, the abdomen can be evaluated thoroughly without surgical exploration. These improvements have reduced the number of biopsies performed to confirm suspected benign diagnoses; allowed more accurate determinations of what tissue requires resection in the active benign lesions and malignant lesions, thus increasing the percent of limb salvage resections performed; and permitted earlier detection and resection of pulmonary metastases. Before CT scans were available, anatomic localization of tumors was less precise, and the oncologic orthopaedic surgeon was forced to be more generous with the resection margin to have an acceptably low incidence of local recurrence. CT scans have improved the accuracy of anatomic localization so that less radical surgery can be performed safely.

The most common error made when requesting a CT scan is not asking specific questions of the radiologist. Radiologists do not know what specific information the orthopaedist wants; only if specific questions are asked is the maximum value of CT scan realized. Ask the radiologist to determine the lesion's location and its density (attenuation coefficient) and vascularity, and search for intralesional characteristics that may provide a diagnostic clue. Have the radiologist include the contralateral normal extremity on the CT scan for comparisons.

The density of a bone or soft tissue mass on a CT scan is called its attenuation coefficient and is measured in Hounsfield units (HU). The density of water is 0 HU; tissues more dense than water have a positive value, and tissues less dense than water have a negative value. The vascularity of a lesion can be evaluated by measuring the increase in the attenuation coefficient of a lesion after intravenous infusion of contrast and comparing this increase to that in an adjacent muscle. Normal muscle has an attenuation coefficient of approximately 60 HU and increases 5 to 10 HU with a bolus of intravenous contrast. Fat has an attenuation coefficient value of approximately -60 HU, and cortical bone is usually more than 1000 HU.

When a hard copy of a CT scan is photographed, the scanner must be adjusted for the upper and lower limits of the Hounsfield units measured. All tissues with an attenuation coefficient above the upper Hounsfield unit selected appear white, and all tissues with an attenuation coefficient below the lower Hounsfield unit appear black. The tissues between these two limits are shades of gray. These upper and lower limits can be adjusted and often are referred to as the window settings. The CT scan should be viewed with window settings to optimize the visualization of the bone and the soft tissue. Adjustments from the standard window setting can be made if necessary and if the radiologist knows in advance what questions need to be answered. This is another reason that it is important to discuss the case with the radiologist prior to obtaining the CT scan, such as in the examination of a patient suspected of having an osteoid osteoma. The osteoid osteoma has a low attenuation coefficient, but it is surrounded by reactive bone, which has a very high attenuation coefficient. If standard bone window settings are used, the nidus may be obscured and the diagnosis missed; if the levels imaged are too far apart, the nidus will be missed. By adjusting the window setting upward and imaging thin slices, the nidus easily is observed, and a diagnosis is made.

The exact location of the lesion can be determined by measurements made on the CT scan. Intraosseous bone lesions without an associated cortical abnormality or a small bone lesion often can be difficult to locate at the time of surgical exploration. Remind the radiologist to measure the distance of the lesion from a palpable anatomic structure, then the lesion can be found when the patient is operated. This reduces the operative dissection necessary for successful biopsy or excision.

Soft tissue lesions are seen best on a CT scan when they are surrounded by normal fat because of the marked difference between tumor and fat attenuation coefficients. CT scans of the trunk and proximal parts of the extremity or in obese patients are better than CT scans of the distal parts of the extremities or in an extremely thin patient. CT scans for soft tissue lesions in the pediatric patient, particularly a lesion in the distal part of the extremity, is less helpful than in adults because of the lack of sufficient intramuscular fat. Intravenous contrast is often helpful in determining the extent of a soft tissue tumor particularly for a soft tissue lesion whose attenuation coefficient is close to that of normal muscle. The neoplasia is almost always more vascular than normal muscle and has an increase in density greater than the normal tissues. In addition, the major veins and arteries can be observed with the infusion of intravenous contrast.

Magnetic Resonance Imaging

Magnetic resonance imaging does not expose the patient to radiation and has proved to be useful in the evaluation of musculoskeletal lesions. MRI produces images of the body in all three plains (axial, sagittal, and coronal) as easily as in a single plain and possesses no known hazards to the patient. The major difficulties are the time required for the examination (an average of 1 hour), the inability to examine a patient who has a ferromagnetic foreign body in the brain or the eye, the artifact caused by ferromagnetic implants, and the claustrophobic conditions of the scanner. The images are produced through a computer program that converts the reactions of tissue hydrogen ions in a strong magnetic field excited by radiowaves. By adjusting excitation variables, images that are T1- and T2-weighted are obtained. A variety of techniques have been used to produce images of improved quality compared with the routine T1- and T2-weighted images. The use of gadolinium as an intravascular contrast agent allows one to judge the vascularity of a lesion, providing even more information about the tumor. Fat suppression images with gadolinium enhancement often are especially useful to demonstrate a soft tissue neoplasia. As is the case with CT scans, it is important for the orthopaedist requesting the MRI to discuss the case with the radiologist. The radiologist can then determine the optimal setting to see the lesion.

Magnetic resonance imaging has become the single most important diagnostic test after physical examination and plain radiographs for evaluating a musculoskeletal lesion. The ability to view the lesion in three planes, determine its intraosseous extent, see the soft tissue component clearly, and have an idea of the tissue type from one diagnostic test is rewarding.

Staging

Patients with neoplasia can be separated into groups based on the extent of their tumor and its potential for metastasis. These groups are called stages. Grouping patients by their stage helps the physician predict a patient's risk of local recurrence and metastasis. This facilitates making treatment decisions about individual patients and helps in the comparison of treatment protocols. Without staging, patients with dissimilar prognoses might be compared, and an erroneous conclusion could be made about a treatment program. Staging systems are based on the histologic grade of the tumor as well as clinical factors, such as the tumor size, location, rate of growth, and presence of regional or distant metastasis. The presence of a metastasis at the time of presentation is the worst prognostic factor, followed by histologic grade and size of the tumor. There are two common staging systems used for musculoskeletal tumors.

The task force on malignant bone tumors of the American Joint Commission on Staging and End Result Studies (AJC) published a staging system for soft tissue tumors in 1977.[45] This system was revised in 1987.[46] Initially, the task force did not propose a staging system for bone tumors, but at the time of the revision of the soft tissue staging system a bone tumor staging system was added. These systems are similar to other staging systems that have been developed by the AJC and are based on the histologic grade (G), local extent, or size (T), whether or not there is involvement of nodes (N) and metastases (M). The tumors are separated into three histologic grades (G1, low grade; G2, medium grade; G3, high grade) and two sizes (T1 ≤ 5 cm, T2 > 5 cm). Patients with nodal involvement are designated N1, and those without nodal involvement are N0. Patients with metastatic disease are designated as M1, and those without as M0. There are four stages with subclasses in each. The patient with stage 1 has the best prognosis, and the patient with stage 4 the worst (Table 12-1).

Enneking and colleagues[44] also proposed a musculoskeletal staging system. This system is different than the one proposed by the AJC. First, it is a surgical staging system to be used by the surgeon planning the treatment. Second, it is used for both bone and soft tissue tumors. This system is used more often by orthopaedists involved in the management of patients with musculoskeletal tumors. It was designed to be

TABLE 12-1 *Revised AJC Staging System for Soft Tissue Sarcoma*

Stage I			
IA—G1, T1, N0, M0	Grade 1 tumor, < 5 cm in diameter with no regional lymph node or distant metastasis	IB—G1, T2, N0, M0	Grade 1 tumor, ≥ 5 cm in diameter with no regional lymph node or distant metastasis
Stage II			
IIA—G2, T1, N0, M0	Grade 2 tumor, < 5 cm in diameter with no regional lymph node or distant metastasis	IIB—G2, T2, N0, M0	Grade 2 tumor, ≥ 5 cm in diameter with no regional lymph node or distant metastasis
Stage III			
IIIA—G3, T1, N0, M0	Grade 3 tumor, < 5 cm in diameter with no regional lymph node or distant metastasis	IIIB—G3, T2, N0, M0	Grade 3 tumor, ≥ 5 cm in diameter with no regional lymph node or distant metastasis
Stage IV			
IVA—G1–3, T1–2, N1, M0	Tumor of any grade or size with histologically verified metastasis to regional lymph nodes but no distant metastasis	IVB—G1–3, T1–2, N0–1	Clinically diagnosed distant metastasis

From Suit H, Mankin HJ, Ward WC, Gebhardt MC, Harmon DC, Rosenberg A. Treatment of the patient with stage M0 soft tissue sarcoma. J Clin Oncol 1988;6:854.

clear cut, straightforward, and clinically practical. The tumors are separated into only two histologic grades (I, low grade; II, high grade) and two anatomic extents (A, intracompartmental; B, extracompartmental). Patients with metastatic disease either in a regional lymph node or a distant site are grouped together as stage III. Each bone was defined as its own separate anatomic compartment. The soft tissue anatomic compartments were defined as muscle groups separated by facial boundaries (Table 12-2). The facial boundaries act as barriers of tumor extension, and by thinking in terms of compartments it is easier to design surgical resections. There are five stages in this system (Table 12-3).

Enneking and colleagues[44] also introduced four terms to indicate the surgical margin of a tumor resection. These terms are commonly used and provide a means of describing the relation between the histologic extent of the tumor and the resection margin. The surgical margins are defined as intralesional, marginal, wide, and radical. An intralesional margin is the surgical margin achieved when a tumor's pseudocapsule is violated and gross tumor is removed from within the pseudocapsule. An incisional biopsy and a curettage are two common examples of an intralesional margin. A marginal surgical margin is achieved

TABLE 12-2 **Surgical Sites**

INTRACOMPARTMENTAL (T₁)	EXTRACOMPARTMENTAL (T₂)
Intraosseous	Extraosseous soft tissue extension
Intraarticular	Extraosseous soft tissue extension
Superficial to deep fascia	Deep fascial extension
Paraosseous	Intraosseous or extrafascial extension
Intrafascial compartments	
Ray of hand or foot	Extrafascial planes or spaces
Posterior calf	
Anterolateral leg	Midfoot and hindfoot
Anterior thigh	Popliteal space
Medial thigh	Groin–femoral triangle
Posterior thigh	Intrapelvic
Buttocks	Midhand
Volar forearm	Antecubital fossae
Dorsal forearm	Axilla
Anterior arm	Periclavicular
Posterior arm	Paraspinal
Periscapular	Head and neck

From Enneking WF, Spanier SS, Goodman MA. A system for the surgical staging of musculoskeletal sarcomata. Clin Orthop 1980; 153:106.

TABLE 12.3 **Surgical Stages**

STAGE	GRADE	SITE
IA	Low (G1)	Intracompartmental (T1)
IB	Low (G1)	Extracompartmental (T2)
IIA	High (G2)	Intracompartmental (T1)
IIB	High (G2)	Extracompartmental (T2)
III	Any (G); regional or distant metastasis	Any (T)

From Enneking WF, Spanier SS, Goodman MA. A system for the surgical staging of musculoskeletal sarcomata. Clin Orthop 1980; 153:106.

when a tumor is removed by dissecting between the normal tissue and the tumor's pseudocapsule. This is a surgical margin obtained when a tumor is "shelled out." A wide surgical margin is achieved when the tumor is removed with a surrounding cuff of normal uninvolved tissue. This is often referred to as en bloc resection. A radical surgical margin is achieved when the tumor and the entire compartment (or compartments) are removed together. This usually is accomplished only with an amputation that is proximal to the joint just proximal to the lesion (e.g., an above-knee amputation for a tibial tumor). As a rule, benign lesions can be managed with an intralesional or marginal surgical margin, but malignant tumors require a wide surgical margin. Radical surgical margins are reserved for recurrent tumors and the most infiltrative malignancy.

Biopsy

Biopsy should be the last step in the evaluation of a patient with a bone or soft tissue tumor and performed only after careful planning.[56] Often, biopsy proves unnecessary after the patient has been thoroughly evaluated, the diagnosis having been made by the clinical setting and radiographic findings. When a biopsy is required, the prebiopsy evaluation improves the chance that adequate and representative tissue will be obtained, the least amount of normal tissue will be contaminated, and the pathologist will make an accurate diagnosis. Biopsies performed without an adequate prebiopsy evaluation are more likely to produce an unsatisfactory result.

The majority of complications of biopsy are due to the biopsy being performed without adequate knowledge of the anatomic extent and exact location of the tumor.[55] The biopsy should not be performed until a thorough evaluation has been completed and should not be performed to justify a thorough workup or a referral to a regional medical center. The patient who is sent unnecessarily for a consultation is more than justified by the limbs and lives saved by the multidisciplinary teams concentrating in the management of musculoskeletal tumors found only in a regional medical center.

The purpose of the biopsy is to confirm the diagnosis suspected by the physician after the evaluation or to determine which diagnosis among a limited differential diagnosis is correct. In addition to making a specific diagnosis, the tissue obtained must be sufficient for histologic grading. It must be representative of the tumor, and because many musculoskeletal tumors are heterogeneous, the specific site from which the tissue is taken is important. The surgeon who is willing to assume the surgical management of the patient, regardless of the diagnosis, should be the one to biopsy the patient's tumor. The biopsy incision and the tissue exposed during the biopsy must be excised with the tumor if a wide surgical margin resection proves to be necessary. If the surgeon who performs the resection has planned and performed the biopsy, the patient has a better chance of a limb salvage and less risk of a local recurrence. The surgeon should consult with the radiologist and the pathologist before performing the biopsy to get their suggestions of the best tissue to obtain. Discussing the case with the pathologist the day before the biopsy also allows the pathologist to be better prepared when he or she is expected to make a diagnosis from a frozen section.

Needle biopsy and fine needle aspirate biopsy often are suggested.[47,48,52,54] Usually, they can be performed without general anesthesia and a hospital admission, saving the patient money and the risk of general anesthesia. It has been suggested that a needle biopsy does not contaminate uninvolved tissue, but this is not true. The needle track can be seeded with tumor and usually needs to be excised at the time of the definitive resection. Needle biopsies and fine needle aspirate biopsies must be planned just as an open biopsy is planned, and the responsible surgeon should decide how the biopsy is performed. Needle biopsies and fine needle aspirate biopsies are most useful for lesions suspected of being metastatic carcinoma or myeloma. These lesions usually are diagnosed easily with a limited amount of tissue and require neither resection or histologic grading. Although an experienced pathologist usually can make the correct diagnosis from a well-done needle biopsy or a fine needle aspirate biopsy, more mistakes are made by these techniques compared with an open biopsy, and histologic grading can be difficult or impossible without an open biopsy. Open biopsy is recommended for most musculoskeletal lesions. A needle biopsy or a fine needle aspirate biopsy are reserved for a limited number of specific clinical circumstances.

Plan the biopsy carefully. Think about possible future treatment, especially a limb salvage resection. The skin incision and deep dissection should be made so that they can be resected with the tumor at the time of a definitive limb salvage operation. Longitudinal skin incisions are better than transverse skin incisions. Transverse incisions are difficult to incorporate into a limb salvage resection, and usually the dissection to obtain a biopsy specimen through a transverse incision contaminates more tissue than does a dissection performed through a longitudinal incision. The dissection should be as limited as possible, flaps should not be raised, and neurovascular bundles should not be exposed. The dissection should be through a muscle, not between muscles. The contaminated muscle needs to be resected with the tumor, but if the biopsy dissection is between two muscles they both must be removed. The tissue obtained should be cut from the tumor. The tumor's pseudocapsule and a portion of the tumor should be excised as a block and sent to the pathologist. A frozen section should be performed even when there are no plans for immediate additional surgery. The pathologist should be sure that adequate and diagnostic tissue is available. Only when dense bone is biopsied is it impossible to perform a frozen section. The pathologist should set aside tissue for subsequent examination with an electron microscope. Some tissue should be kept frozen in the event that immunohistochemistry is required.

I use a tourniquet during the biopsy, but I deflate the tourniquet prior to closure. The use of the tourniquet is controversial. Some believe that the use of the tourniquet increases the risk of the patient developing metastatic disease. It is believed, although not documented, that tumor cells released from the tumor during the biopsy collect in the vein just distal to the tourniquet and are released as a bolus when the tourniquet is deflated. This bolus of tumor cells is believed to present an increased risk to the patient. Surgeons who use a tourniquet do not think that a tourniquet increases the risk of metastasis and believe that the biopsy is safer and the dissection less when the operation is performed in a bloodless field. The tumor should be manipulated as little as possible and do not use a compressive bandage to exsanguinate the extremity but rather elevate the extremity for 3 to 5 minutes before inflating the tourniquet.

Extra care should be taken to obtain hemostasis before closing the wound. The hematoma from the biopsy may contain tumor cells and will require resection if surgery is the treatment. The wound should be drained, but the exit site of the drain must be in line with the incision and close to it. The drain track is resected with the tumor and the biopsy incision.

An excisional biopsy rather than an incisional biopsy occasionally is indicated. An excisional biopsy is appropriate when the lesion is small and easily excised, and a wide excision does not significantly effect the patient's function. An excisional biopsy may be appropriate even when a major resection is required. If the preoperative evaluation strongly supports the diagnosis of a malignancy, particularly one that a frozen section will be difficult to perform or interpret, an excisional biopsy should be considered. The choice between an incisional biopsy and an excisional biopsy usually is easy to make. A clinically obvious exostosis on the proximal tibia should have an excisional biopsy if biopsied at all. A large aggressive lesion in the distal femur invading the adjacent soft tissues should be biopsied incisionally. It is more difficult to decide when the evaluation reveals a small active, possibly low-grade malignancy on the proximal humerus or the distal radius. An incisional biopsy exposes uncontaminated tissues to the tumor, and if the tumor proves to be a malignancy the definitive resection is more complicated. If the lesion can be treated with a curettage or a marginal excision the incisional biopsy leads to the least functional loss. The final decision is made for each patient based on not only the tumor's characteristics but the patient's desires. Some patients want to take the least chances and are willing to accept the possibility of slight overtreatment, whereas others choose to take one step at a time. It is the surgeon's responsibility to inform the patients so an informed decision can be made.

An added advantage of the excisional biopsy is that the pathologist is able to examine the entire lesion, improving the accuracy of the pathologic examination. Musculoskeletal tumors often are heterogeneous, and the amount of tissue obtained with an incisional biopsy always is limited. It can be particularly difficult to distinguish active benign cartilage tumors from low-grade chondrosarcomas. When the entire lesion and especially its interface with the adjacent bone and soft tissue is seen, the distinction is made more easily. Occasionally, even after studying the entire specimen, the pathologist is not able to decide between a benign cartilage tumor and a low-grade chondrosarcoma. In these cases the wide-excision excisional biopsy is particularly appropriate.

A final note of caution is offered with regard to the biopsy: osteomyelitis is more common than bone tumors, especially in children, and osteomyelitis often mimics neoplasia. The reverse also is true; whenever performing a biopsy, even when the diagnosis seems obvious, culture the tumor and biopsy the infection.

SPECIFIC BONE TUMORS

This text is not designed to be a definitive musculoskeletal pathology text, and only those tumors that are common to the practicing orthopaedic surgeon are discussed. I have tried to confine the discussion to pertinent information regarding the tumors, their evaluation, and their treatment. As mentioned previously, the tumors are grouped for discussion by their apparent tissues of origin.

Bone-Forming Tumors

Osteoid Osteoma

Jaffe[66] is credited with the initial description of osteoid osteoma, distinguishing it from a sterile abscess called a Brodie abscess and Garré osteomyelitis. It is a benign tumor and accounts for 11% of the benign bone tumors in Dahlin's series from the Mayo Clinic.[2] The patient is usually a young boy (males are affected more commonly than females at a ratio of 3 to 1; 80% are between 5 and 24 years of age at the time of their initial symptoms) complaining of an intense pain at the site of the lesion.

The pain is an unrelenting, sharp, boring pain, worse at night and, almost without exception, completely relieved by aspirin. If a patient has the typical pain of an osteoid osteoma but is not relieved by aspirin, the diagnosis of an osteoid osteoma should be doubted. The patient may have pain before the plain radiograph is abnormal, and often the patients have had an electromyogram, a myelogram, or an arthrogram before the typical plain radiographic changes are seen. Some patients are suspected of having a psychosomatic disorder before the osteoid osteoma is found.

Osteoid osteoma may arise in any bone, but half of them are found in the femur or the tibia, whereas the other half are distributed throughout the remainder of the skeleton. The proximal femur is a common site. It is also a site in which it may be difficult to find the lesion. Young patients with persistent pain in the groin, the middle thigh, or the knee should be suspected of having an osteoid osteoma. The other common location of an occult osteoid osteoma is the spine. When osteoid osteoma arises in the spine it usually is located in the posterior elements. The osteoid osteoma in the spine does not elicit a significant bony reaction and is very difficult to see on plain radiographs. The patient presents most commonly with a painful scoliosis.[59,67] When a patient with scoliosis complains of back pain, osteoid osteoma should be considered. A technetium bone scan is particularly useful when the clinical presentation suggests an osteoid osteoma but the lesion cannot be found on the plain radiograph. It reveals an area of increased uptake, supporting a diagnosis of osteoid osteoma and showing the lesion's location.

Patients with an osteoid osteoma show few abnormalities on their physical examination, with the exception of scoliosis in patients with osteoid osteoma of the spine. The child may walk with a limp and have atrophy of the involved extremity. If the bone with the osteoid osteoma can be directly palpated, it will be tender. Local erythema or increased temperature are not seen, and joint motion is normal. Serum and urine laboratory values are normal.

The plain radiographic appearance of an osteoid osteoma is of dense reactive bone and usually is diagnostic. The lesion itself (the nidus, <5 mm in diameter) is radiolucent but often is not seen on the plain radiograph because of the density of the intense bone reaction that surrounds it. The nidus may be on the surface of the bone, within the cortex, or on the endosteal surface. Those lesions on the endosteal surface have less reaction than those within or on the cortex. The lesion and the reaction are associated with increased uptake on the radionuclide study (technetium bone scan).[83]

The nidus may be demonstrated with linear tomograms but is better localized with a CT scan.[64] The distance between the CT scan sections should be small (1–2 mm), so that the nidus is not missed. The window settings of the CT scanner should be adjusted so that the dense reaction around the lesion does not obscure the small low-density nidus. When the nidus is found, it helps to have the distance from a bony landmark to the nidus measured on the scan so that the nidus can be found at the time of surgical removal. MRI has been used to examine osteoid osteoma, and the diagnosis can be suspected but the associated edema and reaction make the diagnosis less specific compared with a CT scan. The lesion is better seen on a CT scan.

On gross inspection the nidus of an osteoid osteoma is red and surrounded by dense white bone. The nidus is small, usually not more than 5 to 10 mm in diameter. A lesion with identical histology of the nidus of an osteoid osteoma but larger than 2 cm is called an osteoblastoma. The nidus is composed of numerous vascular channels, osteoblasts, and thin lace-like osteoid seams. Multinucleated giant cells can be seen but are not common (Fig. 12-2).

The pain of an osteoid osteoma can resolve spontaneously.[61] It is believed that osteoid osteoma is a spontaneously healing lesion that eventually involutes over a period of years, and the nidus turns to bone. Occasionally a patient uses aspirin to control the symptoms until the pain disappears, but usually the intensity of pain, the length of time taken for the lesion to spontaneously heal, and the amount of aspirin required is not tolerable, and the patient elects to have surgery. Complete removal of the nidus relieves the patient's pain. Partial removal may provide temporary relief, but the pain will return.[74] Only the nidus needs to be excised, whereas the reactive bone around the nidus does not need to be removed.

There are two surgical methods of removing the nidus. The conventional method is a block resection of the nidus and most of the surrounding reactive bone. The other is a curettage of the nidus. The advantage of the block resection is the greater assurance that all of the nidus is removed, but this technique requires removal of a segment of the cortex and produces a marked reduction in the strength of the bone. The defect created by the excision may need to be bone grafted and the patient's extremity protected for an extended period of time. The advantage of the curettage technique is that the bone is not weakened significantly, and bone grafting is not required. It is more difficult to be certain that all of the nidus is removed.

If curettage is the excision technique used, the nidus must be accurately localized preoperatively and seen intraoperatively. When the nidus cannot be localized accurately preoperatively, or seen intraoperatively, block excision is preferred. Intraoperative radio-

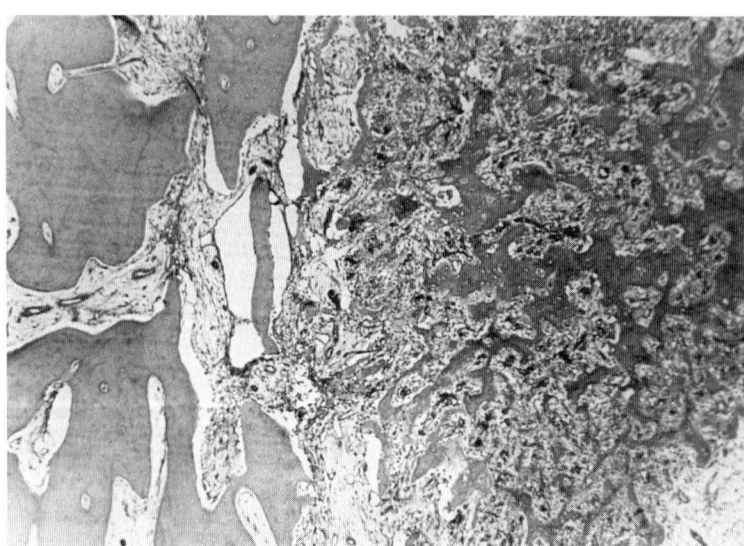

FIGURE 12-2. Histologic appearance of an osteoid osteoma. The bone tissue on the left is reactive trabeculae surrounding the nidus (*right*). The nidus is composed of osteoid, multinucleated giant cells, osteoblasts, and vessels. A thorough curettage of the nidus was done, and the patient's pain resolved completely. (Original magnification ×10.)

nuclide scanning and intraoperative tetracycline-fluorescence demonstration have been reported as a method of finding the nidus in the operating room and assuring the surgeon of its complete removal.[58,60,62,77]

I have not found the use of intraoperative radionuclide scanning or tetracycline-fluorescence helpful. Preoperative planning and careful localization of the nidus is the most important means of insuring that the nidus can be found during the operation. I no longer operate on patients with an osteoid osteoma but treat them with radiofrequency ablation.

I have been experimenting in conjunction with a group of radiologists with a unique treatment technique for osteoid osteoma.[76,85] The procedure is performed under general anesthesia but usually can be done without hospitalization. Using CT to control placement, a needle biopsy is performed to confirm the diagnosis. Then, through the same needle tract, a radiofrequency electrode with an internal thermistor is placed in the nidus. The nidus is heated to 90°C for 4 minutes. Only one of 17 patients who have had this procedure did not have immediate relief, but the follow-up period was less than 2 years in most of these patients. The patients were not protected, nor were their activities limited after the heat ablation, and there have been no complications. This procedure has promise as a treatment for osteoid osteoma. Other closed methods of treatment have been reported.[86]

Osteoblastoma

Osteoblastoma is sometimes called a giant osteoid osteoma because it is histologically identical to an osteoid osteoma but larger. Unlike osteoid osteoma, osteoblastoma is not surrounded by dense reactive bone. Cementoblastoma of the jaw is histologically identical to osteoblastoma. Osteoblastoma is less common than osteoid osteoma, accounting for less than 1% of the primary bone tumors in Dahlin's series.

The typical patient is a boy in the second decade of life (50% of the patients are between 10 and 20 years of age, although the age range is from 5 to 35 years of age) complaining of back pain (approximately 50% of the lesions are in the spine). The pain of an osteoblastoma is not as severe as the pain of an osteoid osteoma, and aspirin does not relieve it. There are no physical findings characteristic of osteoblastoma. When the tumor is in the spine, the patient has decreased motion of the spine in the involved area. Osteoblastomas are tender, and direct palpation often localizes a lesion, even when it cannot be seen on a plain radiograph.

Extremity lesions are usually diaphyseal; the patient often has a limp and mild atrophy and complains of pain directly over the lesion. Blood and urine laboratory examinations are normal. The appearance of osteoblastoma on a radiograph is variable. It is usually a mixed radiolucent, radiodense lesion, more lucent than dense. There is minimal reaction in the surrounding bone. Lesions in the spine may be difficult or impossible to see when initially examining the plain radiograph, but when located by other studies, the subtle abnormality on the plain radiograph can usually be appreciated.

Clues to look for on the plain radiograph indicating the location of an osteoblastoma are an irregular cortex, loss of pedicle definition, and enlargement of the spinous process. As with osteoid osteoma, plain tomography reveals the lesion more clearly, but for best definition the CT scan is preferred. On the CT scan, the lesion usually "expands the bone" and has intralesional stippled ossifications and a high attenuation coefficient (100 HU or more). Osteoblastoma on the radionuclide scan has increased uptake, and a technetium bone scan is an excellent method of initially screening a patient suspected of having an osteoblastoma. The bone scan localizes the lesion, but it is not specific enough for lesions in the spine to plan a surgical resection.

Osteoblastomas should be excised surgically. They continue to enlarge and damage the bone and adjacent structures if left untreated. A wide surgical resection is preferred when practical, but an extended curettage is sufficient for most cases. As much of the surrounding bone should be removed as possible. Most osteoblastomas are controlled by the extended curettage, but recurrence is common, and some can be aggressive locally. Although irradiation has been used in the management of these patients, there is little evidence that it is of benefit.

The histology of osteoblastoma is identical to the nidus of an osteoid osteoma. There should not be abnormal mitoses, although mitotic activity can be observed. There are osteoblasts, multinucleated giant cells, seams of osteoid, and a rich vascular bed. Schajowicz and Lemo[78] suggested that a subset of osteoblastoma be termed malignant osteoblastoma. They believe that this subset has histologic features that are worse than the usual osteoblastoma, more aggressive locally, and more likely to recur after limited surgery. A rare osteoblastoma metastasizes but still meets the histologic definitions of a benign tumor, although these probably should be classified as low-grade osteosarcoma.

Osteosarcoma

Osteosarcoma is defined as a tumor in which malignant spindle cells produce bone. They are two major variances that have significantly different clinical presentations and prognoses. The more common osteosarcoma is called classic high-grade osteosarcoma or conventional osteosarcoma, and the other is called juxtacortical osteosarcoma. Some authors separate juxtacortical osteosarcomas into parosteal and periosteal osteosarcoma. Less common variants of osteosarcoma (e.g., intracortical osteosarcoma, soft tissue osteosarcoma, radiation-induced osteosarcoma, Paget osteosarcoma) are not discussed in this text.

CLASSIC HIGH-GRADE OSTEOSARCOMA. The patient is usually a teenager (about 50% of the patients present during the second decade of life; more than 75% are between the age of 8 and 25 years) complaining of pain and a mass around the knee (Fig. 12-3). Half of the lesions are located in the distal femur or proximal tibia. The proximal humerus, proximal femur and pelvis are the next most common sites. The pain precedes the appreciation of the mass by a few weeks to 2 or 3 months. Boys and girls are affected with equal frequency. The patient does not have systemic symptoms and usually feels well. The mass is slightly tender, firm to hard, and fixed to the bone but not inflamed. The adjacent joint usually has restricted motion.

The remainder of the physical examination is normal except in the rare (<1%) patient who presents with metastases or multiple focal osteosarcoma. One half of the patients have an elevated serum alkaline phosphatase (extremely high serum alkaline phosphatase values indicate a worse prognosis), and approximately one fourth of the patients have an elevated serum lactic dehydrogenase (LDH; an elevated LDH also is associated with a worse prognosis). The remainder of the blood and urine laboratory values are normal.

The plain radiograph of an osteosarcoma is usually diagnostic. The typical lesion is located in the metaphysis, involves the medullary canal, is both lytic (radiolucent) and blastic (radiodense), and has an extraosseous component and a periosteal reaction suggestive of a rapid growth (Codman triangle or sunburst pattern). Many osteosarcomas have a soft tissue component with a fluffy density suggestive of neoplastic bone adjacent to the more obvious bone lesion. Those osteosarcomas that consist primarily of cartilage or fibrous tissue are almost purely radiolucent. Telangiectatic osteosarcoma, a histologic variant of classic high-grade osteosarcoma, may be mistaken on a radiograph for an aneurysmal bone cyst or giant cell tumor.

Linear tomograms reveal the details of the lesion better than a plain radiograph and may be useful in evaluating the extent of cortical destruction and seeing the periosteal reaction, but as is the case with most bone tumors, the CT scan and MRI are more informative. The CT scan should be performed with and without intravenous contrast, and density measurements of the lesion should be made. Density measurements are particularly helpful when determining the intraosseous extent of the tumor. Marrow fat has a negative Hounsfield density, whereas the osteosarcoma, even the most radiolucent, is more dense than water and has a positive Hounsfield value. The CT scan should include the entire bone or at least 10 cm of normal bone proximal and distal to the lesion. MRI has replaced CT as the method of choice for evaluating a suspected osteosarcoma. The lesion's extent is more clearly defined by an MRI, especially the intraosseous component. The lesion can be seen in all three planes, and its soft tissue extension is easily appreciated.

Osteosarcomas should be resected with at least a wide surgical margin, and the anatomic extent of the tumor is the principal determinant of what operation will be required. The MRI is the best method to determine the anatomic extent of an osteosarcoma. The

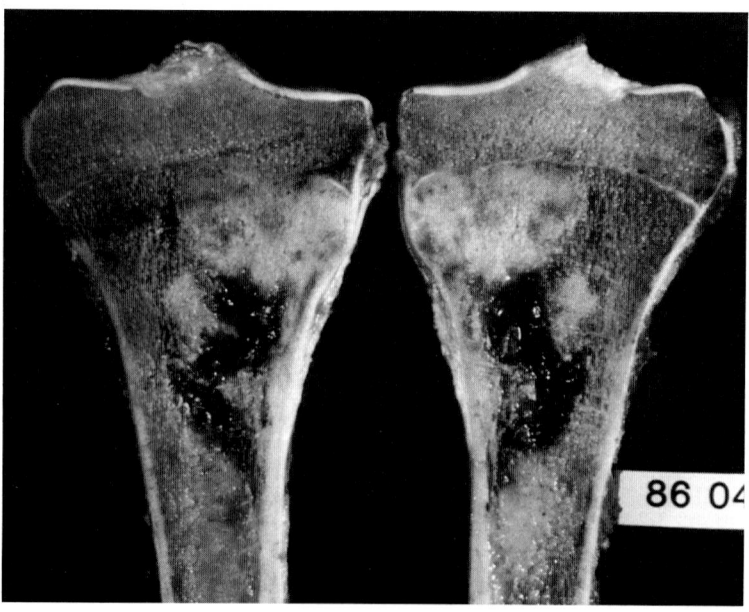

FIGURE 12-3. Classic high-grade osteosarcoma of the proximal tibia. The tibia was bisected for examination. The tumor is composed of an osteoblastic component in the metaphysis that is up to and just through the epiphyseal plate; there also is a more distal cystic component. The tumor has penetrated the cortex and has a small extracortical component. The patient had not received preoperative chemotherapy but was treated successfully with a limb-salvage resection and knee arthrodesis. The patient received postoperative adjuvant chemotherapy and has been continuously disease-free for 4 years.

relation of osteosarcoma to the major neurovascular bundle must be determined. The muscles invaded by the soft tissue extent must be identified. Involvement of the adjacent joint must be looked for, the intraosseous extent measured, and the presence of metastasis noted. Talking to the radiologist before the MRI is performed helps to assure that all this information is obtained.

A chest radiograph and a whole lung tomography or whole lung CT scan is performed because of the relatively high incidence of patients presenting with pulmonary metastasis (10%). Angiography was used prior to the development of CT scanning and MRI but is now only used when the major neurovascular bundle cannot be seen clearly on the MRI or when there is a suggestion that the vessel is encased by the tumor.

The technetium bone scan has increased uptake in the area of the tumor. Occasionally it is useful in determining the intraosseous extent, although MRI scan is more accurate. More importantly, the technetium scan is an excellent screen of the entire skeleton for occult bone lesions. On rare occasions, a lung metastasis is seen on the bone scan, but usually a hot spot in the chest on the bone scan is secondary to involvement of a rib.

There are five major histologic types of conventional osteosarcoma, and each is graded for the degree of malignancy. The histologic type is determined by the predominant cell type of the tumor. Although initially it was thought that the different types had distinct prognoses, it is recognized that if matched for size and histologic grade, all types have the same prognosis. Even the telangiectatic osteosarcoma, which was originally described as having a particularly poor prognosis, is thought to have the same prognosis as the other classic high-grade osteosarcomas.

The five types include osteoblastic, chondroblastic, fibroblastic, mixed, and telangiectatic osteosarcomas. These tumors are graded on a scale of either 1 to 3 or 1 to 4. The higher the number the histologic grade is, the worse the prognosis. Most osteosarcomas are grade 3 or 4 and of the mixed type. The tumor is composed of a mixture of neoplastic cells but must have malignant spindle cells making osteoid. Atypical mitoses are common, and small areas of necrosis are usually seen (Fig. 12-4).

Surgical resection is the treatment of choice for the primary tumor. Before the routine use of adjuvant chemotherapy, amputation was the most frequent operation performed to achieve control. Recently, limb salvage resection has been performed more often, and no increased mortality has been noted. The tumor should be resected with at least a wide surgical margin, and if this can be done without an amputation, a limb salvage operation is usually preferable. The survival with surgery alone was only 20%. In the middle 1970s, chemotherapy, initially methotrexate and later adriamycin and cisplatinum, was introduced, and the number of patients who survived dramatically increased. In the early 1980s there was controversy about the role of adjuvant chemotherapy, and some physicians suggested that osteosarcoma had become less lethal. A controlled multi-institutional study was conducted that demonstrated that adjuvant chemotherapy was important in improving survival of patients with osteosarcoma. In the past few years some studies have demonstrated that adjuvant chemotherapy has raised the overall survival for patients with osteosarcoma to over 50%. The best survival rate is found in patients with more than 90% necrosis in the primary tumor after being treated with preoperative (neoadjuvant) chemotherapy. The group in Bologna[87] report an overall survival of 51% and a disease-free survival rate of almost 70% in the patients who had greater than 90% necrosis after preoperative chemotherapy. The group in New York (Meyers and colleagues)[102] reported similar data, including a 5-year

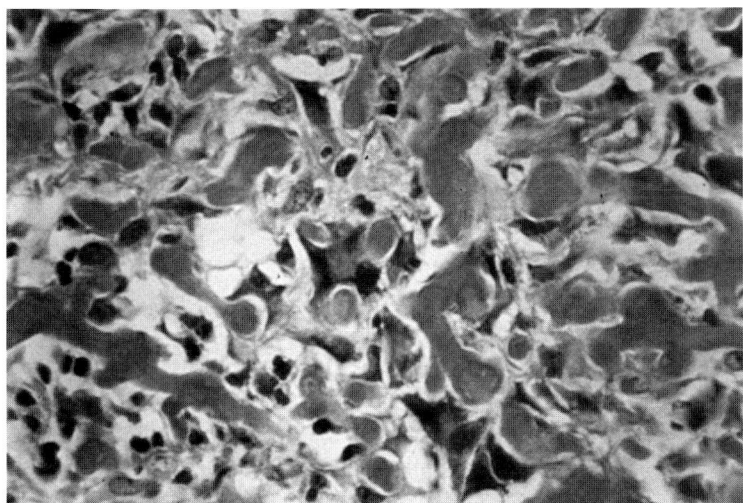

FIGURE 12-4. Histologic appearance of classic high-grade osteosarcoma. The malignant spindle cells are recognized by their abnormal variation in size and shape. No mitotic figures are seen in this photomicrograph, but abnormal mitoses usually are seen in high-grade conventional osteosarcoma. (Original magnification ×40.)

disease-free survival rate of 76% for those patients younger than 21 years who completed the T10 protocol. It is clear that all patients with classic high-grade osteosarcoma should receive adjuvant chemotherapy.

The role of preoperative chemotherapy is being evaluated.[97,102] Preoperative chemotherapy has the advantage of treating the microscopic metastatic disease at the earliest possible date, reducing the extent of the primary disease, possibly resulting in more limb salvage resections, and indicating the effectiveness of the drugs chosen. Preliminary results suggest that limb salvage is more likely to be done after two to four courses of chemotherapy. This may be because of shrinkage of the tumor or the surgeon having more confidence that the patient will not have a local recurrence, even with a close margin. Rapid advances in the management of patients with osteosarcoma are being made, and our treatment protocols are in flux.

Limb salvage surgery has become the usual treatment for all but the largest of osteosarcomas. It is unusual for a patient to need an amputation. Young children, who have not finished growing, with a primary osteosarcoma in the distal femur or proximal tibia are not ideal limb salvage candidates and are usually treated with a rotationplasty or conventional amputation. For older patients, especially those who have completed their growth, limb salvage usually provides them with the same statistical chance of being cured as does a more radical operation. The use of CT and MRI to define the limits of the tumor have made limb salvage safer than when the limits were guessed based on plain radiographs and an angiogram.

The indications for an amputation in a patient with a high-grade sarcoma are a grossly displaced pathologic fracture, encasement of the neurovascular bundle, and a tumor that enlarges during preoperative chemotherapy and is adjacent to the neurovascular bundle. It must be remembered that limb salvage requires a greater investment on the part of the patient, and the complications are greater compared with an amputation. The patient and the patient's family must understand and agree to go through what it takes to save a limb that has a high-grade sarcoma. The more distal a lesion is in the lower extremity, the less benefit a limb salvage has, but in general, a foot that has sensation is better than an artificial one. Limb salvage for osteosarcomas arising in the proximal humerus usually are safely resected without an amputation, and the benefits are obvious.

JUXTACORTICAL OSTEOSARCOMA. Osteosarcomas that arise from or adjacent to the external surface of the bone behave differently from those that arise from within the medullary canal. They are less aggressive locally, have less potential for distant metastasis, and are less common than conventional osteosarcoma. There seems to be two distinct juxtacortical osteosarcomas, parosteal and periosteal, but neither is common and how distinct they are from one another remains a topic of debate.

Geschickter and Copeland[114] were the first to describe osteosarcoma. They thought that there were two distinct lesions, a benign parosteal bone-forming tumor and a malignant bone-forming tumor, but all are defined as malignant and have the potential to metastasize. The patient's age at presentation varies over a greater range (10–45 years) than those with classic high-grade osteosarcoma, and the median age of presentation tends to be slightly older. The patient usually complains of a painless mass that blocks motion in the adjacent joint. This is most often knee flexion because the posterior distal femur is the most common site of a juxtacortical osteosarcoma. Occasionally the patient complains of a mild dull ache in the area of the tumor, but symptoms are minimal. The mass is fixed, hard, and nontender. The adjacent joint may have limited passive and active motion due to the mechanical block from the tumor. Inflammation is not observed. The patient's laboratory values are normal.

The plain radiograph is almost always diagnostic but may be mistaken for an osteocartilaginous exostosis (Fig. 12-5). The lesion arises from the cortex, which may be normal or thickened. The juxtacortical osteosarcoma often wraps around the bone with the periosteum between the tumor and the underlying cortex. This growth pattern (wrapping around the bone) produces the "string sign" on the plain radiograph with a thin radiolucent line between the lesion and the cortex of the bone. The lesion itself is dense and has the pattern of bone. There is increased uptake on the technetium bone scan. The appearance of the lesion on a CT scan is characteristic and distinguishes a juxtacortical osteosarcoma from an exostosis. Juxtacortical osteosarcoma is attached to the cortex growing out into the soft tissue and may invade the cortex, but the normal cortex is intact. An exostosis arises from the cortex, and the cortex of the normal bone becomes the cortex of the exostosis with the medullary canal of the bone communicating with the medullary canal of the exostosis. MRI scan is not necessary unless intraosseous extension is suspected.

An incisional biopsy of a juxtacortical osteosarcoma can be difficult to interpret, and often the lesion is mistakenly called an exostosis. This is particularly true when juxtacortical osteosarcoma is not suspected by the clinician or when the pathologist does not examine the radiograph. This lesion, more than most, is diagnosed by its clinical and radiographic presentation and confirmed by histology, usually obtained by an excisional biopsy. The lesion is composed of regu-

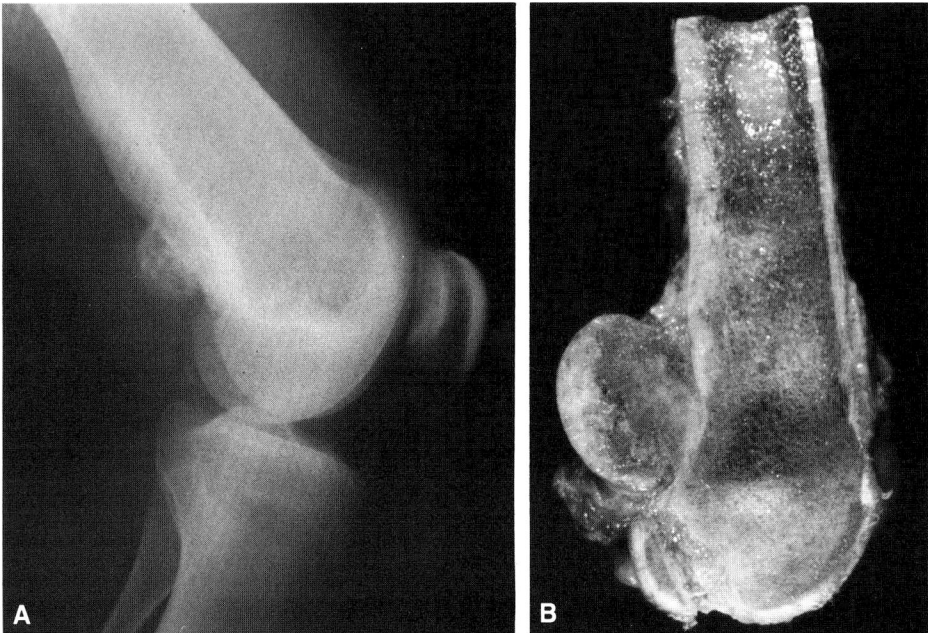

FIGURE 12-5. (A) Lateral radiograph of the distal femur and knee of a patient with a parosteal osteosarcoma. The posterior distal femoral cortex is thickened and slightly irregular. The radiodensity adjacent to the posterior cortex is the central portion of the parosteal osteosarcoma. Surrounding this bony mass is a nonossified component of the tumor composed primarily of fibrous tissue but with some cartilage. This patient was treated with a limb-salvage wide resection of the distal femur and underwent reconstruction with an osteoarticular allograft. No chemotherapy was used, and the patient has remained disease-free for 5 years. (B) The parosteal osteosarcoma is larger than it appears on plain radiograph. The cap of fibrous tissue and cartilage can be seen covering the bony center. The tumor is attached to the cortex but does not extend through it. This gross relation is similar to an exostosis and may lead to a mistaken histologic diagnosis. The gross difference between an exostosis and a parosteal osteosarcoma is that the stalk of an exostosis is cortical bone that blends with the cortex of the host bone and the medullary canal of the stalk and host bone are connected (see Fig. 12-7B). The parosteal osteosarcoma, conversely, is attached to the cortex, but the cortex of host bone is intact, and the medullary canal does not communicate with the parosteal osteosarcoma.

larly arranged bone with a background of usually bland spindle cells and fibrous tissue. A cartilage cap is often present. Recently, parosteal osteosarcomas have been graded histologically on a scale of 1 to 3. Higher grade lesions, especially those with medullary involvement, have a greater risk of metastasizing, usually to the lung, than those of lower grade without medullary extension.

When the diagnosis is made from the preoperative studies a wide excisional biopsy is recommended. The cortical margin should be generous and the tumor pseudocapsule not disturbed. When a lesion from the posterior distal femur is resected, the neurovascular bundle usually can be freed from the lesion without dissecting the pseudocapsule, but the posterior capsule of the knee and the posterior aspect of the femoral condyle should be resected with the tumor. Those lesions that wrap around the bone and have gross invasion of the medullary canal should be resected with the entire end of the bone.

The initial resection is the best opportunity to control the lesion without an amputation. Most patients do not need adjuvant chemotherapy because the cure with surgery alone is approximately 80%. Patients with a histologic grade 3 lesion probably should receive adjuvant chemotherapy, especially if the medullary canal has been invaded, although the data are limited.

The periosteal osteosarcoma is another type of juxtacortical osteosarcoma. It is most common in the anterior proximal tibia, and it tends to be diaphyseal in location. It has a sunburst appearance on the plain radiograph and is composed of malignant cartilage and bone. A wide surgical resection is recommended. The place of adjuvant chemotherapy is controversial and, as with parosteal osteosarcoma, probably only patients with a grade 3 lesion should receive it.

Cartilaginous Tumors

Cartilaginous tumors include enchondroma, exostosis (osteocartilaginous exostosis, osteochondroma), chondromyxofibroma, periosteal chondroma, chondroblastoma, and chondrosarcoma. The benign tumors are common, especially enchondroma and exostosis, whereas chondrosarcoma is extremely rare in the pediatric age group.

Enchondroma

The origin of enchondroma is debatable, and it probably is not a true neoplasia. It may be the result of epiphyseal growth cartilage that does not remodel and persists in the metaphysis, or it may be persistence of the original cartilaginous anlage of the bone. Both have been suggested as an explanation of the cause of this common benign tumor. The majority of patients with a solitary enchondroma present with either a pathologic fracture through a lesion in the phalanx, which is the most common location, or the history that the lesion was an incidental finding on a radiograph taken for another reason (Fig. 12-6). Enchondroma are common lesions and account for 11% of benign bone tumors.

Enchondroma do not need to be removed. The problem they present is one of diagnoses. Usually the diagnosis can be made from the clinical setting and plain radiograph. Forty percent are found in the bones of the hand or feet, usually a phalanx. An enchondroma should not produce symptoms unless there is a pathologic fracture. There are no associated blood or urine abnormalities. The femur and proximal humerus are the next most common sites. Enchondroma are located in the metaphysis and are central lesions in the medullary canal. The bone may be wider than normal, but this is due to the lack of remodeling in the metaphysis and not expansion of the bone by the tumor. The cortex may be thin or normal; the lesion is radiolucent in the pediatric age group but later has intralesional calcifications. There should be no periosteal reaction. In the pediatric patient, unicameral bone cysts have a similar radiographic appearance but are most common in the proximal femur and proximal humerus.

When the findings are typical for an enchondroma, no biopsy is necessary. Repeat plain radiographs and an examination should be performed in approximately 6 weeks and then every 3 to 6 months for 2 years. Although there are reports of solitary enchondroma differentiating into chondrosarcoma, usually late in adult life, it does not occur frequently enough to justify removal of all enchondroma. The patient should be advised that if after age 30 the lesion becomes painful or enlarges it should be considered a low-grade chondrosarcoma and be surgically resected.

Incisional biopsy usually is contraindicated. The pathologists have difficulty distinguishing between active enchondroma (most pediatric age patients have active lesions) and low-grade chondrosarcoma. The clinical course is the best measure of the lesion's significance, and an incisional biopsy alters the status of the lesion and make subsequent evaluation difficult. If the patient or the patient's parents insist on biopsy, it is best that the entire lesion be removed.

Patients with multiple enchondroma are much less common than those with a solitary enchondroma. Multiple enchondroma was originally described in the late 1800s by Ollier.[121] Most patients with Ollier disease have bilateral involvement but with unilateral predominance. These patients have growth deformities, both angular and in length. Their extremity deformities should be managed surgically to maintain function of the limbs without specific regard to the enchondroma. Patients with Ollier disease have an increased risk of developing a secondary chondrosarcoma later in life and should be so advised. The incidence of secondary chondrosarcoma in patients with Ollier disease is not known but may be as high as 25%. The pelvis and shoulder girdle are the most common locations of secondary chondrosarcoma.

Maffucci disease consists of multiple enchondroma and soft tissue hemangioma.[117] These patients have an even greater risk of developing a malignant

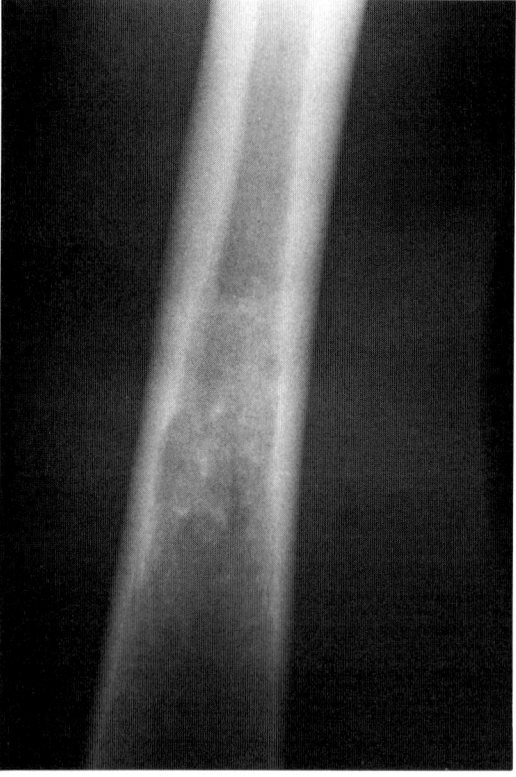

FIGURE 12-6. Anteroposterior radiograph of an enchondroma in the distal femoral shaft. Although this humor is radiolucent in children, intralesional calcification usually occurs later; these flakes of intramedullary calcification are seen in adults. The lesion is spherical, and there is no evidence of periosteal or medullary reaction. In children, enchondromas do not need specific treatment, and malignancy is almost unknown. If there is a pathologic fracture, closed treatment can be used. This patient was not operated on but had no pain or change in the lesion for 3 years after first being seen.

cartilage tumor than patient's with Ollier disease and, more importantly, they have a great risk of developing a carcinoma of an internal organ.[119]

Exostosis

This lesion was first described in the early 1800s. It is very common and accounts for approximately 50% of benign bone tumors. Although the etiology of this lesion is not known, an abnormality or injury to the periphery of the growth plate has been suggested as the cause. It has been shown in an experimental animal study that the periphery of the growth plate can be traumatized and a typical exostosis produced.

The patient with the solitary exostosis usually is brought in by a parent who has just noticed a mass adjacent to a joint. The patient usually has no symptoms. An occasional patient has loss of motion in the adjacent joint due to the size of the mass. The patient often has been aware of the mass for months to years and reports that it has been slowly enlarging. Some patients have pain due to irritation of an overlying muscle, repeated trauma, pressure on adjacent neurovascular bundle, or inflammation in an overlying bursa. On physical examination the mass is nontender, hard, and fixed to the bone. The remainder of the physical examination is normal.

Exostoses are so characteristic on a plain radiograph that they should be diagnosed from their radiographic appearance alone (Fig. 12-7). The mass is a combination of a radiolucent cartilaginous cap with varying amounts of ossification and calcification. The amount of calcification and bone formation increases with age. The base may be broad (sessile exostosis) or narrow (pedunculated exostosis). In both types the cortex of the underlying bone opens to join the cortex of the exostosis so that the medullary canal of the bone is in continuity. This usually can be appreciated on

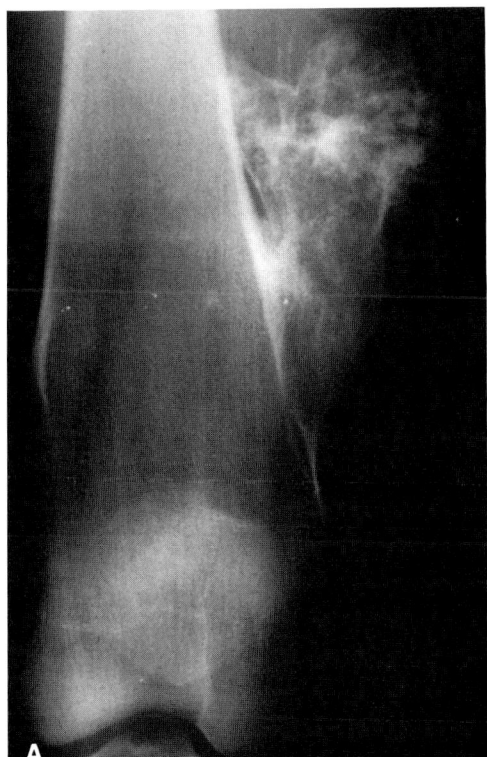
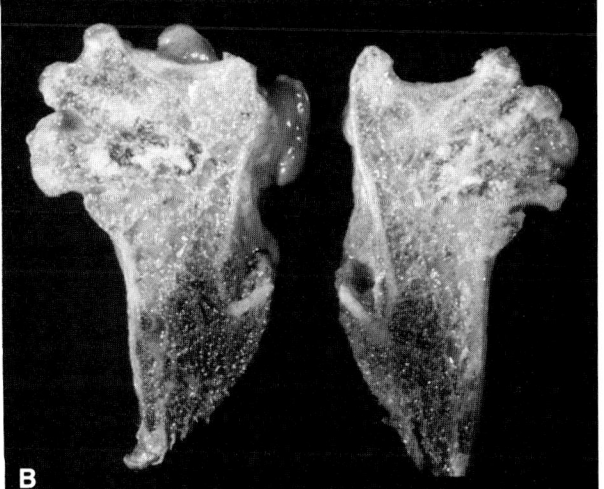

FIGURE 12-7. (A) Anteroposterior radiograph of the distal femur with a typical pedunculated exostosis. The cortex of the lesion blends into the cortex of the femur. The exostosis has an irregular proximal end that is covered by a cartilaginous cap. The pathologic material is the cartilage, but what is seen on a radiograph is the bone formed by enchondral ossification of the cartilage. This patient repeatedly hit the mass while playing football, and it was marginally excised. A small rim of the cortex of the femur was removed along with the exostosis, because ocasionally, any residual cartilage that lies at the base of the stalk can lead to a recurrence. (B) Gross bisected specimen from the patient in **A**. The femoral attachment is inferior, and the cortex of the femur can be seen blending with the cortex of the exostosis. The medullary canal of the femur is filled with hematopoietic marrow and appears dark. The hematopoietic marrow extends into the base of the exostosis, but most of the marrow of the exostosis is fatty. There is a thin, cartilaginous cap. In a child, a cartilaginous cap more than 1 cm thick is of no concern, but in an adult, a cartilaginous cap of more than 1 cm is considered to indicate early malignant degeneration to secondary chondrosarcoma.

the plain radiograph, but if not a CT scan or an MRI establishes this finding and confirms the diagnosis.

In the pediatric age group exostoses should be expected to grow. They may continue to grow well into the third decade of life. The growth rate is not steady, and occasionally a lesion grows more rapidly than expected. Removal of the lesion in a child is indicated only for those patients who have symptoms due to pressure on a neurovascular bundle or irritation of the overlying muscle. Removal in a young child may result in damage to the growth plate and recurrence of the lesion. Malignant degeneration is extremely rare in children and uncommon in adults. Malignant degeneration is more common in lesions in the scapula, the pelvis, and the proximal femur.

Gross examination of an exostosis reveals a lesion that looks like a cauliflower. It has an irregular surface covered with cartilage. The cartilage is usually less than 1-cm thick, except in the young child, in which it may be 2- or 3-cm thick. In an adult, when the cartilaginous cap is thicker than 1 cm, a secondary chondrosarcoma should be suspected. Deep to the cartilaginous cap there is a variable amount of calcification, enchondral ossification, and normal bone with a cortex and cancellous marrow cavity. The microscopic appearance of the cartilaginous cap typically is benign hyaline cartilage.

Some patients have multiple exostoses.[128,130,131] A patient may have three or four lesions but more often has more than 20. Usually the patient has exostoses of all shapes and sizes. They are concentrated in the metaphysis of the long bones but may be in the spine, the ribs, the pelvis, and the scapula. On physical examination they are hard fixed masses adjacent to joints. Patients with multiple exostoses usually are shorter than average but not below the normal range. They have loss of motion in affected joints, especially forearm rotation, elbow extension, hip abduction and adduction, and ankle inversion and eversions.

Multiple hereditable exostosis is transmitted by an autosomal dominant gene with a variable penetrance, and usually half of the children of an affected parent have clinical manifestations. An extensively involved parent may have a child with minimal involvement or vice versa. The majority of patients with multiple hereditable exostoses have a radiographic appearance of the proximal femur, which is diagnostic. The femoral neck is short and broad with multiple bony excrescences.

After the age of 30 years, patients with multiple hereditable exostoses have an increased risk of developing a secondary chondrosarcoma. Secondary chondrosarcoma in the pediatric age group is extremely rare. Occasionally one or more of the exostoses are removed to relieve the pain related to repeated local trauma or improve the motion of the adjacent joint. Those lesions in the pelvis and spine should be observed the closest because they have the greatest risk of undergoing malignant degeneration. I do not recommend removing these lesions simply because they are present.

I advise patients with exostosis, whether single or multiple, to be examined and have a radiograph at least yearly. Patients are told to report symptoms or increasing size immediately. Patients older than 30 years of age with an enlarging exostosis should have it removed as if it were a secondary chondrosarcoma, because this usually is the case.[6]

Chondromyxofibroma

Chondromyxofibroma is a rare tumor. The patient is usually a male (males are more frequently affected than females at a ratio of 2:1) in the second or third decade of life. The patient complains of a dull steady pain that is usually worse at night. The only positive physical finding is tenderness over the involved area, and occasionally a deep mass can be appreciated. Approximately one third of chondromyxofibromas occur in the tibia, usually proximal. It is a radiolucent lesion that involves the medullary canal but is eccentric and erodes the cortex (Fig. 12-8). It may be covered only

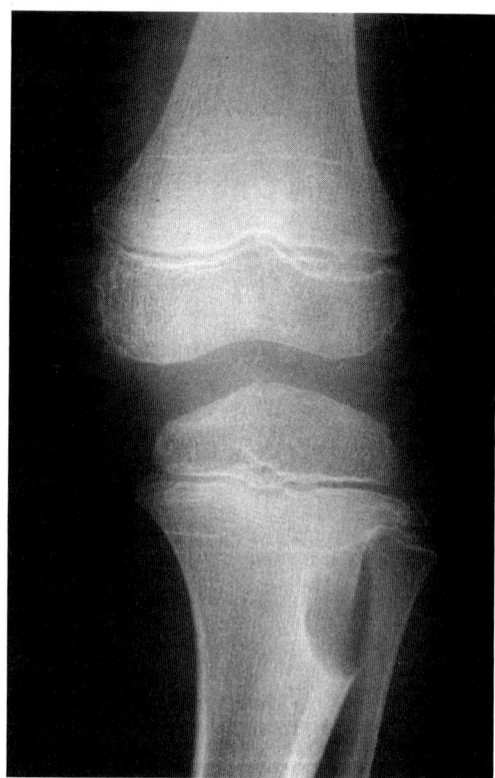

FIGURE 12-8. Anteroposterior radiograph of a chondromyxofibroma of the proximal lateral tibia. The lesion is typically an eccentric, radiolucent abnormality that usually destroys the cortex but is contained by the periosteum. As in this case, the radiographic appearance of chondromyxofibroma is often similar to that of an aneurysmal bone cyst.

by periosteum and is often mistaken for the more common aneurysmal bone cyst. The natural history is not known because of infrequency and usual surgical lesion. A thorough curettage and bone grafting is recommended.

Chondroblastoma

Chondroblastoma, or Codman tumor, initially was thought to be a variant of giant cell tumor of bone. Codman's detailed description in 1931 was of an "epiphyseal chondromatous giant cell tumor."[132] Jaffe and Liechtenstein, in 1941, suggested that it be called "benign chondroblastoma" and separated it from giant cell tumor of bone.[137] Codman was particularly interested in the shoulder, and he thought this lesion was found principally in the proximal humerus (Fig. 12-9). It has since become clear that chondroblastoma is found in many bones, but the proximal humerus is the most common site (approximately 20%).

Chondroblastoma accounts for 1% of bone tumors. The patient with a chondroblastoma is usually in the second decade of life with an open growth plate, but it occurs in older patients as well. The initial symptoms are of pain in the joint adjacent to the lesion, and the patient usually presents with joint complaints. The findings on physical examination also may suggest an intraarticular disorder because most patients have an effusion and diminished motion in the adjacent joint. Frequently the patient is believed to have chronic synovitis; he or she does not have other symptoms or abnormal physical findings. The patient's laboratory data is normal.

The lesion arises in the secondary ossification center. In children it is the most common neoplastic lesion of the secondary ossification center, and in adults only giant cell tumor of bone involves the secondary ossification center more often. On the plain radiograph the lesion is radiolucent, usually with small foci of calcification. The calcification is best seen on linear tomography or a CT scan. There is usually a reactive rim of bone surrounding the lesion and sometimes metaphyseal periosteal reaction. There is increased uptake on a technetium bone scan. Chondroblastoma and osteochondritis dissecans can have a similar appearance on the plain radiograph, but they should not be confused with one another. Osteochondritis dissecans produces an abnormality in the subchondral bone, but the subchondral bone is almost always normal. Patients with chondroblastoma have more of an effusion than patients with osteochondritis dissecans, and their pain is constant and not related to activity, as in patients with osteochondritis dissecans.

The histologic appearance of chondroblastoma is typical and is rarely confused with other diagnoses. It consists of small cuboidal cells, chondroblasts, closely packed together to give the appearance of a cobblestone street. In addition, there are areas with varying amounts of amorphous matrix, which often contains streaks of calcification, and usually there are numerous multinucleated giant cells. Chondroblastoma are not as vascular as osteoblastoma, and there are few if any mitoses and no abnormal mitoses (Fig. 12-10).

Chondroblastomas progress and invade the joint. They should be treated when found. Curettage is the treatment of choice, but it must be a thorough curettage and extend beyond the reactive rim. The lesion should be seen adequately at the time of the curettage, which usually means the joint must be opened. Iatrogenic seeding of a joint is not a significant risk, and an intraarticular surgical exposure is recommended if this facilitates visualization. The majority of recur-

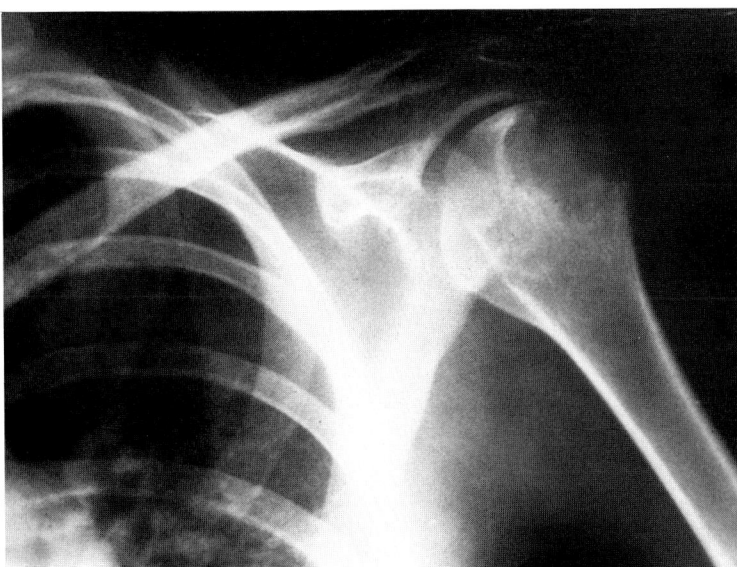

FIGURE 12-9. Radiograph of a chondroblastoma in the proximal humeral epiphysis. This is a typical Codman tumor. The lesion is both epiphyseal and metaphyseal, has an irregular reactive border, and has intralesional calcifications, although these are difficult to see on plain radiographs. Giant cell tumor of bone is similar to chondroblastoma except that there are no intralesional calcifications. This patient was treated with a curettage and bone grafting.

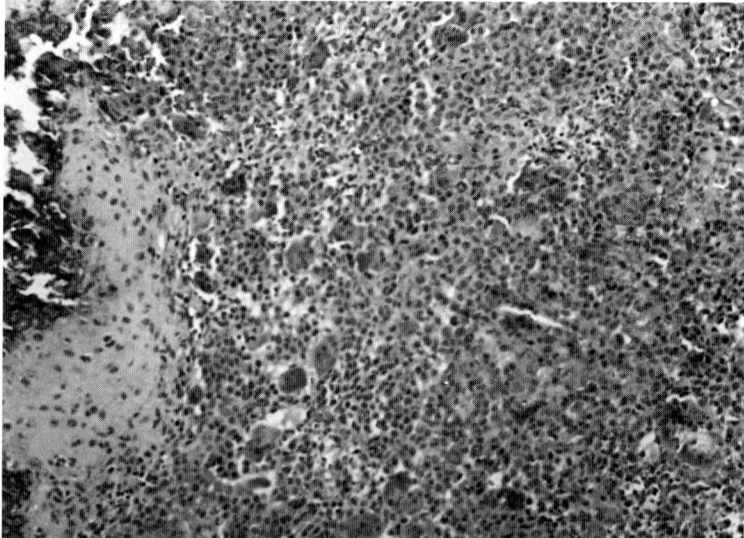

FIGURE 12-10. Histologic appearance of a chondroblastoma. The tumor consists of cuboidal cells (i.e., chondroblasts), varying amounts of amorphous matrix (some of which is calcified), and multinucleated giant cells. Calcification is seen (*left*). The cuboidal cells fit together in such a manner that they have the appearance of cobblestones. (Original magnification ×10.)

rences are cured with a second curettage, but a rare lesion usually is locally aggressive and requires a wide resection.[139] Chondroblastoma of the pelvis frequently behaves more aggressively than those in long bones, and an initial wide excision is recommended.

Most patients are close to skeletal maturity when the diagnosis is made and the risk of growth disturbance from the tumor or its treatment is minimal. When the patient is younger than 10 years old, care should be taken not to damage the growth plate.

Periosteal Chondroma

This is an uncommon lesion that arises from the surface of the cortex, deep to the periosteum. The patient usually complains of pain at the site of the lesion. More than half are found in the proximal humerus, and the others are evenly dispersed through the long bones. The lesion often can be palpated. It is a nontender, hard mass, fixed to the bone. The plain radiograph is typical (Fig. 12-11). It is a scalloped defect on the outer surface of the cortex, occasionally with intralesional calcifications and minimal periosteal reaction. Microscopically periosteal chondroma is benign cartilage but looks more active than an enchondroma. They have been mistaken for chondrosarcoma. A wide excision including the underlying cortex is the treatment of choice.

Lesions of Fibrous Origin

Nonossifying Fibroma

Nonossifying fibroma, which is also known as fibroma of bone, nonosteogenic fibroma, metaphyseal fibrous defect, and fibrous cortical defect, is probably the most common lesion of bone. Up to 40% of children have this lesion, found most often between the ages of 4 and 8 years. Ninety percent are in the distal femur. These are asymptomatic lesions and are found only if a radiograph is taken for another reason or when the patient has a pathologic fracture. The patient has no abnormal physical findings, and the serum and urine chemistries are normal.

Nonossifying fibroma should be recognized based on the clinical presentation and plain radiographic

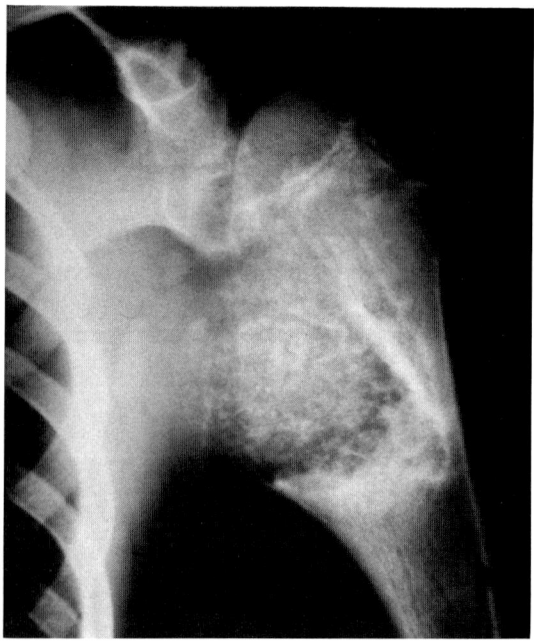

FIGURE 12-11. Radiograph of the shoulder of a 12-year-old boy. The large periosteal chondroma involves the medial aspect of the metaphysis. Most such tumors are smaller. The patient had no symptoms; the lesion was found by the boy's pediatrician on routine physical examination, and an incisional biopsy confirmed the diagnosis. The lesion was only partially removed. The tumor did not change appreciably during 2 years of follow-up.

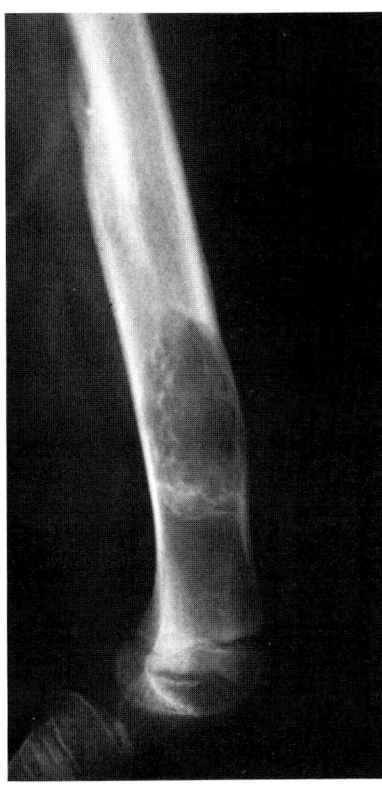

FIGURE 12-12. Lateral radiograph of the distal femur with a large nonossifying fibroma (NOF). The patient had sustained a pathologic fracture that had healed, but the lesion persisted. NOF is usually a metaphyseal, radiolucent, irregular lesion surrounded by a reactive rim of bone. As is often the case, the cortex surrounding a large NOF is thin and appears to be expanded. Although this lesion eventually heals spontaneously, its large size and persistence after pathologic fracture indicated that curettage and bone grafting were necessary. Nonossifying fibromas that replace more than one half of the bone should be curetted and grafted.

mosiderin within the fibroblastic stromal cells and multinucleated giant cells is usual. There is no bone formation within the lesion, and mitoses are not seen.

The small cortical lesion (fibrous cortical defect) needs no treatment but should be observed. Repeat radiographs at 3- to 6-month intervals for 1 to 2 years are suggested. These lesions should heal spontaneously. Nonossifying fibroma may need surgery. Nonossifying fibromas that are less than 50% of the diameter of the bone scan can merely be observed, but they should be curetted and packed with bone graft if they enlarge. Patients with a nonossifying fibroma with larger than 50% of the diameter of the bone probably should have the lesion curetted and packed with bone graft. According to Arata and colleagues[140] these patients have an increased risk of developing a pathologic fracture. Operative treatment also is recommended for the patient around 13 years of age whose lesion does not appear to be healing and who is active in sports.

Patients that present with a pathologic fracture should have the fracture treated nonoperatively if possible. The fracture should heal without difficulty in a normal length of time. There is no evidence that the healing of the fracture increases the chances of spontaneous healing of a nonossifying fibroma or of any other benign lesion. Nonossifying fibroma usually heals spontaneously, which may happen after the fracture, but usually the fracture callus obscures the radiolucent lesion, and the physician is fooled into thinking that the lesion is healing. When the callus has remodeled and the cortices become distinct on the radiograph, the lesion can be seen again. Patients with

findings. Biopsy for diagnosis is rarely necessary. There are two radiographic appearances seen. The more common fibroma is a small (<0.5 cm) radiolucent lesion within the cortex with a sharply defined border. Most authors call this lesion a fibrous cortical defect. There is little or no increased uptake on the technetium bone scan.

The other appearance is that of a metaphyseal lesion eccentrically located (Fig. 12-12). This lesion probably started out as a fibrous cortical defect but continued to enlarge. It appears to have arisen from within the cortex expanding into the medullary cavity and rising the periosteum. The lesion is surrounded by a well-defined thin rim of reactive bone. There should be no acute periosteal reaction unless there has been a fracture. There may be slight increased uptake on the technetium bone scan. This lesion is called a nonossifying fibroma.

Both lesions consists of benign, spindle, fibroblastic cells arranged in a storiform pattern (Fig. 12-13). Multinucleated giant cells are common, and areas of large lipid laden macrophages often can be seen. He-

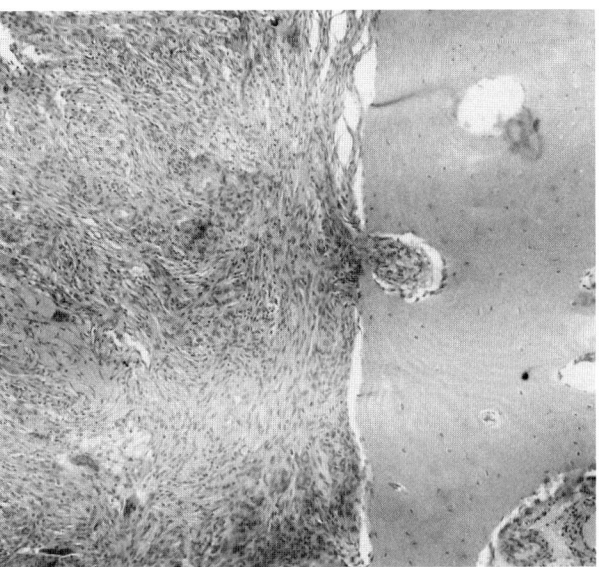

FIGURE 12-13. Low-power histological view of a typical nonossifying fibroma. The fibroma is composed of benign fibrous tissue and multinucleated giant cells. Hemosiderin is often present. The nonossifying fibroma is invading cortical bone (*right*). (Original magnification ×10.)

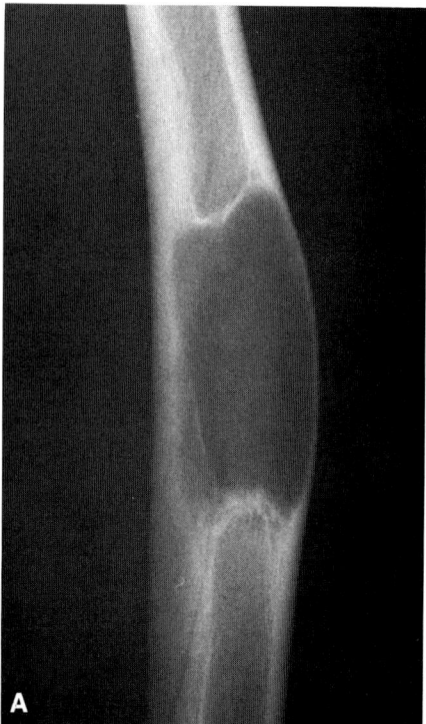

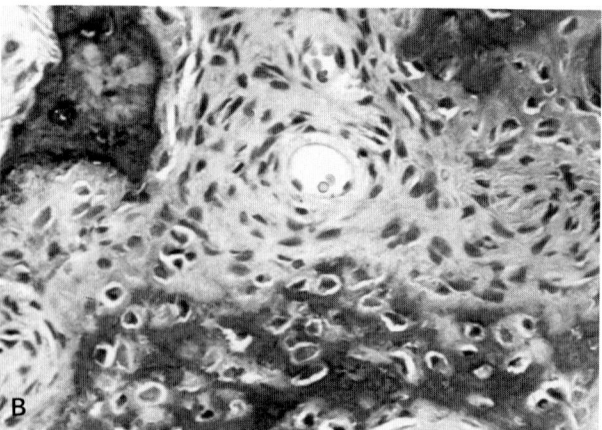

FIGURE 12-14. (A) Radiograph of a fibrous dysplasia in the diaphysis of a long bone. The ground-glass appearance, the thin cortex, and the angular deformity of the bone are all typical features of fibrous dysplasia. Because this lesion was large and the patient had an angular deformity, a cortical bone graft was placed within the cortex to increase the strength of the bone. Curettage of the lesion probably does not increase local control but should be performed if it can be carried out easily. Fibrous dysplastic bone is structurally weak, and cortical grafts are more likely to improve the strength of the bone and not be resorbed by the host. (B) Histologic appearance of fibrous dysplasia. The tumor is mostly fibrous tissue composed of collagen and fibroblast. Small bits of bone and osteoid, often having a C or O shape, seem to have been sprinkled on the fibrous tissue. Osteoblasts are not seen, and the bone seems to be produced by the fibroblastic cells. (Original magnification × 40)

pathologic fractures must be followed until the callus has remodeled sufficiently so that a final determination can be made about the status of the underlying nonossifying fibroma. If it persists after the fracture has healed, curettage and bone grafting is suggested.

Fibrous Dysplasia

Fibrous dysplasia probably is not a true neoplasia but a developmental abnormality. It is a common disorder that produces a variety of complaints and physical findings. The majority of patients (approximately 85%) have a single skeletal lesion, monostotic fibrous dysplasia, whereas the remainder have numerous lesions (polyostotic fibrous dysplasia). The patients with polyostotic fibrous dysplasia may have only two or three small areas of involvement or may have extensive skeletal abnormalities with grossly deformed bones.

The patient with monostotic fibrous dysplasia usually presents without symptoms, and the lesion found when a radiograph is taken for unrelated reasons. Occasionally the child presents with a pathologic fracture or angular deformity. A rib is the most common location of monostotic fibrous dysplasia, but any bone can be involved. There are no physical findings associated with monostotic fibrous dysplasia, and the cafe-au-lait lesions and endocrine abnormalities sometimes found in patients with polyostotic fibrous dysplasia are extremely rare in those with the monostotic variant. Serum and urine chemistries are normal in patients with fibrous dysplasia.

The plain radiograph is often diagnostic, although the radiographic appearance of fibrous dysplasia is variable (Fig. 12-14A). It is a medullary process that is less dense than cortical bone, typically producing a ground glass appearance on the radiograph. The lesion is usually diaphyseal. The diaphysis is larger than normal, and the ground glass appearance of the medullary canal blends into the thinned cortex so that it is difficult to define the border between the medullary canal and the cortex. There may be an angular deformity in the bone, especially when the lesion is large. The lesions may mature with age and become radiodense or cystic. Fibrous dysplasia has excessive uptake on a technetium bone scan, out of proportion to what one might predict from the plain radiographic appearance.

The patient with polyostotic fibrous dysplasia usually presents around the age of 10 years, complaining of an angular deformity of a bone. The most common deformity is varus of the proximal femur, or shepherd's crook deformity. Their patients have light brown skin lesions with an irregular border. These are called coast of Maine café-au-lait spots. The smooth bordered lesions associated with neurofibromatosis are called "coast of California café-au-lait spots."

Hyperthyroidism and diabetes mellitus have been reported as associated endocrinopathies, and vascular tumors have been seen in association with fibrous dysplasia. Albright syndrome is a triad of fibrous dysplasia, café-au-lait spots, and precocious puberty.[143] The lesions in polyostotic fibrous dysplasia tend to be more unilateral than bilateral. The radiographic appearance of the lesion is the same as in patients with monostotic disease. The structural strength of the bones with fibrous dysplasia is reduced as a result of the poorly organized trabecular pattern and the thinned cortex. The weakness of the bones leads to the deformities usually present.

Microscopically, fibrous dysplasia, both the monostotic and polyostotic forms, is composed of fibrous tissue with normal-appearing nuclei and irregularly shaped strands of osteoid and bone (Fig. 12-14B). There are few if any osteoblasts present, and the osteoid and bone seem to arise directly from the background fibrous stoma. The bone is irregularly organized and is often C-shaped or O-shaped.

Multinucleated giant cells are rare in fibrous dysplasia, and there should be few mitoses, and none of these cells should be abnormal. Nodules of cartilage may be present in typical fibrous dysplasia.

Treatment should be directed toward providing sufficient strength for the skeleton to function. Many of the monostotic lesions need no treatment because they pose no problems for the patient. Angular deformity should be straightened and the bone augmented with cortical bone graft with or without internal fixation. The proximal femoral neck is a common location for these patients, and they often have hip pain secondary to fatigue fractures. Enneking and Gearen[144] recommend a cortical strut graft to strengthen the bone and relieve the patient's symptoms. Internal fixation can be added, if necessary. There probably is no benefit in removing the dysplastic bone, and no extra effort should be made to do so. Cortical bone graft is preferred to cancellous bone because it is less likely to be remodeled by the host. The patient replaces cancellous bone graft with dysplastic bone. Allograft may be superior to autogenous graft because it is resorbed even more slowly.

Osteofibrous Dysplasia

Kempson[154] described the osteofibrous dysplasia lesion, which is found in the mandible and the anterior cortex and the tibia of children. It is benign but may be locally aggressive. It is *not* a healing nonossifying fibroma. The patients usually do not have symptoms and usually are brought to the physician's attention by a parent who has noticed an anterior bowing or mass in the tibia. The lesion is located within the anterior cortex and is best seen on the lateral radiograph (Fig. 12-15). There are usually numerous radiolucent lesions with a rim of reactive bone. There is increased uptake on the technetium bone scan in the area of the lesion.

Although Kempson[154] suggested the name ossifying fibroma, the more commonly used term is osteofibrous dysplasia. Some authors believe osteofibrous dysplasia is a type of fibrous dysplasia, but this is con-

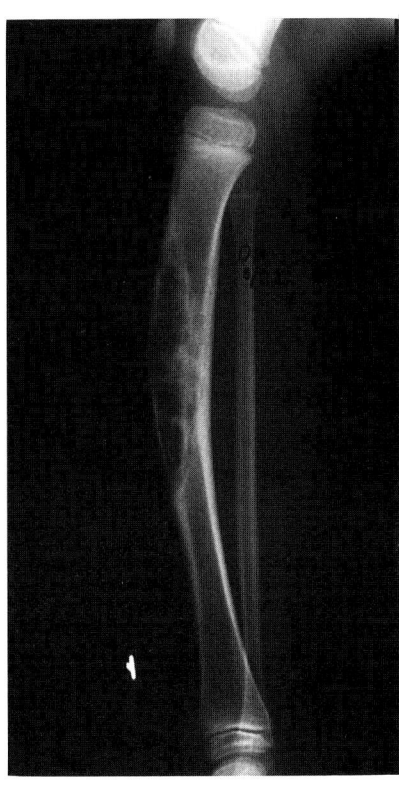

FIGURE 12-15. Lateral radiograph of the leg of a patient with an ossifying fibroma. Found almost exclusively in the tibia, the lesions involve the anterior cortex and can extend into the medullary canal. The tibia commonly has an anterior bow.

troversial. Fibrous dysplasia has numerous characteristics that osteofibrous dysplasia does not have. Fibrous dysplasia arises from the medullary canal and rarely produces bowing of the tibia. It rarely recurs after curettage and is not an aggressive lesion unless the patient has polyostotic disease. Osteofibrous dysplasia, on the other hand, arises from the cortex and involves the medullary canal late. It usually is associated with a bowed tibia and quickly recurs if curetted. It usually requires a resection for control. There have been few studies of patients with osteofibrous dysplasia with adequate follow-up, but the evidence is that most are eventually resected.

I recommend observation of the lesion when it is found in a patient younger than 10 years of age. Bracing may not prevent progressive bowing but can be tried if there is an angular deformity. If the lesion progresses, resection is suggested. If the patient presents after the age of 10 years, especially if the lesion is large or has aggressive features on the plane radiographs, a biopsy is suggested to rule out an adamantinoma. An adamantinoma probably requires a wider resection than does an enlarging osteofibrous dysplasia.

Adamantinoma has a similar clinical presentation to osteofibrous dysplasia. In adamantinoma, however, usually the patient is older (third decade of life), and the lesion appears more aggressive in the radiographs (e.g., soft tissue extension, acute periosteal reaction, large, involvement of the medullary canal), but this is not always the case. It has been suggested that there is another type of adamantinoma that looks extremely similar to osteofibrous dysplasia, even with examination of the histology. One must be suspicious of the diagnosis of osteofibrous dysplasia, especially in a progressive lesion in a patient over 10 years of age.[153]

If a lesion suspected of being an osteofibrous dysplasia is going to be observed the patient should have a radiograph at least every 6 months until it heals or until it is resected. Typical adamantinoma has a risk of metastasizing, but it is not known if the adamantinoma that looks like osteofibrous dysplasia can metastasize.

Miscellaneous Lesions

Eosinophilic Granuloma

In 1941, Farber suggested that eosinophilic granuloma, Hand-Schüller-Christian disease, and Letterer-Siwe disease were related.[196] Lichtenstein and Jaffe believed that this concept was ill-founded. Lichtenstein published an article agreeing with Farber and suggested the term histiocytosis X.[198] Langerhans cell histiocytosis is another term that is used.[200,201] This is a disorder of the histiocytes and, although they are a common component of the lesion, eosinophils are not necessary for the diagnosis (Fig. 12-16).

Eosinophilic granuloma usually occurs in patients between the ages of 5 and 15 years. The skull is the most commonly involved bone. Many of the skull lesions probably are not diagnosed because the only abnormality is a painless, small, spontaneously resolving lump in the scalp. The vertebral bodies and the ilium are then next most common sites of involvement. Those lesions in long bones may weaken the bone sufficiently that the patient presents with activity related pain suggestive of a fatigue fracture, or they present with a pathologic fracture. The lesion is a radiolucent abnormality with sharp borders of transition and often no reaction by the host bone. An apparent central sequestrum of bone may be seen. Eosinophilic granuloma usually results in an increased uptake on a technetium bone scan.

It was believed that eosinophilic granuloma needed to be treated, and many children received irradiation, curettage, or an excision. At present, it is believed that the majority of the lesions are self healing, and no specific treatment is necessary.[200] Intralesional injection of corticosteroids has been recommended by some physicians. Patients with Hand-Schüller-Christian disease should be treated with systemic corticosteroids or chemotherapy.

Despite anecdotal reports, there are no documented cases of eosinophilic granuloma progressing to Hand-Schüller-Christian syndrome. Such reports may be the result of inadequate evaluation of some patients at the time of their initial presentation. When a patient with eosinophilic granuloma is being evaluated, it is best to obtain a radiograph of the skull and collect a first-voided urine specimen after overnight fluid restriction to test the patient's ability to concentrate urine.

Unicameral Bone Cysts

Unicameral bone cysts are not always unicameral. They also are called simple bone cysts, but they may not be simple to treat. These common lesions usually are found when the patient sustains a pathologic frac-

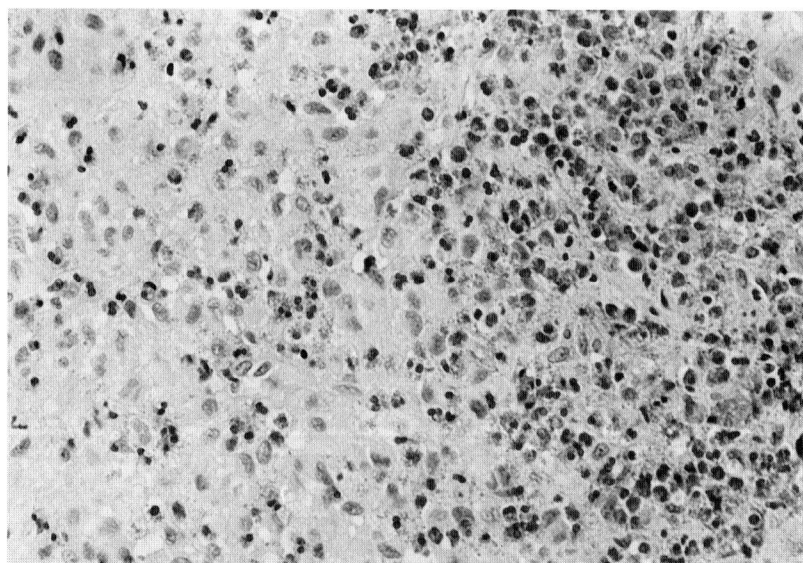

FIGURE 12-16. Low-power view of an eosinophilic granuloma (Langerhans granuloma). The eosinophils are numerous, but it is the presence of histiocytes that define this tumor. The histiocytes are large cells with a clear folded nucleus and a prominent nucleolus. (Original magnification ×10.)

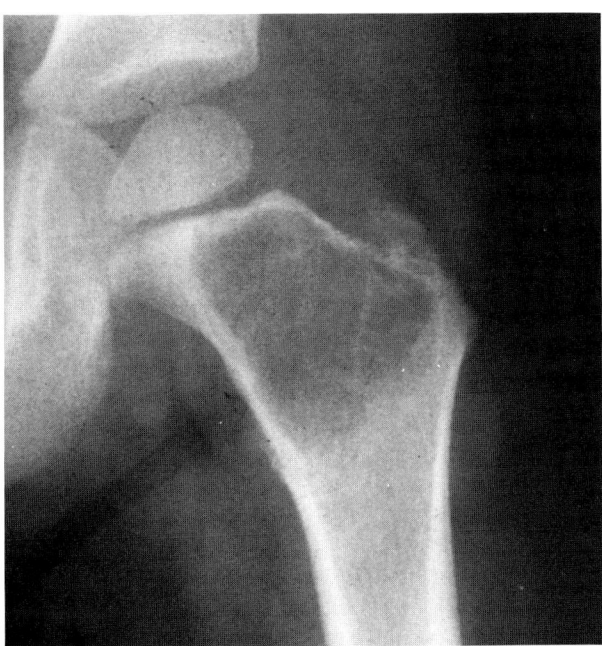

FIGURE 12-17. Anteroposterior radiograph of a proximal femoral unicameral bone cyst (UBC). UBCs are radiolucent lesions immediately adjacent to the growth plate that extend into the metaphysis. This UBC is considered active because it is immediately adjacent to the growth plate and the patient is younger than 10 years old. Large lesions in the proximal femur should be treated because of the risk of pathologic fracture. Initial treatment should be a corticosteroid injection.

ture. Their radiographic appearance is so typical that most can be diagnosed without a biopsy (Fig. 12-17). The proximal humerus and the proximal femur account for 90% of unicameral bone cysts. The cysts seem to arise from the epiphyseal plate and are immediately adjacent to the plate extending into the metaphysis. The metaphyseal bone does not remodel, and the metaphysis is broader than normal but not broader than the width of the epiphyseal plate. A thin rim of bone borders the unicameral bone cyst. The surrounding bone is not reactive, and there is no acute periosteal reaction. When the cyst becomes mature (latent), usually after the patient reaches the age of 10, the epiphysis grows away from the lesion. The unicameral bone cyst eventually heals spontaneously and fills in with bone. No evidence of its previous existence is seen.

Treatment is to prevent a pathologic fracture. Some lesions remain small and do not present a significant risk to the patient. Other lesions are so large (e.g., proximal humeral lesions), in high-stress anatomic sites (e.g., the femoral neck), or persist after the patient has become a young adult that treatment is indicated. Only those patients who have a unicameral bone cyst that is at risk for a pathologic fracture should be treated. Injection is recommended rather than an operative procedure because the results of injection are equal to curettage and bone grafting, whereas the risk, recovery, and cost are less. Intracyst injection of corticosteroids is the treatment of choice as an initial means of stimulating the cyst to heal.[163,164] Prior to the common use of corticosteroid injections, curettage and autogenous bone graft had been the most common treatment. Numerous other methods have been used but none have been universally successful. Operative treatment with curettage and autogenous bone graft is reserved for those lesions that do not respond to repeated injections of corticosteroid. The injection of autogenous bone marrow is a new technique that has not been completely evaluated.

The injection of corticosteroid was introduced by Scaglietti.[164] It has been used extensively and is an established method of treatment of a unicameral bone cyst. It should be performed with anesthesia (usually general anesthesia) and with the aid of fluoroscopic visualization. An 18- or 20-gauge spinal needle is passed percutaneously into the cyst. The wall of the cyst is penetrated easily by an 18-gauge needle with the stylet in place. Rotating the needle as it is pushed through the bone often helps it penetrate the cortex. Clear yellow or slightly bloody fluid should be obtained. If no fluid is aspirated, the diagnosis of unicameral bone cyst should be questioned and the lesion biopsied.

Once the fluid has been withdrawn, a second needle is introduced into the cyst as far from the first as possible.[7] A radiopaque dye (usually Renografin 60) is injected into the cyst to confirm that it is unicameral and that all parts are filled with dye. Frequently the draining veins are seen shortly after the cyst is injected. If the cyst has more than one cavity each should be injected.

It is not known if the type of corticosteroid used is important, but I use methylprednisolone acetate (Depo-Medrol). There is no standard amount of corticosteroid. Usually 80 mg is sufficient for a small cyst, and up to 160 mg may be used for large cysts. There are two techniques for corticosteroid injection. One is to inject the corticosteroid under pressure, with the second needle occluded, to rupture the cyst wall. The other is to inject the corticosteroid without pressure, using the second needle as a vent. It is unclear which method is better, but injecting under pressure may be dangerous and I do not use this technique.

A repeat radiograph is taken in 1 month, and if there is no evidence of early healing (e.g., increased thickness of the reactive wall) a repeat injection is done. I do not inject lesions more than 3 times, but some physicians have injected cysts 8 to 10 times.

The rare unicameral bone cyst that requires operative treatment should be curetted and packed with bone graft. When the cyst is adjacent to the growth plate, care should be taken not to damage the epiphyseal cartilage during the curettage. Autogenous bone or allograft cortical cancellous bone can be used to pack the cavity. Freeze-dried cortical cancellous allograft is particularly advantageous because it is associated with an excellent healing rate and little if any incidence of complications, and no secondary incision is required to obtain the autogenous bone graft.

Aneurysmal Bone Cysts

Aneurysmal bone cyst is a controversial lesion. Some believe that this lesion occurs only in association with another bone tumor, whereas others recognize aneurysmal bone cysts as a primary diagnosis. Aneurysmal bone cysts often occur in association with a number of benign tumors (e.g., giant cell tumor, chondroblastoma, osteoblastoma) or with osteosarcoma. When it is a secondary lesion the primary lesion usually is obvious, and the aneurysmal bone cyst component is limited to only a small portion of the tumor. Secondary aneurysmal bone cysts are classified with their underlying diagnosis. The presence of a secondary aneurysmal bone cyst does not change the therapy or prognosis of the underlying primary tumor.

Primary aneurysmal bone cyst occurs most commonly in teenagers (80%). More than 50% of these cysts arise in large tubular bones, and almost 30% occur in the spine. The patient usually complains of a mild dull pain, and only rarely is there a clinically apparent pathologic fracture. The patient's physical examination is usually normal and there are no abnormal laboratory findings associated with aneurysmal bone cyst.

On the plain radiograph aneurysmal bone cyst is a radiolucent lesion arising in the medullary canal of the metaphysis (Fig. 12-18). It resorbs the cortex and elevates the periosteum. Usually there is a thin shell of reactive periosteal bone, but occasionally this bone cannot be seen. When anneurysmal bone cyst arises in a long bone it is metaphyseal. When it arises in the spine it originates in the posterior elements but may extend into the body. Giant cell tumor of the bone and telangiectatic osteosarcoma may have identical radiographic appearances as aneurysmal bone cyst. The periosteal reaction has an aggressive appearance, and the lesion can be mistaken for an aggressive or malignant tumor. Aneurysmal bone cyst can arise in the cortex and elevate the periosteum with or without involving the medullary canal.

The CT scan is helpful in making the diagnosis of aneurysmal bone cyst. The lesion should have a density of approximately 20 HU, and this does not increase with intravenous contrast injection. When the patient lies still for 20 to 30 minutes the cells in the fluid within the cyst cavity settle, and a fluid level can be seen.[167] Similar findings can be seen on the MRI. Aneurysmal

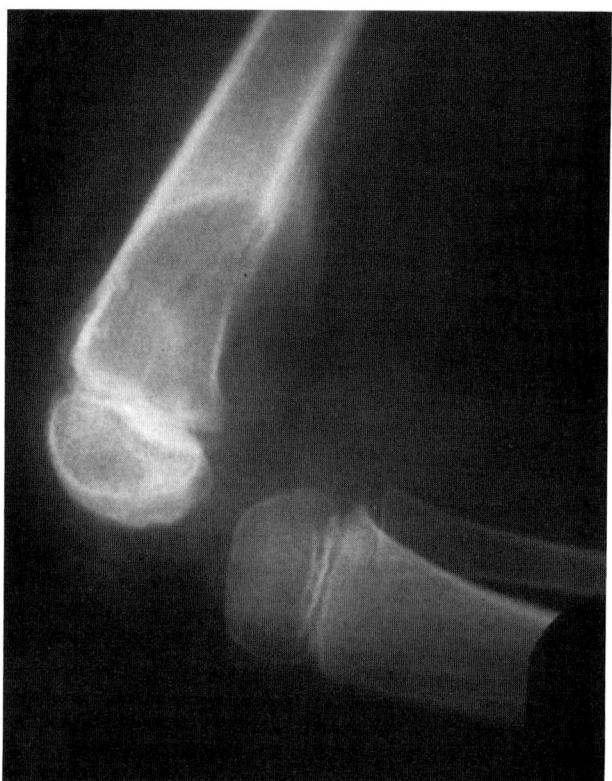

FIGURE 12-18. Radiograph of a distal femur with an aneurysmal bone cyst involving the distal metaphysis and extending through the posterior cortex. As in this patient, an aneurysmal bone cyst can have the appearance of an aggressive tumor. When the cyst erodes through the cortex, it usually is contained by the periosteum, which reacts and produces bone. The differential diagnosis should include the aneurysmal bone cyst, osteosarcoma (telangiectatic variant), Ewing sarcoma, and osteomyelitis. The patient was successfully treated with curettage and bone grafting.

bone cyst has an increased uptake of technetium on the bone scan, but often the scan has a central area of decreased uptake.

Aneurysmal bone cysts should be biopsied to establish the diagnosis and then curetted and packed with bone graft. The pathologist should be advised in advance and the possibility of a telangiectatic osteosarcoma discussed. It is uncommon for the histology of an aneurysmal bone cyst to be confused with that of a telangiectatic osteosarcoma, although the radiograph and gross appearance can be identical. On gross inspection an aneurysmal bone cyst is a cavitary lesion with a villous lining. Microscopic examination reveals the lining to be composed of hemosiderin-laden macrophages, multinucleated giant cells, a fibrous stroma, and usually small amounts of woven bone (Fig. 12-19).

The microscopic appearance of the lining of the aneurysmal bone cyst is similar to that of a giant cell tumor of bone. The majority of aneurysmal bone cysts are treated successfully with curettage and packing of bone graft. The first recurrence can be recuretted and

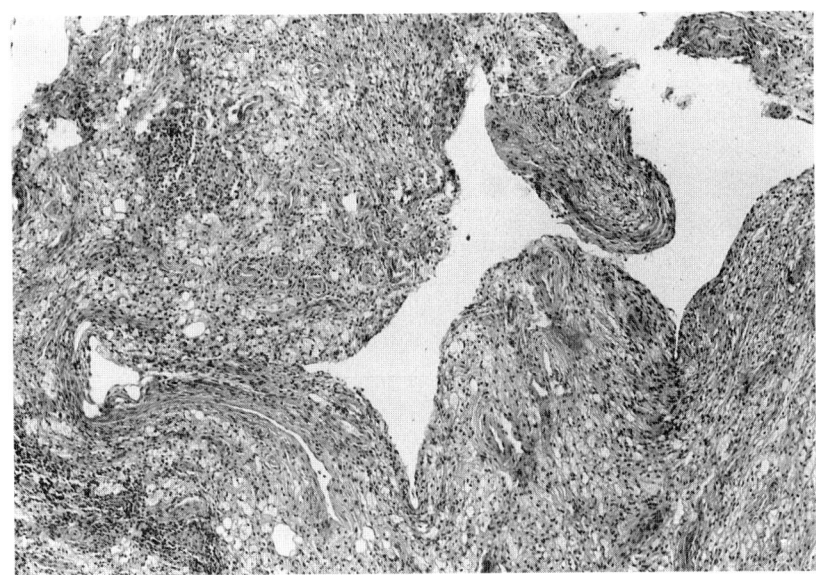

FIGURE 12-19. Low-power view of the tissue lining an aneurysmal bone cyst. The lining is composed of fibrous tissue with multinucleated giant cells, foamy histiocytes, hemosiderin, and often, spicules of immature bone (not seen). The fronds and spaces are typical. (Original magnification ×10.)

grafted. A definitive resection can be performed when the consequences of the resection are minimal but is only absolutely necessary when the lesion has a particularly aggressive clinical growth pattern.

Aneurysmal bone cyst of the spine (≤30%) can present a particularly challenging problem. The lesion always involves the posterior elements but can also involve the vertebral body.[166] The patients complain initially of pain at the site of the lesion, but the aneurysmal bone cyst often is not found until the patient has nerve root or cord compression. Radiotherapy has been used in the management of patients with aneurysmal bone cyst of the spine, but surgery is recommended for all patients as the initial means of treatment. Most cases are controlled with a simple curettage. Usually the posterior elements are resected, and involvement of the pedicles or the body is curetted. If a complete laminectomy is performed a short posterior fusion is advised. Radiotherapy can be used in the postoperative period but usually is reserved for the rare case of rapid recurrence with soft tissue infiltration. A postoperative MRI or CT scan is recommended to be used as a baseline study with which to compare any later scans.

Giant Cell Tumor of Bone

Giant cell tumor bone is rare in the patient with an open epiphysis and occurs predominantly in the late teenage years or during the third or fourth decade (85% > age 19 years). When it occurs in a child with an open epiphyseal plate, it is located in the metaphysis.[179] Giant cell tumor of bone is common and represents 18% of all benign tumors of bone.

The patient complains of a mild, dull pain and often has symptoms suggestive of an internal derangement of the adjacent joint. It is not uncommon to see a patient with a pathologic fracture through the lesion. Usually the patient provides a history of a few months of mild pain that had been ascribed to arthritis. It is common to see patients who have been treated for joint sprain or torn meniscus. The patient is more likely to be a girl with symptoms in the knee (more than 50% arise in the distal femur, proximal tibia, or proximal fibula). The distal radius and the sacrum are other common sites, but giant cell tumor of bone may occur in any bone. Radiolucent lesions in the body of a vertebra in a young patient are usually giant cell tumors.

On physical examination, atrophy of the muscles that control the joint adjacent to the tumor is found. The range of motion in that joint is decreased, and an effusion may be present. Frequently, especially in those lesions arising from the distal radius, an extraosseous mass can be palpated. This mass is warm, firm, slightly tender, and may be pulsatile. The entire skeleton should be examined because giant cell tumor of bone may (<1%) present with multiple lesions. The patient's parathyroid glands should be examined because hyperparathyroidism may produce brown tumors that are radiographically and histologically similar to giant cell tumor of bone. The parathormone levels can be measured to exclude hyperparathyroidism, and a serum calcium and serum phosphorus as well as an alkaline phosphatase should be obtained. The laboratory data is normal in patients with giant cell tumor of bone.

The plain radiograph of a giant cell tumor is almost diagnostic (Fig. 12-20). The tumor is a radiolucent lesion that involves the epiphysis and metaphysis of a long bone. It invariably extends to and sometimes through the subchondral bone. Giant cell tumor of

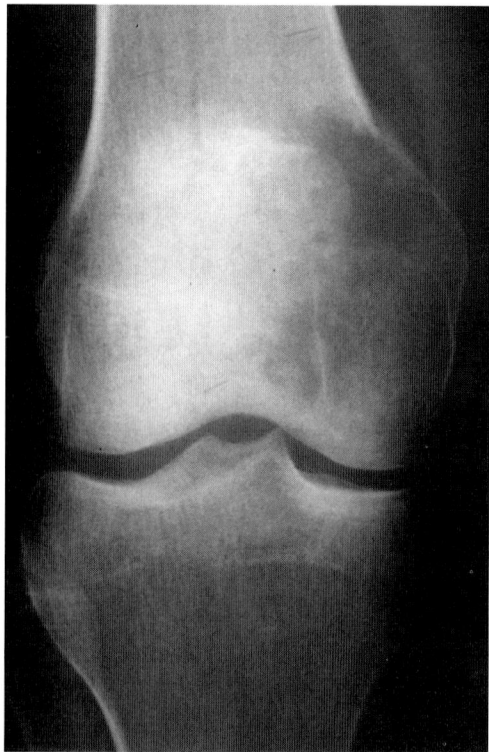

FIGURE 12-20. Anteroposterior radiograph of a typical giant cell tumor of bone in the distal femur. The lesion is eccentric and involves the metaphysis and epiphysis. There is minimal reaction of the host bone, the border of transition is narrow, and there are no radiodensities within the lesion.

bone is unique in its ability to invade articular cartilage. There are no intralesional densities. There is a narrow border of transition between the tumor and surrounding bone and little if any endosteal or periosteal reaction is present. An angiogram demonstrates the hypervascularity of this lesion but not otherwise add to the evaluation. The CT and MRI scan show the extent of the tumor better than the plain films and demonstrate cortical destruction more accurately, but the radiographic diagnosis is made from the plain radiograph. Giant cell tumor of bone has an increased uptake on the technetium bone scan.

Giant cell tumor of bone is composed of multinucleated giant cells, background of fibrous tissue, and small single nucleated cells whose nuclei are similar to those of the multinucleated giant cells (Fig. 12-21). Mitoses are common, but they should be normal in appearance. Abnormal-appearing mitotic figures are strong evidence that the tumor is malignant. Giant cell tumor of bone is one of the few benign bone tumors that commonly has areas with spontaneous necrosis.

In the past, the majority of giant cell tumors of bone were treated by simple curettage and bone grafting. The local recurrence rate was high (>35%). In the 1940s and 1950s, pathologists believed that they could grade giant cell tumors of bone and predict which tumors would be the most aggressive. The histologic grading system was suggested by Lichenstein and Jaffe.[174] They based the grade on the appearance of the background cells, not the multinucleated giant cells. Unfortunately the histologic grade system proved not to be predictive. Campanacci[171] suggested a grading system based on the radiographic appearance, but this too has not proven of sufficient predictive value to be useful. Because of the frequency of local recurrence and the inability to predict the behavior of giant cell tumor surgical resection became popular in the 1960s through the early 1980s. Although these resections controlled giant cell tumor better than curettage, the loss of function was too great, and for the past 10 years less aggressive treatment has been used as an initial management. Resections are reserved for the neglected large lesion, the lesion with a displaced patho-

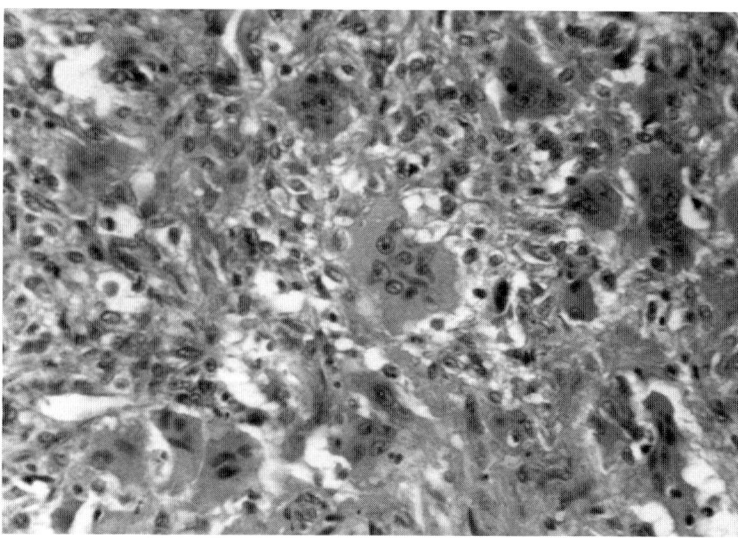

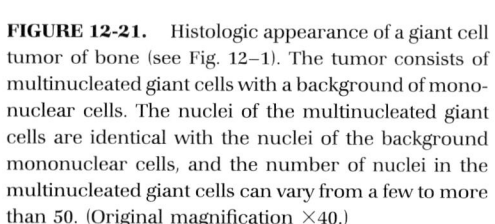

FIGURE 12-21. Histologic appearance of a giant cell tumor of bone (see Fig. 12–1). The tumor consists of multinucleated giant cells with a background of mononuclear cells. The nuclei of the multinucleated giant cells are identical with the nuclei of the background mononuclear cells, and the number of nuclei in the multinucleated giant cells can vary from a few to more than 50. (Original magnification ×40.)

logic fracture, or the rapidly recurrent giant cell tumor.

Numerous adjuvant treatments to reduce the local recurrence have been tried.[175] The most popular treatment method is an extended curettage with the use of a high-speed burr and packing with polymethyl methacrylate (PMMA). The most important part of the curettage is to see the entire cavity at the time of the operation. A wide opening in the bone must be made, and the curettage must be complete beyond the reactive rim of bone surrounding the lesion.

Some authors irrigate the bone cavity with phenol after the extended curettage, and others cauterize the cavity surface. Cryosurgery (freezing of the lesion) has been used and has been successful in eradicating the tumor but has a high incidence of complications, even in the hands of the experienced cryosurgeon. I recommend a wide curettage with a high-speed burr, pulsed lavage with saline, and packing with PMMA.

Approximately 5% of patients with giant cell tumor of bone develop a pulmonary metastasis. The tumor is considered benign if the pulmonary lesions are histologically benign. The patient with metastatic giant cell tumor of bone usually is cured by surgical resection, although irradiation also has been used.

Ewing Sarcoma

Ewing sarcoma was the most lethal of all primary bone tumors prior to the routine use of adjuvant chemotherapy with a 5-year survival of approximately 15%. Before the use of adjuvant chemotherapy, most patients were treated with irradiation alone. With improved survival associated with adjuvant chemotherapy, the role of surgery is being reevaluated, and there is evidence, albeit only from retrospective studies, that surgical resection combined with chemotherapy produces an improved survival compared with the survival after irradiation and chemotherapy.

The patient with a Ewing sarcoma initially complains of pain. Some have generalized symptoms with fever, weight loss, and malaise, but this is not the usual presentation. Males are affected at a 3:2 ratio over females, and most patients are between the age of 5 and 30 years. Any bone may be affected. The femur is the most common site of origin (20%); the pelvis and the humerus are also common sites. There is usually a soft tissue mass associated with the bone lesion, and on physical examination this mass often can be palpated. The mass is warm, firm, and tender, and it may be pulsatile. There are no specific abnormal laboratory values diagnostic of Ewing sarcoma, but the sedimentation rate often is increased. An elevated LDH is a poor prognostic sign.

The typical plain radiograph of a Ewing sarcoma reveals diffuse destruction of the bone, extension of the tumor through the cortex, a soft tissue component, and a periosteal reaction (Fig. 12-22). The periosteal reaction may produce a Codman triangle, an "onion-skin" appearance, or a sunburst appearance. These suggest an aggressive lesion that has rapidly penetrated the cortex and elevated the periosteum. The extraosseous soft tissue mass and medullary canal involvement can be seen on CT and MRI scans and usually is beyond that expected from the plain radiograph.

The MRI has proved to be more accurate in determining the intramedullary extent of Ewing sarcoma than the CT scan. The inflammation around the tumor is seen on the MRI more easily than other studies, and its extent is often more than expected from the other test. The technetium bone scan is most useful in finding occult bone metastasis. Approximately 5% of the patients present with pulmonary metastasis.

The histologic appearance of Ewing sarcoma is that of a small round cell tumor (see Fig. 12-22). The Ewing cell has a distinct nuclei with minimal cytoplasm and an indistinct cytoplasmic border. The cells are similar, and mitoses are uncommon. Necrotic areas usually are seen. There are glycogen granules in the cytoplasm, and these produce the positive periodic acid–Schiff (PAS) stain on routine histology. The intracellular glycogen granules are diastase positive (i.e., exposure to diastase will break the glycogen down, eliminating PAS staining). The glycogen can be seen as dense cytoplasmic granules on the electron microscopic photographs. Ewing sarcoma and peripheral neuroectodermal tumor have a somatic genetic defect [t(11;22)(q24;q12)] that is thought to be a marker of these two tumors.

Conventional treatment is irradiation (approximately 5500 cGy) to the primary lesion and adjuvant multidrug chemotherapy. More recent therapeutic protocols start with two or four courses of multidrug chemotherapy regimen and then irradiation or a surgical resection followed by more chemotherapy. The primary tumor usually shrinks dramatically, and often the entire extraosseous component resolves. Since the use of adjuvant chemotherapy, survival has improved and is better than 50% at 5 years.

In 1975, a retrospective analysis of patients with Ewing sarcoma who had received adjuvant suggested that surgical resection resulted in an improved survival when compared to irradiation.[183] Since then numerous other retrospective studies have supported this view but there have been no prospective studies to confirm that surgical resection is better than irradiation. Despite the lack of data to indicate that a surgical resection is better than irradiation, surgeons increasingly have resected the residual abnormal tissues after preoperative chemotherapy. This is especially advantageous when the resection does not produce a sig-

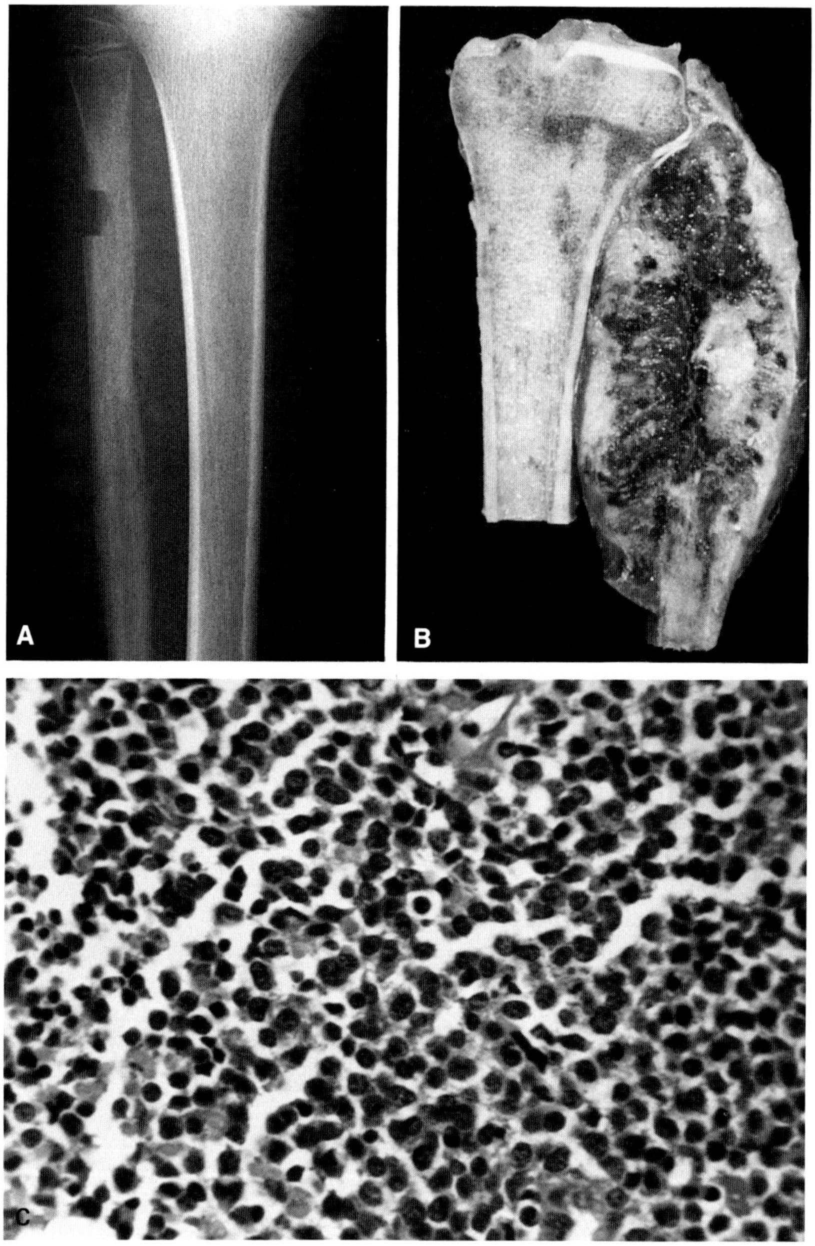

FIGURE 12-22. (A) Anteroposterior radiograph of the proximal tibia and fibula of a patient with Ewing sarcoma involving the proximal fibula. The fibular cortical detail is lost, and erosion of the medial surface, soft tissue mass, and periosteal reaction—typical findings of Ewing sarcoma—are present. The combination of these findings are indicative of an aggressive process. Acute osteomyelitis may have this appearance, but the patient usually has other signs of infection. The defect in the lateral aspect of the fibula is due to an incisional biopsy of the bone. The bone should not be biopsied if there is sufficient soft tissue extension. This will lessen the chance of pathologic fracture. In addition, the extraosseous tumor is usually more easily cut, and the histologic appearance is better. (B) Gross specimen of Ewing sarcoma of the proximal fibula, similar to the case in **A**. The tumor has replaced the proximal fibula, and there is a large soft tissue mass with invasion of surrounding muscles and no involvement of the tibia. This patient chose to have an immediate amputation, although this is not standard treatment. (C) Histologic appearance of Ewing sarcoma. The nuclei are easily seen, and there are nucleoli within the nucleus. The cells are small and round with very little variation in nuclear appearance. Mitoses are rare. The cytoplasm is faint and difficult to see, and the cytoplasmic borders are poorly defined. (Original magnification ×10.)

nificant function deficit (e.g., proximal fibula, rib, or clavicle lesions), and the patient can be spared irradiation. There is a low but significant incidence of radiation associated with malignancies in children who have had chemotherapy and irradiation. Whether a more important bone (e.g., proximal femur, acetabulum, distal femur) should be resected is unresolved. Many centers recommend that all Ewing sarcomas be resected regardless of the bone of origin; it soon may be known whether this recommendation is appropriate.

Scully and associates[184] reviewed a series of patients with Ewing sarcoma of the pelvis. There were 39 patients with a pelvic Ewing sarcoma treated between 1975 and 1991. Nineteen had a surgical resection, and 20 did not. There was improved survival among those that had a surgical resection, but the differences were not significant. There are probably too few patients to show a small but significant improvement in survival, but this theory will not be confirmed until more patients are treated.

Soft Tissue Tumors

The majority of soft tissue tumors in children are benign. Only rhabdomyosarcoma in the younger age group and synovial cell sarcoma in teenagers and older patients occur with any frequency, and they are both rare tumors. Hemangioma, the fibromatoses, neurolemma, and neurofibroma are more common.

The physician must be aware of the possibility of malignant soft tissue tumor in the child and evaluate any lump carefully.

Hemangioma

Hemangioma may be be a true neoplasia, a hamartoma, or an arteriovenous fistula. Its origin is controversial. It is important that the abnormality is recognized as a benign lesion that in certain circumstances spontaneously regresses and in others infiltrates the muscle and occasionally bone. Hemangiomas are the most common tumors in infancy and childhood and account for 7% of benign soft tissue tumors in all age groups. They are most common in the head and neck regions but may be found in internal organs, especially the liver. Often an intrahepatic hemangioma can be seen on a CT scan on the abdomen taken for another reason, and their existence is of little concern.

Enzinger and Weiss[4] provide a classification of vascular tumors of soft tissue. The borderline malignant and malignant vascular tumors are not pertinent to this discussion; therefore only the benign tumors are included.

> Localized hemangioma
> Capillary hemangioma (including juvenile type)
> Cavernous hemangioma
> Venous hemangioma
> Arteriovenous hemangioma (racemose hemangioma)
> Epithelioid hemangioma (angiolymphoid hyperplasia, Kimura disease)
> Hemangioma of granulation tissue type (pyogenic granuloma)
> Miscellaneous hemangiomas of deep soft tissue (synovial, intramuscular, neural)
> Angiomatosis (diffuse hemangioma)

Capillary hemangioma constitutes the largest group of benign vascular tumors. The juvenile hemangioma variant of capillary hemangioma occurs 1 every 200 live births. They may be cutaneous or deep and usually are seen within the first few weeks of life, often enlarging for the first 6 months but then regressing and becoming 75% to 95% involute by the age of 7 years. Capillary hemangiomas do not require treatment.

Cavernous hemangioma are not as common as the capillary type but do not spontaneously regress and may require treatment. They most commonly arise within muscle and invade tissue planes extensively. The patient often presents with complaints of swelling, tenderness, and inflammation secondary to thrombophlebitis within the hemangioma. This inflammation resolves within a few days and can be treated with local heat and oral aspirin. The noninflamed hemangioma is soft and ill defined. The patient may have no symptoms or have the sensation of heaviness or a tight feeling in the extremity. On the plain radiograph there are often small smooth round calcifications called phleboliths. The appearance of hemangiomas on MRI is virtually diagnostic because they are composed of smooth regular blood vessels and normal fat.

The cavernous hemangiomas have an indirect communication with the major vascular tree and are not easily filled with contrast on an angiogram or venogram (Fig. 12-23). Occasionally a tourniquet proximal to the hemangioma permits filling of the tumor veins at the time of a venogram or angiogram. If an intravenous injection does not demonstrate the hemangioma, the dye can be injected directly into the hemangioma. The CT scan, particularly if performed with intravenous contrast, is almost always diagnostic. The hemangioma has varying densities with multiple dye-filled areas. Biopsy is performed only to confirm the diagnosis, and resection is not necessary unless the patient has repeated bouts of inflammation or complaints of discomfort (usually a full or tight feeling) or the parents are anxious about the mass.

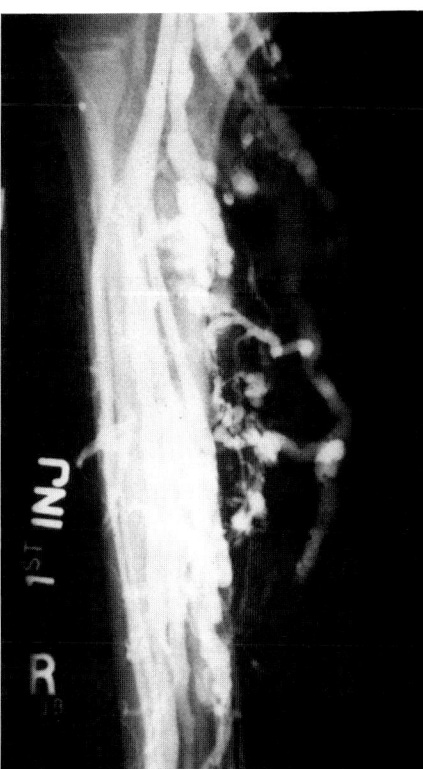

FIGURE 12-23. Venogram of a patient with a hemangioma of the calf. The hemangioma communicated with the deep venous system and was easily filled when the normal veins were injected with contrast; this is not always the case. This patient had two pulmonary emboli, and the hemangioma was confined to the gastrocnemius muscle. Therefore, the entire gastrocnemius muscle was resected.

Surgical excision usually is not required. When performed the hemangioma often recurs unless the entire muscle or muscles involved are resected. These lesions are probably best considered congenital abnormalities that involve most of the veins in the extremity. When the grossly involved veins are resected the surrounding vessels dilate resulting in a clinical recurrence. Hemangiomas do not undergo malignant degeneration, and although they can produce significant abnormalities in the extremity, surgical resection is rarely curative, although it may reduce the symptoms. Irradiation has been used with varying benefit. Embolization also has been used for patients who have severe pain.

Hemangioma of bone, either solitary or diffuse, is a hamartoma and not a true neoplasia. The solitary lesions are more frequent, especially in the vertebral bodies, where they are almost a normal variant (Fig. 12-24). Solitary lesions may occur in any bone, but the skull is the second most common site. These lesions do not produce symptoms and usually are found when a radiograph is taken for another reason. The radiograph and CT scan are diagnostic. The bone has a honeycomb appearance with increased trabecular markings around radiolucencies.

Patients with multiple lesions are more likely to present during the first or second decade of life with either mild discomfort or a pathologic fracture. These patients can have involvement of their viscera and skin. When multiple sites are involved they often involve the long bones of the extremities and the short bones of the hands and feet. Treatment should be symptomatic with curettage and bone grafting for lesions that weaken the bone. Those lesions not producing symptoms or at risk for fracture should be observed. They should resolve with time.

Fibromatoses

Benign fibrous lesions in children are relatively common and rarely malignant. Extraabdominal desmoid, or aggressive fibromatosis, is the most common benign fibrous lesion seen in children.[8] The less common lesions are not discussed in this text. Enzinger and Weiss[4] discuss these elsewhere.[4]

Extraabdominal desmoid or aggressive fibromatosis is the most common benign fibrous tumor seen in patients over 10 years of age. The patient presents with mild pain and a slowly enlarging mass. The mass is deep, firm, and slightly tender, but it is not inflamed. The adjacent joint is normal. A soft tissue mass can be seen on a plain radiograph, but there are no distinguishing features. Calcifications within the mass are not expected.

There is usually increased activity in the lesion on the technetium bone scan, although some large masses will not display increased uptake. Often, even when the lesion is immediately adjacent to the bone, there is no increased uptake of technetium. The mass has a density similar to that of muscle on the CT scan but usually is more vascular and can be distinguished best from the surrounding tissue by performing the CT scan while the patient is infused with intravenous contrast. The classic collagen bundles produce a relative signal void (dark on T1- and T2-weighted images) on the MRI, but because the cellularity varies fibromatoses may have a similar appearance on MRI as any soft tissue neoplasia.

Histologically, fibromatosis has the appearance of scar tissue. It is composed of dense bundles of collagen with evenly dispersed benign cells (Fig. 12-25). The cell of origin is believed to be the myofibroblast. The histologic appearance and cell of origin of fibromatosis are identical with those of plantar fibromatosis and Dupuytren contracture, but the latter conditions are not as clinically aggressive as fibromatosis. Although they recur, they do not extend proximally out of the feet or hands, as seen in aggressive fibromatosis.

Aggressive fibromatosis is an infiltrative lesion, and local excision rarely removes the entire tumor even when the surgeon is convinced that the margin is wide. The presence of a positive margin at the initial resection does not always lead to a local recurrence. On the other hand, lesions that have recurred must be widely excised if local control is to be expected. Patients younger than 10 years of age have a greater risk of developing a local recurrence than older patients. Irradiation and surgery have been combined to control recurrent fibromatosis, but the long-term

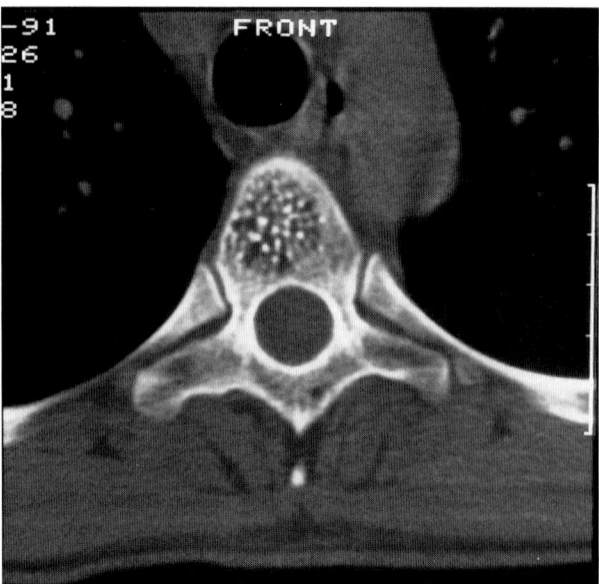

FIGURE 12-24. Computed tomographic scan of a typical hemangioma of the vertebral body. The small foci of increased density are thickened trabeculae of bone, and the low-density areas are filled with the hemangiomatous tissue.

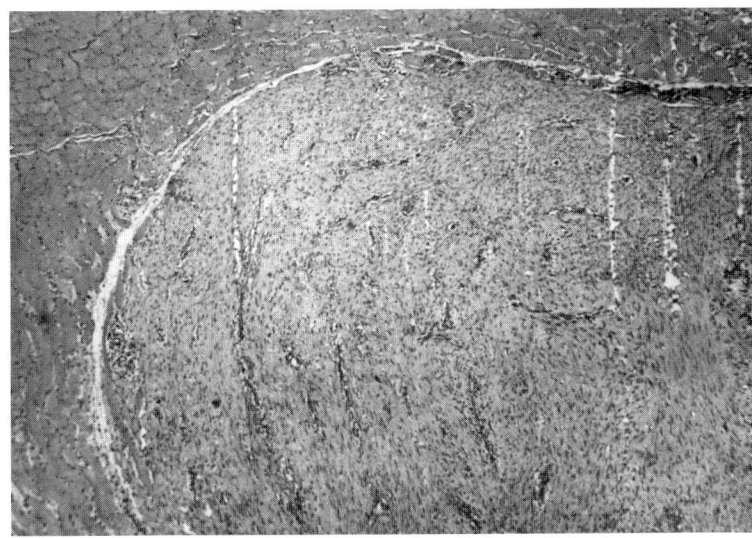

FIGURE 12-25. Histologic appearance of fibromatosis. The lesion infiltrates a muscle and is more cellular than the typical fibromatosis. A wide resection was attempted, but this patient had a microscopically positive margin. One year later, the patient had not had a recurrence. (Original magnification ×10.)

results are not known. Whenever possible, initial treatment should be a wide resection. Observation is suggested after the surgery for those patients whose resection had a negative margin. There is no consensus about how to treat the patient with a positive margin. Most do not recur; if the patient develops a recurrence, either a more aggressive resection can be performed or limited surgery combined with irradiation is recommended. A variety of chemotherapeutic agents have been tried, but none has proved clinically useful.

Benign Tumors of Nerve Origin

There are two common benign tumors that arise from nerves: neurilemoma and neurofibroma. Neurilemomas, or schwannomas, arise from the nerve sheath. They occur most often in early adulthood and usually are solitary and slow growing. The patient usually presents with a painless mass and has a Tinel sign when the mass is tapped. The mass may be from any nerve, but it is often in the superficial tissue arising from a small sensory nerve. When arising from a spinal nerve root, the foramen may be enlarged because of the pressure of the tumor on the bone. Nerve dysfunction is uncommon and is seen only when the nerve is compressed between the tumor and an adjacent rigid structure. Patients with superficial nerve lesions usually present early with small-sized tumors, but deep-seated lesions may be large before they are discovered. Neurilemoma rarely are seen in patients with von Recklinghausen disease because neurofibroma are the common type in these patients. Neurilemoma are uninodular masses with a distinct capsule and are easily separated from the nerve of origin. Their microscopic appearance is a combination of a cellular area (Antoni A) and a myxoid area (Antoni B). The Antoni A area is composed of benign spindle cells that tend to have their nuclei stacked with intervening cytoplasm (Fig. 12-26). The nuclear stacking is called a palisaded appearance, and the arrangement of alter-

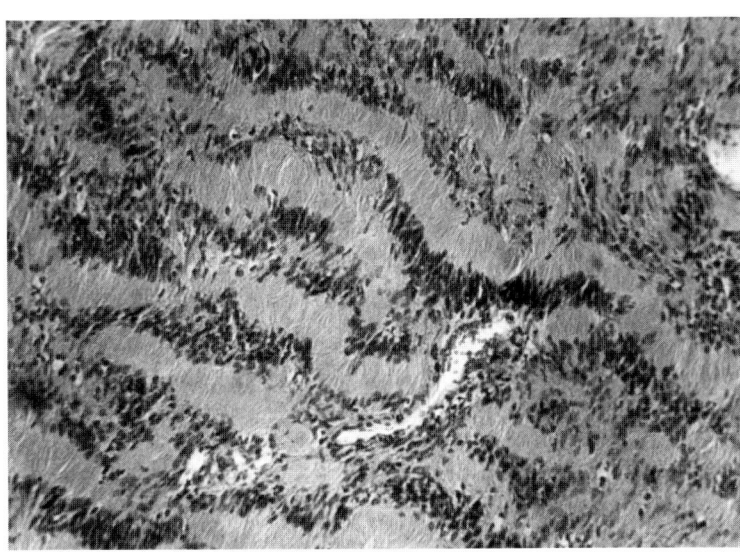

FIGURE 12-26. Histologic appearance of a neurilemoma (Antoni A area). The nuclei are stacked, giving the lesion a palisaded appearance. (Original magnification ×10.)

nating nuclei and cytoplasm is called a Verocay body. Antoni B area is composed of myxomatous tissue with less cellularity than the Antoni A areas. Neurilemomas are treated by a marginal excision without sacrificing the affected nerve. Neurilemomas should not recur.

Neurofibromas may arise as a solitary lesion or multiple lesions. The majority, maybe as many as 90%, are solitary and are not characteristic of von Recklinghausen disease. They may arise in the skin or be associated with a recognizable peripheral nerve. As with neurilemomas they usually present as a painless mass with a Tinel sign. Unlike neurilemomas they tend to be intimately associated with the nerve fibers. Fortunately, most arise from small cutaneous nerves and can be removed without loss of nerve function. Histologically, neurofibromas are not encapsulated and invade the nerve fibers and, rarely, the adjacent soft tissue. The cells are elongated, wavy, and have dark-staining nuclei. There is a collagen matrix composed of stringy appearing fibers. Neurites usually are seen within the lesion. Surgical resection is recommended for those lesions that are solitary and not associated with a major nerve. Those arising from a major nerve can be resected, but the nerve fascicles must be split and the neurofibroma removed from between them. Neither solitary neurilemomas nor neurofibromas have a significant incidence of malignant degeneration, although patients with neurofibromatosis have a small risk of developing a neurofibrosarcoma.

Rhabdomyosarcoma

Rhabdomyosarcoma is a malignant tumor of muscle. It was once thought to occur in adults and children with almost equal frequency, but since the middle 1970s most of the adult tumors once called rhabdomyosarcoma have been reclassified as malignant fibrous histiocytoma. Rhabdomyosarcoma is believed to be extremely rare in adults but is the most common malignant soft tissue tumor in patients younger than 15 years of age. It accounts for approximately 3.5% of children's malignancies, and there are approximately 350 new cases per year in the United States. There are four histologic patterns: embryonal, botryoid type, alveolar, and pleomorphic.

Botryoid type rhabdomyosarcoma is histologically identical to the embryonal pattern but is separated because of its gross appearance. A botryoid rhabdomyosarcoma is an embryonal cell type that involves a hollow viscus. Pleomorphic rhabdomyosarcoma is a histologic type seen in adults and is the least common. Embryonal rhabdomyosarcoma is the most common type but usually arises in the head, the neck, the genitourinary tract, and the retroperitoneum. It is rare in the extremities. Botryoid rhabdomyosarcoma tends to occur in the first decade of life. The current treatment is a combination of chemotherapy, surgery, and if not totally excised, irradiation. When chemotherapy is given preoperatively, the surgery required is less radical, and adequate surgical margins are more easily achieved.

Alveolar rhabdomyosarcoma is more common in the extremities than the trunk and is seen in the older child, usually between 10 and 25 years of age. The patient presents with a rapidly growing painless mass deep within the muscle. This occurs with equal frequency in the upper and lower extremities. There are no clinical or laboratory findings that distinguish rhabdomyosarcoma from other soft tissue tumors. As with the embryonal type, treatment is a combination of chemotherapy and surgery. If the lesion is small it should be totally resected initially, but more often preoperative chemotherapy is appropriate to reduce the size of the tumor so that it can be widely resected. A wide surgical margin is recommended, and the muscle involved should be excised from its origin to insertion. Preoperative irradiation is reserved for lesions that would require an amputation to obtain a wide margin. Postoperative irradiation is used when no preoperative irradiation was given and the surgical margins are positive for tumor.

The histologic appearance of embryonal rhabdomyosarcoma can vary. It consists of poorly differentiated rhabdomyoblasts with a limited collagen matrix. The rhabdomyoblasts are small, round to oval cells with dark-staining nuclei and limited amounts of eosinophilic cytoplasm. Cross-striations are not seen regularly. Alveolar rhabdomyosarcoma is composed of small, round to oval tumor cells loosely arranged together in groups by dense collagen bundles. This arrangement of the cells in groups produces an alveolar appearance and hence the name.

Because rhabdomyosarcoma is rare, most patients are treated on a protocol developed by a multi-institutional group referred to as the Intergroup Rhabdomyosarcoma Committee, with representation from both the Pediatric Oncology Group and the Children's Cancer Study Group. They have developed a new staging system for patients with rhabdomyosarcoma to replace the one used before 1992[186] (Table 12-4).

Survival of the patient is related to the anatomic site, its size at presentation, the presence of metastatic disease, the ability for it to be totally removed, and its response to chemotherapy.

Malignant Fibrous Histiocytoma

Malignant fibrous histiocytoma can occur in bone or the soft tissues. It is more common in the soft tissues and is the single most common soft tissue sarcoma seen in adults. This is a diagnosis that rarely was made before 1970. Most of the lesions that would be called MFH that were diagnosed before the middle

TABLE 12.4 *Intergroup Rhabdomyosarcoma Staging System*

STAGE	SITE	SIZE	NODES	METS
1	Orbit Head and neck Genitourinary (not bladder or prostate)	Any	Any	None
2	Bladder and prostate Extremity Cranial parameningeal Other	≤ 5 cm	None or unknown	None
3	Bladder and prostate Extremity Cranial parameningeal Other	≤ 5 cm ≥ 5 cm	Clinically involved Any	None None
4	All	Any	Any	Present

1970s were called rhabdomyosarcoma. Rhabdomyosarcoma is a diagnosis that occurs almost exclusively in children and teenagers. Malignant fibrous histiocytoma of bone is uncommon but occurs in adults and children with a peak in both the teenage years and after 50 years of age. In the pediatric age group it is similar to osteosarcoma in its presentation and treatment.

Malignant fibrous histiocytoma of soft tissue, like other soft tissue sarcomas, are most common in the thigh. Usually, the patient has no or minimal pain and presents with an enlarging mass. The evaluation reveals a deep-seated soft tissue lesion. It is usually firm but without other typical characteristics. On the plain radiograph only a soft tissue density is seen. The MRI is the diagnostic test of choice, and most soft tissue MFHs are revealed as inhomogenous lesions with areas of necrosis and increased vascularity. They can arise from the subcutaneous tissue or within muscles, deep within a compartment.

The histologic characteristics of malignant fibrous histiocytoma (both bone and soft tissue) is a storiform pattern made by the fibrous component and large, bizarre, malignant tumor cells (Fig. 12-27). The mitotic rate is usually high, and areas of necrosis are common. Most of these lesions are of high histologic grade.

The treatment of a soft tissue malignant fibrous histiocytoma is a wide surgical resection with or without adjuvant chemotherapy, depending on the size and grade of the lesion and the local protocol. If a wide margin cannot be achieved without an amputation it is common for these patients to have irradiation combined with a limited surgical margin. The most likely site of distant spread is the lung, and overall the survival rate of patients with malignant fibrous histiocytoma is approximately 60%. The prognosis is

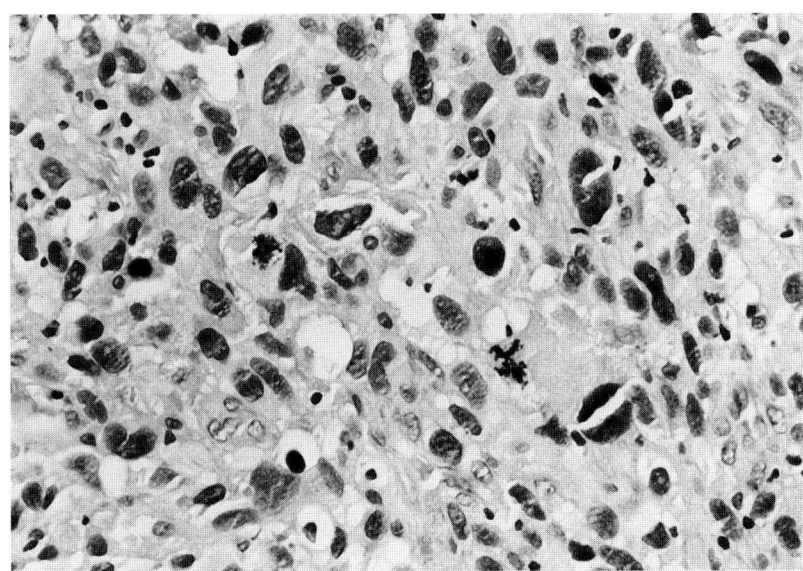

FIGURE 12-27. High-power view of a malignant fibrous histiocytoma. Abnormal mitoses are numerous, as are other bizarre-appearing cells. The storiform pattern seen at lower-power magnification is not appreciated at this power. (Original magnification ×40.)

dependent on size and grade with larger tumors with a higher histologic grade doing worse compared with smaller ones with a lower histologic grade.

Synovial Cell Sarcoma

Synovial cell sarcoma is a malignant tumor of soft parts whose cellular characteristics suggest that the tumor arises from primitive synovial cells, but it rarely occurs within a joint. Unlike other soft tissue sarcomas, synovial cell sarcomas occur frequently in the hand and foot. They usually are in the deep soft tissues near a joint. These tumors account for 10% of all soft tissues near a joint and 10% of all soft tissue sarcomas. Most patients are between 15 and 35 years of age, and males predominate slightly. Patients with a synovial cell sarcoma often complain of pain before they have a palpable mass, and many patients provide a history of having complained of pain for 2 to 4 years before the lesion was found. Synovial cell sarcoma, although rare, may be the explanation of persistent pain in a young patient.

The usual physical finding is the firm, slightly tender mass. Up to 25% of the patients have metastasis to regional lymph nodes, and the lymph nodes should be examined carefully. The patient's blood and urine laboratory values are normal.

The lesion occurs in all parts of the body. The head, the neck, and the trunk account for approximately 15% of the lesions, whereas the upper and lower extremities account for just over half. Almost 10% arise in the hands or feet.

Synovial cell sarcomas may have calcifications or ossification within the tumor, and these often are seen on a plain radiograph. The radiodensities are usually very small. Small irregular calcific foci, or irregular ossification within a soft tissue tumor, should suggest the diagnosis of a synovial cell sarcoma. The CT scan demonstrates a soft tissue mass with these calcified densities deep within the tumor. Although the small foci of calcification or mineralization are not seen as well on MRI as a CT scan, MRI is preferred over CT as the staging test. This is true for all soft tissue masses. Neurofibrosarcoma and fibrosarcoma also can have intralesional calcification, but synovial cell sarcoma is the most common tumor with intralesional densities.

The characteristic histologic findings are of a biphasic tumor with areas of epithelioid or glandular appearance mixed with areas having spindle cell appearance. Usually the spindle cell component predominates (Fig. 12-28). Some of the synovial cell sarcomas have only the spindle cell component and are called monophasic synovial cell sarcoma. There seem to be no clinically significant differences between the two types. Mitoses are usually present, but the tumor is more difficult to grade histologically than other soft tissue sarcoma. Synovial cell sarcoma is almost always a high-grade soft tissue sarcoma.

Surgical resection is and has been the principal treatment of synovial cell sarcoma. Adjuvant chemotherapy is used, but the data regarding the efficacy in synovial cell sarcoma are equivocal at best. In adults and older children with a synovial cell sarcoma, as in other soft tissue sarcomas, preoperative radiotherapy is used in conjunction with less than radical surgery in an attempt to salvage more extremities. Approximately 15% of synovial sarcomas occur in the foot. It was believed that the scarring from irradiation precluded its use in the feet and hands, but with modern techniques adjuvant irradiation and a marginal resection can be performed in the majority of sarcomas of the feet or hands with the preservation of a functioning

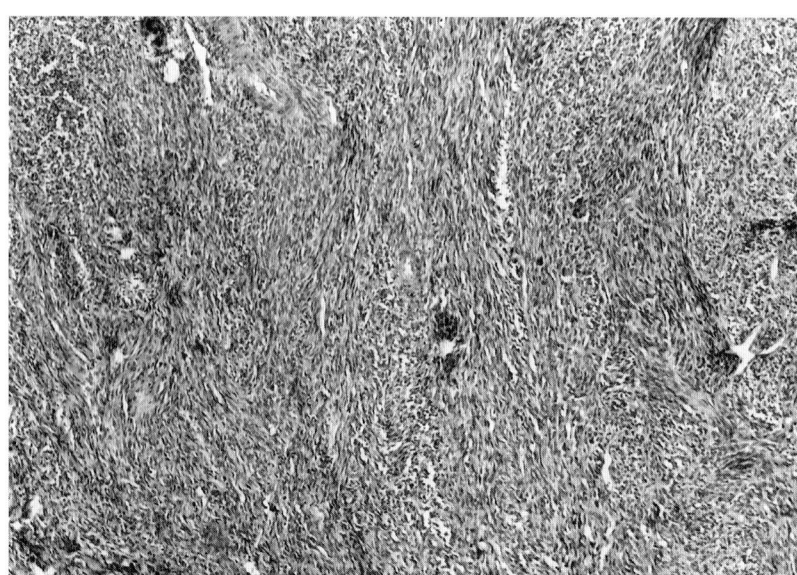

FIGURE 12-28. Low-power view of the spindle component of a synovial cell sarcoma. It is composed of malignant spindle cells with a minimal amount of matrix. At a higher power, mitotic figures are seen. Other areas of this tumor have a glandular appearance, which is the reason this synovial cell sarcoma is a biphasic tumor. (Original magnification ×10.)

extremity. Preoperative irradiation and surgery are recommended for most soft tissue sarcomas of the feet. This has been successful in saving extremities and controlling the disease locally, but the incidence of metastatic disease remains high, at slightly over 50%.[10]

Synovial Tumors

There are only two neoplasias that arise from the synovial lining of a joint. Synovial cell sarcoma has been reported to have arisen from within a joint but this is decidedly rare, and the majority of synovial sarcomas arise within periarticular soft tissues and do not invade joints. Synovial chondromatosis and PVNS arise from synovial tissue and are found in joints, bursa, and tendon sheaths. They are the only two neoplasia that commonly occur in the joint.

SYNOVIAL CHONDROMATOSIS. Synovial chondromatosis is a disorder of the synovial tissues. It is most common in the knee but can arise in any joint, a tendon sheath, or a bursa. Its cause is unknown, and it has no recognized familiar pattern of occurrence. The subliminal lining of the joint produces small nodules of hyaline appearing cartilage that are extruded from the synovial lining to become loose bodies within the joint (Fig. 12-29). The cartilage may become necrotic, if they become large, or they may undergo enchondral ossification, if they have a blood supply. In both cases, they can be seen on plain radiographs. Without the calcification or the ossification the cartilage are radiolucent and not visible on routine radiographs.

The disease is rare in children and presents most commonly between the ages of 20 and 50 years. The most common joint involved is the knee, with the elbow next in frequency and the hip third. The patient usually presents with mild discomfort, minimal loss of motion, and a joint effusion. There may be a history of locking. The knee may be normal on examination, but usually there is a moderate to large effusion, limited motion, and a boggy synovium. The plain radiographs are normal or have small intraarticular calcified bodies. The arthrogram is diagnostic with an irregular synovial surface and normal to thinned synovial fluid. The MRI is usually diagnostic.

Most patients have sufficient symptoms and require removal of loose bodies. Usually a synovectomy is performed, but recurrence is common as the synovial lining is regenerated. The process seems to have a limited natural history, and the production of new loose bodies ceases after 1 or 2 years.

PIGMENTED VILLONODULAR SYNOVITIS. PVNS is a rare disorder of the synovial tissues that may be a true neoplasia, although it has been suggested that it is caused by an infectious process. The synovial lining becomes proliferative and hypertrophic. It can involve a joint (most commonly the knee) or a tendon sheath. When tendon sheaths are involved, PVNS usually occurs in the hand or the foot. The patient presents with a swollen joint that is usually painless. The synovial tissue is boggy to examination. The joint fluid has old dark blood in it, and it is common for the diagnosis to be suspected first when the joint is aspirated just prior to the injection of contrast material for an arthrogram. The arthrogram is diagnostic with a thickened shaggy lining.

The majority of the patients with PVNS are between 20 and 40 years of age. The plain radiograph is usually normal except for the soft tissue swelling, but occasionally the proliferative synovial tissues invade

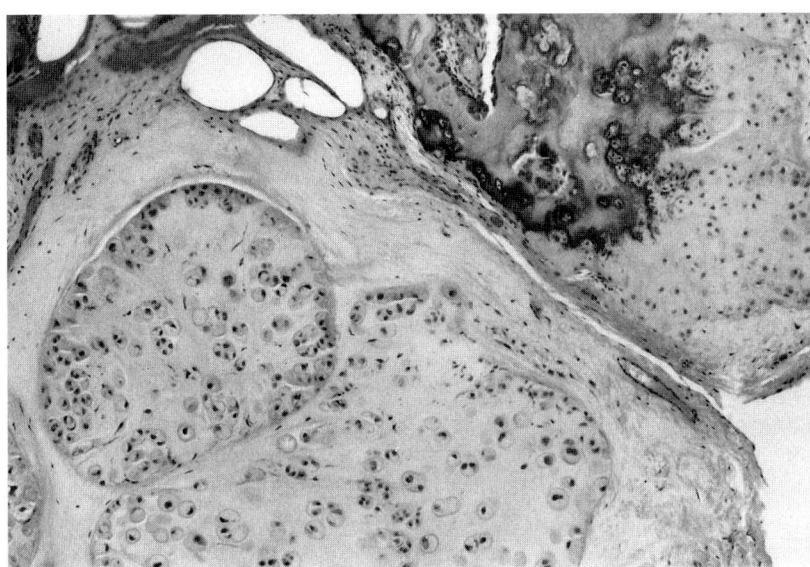

FIGURE 12-29. Low-power view of synovial chondromatosis. The nodules of cartilage are formed within the synovial lining and extruded into the joint to produce loose bodies. The nodules can undergo enchondral ossification if they have a blood supply (*top right*).

the bones adjacent to the joint. This happens most frequently when the hip joint is involved. A synovectomy is the treatment of choice, but there is a high incidence of recurrence (>50%). Intraarticular injection of radioactive materials (dysprosium or yttrium) has been used as a means of controlling recurrent disease with success. Some patients have minimal symptoms with their recurrence and accept the chronic swelling. As long as the bones remain uninvolved there is no absolute indication for surgical removal.

CHEMOTHERAPY FOR MUSCULOSKELETAL TUMORS

It was not until the 1970s that chemotherapy was believed to be effective for malignant tumors of the musculoskeletal system; before that time chemotherapy had been used only for patients with documented metastasis. The extremely high incidence of metastatic disease in patients with osteosarcoma (>80%) and Ewing sarcoma (>85%) and some promising results in patients with metastatic sarcoma prompted the use of adjuvant chemotherapy in patients who did not have documented disease but in whom the risk of having subclinical metastasis was high. The early results were exciting, and even the use of what consider minimal amounts of less-than-optimal drugs improved survival. These early studies lead to the acceptance of adjuvant chemotherapy for Ewing sarcoma, osteosarcoma, and rhabdomyosarcoma. There are no chemotherapeutic agents believed to be effective for chondrosarcoma, and the use of chemotherapy for soft tissue sarcomas remains controversial.

In the 1980s preoperative chemotherapy was introduced and is the accepted timing for the administration of the initial chemotherapy for patients with Ewing sarcoma, osteosarcoma, and rhabdomyosarcoma. Neoadjuvant chemotherapy is a term used to indicate that the patient receives chemotherapy before the definitive treatment of the primary lesion. This was initially used as a means of treating patients with osteosarcoma who were waiting for the production of a custom prosthesis. The effect of chemotherapy on the tumor was significant and of prognostic significance, leading to the routine use of preoperative chemotherapy.

There are numerous chemotherapeutic protocols for the three skeletal malignancies for which chemotherapy is used (Ewing sarcoma, osteosarcoma, and rhabdomyosarcoma). All use more than one drug, usually three to five. Most protocols are between 9 and 12 months long. Approximately one third is given preoperatively and the remainder after surgery.

The drugs used for musculoskeletal tumors include

Doxorubicin (Adriamycin), a cytotoxic anthracycline antibiotic that passively enters the cell to diffuse into the nucleus, where it binds nucleic acids and prohibits DNA synthesis. It is cardiotoxic, myelosuppressive, and produces alopecia. It is given intravenously in divided doses over 6 months with 450 mg/m^2 recommended as the maximum.

Methotrexate is an antimetabolite that inhibits dihydrofolic acid reductase. This interferes with DNA synthesis and repair and alters cellular replication. When administered in high doses (12 mg/m^2 intravenously) leucovorin, or citrovorum factor, is given to the patient to rescue the normal cells. Leucovorin is a chemically reduced derivative of folic acid and is used by the cells to complete the normal cell functions without the need of dihydrofolic acid reductase. Tumor cells seem less able to use leucovorin than normal cells, and this difference allows methotrexate to be effective against malignant tumors. The primary side effects of methotrexate are gastrointestinal, including nausea, vomiting, and loss of appetite.

Cisplatin is a heavy metal that is thought to cause intrastrand cross-links in DNA and therefore interference with the DNA. It is given intravenously in doses of 75 to 100 mg/m^2 repeatedly over the course of the treatment. The principle side effect of cisplatin is nephrotoxicity.

Cyclophosphamide (Cytoxan) is a synthetic drug chemically related to nitrogen mustard. It cross-links DNA and interferes with DNA functions. It is given intravenously at a dose of 40 to 50 mg/Kg in divided doses over 4 to 5 days. The major side effects of cyclophosphamide are gastrointestinal disorders and myelosuppression.

Ifosfamide is a synthetic analog of cyclophosphamide with similar actions. It is given intravenously at 1.2 g/m^2/day for 5 days.

Vincristine is an alkaloid from the periwinkle plant. It is thought to arrest dividing cells in metaphase state by inhibiting microtubule formation in the mitotic spindle. It is given intravenously at weekly intervals at a dose of 1.4 mg/m^2 in adults and 2.0 mg/m^2 in children. The major side effect of vincristine is peripheral neuropathy.

Bleomycin is a cytotoxic glycopeptide antibiotic from a strain of *Streptomyces verticillus*, which inhibits DNA synthesis. It also probably inhibits RNA and protein synthesis. It is given intravenously at 0.25 to 0.50 U/Kg once or twice a week. The most serious side effect of bleomycin is a 10% incidence of severe pulmonary fibrosis.

Actinomycin D (Dactinomycin) is one of a number of actinomycin antibiotics from the *Streptomyces* family. It binds to DNA by intercalation with the phenoxazone ring. This inhibits the DNA from being a template for RNA and synthesizing itself. It is given intravenously at 0.5 mg every day for 5 days. Dactinomycin produces nausea and vomiting and is myelosuppressive.

These drugs are given in various combinations and doses depending on the specific diagnosis, the protocol, the response of the patient, and the aggressiveness of the medical oncologist.

References

1. Campanacci M. Bone and soft tissue tumors. Bologna: Aulo Gaggi Editore, 1990.
2. Dahlin DC. Bone tumors. 3rd ed. Springfield, IL: Charles C Thomas, 1978.
3. Enneking WF. Musculoskeletal tumor surgery. New York: Churchill Livingstone, 1983.
4. Enzinger FM, Weiss SW. Soft tissue tumors. St. Louis: CV Mosby, 1983.
5. Hajdu SI. Pathology of soft tissue tumors. Philadelphia: Lea & Febiger, 1979.
6. Hudson TM. Radiologic-pathologic correlation of musculoskeletal lesions. Baltimore: Williams & Wilkins, 1987.
7. Huvos AG. Bone tumors: diagnosis, treatment and prognosis. Philadelphia: WB Saunders, 1979.
8. Jaffe H. Tumors and tumorous conditions of bones and joints. Philadelphia: Lea & Febiger, 1958.
9. Lewis MM. Bone tumors: evaluation and treatment. Orthop Clin North Am 1989;20:273.
10. Lichtenstein L. Bone tumors. 5th ed. St. Louis: CV Mosby. 1977.
11. Schubiner JM, Simon MA. Primary bone tumors in children. Orthop Clin North Am 1987;18:577.

Etiology

12. Bishop JM. Molecular themes in oncogenesis. Cell 1991; 64:235.
13. Bishop JM. The molecular genetics of cancer. Science 1987;235:305.
14. Diller L, Kassel J, Nelson CE, et al. p53 functions as a cell cycle control protein in osteosarcoma. Mol Cell Biol 1990;10:5772.
15. Fidler IJ, Radinsky R. Genetic control cancer metastasis. J Natl Cancer Inst 1990;82:166.
16. Knudson AG. Mutation and cancer: statistical study of retinoblastoma. Proc Natl Acad Sci USA 1971;68:820.
17. Marshall CJ. Tumor suppressor genes. Cell 1991;64:313.

Planning

18. Barbera C, Lewis MM. Office evaluation of bone tumors. Orthop Clin North Am 1988;19:821.
19. Lodwick GS. A systematic approach to the roentgen diagnosis of bone tumors. Chicago: Year Book Medical, 1965:49.
20. Merkel KD, Springfield DS: Rotationplasty as a reconstructive operation after tumor resection. Clin Orthop 1991;270:231.
21. Picci P, Boriani S. Diagnostic approach to bone tumours. Ital J Orthop Traumatol 1986;12:327.
22. Simon MA, Finn HA. Diagnostic strategy for bone and soft-tissue tumors. J Bone Joint Surg [Am] 1993;75:622.
23. Springfield DS: Limb salvage in the treatment of musculoskeletal tumors. Orthop Clin North Am 1991;22.

Scintigraphy

24. Bastaille R, Chevalier J, Ross M, Sany J. Bone scintigraphy in plasma-cell myeloma. Radiology 1982;145:801.
25. Crone-Munzebrock W, Brassow F. A comparison of radiographic and bone scan findings in histiocytosis-X. Skeletal Radiol 1983;9:170.
26. Hudson TM. Schakel MII, Springfield DS, et al. The comparative value of bone scintigraphy and computed tomography in determining bone involvement by soft tissue sarcomas. J Bone Joint Surg [Am] 1984;66:1400.
27. Kirchner PT, Simon MA. The clinical value of bone and gallium scintigraphy for soft tissue sarcomas of the extremities. J Bone Joint Surg [Am] 1984;66:319.
28. Parker BR, Pinkney L, Etcubanas E. Relative efficacy of radiographic and radionuclide bone surveys in the detection of the skeletal lesion of histiocytosis-X. Radiology 1980;134:377.
29. Siddiqui AR, Tashjian JH, Lazarus K, et al. Nuclear medicine studies in evaluation of skeletal lesion in children with histiocytosis-X. Radiology 1981;140:787.
30. Simon MA, Kirchner PT. Scintigraphic evaluation of primary bone tumors. J Bone Joint Surg [Am] 1980;62:758.
31. Stark DD, Moss AA, Brasch RC, et al. Neuroblastoma: diagnostic imaging and staging. Radiology 1983;148:101.
32. Woolfenden JM, Pitt MJ, Durie BGM, Moon TE. Comparison of bone scintigraphy and radiography in multiple myeloma. Radiology 1980;134:723.

Angiography, Computed Tomography, Magnetic Resonance Imaging

33. Armstrong SJ, Watt I. Imaging of soft tissue tumors. Curr Opin Radiol 1992;4:39.
34. Bohndorf K, Reiser M, Lochner B, Feaux deLacroix W, Steinbrich W. Magnetic resonance imaging of primary tumours and tumour-like lesions of bone. Skeletal Radiol 1986;15:511.
35. Dalinka MK, Zlatkin MB, Chao P, Kricun ME, Kressel HY. The use of magnetic resonance imaging in the evaluation of bone and soft-tissue tumors. Radiol Clin North Am 1990;28:461.
36. Hogeboom WR, Hoekstra HJ, Mooyaart EL, et al. MRI and CT in the preoperative evaluation of soft tissue tumors. Arch Orthop Trauma Surg 1991;110:162.
37. Hudson TM, Hass G, Enneking WF, Hawkins EF. Angiography in the management of musculoskeletal tumors. Surg Gynecol Obstet 1975;141:11.
38. Kransdorf MJ, Jelinek JS, Moser RP Jr. Imaging of soft tissue tumors. Radiol Clin North Am 1993;31:359.
39. Pettersson H, Gillespy T III, Hamlin DJ, et al. Primary musculoskeletal tumors: examination with MR imaging compared with conventional modalities. Radiology 1987;164:237.
40. Sundaram M, McGuire MH. Computed tomography or magnetic resonance for evaluating solitary tumors or tumorlike lesions of bone? Skeletal Radiol 1988;17:393.

41. Zimmer WD, Berquist TH, McLeod RA, et al. Bone tumors: magnetic resonance imaging versus computed tomography. Radiology 1985;155:709.

Laboratory Evaluation

42. Simon MA, Schaaf HW, Metz CE. Clinical utility of the erythrocyte sedimentation rate in preoperative evaluation of solitary skeletal lesions. J Orthop Res 1984;2:262.
43. Thorpe WP, Reilly JJ, Rosenberg SA. Prognostic significance of alkaline phosphatase measurements in patients with osteogenic sarcoma receiving chemotherapy. Cancer 1979;43:2178.

Staging

44. Enneking WF, Spanier SS, Goodman MA. A system for the surgical staging of musculoskeletal sarcomata. Clin Orthop 1980;153:106.
45. Russell WO, Cohen J, Enzinger F, et al. A clinical and pathological staging system for soft tissue sarcomas. Cancer 1977;40:1562.
46. Suit H, Mankin HJ, Wood WC, Gebhardt MC, Harmon DC, Rosenberg A. Treatment of the patient with stage M0 soft tissue sarcoma. J Clin Oncol 1988;6:854.

Biopsy

47. Akerman M, Rydholm A, Persson BM. Aspiration cytology of soft tissue tumors. The 10-year experience at an orthopaedic oncology center. Acta Orthop Scand 1985;56:407.
48. Ball ABS, Fisher C, Pittam M, Watkins RM, Westbury G. Diagnosis of soft tissue tumours by Tru-cut biopsy. Br J Surg 1990;77:756.
49. Brostrom LA, Harris MA, Simon MA, Cooperman DR, Nilsonne U. The effect of biopsy on survival of patients with osteosarcoma. J Bone Joint Surg [Br] 1979;61(2):209.
50. Clark CR, Morgan C, Sonstegard DA, Matthews LS. The effect of biopsy-hole shape and size on bone strength. J Bone Joint Surg [Am] 1977;59:213.
51. Enneking WF. The issue of the biopsy (editorial). J Bone Joint Surg [Am] 1982;64:1119.
52. Ghelman B, Lospinuso MF, Levine DB, Oleary PF, Burke SW. Percutaneous computed tomography guided biopsy of the thoracic and lumbar spine. Spine 1991;16:736.
53. Joyce MJ, Mankin HJ. Caveat athroscopos: extra-articular lesions of bone simulating intra-articular pathology of the knee. J Bone Joint Surg [Am] 1983;65:289.
54. Kissin MW, Fisher C, Carter R, Horton LWL, Westbury G. Value of Tru-cut biopsy in the diagnosis of soft tissue tumours. Br J Surg 1986;73:742.
55. Mankin HJ, Lange TA, Spanier SA. The hazards of biopsy in patients with malignant primary bone and soft tissue tumors. J Bone Joint Surg [Am] 1982;64:1121.
56. Simon MA. Biopsy of musculoskeletal tumors. J Bone Joint Surg [Am] 1982;64:1253.
57. Simon MA, Biermann JS. Biopsy of bone and soft-tissue lesions. J Bone Joint Surg [Am] 1993;75:616.

Osteoid Osteoma and Osteoblastoma

58. Ayla AG, Murray JA, Erling MA, Raymond AK. Osteoid osteoma: intraoperative tetracycline-fluorescence demonstration of the nidus. J Bone Joint Surg [Am] 1986;68:747.
59. Freiberger RH. Osteoid osteoma of the spine. A cause of backache and scoliosis in children and young adults. Radiology 1960;75:232.
60. Ghelman B, Thompson FM, Arnold WD. Intraoperative radioactive localization of an osteoid-osteoma. J Bone Joint Surg [Am] 1981;63:826.
61. Golding JSR. The natural history of osteoid osteoma with a report of twenty cases. J Bone Joint Surg [Br] 1954;36:218.
62. Gore DR, Mueller HA. Osteoid osteoma of the spine with localization aided by 99mTc-polyphosphate bone scan. Case report. Clin Orthop 1975;113:132.
63. Healey JH, Ghelman B. Osteoid osteoma and osteoblastoma. Current concepts and recent advances. Clin Orthop 1986;204:76.
64. Herrlin K, Ekelung L, Lovdahl R, Persson B. Computed tomography in suspected osteoid osteomas of tubular bones. Skeletal Radiol 1982;9:92.
65. Jaffe HL. Benign osteoblastoma. Bull Hosp Joint Dis 1956;17:1441.
66. Jaffe HL. "Osteoid osteoma": a benign osteoblastic tumor composed of osteoid and atypical bone. Arch Surg 1935;31:709.
67. Keim HA, Reina EG. Osteoid osteoma as a cause of scoliosis. J Bone Joint Surg [Am] 1975;57:159.
68. Lichtenstein L. Benign osteoblastoma: category of osteoid and bone forming tumors other than classical osteoid osteoma which may be mistaken for giant-cell tumor or osteogenic sarcoma. Cancer 1956;9:1044.
69. Makely J. Prostaglandins—a mechanism for pain mediation in osteoid osteoma. Orthop Trans 1982;6:72.
70. Marcove RC, Heelan RT, Huvos AG, Healey J, Lindque BG. Osteoid osteoma. Diagnosis, localization, and treatment. Clin Orthop 1991;267:197.
71. Marsh BW, Bonfiglio M, Brady LP, et al. Benign osteoblastoma-range of manifestations. J Bone Joint Surg [Am] 1975;57:1.
72. Mcleod RA, Dahlin DC, Beabour JW. The spectrum of osteoblastoma. AJR 1976;126:132.
73. Mobey E. The natural course of osteoid osteoma. J Bone Joint Surg [Am] 1951;33:166.
74. Norman A. Persistance or recurrence of pain: a sign of surgical failure in osteoid osteoma. Clin Orthop 1978;130:263.
75. Pettine KA, Klassen RA. Osteoid-osteoma and osteoblastoma of the spine. J Bone Joint Surg [Am] 1976;68:354.
76. Rosenthal DI, Alexander A, Rosenberg AE, Springfield D. Ablation of osteoid osteomas with a percutaneously placed electrode: a new procedure. Radiology 1992;183:29.
77. Rinsky LA, Goris M, Bleck EE, Halpern A, Hirshman P. Intraoperative skeletal scintigraphy for localization of osteoid osteoma in the spine. Case report. J Bone Joint Surg [Am] 1980;62:143.
78. Schajowicz F, Lemos C. Malignant osteoblastoma. J Bone Joint Surg [Br] 1976;58:202.
79. Schulman L, Dorfman HD. Nerve fibers in osteoid osteoma. J Bone Joint Surg [Am] 1970;52:1351.
80. Sherman MS. Osteoid osteoma: review of the literature and report of 30 cases. J Bone Joint Surg [Am] 1947;29:918.
81. Sherman MS, McFarland GF. Mechanism of pain in osteoid osteoma. South Med J 1965;58:163.
82. Sims FH, Dahlin DC, Beabou JW. Osteoid-osteoma: diagnostic problem. J Bone Joint Surg [Am] 1975;57:154.
83. Smith FW, Gilday DL. Scintigraphic appearances of osteoid osteoma. Radiology 1980;137:191.
84. Subanas AO, Bickel WH, Moe JH. Natural history of osteoid osteoma of the spine. Revew of the literature and report of three cases. Am J Surg 1956;91:880.
85. Tillotson CL, Rosenberg AE, Rosenthal DI. Controlled thermal injury of bone. Report of a percutaneous technique using

radio-frequency electrode and gererator. Invest Radiol 1989;24:888.
86. Voto SJ, Cook AJ, Winer DS, Ewing JW, Arrington LE. Treatment of osteoid osteoma by computed tomography guided excision in the pediatric patient. J Pediatr Orthop 1990;10:510.

Osteosarcoma

87. Bacci G, Picci P, Ruggieri P, et al. Primary chemotherapy and delayed surgery (neoadjuvant chemotherapy) for osteosarcoma of the extremities. Cancer 1990;65:2539.
88. Cortes EP, Holland JF, Wang JJ, et al. Amputation and adriamycin in primary osteosarcoma. N Engl J Med 1974;291:998.
89. deSantos LA, Bernardino ME, Murray JA. Computed tomography in the evaluation of osteosarcoma:experience with 25 cases. AJR 1979;132:535.
90. Destouet JM, Guild LA, Murphy WA. Computed tomography of long bone osteosarcoma. Radiology 1979;131:439.
91. Eilber F, Giuliano A, Eckhardt J, Patterson K, Moseley S, Goodnight J. Adjuvant chemotherapy for osteosarcoma: a randomized prospective trial. J Clin Oncol 1987;5:21.
92. Enneking WF, Springfield DS. Osteosarcoma. Orthop Clin North Am 1977;8:785.
93. Hudson TM, Schiebler M, Springfield DS, et al. Radiologic imaging of osteosarcoma: role in planning surgical treatment. Skeletal Radiol 1983;10:137.
94. Huvos AG, Rosen G, Marcove RC. Primary osteogenic sarcoma: pathologic aspects in 20 patients after treatment with chemotherapy, en bloc resection, and prosthetic bone replacement. Arch Pathol Lab Med 1977;101:14.
95. Jaffe N, Frei E III, Traggis D, et al. Adjuvant methotrexate citrovorum factor treatment of osteosarcoma. N Engl J Med 1974;291:994.
96. Jaffe N, Frei E III, Watts H, Traggis D. High-dose methotrexate in osteogenic sarcoma: a 5-year experience. Cancer Treat Rep 1978;62:259.
97. Link MP, Goorin AM, Horowits M, et al. Adjuvant chemotherapy of high-grade osteosarcoma of the extremity. Updated results of the multi-institutional osteosarcoma study. Clin Orthop 1991;270:8.
98. Link MP, Goorin AM, Miser AW, et al. The effect of adjuvant chemotherapy on relapse-free survival in patients with osteosarcoma of the extremity. N Engl J Med 1986;134:1600.
99. Marcove RC. En bloc resection for osteogenic sarcoma. Cancer Treat Rep 1978;62:225.
100. Marcove RC, Mike V, Hajek JV, et al. Osteogenic sarcoma under age of twenty-one: a review of one hundred and forty-five operative cases. J Bone Joint Surg [Am] 1970;52:411.
101. Matsuno T, Unni KK, McLeod RA, et al. Telangiectatic osteogenic sarcoma. Cancer 1976;38:2538.
102. Meyers PA, Heller G, Healey J, et al. Chemotherapy for nonmetastatic osteogenic sarcoma: the Memorial Sloan-Kettering experience. J Clin Oncol 1992;10:5.
103. Rosen G, Capanos B, Huvas AG, et al. Preoperative chemotherapy for osteogenic sarcoma: selection of postoperative adjuvant chemotherapy based on the response of the primary tumor to preoperative chemotherapy. Cancer 1982;49:1221.
104. Rosen G, Murphy ML, Huvos AG, et al. Chemotherapy, en bloc resection, and prosthetic bone replacement in the treatment of osteogenic sarcoma. Cancer 1976;37:1.
105. Spanier SS, Shuster JJ, VanderGriend RA. The effect of local extent of the tumor on prognosis in osteosarcoma. J Bone Joint Surg [Am] 1991;73:789.
106. Springfield DS, Schmidt R, Graham-Pole J, Marcus R Jr, Spanier S, Enneking WF. Surgery for osteosarcoma. J Bone Joint Surg [Am] 1988;70:1124.
107. Sundaram M, McGuire MH, Herbold DR. Magnetic resonance imaging of osteosarcoma. Skeletal Radiol 1987;16:23.
108. Taylor WF, Ivins JC, Unni KK, Beabout JW, Golenzer HJ, Black LE. Prognostic variables in osteosarcoma: a multi-instiutional study. J Natl Cancer Inst 1989;81:21.
109. Winzler K, Beron G, Kotz R, et al. Neoadjuvant chemotherapy for osteogenic sarcoma: results of a cooperative German/Austrian study. J Clin Oncol 1984;2:617.

Juxtacortical Osteosarcoma and Chondrosarcoma

110. Ahuja SC, Villacin AB, Smith S, et al. Juxtacortical (parosteal) osteogenic osteosarcoma. Histologic grading and prognosis. J Bone Joint Surg [Am] 1977;59:632.
111. Bertoni F, Boriani S, Laus M, et al. Periosteal chondrosarcoma and periosteal osteosarcoma. Two distinct entities. J Bone Joint Surg [Br] 1982;64:370.
112. Campanacci M, Picci P, Gherlinzoni F, et al. Parosteal osteosarcoma. J Bone Joint Surg [Br] 1984;66:313.
113. deSantos LA, Murray JA, Finklestein JB, et al. The radiographic spectrum of periosteal osteosarcoma. Radiology 1978;127:123.
114. Geschickter CF, Copeland MM. Parosteal osteoma of bone: a new entity. Ann Surg 1951;133:790.
115. Schajowicz F. Juxtacortical chondrosarcoma. J Bone Joint Surg [Br] 1977;59:473.
116. Unni KK, Dahlin DC, Beabout JW. Periosteal osteogenic sarcoma. Cancer 1976;37:2476.

Enchondroma

117. Bean WB. Dyschondroplasia and hemangiomata (Maffucci's syndrome). Arch Intern Med 1955;95:767.
118. Elmore SM, Cantrell WC. Maffucci's syndrome. Case report with a normal karyotype. J Bone Joint Surg [Am] 1966;48:1607.
119. Lewis RJ, Ketcham AS. Maffucci's syndrome: functional and neoplastic significance. Case report and review of the literature. J Bone Joint Surg [Am] 1973;55:1465.
120. Noble J, Lamb DW. Enchondromata of bones of the hand. A review of 40 cases. Hand 1974;6:275.
121. Olller M. Exostoses osteogeniques multiples. Lyon Med 1898;88:484.
122. Schwartz HS, Zimmerman NB, Simon MA, Wroble RR, Miller EA, Bonfiglio M. The management of enchondromatosis. J Bone Joint Surg [Am] 1987;69:269.
123. Sun Te-ching, Swee RG, Shives TC, Unni KK. Chondrosarcoma in Maffucci's syndrome. J Bone Joint Surg [Am] 1985;67:1214.

Periosteal Chondroma

124. Boriani S, Bacchini P, Bertoni F, Campanacci M. Periosteal chondroma. J Bone Joint Surg [Am] 1983;65:205.
125. Lichtenstein L, Hall JE. Periosteal chondroma. A distinctive benign cartilage tumor. J Bone Joint Surg [Am] 1952;34:691.
126. Rockwell MA, Saiter ET, Enneking WF. Periosteal chondroma. J Bone Joint Surg [Am] 1972;54:102.

Exostosis

127. Hudson TM, Chew FS, Manaster BJ. Scintigraphy of benign exostoses and exostotic chondrosarcomas. AJR 1933;10:581.
128. Jaffe HL. Hereditary multiple exostosis. Arch Pathol 1943;36:335.

129. Lange RH, Lange TA, Rao BK. Correlative radiographic, scintographic, and histologic evaluation of exostoses. J Bone Joint Surg [Am] 1984;66:1454.
130. Shapiro F, Simon S, Glimcher MJ. Hereditary multiple exostosis. J Bone Joint Surg [Am] 1979;61:815.
131. Solomon L. Hereditary multiple exostosis. J Bone Joint Surg [Br] 1963;45:292.

Chondroblastoma

132. Codman EA. Epiphyseal chondromatous giant cell tumors of the upper end of the humerus. Surg Gynecol Obstet 1931;52:543.
133. Dahlin DC, Ivins JC. Benign chondroblastoma. A study of 125 cases. Cancer 1972;30:401.
134. Gardner DJ, Azouz EM. Solitary lucent epiphyseal lesions in children. Skelet Radiol 1988;17:497.
135. Green P, Whittaker RP. Benign chondroblastoma. Case report with pulmonary metastasis. J Bone Joint Surg [Am] 1975;57:418.
136. Huvos AG, Marcove RC. Chondroblastoma of bone. A critical review. Clin Orthop 1973;95:300.
137. Jaffe HJ, Lichtenstein L. Benign chondroblastoma of bone. A reinterpretation of the so-called calcifying or chondromatous giant cell tumor. Am J Pathol 1942;18:969.
138. McLeod RA, Beabout JW. The roentgenographic features of chondroblastoma. AJR 1973;118:464.
139. Springfield DS, Capanna R, Gherlinzoni F, Picci P, Campanacci M. Chondroblastoma. A review of seventy cases. J Bone Joint Surg [Am] 1985;67:748.

Nonossifying Fibroma

140. Arata MA, Peterson HA, Dahlin DC. Pathological fractures through non-ossifying fibromas. J Bone Joint Surg [Am] 1981;63:980.
141. Brower AC, Culver JE Jr, Keats TE. Histological nature of the cortical irregularity of the medical posterior distal femoral metaphysis in children. Radiology 1971;99:389.
142. Dunham WK, Marcus NW, Enneking WF, Haun C. Developmental defects of the distal femoral metaphysis. J Bone Joint Surg [Am] 1980;62:801.

Fibrous Dysplasia

143. Albright F, Butler AM, Hampton AO, Smith P. Syndrome characterized by osteitis fibrosa disseminata, area of pigmentation and endocrine dysfunction, with precocious puberty in females. N Engl J Med 1937;216:727.
144. Enneking WF, Gearen PF. Fibrous dysplasia of the femoral neck. Treatment by cortical bone-grafting. J Bone Joint Surg [Am] 1986;68:1415.
145. Grabias SL, Campbell CJ. Fibrous dysplasia. Orthop Clin North Am 1977;8:771.
146. Harris WH, Dudley HR Jr, Barry RJ. The natural history of fibrous dysplasia. An orthopaedic, pathological, and roentgenographic study. J Bone Joint Surg [Am] 1962;44:207.
147. Henry A. Monostotic fibrous dysplasia. J Bone Joint Surg [Br] 1969;51:300.
148. Lichtenstein L. Polyostotic fibrous dysplasia. Arch Surg 1938;36:874.
149. Stephenson RB, London MD, Hankins FM, Kaufman H. Fibrous dysplasia. An analysis of options for treatment. J Bone Joint Surg [Am] 1987;69:400.
150. Steward MJ, Gilmer WS, Edmunson AS. Fibrous dysplasia of bone. J Bone Joint Surg [Br] 1962;44:302.

Osteofibrous Dysplasia

151. Campanacci M, Laus M. Osteofibrous dysplasia of the tibia and fibula. J Bone Joint Surg [Am] 1981;63:367.
152. Campbell CJ, Hawk T. A variant of fibrous dysplasia (osteofibrous dysplasia). J Bone Joint Surg [Am] 1982;64:231.
153. Hazelbag HM, Taminian AHM, Fleuren GJ, Hogendoorn PC. Adamantinoma of the long bones. A clinicopathological study of thirty-two patients with emphasis on histological subtypes, precursor lesions, and biological behavior. J Bone Joint Surg [Am] 1994;76:1482.
154. Kempson RL. Ossifying fibroma of the long bones. Arch Pathol 1966;82:218.

Unicameral Bone Cyst

155. Campanacci M, Capanna R, Picci P. Unicameral and aneurysmal bone cysts. Clin Orthop 1986;204:25.
156. Capanna R, Albisinni U, Caroli GC, et al. Constrast examination as prognostic factor in the treatment of solitary bone cyst by cortisone injection. Skeletal Radiol 1984;12:97.
157. Chigira M, Maecharu S, Arita S, Udagawa E. The aetiology and treatment of simple bone cysts. J Bone Joint Surg [Br] 1983;65:633.
158. Cohen J. Unicameral bone cysts. A current synthesis of reported cases. Orthop Clin North Am 1977;8:715.
159. Cohen J. Etiology of simple bone cysts. J Bone Joint Surg [Am] 1970;52:1493.
160. Kruls HSA. Pathological fractures in children due to solitary bone cyst. Reconst Surg Trauma 1979;17:133.
161. Makley JT, Joyce MJ. Unicameral bone cyst. Orthop Clin North Am 1989;20:407.
162. Neer CS II, Francis KC, Marcove RC, Terez J, Carbonara PN. Treatment of unicameral bone cyst. A follow-up study of 175 cases. J Bone Joint Surg [Am] 1966;48:731.
163. Oppenheim WL, Galleno H. Operative treatment versus steroid injection in the management of unicameral bone cysts. J Pediatr Orthop 1984;4:1.
164. Scaglietti O, Marchetti PG, Bartolozzi P. Final results obtained in the treatment of bone cyst with methylprednisolone acetate (Depo-Medrol) and a discussion of results achieved in other bone lesions. Clin Orthop 1982;165:33.

Aneurysmal Bone Cyst

165. Biesecker JL, Marcove RC, Huvos AG, Mike V. Aneurysmal bone cysts. Cancer 1970;26:615.
166. Capanna R, Albisinne U, Picci P, Calderoni P, Campanacci M, Springfield D. Aneurysmal bone cysts of the spine. J Bone Joint Surg [Am] 1985;67:527.
167. Hudson TM. Fluid levels in aneurysmal bone cyst: a CT feature. AJR 1984;141:1001.
168. Lichtenstein L. Aneurysmal bone cysts. Cancer 1950;3:279.
169. Martinez V, Sissons HA. Aneurysmal bone cyst. A review of 123 cases including primary lesions and those secondary to other bone pathology. Cancer 1988;61:2291.
170. Tillman BP, Dahlin DC, Lipscomb PR, et al. Aneurysmal bone cyst: an analysis of ninety five cases. Mayo Clin Proc 1968;43:478.

Giant Cell Tumor of Bone

171. Campanacci M, Giunti A, Olmi R. Giant cell tumors of bone. A study of 209 cases with long-term follow-up with 130. Ital J Orthop Traumatol 1975;1:249.
172. Fain JS, Unni KK, Beabout JW, Rock MG. Nonepiphyseal giant cell tumor of long bones. Cancer 1993;71:3514.

173. Goldenberg RR, Campbell CJ, Bonfiglio M. Giant-cell tumor of bone. An analysis of two hundred and eighteen cases. J Bone Joint Surg [Am] 1970;52:619.
174. Jaffe HL, Lichtenstein L, Portis RB. Giant cell tumor of bone, its pathologic appearance, grading, supposed variants and treatment. Arch Pathol 1940;30:993.
175. Marcove RC, Lyden JP, Huvos AG, Bullough PG. Giant cell tumor treated by cryosurgery: 25 cases. J Bone Joint Surg [Am] 1973;55:1633.
176. Marcove RC, Weis L, Vaghaiwalla MP, Pearson R. Cryosurgery in the treatment of GCT of bone: 52 consecutive cases. Clin Orthop 1978;134:275.
177. McDonald DJ, Sim FH, McLeod RA, Dahlin DC. Giant-cell tumor of bone. J Bone Joint Surg [Am] 1986;68:235.
178. Persson BM, Wouters HW. Curettage and acrylic cementation in surgery of GCT of bone. Clin Orthop 1976;120:125.
179. Picci P, Manfrini M, Zucchi V, et al. Giant-cell tumor of bone in skeletally immature patients. J Bone Joint Surg [Am] 1983;65:486.

Ewing Sarcoma

180. Chan RC, Sutow WW, Lindberg RD, Samuels ML, Murray JA, Johnston DA. Management and results of localized Ewing's sarcoma. Cancer 1979;43:1001.
181. Frassica FJ, Frassica DA, Pritchard DJ, Schomberg PJ, Wold LE, Sim FH. Ewing sarcoma of the pelvis. J Bone Joint Surg [Am] 1993;75:1457.
182. Kissane JM, Aslzin FB, Foulkes M, Stratton LB, Shirley SF. Ewing's sarcoma of bone: clinicopathologic aspects of 303 cases from the intergroup Ewing's sarcoma study. Hum Pathol 1983;14:773.
183. Pritchard DJ, Dahlin DC, Dauphine RT, Taylor WF, Beabout JW. Ewing's sarcoma: a clinicopathological and statistical analysis of patients surviving five years or longer. J Bone Joint Surg [Am] 1975;57:10.
184. Scully S, Temple HT, OKeefe RJ, Scarborough MT, Mankin HJ, Gebhardt MC. The role of surgical resection in pelvic Ewing's sarcoma. AAOS, New Orleans, LA, 1990.

Soft Tissue Tumors

185. McCoy DM, Levine EA, Ferrer K, Das Gupta TK. Pediatric soft tissue sarcomas of nonmyogenic origin. J Surg Oncol 1993;53:149.
186. Tsokus M, et al. Rhabdomyosarcoma: a new classification scheme related to prognosis. Arch Pathol Lab Med 1992;116:847.

Synovial Disorders

187. Beguin J, Locker B, Vielpeau C, Souguieres G. Pigmented villonodular synovitis of the knee: results from 13 cases. Arthroscopy 1989;5:62.
188. Butt WP, Hardy G, Ostlere SJ. Pigmented villonodular synovitis of the knee: computed tomographic appearance. Skeletal Radiol 1990;19:191.
189. Flandry F, Hughston JC, McCann SB, Kurtz DM. Diagnostic features of diffuse pigmented villonodular synovitis of the knee. Clin Orthop 1994;298:212.
190. Goldman AB, Dicarlo EF. Pigmented villonodular synovitis. Diagnosis and differential diagnosis. Radiol Clin North Am 1988;26:1327.
191. Shpitzer T, Ganel A, Engelberg S. Surgery for synovial chondromatosis. Acta Orthop Scand 1990;61:567.
192. Steinbach LS, Neumann CH, Stoller DW, et al. MRI of the knee in diffuse pigmented villonodular synovitis. Clin Imaging 1989;13:305.

Histiocytosis X

193. Crone-Munzebrock W, Brassow F. A comparison of radiographic and bone scan findings in histiocytosis X. Skeletal Radiol 1981;9:170.
194. David R, Oria RA, Kumar R, et al. Radiologic features of eosinophilic granuloma of bone. AJR 1989;153:1021.
195. Egeler RM, Thompson RC Jr, Voute PA, Nesbit ME Jr. Intralesional infiltration of corticosteroids in lodalized Langerhans' cell histiocytosis. J Pediatr Orthop 1992;12:811.
196. Farber S. The nature of "solitary or eosinophilic granuloma" of bone. Am J Path 1941;17:625.
197. Greis PE, Hankin FM. Eosinophilic granuloma. The management of solitary lesions of bone. Clin Orthop 1990;257:204.
198. Lichtenstein L. Histiocytosis X. Integration of eosinophilic granuloma of bone, "Letterer-Siwe disease," and "Schüller-Christian disease" as related manifestations fo a single nosologic entity. Arch Pathol 1953;56:84.
199. Mackenzie WG, Morton KS. Eosinophilic granuloma of bone. Can J Surg 1988;31:264.
200. Sessa S, Sommelet D, Lascombes P, Prevot J. Treatment of Langerhans-cell histiocytosis in children. Experience at the Children's Hospital of Nancy. J Bone Joint Surg [Am] 1994;76:1513.
201. Stull MA, Kransdorf MJ, Devaney KO. Langerhans cell histiocytosis of bone. Radiographics 1992;12:801.
202. VanderWilde RS, Wold LE, McLeod RA, Sim FH. Eosinophilic granuloma. Orthopedics 1990;13:1301.

Chapter 13

Cerebral Palsy

Thomas S. Renshaw

Basic Brain Development
Etiology
Prevalence
Classification
    Neuropathic Types
    Anatomic Patterns
Associated Problems in Other Systems
    Central Nervous System
    Gastrointestinal System
    Genitourinary System
Diagnosis
    History
    Physical Examination
    Other Tests
Common Types of Cerebral Palsy
    and Their Management
    Spastic Quadriplegia
    Spastic Diplegia
    Spastic Hemiplegia
    Athetoid Cerebral Palsy
Upper Extremity Involvement
    Nonsurgical Treatment
    Surgical Treatment

Cerebral palsy is a generic term that is used to describe various clinical syndromes whose common feature is the abnormal control of motor function by the brain. The abnormal control results in a disorder of movement, posturing, and sometimes sensory functioning, the manifestations of which often change with growth, development, and maturation.

The etiologic agents of cerebral palsy afflict the immature brain and usually produce neuropathologic lesions that do not progress. Although some parts of brain development continue throughout childhood, Gage has defined the "immature brain" as being younger than age 2 years. He classifies lesions occurring after that as producing static encephalopathy instead of cerebral palsy.[61]

BASIC BRAIN DEVELOPMENT

An excellent overview of brain development has been provided by Goldberg.[66] During the first trimester of embryonic life, the brain grossly differentiates into a recognizable cerebrum, cerebellum, and other structures. An insult during this period usually produces a structural lesion that is detectable by magnetic resonance imaging (MRI).

Neurons begin to develop early in the second trimester, originating in the periventricular regions and migrating toward the surface of the cerebral cortex. By the 15th week of gestation, fetal reflex movements can be detected. At the end of the second trimester, all neurons have been formed and any damage or loss cannot be replaced.

Synaptic connections begin to be established early in the third trimester and intensify after birth. Glialization, which begins in the second trimester, occurs at least until age 2 years.[169] Myelination in the brain does not begin until late in the third trimester but it continues into adolescence in a well-defined pattern. As more pathways become myelinated, prime reflexes drop out, mostly during the first 6 months after birth, and normal postural reflexes appear. As myelination continues, pathology in the brain becomes apparent. Overall brain morphologic maturation, as detectable by MRI, has been reported to continue through at least age 10 years.[184]

As Goldberg points out, only after the neuronal pathways from brain lesions have become myelinated and can be tested and found to be abnormal can such lesions be detected. For this reason, because different pathways are myelinated at different times, spastic diplegia usually is not detected until at least 8 to 10 months of age, hemiplegia usually at about 20 to 24 months, and athetosis usually after 24 months.[66] Once the lesions are apparent, their manifestations can change with further growth and maturation of the child.

ETIOLOGY

The cause of many cases of cerebral palsy remains unknown and is not necessarily the result of a static brain lesion that occurred in the prenatal or perinatal period. Only about 10% to 15% of patients in one large group had documented perinatal hypoxia or other problems.[139] It is not solely the result of prematurity because 60% to 65% of children with cerebral palsy are born at full term.[61] Other factors, genetic abnormalities, or teratologic agents sometimes may play a causative role.[50,148] Some patients probably have multiple etiologic factors.

The etiologic insult can occur in the prenatal period as the result of undetected agents or from a lesion caused by such problems as maternal infection, maternal drug or alcohol abuse, or congenital malformations of the child's brain.[228] Maternal epilepsy, hyperthyroidism, severe toxemia, an incompetent cervix, and third trimester bleeding have also been implicated.[184]

The insult can happen in the perinatal period because of trauma, placental complications, hypoxia, or anoxia. Low birth weight for gestational age and prematurity are commonly associated with the development of cerebral palsy, particularly the spastic diplegic type.[7] Breech presentation has been associated with increased risk.[61]

Postnatally, an insult to the brain can come from head trauma,[53] vascular accidents in the brain, central nervous system infections, kernicterus, hypoxia or anoxia from such causes as near drowning, suffocation and cardiac arrest, and other problems. The long-term manifestations of cerebral palsy caused by specific agents have not been extensively comparatively studied but there is some evidence that postnatal infectious causes commonly produce more severe orthopaedic deformities than do many other agents.[113]

The brain lesion is permanent and nonprogressive. Nevertheless, the natural history of cerebral palsy is not static. The effects of growth and maturation of not only the central nervous system but also the whole patient often cause changing musculoskeletal problems in the child.

PREVALENCE

Cerebral palsy is found in from 1 to 7 per 1000 children throughout most of the world, theoretically being more common in areas where prenatal maternal and perinatal infant care are poor.[138,169] In areas where sophisticated neonatal intensive care units exist, the risk of brain damage may be reduced by early treatment of certain problems, and the lives of very premature infants and those with other life-threatening problems are often saved. Overall, this only slightly reduces the incidence of cerebral palsy.[169]

Twin pregnancies result in a child with cerebral palsy about 12 times more commonly than do singleton pregnancies. This is largely related to low birth weight.[73]

The prevalence of the neuropathic types and anatomic patterns of cerebral palsy varies greatly in many reports because of the widely differing populations studied. For example, a study containing the residents of state institutions shows many more severely involved individuals than does a study derived from a large private practice.

CLASSIFICATION

Cerebral palsy is classified by the neuropathic type of motor abnormality and by the anatomic region of involvement.

Neuropathic Types

Spastic

Spasticity is an imprecise global term for an upper motor neuron syndrome. Lesions of the pyramidal system of the brain result in spasticity. The syndrome includes a velocity-dependent increase in tonic stretch reflexes (muscle tone) with exaggerated tendon jerks resulting from hyperexcitability of the stretch reflex. It may also include weakness, loss of muscle control or dexterity, interference with balance, fatigability, and often, the simultaneous contracting of antagonistic muscles.[233] Severe spasticity is often referred to as rigidity. Joint contractures are common in spastic cerebral palsy.

Athetoid

Athetosis is a type of dyskinesia (i.e., abnormal movement) caused by an extrapyramidal lesion and is distinguished by purposeless writhing movements that become aggravated when the child is frightened or excited. With pure athetosis, joint contractures are uncommon and muscle tone may not be increased. Tendon lengthenings in children with athetosis are often unpredictable and may result in creation of an opposite deformity that is more difficult to treat. Decades ago, athetosis comprised about 25% of cases of cerebral palsy because a major cause, Rh incompatibility with resulting kernicterus, was not easily detected and prevented.

Dystonia can occur together with athetosis. These children usually have increased general muscle tone, characterized by distorted postures and positions that are induced by voluntary movements.

Mixed

Children with mixed cerebral palsy have both pyramidal and extrapyramidal motor control involvement. Variable amounts of spasticity and athetosis usually occur together in the mixed form. Sometimes the athetoid component is barely detectable but may nevertheless make surgical treatment less predictable.

Ataxic

Ataxic cerebral palsy is uncommon. It is a disturbance of coordinated movement, most notable when walking, and is usually the result of cerebellar dysfunction. A mild intention tremor may be present, contractures are rare, and except for the treatment of scoliosis and hip dysplasia, surgery is rarely necessary.

Hypotonic

This is most often a stage through which an infant who eventually develops spastic cerebral palsy passes before having overt spasticity. The brain lesion is present but masked by lack of myelination of the pathways that will carry its abnormal messages. Occasionally, mentally retarded children are erroneously referred to as having hypotonic cerebral palsy.

Anatomic Patterns

Quadriplegia

Quadriplegia, also known as tetraplegia, implies involvement of all four limbs. Many of these children have global involvement, with mental retardation; bulbar dysfunction, manifested by drooling, dysarthria, and dysphagia; and seizures. The usual cause is severe hypoxia; after initially presenting as a floppy baby, the child shows delayed developmental milestones. The spectrum of severity is variable, from having no sitting ability or head control to being able to walk independently.

Diplegia

With diplegia, both lower extremities are involved and to a greater extent than the uppers, which are always affected to some degree. A substantial percentage of diplegia results from prematurity, which often has an associated periventricular hemorrhage in and around the third ventricle, producing the characteristic lesion of diplegia in the motor fibers to the lower extremities before they enter the internal capsule.[61] Intelligence is usually normal.

Hemiplegia

In hemiplegia, one side of the body is involved, the upper limb being more affected than the lower. The diagnosis is usually not made until after walking has begun or fine motor hand control is noted to be deficient. A focal traumatic, vascular, or an asymmetric infectious lesion is likely to be the cause of hemiplegia.

Seizure disorders are most frequently seen in this type of involvement, probably because of the focal brain lesion.[184] The seizures usually develop in the first 2 years of life.[40] Children with hemiplegia are also more likely to have homonymous hemianopsia and stereognostic deficits than those with other types of involvement.[184] Asymmetry of upper and lower limb growth, with the involved side being smaller, is also a common finding and is related to the trophic factor of sensory loss.[6]

Other Types

Anatomic patterns of involvement are not always clear cut, and some patients do not fit these common types. Blair and Stanley found only 55% intraobserver agreement in a cerebral palsy classification study.[21]

Double hemiplegia refers to bilateral and symmetric involvement, with the upper extremities being more afflicted than the lower extremities. Triplegia implies difficulty with any three limbs, usually both lower and one upper. Monoplegia means only one limb is affected.

Paraplegia is used to describe involvement of the lower extremities only. This is a rare occurrence as the result of a brain injury, and such a pattern of motor dysfunction should alert the physician to the possibility of pathology in the spinal cord or canal.

ASSOCIATED PROBLEMS IN OTHER SYSTEMS

Central Nervous System

Other central nervous system problems occur as the result of global brain involvement, with the spinal cord usually being spared. Seizures afflict about 30% of children with cerebral palsy and are most often seen in hemiparesis and quadriparesis, in patients with mental retardation, and in postnatally acquired cerebral palsy.[65]

Mental retardation, defined as IQ less than 50, occurs in 30% to 65% of children with cerebral palsy.[65,139] It is most prevalent in those with spastic quadriplegia. Other problems include behavioral and emotional difficulties; learning disorders; bulbar involvement with drooling, difficulty swallowing, and speech impairment; sensory deafness; and visual difficulties, such as perceptual problems, strabismus, nystagmus, and cortical blindness. Visual problems affect about 50% of children with cerebral palsy[61] and therefore, visual screening examinations are important for young children.

Gastrointestinal System

Problems with this system are particularly common in more severely involved children. Constipation and fecal impaction are common problems in children with global involvement.

Impaired swallowing, vomiting, esophageal reflux, and hiatal hernia can cause aspiration and the risk of severe pneumonia, epigastric pain, profound feeding problems, and poor nutrition.[33] Children with cerebral palsy who are malnourished have soft tissue wasting and interference with growth.[57,158] When they undergo surgery, they are at higher risk for postoperative infections.[100]

Assessment of nutrition includes composition of the diet, especially regarding calorie and protein intake, and the feeding history. Can the child feed him or herself and if not, who is the feeder? Is the swallowing competent or does frequent aspiration occur? A radiologic contrast study of swallowing and to rule out gastroesophageal reflux may be helpful. Nutritional status can be poor despite obesity, and therefore, studies such as total serum proteins and albumen; iron, iron-binding capacity, and transferrin levels; hemoglobin and erythrocyte mean corpuscular volume; and total lymphocyte count may be helpful as a indication of poor nutritional status.[99,116,230] Keep in mind, however, that no single study is an absolute indicator of malnutrition.

Correction of malnutrition is best accomplished by enteric feeding augmentation, if possible. If swallowing is impaired, a tube feeding program likely is necessary. When oral or tube feeding supplementation is not feasible, the child should be referred to an appropriate surgeon for consideration for a feeding gastrostomy or jejunostomy. Gastroesophageal reflux sometimes can be managed successfully by medical means but may require surgical fundoplication to improve alimentation and nutritional status.

Genitourinary System

Bladder dysfunction and urinary incontinence are common in severely afflicted children. They also have a higher incidence than the normal population of urinary tract infections, which may relate to bladder dysfunction and retrograde colonization from frequent diaper soiling and urolithiasis, probably caused by dehydration and urinary stasis.

McNeal and colleagues, in a study of cerebral palsy patients, noted that 28% complained of enuresis, 26% had stress incontinence, 18% had urgency, and 36% had more than one symptom.[125]

DIAGNOSIS

The diagnosis usually is established by a pediatrician or a neurologist before the child has had occasion to visit the orthopaedic surgeon. In some instances, however, an unexplained abnormal posturing, limp, toe walking, limb asymmetry, joint tightness, developmental delay, or other finding enables the orthopaedist to make the diagnosis of cerebral palsy.

History

Except for familial spastic paraparesis, which is an inherited condition, cerebral palsy is not a genetic disease. Relevant history begins with a search for possible etiologies, including environmental factors, any abnormal events during the pregnancy, the details of the birth, and assessment of the early neonatal and infantile periods. Next, it is important to assess some benchmark physical developmental milestones, such as sitting, crawling, cruising, and walking (Table 13-1). These may be normal with hemiplegia. The review of systems should be thorough to detect any of the commonly related problems. A history of previous treatment, including surgery, is essential.

Physical Examination

There are five main goals of the physical examination. They are:

1. To determine the grades of muscle strength and selective control
2. To evaluate the muscle tone and determine whether it is spastic, athetoid, or mixed
3. To evaluate the degree of deformity or muscle contracture at each of the major joints
4. To assess linear, angular, and torsional deformation of the spine and long bones and fixed hand or foot deformities
5. To appraise balance, equilibrium, and standing or walking postures.[61]

Physical assessment begins with observation of the child while taking the history. Next, as a dynamic examination, evaluate the head control, sitting balance, the ability to crawl, the ability to pull up to stand, standing posture and balance, and the ability to walk. Observational gait assessment is imperative in those who can walk. The remainder of the examination is performed on the examining table or, better yet, on the parent's lap if appropriate. Evaluation of the primitive neurologic reflexes and of muscle strength, muscle tone, joint range of motion, contractures, and torsional abnormalities should be assessed.[23,61,222] Motor dysfunction in the extremities can also be a manifestation of a brain or spinal cord tumor, infection, or other problem.

At the end of the initial history and physical examination, it is useful to formulate an overall general functional assessment of the patient, particularly for documentation at that time and when communicating with other health care professionals. The following is an example of such an assessment: "The patient is a 5-year-old boy with spastic quadriplegic cerebral palsy. He is the product of a 32-week uncomplicated pregnancy and was delivered by emergency cesarean section because of uncontrolled uterine bleeding. He has fair head control, poor sitting balance, and has never pulled to stand or walked. He is able to communicate discomfort only and does not participate in any activities of daily living."

Other Tests

Highly specialized gait analysis, valuable in the management of certain patients with cerebral palsy, is rarely necessary for diagnostic purposes. It may be useful in differentiating between idiopathic toe walking and mild spastic diplegia.[83,101,157]

The diagnosis of such conditions as dysmorphic syndromes or congenital metabolic, neurologic, and muscular diseases usually can be differentiated from global involvement with cerebral palsy by chromosomal analysis. Special imaging techniques, including MRI, positron-emission tomography, and computed tomography are useful in the evaluation of intracranial pathology.

Plain radiographs may be important. If there is any sign of a spinal deformity, radiographs in the coronal or sagittal planes or both document the degree and sometimes the cause (e.g., a congenital vertebral anomaly) of the deformity. It can be cogently argued that a periodic (every 6–12 months) coronal plane radiograph of the pelvis is necessary for the early detection of hip pathology in children with spastic diplegia or quadriplegia who are not walking (Fig. 13-1). Weight-bearing radiographs of the feet and ankles, in the anteroposterior and maximally dorsiflexed lateral projections, document the status of foot deformities when surgical intervention is being considered.

COMMON TYPES OF CEREBRAL PALSY AND THEIR MANAGEMENT

The remainder of this chapter uses the formats of spastic quadriplegia, diplegia, and hemiplegia; athetoid cerebral palsy; and the upper extremity to discuss the principles and techniques of management of the most common problems faced by the child with cerebral palsy.

Many centers have developed cerebral palsy management programs conducted by teams of knowledgeable specialists. Team members usually include a pediatrician, orthopaedic surgeon, neurologist, consultant neurosurgeon, clinical nurse specialist, physical therapist, occupational therapist, speech-language specialist, social worker, educator, and psychologist.[184] It is especially important for the team members to frequently communicate and confirm that they are in agreement, at least substantially, so that the family does not receive mixed or conflicting messages about their child's problems or care. The family is the most important member of the team.

Spastic Quadriplegia

The example for this section is a patient with global involvement, who is unable to walk, and who requires

TABLE 13-1 Simple Developmental Milestones

MILESTONE	AVERAGE AGE ACHIEVED (mo)	95th PERCENTILE (mo)
Head control	3	6
Independent sitting	6	9
Crawling	8	Some never do
Pull up to stand	8	12
Independent walking	12	17

From Rang M. Cerebral palsy. In: Morrissy RT, ed. Lovell and Winter's pediatric orthopaedics, ed 3. Philadelphia: JB Lippincott, 1990.

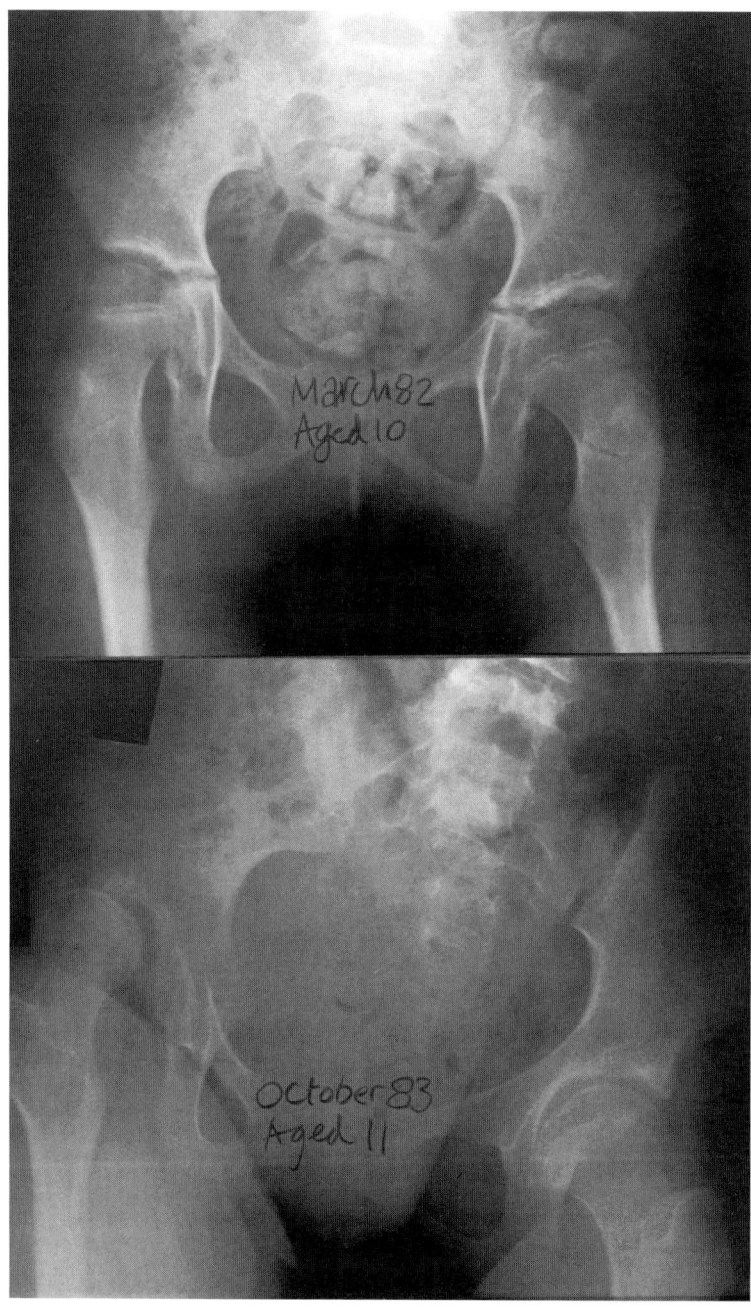

FIGURE 13-1. Radiographs showing substantial changes in the right hip, including dislocation, which developed over a few months at age 10 years. Annual hip evaluations, including radiographs, are important in detecting such problems.

nearly total care. Of paramount importance are the priorities of such a patient, which are, in order of importance: communication with others; the ability to take care of activities of daily living, especially personal hygiene; mobility in the environment; and walking.[23] Only about 20% of the children with spastic quadriplegia eventually walk.

Given that most people in this group will not be walking, realistic goals for their orthopaedic care are directed toward maintaining balanced, comfortable sitting. The specific objectives are achievement and maintenance of:

- a straight spine and a level pelvis
- located, mobile, painless hips that flex to at least 90 degrees for comfortable sitting and extend to at least 30 degrees of flexion to accomplish pivot transfers
- mobile knees that flex for sitting and can extend enough (to ~20 degrees or less of flexion) to be controlled by orthoses for transfers
- plantigrade feet for wearing of shoes and for comfort on the footplates of wheelchairs
- an appropriate wheelchair
- management of problems in the other systems, such as malnutrition, seizures.

It is important to understand that it is in the wheelchair that the patient with spastic quadriplegia will spend most waking hours. This chair should be

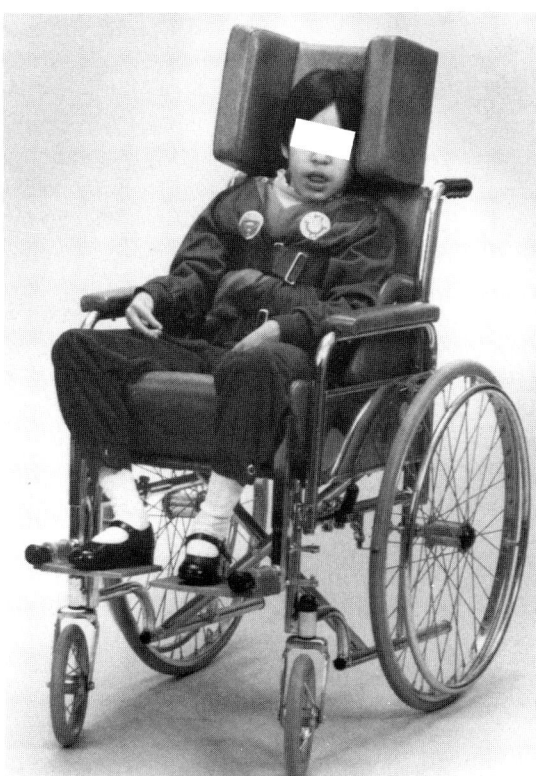

FIGURE 13-2. An appropriately fitted wheelchair provides proper body positioning, including head control.

thought of as a total body orthosis, to be fitted and maintained by an expert (Fig. 13-2). It is beneficial for all concerned to have a physical therapist who is experienced in dealing with wheelchairs collaborate in developing the wheelchair prescription. The following should be considered in wheelchair design:

Foot rests
Should be long enough for the shoes
Should support the entire foot in its position
Should be able to swing out of the way for entering and exiting the chair
Should accommodate foot restraint straps if needed.

Seat
Height must allow the feet to correctly contact the foot rests
Depth should entirely support each of the thighs, which may not be of equal lengths, but not compress the popliteal area
Width should not compress the trochanters but should also not allow lateral shifting or excessive tilting of the pelvis
Firmness should be as much as tolerated by the patient, to provide maximum pelvic stability but without creating excessive skin pressure over bony prominences
Contour should be incorporated if necessary for comfort

Chairback
Height should support the patient's trunk from the pelvis to the midscapular region
Width should accommodate the trunk and any needed thoracic support pads
Firmness should be a much as comfortable, to aid in preventing collapsing kyphosis
Contouring should be incorporated if necessary to accommodate scoliosis
Reclining feature may be a necessary feature
Restraint components
May be necessary for foot, leg, pelvic, trunk, arm or head control
Portability
Necessary if transportation in the community is desired
Propulsion method
The patient's arms
An attendant
Motorization.

The method of propulsion is of paramount importance. The ability to independently transfer in and out of a wheelchair greatly facilitates the ability to live in a group-home setting for an adult with spastic quadriplegia.

Because the child's waking activities are performed while sitting, the spine and hips are of prime importance and are often the site of major problems in spastic quadriplegia. Other lower extremity problems specific to the patient with spastic quadriplegia who can walk are addressed in the section on spastic diplegia.

Hyperlordosis

Increased lordosis in the lumbar spine is almost never a primary deformity in patients with cerebral palsy. It is usually secondary to hip flexion contractures, and in this situation, it responds to correction of those contractures by appropriate means such as stretching or, more often, surgical lengthening of the psoas tendon. Hyperlordosis can also be a compensatory deformity below a rigid thoracic hyperkyphosis, and it usually responds to correction of the primary problem. When surgical spinal fusion is necessary to correct severe scoliosis, it is essential to consider the sagittal plane spinal balance and preserve adequate lumbar lordosis by avoiding overdistraction across the lumbar spine.

Hyperkyphosis

Hyperkyphosis is most commonly seen in the young child with cerebral palsy who has weak spinal extensor musculature and a resultant long, C-shaped kyphosis posturing of the entire spine. This is almost always flexible and corrects fully on prone lying. It is best controlled by proper seating adaptation, such as restraint straps on the wheelchair or less often by a thoracolumbosacral orthosis to provide sitting support. There is debate regarding whether increasing the sitting support inhibits the function in the spinal extensor muscles and weakens them further and whether physical therapy or muscle stimulation is helpful in maintaining or enhancing spinal extensor muscle strength. In all likelihood, such treatment is not of any functional benefit.

Kyphosis occasionally occurs in the lumbar spine as the result of overly tight hamstring muscles. This kyphosis disappears with proximal lengthening of the hamstrings.

Children with cerebral palsy are not immune to the spinal deformities that afflict normal children, and thoracic hyperkyphosis as the result of Scheuermann condition or postural juvenile kyphosis may also occur. Indications for orthotic treatment in these kyphotic conditions are similar to those in normal children but spinal orthotics are not likely to be as well tolerated.

Scoliosis

Scoliosis is more prevalent in all types of cerebral palsy when compared with the general population and varies directly with the severity of motor involvement. In patients with mild hemiplegia, scoliosis occurs in probably in fewer than 5%; in patients with severe spastic quadriplegia, it is higher; overall, in all cerebral palsy patients, it is about 25%. Specific increased risk factors for curve progression are quadriplegia, younger age, poor sitting balance, pelvic obliquity, and the presence of multiple curves.

Scoliosis in cerebral palsy is different from idiopathic scoliosis. It develops earlier; is more likely to be progressive; progresses beyond skeletal maturity, especially when the curve exceeds 40 degrees; is markedly less responsive to orthotic control; and is more likely to require surgical treatment.

As with idiopathic or other types of scoliosis, there are only three appropriate options for management. These are observation with documentation, orthotic treatment, or surgical stabilization. Observation alone is indicated for a curve that is of insufficient magnitude to require treatment (<25–30 degrees) or is present in a patient whose best interests may not be served by active surgical intervention. The latter category is difficult to define; it would include the most severely involved individuals who are unable to perceive or interact with their environment in any meaningful fashion, based on severe and global compromise of their cognitive and sensory perception abilities. Only careful study by many members of the cerebral palsy team and the patient's family can lead to this assessment. In such cases, the overall management goals are the patient's safety and comfort.

The orthotic treatment of scoliosis in quadriplegic cerebral palsy was based mostly on hope and empiricism until two studies showed that it rarely succeeds in controlling a curve.[126,174] Most quadriplegic patients from each center did not experience any meaningful curve control from orthotic treatment. In some cases, however, an orthosis may slow curve progression, particularly in curves of 30 to 60 degrees, allowing beneficial growth in an immature spine before definitive surgical stabilization. At best, no more than 15% of brace-treated curves stop progressing. This may simply reflect the natural history of some cases of scoliosis in cerebral palsy.[175] Ambulatory patients with spastic diplegia may develop idiopathic-type scoliotic curves. In these milder cases of cerebral palsy, brace control may be successful. Orthoses and other types of external devices for trunk support may be of value in improving sitting balance, particularly for those patients in whom surgery is not indicated and for those who still have significant spinal imbalance after surgical treatment. If the patient can tolerate a total contact low-profile orthosis, this is the most effective and economical means of providing improved trunk support, even if it is a relatively soft orthosis.[112] This is often not the case, however, and a custom-molded trunk or total-body–supporting wheelchair insert is required. These devices are difficult to fit properly, often quickly outgrown, and expensive. They must provide adequate pelvic support, trunk control, and head control.[170] Nevertheless, the ability to sit as erectly and comfortably as possible is essential for a totally involved patient. Good sitting improves the patient's mental outlook, communication ability, respiratory function, ease of feeding, gastrointestinal function, hand usage, and mobility in the environment.[142]

Surgical stabilization of progressing scoliosis is the only way to stop such a curve in most cases.[64,220] The benefit of a procedure of this magnitude and expense has been questioned by some,[103] but most orthopedic surgeons strongly believe that the surgery is worthwhile, particularly in preventing loss of the ability to sit. Postoperative patients with reasonably balanced nonprogressive scoliosis have better endurance for sitting and, according to their caregivers, are easier to feed, dress, and transport than those with severe untreated scoliosis. Perhaps after fusion they have less back discomfort, better pulmonary function and resistance to respiratory infections, and less decubitus skin ulceration than similarly involved patients with severe, untreated scoliosis, but this is difficult to prove.[69]

Once a curve exceeds 40 degrees magnitude, it is likely to continue progressing and surgery is usually indicated. Posterior internal fixation with a segmental system, such as double rods with cross-links connected to the spine by multiple hooks; sublaminar wires; interspinous wires; or combinations of these techniques and an adequate posterior fusion mass is usually all that is needed to achieve a balanced spine over a reasonably level pelvis, the objective of such surgery.[4,64,114,201] Whenever possible, a larger and more rigid rod is preferable to provide better correction, resist deforming forces, and promote a solid arthrodesis. It is essential to achieve spinal balance in both the coronal and sagittal planes to maximize sitting balance. An abundance of banked allograft bone should be available to generate the adequate fusion mass.

Fusion limits are usually from the upper thoracic region (T1–T3) to L5 or more commonly to the pelvis. When the fusion does not extend to the upper thoracic region, there is the risk of developing a substantial junctional kyphosis cephalad to it, and this may interfere with the ability of the patient to see at or above the horizontal or require constant and eventually painful neck hyperextension to do so. Applying a bilateral two-level clawed hook configuration at the cephalad end of the rods (Fig. 13-3) preserves the uppermost posterior ligaments and may help to prevent a junctional kyphosis. Nevertheless, no matter how cephalad the upper fusion level or what type the fixation, some patients still develop a junctional kyphosis.

Fusions should include the pelvis if pelvic obliquity exceeds 10 degrees from the intercrestal iliac line to the top of L5 or L4 when measured on a sitting anteroposterior radiograph. Otherwise, pelvic obliquity may continue to progress and make sitting more difficult. Various techniques for pelvic fixation are available, including hooks, rods, and screws anchored to various bones, but none have withstood the test of time better than the Galveston technique.[5]

Routine anterior spinal surgery is not necessary in cerebral palsy. The most common indication for anterior spinal surgery in cerebral palsy is to improve curve correctability. This increased correction may be needed to level the pelvis when pelvic obliquity is rigid and severe; to balance the spine in large, rigid curves that do not correct to less than 60 degrees during supine bending or maximum traction radiographs; to release the anterior tether of a kyphos; or to attempt to improve respiratory function or decrease the likelihood of the development of a pseudarthrosis in severe curves. In such cases, release of deforming structures is accomplished by dividing the anterior longitudinal ligament, excising the annulus fibrosis and removing all of the disc material back to the posterior annulus and longitudinal ligament, removing the vertebral end plates to subchondral or cancellous bone, and packing bone graft into the disc spaces. Anterior internal fixation is rarely necessary when strong, rigid posterior fixation is performed. Most surgeons prefer to accomplish both the anterior and the posterior operations at the same surgical setting rather than to stage them several days or weeks apart.[116]

There are several other important considerations when managing a spinal deformity by surgical means in a patient with cerebral palsy. Many of the patients are malnourished and may have gastroesphageal reflux, as discussed earlier. Detecting and correcting these conditions preoperatively helps prevent postoperative wound infection and healing problems by improving the patient's nutritional status.[55] Intraoperative blood loss should be calculated carefully, expressed in terms of percentage of blood volume, and appropriately replaced to avoid hypovolemia or dangerous coagulopathies, especially when blood loss nears 50% of the blood volume. With this method, preoperative blood volume must be accurately estimated and suctioned blood loss plus blood in weighed sponges carefully measured. Another means of monitoring blood loss and replacement is by calculating erythrocyte mass and considering hematocrit measurements in the lost blood as well as in the replacement source.

Postoperative pulmonary problems such as hypoventilation, atelectasis, aspiration pneumonia, and the adult respiratory distress syndrome may occur and every preventive effort, including rapid mobilization of the patient, must be undertaken.

Spondylolysis and Spondylolisthesis

Although spondylolysis and spondylolisthesis do not occur in nonambulatory patients, they have been reported in ambulatory patients with cerebral palsy with an incidence similar to that in the general population. No increased severity of symptoms or relation to hip flexion contractures has been noted.[81]

Hip Problems

There is a spectrum of hip problems commonly seen in spastic quadriplegia, including limitation of motion, contractures, hip at risk, subluxation, and dislocation of the hip.

The hip at risk has increased valgus and anteversion and a shallow acetabulum but no subluxation. Tightness and contractures in the adductor and flexor muscles are usually present, and concern for progressive hip instability is particularly warranted with less than 30 degrees of abduction in flexion or extension and greater than 20 to 25 degrees of flexion contracture.

Causative factors of hip problems are probably combinations of muscle imbalance, acetabular dyspla-

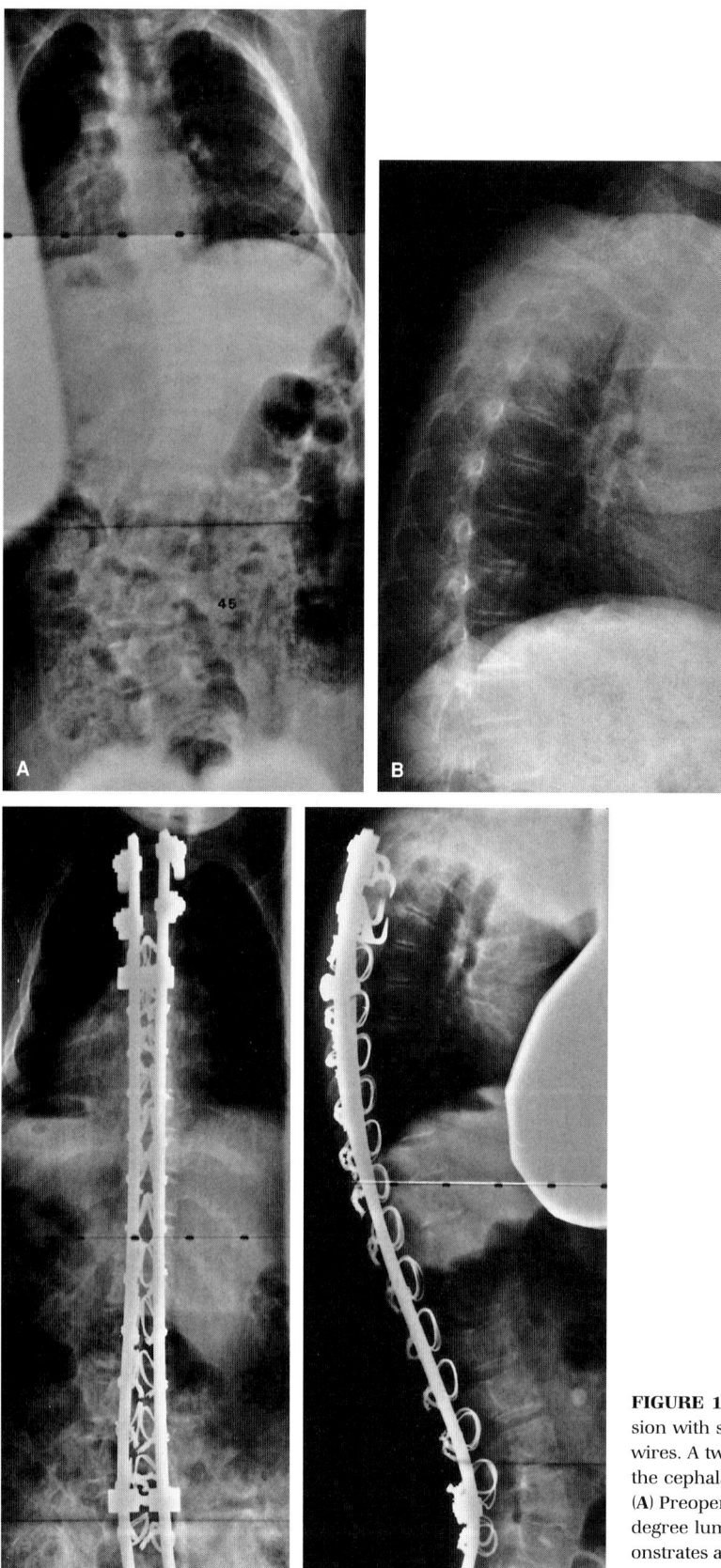

FIGURE 13-3. Treatment of scoliosis by posterior spinal fusion with segmental instrumentation, using mostly sublaminar wires. A two-level transverse process–pedicle claw was used at the cephalad end in an attempt to prevent junctional kyphosis. (**A**) Preoperative posteroanterior radiograph demonstrates a 45-degree lumbar curve. (**B**) Preoperative lateral radiograph demonstrates associated thoracic kyphosis. (**C**) Postoperative posteroanterior radiograph. (**D**) Postoperative lateral radiograph demonstrates the cephalad claw configuration of the hooks.

sia, pelvic obliquity, excessive femoral anteversion, increased femoral neck valgus, lack of weight bearing, and maldirected resultant force vectors across the hip joint. Femoral anteversion is greater at all age levels in children with cerebral palsy than in the normal population. It does not change significantly after age 6 years[111] and is greater in ambulatory children than in nonwalkers.[1]

Because of increased muscle tone and some contracture, it can be difficult to detect even substantial hip abnormalities by routine physical examination. For this reason, it is wise to obtain an annual screening radiograph of the hips in children with spastic quadriplegia and in patients with spastic diplegia who do not walk. Hip subluxation or dislocation, although more common before the age of 6 years, may occur at any age. Children particularly at risk are those with less than 30 degrees of hip abduction in flexion or extension and those with hip flexion contractures of greater than 20 degrees.

In all but the most severely involved children, it is wise to prevent hip dislocation. Although hips at risk and hips that are subluxated rarely cause discomfort, dislocation can lead to pain. Studies have reported pain in about 50% of cerebral palsy patients with dislocated hips,[41,131] and the associated increased contractures may make care more difficult and worsen sitting balance. One study, however, found that surgical reduction of dislocated hips did not improve pain or sitting ability.[168] Until more studies with longer follow-up regarding treatment of dislocated hips in cerebral palsy are available, most surgeons follow the management described in the following section.

Hip Management

HIP AT RISK. Hips at risk often progress to subluxation or dislocation unless treated. Such progression may be slow (months to years) or occur in a period of days to weeks. It is not possible, however, to predict the natural history of every hip at risk in cerebral palsy. Indeed, the literature lacks valid data regarding the likelihood of such hips worsening. That leaves the surgeon with the options of closely following hips at risk or intervening; most intervene, unless the patient is so cerebrally compromised as to preclude surgical treatment, while realizing that at least in some cases the hip pathology would not have been progressive.

Treatment of the hip at risk consists of surgical lengthening and weakening of the tight adductors and flexors.[144,166,198] The adductor longus and often part or all of the adductor brevis and the gracilis should always be released or transferred, and tenotomy or elongation of the psoas tendon, sparing the iliacus fibers, should be performed. The issue of whether to release or transfer the adductors is discussed in the section on spastic diplegia. Psoas tenotomy in a nonambulatory patient with spastic quadriplegia may be performed either at the pelvic brim or just above the lesser trochanter. The more caudal site produces more weakness in the iliopsoas muscle complex, a situation of no consequence to a nonwalker but one that may be detrimental to an ambulatory patient who needs adequate hip flexor power to lift the limb for step climbing.[66]

Postoperatively, many surgeons use abduction splinting, applied at night and always within the child's range of comfortable abduction, for several months in an attempt to avoid recurrent contractures. The value of such splinting is debatable and a controlled study proving that splinting prevents recurrent contractures would be beneficial but difficult.

In the past, anterior branch or even complete obturator neurectomy has been performed to denervate the adductor muscles in addition to lengthening them. This is not common because most surgeons believe that it is unnecessary when an adequate adductor release (i.e., allowing ≥60 degrees of passive abduction) has been performed. If the child has an athetoid component in addition to the spasticity, obturator neurectomy can result in a severe, disabling, problematic abduction contracture.

The use of stretching exercises alone as treatment for hips at risk is rarely successful. In cases of hips at risk in which muscle tightness is absent, night splinting, in an attempt to improve acetabular depth, is an option that most surgeons would choose.

SUBLUXATION. Hip subluxation is defined as uncovering of more than a third of the femoral head[69,194] and a break in the Shenton line but with the femoral head maintaining at least some contact with the acetabulum. Surgical treatment of the subluxation can prevent subsequent dislocation.[8,90]

Although soft tissue releases and prolonged splinting can occasionally be successful, the subluxated hip most often has increased valgus, anteversion, or both and requires corrective proximal femoral osteotomy.[90,94,102,115] To stabilize the hip joint, varus of the femoral neck is usually reduced to about 115 degrees in an ambulatory child, sometimes more in a nonambulator, and derotation of the excessive femoral anteversion to about 20 degrees is performed, in addition to appropriate tendon releases.

If acetabular dysplasia is present (acetabular index > 25 degrees),[136] it should also be corrected, when severe, in a child younger than 4 or 5 years and almost always in older children. Older children have less potential for biologic remodeling to normalize the acetabulum after varization and derotation, as can happen in the younger children. The dysplasia is corrected by choosing the appropriate procedure and being certain that its prerequisites are met. The Salter, Steel, and Sutherland types of acetabular redirection, the Pemberton procedure, the Dega osteotomy, Chiari medializing osteotomy, and shelf augmentation of the acetabular rim all have appropriate indications in cerebral palsy[38,69,150,162,203,205,214,234] and arthrographic evaluation and when available, three-dimensional reformatted CT scanning images are often helpful in the decision-making process.[1,79] Before age 9 years, unilateral subluxation may best be treated by bilateral surgery because the other hip is usually at least somewhat abnormal or likely will become so when only unilateral surgery is done.[37]

The dysplastic acetabulum in cerebral palsy is shallow and associated with an increase in the femoral neck-shaft angle and femoral anteversion. In nonambulators, the acetabular deficit is superior and posterior, whereas in ambulatory patients, acetabular dysplasia may be less severe but femoral anteversion is greater than for nonambulators.[1]

After careful evaluation of the pathoanatomy, most patients are found to need a femoral varization and derotational osteotomy. The derotation should preserve 5 to 15 degrees of anteversion[31] or 30 to 45 degrees of passive internal hip rotation to prevent postoperative posterior subluxation.[27] Varization should always restore normal anatomy, with preservation of a neck-shaft angle of about 120 to 125 degrees,[31] although greater amounts of varization are acceptable in nonambulatory children (Fig. 13-4).

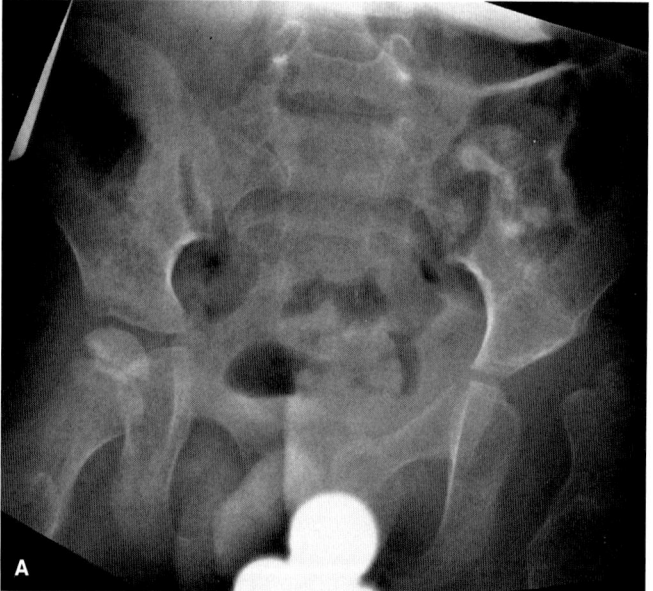
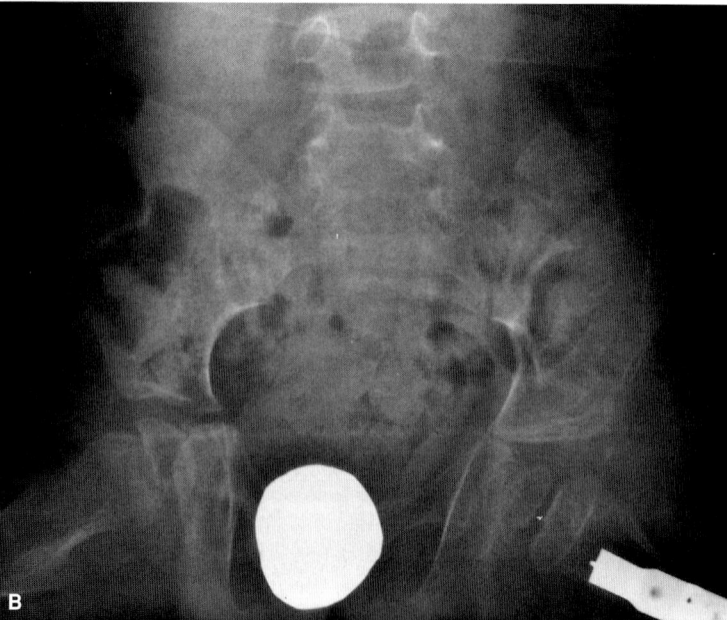

FIGURE 13-4. Dislocation of the left hip in this patient with spastic quadriplegia was treated by varization-derotation osteotomy and innominate osteotomy.

If the acetabulum is found to be deficient superiorly and anteriorly (rare) or purely superiorly, an anterolateral rotational osteotomy such as a Pemberton, Salter, Steel, or Sutherland procedure is appropriate. More often, there is superior and posterior deficiency, in which restoration of posterior coverage by a shelf-augmentation procedure, a Dega procedure,[48] or a pericapsular osteotomy[136] is more appropriate. The Chiari osteotomy can be performed if the superior acetabular rim has not been so proximally eroded that the cut will enter the sacroiliac joint; however, in younger patients (i.e., bone ages younger than 12 years) the pericapsular acetabuloplasty hinges at the triradiate cartilage and provides good coverage of the femoral head by original acetabular cartilage.[27,136]

DISLOCATION. Hip dislocation may be addressed by relocation procedures,[76] by accepting the dislocation, by proximal femoral resection,[39] or less commonly, by hip arthrodesis or total hip replacement arthroplasty.[106,177] If the dislocation occurred within 1 year, most surgeons elect to perform anterior open reduction, combined with appropriate soft tissue releases (usually adductors and psoas tendon) and proximal femoral shortening, varization, and derotation osteotomy. Often, some degree of acetabular dysplasia is associated with the dislocation, and it is wise to correct this at the same time. The pelvic procedure should be tailored to the situation, as described in the previous discussion of the subluxated hip, and such operations as the pericapsular osteotomy,[136] Chiari osteotomy,[38,150] the Pemberton procedure,[162] rotational innominate osteotomies,[205,214] and shelf-augmentation procedures[203,233] have all been successfully applied in cerebral palsy.

If the hip has been dislocated for longer than 1 year, achieving a painless, mobile, stable hip from open reduction and other surgery is less likely because of joint incongruity and eroded articular cartilage on the femoral head. When such a hip is painless, no treatment is required. When the hip is painful, proximal femoral resection with muscle interposition, as described by Castle,[39,122] has a high success rate. This resection is performed at the subtrochanteric level, and muscle cuffs are sewn over the acetabulum and the femoral stump (Fig. 13-5). Postoperative management should consist of either abduction bracing, abduction cylinder casts, or comfortable but effective hip range of motion exercises to assure maintenance of the desired hip motion (i.e., minimal flexion contracture, at least 100 degrees of flexion, neutral rotation, and abduction to at least 20 degrees). Postoperative traction or external fixators are rarely necessary. The result is usually good motion, good pain relief, and definite thigh shortening, which must be accommodated in the seat of the wheelchair. Another option for the long-standing painful dislocated hip is arthrodesis, as discussed in the following section.

OSTEOARTHRITIS. The located osteoarthritic hip in cerebral palsy need not be treated surgically unless it is painful and nonsurgical methods have been

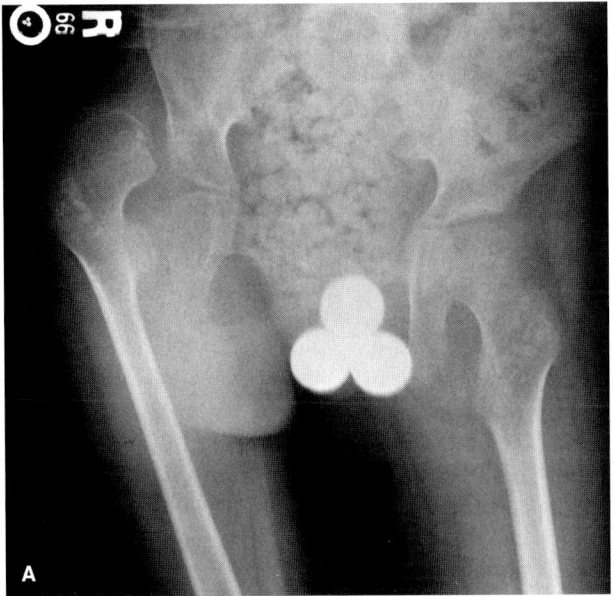
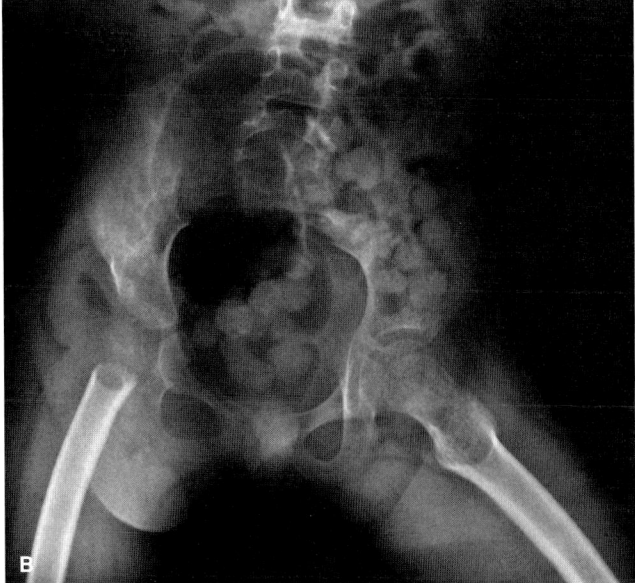

FIGURE 13-5. This nonambulatory child's painful dislocated right hip was treated by resection of the proximal femur just distal to the lesser trochanter and oversewing muscle flaps. This is known as the Castle procedure. His pain was relieved. (**A**) Preoperative anteroposterior radiograph shows the dislocated right hip with femoral head deformity and acetabular dysplasia. (**B**) Posterative radiograph. The proximal femur has been resected at the distal end of the lesser trochanter.

unsuccessful. In that case, arthrodesis and replacement arthroplasty have both been successful, the latter being preferred because of less postoperative morbidity and easier management.[178] Arthrodesis in usually performed in a position appropriate for walking, sitting, and lying: 20 to 30 degrees of flexion, 5 to 10 degrees abduction, and neutral rotation for an ambulatory patient and 45 degrees of flexion for a nonambulator. Leg length equalization should be considered in walking patients because it may defer the development of back pain.[17] Arthrodesis may be more difficult to accomplish in nonambulatory patients with severe spasticity; when enough flexion is provided to make sitting comfortable, it may limit the ability to lie supine comfortably. Arthrodesis, therefore, is not often performed.

The reported experience with replacement arthroplasty for painful dislocated hips is small.[178] This procedure is indicated for the ambulatory adult with mild to moderate spasticity and severe degenerative arthritis of the hip.

EXTENSION CONTRACTURE AND EXTENSOR THRUST. Extension contracture of the hip occasionally occurs in the severely spastic child with quadriplegia. It is caused by tight, contracted hamstrings, which are hip extensors as well as knee flexors, and it can greatly interfere with comfortable sitting because the extension contracture does not allow adequate hip flexion. The treatment of extension contracture is lengthening of the proximal hamstrings.[57,69] When this is not adequate, posterior capsulotomy of the hip and release of the external rotator muscles may also be necessary. A more common situation is extensor thrust, rigid and sustained hip extension that literally almost throws the child out of the wheelchair. Treatment options are proximal lengthening of the hamstrings or injections into the hamstrings of neuromotor blocking agents, a method with which this author has had no experience.

EXTENSION AND ABDUCTION CONTRACTURE. Extension and abduction contracture of the hip is not common. It most often occurs after injudicious release of the flexors and adductors in patients with athetosis and is also seen after aggressive flexor and adductor releases in patients with severe rigidity and spasticity plus previously undetected cospasticity in the hip extensor and abductor muscles.

Cospasticity is the simultaneous existence of spasticity in both the agonist and antagonist muscles controlling a joint. The spasticity may or may not be of equal magnitude. It can be difficult to detect, even by careful physical examination, but when severe both flexion and extension of the joint are substantially limited. Gait analysis with kinematics and telemetered electromyographic monitoring detects cospasticity in ambulatory patients.

Fortunately, patients with profound athetosis, because of their writhing movements, rarely develop contractures that require surgical releasing. The problem is in the mixed spastic-athetoid patient, in whom the surgeon cannot precisely know just how much spastic muscle to weaken. It is definitely better to err on the side of underrelease.

Treatment of mild cases of extension and abduction contracture of the hip consists of stretching exercises and proper seating in the wheelchair. With more severe involvement, surgical treatment is necessary. This involves release of the proximal hamstrings, the femoral and iliotibial band insertions of the gluteus maximus, the external rotator muscles, and even posterior capsulotomy of the hip joint if necessary. In long-standing severe contractures, femoral shortening may be necessary to prevent overstretching of the sciatic nerve.[216]

Spastic Diplegia

Most children with spastic diplegia walk, although late walking is the rule and it is not unusual for a diplegic child not to begin ambulation until age 4 years or even later.[140] Motor improvement, however, usually reaches a plateau at about age 7 years, so that if a child is not walking by then, there is little likelihood that he or she will walk.[16,23] The severity of lower extremity involvement is the most important factor in walking ability. A seizure disorder, marked flaccidity, persistent abnormal primitive reflexes, or a dislocated hip are significant deterrents to walking, whereas intelligence, upper extremity severity index, or birth weight do not correlate closely with walking prognosis.[16] Mental retardation has little or no effect on walking ability.[23,130]

Bleck (Table 13-2) and Beals (Table 13-3) have described criteria for predicting the likelihood of walking in children with cerebral palsy,[16,22,25] and Campos da Paz studied 272 children with cerebral palsy and found that achievement of head balance before age 9 months, independent sitting by 24 months, and crawling by 30 months were good prognostic indicators for walking, whereas lack of head control by age 20 months indicated a poor prognosis.[34] Conversely, Molnar and Gordon, in a study of 233 children with cerebral palsy, found that in children younger than age 2 years, independent sitting was not a good predictor for walking ability, but that after age 4 years, inability to sit predicted nonambulation.[130]

Hoffer and colleagues classified ambulation for meningomyelocele into four functional levels. This classification is often used in children with cerebral palsy:

TABLE 13-2 Bleck's Walking Prognosis Criteria

1. Asymmetric tonic neck reflex (ATNR)
2. Neck-righting relfex (NRR)
3. Moro reflex (MR)
4. Symmetric tonic neck reflex (STNR)
5. Parachute reaction (PR)
6. Foot-placement reaction (FPR)
7. Extensor thrust (ET)

These tests are performed in order on nonambulatory children after the age of 12 months. When one of the following is present (ATNR, NRR, MR, STNR, ET) or absent (PR, FPR), one point is given. A score of zero gives a good prognosis for walking; patients with one point has a guarded prognosis; and two or more points indicates a poor prognosis.

From Bleck EE. Orthopaedic management of cerebral palsy. Philadelphia: WB Saunders, 1979.

1. Community ambulators: these patients walk indoors and outdoors for most of their activities and may need crutches, braces, or both. They use a wheelchair only for long trips out of the community.
2. Household ambulators: these patients walk only indoors and with apparatus. They are able to get in and out of the chair and bed with little or no assistance. They may use the wheelchair for some indoor activities at home and school and for all activities in the community.
3. Nonfunctional ambulators: walking for these patients is a therapy session at home, in school, or in the hospital. Afterward, they use their wheelchairs to get from place to place and to satisfy all their needs for transportation.
4. Nonambulators: these patients are wheelchair-bound but usually can transfer from chair to bed.[86]

Children with spastic diplegia are less often afflicted with scoliosis, seizures, speech impediments, and major problems in other systems than are those with quadriplegia. Hip dislocation is also less likely but excessive valgus and anteversion of the proximal femur, acetabular dysplasia, and hips at risk or subluxated are not uncommon.

Treatment and diagnostic modalities for patients with spastic diplegia include drugs, physical therapy, intramuscular injections, manipulation and casting, orthotics, selective dorsal rhizotomy, gait analysis, and musculoskeletal surgery. These modalities are discussed in this section.

Treatment Methods

DRUGS. Ideally, a systemic, orally administered medication would appropriately temper spasticity and allow nearly normal voluntary muscle control to occur over the long term. Unfortunately, such an agent does not exist. Many types of systemic muscle relaxants, antispasmodics, and neuroinhibitory medications have been tried to little or no avail. Pharmacotherapy widely accepted as effective for problems in cerebral palsy has been limited to anticonvulsants for seizures; diazepam for superimposed postoperative myospasms, by its probable effect of increasing presynaptic inhibition[232] and perhaps for its tranquilizing effect on pain perception; and locally injected nerve or muscle blocking agents such as local anesthetics, alcohol, phenol, and botulinum-A toxin, which are discussed in the section on intramuscular injections.

The intrathecal injection of baclofen, an agonist of the inhibitory neurotransmitter γ-aminobutyric acid, which interferes with release of excitatory transmitters,[232] has shown some ability to decrease lower extremity spasticity for about 8 hours without an effect on upper extremity tone. This drug is thought to act on spinal cord synaptic reflexes.[61] It has not been effective when given orally. Large long-term studies of its benefits when administered by indwelling intrathecal catheter are not yet available. It may be of some benefit in assessing the potential benefit of selective posterior rhizotomy.[3]

PHYSICAL THERAPY. There are several possible roles for physical therapy in cerebral palsy, some generally well accepted and some not. Regarding the latter, several attempts to modify the central nervous system by externally applied stimuli have been exhaustively tried over the past several decades. These include neurodevelopmental therapy, sensory integration therapy, patterning, conductive education, pressure-point stimulation, bracing and stretching, and many recreation-based therapies.[179] The benefits of most of these methods continue to be debated.[82,104,155,167,231] For them to succeed, the central ner-

TABLE 13-3 Beals Walking Prognosis Criteria

SEVERITY INDEX*	WALKING PROGNOSIS
>8	Free walking by age 3
12–18	Free walking by age 7
10–11	Free or crutch walking by age 6
0–9	Crutch or no walking

* The severity index is defined as the motor age in months at the chronologic age of 3 years.

From Beals R. Spastic paraplegia and diplegia: an evaluation of the non-surgical and surgical factors influencing the prognosis for ambulation. J Bone Joint Surg [Am] 1966;48:827.

vous system probably has to be modified or reprogrammed to make new connections that function almost as well as those the brain originally made,[66] and this may not be possible.

There is considerable difference of opinion regarding the role and value of such types of therapy in attempts to reduce muscle tone and increase voluntary control. Debate in this area covers which modalities should be employed, at what age, how often (from once per week to virtually continuous therapy for 18 hours a day), by whom, and how the results are to be measured, documented, and assessed. Some published studies suggest that certain physical therapy programs can improve a cerebral palsy child's joint contractures, motor status, and social motivation,[154,184,186] whereas others suggest that they do not.[155,231] Significant problems with the literature include small, heterogenous samples, nonrandomized treatment, and patient attrition from many studies.[155] In many instances, it is difficult or impossible to determine whether the therapy was of benefit or whether improvement in motor skills was the result of the child's obligatory neurologic maturation and learning experiences, completely independent from any actual restructuring of neurocentral control patterns. Nevertheless, most parents like their children to have lots of physical therapy and many develop strongly bonded and trusting relationships with a particular therapist.

Whenever practical, it is beneficial when a parent can perform as much of the physical therapy as possible and not rely totally on the physical therapist.[184] This saves professional fees, minimizes trips to the therapist or interference with school time, and positively involves parents and even siblings with the child. Many parents, however, decline such involvement because of other family or career demands or simply because they are too tired to commit the time and effort necessary.

Frequent physical therapy sessions and protracted therapy programs are expensive, time-consuming, and generate hopes and expectations for all involved. If not of benefit or if ineffective modalities are employed, the therapy process can raise false hopes, increase frustrations for the child and the family, and sometimes unbalance interactions among the members of the family unit.[82,184,229]

There is general agreement that postoperative rehabilitative physical therapy is not only helpful but usually essential to maximize the benefits of most types of orthopaedic surgery in cerebral palsy. The goals are to maintain or improve joint range of motion, regain preoperative muscle strength, maximize ambulation, and improve function if possible. How long should the postoperative therapy continue, and how frequently should it be done? This varies with the magnitude of the surgery performed. It may be necessary for as little as 1 or 2 weeks or as long as several months, with as much of the therapy as possible being undertaken by the family. The family can provide the treatments on a daily basis. If all treatments must be provided by the therapist, two or three times per week is standard.

Another potential benefit of physical therapy is the prevention of joint contractures by the supervision of a daily range of joint motion program for those who lack the motor strength and voluntary control to maintain their own ranges. This type of program usually can be done by a parent, an aide, or a caretaker and not require the services of a physical therapist, other than to develop and monitor the program. As previously noted, however, data proving the benefit of such a program are lacking. In some severely involved children, it is impossible to prevent contractures, no matter how aggressive the treatment.

An unresolved issue is the duration of maintenance physical therapy. Although some parents want and even demand therapy two or three times a week for the life of their child, there is no evidence that any type of physical therapy can have a beneficial, lasting effect on motor function beyond early to middle childhood (age 4–8 years). Children older than this no doubt benefit more by devoting their time (and their families' and society's resources) to the development of communication, cognitive, and recreational skills instead of endless therapy sessions.

It is irrefutable that the physical therapist can be of great benefit to the child and family. She or he is a patient resource and sometimes a case manager for adaptive and therapeutic equipment, including seating systems, fabricating some types of splints and basic orthotics, educating the family about cerebral palsy and the child's deficits and potential, advising the family regarding modifications in the home, using community resources, acting as liaison with the school and as a realistic, supportive health care professional. The physical therapist is also a resource for educating school teachers and other personnel.[210]

Of great importance is a good two-way communication pathway between the therapist and the physician. The therapist is often the primary person who documents the child's neuromotor status, monitors progress, and may recommend surgery or other treatments. In this regard, it is important that motor function be accurately documented by the therapist periodically during the child's early growth years.

A different and interesting therapy approach, described in a pilot study, is that of using low-intensity transcutaneous electric stimulation in an attempt to strengthen weaker antagonistic lower extremity muscles. The treatment is applied only at night. In a small group of patients, motor improvement was noted but was lost after the stimulation was withdrawn.[156] More investigation of this approach is necessary before its clinical relevance is determined.

INTRAMUSCULAR INJECTIONS. The purpose of injecting various substances into muscles or around nerves is to weaken a muscle and thereby help to balance the forces across a joint. This is usually a temporary objective, but in some cases it may be of value to allow a stretching and strengthening physical therapy program to perhaps avoid or, more likely, defer the need for surgery. The most common muscle injected is the gastrocnemius, to reduce equinus deformity. Other common sites are the hamstrings and hip adductors. Repeated injections may be necessary to achieve the desired effect, and these injections are painful unless general anesthesia is used. In addition, the effect is not permanent, so that most surgeons, myself included, prefer surgical methods of muscle balancing, especially when more than one pair of muscle groups need treatment.

The shortest-acting drug is a local anesthetic agent, injected in the immediate vicinity of a specific nerve to block its motor fibers and allow the physician to observe the effect. If the effect is beneficial, then repeating the injection with another longer-acting agent, such as 45% alcohol, may reproduce the effect.[35] If the goal is to make the effect permanent, phenol is used to destroy the nerve fibers.

Another means of weakening the muscle is to inject 45% alcohol into its fibers in a more regional distribution to inhibit nerve transmission and thereby, muscle contraction. This is painful and therefore requires general anesthesia. When successful, the effect of alcohol injection lasts for a variable period but usually about 6 weeks.[23,36]

A newer agent for injection to block the myoneural junction is botulinum-A toxin. This agent is injected without local or general anesthesia using 23-gauge needles into sites of nerve arborization in the muscles and blocks the release of acetylcholine from synaptic vesicles at the myoneural junction. It has been shown to be a safe technique, whose beneficial effects on paraspinal and extremity muscles begin in 12 to 72 hours and may last for 3 to 6 months.[42,108] Injections may be repeated after 2 or more weeks, and up to six injections may be given at a site until the desired response in muscle tone reduction has been achieved. This treatment is contraindicated in the presence of fixed joint contractures. It is likely to be most useful in very young patients when the surgeon wishes to defer surgical intervention until the child is older, has a stabilized gait pattern, and other components of the child's problem can be more precisely identified and addressed. A double-blind trial in 12 patients with equinovarus or equinovalgus foot deformities showed improvement in five of six treated patients and improvement in two of six placebo-injected patients.[109]

MANIPULATION AND CASTING. Obtaining beneficial elongation of tight or contracted musculotendinous units or joint capsules can sometimes be accomplished by gentle, nonpainful, repeated passive stretching, followed by maintaining the correction with casts, splints, or adjustable orthotic devices. This treatment method has the potential to cause pain to the child and raise false hopes for improvement when applied to more than mild spasticity, tightness, or contractures or when used in patients who are unable to accurately communicate their discomfort.

With properly selected patients, manipulation and casting can sometimes improve at least temporarily[26] contractures of the ankle, knee, elbow, wrist, or hand. The process may be repeated from every few days to a week, and various casting materials, dropout casts, removable splints, and orthotics with dial lock or ratchet hinges may be used. The use of nerve or muscle blocks as an adjunct may sometimes be worthwhile.

Another method known as inhibition casting has been employed for several years. This treatment is applied to the lower extremities by carefully molding bilateral plaster below-knee casts in an attempt to inhibit certain normal tonic plantar reflexes, especially grasp, and thus reduce overall lower extremity tone. A probable added benefit is stabilization of the foot and ankle by the well-molded cast. The casts are either left in place or changed weekly for 3 or 4 weeks, during which time intensive physical therapy is performed. Hinged ankle-foot orthoses (AFOs) are then substituted for the casts. This method has reportedly been successful in some hands,[44,56,151,209,211] but because the noted improvement may not be maintained for more than a few months, others have not considered it to be of value.[227]

ORTHOTICS. Orthotic devices are classically used to prevent deformity, to improve function by substituting for a weakened muscle, or to protect a weakened part. In cerebral palsy, they are most commonly used in the lower extremities to stabilize feet, ankles, and knees; to maintain nighttime hip abduction to prevent subluxation; to possibly slow the progression of spinal deformity to obtain beneficial growth or improve sitting balance; and as night splints to prevent hand and wrist deformity.

Progress has been made in understanding the biomechanics of the lower extremities in cerebral palsy and developing strong, lightweight, comfortable new materials for the orthoses. It is uncommon for lower extremity orthotics to have to extend above the knee in patients with spastic diplegia.[183]

Commonly used lower extremity orthotics include those for foot control, such as the UCBL orthosis (University of California Biomechanics Laboratory), which can maintain forefoot, hindfoot, and subtalar alignment in a supple but not in a rigid foot, and various types of AFOs. These include the solid ankle type, to control the entire foot, provide mediolateral ankle stability, and maintain the ankle in a rigid plantigrade position. The solid ankle AFO is the best choice for the spastic foot and can be used in almost any instance. Modifications to the solid ankle AFO have been made to improve foot and ankle function. An example is the posterior leaf spring AFO, which does not provide mediolateral ankle stability but allows some plantar flexion and dorsiflexion from neutral while preventing footdrop. This type is used when spasticity is minimal. Articulated AFOs have hinged ankles and plantar flexion stops, which prevent equinus and excessive extensor thrust while allowing free dorsiflexion during gait and also allowing more tibialis anterior muscle function. Although articulated AFOs better allow dorsiflexion activities such as bending over and stair climbing, they provide less ankle support, are bulky and do not fit into shoes well, and are more likely to cause heel irritation. Another type of AFO is the floor-reaction type, of which there are several varieties. It uses the plantar flexion–knee extension couple to prevent knee flexion crouch and gain appropriate stance-phase knee extension during gait, provided that the foot is plantigrade, no significant knee flexion contracture is present (>10 degrees), hip extension is full, and no major rotational malalignments are present in the limb.[48] This approach has essentially eliminated the need to ever prescribe a KAFO (knee-ankle-foot orthosis) in an ambulatory child with cerebral palsy. The main indication for KAFOs is to brace the lower limbs for transfer ease in a nonambulatory patient.

SELECTIVE POSTERIOR RHIZOTOMY. This procedure has been employed for several decades[147] but only in the past 10 years has it been widely used in North America.[160,161] Unlike earlier attempts to surgically or electrically alter the central nervous system beneficially (e.g., cerebellar stimulation),[47] it has met with growing acceptance. The principle of selective posterior rhizotomy is to reduce spasticity by balancing muscle tone by the control exhibited by the anterior horn cells in the spinal cord. The normal inhibitory influences on the gamma efferent system, produced by higher centers in the brain and carried to the anterior horn cell by long intraspinal tracts, are deficient in cerebral palsy, as is the ability to coordinate movement as mediated through the extrafusal fibers from the alpha motor neurons. Selective posterior rhizotomy attempts to limit the stimulatory inputs from the muscle spindles in the lower limbs that arrive by the afferent fibers in the dorsal roots. This is done by sectioning only those dorsal rootlets that exert excessive faciliatory influence on the anterior horn cell and thereby better balance these influences.

The operation is performed under general anesthesia without relaxants. The lumbar laminae and the intervening ligaments are removed as an en bloc laminoplasty from L1 to S1, preserving the facet joints and carefully dissecting out individual posterior rootlets from the L1 to S1 posterior roots, stimulating the rootlets, noting the electromyographic and physical response, and surgically dividing those that supply the offending muscles. Rootlets are spared if they show decremental and squared-type electromyographic responses. They are divided if the responses are incremental, clonic, multiphasic, sustained, or contralateral, although this determination is not always easy. In most cases, up to 70 rootlets per root are stimulated and 25% to 50% are sectioned. The laminae and ligament complex are then replaced. The theoretic advantages of laminoplasty over laminectomies at each level are that it is faster, may result in less scarring in the spinal canal, and replacement of the intact laminae may prevent some cases of lumbar instability or deformity.

The patient best served by selective posterior rhizotomy is the young child (age 3–8 years) with spastic diplegic involvement, voluntary motor control, reasonable intelligence and motivation, no fixed contractures, good trunk control, the ability to walk with good underlying strength and balance, and who has severe, pure spasticity, and was preterm or of low birth weight.[204] Full-term children are more likely to have rigidity plus spasticity and therefore may not respond as favorably to selective posterior rhizotomy.[61,147] Availability for and cooperation with postoperative physical therapy are prerequisites for the procedure. The procedure is not indicated in children with athetosis, ataxia, rigidity, dystonia, antigravity muscle and truncal weakness or hypotonia, overlengthened tendons, and severe fixed contractures. Information regarding any benefits in those with spastic quadriplegia is limited.[29] The results of unilateral rhizotomy in spastic hemiplegia are not available, but at least one source does not recommend it.[147]

In the early postoperative period, the patient is weaker than before surgery and requires intensive physical therapy, but once the acute rehabilitation is complete, improvement in the lower extremities may be dramatic and perhaps lasting. Sometimes, even improvement in upper extremity function, seizure control, bladder function, swallowing, speech, and personality is seen after an overall reduction in muscle tone.[146] Results thus far show lasting reduction in spasticity; increased hip, knee, and ankle range of motion; often a plantigrade foot in stance; increased stride length and walking speed; and no increase in sensory deficits.[19,28,146,147,164,224] Although this procedure reduces spasticity and tone, it does not affect joint contractures or the overly contracted musculotendinous unit. These must be treated by orthopaedic surgical procedures after rehabilitation from the rhizotomy, and it is estimated that about 50% of patients require additional procedures.[147]

Selective posterior rhizotomy can be beneficial, but it is not a miracle procedure, nor does it cure cerebral palsy. The patient will still have poor motor control and balance, muscle weakness, contractures, sensory involvement, and persisting primitive reflexes if he or she did so preoperatively.

As with virtually everything else in medicine, there are some caveats. An occasional patient develops rapid and severe hip subluxation or dysplasia after this type of rhizotomy.[72] Heterotopic ossification about the hip has been reported to occur after varus derotation osteotomy of the proximal femur in patients with spastic quadriplegia who have previously had selective posterior rhizotomy.[159] Patients with preexisting lumbar lordosis of more than 60 degrees on a sitting lateral radiograph are at risk for the development of postoperative lumbar hyperlordosis.[127] Another study noted some increase in sagittal plane anterior pelvic tilt in independent ambulators after rhizotomy as being its only consistent negative effect.[28]

Long-term results with many patients followed over several decades are not yet available, but thus far, an increased risk of developing spinal deformity has not been reported. Another question remaining to be answered is whether late neuropathic arthropathy will occur, but this seems unlikely.

Selective posterior rhizotomy is a demanding procedure for the patient, the family, and the professional staff. Although there is little risk involved, it is expensive, long-term results are unknown, and careful patient selection and surgical technique are mandatory. Nevertheless, it can be of substantial benefit to many children.

GAIT ANALYSIS. Gait analysis in cerebral palsy is a valuable and well-established method of documentation that allows the careful study of the various components of the pathologic gait of these children, the energy expended,[180] and the results of treatment protocols. Gait analysis is discussed in another chapter in this textbook and in others devoted exclusively to the subject.[61]

Although formal preoperative gait analysis is theoretically desirable, it is neither possible nor necessary for every child who undergoes surgery. Nevertheless, every surgeon who treats children with cerebral palsy should have a good knowledge of normal (Fig. 13-6)[212] and pathologic human gait and understand gait analysis and pattern recognition. The application of his or her observational gait analysis therefore will be more accurate.

The prerequisites for normal gait are:

- stability of the foot and entire lower extremity in stance phase
- clearance of the ground by the foot in swing phase
- appropriate prepositioning of the foot at the end of swing phase
- adequate step length
- maximization of energy conservation.[61]

Observational gait analysis is done by watching the child walk repeatedly while viewing the gait from the front, back, and side. Study only one component at a time (e.g., cadence, stride length, the foot, the knee, the hip, lower extremity rotational alignment, the pelvis, the trunk), recognizing that often there are differences between the sides. Gage has described observational gait analysis in detail.[61] For a given child, intraobserver observations are more accurate than interobserver observations.[110] In either situation, the opportunity to study a videotape of the gait from the front, back, and sides, with zoom capability for the feet, increases accuracy.

Pattern recognition allows the surgeon to observe the gait cycles of the walking child, look for the priorities of gait and deviations from normal, and correlate this information to the findings on static physical examination. If all this information is consistent with a recognized standard pattern (e.g., one of the types of

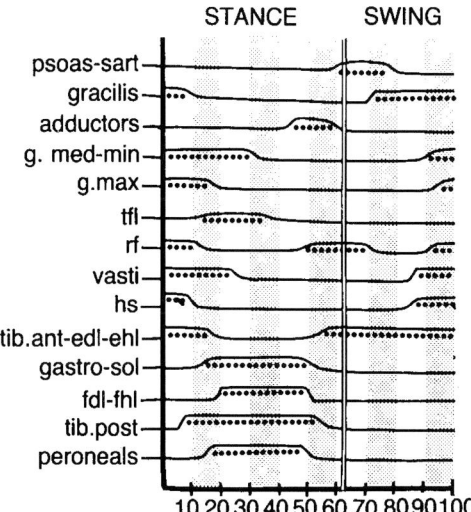

FIGURE 13-6. Chart of normal muscle-firing patterns (*dotted lines*) for the lower extremities. The patterns of a child with cerebral palsy are compared with this normal data.

hemiplegia or a diplegic gait with equinovalgus feet, tight hamstrings, tight hip flexors and adductors, increased femoral anteversion), there is a strong likelihood of success after applying the proper surgical procedures to address each problem.

Whereas it would be ideal, if cost and accessibility to sophisticated gait labs were not a problem, to review a high-tech gait analysis on every ambulatory cerebral palsy patient preoperatively, surgeons who must prioritize their patients will be most comfortable without gait analysis with those patients who have apparently straightforward patterns of gait pathology. Nevertheless, gait analysis provides a more precise definition of the gait abnormality in more complex cases, such as those of severe diplegia and in those who have had previous surgery with little success.

SURGERY. Surgical treatment is the most rapid and dramatic means of altering the structure and function of the musculoskeletal system in children with cerebral palsy.

Treatment of Specific Problems

The following are recommendations for the treatment of the most common problems and deformities in spastic diplegia. It is assumed that the patient in each instance is ambulatory.

In most cases, the patient has several abnormal elements in the disturbed gait. Best results are obtained from surgery if all of the abnormalities are identified preoperatively and corrected during the same surgical setting,[30,141] requiring only one rehabilitation period. No benefit is derived by simply performing one procedure, such as a triceps surae lengthening, and waiting to assess its effect on other abnormal elements of the child's gait before proceeding to correct them. This strategy does not improve the final result and inflicts unnecessary discomfort, hospitalization, and rehabilitation on the child.

The best age to perform the surgery varies with the patient and his or her problems but almost always is after the child is at least cruising or ambulating in some fashion, after age 4 or 5 years but before age 8 years, although surgery can be successful in older children and adults. In cases in which the hips are at risk for dislocation or progressive acetabular dysplasia, surgery should not be delayed, regardless of age.

In the immediate postoperative period, the major concerns related to the orthopaedic surgical procedures are pain management, relief of superimposed myospasms, and minimization of the child's anxiety. Giving the analgesic medication through the existing intravenous access line, using patient-controlled analgesia when possible, routinely administering diazepam for about 72 hours to lessen myospasms, providing continuous caudal analgesia through a small catheter, and the presence of kind, supportive personnel are most helpful to the child.

Overall, the postoperative management is aimed at restoration of joint motion, muscle strength, and improved gait as rapidly as possible. During this period, it may be beneficial to use night splints for comfort and to prevent joint positioning that could contribute to recurrent contractures. Such splinting should never exceed the comfort tolerance of the child. In this regard, it is sometimes necessary to alternate control of one ankle and the opposite knee on successive nights or use splinting only during the day, when it can be effectively monitored. The value of night splinting is not universally accepted, and valid well-controlled studies proving its efficacy are lacking. It is expensive and can be burdensome and uncomfortable for the patient because of malfitting splints, the frustration of substantially restricted mobility, or maintenance of a continuous overstretch on muscles.

If osteotomies or subtalar arthrodeses have been performed, partial weight bearing, if the patient can comply, may begin as soon as 3 weeks postoperatively, assuming that the internal fixation is adequate. Full unrestricted weight bearing should probably be deferred until radiographic evidence of adequate early bony healing is seen, usually by about 6 weeks. It may take at least 3 months and sometimes longer to regain the preoperative level of strength after most multiple lower extremity surgical procedures in patients with spastic diplegia.

HALLUX VALGUS. Hallux valgus and bunions occur commonly in cerebral palsy, most likely because of a combination of muscle imbalance with adductor hallucis overactivity and externally applied forces resulting from equinovalgus deformity of the foot and ankle forcing the phalanges of the great toe into valgus.[93,174] Equinus and particularly valgus of the foot must be corrected first, to achieve a lasting good result from hallux valgus surgery in cerebral palsy.

Indications for surgery in this condition are pain and difficulty with proper shoeing; rarely is cosmesis alone an indication. There are myriad operations for the correction of hallux valgus, and most have been used with varying degrees of success in cerebral palsy. When spasticity is mild, such procedures as ostectomy, capsulorrhaphy, adductor hallucis release or transfer, and proximal or distal first metatarsal osteotomy can be successful.[11,24,80,117,191] With recurrence or in patients with more severe spasticity, the McKeever metatarsophalangeal arthrodesis,[124] with the joint in a few degrees of valgus and 10 degrees of dorsiflexion, is an excellent procedure.[174]

ANKLE EQUINUS. Pure equinus of the ankle, without associated valgus or varus, is not common. It is the result of overactivity or contracture of the triceps surae group, which is normally six times stronger than the ankle dorsiflexors.[197] Most of the overactivity is in the gastrocnemius muscle. The soleus is usually not the major problem. The equinus deformity can be treated by serial manipulation and casting, which is most successful in patients who are young, have less spasticity, and whose equinus in mild. Recurrence of the equinus deformity after several months is not uncommon after manipulation and casting.

Lasting correction most often requires surgical elongation of the gastrocnemius unit, which if performed as an isolated procedure can usually be done as outpatient surgery.[71,132] Elongation is most commonly done by lengthening the Achilles tendon (which also lengthens the soleus) by either multiple partial tenotomies, the Hoke triple cut[92] or White double cut[67,229] techniques (either percutaneously or open), or by an open step-cut lengthening. When percutaneous techniques are employed, care should be taken to avoid completely dividing the Achilles tendon. Some surgeons have advocated methods of attempting to quantify the exact amount of lengthening necessary.[62,63] These methods have not gained wide acceptance.

Some authors advocate the Baker[9,10] or Vulpius[98,225] fascial division type of lengthening of the gastrocnemius aponeurosis alone. This method has the advantage of not only preserving but actually generating more soleus strength for pushoff.[181] Whether it results in a higher recurrence rate is debatable.[143] Similar results have been reported in studies comparing tendon lengthening with muscle lengthening in the treatment of equinus deformity.[58,193]

Another less popular method is Achilles tendon advancement anteriorly (i.e., closer to the talus) on the calcaneus to decrease its power by decreasing its lever arm.[207,208,223] This procedure is more complex than the tendon lengthenings and has not been demonstrated to be superior. Its best results occur when it is combined with other procedures.[207]

Regardless of the surgical technique selected, the result is usually good.[68] Recurrence rates are inversely proportional to the age of the child at the time of surgery; lower rates are seen in older children. Before age 4 years, the recurrence rate is about 25%, whereas it approaches zero when the surgery is done after age 8 years.[171,218] After surgical lengthening, some believe it is beneficial to control the ankle with a night splint and an orthosis to prevent recurrent deformity and improve function.[12] Others have shown that orthotics do not prevent recurrent deformity.[171] A reasonable approach is to use an AFO to improve functional stability or control weakness in those who need it and reserve night splinting for those who show signs of early recurrent tightness. If the patient has voluntary active foot dorsiflexion to more than 10 degrees postoperatively, there is a good likelihood that an AFO will not be necessary.

Triceps surae elongation is treated with a below-knee cast for 2 to 3 weeks if only the gastrocnemius aponeurosis has been lengthened or an incomplete Achilles tenotomy (e.g., the Hoke technique) has been done. The below-knee cast is left in place for 4 to 6 weeks after step-cut lengthening of the Achilles tendon. If necessary, the appropriate AFO is then applied, the mold for which may be obtained at the time of surgery if convenient.

A problem to be avoided is the postoperative development of a calcaneus deformity from overlengthening the heel cord. Other causes of calcaneus deformity are injudicious transfer of a tibialis posterior tendon that is spastic throughout the gait cycle through the interosseous membrane to the dorsum of the foot and lengthening the Achilles tendon in a patient with athetosis. Treatment for an overlengthened heel cord is difficult, but Roberts has had some success with shortening the Achilles tendon by surgical reattachment or imbrication,* and Tardieu suggests a period of casting the ankle in plantar flexion, followed by orthotic control at plantigrade during the day and in equinus at night.[217]

FOOT AND ANKLE EQUINOVARUS. Ankle equinus, varus of the hindfoot, and often varus and supination of the forefoot are present in this deformity; it is most often seen in hemiplegia but may occur in children with diplegia and quadriplegia also. The hindfoot varus is most likely caused by overactivity of the tibialis posterior muscle, whereas varus and supination of the forefoot are more likely caused by overactivity of the tibialis anterior muscle, which may also contribute to hindfoot varus.

For treatment of hindfoot equinovarus, correction of the equinus, as described above, must be combined with lengthening or split transfer of the tibialis posterior tendon. Lengthening may be by the step-cut method or by intramuscular tenotomy cephalad to the musculotendinous junction, which is also known as the Frost procedure.[118,183] Some surgeons prefer to split the tendon and transfer the lateral half to the peroneus brevis tendon,[70,105] so as to not weaken the muscle as much as a lengthening would. Others believe that some weakening is desirable. There are several reports of good results with this split transfer, and many indicate that preoperative gait analysis is not necessary for a successful outcome.[200]

Although anterior transfer of the tibialis posterior tendon has been advocated,[20,179] it probably should not be transferred through the interosseous membrane to the dorsum of the foot in cerebral palsy patients. This approach can result in an eventual calcaneovalgus deformity that is difficult to correct.[187]

---

* Roberts JM, personal communication, February 1994.

In varus and supination foot deformities caused by overactivity of the tibialis anterior muscle, a split transfer of the lateral half of its tendon to the cuboid bone usually successfully balances the foot.[85] DeGnore and Greene use hindfoot varus that occurs in the swing phase of gait and a positive confusion test as their indication for split anterior tibialis tendon transfer.[49] The validity of the confusion test, however, has been questioned because it does not predict ankle kinematics in the swing phase of gait.[46]

Nonfixed varus of the hindfoot often occurs with varus and supination of the forefoot. In this situation, split anterior tibialis tendon transfer combined with posterior tibialis tendon lengthening is appropriate.

When the hindfoot varus is fixed, bony surgery, in addition to addressing the triceps surae and tibialis posterior units, is necessary to correct the deformity.[195] This is done by either a laterally based closing wedge osteotomy of the calcaneus with staple or screw fixation, which is sometimes technically difficult to reduce and adequately fix, or by obliquely dividing the calcaneus in the coronal plane, posterior and parallel to the peroneal tendons, sliding the posterior fragment laterally and fixing it with a cannulated or cancellous screw or pins. I prefer the latter procedure. Assuming adequate internal fixation with either procedure, a below-knee cast is necessary until bony healing has occurred (usually 6–8 weeks). Orthotic control of the foot and ankle is then usually appropriate.

FOOT AND ANKLE EQUINOVALGUS. This is the more common situation in patients with diplegia. Its cause is probably muscle imbalance with triceps surae overactivity and weakness of the tibialis posterior muscle, with relative overpull of the peroneal musculature.[18] The equinus is addressed as described above. It should not be assumed that the valgus originates at the subtalar joint. It may be coming from the ankle, and appropriate weight-bearing radiographs of the ankle should be studied as part of surgical planning. If the ankle valgus is really in the distal tibia, it may be corrected by osteotomy or in some cases by hemi-epiphyseodesis or stapling of the medial side of the physis if sufficient growth remains.

If the subtalar valgus is mild and supple, it can be controlled by an orthosis, either an AFO or a UCBL type. This may be augmented by intramuscular lengthening of the peroneus brevis tendon, which decreases the power of the muscle by one grade.[137] The peroneus longus tendon should not be lengthened, because a varus deformity may ensue. Transfer of the peroneus brevis to the tibialis posterior tendon has been performed, but published large series with evaluations of results are lacking.[18]

With more severe valgus that is passively correctable, stabilization or fusion of the subtalar joint is usually required because orthotic control rarely succeeds in severe valgus. The indication for surgery is failure of an orthosis to control the hindfoot valgus, such that painful calluses and blisters result on the medial side of the foot.

Most surgeons prefer subtalar arthrodesis, using internal fixation and bone grafting (Fig. 13-7).[52] This method rigidly fixes the subtalar joint and yields a higher fusion rate than the classic Grice procedure or modifications thereof, which rely on bone graft alone.[13,74,121,133,190] Stabilization also may be accomplished by arthroereisis, using a staple or an inert plastic block.[43] This technique may be effective in some very young children, but it is not widely accepted. It

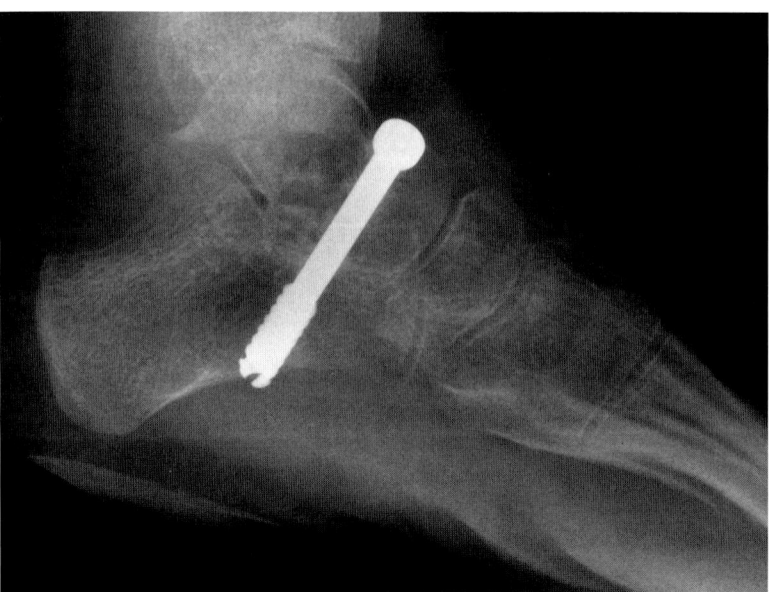

FIGURE 13-7. Postoperative lateral radiograph of a subtalar arthrodesis stabilized by a cannulated screw and augmented by iliac autograft bone.

has been used by few surgeons, and multiple series with adequate long-term follow-up are lacking.

Another method of correcting a supple valgus hindfoot deformity is by medial displacement of an oblique osteotomy of the calcaneus with screw or pin fixation. Although limited experience with this procedure has been reported, the osteotomy heals rapidly, preserves subtalar motion, and is easy to perform.[107,188]

When fixed hindfoot valgus is present, the options are a sliding medial displacement calcaneal osteotomy, a Dillwyn Evans lateral opening wedge lengthening osteotomy of the distal calcaneus,[59,134] a lateral opening wedge or medial closing wedge osteotomy of the proximal calcaneus, or a triple arthrodesis. Triple arthrodesis provides correction[219] but is best avoided if possible in very young patients in whom growth of the foot will be substantially inhibited. For this reason, it probably should be not be performed on a child who is not within about 2 years from the end of growth. Triple arthrodesis appears to be successful over the long term in patients with otherwise mild involvement who are community ambulators and does not increase the risk of later development of midfoot and ankle osteoarthritis as the result of increased and mechanically abnormal forces being transferred to those joints over a long period.[2] It is always important to achieve the best possible muscle balance at the foot and ankle; otherwise, even a triple arthrodesis may deform in time.

EXTERNAL TIBIAL TORSION. Profound external tibial torsion substantially shortens the lever arm effect of the foot in generating the plantar-flexion–knee-extension couple, which facilitates knee extension in the midstance and late stance phases of gait and helps to prevent crouch. Stance phase is often shortened and pushoff power is compromised. The solution to this problem is distal derotational osteotomies of the tibia and fibula at the supramalleolar level to align the ankle and foot progression angle with the direction of gait and the axis of the knee. The fibula is divided transversely just proximal to the syndesmosis, and the tibia is divided about 2.5 cm above the physis. Fixation by crossed smooth Steinmann pins, cut and bent extracutaneously, and an above-knee cast is adequate. The pins are removed and the cast changed to below-knee at 6 weeks. As with any surgical procedure near to an open physis, care must be taken to avoid inadvertent damage to the growth plate.

KNEE FLEXION DEFORMITY. This problem is most often associated with hip flexion contracture and a crouched gait. It may also be the result of calcaneus deformity (hyperdorsiflexion) at the ankle. It is therefore essential to assess and address all factors to appropriately manage a crouched gait.

The knee flexion deformity may be a true flexion contracture but is more often simply caused by spastic and tight hamstring muscles, without fixed capsular contracture.[45] The medial hamstrings are more often the major offenders.[213]

Another commonly associated finding is cospasticity of the rectus femoris muscle and the hamstrings. In this situation, when the hamstrings alone are lengthened, a stiff-knee gait results, which lacks adequate knee flexion in swing phase and interferes with foot clearance.[163] This problem is prevented by concomitant transfer of the distal rectus femoris tendon, usually medially if there is associated internal rotation from the hip or laterally if there is external rotation. The transfer does not affect gait abnormalities in the transverse plane (i.e., in-toeing or out-toeing) and it makes no difference whether the transfer is attached to the sartorius, gracilis, semitendinosus, or iliotibial band.[152] This transfer has been successful in restoring good knee motion in both the stance and swing phases of gait. It has been shown that transfer is necessary to accomplish this, not just tenotomy of the distal rectus femoris tendon. The indication for distal rectus femoris tendon transfer is a preoperative range of knee motion during gait of less than 80% of normal and hamstring–rectus femoris cospasticity.[60,153,215]

As a general rule, the hamstrings require lengthening when straight-leg raising cannot exceed 70 degrees above the horizontal or when the popliteal angle (i.e., the femorotibial sagittal angle with maximum knee extension, the patient supine, and the hip first flexed to 90 degrees) is less than 135 degrees (i.e., 45 degrees short of full extension). Lengthening of the medial hamstrings is performed by incising the fascial aponeurosis of the semimembranosis muscle at a minimum of two levels and step-cut lengthening or tenotomizing the semitendinosis and gracilis tendons. If after these procedures the lateral hamstrings are still tight, they may also require lengthening.[96,172]

Hamstring lengthenings, with or without distal rectus femoris transfers, are managed in removable knee-immobilizer splints, which can easily fit over a below-knee cast. Passive range of motion exercises may begin on the third or fourth postoperative day. If no bony surgery has been performed, walking training may begin as early as the fifth postoperative day. When adequate quadriceps strength has been regained, usually by the fourth postoperative week, the knee immobilizers may be discarded or used as night splints. Between physical therapy sessions, sitting should be done with the knees alternately in extension and flexion.

Good results can also be obtained by lengthening the hamstrings proximally.[192] It has been found, however, that lumbar lordosis may increase after this procedure because of the overactive hip flexors; also, the desired effect on the distal hamstring tightness may not be achieved.[54]

It must be remembered that the hamstrings are also hip extensors, sometimes contributing up to a third of the extensor torque.[91,226] Therefore, hip extensor power is somewhat lessened by hamstring lengthening, especially proximal hamstring lengthening. Therefore, this procedure may increase a preexisting hip flexion contracture and also increase the lumbar lordosis if the iliopsoas unit is not addressed concomitantly. To preserve some of the hip extensor power of the hamstrings, Gage recommends transfer of the distal semitendinosis to the lateral femoral metaphysis. This may minimally augment external rotation at the hip.[61]

HIP ADDUCTION CONTRACTURE. Tightness in the hip adductors can result in a scissoring type of gait pattern and predispose the patient to hip dysplasia or subluxation. Generally, when the hips cannot be abducted beyond 30 degrees in flexion or extension, adductor release or transfer posteriorly to the ischial tuberosity, which has its advocates,[14,177] is indicated. There seems to be little difference in the results from release or transfer,[75,173] but one study reports a high incidence of pelvic obliquity and hip subluxation after adductor transfer.[189] Neurectomy of the anterior branch of the obturator nerve is rarely indicated in diplegic patients who can walk because it excessively weakens the adductor brevis muscle and can result in a wide-based gait with hyperabduction of the hips.[120] The hip adductors function to stabilize the hip against excessive abduction during gait, running, and in activities such as skiing, skating, and horseback riding. The gait stability they provide allows more effective hip flexor and extensor activity. Thus, it is important not to "go for broke" and overlengthen or overweaken the adductors in ambulatory patients.

Release of the tight adductors is performed with the patient supine, through either a longitudinal or transverse incision, depending on the preference of the surgeon. The adductor longus is always completely divided; occasionally, this is adequate to allow at least 60 degrees of passive abduction on each side with the hip and knee flexed to 90 degrees or at least 45 degrees of passive abduction with the hip and knee extended (the medial hamstrings are also hip adductors), the objective of adductor release for most surgeons. Often, some or most of the adductor brevis may also need to be released or it may be necessary to divide the gracilis muscle to achieve the desired abduction.

HIP FLEXION CONTRACTURE. Hip flexion contracture is best detected by the Thomas test, the prone extension test, or both, as described by Staheli.[202] When the contracture exceeds about 20 to 25 degrees, it should be released. Most contractures are caused by a spastic, contracted iliopsoas unit, but when the contracture is severe and of long standing, nearly all soft tissues anterior to the hip joint may be involved.

In ambulatory children, release of the iliopsoas tendon by tenotomy at the lesser trochanter weakens hip flexor power excessively and may prohibit enough hip flexion strength to lift the limb in climbing stairs.[119] Ambulatory children should have tenotomy of the psoas tendon alone, not the iliacus fibers, performed over the brim of the pelvis at the level of the superior pubic ramus. This is accomplished through an anterior incision with intrapelvic extraperiosteal dissection. Care must be exercised to differentiate the psoas tendon from the femoral nerve.

Hip flexor releases are treated by lying prone several times per day, by skin traction in extension, or by both. Painful muscle spasms are particularly common in the first few days after hip surgery and may be treated with diazepam and analgesics. It is desirable to begin gentle passive range of motion exercises by the third or fourth day after flexor or adductor releases, and gait training may begin at 5 to 7 days postoperatively. After 3 weeks, more vigorous muscle strengthening exercises are tolerated.

LUMBAR HYPERLORDOSIS. Hyperlordosis is usually the result of compensation for bilateral hip flexion contractures; correcting the contractures corrects the excessive lordosis. It should be remembered that other conditions can also produce lumbar hyperlordosis, such as compensation for a rigid thoracic kyphosis.

IN-TOEING. In-toeing is most commonly the result of excessive femoral anteversion but occasionally is caused by increased spasticity in the internal rotator muscles of the hip (the medial hamstrings or the anterior fibers of the tensor fascia lata and gluteus medius).[213] Derotational osteotomy of the femur is the treatment for increased femoral anteversion. Excessive femoral anteversion causing in-toeing rarely exists as an isolated finding in spastic diplegia but is usually accompanied be lower extremity musculotendinous tightness or contractures that also require correction. The appropriate age for derotation osteotomy is whenever other lower extremity surgery is being done. This usually means after age 4 years. The derotation may be at the supracondylar region in younger children with mild to moderate spasticity and fixed with crossed Steinmann pins or protruding parallel pins and either a cylinder[69] or a hip spica cast. In older children and in anyone with substantial spasticity, it is best to perform the osteotomy at the intertrochanteric level and preserve the attachment the iliopsoas. Fixation with a strong blade-plate avoids the need for a postoperative spica cast in patients with adequate bone stock and allows early hip motion. Such strong internal fixation obviates the problems of loss of fixation and malunion, which occasionally occur after the pin and cast fixation of distal femoral osteotomies. The proximal osteotomy operation is facilitated by placing the patient in the prone position and using the approach described by Root and Siegal.[176] Another option for derotation in children older than age 10 years is in the subtrochanteric region, with fixation by a locked intramedullary rod.

Femoral derotational osteotomies to correct excessive anteversion require external rotation of the distal segment, which tightens the medial hamstrings. To prevent this increased medial hamstring tightness, which may actually increase internal rotation, these hamstrings usually need to be lengthened when femoral derotation is performed.

Other methods of treating in-toeing gait in children with cerebral palsy have been advocated. These include transfer of the semitendinosus tendon to the distal lateral femur,[61] transfer of the distal tendon of the rectus femoris to the gracilis or sartorius, and transfer of the greater trochanter with its attached gluteus medius muscle to the anterior proximal femur, so that it may function as an external rotator as well as an abductor.[206] The first two of these techniques have not been shown to be effective.[152] It must be understood that although transfer of the distal tendon of the rectus femoris either medially or laterally has negligible rotatory effect on the limb, this transfer definitely improves the swing phase of gait knee flexion for foot clearance.[152] The abductor transfer, although sometimes successful, can produce an abductor weakness–type gait and has not been widely adopted.[69]

Spastic Hemiplegia

Children afflicted with spastic hemiplegia classically have involvement of one side of the body, with the arm and hand more severely involved than the lower extremity. On closer evaluation, mild involvement on the contralateral side often is also found, especially in those with more severe affliction.[61]

The hemiplegia type comprises about 30% of all cerebral palsy cases. About 1 in 3 patients have a seizure disorder, and almost one half have some degree of mental retardation.[169] More common than mental retardation is an attention deficit, learning, or behavioral disorder.[196] A history of head trauma or intracranial hemorrhage is frequently found in this type of involvement. Virtually all are community ambulators, although only about half can walk by age 18 months.[169] Some limb length inequality and a difference in foot size are the rule but rarely require any treatment.

The stereotypic picture of the patient with hemiplegia is someone with equinovarus at the foot and ankle, flexion at the knee and hip, internal rotation of the lower limb, internal rotation at the shoulder, flexion at the elbow, pronation of the forearm, flexion and ulnar deviation at the wrist, and thumb-in-palm with finger flexion in the hand. Actually, the degree of involvement with spastic hemiplegia is a spectrum, which has been separated into four subtypes.[231] It is essential in planning treatment to quantify the involvement. Surgical results are predictable and good in spastic hemiplegia.

Type I hemiplegia is characterized by weakness of the tibialis anterior muscle, and the triceps surae group is not tight. This type is manifest as a footdrop and a steppage gait, with plantar flexion disappearing during stance phase. It is easily treated with an appropriate AFO, usually a posterior leaf spring or an articulated ankle type. The most difficult part of management is to get the child to wear the orthosis, if he or she has no other noticeable variation from normality. One reported surgical approach to this type of hemiplegic problem has been transfer of the flexor digitorum longus and flexor hallucis longus tendons to the dorsum of the foot.[84] Experience with this technique is limited, and meaningful long-term results are not available.

Type II hemiplegia has tibialis anterior muscle weakness plus spasticity in the triceps surae group and usually some spasticity in the tibialis posterior muscle. This results in equinovarus deformity of the foot and ankle, which persists throughout all phases of gait and may produce some knee hyperextension in the late stance phase. Correction is accomplished by lengthening the gastrocnemius aponeurosis or Achilles tendon, lengthening or performing a split transfer of the tibialis posterior tendon,[70,105] and providing an AFO, as in type I. The split posterior tibial tendon transfer is indicated for correction of the varus heel in stance phase when there is no fixed deformity and the muscle is firing in phase, which is during stance. If the tibialis posterior is active throughout the gait cycle, it is probably better to lengthen its tendon rather than to perform the split transfer.[169] If the tibialis anterior muscle, instead of being weak, is overactive during the swing phase of gait, a split anterior tibialis tendon transfer can be effective in achieving transverse plane balance of the foot.[85] This is usually combined with tibialis posterior tendon lengthening.

An orthosis is used to assist a weak tibialis anterior or aid in preventing recurrent equinus deformity. In this regard, an ankle-foot night splint may also be beneficial. Some children are orthosis-free after the surgery. The risk of recurrence of the equinus deformity in hemiplegia decreases as the child grows older, being reported at about 25% below the age of 4 years and 12% thereafter.[169]

In type III hemiplegia, not only are the triceps surae and tibialis posterior muscles spastic and usually contracted but hamstring involvement, often with cospasticity of the rectus femoris, produces a stiff-knee gait with an equinovarus foot and ankle deformity. Successful treatment includes the tendon elongations discussed for type II and the addition of medial hamstring lengthenings and usually a distal rectus femoris tendon transfer, as described in the section on spastic diplegia. Again, the appropriate AFO is usually necessary postoperatively, sometimes temporarily and sometimes permanently.

Type IV hemiplegia has the features of type III, with the addition of hip flexor and adductor spasticity or contracture. Iliopsoas lengthening by release of the psoas tendon over the pelvic brim and appropriate adductor releases are added to the treatment recommended for those with type III involvement.

This classification is helpful in the management of most patients with spastic hemiplegia. It is not infallible, however, and patients occasionally are encountered who have profound equinus, with little or no varus; who have increased ipsilateral femoral anteversion in addition to type IV involvement; or who have other abnormalities.

Athetoid Cerebral Palsy

Children with athetoid cerebral palsy have dyskinesia (i.e., abnormal muscle tension and tone) and assume abnormal postures. Their limb movements are involuntary and almost continuously changing. The movements are coarse, irregular, and often give the child the appearance of squirming or writhing, and extensor tone predominance is the rule. The movements disappear during sleep.[51]

The muscle tension often changes with the emotional state. The athetoid movements are greater in the more distal parts of the limbs and often rapidly flow from flexion to extension, adduction to abduction, and pronation to supination. Because of the almost constant motion, most of the joints are put through a full range of motion and contractures are not common unless there is an asymmetric component of mixed spasticity present.

Most children with substantial athetosis are not able to walk. Their mobility is by power wheelchair, often with an adapted steering mechanism. Therapeutic focus for these children should be on communication methods, facilitating their control over activities of daily living, and wheelchair mobility.[32]

The gait pattern of those patients with athetosis who can walk is random, inconsistent, and influenced by many external stimuli. Without a consistent baseline, the results of soft tissue surgery are unpredictable. Soft tissue surgery, especially tenotomies and muscle releases, should be done infrequently in patients with significant athetosis because often the result is a severe, almost untreatable deformity opposite the one originally addressed.

Scoliosis is not uncommon in athetoid patients and responds well to the internal fixation and spinal fusion techniques described earlier. Adult athetoid patients may develop profoundly painful degenerative spondylosis and sometimes instability in the cervical spine. One study identified two thirds of athetoid patients by age 44 years and all patients older than age 55 years with moderate or severe cervical disc degeneration.[77] The most common level is C5–C6. This usually responds well to anterior cervical fusion.[185]

UPPER EXTREMITY INVOLVEMENT

The upper extremity is most abnormally involved in spastic cerebral palsy in patients with hemiplegia and quadriplegia. In these patients, it is essential to consider the function of the entire upper limb, not just a part of it, when considering treatment. The problems of spasticity, weakness, poor motor control, poor proprioception and stereognosis, and joint contractures reduce or eliminate the possible benefits of tendon lengthenings, transfers, or other surgical treatment in most cases. Mental retardation, visual deficits, behavioral problems, and particularly dyskinetic involvement may contraindicate upper extremity surgery. Fewer than 5% of patients are appropriate candidates for such surgery.[199] Nevertheless, patients with mild hemiplegic involvement may functionally benefit, and major cosmetic improvement or facilitation of care such as dressing and gloving can be achieved in more severely involved patients. Patients with hemiplegia usually do better than those with quadriplegia and postoperative function is usually better with right hemiplegia than with left.[149]

Patients who are most likely to benefit from upper extremity surgery in cerebral palsy are those with good intelligence; a stable trunk and body position; good hand proprioception, stereognosis, and other sensations; adequate passive range of motion of all upper extremity joints; and good hand placement capability, with voluntary control.[129] In many instances, the use of preoperative dynamic electromyographic studies aids in decision-making regarding lengthening or transferring musculotendinous units.[89,135,165]

An important indication for surgical correction of wrist and elbow contractures can be cosmesis. Older children and adolescents with reasonable intelligence who function well in public may have a negative body image with a rigid, contracted wrist and elbow. This may also have a negative effect on peer group acceptance. In such cases, correction of those deformities, although having no beneficial effect on upper extremity function, can be of immense psychologic value to the patient.

Nonsurgical Treatment

Nonsurgical treatment modalities include passive range of motion exercises and passive night splinting to attempt to prevent contractures, and serial casting or judiciously applied dynamic splinting to attempt correction of mild contractures in the absence of much spasticity. The daytime use of orthoses in attempts to improve function almost always meets with failure in hands with poor sensation and control.

Surgical Treatment

Some common surgical procedures and their indications in spastic patients follow. Those patients with athetosis almost never have enough voluntary control to benefit from upper extremity surgery.

Shoulder

Although it is rarely necessary to operate on the shoulder, with severe spasticity, an adduction and internal rotation contracture may develop, caused by contractures of the subscapularis and pectoralis major muscles. If hand function is reasonable but the ability to position the hand in space is compromised, correction of shoulder contractures is appropriate. This is performed by releasing the tendon of the subscapularis and lengthening the tendon of the pectoralis major. If this does not provide the needed correction, a proximal humeral derotational osteotomy, fixed with a compression plate, usually solves the problem.[129,199]

Elbow

The elbow is prone to develop flexion and pronation contractures in children with substantial spasticity. Although serial casting, dropout casts (long arm casts with the posterior plaster above the elbow removed to allow further extension while blocking further flexion), and dynamic splints may occasionally succeed, surgery is usually necessary to gain lasting correction.[105] The indications are to improve the ability to position a functional hand in space, to improve hygiene or prevent skin breakdown, and to improve cosmetic apperance.

Most flexion contractures of the elbow can be corrected by division of the lacertus fibrosus and brachialis aponeurosis and lengthening of the biceps tendon.[128] Occasionally, anterior capsulotomy of the elbow is also necessary.[199]

Pronation contracture of the elbow is the result of overactivity of the pronator teres, perhaps the pronator quadratus, and weakness of supination. When combined with a flexion contracture in a young child, dislocation of the radial head may occur. Surgical treatment of pronation contracture consists of distal release of the pronator teres muscle.[199] If passive supination is full, some advocate transfer of the pronator teres tendon posterior to the radius to an anterolateral insertion, so that it can function as a supinator.[149] Results of this transfer are not always good, and a fixed supination deformity is a larger problem than a pronation deformity.[149] Release of the pronator alone is usually successful and is preferred by most surgeons.

Wrist

Flexion deformity or contracture with some ulnar deviation is the usual finding at the wrist in spastic upper extremities and is usually associated with pronation of the forearm and weakness of the wrist extensor muscles. If flexor spasticity is minimal and finger extension is good, simply lengthening the flexor carpi ulnaris or the flexor carpi radialis but not both and, if necessary, the flexor digitorum sublimis and profundus muscles by complete transverse circumferential release of their aponeuroses in the proximal third of the forearm may be adequate.

Another usually effective means of weakening spastic wrist and finger flexors is the flexor pronator release procedure.[97,129] The disadvantage of this operation is that it is nonselective, releasing all wrist and finger flexors and the pronator teres from the medial epicondyle of the distal humerus.[69]

Often, flexor spasticity is very severe and extensor weakness is profound. In such cases, flexor carpi ulnaris transfer is recommended.[145,221] Before transfer, an electromyogram can be performed to determine the phase of the muscle if it cannot be determined by clinical examination. Transfer of the flexor carpi ulnaris tendon around the ulnar border of the wrist and into the extensor carpi radialis brevis is indicated if the transferred muscle is active during grasp and the patient has poor wrist extension and poor grasp but can actively extend the fingers with the wrist in neutral or dorsiflexion (Fig. 13-8).[15,148] If the flexor carpi ulnaris muscle is active during release and there is adequate grasp but poor release, it is transferred to the extensor digitorum comminus tendons. At least one long-term follow-up study has indicated that transfer to the wrist extensor is less predictable than

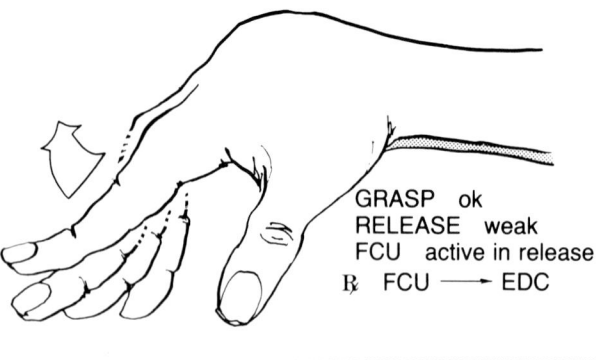

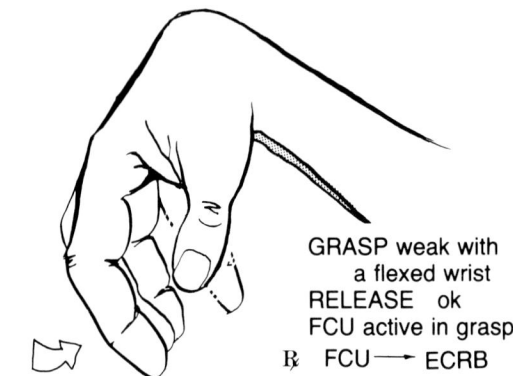

FIGURE 13-8. The spastic hemiplegic hand. The hand at *top* will benefit from transfer of the flexor carpi ulnaris to augment the extensor digitorum communis. At the *bottom*, the hand needs augmentation of wrist extension by transferring the flexor carpi ulnaris to the extensor carpi radialis brevis.

transfer to the finger extensors.[87] Regardless of the site of transfer, the flexor carpi radialis tendon should not be lengthened in association with flexor carpi ulnaris transfer because that likely overly weakens wrist flexion.

Wrist arthrodesis eliminates any useful compensatory or functional motion of the wrist and prevents the wrist from any helpful participation, by tenodesis effect of the extrinsic muscles, in grasp and release. It is therefore most often indicated only in severely involved patients for hygienic or cosmetic reasons, such as putting the hand through a sleeve or into a pocket or a glove.

Ulnar deviation of the wrist is thought to be caused by overactivity in the extensor carpi ulnaris muscle with volar displacement of its tendon. Split transfer of its tendon to the extensor carpi radialis brevis has been recommended.[129]

Hand

The common hand deformities are flexion and adduction of the thumb and either clawing with hyperextension of the finger metacarpophalangeal joints with flexion contractures of the distal finger joints, full flexion at all finger joints, or swan neck deformities of the fingers. Thumb-in-palm deformities are often complex and require careful assessment before the appropriate treatment can be recommended. In most cases, the adductor pollicis and first dorsal interosseus muscles overpower the abductor pollicis longus and the extensor pollicis longus and brevis muscles. Common patterns of deformity are thumb-carpometacarpal joint adduction contracture associated with contracture of the skin of the first web, and either metacarpophalangeal flexion contracture, with or without interphalangeal flexion deformity, or hyperextension contracture of the metacarpophalangeal joint. There are many ways to surgically treat these deformities, but in principle, all involve release of contractures of the skin, joints, and spastic muscles; joint stabilization; and augmentation of the weakened muscles (Fig. 13-9).[95,129,199] Thumb adduction contracture is often treated by release of the adductor pollicis brevis muscle from its origin on the third metacarpal diaphysis plus either transfer of the brachioradialis tendon to the abductor pollicis longus tendon or tenodesis of the latter tendon to the distal radius. Hoffer and colleagues recommend only partial myotomy if selective control of the adductor muscle is present during grasp or release.[88] Lengthening of the flexor pollicis longus tendon is the most common treatment for flexion deformity of the thumb. It may be advisable also to reroute the extensor pollicis longus tendon from the third to the first dorsal compartment. Arthrodesis of either the metacarpophalangeal or interphalangeal joint of the thumb corrects gross instability.

Often the problem in the claw hand, with wrist

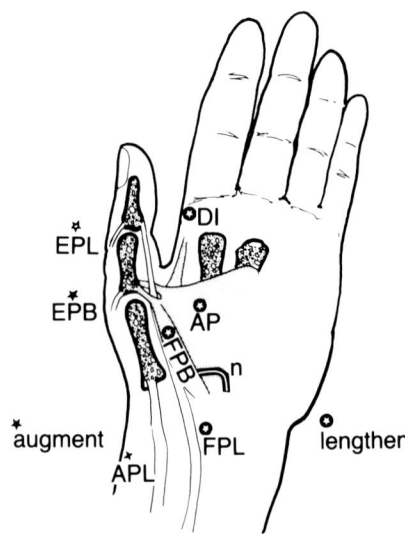

FIGURE 13-9. The repertoire of operations for the thumb-in-palm deformity. Shortened muscles should be lengthened, and weak long muscles should be shortened and augmented. An unstable metacarpophalangeal joint should be stabilized. (AP, adductor pollicis; APL, abductor pollicis longus; DI, first dorsal interosseous; EPB, extensor pollicis brevis; EPL, extensor pollicis longus; FPB, flexor pollicis brevis; FPL, flexor pollicis longus.

flexion and metacarpophalangeal hyperextension, is wrist flexor–wrist extensor imbalance. This is usually treated by transferring either the flexor carpi radialis or the flexor carpi ulnaris to the extensor carpi radialis brevis.[129]

In tightly flexed fingers that cannot be extended even with the wrist flexed, an effective treatment is tenotomies of the flexor digitorum profundus and sublimis tendons at different levels in the distal forearm. With the fingers extended, the proximal ends of the sublimis tendons are then sutured to the distal ends of the profundus tendons. Tenotomies of the wrist flexors usually are also necessary. Less commonly, proximal row carpectomy can be used to gain additional "length" in the soft tissues.

The often seen swan neck deformities of the fingers result from extensor overpull, partly caused by the wrist flexion deformity, by compensation for weak wrist extensors, or by both, with resultant overpull on the central slip of the extensor mechanism. With time, the volar plate becomes incompetent, and the proximal interphalangeal joint may subluxate and become fixed. In the latter situation, it is unlikely that function can be improved with surgery. If the hyperextended proximal interphalangeal joint is stable and mobile, tenodesis of the flexor digitorum sublimis to the neck of the proximal phalanx and volar capsulorrhaphy may be successful.[129,199]

Appropriate postoperative care, especially after tendon transfers, is essential to the success of hand and upper extremity surgery in cerebral palsy. Recommended treatment for most patients is 4 weeks of complete immobilization and then an intensive exercise program with emphasis on reach, grasp, and release. Removable splints are used for several months during the day and often at night for several years.[199]

The importance of nonsurgical treatment becomes clear when it is realized that only a small percentage of children with spastic cerebral palsy benefit from upper extremity surgery. Those who benefit have either a reasonable degree of intelligence but severe deformity and appreciate the cosmetic improvement, or have good voluntary control of their hands; good sensation of touch, stereognosis, and proprioception; good range of motion of the joints; and motivation.

References

1. Abel MF, Wenger DR, Mubarak SJ, Sutherland DH. Quantitative analysis of hip dysplasia in cerebral palsy: a study of radiographs and 3-D reformatted images. J Pediatr Orthop 1994;14:283.
2. Aiona M. Triple arthrodesis in cerebral palsy: long-term results (abstract). Orthop Trans 1993;16:626.
3. Albright AL, Cervi A, Singletary J. Intrathecal baclofen for spasticity in cerebral palsy. JAMA 1991;265:1418.
4. Allen BL, Ferguson RL. Technique: L-rod instrumentation for scoliosis in cerebral palsy. J Pediatr Orthop 1982;2:87.
5. Allen BL, Ferguson RL. The Galveston technique for L-rod instrumentation of the scoliotic spine. Spine 1982;7:276.
6. Aram DM, Ekelman BL, Satz P. Trophic changes following early unilateral injury to the brain. Dev Med Child Neurol 1986;28:165.
7. Atkinson S, Stanley FJ. Spastic diplegia among children of low and normal birthweight. Dev Med Child Neurol 1983;25:693.
8. Bagg MR, Farber J, Miller F. Long-term follow-up of hip subluxation in cerebral palsy patients. J Pediatr Orthop 1993;13:32.
9. Baker LD, Hill LM. Foot alignment in the cerebral palsy patient. J Bone Joint Surg [Am] 1964;46:1.
10. Baker LD. A rational approach to the surgical needs of the cerebral palsy patient. J Bone Joint Surg [Am] 1956;38:313.
11. Ball J, Sullivan JA. Treatment of the juvenile bunion by Mitchell osteotomy. Orthopedics 1985;10:1249.
12. Banks HH. Equinus and cerebral palsy—its management. Foot Ankle 1983;4:149.
13. Barrasso JA, Wile PB, Gage JR. Extra-articular subtalar arthrodesis with internal fixation. J Pediatr Orthop 1984;4:555.
14. Baumann J, Meyer E, Schurmann E. Hip adductor transfer to the ischial tuberosity in spastic and paralytic hip disorders. Arch Orthop Trauma Surg 1978;92:107.
15. Beach W, Strecker WB, Coe J, et al. Use of the Green transfer in treatment of patients with spastic cerebral palsy: 17 year experience. J Pediatr Orthop 1991;11:731.
16. Beals R. Spastic paraplegia and diplegia: an evaluation of the non-surgical and surgical factors influencing the prognosis for ambulation. J Bone Joint Surg [Am] 1966;48:827.
17. Benaroch TE, Richards BS, Haideri N. Intermediate follow-up of a simple method of hip arthrodesis in adolescent patients. Paper 477. New Orleans: American Academy of Orthopaedic Surgeons, 1994.
18. Bennet GC, Rang M, Jones D. Varus and valgus deformities of the foot in cerebral palsy. Dev Med Child Neurol 1982;24:499.
19. Berman B, Peacock WJ, Vaughan CL, Bridger RS. Assessment of patients with spastic cerebral palsy before and after rhizotomy (abstract). Dev Med Child Neurol Suppl 1987;55:24.
20. Bisia RS, Louis HJ, Albano P. Transfer of tibialis posterior tendon in cerebral palsy. J Bone Joint Surg [Am] 1976;58:497.
21. Blair E, Stanley FJ. An epidemiologic study of cerebral palsy in Western Australia, 1956–1975. III: postnatal aetiology. Dev Med Child Neurol 1982;27:615.
22. Bleck EE. Locomotor prognosis in cerebral palsy. Dev Med Child Neurol 1975;17:18.
23. Bleck EE. Orthopaedic management of cerebral palsy. Philadelphia: WB Saunders, 1979.
24. Bleck EE. Forefoot problems in cerebral palsy—diagnosis and management. Foot Ankle 1984;4:188.
25. Bleck EE. Orthopaedic management in cerebral palsy. Clin Dev Med 1987;99/100:17.
26. Bleck EE. Management of the lower extremities in children who have cerebral palsy. J Bone Joint Surg [Am] 1990;72:140.
27. Bleck EE. I. Cerebral palsy hip deformities: is there a consensus? (editorial). J Pediatr Orthop 1994;14:281.
28. Boscarino LF, Ounpuu S, Davis RB III, et al. Effects of selective dorsal rhizotomy on gait in children with cerebral palsy. J Pediatr Orthop 1993;13:174.
29. Bretas CT, Dias LS, Gaebler-Spira D. Selective posterior rhizotomy in spastic quadriplegia: results (abstract). Orthop Trans 1993;16:627.
30. Browne AO, McManus F. One-session surgery for bilateral correction of lower limb deformities in spastic diplegia. J Pediatr Orthop 1987;7:259.
31. Brunner R, Baumann JU. Clinical benefit of reconstruction of dislocated or subluxated hip joints in patients with spastic cerebral palsy. J Pediatr Orthop 1994;14:290.
32. Butler C. Effects of powered mobility on self initiated behav-

iors of very young children with locomotor disability. Dev Med Child Neurol 1986;28:325.
33. Cadman D, Richards J, Feldman W. Gastro-esophageal reflux in severely retarded children. Dev Med Child Neurol 1978; 20:95.
34. Campos da Paz A Jr. Walking prognosis in cerebral palsy: a 22-year retrospective. Presented at the American Orthopaedic Association 107th Annual Meeting, Sun Valley, Idaho, June 1994.
35. Carpenter EB. Role of nerve blocks in the foot and ankle in cerebral palsy: therapeutic and diagnostic. Foot Ankle 1983;4:164.
36. Carpenter EB, Seltz DB. Intramuscular alcohol as an aid in management of spastic cerebral palsy. Dev Med Child Neurol 1980;22:497.
37. Carr C, Gage JR. The fate of the non operated hip in cerebral palsy. J Pediatr Orthop 1987;7:262.
38. Chiari K. Medial displacement osteotomy of the pelvis. Clin Orthop 1974;98:55.
39. Castle ME, Schneider C. Proximal femoral resection-interposition arthroplasty. J Bone Joint Surg [Am] 1978;60:1051.
40. Cohen ME, Duffner PK. Prognostic indicators in hemiparetic cerebral palsy. Ann Neurol 1981;9:953.
41. Cooperman DR, Bartucci E, Dietrick E, Millar EA. Hip dislocation in spastic cerebral palsy: long term consequences. J Pediatr Orthop 1987;7:268.
42. Cosgrove AP, Graham HK. Botulinum toxin-A in the management of children with cerebral palsy (abstract). Orthop Trans 1993;16:625.
43. Crawford AH, Kucharzuk D, Roy DR, Blibo J. Subtalar stabilization of the planovalgus foot by staple arthroereisis in young children who have neuromuscular problems. J Bone Joint Surg [Am] 1990;72:840.
44. Cusick B, Sussman M. Short leg casts: their role in the management of cerebral palsy. Phys Occup Ther Pediatr 1982;2:93.
45. Damron T, Breed A, Roecker E. Hamstring tenotomies in cerebral palsy: long-term retrospective analysis. J Pediatr Orthop 1991;11:514.
46. Davids JR, Holland WC, Sutherland DH. Significance of the confusion test in cerebral palsy. J Pediatr Orthop 1993;13:717
47. Davis R, Schulman J, Delahanty A. Cerebellar stimulation for cerebral palsy: double blind study. Acta Neurochir Suppl 1987;39:126.
48. Dega W. Osteotomia trans-iliakalne w leczeniu wrodzonej dysplazji biodra. Chir Narz Ruchu Ortop Polska 1974;39:601.
49. DeGnore LT, Greene WB. Split anterior tibialis tendon transfer in cerebral palsy (abstract). Orthop Trans 1993;16:785.
50. Delong MR. Possible involvement of central pacemakers in clinical disorders of movement. Fed Proc 1978;37:2171.
51. DeJong RN. The neurologic examination. New York: Hoeber-Harper, 1958.
52. Dennyson WG, Fulford GE. Subtalar arthrodesis by cancellous grafts and metallic internal fixation. J Bone Joint Surg [Br] 1976;58:507.
53. Diamond LJ, Jaudes PK. Child abuse in a cerebral palsied population. Dev Med Child Neurol 1983;25:169.
54. Drummond DS, Rogala E, Templeton J, Cruess R. Proximal hamstring release for knee flexion and crouched gait in cerebral palsy. J Bone Joint Surg [Am] 1974;56:1598.
55. Drvaric DM, Roberts JM, Burke SW, et al. Gastroesophageal evaluation in totally involved cerebral palsy patients. J Pediatr Orthop 1987;7:187.
56. Duncan W, Mott D. Foot reflexes and the use of the "inhibitive cast." Foot Ankle 1983;4:145.
57. Elmer E, Wenger DR, Mubarak SJ, Sutherland DH. Proximal hamstring lengthening in the sitting cerebral palsy patient. J Pediatr Orthop 1992;12:329.
58. Etnyre B, Chambers CS, Scarborough NH, Cain TE. Preoperative and postoperative assessment of surgical intervention for equinus gait in children with cerebral palsy. J Pediatr Orthop 1993;13:24.
59. Evans D. Calcaneo-valgus deformity. J Bone Joint Surg [Br] 1975;57:270.
60. Gage JR, Perry J, Hicks RR, et al. Rectus femoris transfer to improve knee function of children with cerebral palsy. Dev Med Child Neurol 1987;29:159.
61. Gage JR. Gait analysis in cerebral palsy. London: MacKeith Press, 1991.
62. Gaines RW, Ford TB. A systematic approach to the amount of Achilles tendon lengthening in CP. J Pediatr Orthop 1985; 4:448.
63. Garbarino JL, Clancy M. A geometric method of calculating tendo Achillis lengthening. J Pediatr Orthop 1985;5:573.
64. Gersoff W, Renshaw TS. Treatment of scoliosis in CP by posterior spinal fusion with Luque-rod segmental instrumentation. J Bone Joint Surg [Am] 1988;70:41.
65. Gibbs FA, Gibbs EL, Perstein MA, Rich CL. Electroencephalographic and clinical aspects of cerebral palsy. Pediatrics 1963;32:73.
66. Goldberg MJ. Measuring outcomes in cerebral palsy. J Pediatr Orthop 1991;11:682.
67. Graham HK, Fixsen JA. Lengthening of the calcaneal tendon in spastic hemiplegia by the White technique: a long term review. J Bone Joint Surg [Br] 1988;70:472.
68. Grant AD, Feldman R, Lehman WB. Equinus deformity in CP. A retrospective analysis of treatment and function in 39 cases. J Pediatr Orthop 1985;5:678.
69. Green NE. Cerebral palsy. In: Canale ST, Beaty JH, eds. Operative pediatric orthopaedics. St. Louis: Mosby-Year Book, 1991:611.
70. Green NE, Griffin PP, Shiavi R. Split posterior tibial tendon transfer in spastic cerebral palsy. J Bone Joint Surg [Am] 1983;65:748.
71. Greene WB. Achilles tendon lengthening in cerebral palsy: comparison of inpatient versus ambulatory surgery. J Pediatr Orthop 1987;7:256.
72. Greene WB, Dietz FR, Goldberg MJ, et al. Rapid progression of hip subluxation in cerebral palsy after selective posterior rhizotomy. J Pediatr Orthop 1991;11:494.
73. Grether JK, Nelson KB, Cummins SK. Twinning and cerebral palsy: experience in four northern California counties, births 1983 through 1985. Pediatrics 1993;92:854.
74. Grice DS. The role of subtalar fusion in the treatment of valgus deformities of the feet. Instr Course Lect 1959;16:127.
75. Griffin PP, Wheelhouse WW, Shiavi R. Adductor transfer for adductor spasticity: clinical and EMG gait analysis. Dev Med Child Neurol 1979;19:783.
76. Gross MS, Ibrahim K, Wehner J, Dvonch V. Combined surgical procedure for treatment of hip dislocation in CP (abstract). Dev Med Child Neurol 1984;26:255.
77. Harada T, Ebara S, Kajiura I, et al. Cervical spondylosis in patients with athetoid cerebral palsy (abstract). Orthop Trans 1993;16:790.
79. Heinrich S, MacEwen GD, Zembo M. Hip dysplasia, subluxation, and dislocation in cerebral palsy: an arthrographic analysis. J Pediatr Orthop 1991;11:488.
80. Helal B. Surgery for adolescent hallux valgus. Clin Orthop 1981;157:50.
81. Hennrikus WL, Rosenthal RK, Kasser JR. Incidence of spondylolisthesis in ambulatory cerebral palsy patients. J Pediatr Orthop 1993;13:37.
82. Herndon WA, Troup P, Yngve DA, Sullivan JA. Effects of neurodevelopmental treatment on movement patterns of children with cerebral palsy. J Pediatr Orthop 1987;7:395.

83. Hicks R, Durinick N, Gage JR. Differentiation of idiopathic toe-walking and cerebral palsy. J Pediatr Orthop 1988;8:160.
84. Hiroshima K, Hamada S, Shimizu N, et al. Anterior transfer of the long toe flexors for the treatment of spastic equinovarus and equinus foot in cerebral palsy. J Pediatr Orthop 1988; 8:164.
85. Hoffer MM, Barakat G, Koffman M. 10 year follow-up of split anterior tibial tendon transfer in cerebral palsied patients with spastic equinovarus deformity. J Pediatr Orthop 1985;5:432.
86. Hoffer MM, Felwell E, Perry R, et al. Functional ambulation in patients with myelomeningocele. J Bone Joint Surg [Am] 1973;55:137.
87. Hoffer MM, Lehman M, Mitani M. Long-term follow-up on tendon transfers to the extensors of the wrist and fingers in patients with cerebral palsy. J Hand Surg 1986;11:836.
88. Hoffer MM, Perry J, Garcia M, Bullock D. Adduction contracture of the thumb in cerebral palsy. J Bone Joint Surg [Am] 1983;65:755.
89. Hoffer MM, Perry J, Melkonian G. Dynamic EMG and decision-making for surgery in the upper extremity of patients with cerebral palsy. J Hand Surg 1979;4:424.
90. Hoffer MM, Stein GA, Koffman M, Prietto M. Femoral varus-derotation osteotomy in spastic cerebral palsy. J Bone Joint Surg [Am] 1985;67:1229.
91. Hoffinger SA, Rab GT, Abou-Ghaida H. Hamstrings in cerebral palsy crouch gait. J Pediatr Orthop 1993;13:722.
92. Hoke M. An operation for stabilizing paralytic feet. J Orthop Surg 1921;3:494.
93. Holstein A. Hallux valgus: an acquired deformity of the foot in cerebral palsy. Foot Ankle 1980;1:33.
94. Houkom JA, Roach JW, Wenger DR, et al. Treatment of acquired hip subluxation in CP. J Pediatr Orthop 1986;6:285.
95. House J, Gwathmey G, Fidler M. A dynamic approach to the thumb-in-palm deformity in cerebral palsy. J Bone Joint Surg [Am] 1981;63:216.
96. Hsu L, Helena L. Distal hamstring elongation in the management of spastic cerebral palsy. J Pediatr Orthop 1990;10:378.
97. Inglis AE, Cooper W. Release of the flexor-pronator origin for flexion deformities of the hand and wrist in spastic paralysis. J Bone Joint Surg [Am] 1966;48:847.
98. Javors JR, Klaaren HE. The Vulpius procedure for correction for equinus deformity in CP. J Pediatr Orthop 1987;7:191.
99. Jensen JE, Jensen TG, Smith TK, et al. Nutrition in orthopaedic surgery. J Bone Joint Surg [Am] 1982;64:1263.
100. Jevsevar DS, Karlin LI. The relationship between preoperative nutritional status and complications after an operation for scoliosis in patients who have cerebral palsy. J Bone Joint Surg [Am] 1993;75:880.
101. Kalen V, Adler N, Bleck EE. Electromyography of idiopathic toe walking. J Pediatr Orthop 1986;6:31.
102. Kalen V, Bleck EE. Prevention of spastic paralytic dislocation of the hip. Dev Med Child Neurol 1985;27:17.
103. Kalen V, Conklin M, Sherman F. Untreated scoliosis in severe cerebral palsy. J Pediatr Orthop 1992;12:337.
104. Kanda T, Yuge M, Yamori Y, et al. Early physiotherapy in the treatment of spastic diplegia. Dev Med Child Neurol 1984;26:438.
105. Kling TF, Kaufer HA, Hensinger RN. Split posterior tibial tendon transfers in children with cerebral spastic paralysis and equinovarus deformity. J Bone Joint Surg [Am] 1985;67:186.
106. Koffman M. Proximal femoral resection or THR in severely disabled cerebral spastic patients. Orthop Clin North Am 1981;12:91.
107. Koman LA, Mooney JF, Goodman A. Management of valgus hindfoot deformity in pediatric cerebral palsy patients by medial displacement osteotomy. J Pediatr Orthop 1993;13:180.
108. Koman LA, Mooney JF, Smith B, Goodman A, Mulvaney T. Management of cerebral palsy with botulinum-A toxin: preliminary investigation. J Pediatr Orthop 1993;13:489.
109. Koman LA, Mooney JF, Smith BP, et al. Management of spasticity in cerebral palsy with botulinum-A toxin: report of a preliminary, randomized, double-blind trial. J Pediatr Orthop 1994;14:299.
110. Krebs DE, Edelstein JE, Fishman S. Reliability of observational kinematic gait analysis. Phys Ther 1985;65:1027.
111. Laplaza FJ, Root L, Tassanawipas A, Glasser DB. Femoral torsion and neck-shaft angles in cerebral palsy. J Pediatr Orthop 1993;13:192.
112. Letts RM, Rathbone MD, Yamashita T, et al. Soft Boston orthosis in management of neuromuscular scoliosis: a preliminary report. J Pediatr Orthop 1992;12:470.
113. Loder RT. Orthopaedic aspects of children with infectious (central nervous system) postnatal cerebral palsy. J Pediatr Orthop 1992;12:527.
114. Lonstein JE, Akbarnia BA. Operative treatment of spinal deformities in patients with cerebral palsy or mental retardation. J Bone Joint Surg [Am] 1983;65:43.
115. Lonstein JE, Beck K. Hip dislocation and subluxation in CP. J Pediatr Orthop 1986;6:521.
116. Lonstein JE. Cerebral palsy. In: Weinstein SL, ed. The pediatric spine—principles and practice. New York: Raven Press, 1994.
117. Luba R, Rosman M. Bunions in children—treatment with a modified Mitchell osteotomy. J Periatr Orthop 1984;4:44.
118. Majestro TC, Ruda R, Frost HM. Intramuscular lengthening of the posterior tibialis tendon. Clin Orthop 1963;79:59.
119. Matsuo T, Hara H, Tada S. Selective lengthening of the psoas and rectus femoris and preservation of the iliacus for flexion deformity of the hip in cerebral palsy patients. J Pediatr Orthop 1987;7:690.
120. Matsuo T, Tada S, Hajime T. Insufficiency of the hip adductor after anterior obturator neurectomy in 42 children with cerebral palsy. J Pediatr Orthop 1986;6:686.
121. McCall RE, Lillich JS, Harris JR, Johnston FA. The Grice extra-articular arthrodesis: a clinical review. J Pediatr Orthop 1985;5:442.
122. McCarthy RE, Simon S, Zawacky R, Reese N. Proximal femoral resection to allow adults who have severe cerebral palsy to sit. J Bone Joint Surg [Am] 1988;70:1011.
124. McKeever DC. Arthrodesis of the first metatarsophalangeal joint for hallux valgus, hallux rigidus, and metatarsus primus varus. J Bone joint Surg [Am] 1952;34:129.
125. McNeal DM, Hawtrey CE, Wolraich MG. Symptomatic neurogenic bladder in a cerebral palsied population. Dev Med Child Neurol 1983;25:612.
126. Miller AR, Miller F, Temple T. Impact of orthoses on the rate of scoliosis progression in children with cerebral palsy. Paper 81. San Francisco: American Academy of Orthopaedic Surgeons, 1993.
127. Millis MB. Rapidly progressive lumbar hyperlordosis following selective posterior rhizotomy for spastic quadriplegia (abstract). Orthop Trans 1993;16:10.
128. Mital MA. Lengthening of the elbow flexors in cerebral palsy. J Bone Joint Surg [Am] 1979;61:515.
129. Mital MA, Sakellarides HT. Surgery of the upper extremity in the retarded individual with spastic cerebral palsy. Orthop Clin North Am 1981;12:127.
130. Molnar GE, Gordon SV. Predictive value of clinical signs for early prognostication of motor function in cerebral palsy. Arch Phys Med 1976;57:153.
131. Moreau MJ, Drummond DS, Rogala E, et al. Natural history of the dislocated hip in spastic cerebral palsy. Dev Med Child Neurol 1979;21:749.

132. Moreau MJ, Lake DM. Outpatient percutaneous heel cord lengthening in children. J Pediatr Orthop 1987;7:253.
133. Moreland JR, Westin WG. Further experience with Grice subtalar arthrodesis. Clin Orthop 1986;207:113.
134. Mosca V. Calcaneal neck lengthening for severe abductovalgus flat hindfoot deformity in children (abstract). J Pediatr Orthop 1992;12:817.
135. Mowery CA, Gelberman RH, Rhoades C. Upper extremity tendon transfers in cerebral palsy: electromyographic and functional analysis. J Pediatr Orthop 1985;5:69.
136. Mubarak SJ, Valencia FG, Wenger DR. One-stage correction of the spastic dislocated hip. J Bone Joint Surg [Am] 1992;74:1347.
137. Nather A, Fulford GE, Stewart K. Treatment of valgus hindfoot in cerebral palsy by peroneus brevis lengthening. Dev Med Child Neurol 1984;26:335.
138. Nelson KB, Ellenberg JH. Epidemiology of cerebral palsy. In: Schoenberg BS, ed. Advances in neurology. vol. 19. New York: Raven Press, 1978:421.
139. Nelson KB, Ellenberg JH. Antecedents of cerebral palsy II. Multivariate analysis of risk. N Engl J Med 1986;315:81.
140. Norlin R, Odenrick P. Development of gait in spastic children with CP. J Pediatr Orthop 1986;6:674.
141. Norlin R, Tkaczuk H. One-session surgery for correction of lower extremity deformities in children with cerebral palsy. J Pediatr Orthop 1985;5:208.
142. Nwaobi OM, Smith PD. Effect of adaptive seating on pulmonary function of children with CP. Dev Med Child Neurol 1986;28:351.
143. Olney BW, Williams PF, Menelaus MB. Treatment of spastic equinus by aponeurosis lengthening. J Pediatr Orthop 1988;8:422.
144. Onimus M, Allamel G, Manyone P, Laurain JM. Prevention of hip dislocation in cerebral palsy by early psoas and adductors tenotomies. J Pediatr Orthop 1991;11:432.
145. Ono CM, Lipp EB. Green-Banks flexor carpi ulnaris transfer to wrist extensors for spastic cerebral palsy (abstract). Orthop Trans 1993;16:325.
146. Oppenheim WL. The case for selective posterior rhizotomy. Presented at pediatric specialty day meeting, American Academy of Orthopaedic Surgeons, New Orleans, 1990.
147. Oppenheim WL, Peacock WJ. Selective dorsal rhizotomy (abstract). J Pediatr Orthop 1991;11:690.
148. Orthopaedic knowledge update 3. Park Ridge, IL: American Academy of Orthopaedic Surgeons, 1990:286.
149. Orthopaedic knowledge update 2. Park Ridge, IL: American Academy of Orthopaedic Surgeons, 1987:191.
150. Osterkamp J, Caillouette JT, Hoffer MM. Chiari osteotomy in cerebral palsy. J Pediatr Orthop 1988;8:274.
151. Otis JC, Root L, Kroll MA. Measurement of plantar flexor spasticity during treatment with tone-reducing casts. J Pediatr Orthop 1985;5:682.
152. Ounpuu S, Mulk E, Davis RB III, et al. Rectus femoris surgery in children with cerebral palsy. Part I: the effect of rectus femoris transfer location on knee motion. J Pediatr Orthop 1993;13:325.
153. Ounpuu S, Mulk E, Davis RB III, et al. Rectus femoris surgery in children with cerebral palsy. Part II: a comparison between the effect of transfer and release of the distal rectus femoris on knee motion. J Pediatr Orthop 1993;13:331.
154. Paine RS. On the treatment of cerebral palsy: the outcome of 177 patients, 74 totally untreated. Pediatrics 1962;29:605.
155. Palmer FB, Shapiro BK, Wachtel RC, et al. The effects of physical therapy on cerebral palsy: a controlled trial in infants with spastic diplegia. N Engl J Med 1988;318:803.
156. Papariello SG, Skinner SR. Dynamic electromyography analysis of habitual toe walkers. J Pediatr Orthop 1985;5:171.
157. Pape KE, Kirsch SE, Galil A, et al. Neuromuscular approach to the motor deficits of cerebral palsy: a pilot study. J Pediatr Orthop 1993;13:628.
158. Patrick J, Boland M, Stoski D, Burray GE. Rapid correction of wasting in children with CP. Dev Med Child Neurol 1986;28:734.
159. Payne LZ, DeLuca PA. Heterotopic ossification after rhizotomy and femoral osteotomy. J Pediatr Orthop 1993;13:733.
160. Peacock WJ, Arlens L, Berman B. CP spasticity: selective posterior rhizotomy. Pediatr Neurosci 1987;13:61.
161. Peacock WJ, Staudt LA. Functional outcomes following selective posterior rhizotomy in children with cerebral palsy. J Neurosurg 1991;74:380.
162. Pemberton PA. Pericapsular osteotomy for congenital dislocation of the hip. J Bone Joint Surg [Am] 1965;47:65.
163. Perry J. Distal rectus femoris transfer. Dev Med Child Neurol 1987;29:153.
164. Perry J, Adams J, Cahan LD. Foot-floor contact patterns following selective dorsal rhizotomy (abstract). Dev Med Child Neurol Suppl 59 1989;31:19.
165. Perry J, Hoffer MM. Preoperative and postoperative dynamic EMG as an aid in planning tendon transfers in children with cerebral palsy. J Bone Joint Surg [Am] 1977;59:531.
166. Phelps W. Prevention of acquired dislocation of the hip in cerebral palsy. J Bone Joint Surg [Am] 1959;41:440.
167. Piper MC, Kumos VI, Willis DM, et al. Early physical therapy effects on the high risk infant: a randomized control trial. Pediatrics 1986;78:216.
168. Pritchett JW. Treated and urtreated unstable hips in severe cerebral palsy. Dev Med Child Neurol 1990;32:3.
169. Rang M. Cerebral palsy. In: Morrissy RT, ed. Lovell and Winter's pediatric orthopaedics. 3rd ed. Philadelphia: JB Lippincott, 1990.
170. Rang M, Douglas G, Benner GC, Koreska J. Seating for children with cerebral palsy. J Pediatr Orthop 1981;1:279.
171. Rattey TE, Leahey L, Hyndman J, et al. Recurrence after Achilles tendon lengthening in cerebral palsy. J Pediatr Orthop 1993;13:184.
172. Relmers J. Contracture of the hamstrings in spastic cerebral palsy. A study of three methods of operative correction. J Bone Joint Surg [Br] 1974;56:102.
173. Reimers J, Poulsen S. Adductor transfer versus tenotomy for stability of the hip in spastic cererbral palsy. J Pediatr Orthop 1984;4:52.
174. Renshaw TS, Sirkin RB, Drennan JC. The management of hallux valgus in cerebral palsy. Dev Med Child Neurol 1979;21:202.
175. Renshaw TS, Larkin J. Results of orthotic treatment of scoliosis in cerebral palsy (abstract). Orthop Trans 1987;11:38.
176. Root L, Siegal T. Osteotomy of the hip in children: posterior approach. J Bone Joint Surg [Am] 1980;62:571.
177. Root L, Spero C. Hip adductor transfer compared with adductor tenotomy in cerebral palsy. J Bone Joint Surg [Am] 1981;63:767.
178. Root L, Goss JR, Mendes J. The treatment of the painful hip in cerebral palsy by total hip replacement or hip arthrodesis. J Bone Joint Surg [Am] 1986;68:590.
179. Root L, Miller SR, Kirz P. Posterior tibial tendon transfer in patients with cerebral palsy. J Bone Joint Surg [Am] 1987;69:1133.
180. Rose J, Medeiros JM, Parker R. Energy cost index as an estimate of anergy expenditure of CP children during assisted ambulation. Dev Med Child Neurol 1985;27:485.
181. Rose SA, DeLuca PA, Davis RB III, et al. Kinematic and kinetic evaluation of the ankle after lengthening of the gastrocnemius fascia in children with cerebral palsy. J Pediatr Orthop 1993;13:727.
182. Rosenthal RK, Deutsch SD, Miller W, et al. A fixed-ankle,

below-the-knee orthosis for the management of genu recurvatum in spastic cerebral palsy. J Bone Joint Surg [Am] 1975;57:545.
183. Ruda R, Frost HM. Cerebral palsy: spastic varus and forefoot adductus treated by intramuscular posterior tibial tendon lengthening. Clin Orthop 1971;79:61.
184. Russman BS, Gage JR. Cerebral palsy. Curr Probl Pediatr 1989;19:65.
185. Samilson RL. Orthopaedic aspects of cerebral palsy. Clin Dev Med 1975;52/53:142.
186. Scherzer AL, Mike V, Ilson J. Physical therapy as a determinant of change in the cerebral palsied infant. Pediatrics 1976;58:47.
187. Schneider M, Balon K. Deformity of the foot following anterior transfer of the posterior tibial tendon and lengthening of the Achilles tendon for spastic equinovarus. Clin Orthop 1977;125:113.
188. Schwend RM, Millis MB, Hall JE. Calcaneal displacement osteotomy for correction of hindfoot deformities. Presented at the American Academy of Orthopaedic Surgeons 60th annual meeting, San Francisco, 1993.
189. Scott A, Chambers C, Cain TE, Hadley NA. Adductor transfers in cerebral palsy: long-term results studied be gait analysis (abstract). Orthop Trans 1993;16:626.
190. Scott SM, Janes PC, Stevens PM. Grice subtalar arthrodesis followed to skeletal maturity. J Pediatr Orthop 1988;8:176.
191. Scranton PE, Zuckerman JD. Bunion surgery in adolescents—results of surgical treatment. J Pediatr Orthop 1984;4:39.
192. Sharps CH, Clancy M, Steel HH. A long term retrospective study of proximal hamstring release for hamstring contracture. J Pediatr Orthop 1984;4:443.
193. Sharrard WJW, Bernstein S. Equinus deformity in cerebral palsy: a comparison between elongation of the tendo calcaneus and gastrocnemius recession. J Bone Joint Surg [Br] 1972;54:272.
194. Sharrard WJW, Allen MH, Heany SH, Prendiville GRG. Surgical prophylaxis of subluxation and dislocation of the hip in cerebral palsy. J Bone Joint Surg [Am] 1975;57:160.
195. Silver CM, Simon SD, Lichtman HM. Long-term follow-up observations on calcaneal osteotomy. Clin Orthop 1974;99:181.
196. Silver LB. Controversial approaches to treating learning disabilities and attention deficit disorders. Am J Dis Child 1986;140:1045.
197. Silver RL, de la Garza J, Rang M. The myth of muscle imbalance: a study of relative strengths and excursions of normal muscles about the foot and ankle. J Bone Joint Surg [Br] 1985;67:432.
198. Silver RL, Rang M, Chan J, de la Garza J. Adductor release in non ambulant children with cerebral palsy. J Pediatr Orthop 1985;5:672.
199. Skoff H, Woodbury DF. Current concepts review: management of the upper extremity in cerebral palsy. J Bone Joint Surg [Am] 1985;67:500.
200. Snyder M, Kumar SJ, Stecyk MD. Split tibialis posterior tendon transfer and tendo-Achilles lengthening for spastic equinovarus feet. J Pediatr Orthop 1993;13:20.
201. Sponseller PD, Whiffen JR, Drummond DS. Interspinous process segmental spinal instrumentation for scoliosis in cerebral palsy. J Pediatr Orthop 1986;6:559.
202. Staheli LT. The prone hip extension test. Clin Orthop 1977;123:12.
203. Staheli LT. Technique: slotted acetabular augmentation. J Pediatr Orthop 1981;1:321.
204. Staudt LA, Peacock WJ. Selective posterior rhizotomy for the treatment of spastic cerebral palsy. In: Long T, ed. Pediatric physical therapy. vol. 1. Baltimore: Williams & Wilkins, 1989:3.
205. Steel HH. Triple osteotomy of the innominate bone. Clin Orthop 1977;122:116.
206. Steel HH. Gluteus medius and minimus insertion advancement for correction of internal rotation gait in cerebral palsy. J Bone Joint Surg [Am] 1980;62:919.
207. Stevens DB, Opfell AR, Stanley N, Walker JL. Heel cord advancement for treatment of spastic equinus deformity in children (abstract). Orthop Trans 1993;16:625.
208. Strecker WB, Via MW, Oliver SK, Schoenecker PL. Heel cord advancement for treatment of equinus deformity in cerebral palsy. J Pediatr Orthop 1990;10:105.
209. Sussman MD. Casting as an adjunct to neurodevelopmental therapy in cerebral palsy. Dev Med Child Neurol 1983;25:804.
210. Sussman MD. Role of the physical therapist in treatment of children with cerebral palsy (abstract). J Pediatr Orthop 1991;11:688.
211. Sussman MD, Cusick B. The role of short-leg, tone reducing casts as an adjunct to physical therapy of patients with cerebral palsy. Johns Hopkins Med Bull 1979;145:112.
212. Sutherland DH, Oishen R, Cooper L, Woo SL-Y. The development of mature gait. J Bone Joint Surg [Am] 1980;62:336.
213. Sutherland DH, Schottstaedt ER, Larsen LJ, et al. Clinical and EMG study of seven spastic children with internal rotation gait. J Bone Joint Surg [Am] 1969;51:1070.
214. Sutherland DH, Greenfield R. Double innominate osteotomy. J Bone Joint Surg [Am] 1977;59:1082.
215. Sutherland DH, Santi M, Abel MF. Treatment of stiff-kneed gait in cerebral palsy: a comparison by gait analysis of distal rectus femoris transfer versus proximal rectus release. J Pediatr Orthop 1990;10:433.
216. Szalay EA, Roach JW, Houkom JA, et al. Extension-abduction contracture of the spastic hip. J Pediatr Orthop 1986;6:1.
217. Tardieu G, Tardieu C. Cerebral palsy: mechanical evaluation and conservation correction of limb joint contractures. Clin Orthop 1987;219:63.
218. Taussig G, Pilliard D. Triceps lengthening in children with cerebral palsy performed before the age of six years. Results at the end of growth. Rev Chir Orthop 1988;74:79.
219. Tenuta J, Shelton YA, Miller F. Long-term follow-up of triple arthrodesis in patients with cerebral palsy. J Pediatr Orthop 1993;13:713.
220. Thometz JG, Simon SR. Progression of scoliosis after skeletal maturity in institutionalized adults who have cerebral palsy. J Bone Joint Surg [Am] 1988;70:1290.
221. Thometz JG, Tachdjian MO. Long term follow-up of the flexor carpi ulnaris transfer in spastic hemiplegia children. J Pediatr Orthop 1988;8:407.
222. Thompson G, Rubin I, Bilenker R. Comprehensive management of cerebral palsy. New York: Grune & Stratton, 1983.
223. Throop FB, DeRosa GP, Reeck C, Waterman S. Correction of equinus in cerebral palsy by the Murphy procedure of tendo calcaneus advancement: a preliminary communication. Dev Med Child Neurol 1975;17:182.
224. Tippets RH, Walker ML, Liddell KL. Long-term follow-up of selective dorsal rhizotomy for relief of spasticity in cerebral-palsied children (abstract). Dev Med Child Neurol Suppl 1989;31(59):19.
225. Vulpius O, Stoffel A. Orthopaedische Operationslehre. Stuttgart: Ferdinand Enke, 1913.
226. Waters RL, Perry J, McDaniels JM, House K. The relative strength of the hamstrings during hip extension. J Bone Joint Surg [Am] 1974;56:1592.
227. Watt J, Sims D, Harckham F, et al. A prospective study of inhibitive casting as an adjunct to physiotherapy for cerebral palsied children. Dev Med Child Neurol 1986;28:480.
228. Weindling AM, Rochefort MJ, Claverty SA, et al. Development

of cerebral palsy after ultrasonographic detection of periventricular cysts in the newborn. Dev Med Child Neurol 1985;27:800.
229. White JW. Torsion of the Achilles tendon: its surgical significance. Arch Surg 1943;46:784.
230. Winter S. Preoperative assessment of the child with neuromuscular scoliosis. Orthop Clin North Am 1994;25:239.
231. Winters TF, Gage JR, Hicks R. Gait patterns in spastic hemiplegia in children and young adults. J Bone Joint Surg [Am] 1987;69:437.
232. Wright T, Nicholson J. Physiotherapy for the spastic child: an evaluation. Dev Med Child Neurol 1973;15:146.
233. Young RR, Wiegner AW. Spasticity. Clin Orthop 1987;219:50.
234. Zuckerman JD, Staheli LT, McLaughlin JF. Acetabular augmentation for progressive hip subluxation in CP. J Pediatr Orthop 1984;4:436.

Chapter 14

Myelomeningocele

Richard E. Lindseth

Classification and Pathology
Neurologic Abnormality
Genetics, Etiology, and Prenatal Diagnosis
Natural History
    Hydrocephaly
    Arnold-Chiari Deformity
    Tethered Cord Syndrome
    Latex Hypersensitivity
Effect of Myelomeningocele on
    Developmental Sequence

Treatment
    Spine
    Hip
    Thoracic Paraplegia
    Upper Lumbar Paraplegia
    Middle and Lower Lumbar Paraplegia
    Knee
    Foot
    Orthotic Devices

Myelomeningocele is the most complex treatable congenital malformation of the central nervous system. Its effect on the child, the parents, and the medical community may be devastating. The initial treatment, which consists of closure of the meningocele and insertion of a ventriculoperitoneal shunt, is straightforward and well within the capability of most neurosurgeons. The child is then referred to the orthopaedist for rehabilitation. Family members are grief stricken, confused, and angry. They fully expect that the medical treatment prescribed will make the child normal.

The orthopaedist faced with a child with multiple physical deformities and neurologic dysfunction may react in one of several ways. He or she may be overwhelmed by the situation and project a pessimistic prognosis to the family, further increasing the depression and hopelessness of the parents. The orthopaedist may respond in an overly positive way, making use of the principles learned in the treatment of idiopathic clubfoot, congenital dislocation of the hip, idiopathic scoliosis, and cerebral palsy. The disease process of myelomeningocele is different, however, from that of the other conditions, and the recommended treatment programs often result in failure. This also angers and depresses the family. It is better to be supportive of the family in its grief without being too optimistic and positive about what can be done to help the child.

The orthopaedic care of these patients is strongly influenced by factors beyond our control, including changes in the neurologic system, urologic abnormalities, societal pressures, education, and the availability of medical resources. It is almost impossible to carry out the necessary treatment program without a coordinated interdisciplinary team consisting of a neurosurgeon, an orthopaedist, a urologist, a social worker, physical and occupational therapists, educators, a pediatrician, and a nurse specialist. If these services cannot be provided, the child should be referred to a clinic that can provide them.

CLASSIFICATION AND PATHOLOGY

The pathologic description of spina bifida and associated neurologic abnormalities was made by von Recklinghausen in 1886.[133] His observations remain current, and only recently have we begun to understand the pathologic processes that lead to the formation of myelomeningocele and other associated diseases.

Neural tube defects are grouped together under the generic terms *myelodysplasia*, *spinal dysraphia*, and *spina bifida aperta*. These are not to be confused with *spina bifida occulta*, which is a common radiographic finding of a lack of fusion of the spinous process of the lower lumbar and sacral spine without neurologic abnormalities. Neural tube defects can be divided into four subtypes: meningocele, myelomeningocele, lipomeningocele, and rachischisis.

A cyst involving only the meninges but not any neural elements is called a *meningocele*. It often requires surgical excision and closure by a neurosurgeon. However, it does not cause neurologic or orthopaedic abnormalities, and further treatment is not needed.

A myelomeningocele includes the abnormal neural elements as a part of the sac (Fig. 14-1). The sac may assume any size, form, or location along the spine. It is less likely to be epithelialized than a meningocele sac. The neural elements are abnormal, and pronounced peripheral neurologic deficits are common. Central nervous system abnormalities, including Arnold-Chiari deformity and hydrocephalus, are common.

A *lipomeningocele* is a lesion in which the sac contains a lipoma that is intimately involved with the sacral nerves. These lesions often are epithelialized at birth. Children with lipomeningocele may not have hydrocephaly or other central nervous system abnormalities. Neurologic function, which is almost normal at birth, may become impaired with growth. This abnormality is similar to other abnormalities of the spine, including dermoid sinus, dermoid cyst, and diastematomyelia. When paralysis occurs, it rarely extends above the lumbosacral area. Progressive neurologic loss should be the major concern in the treatment of these children.

Rachischisis is a complete absence of the skin and sac, with exposure of the muscle and the presence of a dysplastic spinal cord without evidence of a covering. Occasionally, even the bone is exposed, but usually there is a thin covering of muscle.

The embryologic development of myelomeningocele is unknown. There are two opposing schools of thought that have existed since the initial description of the disease[133]: von Recklinghausen's hypothesis that the defect was caused by lack of closure of the spine, and Morgagni's proposal that it was caused by a rupture of a previously closed neural tube.[43–47,100] Proponents of each theory have gained prominence.

The formation of the myelomeningocele occurs early in life, probably between the third and fourth weeks of gestation. This has two implications. The first is that if myelomeningocele is to be prevented by eliminating teratogenic factors and providing a nutritional supplement, it must be done very early, almost before the mother is aware that she is pregnant. The second implication is that the lesion has occurred before limb bud development, yet most often the limb bud of the lower extremity is essentially normal. This seems to suggest that, at least initially, neurologic function is normal and remains so until late in prenatal development. This has led some investigators to evaluate the benefit of delivery by cesarean section when maturity of the lungs permits, avoiding the trauma to the neural plate caused by the decrease in amniotic fluid as maturity progresses and the birth process itself.[118] However, the studies are inconclusive.

The roof of the myelomeningocele is composed of the spinal cord. It is open from the central canal posteriorly through the dorsal columns (see Fig. 14-1). The anterior roots are intact, whereas the posterior roots to the dorsal cord are more likely to be involved in the pathologic process. The central canal of the cord is open and communicates with the fourth ventricle of the brain; this allows the cerebral spinal fluid to flow to the outside. Because of the probable

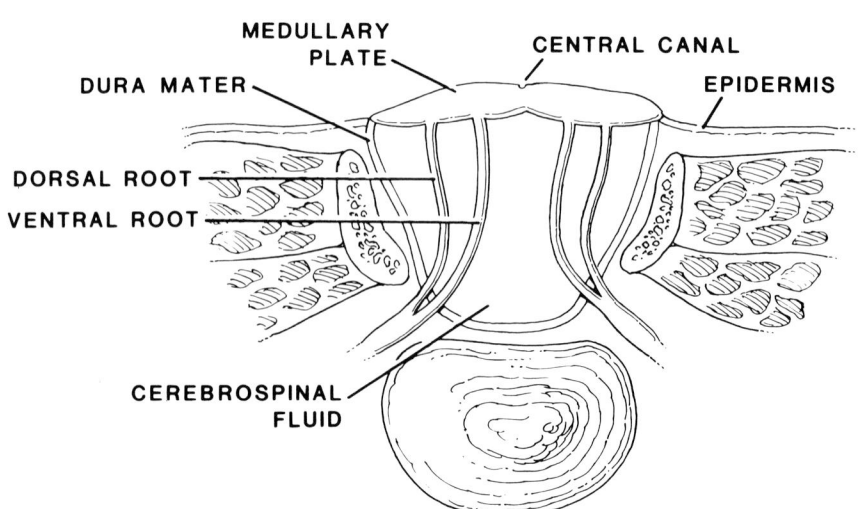

FIGURE 14-1. Cross section of myelomeningocele. The abnormal cord is part of the sac and is elevated out of the canal.

involvement of the posterior columns, sensory and proprioception abnormalities probably are worse than the motor abnormalities. This abnormality of sensory feedback and crossing nerve fibers around the central cord may explain the lack of coordinated reciprocal functioning and the presence of spasticity frequently observed in children with myelomeningocele.

The attachment of the spinal cord to the meningocele sac prevents the normal upward migration of the spinal cord with growth. This produces the tethered cord. Even with surgical release of the spinal cord from all adhesions at the time of sac closure there is a likelihood of reattachment of the cord during the healing process with recurrence of tethered cord syndrome later in life. The incidence of symptomatic re-tethering is unknown. However, it seems that the more we look for it, the more common it becomes.

Because of tethered cord or hydrocephaly, almost all children with myelomeningocele have displacement of the brain stem through the foramen magnum into the cervical neural canal, Arnold-Chiari type II malformation. The extent of the displacement determines the type of deformity. Type I malformation has minimal deformity; type II deformity consists of the displacement of the medulla oblongata and the spinal cord to the extent that the cervical nerve roots must take an upward course to reach their outlet foramina (Fig. 14-2). This is the most common deformity in myelomeningocele. The type III deformity is more severe in displacement and includes part of the cerebellum.

The final pathologic abnormality is hydrocephaly, which consists of excessive cerebral spinal fluid in the ventricles of the brain. Almost 90% of children with myelomeningocele develop hydrocephaly, which communicates to a persistently open central canal of the cord, which in turn communicates with the meningocele sac. This open communication of the central canal and the fourth ventricle permits the outflow of the cerebral spinal fluid, decompresses the ventricular pressure, and relieves the hydrocephaly. However, at the time of sac closure the fluid flow from the central canal is stopped and hydrocephaly returns. If hydrocephaly is not shunted, the fluid pressure increases in the brain and the spinal cord, which causes brain atrophy, hydromyelia, and eventually syringomyelia.

NEUROLOGIC ABNORMALITY

The neurologic abnormality defies simple classification[87] because of the complex abnormalities of the central nervous system, which include hydrocephaly, Arnold-Chiari defect, hydrosyringomyelia, tethered cord, and injury to the posterior column of the spinal cord. Attempts to classify the level of paralysis by muscle function as though the defect is similar to a spinal cord injury seen in vertebral fractures are unsuccessful. Sharrard[114] initially formulated the classification by lumbar segmental levels based on motor segmental innervation using anterior level of the anterior horn cells in the spinal cord. This classification does not match the clinical observation of function in the lower extremities. For example, there is confusion in the literature about what is an L4 versus an L5 level of

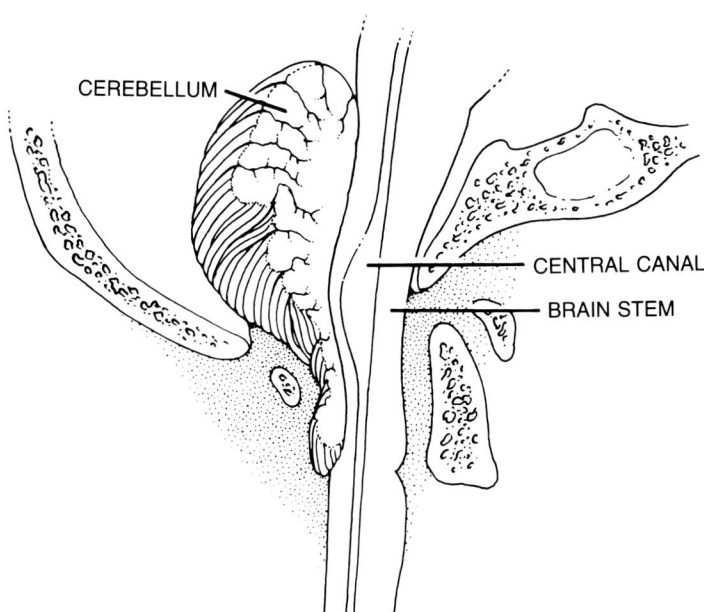

FIGURE 14-2. Arnold-Chiari type II malformation of the brain stem. This is the most common type of malformation seen in myelomeningocele. The medulla oblongata is displaced distally through the foramen magnum into the cervical neural canal. The ventricle communicates with the still open central canal of the cord.

paralysis. The problem is using motor function to describe the level of paralysis when central nervous system dysfunction is common. If sensation, the most severely damaged nerve function, is used to describe the level of paralysis, the classification better describes what is seen clinically. Muscles that can communicate with the brain through sensory feedback are functional. Muscles that cannot do this may be ignored by the brain and become flaccid or spastic and function only by reflex. I recommend that classification of function be made by sensory level rather than motor level because it will be more consistent between patients and different observers.

Another confounding variable is abnormality of coordinated muscle function due to brain stem abnormalities. On manual testing, the muscles contract to simple commands, such as "Extend (or flex) the knee." However, on complex coordinated activities, such as walking, the leg muscles do not contract as expected but contract and relax simultaneously in a co-contraction rather than sequentially, as seen in normal gait (Fig. 14-3). This dynamic co-contraction is very common in the L3 to L5 level of paralysis and may explain the knee flexion contractures in these patients despite normal quadriceps strength. I observed this phenomenon in a child with hydrocephalus and Arnold-Chiari malformation without myelomeningocele. This may suggest that it is related to the brain stem rather than the meningocele itself.

Other neurologic defects that are not well understood but common are decreased perceptual motor function of the hands and attention deficit disorder manifested by short attention span at school.[139]

GENETICS, ETIOLOGY, AND PRENATAL DIAGNOSIS

About 6000 infants in the United States are born each year with neural tube defects. This includes anencephaly, myelomeningocele, and related abnormalities. A gradual decrease in incidence worldwide has occurred over the last 30 years.[120] The reason for this fluctuation is not clear and probably involves both genetic and environmental factors.

Most neural tube defects occur as isolated malformations caused by a variety of factors, both inherited and acquired.[21,126] This pattern is known as *multifactorial inheritance*. In the United States, the overall incidence of neural tube defects is 0.15% among Caucasians and 0.04% among African Americans. After the birth of one affected child, the risk of a second affected child is higher.[21,69] In the United States, the occurrence of a neural tube defect in first-degree relatives of an affected member was 3.2%, in second-degree relatives, 0.5%, and in third-degree relatives, 0.17%.[126]

Not all neural tube defects are multifactorially inherited; some are caused by chromosome abnormalities, and others are caused by single-gene abnormalities. Usually, children with chromosomal or single-gene abnormalities have other birth defects. Some cases of spina bifida and anencephaly entirely are produced environmentally. These abnormalities are caused by exposure during pregnancy to teratogenic agents, such as valproic acid taken for seizure control.[23]

Yates and colleagues[140] have shown an association between susceptibility of offspring with neural tube

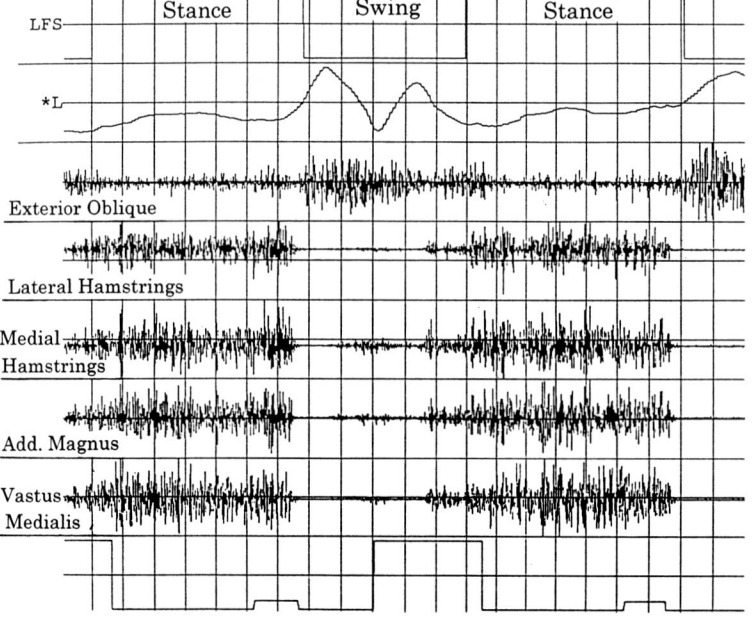

FIGURE 14-3. Dynamic electromyograms taken during a gait assessment analysis of a 5-year-old child with an L4 level of paraplegia and a type II Arnold-Chiari malformation. Surface electrodes were used during this analysis. The external oblique muscle is a swing phase muscle. The medial and lateral hamstrings, the adductor magnus, and the vastus medialis contract simultaneously throughout the stance phase. This observation has been checked using fine wire electrodes, which show that the simultaneous contraction is not caused by cross talk between the surface electrodes.

defects and depressed red cell folate levels, which cannot be attributed entirely to low dietary intake of folate. They postulate that a factor that predisposes a person to the current neural tube defect is an inherent disorder of folate metabolism. This theory is supported by a study by Sellar and Nevin,[111] in which a decreased incidence of neural tube defects was found in children of mothers taking periconceptional vitamin supplementation. The FDA recommends that all women of child-bearing age receive 0.4 mg folate before conception and during early pregnancy. The Centers for Disease Control and Prevention[23] recommends that women who fall in the high-risk group of bearing a child with a neural tube defect because of giving birth to a prior affected child or a first-degree relative with a neural tube defect receive a larger dose of folate, 4.0 mg/day.

Prenatal diagnosis of a neural tube defect allows the family in consultation with the medical community to make informed decisions about its child. These decisions range from termination of pregnancy to attempts to improve the outcome of pregnancy by improved perinatal care in institutions medically prepared to provide optimal care for the child. The aim of any prenatal screen for open neural tube defect is to be able to pinpoint women with a sufficiently high risk of having an affected infant to justify carrying out special diagnostic procedures, such as amniocentesis for amniotic fluid, alpha-fetoprotein and acetylcholinesterase determinations, and detailed ultrasonography for examination of the fetus.[1] Women who have had an infant with a neural tube defect carry enough risk of having another affected child to justify undergoing amniocentesis. Longitudinal ultrasound examination of the fetal spine provides vital information about the presence or absence of neural tube defect. The sensitivity of ultrasound examination is excellent for studying women at high risk for carrying a fetus with neural tube defect. In almost all fetuses with anencephaly and at least 80% of fetuses with open spina bifida, diagnoses are correct. When no abnormalities are found on detailed ultrasound examination, amniocentesis is recommended for evaluation for alpha-fetoprotein and acetylcholinesterase.[70]

NATURAL HISTORY

Most children born with myelomeningocele die in early infancy if left untreated. This has been documented in several series of untreated children in the late 1950s and early 1960s. The mortality rates range from 90% to 100%.[58,83] The cause of death in most infants is meningoventriculitis. Surgical treatment is not necessary for survival if antibiotics are administered and nutrition is maintained. However, the surviving children are disabled further by a high level of paralysis and increased mental retardation resulting from the continued trauma to the spinal cord and the uncontrolled hydrocephaly, which would not have been present if surgical treatment had been carried out.

During the 1970s there was an attempt to select patients for treatment according to the criteria suggested by Lorber.[83] However, most neurosurgeons have had great difficulty in withholding all forms of treatment from selected infants with myelomeningocele. They are performing initial sac closure and ventriculoperitoneal shunts on most infants with myelomeningocele.

Because most patients are treated with initial closure and ventriculoperitoneal shunt, a new and different natural history of the disease following this early treatment is being studied and documented. This is a difficult task because our initial treatment and understanding of the disease processes constantly are improving. Studies conducted in the 1960s cannot be equated with the disease course of the children of this decade.

An important discovery about the nature of myelomeningocele during the last 15 years is that the disease is not static but may undergo progressive neurologic degeneration manifested by increasing levels of paralysis and decreasing upper extremity function.[15,52,110] Neurologic deterioration can be sudden and dramatic or very slow and insidious. It is extremely important that the orthopaedist carry out a detailed neurologic evaluation, including upper and lower extremities and motor function, at each clinic visit, and any change in function requires a referral to the neurosurgeon for appropriate diagnosis and treatment. Three major areas of deterioration of the central nervous system have been found: hydrocephaly and associated hydrosyringomyelia, Arnold-Chiari deformity, and tethered cord syndrome.

Hydrocephaly

Hydrocephaly is a common disabling abnormality found in myelomeningocele due to obstruction of fluid movement by complex deformities of the posterior fossa and brain stem. In 1974, Lorber showed that of patients *without* hydrocephaly, 30% had IQs above 100, 50% had IQs between 80 and 99, 12% had IQs between 60 and 79, and 8% had IQs under 60. In contrast, of patients *with* hydrocephaly, only 20% had IQs above 100, 30% had IQs between 80 and 99, 30% had IQs between 60 and 79, and 20% had IQs under 60.[83] Perceptual motor abnormalities appeared to be the biggest factor in intellectual function. Most of these children perform well in their verbal scores but are considerably below average in their perceptual motor and hand function scores.

Although in some children with myelomeningocele the hydrocephaly becomes arrested in infancy without evidence of increasing head size or symptoms of acute intracranial pressure, most children require a ventriculoperitoneal or ventriculoatrial shunt.[54] Considerable improvements in the design and construction of the shunt have been achieved; however, it is still an unsophisticated device for controlling the right amount of ventricular pressure. Shunt failure can occur at any age and must be evaluated at each clinic visit.

In the young child, shunt failure is accompanied by the typical symptoms of hydrocephaly. However, in the older age groups, shunt malfunction rarely is associated with signs of acute hydrocephaly, such as nausea, vomiting, and severe headache. More likely it is associated with increased irritability, decreased perceptual motor function, short attention span, intermittent headaches, increasing scoliosis, and increased paralysis.[52-54]

Because of the communication of the fourth ventricle with the persistent central canal of the cord, increased hydrocephaly results in fluid entering the central canal, causing dilation and pressure in the cord.[47] If left unresolved, this eventually causes the formation of hydrosyringomyelia. Three problems have been shown to result from hydrosyringomyelia. The first problem is increasing paralysis of the lower extremities, occasionally associated with increased spasticity and, to a lesser extent, back pain. This problem is seen usually when the child is in his or her early school-age years. The second problem is progressive scoliosis, which may occur as early as 5 years of age but is more likely to be seen in the 7- to 10-year-old group.[53,54] The third problem is weakness of the hands and upper extremity.[52] This occurs when the child is in the teenage years. Most of these symptoms are resolved by early correction of the hydrocephalus by shunt replacement.

Arnold-Chiari Deformity

Associated with hydrocephaly is the Arnold-Chiari deformity, which is classified into three types according to the degree of displacement of the brain stem and hindbrain through the foramen magnum. Most of these affected children have a type II anomaly, which is characterized by displacement of the medulla oblongata into the cervical neural canal through the foramen magnum, requiring the cervical roots to take an upward course to reach their outlet foramina (see Fig. 14-2). Occasionally type III malformation is present, in which the cerebellum is also a part of the herniation.

The symptoms of an Arnold-Chiari type II malformation in infants includes periodic apnea, stridor, nystagmus, weak or absent cry, and upper extremity spasm and weakness. Symptoms come in episodes between which the infant may show minimal involvement. The cause of the episodic nature of the symptoms is not determined. During childhood, symptoms include spastic weakness of the upper extremities and occasionally leg involvement. Children also have nystagmus, stridor, difficulties in swallowing, and depressed or absent cough reflex. Symptoms in older patients still are being determined and probably include scoliosis, decreased upper extremity function, neck pain, and decreased respiratory function. The most serious difficulties appear to be present in infancy and decrease as the child matures.

In many children, following initial placement of the ventriculoperitoneal shunt to control hydrocephalus, brain stem symptoms resolve on their own and do not require surgical decompression procedures. In a few infants and children in whom the brain stem compressive symptoms persist or progress, the posterior fossa and upper spinal region are decompressed surgically. The effect of aggressive treatment of Arnold-Chiari deformity on overall survival and function has yet to be determined.

Tethered Cord Syndrome

Tethered cord syndrome is another major cause of decreased nerve function.[56] During the formation of the myelomeningocele, the open neural elements are attached to the ectoderm at its periphery. This prevents it from migrating cephalad during the growth of the fetus Consequently, all children with myelomeningocele have a degree of tethered cord at the time of birth. During closure of the sac, the everted spinal cord is dissected from the skin and allowed to fall back inside the neural canal. If any dermal elements are left attached to the spinal cord, dermoid cysts may develop and eventually cause decreasing function in the lumbosacral roots by direct pressure on the nerve elements.

After sac closure, there still is a tendency for the spinal cord to become adherent to the meningocele repair. As the child grows, this adherence again produces a tethered cord and prevents the spinal cord from migrating cephalad during growth. Although many children have a tethering of their spinal cord, only a few actually have symptoms of the condition and require surgical release. Because the posterior part of the spinal cord is adherent to the meningocele repair and the cord proximal to the meningocele is held posteriorly, where it is compressed by the posterior neural arch in the area of the lumbar lordosis, most symptoms are associated with posterior column abnormalities.

Pain appears to be a prominent symptom of the tethered cord syndrome and may occur in the lower lumbar spine, in the area of the myelomeningocele, or the sacral roots, with pain in the buttock and the posterior thigh. The pain is also activity related and becomes worse after walking long distances. In addition, increasing spasticity and decreasing function of the lower extremities are frequently present. Occasionally, there is an associated progressive scoliosis associated with marked lordosis. Changes in dermatomal somatosensory evoked potentials are present and are helpful in making the diagnosis if serial examinations have been made.[109] Changes in bladder function are common. The diagnosis of tethered cord syndrome is made on clinical evaluation, not by the presence or absence of a tethered cord on radiographic MRI study. The MRI describes the nature of the tether and confirms the diagnosis. The diagnosis of tethered cord syndrome in thoracic level paraplegics is rare and becomes more common the lower the level of paralysis. In my experience, surgical release of the tethered cord rarely provides complete return of lost function. The diagnosis must be made early, and appropriate care must be provided before major loss occurs.

Latex Hypersensitivity

During the past 10 years there have been increasing reports of severe immediate-type allergic reactions to latex exposure.[127] Although anyone may become sensitized to latex, three groups appear to have a high risk: children with myelomeningocele, health care workers, and workers in the latex industry. The reported incidence is as high as 34% in myelomeningocele children and may increase in the future.[3]

All patients should be questioned about a history of latex allergy. A history suggesting sensitivity includes swelling or itching of the lips from blowing up balloons or after dental examinations, and swelling or itching of the skin after contact with any rubber products. Other information that may suggest increased risk of latex allergy includes hand eczema; oral itching after eating bananas, chestnuts, or avocados; and multiple surgical procedures in infancy.

There is no standard test for latex allergy. Skin testing with a latex extract or glove extract may be the best test available. However, anaphylaxis has occurred in spina bifida patients during skin testing. In vitro tests may not be sensitive enough to detect all persons who may be at risk for latex contact.

Because of the high incidence of latex allergy in myelomeningocele, it is recommended that all patients regardless of history should have their surgery performed in a latex-free environment. There have been several lists published of latex-containing items. However, they are being revised almost daily, and no list should be considered complete. Some things that are labeled "latex," such as latex paint, are not latex based. It is best to ask the manufacturer if there is any question. If the child is known to be allergic, the parents will be able to tell what things need to be avoided in the hospital environment. However, in surgery it must be assumed that the child is sensitive to all latex material. A latex-free environment is one in which no latex gloves are used by any personnel in the operating room, and there should be no latex accessories (e.g., catheters, adhesives, tourniquets, anesthesia equipment) that come into direct contact with the patient.

EFFECT OF MYELOMENINGOCELE ON DEVELOPMENTAL SEQUENCE

The normal child undergoes a sequential development of fine motor, gross motor, personal, social, language, and cognitive skills, which are the result of the child's physical abilities and his or her interaction with the environment.[139] Three major areas that interfere with normal development face the myelomeningocele child: residual physical deformity, iatrogenic factors, and restrictions by society.

Our medical treatment of children with myelomeningocele contributes greatly to their delayed development. Prolonged and frequent hospitalization during the first years of life, although often necessary, considerably interfere with the learning experiences of the child. Hostler[61] pointed out that because of this environmental deprivation, a 1-month-old infant with myelomeningocele frequently cannot follow a light to a midline, fix both eyes on the light, and respond to the sound of a rattle.

Along with the frequent shunt malfunctions and repeated hospitalizations, the child also is placed in casts and splints to treat physical deformity, which further interferes with mobility and physical contact with parents and prevents parent-child bonding. As the child becomes older, individuality often is denied as he or she is treated as a disease entity rather than a person. In the clinic, the children frequently are undressed to their diapers and then paraded before members of the clinic, without regard for their embarrassment. The tendency is to treat them as asexual beings. If it is necessary to present a physical function abnormality to a group for discussion or education, a picture or a video recording should be used.

The last impediment to normal development is the resistance of society to accept and accommodate handicapped persons. Although there have been considerable improvements in treatment of children with myelomeningocele during the last 10 years, there still are considerable societal barriers to these children. For example, access to schools, playgrounds, amusement parks, sporting events, movie theaters, and private homes are limited to some extent. Also, acceptance of handicapped people in the employment market is restricted.

Although many previously mentioned factors are beyond our control, these myelomeningocele patients can be helped to overcome their handicap. We must plan our hospitalization and treatment programs to interfere as little as possible with the normal developmental sequence, particularly in infancy. We must work within the clinics, schools, and to a larger extent, society to promote acceptance of these patients as individuals and help them carry out the four principle tasks of childhood and adolescence: establishment of a stable self-image, acceptance of an adult sexual role, development of independence, and choice of a career.[55]

Development of a positive self-image and adult sexuality is a difficult task. Because of the physical impairment of children with myelomeningocele, personal interactions among peers is severely restricted, beginning in early childhood and extending into adolescence. The child with myelomeningocele looks different because of braces, orthopaedic shoes, wheelchairs, and deformities; these are barriers to peer acceptance. These feelings of being different may never be erased even if the cause of these feelings is eliminated.[65] Sexual information for these patients often is avoided or erroneous. Shurtleff[118] showed that many adults with myelomeningocele could have sexual relationships, including procreation; however, knowledge about the specific problems in myelomeningocele is meager, and a local resource person may be difficult to find.

Development of independence is a complex issue between the parents and their dependent handicapped child. The parents are often overprotective of the child. This protective attitude is also present in school and in society at large, especially if the child is confined to a wheelchair.

The choice of a career is also difficult. High school counselors are not trained to advise disadvantaged children, especially those with perceptual motor abnormalities of the hands. Government programs are not available until the patient is 18 years old or has graduated from high school. This is too late. Employment opportunities also are limited by the lack of ability to get health insurance.

TREATMENT

Treatment of children with myelomeningocele is not a matter of what can be done but what should be done for each child. The decision-making may begin prenatally if the diagnosis is made by alpha-fetoprotein testing or ultrasound examination. The option to continue or terminate the pregnancy can be made at this time. If it is continued, decisions must be made on how to improve the prognosis of the child. These include referral to a center experienced in the care of these children before delivery so that adequate planning and preparation for the family can be carried out. If the diagnosis is made after birth, then the next decision is whether the meningocele should be closed and the child treated. Most children are treated unless there are other deformities present that are not compatible with life, such as anencephaly, congenital heart disease, pulmonary insufficiency, and other congenital malformations. In some cases, the lesion may be surgically untreatable.

Orthopaedic treatment is intertwined with the neurosurgical treatment. It is also tied in with urologic treatment. Almost all of these children have urologic abnormalities that require bladder drainage by conduits or intermittent catheterization. Frequent infection may spread to orthopaedic surgical areas, and the orthopaedic treatment of spine deformity influences the ability of the patient for self-catheterization.

Orthopaedic treatment of myelomeningocele has three major goals. The first goal is to provide for maximal use of residual ability to maintain range of motion and stability of the spine and extremities. The second is to provide for mobility, by means of a wheelchair and other wheeled devices or by ambulation. The third goal is to prevent deterioration of neurologic function. Although it is true that the actual treatment of the central nervous system is performed by the neurosurgeon, the diagnosis of decreased function is made by the orthopaedist from observations of the spine and extremities. It cannot be assumed that because these patients are being seen and followed-up by neurosurgeons that subtle changes in function are going to be observed. Teamwork is essential in treatment of children with myelomeningocele.

The ability to walk is important and often necessary in our society despite recent advances in wheelchair design and wheelchair accessibility in the community. It also is the desire of every child with spina bifida. Although it is possible for most paraplegics children to walk to some degree during preschool and school age, many adults are not able to continue walking. Abnormalities of the spine and legs are often the cause for this inability. There are four necessary requirements of walking: 1) alignment of trunk and legs; 2) range of motion; 3) control of the hip, knee, and ankle joints; and 4) power to provide forward motion.

The alignment of the spine and the legs must be such that the center of gravity passes through the joints of the pelvis, the hip, the knee, and the foot. Deformities of the spine, such as scoliosis, kyphosis, and pelvic obliquity, prevent the center of gravity from passing through the center of the hip joint. Contractures of the hip or knee also will prevent stable weight bearing.

Motion of the lumbosacral spine and the hip are essential for functional walking. Motion of the knee is less important and is useful only in clearing the swing leg. Mobility of the spine must allow the center of gravity to be shifted from side to side over the stance leg. Motion of the hip is the most important part of walking. Analysis of spina bifida children who maintain walking ability has shown normal flexion/extension of the hip. Thirty degrees of motion is necessary for forward progression. If there is less motion than this, then pelvic motion must help compensate for this decreased motion.

The child must be able to control the position of the trunk and hip, knee, and ankle joints during the gait cycle. If this cannot be performed by muscle activity, then it must be provided by an orthotic device. The determination of available muscles to control the joints is dependent upon the level of paralysis.

The *thoracic level paraplegic* has no active muscle contraction across the hip joint and no feeling below the groin or in the hip. The child has no control of the hip and the hip is unstable, even though it may be reduced and appear stable on radiograph examination. Stability for walking can only be provided by an orthosis that crosses the hip joint.

The *upper lumbar paraplegic* child has several muscles crossing the hip joint. These muscles include the hip flexors and the hip adductors. These children have some sensation crossing the hip joint. Contraction of the hip flexors causes the hip to flex, pitching the child forward. In order to keep from falling, it is necessary to place most of his or her weight on the arms and crutches or walker. This is not a useful posture for walking and must be corrected. There is no way of surgically providing stability to this hip and, similar to the thoracic level paraplegic, the stability must be provided by an orthosis.

The *middle and lower lumbar paraplegic* child has hip flexors and adductors, knee extensors, and weak knee flexors. These children do not have normal hip extension or hip abduction, which are the most important muscles for standing and walking. Their weak hamstring muscles have a tendency to extend the hip and make these children walk without the need for orthotic control of the hip. The result of this is knee flexion contracture. The force imbalance around the hip results in eventual hip dislocation. Increased stability and control of the hip can be obtained only by moving muscles to a more functional position or by adding muscles to the hip. Muscles available for transfer include the iliopsoas, the abdominal muscles, and the adductor muscles. Control of the hip and knee can be achieved by muscle activity; however, the ankle requires an orthosis.

The *sacral level paraplegic* child has sufficient muscle control around the hip, the knee, and the ankle to provide the necessary stability.

The force necessary to move forward is beyond the muscle contraction needed to control the joint. In normal individuals, it is provided by the calf muscle, which pushes people forward into their next step, and the hip extensors, which pull forward after the foot hits the floor. Both of these muscles have sacral level innervation and are paralyzed in almost all spina bifida children. In the thoracic and upper lumbar levels of paraplegia, the arms become the power producers to move forward. The arms are not designed for this activity and are inefficient. Consequently, it takes increased energy to walk, and the walking pace is much slower than normal. Eventually, most thoracic and upper lumbar level paraplegic people discover that the wheelchair is a much more efficient means of transportation.

The middle and lower lumbar level paraplegics substitute trunk shift and sway to produce the forward motion. Much of the motion is from side to side rather than forward. This also is an inefficient method of walking, and some children abandon it for a wheelchair when they become adults. The use of muscle transfers to increase hip extension does aid in the efficiency of walking and may keep the patient walking longer.

Spine

Spine deformity is so common in myelomeningocele that it should be considered part of the disease complex.[62] The spine deformities usually are progressive and may cause severe disability, interfere with rehabilitation, and negate previous treatment to maintain ambulation.

The most obvious and consistent abnormality of myelomeningocele spinal deformity is the incomplete posterior arch in the lumbosacral spine. This abnormality affects many aspects of scoliosis and kyphosis treatment. Other congenital malformations also may be present.[12] Hemivertebrae and diastematomyelia may occur at any level along the spine. Similarly, unsegmented bars may occur at any level. They are particularly difficult to identify and evaluate if they occur in the area of the spina bifida where the facet joints, lamina, and spinous processes are difficult to identify on standard radiographs.

The spinal curvature often appears at a younger age than that typical for most developmental abnormalities. It may be present by 2 to 3 years of age, becoming severe by age 7. Because of the early onset of the deformity, treatment plans need to anticipate growth of the spine. However, the projections for growth in children with myelomeningocele are different from those for children with normal growth potential. Children with myelomeningocele may have slow growth due to growth hormone deficiency and mature earlier than usual, often by 9 to 10 years of age in girls and 11 to 12 in boys. The cause of the hormonal abnormalities has not been discerned, but they are treatable if it is necessary for the overall management of the child.

Another factor that needs to be considered in the surgical treatment of these patients is the high infection rate.[34,62,104,119] These patients are subject to frequent septicemias due to urinary tract infections. Most of these children have chronic contamination of the urinary tract, which always has the potential to progress into an infection. During surgical procedures, adequate drainage of the bladder and appropriate antibiotics should be a routine part of the surgical management. The skin in the area of the meningocele repair is often of poor quality and gives minimal coverage to the instrumentation.

These children also have deformity of the pelvis and hips that affects spine balance. For example, asymmetric hip contractures may cause lumbar scoliosis, pelvic obliquity, and abnormal lordosis in the standing or sitting position. Similarly, correction of the spine in the treatment of scoliosis can position the legs in a way that prevents functional sitting or standing.

As with all children with spinal deformities, the goals of treatment are the prevention of further deformity and the creation of a stable, balanced spine. Children with myelomeningocele, however, require more precise correction of the deformities. Residual deformity may prevent them from sitting, standing, or walking. Pressure sores are likely to develop if pelvic obliquity remains, and their sagittal plane alignment must allow them to perform intermittent self-catheterization.

Scoliosis and Lordosis

Scoliosis occurs in almost 100% of patients with thoracic level paraplegia.[92] Eighty-five percent of these curves are greater than 45 degrees. As the paralysis level lowers, so does the incidence of scoliosis. At the fourth lumbar level of paraplegia, the instance of curvature decreases to about 60%, with only 40% requiring surgical intervention (Fig. 14-4).[92] Lordosis without concurrent scoliosis is rare and usually is caused by hip flexion contractures. Historically it has been seen after spinal-peritoneal shunting for hydrocephalus; however, this procedure is rarely performed.

Several causes have been identified for the scoliosis. A C-shaped scoliosis is usually caused by muscle weakness associated with high level paraplegia. It also may be associated with asymmetric levels of paralysis or a spastic hemiplegia due to the hydrocephalus. This type of scoliosis may be associated with kyphosis rather than lordosis. Typically, this curve pattern oc-

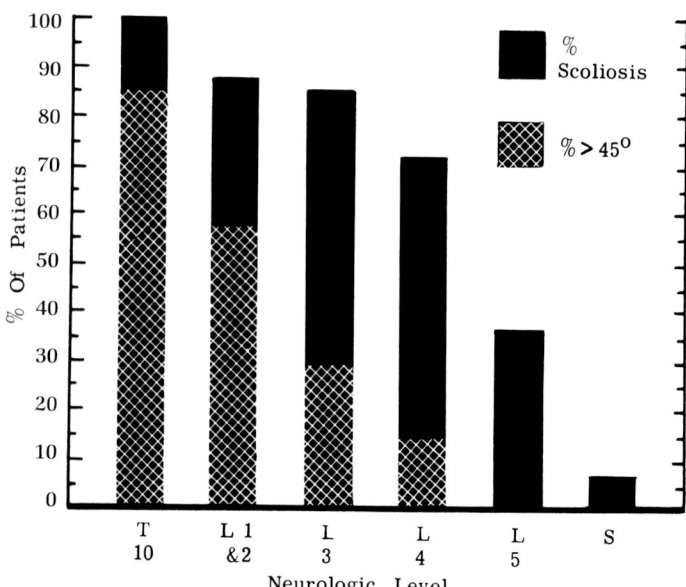

FIGURE 14-4. Incidence and severity of scoliosis based on the level of paraplegia. (From Lindseth RE. Scoliosis etiology and conservative treatment. In: McLaurin RL, et al. eds. Spina Bifida: a multidisciplinary approach. New York: Praeger, 1986:439.)

curs at a young age, often in infancy, and is usually progressive. If severe spasticity is present, an intraspinal rhizotomy or cordectomy may be necessary.[89]

Hydromyelia or hydrosyringomyelia associated with uncompensated hydrocephalus can cause scoliosis.[52–54] The scoliosis is usually in the thoracic or the thoracolumbar region, and it is typically S shaped. Because of stiffness in the area of the myelomeningocele in the lumbar spine, the compensation for the major curve may be incomplete and associated with pelvic obliquity. Scoliosis may be the only clinical sign of shunt malfunction or progressive hydromyelia and may occur at any age, even early in childhood. Headache, nausea, vomiting, and vision changes—the usual signs of hydrocephalus—may be absent. Other symptoms of hydromyelia are back pain, weakness of the upper extremities, and increasing paralysis of the legs. It has been shown that reinserting a functional shunt may decrease the scoliosis if it is less than 50 degrees.[53]

Another cause of scoliosis is the tethered cord syndrome.[15,56,90] This abnormality is caused by attachment of the spinal cord to the area of the myelomeningocele, preventing its upward migration with growth. This syndrome may be associated with other intraspinal pathologies, such as dermoid tumors, lipomas, and diastematomyelia. The scoliosis is usually in the dorsal lumbar or lumbar spine with a marked increase in lumbar lordosis. Results of releasing the tethered cord are variable, but frequently curve progression is stopped; in a few cases, it improves. If the curve is more than 50 degrees, the scoliosis should be corrected and stabilized with spine fusion.

Congenital malformations, including the lack of formation and the lack of segmentation,[12,138] may exist in combination with hydromyelia, tethered cord, or muscle paralysis. When evaluating a child with scoliosis, the physician must consider each component of the scoliosis in the treatment program. Because of the high number of neurologic abnormalities associated with scoliosis, a referral to a neurosurgeon should be made at the first sign of increasing scoliosis. It may be necessary to reinsert the shunt, untether the spinal cord, and treat the congenital scoliosis, if all are present.

DIAGNOSTIC STUDIES. At each visit, a thorough neurologic examination of muscle strength, levels of sensation, and reflex activity of the upper and lower extremities should be carefully documented. If scoliosis is developing, the documented changes in neurologic function are of major diagnostic importance as to the etiology of the scoliosis.

Radiographic evaluation should be carried out annually from the age of 1 year. These radiographs should be taken while the child is sitting, when the child can do so. This eliminates the problems related to hip flexion contracture and asymmetric abduction and adduction. If there is documented progressive scoliosis, additional radiographic examination is indicated. Magnetic resonance imaging (MRI) probably gives the most information without requiring invasive studies.[11] MRI of the head and cervical spine evaluates the hydrocephalus and the degree of Arnold-Chiari malformation. The cervical, thoracic, and lumbar spine also should be scanned. The cervical and thoracic spine are evaluated for the appearance of syrinx or hydromyelia. The scan of the lumbar spine provides information on the posterior displacement of the conus and the presence of intraspinal tumors, such as lipoma or dermoid cysts. The MRI studies must be interpreted in association with the clinical findings to determine the cause of the scoliosis. The presence of a tethered cord is common, and it alone may not be the cause of the deformity. In my experience, the scoliosis is in the lumbar spine with the apex at the last intact neural arch, the lordosis is in excess of 90 degrees, and other signs of tethered cord, such as changes in bladder function and neurologic function of the legs, are present.

Computed tomography (CT) also can be used. However, to get the maximum benefit from the study, contrast material is usually necessary for evaluation of the spinal cord. Both MRI and CT studies usually require sedation or anesthesia in young children.

TREATMENT. If the scoliosis continues to progress after neurologic problems have been corrected, orthopaedic treatment is indicated. If the spine is balanced and the curve is 30 degrees or less, observation probably is indicated. However, if the curve is unbalanced or greater than 30 degrees the center of gravity falls outside of the pelvic base of support, the spine will become unstable, and progression of the deformity is almost assured. A trial of bracing is indicated in children younger than the age of 7 years if the curve is supple and can be corrected easily. However, because bracing in paralytic scoliosis is passive, the brace tends to deform the rib cage and produce pressure sores in the area of insensate skin. In infants special care is needed to avoid abdominal compression, which may make it difficult for the child to breathe and eat. Although the use of a brace is only temporary, it may delay the necessity of surgery until the child is 8 or 9 years old, when many of these children are beginning adolescence.[12,13]

The most effective spinal orthosis is a two-piece, polypropylene, bivalved, molded body jacket. This design allows the brace to be expanded or contracted throughout the day to allow for eating and allows some adjustability for growth. Meticulous care is required because pressure sores are frequent, and once they develop, it is almost impossible to continue using the brace for control of the curve. In general, the child begins orthosis wear slowly, starting at 1 hour intervals, after which the skin should be inspected. If any redness does not disappear within 4 hours, the orthosis must be modified. The time in the brace is gradually increased over 2 to 3 weeks until the child is wearing it throughout the day except for naps and nighttime. If the family or caregivers are unable to provide this degree of care, an orthosis is probably not indicated.

Most of these children require surgical correction and spinal fusion. Levels of fusion depend on the age of the child, the location of the curve, the level of paralysis, and the ambulatory status.

The treatment of the tethered cord, even if it is not symptomatic when correction of the scoliosis is performed, is an unsettled issue. Correction of the scoliosis lengthens the posterior spine and puts the tethered cord on stretch. This may produce neurologic changes, even if they were absent before. Therefore, the neurosurgeons at our clinic believe that the tethered cord should be released either before or during the scoliosis surgery. If it is done before, the time between release and the spine surgery should probably be no more than 6 months because of the frequent retethering. I prefer to do it at the same time as the scoliosis surgery.

Generally, the same guidelines for instrumentation and fusion of idiopathic scoliosis are applicable to the myelomeningocele spine. The fusion should go from neutral vertebra to neutral vertebra, and the end vertebra should be located within the stable zone. This holds true for thoracic and the thoracolumbar curves. However, in double curves, uncompensated curves, and primary lumbar curves, the decision becomes more difficult. The guidelines for fusion and instrumentation in these cases differ from those for idiopathic scoliosis. In general, it is a mistake to fuse short; if there is a question, fuse long. A compensatory thoracic curve should be fused for its entire length, and the fusion should not end in the middle of a sagittal curve or at a junctional kyphosis.

The selection of the level at the distal end usually is complicated by the open vertebral arch, which prevents attachment of the instrumentation to the end vertebra. Lumbar hyperlordosis usually is present, compounding the problem of deciding on the distal level of fusion. In the past, the instrumentation was extended to the pelvis because of the difficulty getting a firm attachment to the lower lumbar vertebrae.[2] With the newer methods of pedicle fixation, it may be possible to control some curves without fusing the lumbosacral joint. The indications for extending the fusion mass to the sacrum are not well established. Lumbosacral arthrodesis is difficult to obtain because of the lack of posterior vertebral arch to fuse. Consequently, pseudoarthroses and instrumentation failures are common.[119] Attempts to correct these problems require repeated surgical procedures and have an uncertain outcome. If a successful fusion to the sacrum is obtained, it may deprive ambulatory patients of the ability to walk.[95] In wheelchair-bound patients, a lumbosacral fusion may cause difficulty because of increased occurrence of pressure sores if the residual pelvic obliquity is 15 degrees or greater. Movement in the lumbosacral spine absorbs much of the angular and rotational movements of the trunk during wheelchair activities. If the lumbosacral spine is fused, these torsional movements are transmitted to the pelvis, creating increased shear between the pelvis, the skin, and the wheelchair seat.

If the lumbosacral joint is not fused, the scoliosis tends to increase unless the lumbar scoliosis can be corrected to less than 20 degrees and the pelvic obliquity to less than 15 degrees. Therefore, it is important to treat the scoliosis while the curve is small and can be corrected to less than a 20-degree lumbar curve and a 15-degree pelvic obliquity, whether fusion to the sacrum is planned or not. The delay of surgical correction of the scoliosis to allow the spine to grow may lead to an unsatisfactory correction. After spine correction, residual pelvic obliquity greater than 15 degrees can be corrected by a bilateral posterior iliac osteotomy with transfer of a wedge of bone from the long side to the short side.[74]

Children with a thoracic or upper lumbar level of paraplegia should be fused to the sacrum (Fig. 14-5). In children with low lumbar and sacral levels of paraplegia, the lumbosacral joint should be spared if they are walkers, and the spine can be aligned satisfactorily (Fig. 14-6).

The sagittal deformity also must be evaluated because increased lumbar lordosis is a common deformity. Assessment of sitting, supine, and standing posture must be made before correcting the lumbar lordosis. These children often require a greater degree of lordosis than normal. Restoring the lumbar lordosis to the normal range may uncover a hip flexion contracture and prevent the child from standing or walking. If too much lordosis is fused into the lumbar spine of a female patient, she may not be able to carry out intermittent self-catheterization. The degree of lordosis left in the spine after fusion needs to be tailored to each patient. It is best to treat the hip contractures before correcting the spine. If the hip deformity is not corrected first, positioning of the spine on the operating table will be difficult and torque the spine postoperatively, leading to instrument failure and pseudoarthrosis.

Ischial pressure sores also should be treated before spinal fusion to lessen the chance of infection.

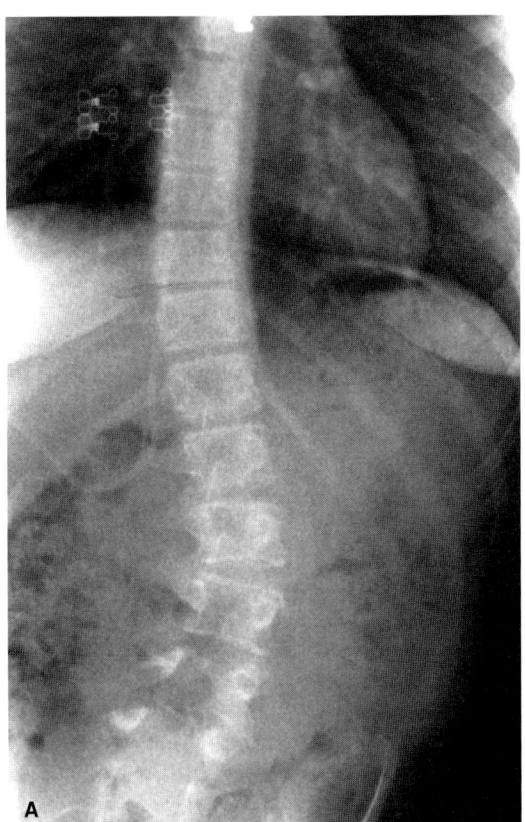
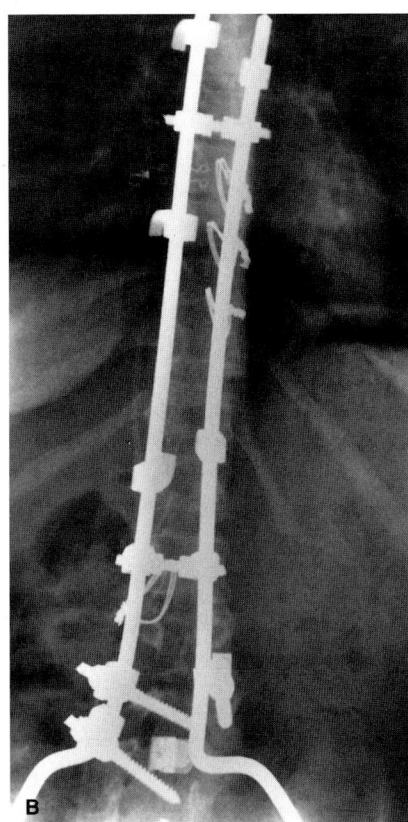
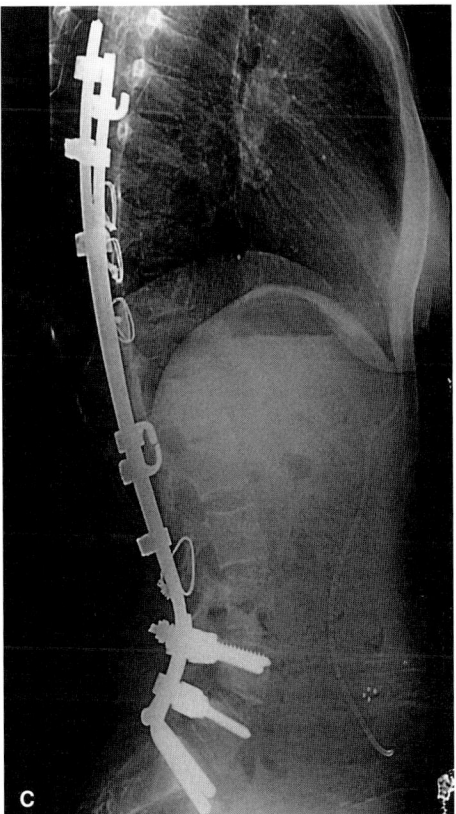

FIGURE 14-5. A 13-year-old girl has an L3 level paraplegia but is not ambulatory. She is obese and has a progressive lumbar scoliosis and pelvic obliquity. A tethered spinal cord previously was released. (A) Anteroposterior radiograph shows a 50-degree uncompensated lumbar scoliosis resulting in 35-degrees of pelvic obliquity. There is excessive lumbar lordosis. (B) Postoperative anteroposterior radiograph shows complete correction of the scoliosis. The sacrum was included in the fusion because the lumbar scoliosis included the first sacral vertebra and the child was not ambulatory. Pedicle screws were used to secure the segmental instrumentation to L4 and L5. Anterior interbody fusion was performed from T10 to the sacrum. (C) Postoperative radiograph shows restoration of normal sagittal alignment. Lumbar lordosis now measures 55 degrees. The patient has full extension of her hips and is able to perform intermittent self-catheterization. (From Lindseth RE. Myelomeningocele spine. In: Weinstein SL, ed. The pediatric spine: principles and practice. New York: Raven Press, 1994:1053.)

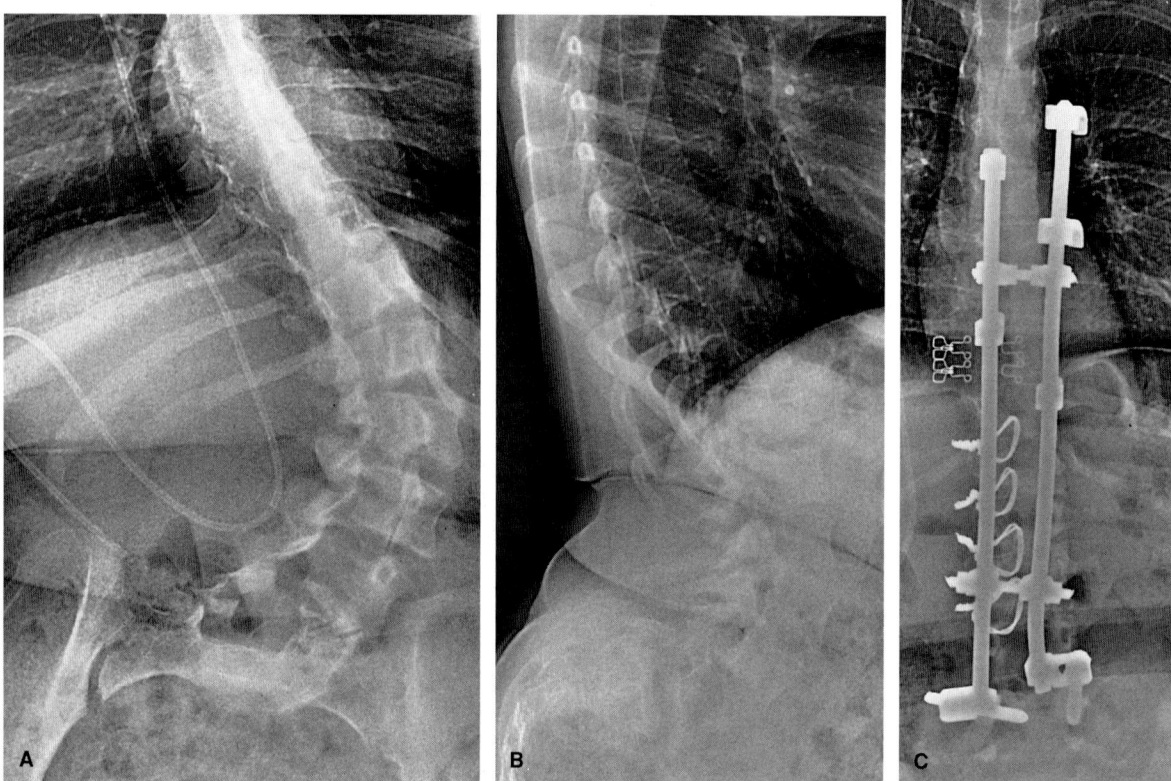

FIGURE 14-6. A mature 12-year-old girl with progressive lumbar scoliosis is an L4-level paraplegic and is a community walker with ankle-foot orthoses and crutches. **(A)** Anteroposterior radiograph shows 55-degree lumbar scoliosis from T10 to L3. There is a 20-degree compensatory curve from L4 to the sacrum. There is residual 30-degree pelvic obliquity. The last intact vertebral arch is L2. **(B)** Lateral radiograph shows severe 120-degree lordosis, which is typical of the deformity associated with tethered cord. **(C)** Anteroposterior radiograph shows correction of the scoliosis and pelvic obliquity. Pelvic screws are used to fix the distal end vertebrae at L5. The lumbosacral joint was left unfused to allow the patient enough pelvic mobility to continue walking. Release of the tethered cord was performed at the same time as the spine fusion. An anterior interbody fusion was performed from T9 to L5 without instrumentation. **(D)** Lateral radiograph shows correction of the lordosis to 45-degree and the achievement of a normal sagittal alignment. (From Lindseth RE. Myelomeningocele spine. In: Weinstein SL, ed. The pediatric spine: principles and practice. New York: Raven Press, 1994:1053.)

This is often difficult to do because the pelvic obliquity is a major cause of the ulceration, and unless it is corrected, pressure cannot be relieved from the ulcer. In this circumstance, a gluteus maximus myocutaneous flap can be used to promote primary healing. The patient is maintained on an air mattress bed until the spinal correction can be performed. This may seem extreme but is much less of a problem than an infected spinal fusion that requires instrument removal.

The age of the child at the time of surgery is an important consideration. If the child has not yet reached adolescence, as determined by the beginning of the appearance of pubic hair and a Risser sign of I, there is an almost 100% assurance that the curve will continue to progress despite posterior fusion unless the anterior spine is fused to the same level. The lumbar spine usually is fused anteriorly as well as posteriorly because of the deficient posterior vertebral arch, but if the posterior fusion extends up into the thoracic spine, it must be fused anteriorly as well.

In a child with a progressive curve that cannot be controlled by a brace and who is younger than 8 years old, the preferred treatment is segmental Luque instrumentation without spinal fusion. Distal fixation of the rods in the area of the open spine is difficult. I prefer use of the first sacral foramen as the anchor point. However, the ilium is also a possibility, although I have experienced loosening of the rod in the ilium with loss of fixation and erosion of the rod through the skin. Postoperative brace treatment is still indicated, and complications from this approach include rod breakage, wire breakage, and spontaneous fusion. To provide a definitive solution, reoperation is often necessary when the child reaches maturity.

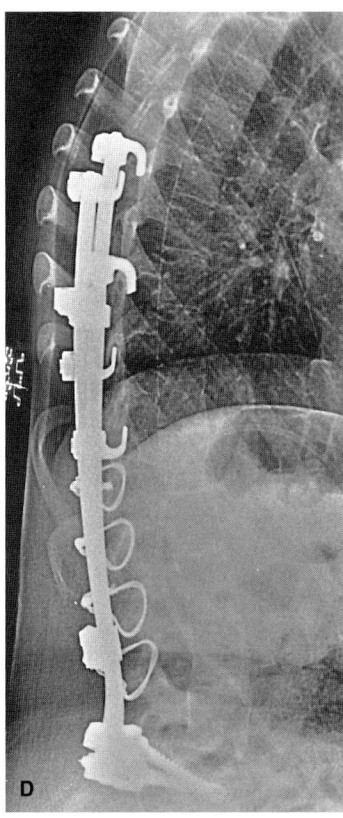

FIGURE 14-6. (Continued).

INSTRUMENTATION. Spinal fusion is still the most important part of surgical treatment of scoliosis despite the recent advances in spinal instrumentation. The role of the instrumentation is to improve spinal alignment and the fusion rate and reduce the need for recumbency or postoperative immobilization. Whatever the instrumentation used, the degree of correctability of the curve is limited. It is important to carry out an early fusion when the deformity is manageable. The amount of correction that is possible is probably limited to about 60 degrees, despite the size of the curve. Occasionally, it is possible to produce amazing degrees of correction, but this is not the rule. It is better to correct completely a 60-degree curve than to correct a 120-degree curve to 60 degrees.

It is agreed that anterior and posterior fusion is necessary in the area of the lumbar spine.[8,92,96,102] However, there is no agreement about whether the anterior spine needs to be instrumented. The more severe the deformity to be corrected, the greater the indication for using anterior instrumentation, but there is still a great risk of producing kyphosis of the lumbar spine or at least flattening the normal lumbar lordosis. Anterior instrumentation to the sacrum is difficult, and it is questionable whether an anterior interbody fusion of L5–S1 is necessary. Normally, this is a very stable joint, and adequate posterior fusion can be obtained by grafting from the lamina and transverse process of L5 to the sacral ala. However, if the anterior longitudinal ligament is destroyed along with the annulus fibrosis, instability and severe deformity of this joint may occur if the child develops a pseudoarthrosis of the lumbosacral joint. Because repair of this deformity and pseudoarthrosis can be difficult, it is preferable to end the anterior instrumentation at L4 in those patients who have a dorsal lumbar curve that ends or is stable at L3–L4. If it is necessary to extend the fusion down to the pelvis, perform an anterior fusion only down to L5 and posteriorly to the pelvis.

Posterior instrumentation has evolved considerably over the last 20 years. Initially, Harrington instrumentation was used, but because of the lack of posterior vertebral arch, distal fixation of the fusion was difficult unless the instrumentation was extended down to the sacral ala. The alar hooks frequently became displaced, and the pseudoarthrosis and complication rates were unacceptably high.[102] The child also required postoperative immobilization, which increased the occurrence of pressure sores.

Luque instrumentation has become the standard instrumentation for these children.[2] Because of the segmental fixation to each vertebra, there is much better control over the spine, and postoperative immobilization is not required. However, it does not fix the length of the spine as a rod with hooks does; therefore, the spine may settle or collapse along the rod, with loss of some correction in the immediate postoperative period. If the rod is contoured to maintain a normal sagittal alignment, there is a tendency for the rod to twist into the coronal plane deformity, with loss of correction. This is lessened by the use of the unit rod or multiple transverse rod connectors. Fixation to the open posterior spine in the lumbar area by wires around the pedicle is weak, and extension of the instrumentation to the ilium is usually necessary. Even this distal attachment of the Luque rods is weak because there may be significant osteoporosis of the pelvis. Loosening of the instrumentation and pseudoarthrosis of the lumbosacral joint is frequent. Although this is not usually symptomatic, I have observed increased scoliosis, pelvic obliquity, and pressure sores.

The development of instrumentation that allows segmental fixation, distraction, and compression on the same rod, along with the use of pedicle screws, may solve many problems of instrumentation of the distal spine. The pedicle screws allow the end vertebra to be positioned in three planes and provide stable segmental instrumentation. This instrumentation may lessen the desirability of anterior instrumentation. Long-term studies have not yet been performed, but early experience indicates that satisfactory results can be obtained (see Figs. 14-5 and 14-6).

Whatever the instrumentation used posteriorly, it should be low-profile in design. In the area of the meningocele sac, there is poor skin and soft tissue coverage. Prominence of hardware invariably leads to ulceration over the hardware, eventual infection, and the need to remove the instrumentation.

Congenital Scoliosis

Congenital scoliosis may occur anywhere along the spine, including the cervical, the thoracic, and the lumbosacral spines. Congenital malformations may be caused by the lack of formation or segmentation or a combination of the two. If the malformation occurs in the lumbosacral area, the progression of deformity is usually rapid and uncompensated, causing severe pelvic obliquity. Nonoperative methods of treatment do not correct congenital scoliosis or even prevent it from worsening. These children, because of their neurologic abnormalities, are unable to tolerate an unbalanced spine. Therefore, it is important that treatment be carried out in infancy, when the deformity is small, rather than waiting until the child is older and heroic measures are needed to obtain satisfactory alignment.

Posterior fusion of the malformation is rarely successful in preventing progression. Anterior and posterior fusion is the procedure of choice, and it should be performed when a diagnosis of progressive scoliosis is made, usually at 1 year of age. The spine may be approached in staged or separate anterior and posterior procedures, or anterior and posterior interbody fusions may be performed through a posterior approach, using the pedicle as the access conduit to the anterior spine.[79] The posterior approach is useful when the malformation is in the upper thoracic spine, where the anterior approach is difficult. If the lumbar curve is already so severe that the pelvic obliquity is greater than 15 degrees, an osteotomy of the spine to correct the deformity should be considered. Another possibility in a child over 10 years of age is to perform a bilateral posterior iliac osteotomy to balance the pelvis after the spine has been fused.[74]

Kyphosis

Lumbar kyphosis is a major deformity that occurs in 8% to 15% of patients with myelomeningocele.[32,38,60,80,104,113] It often measures 80 degrees or more at birth and usually progresses with growth. Children with extensive kyphosis are unable to wear braces, have trouble sitting in a wheelchair, and often have ulcerations over the prominent kyphos. Progression of the kyphosis may lead to breathing difficulty because the abdominal contents are crowded into the chest cavity by increasing upward pressure on the diaphragm. These children also have difficulty eating because of loss of abdominal size, which results in a failure to thrive. They are underweight and short in stature. The increased flexion of the trunk also may interfere with drainage of urine if the child has a urethrostomy, a vesicotomy, or an ileostomy.

Kyphosis is almost always progressive, and attempts to delay definitive treatment until the child is older leads to a more severe deformity.[6,100] The aorta and the vena cava do not follow the anterior border of the spine across the kyphosis[82]; they take the short route like a bowstring, limiting the amount of surgical correctability. Therefore, it is important to carry out treatment early even though it may be only a temporizing procedure. A more definitive procedure can be performed later.

The goal of treatment is to increase abdominal height to allow more room for the abdominal contents and relieve pressure on the diaphragm and the lungs. In addition, the kyphosis must be minimized to lessen the incidence of pressure sores and move the center of gravity posteriorly to center it over the ischium. This improves the child's ability to sit without using the arms for support.

The kyphosis deformity can be divided into two types (Fig. 14-7).[77] The first type is a collapsing kyphosis; it is often C shaped and supple, at least during the initial stages. The apex may occur anywhere from the lower dorsal spine to the lumbosacral joint. The second type is a rigid S-shaped lumbar kyphosis with a proximal dorsal lordosis. The kyphosis is usually centered at L2 and the proximal rigid lordosis at about T10. This is the most common variety of congenital kyphosis.

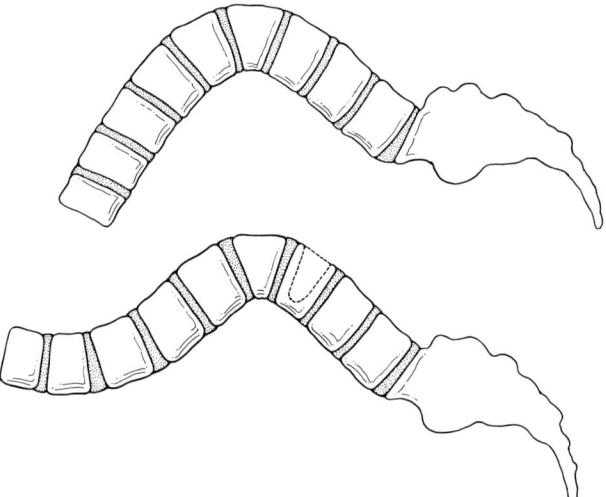

FIGURE 14-7. Two types of lumbar kyphosis: the C-shaped collapsing curve (*top*) and the S-shaped curve (*bottom*). (From Lindseth RE. Myelomeningocele spine. In: Weinstein SL, ed. The pediatric spine: principles and practice. New York: Raven Press, 1994:1058.)

COLLAPSING KYPHOSIS. Conservative treatment, which consists of observation, is usually futile. The curve progresses rapidly, and it is not unusual to see a 2- or 3-year-old child with a kyphosis greater than 100 degrees. In those few instances in which the collapsing curve does not progress rapidly and is less than 20 to 30 degrees, an initial period of observation may be worthwhile. If the curve is supple and the skin is in excellent condition, a brace can be tried. However, because any orthotic device must push over the apical vertebra posteriorly and against the protuberant abdomen anteriorly, it may lead to pressure sores over the gibbus and increased pressure on the abdominal contents. The kyphosis almost always requires surgical correction; this should not be delayed if brace treatment is unsatisfactory.

Collapsing scoliosis in the immature child is difficult to treat surgically. Posterior spinal fusion without instrumentation usually fails because of tension forces in the fusion mass. When instrumentation is used, instrument failure is common. Attempts to provide stability by anterior strut fusion with a strut graft also tend to fail in young patients. The fusion creates an anterior unsegmented bar, with growth potential remaining posteriorly. As the child grows, the kyphosis increases. If the surgeon waits until the child is older to carry out anteroposterior fusion with instrumentation along the dorsal lumbar spine, the curve is often so severe that satisfactory correction is difficult if not impossible to obtain. If the anteroposterior fusion is carried out in infancy, the resulting spine is too short to allow sufficient room for abdominal volume and respiratory sufficiency.

The anterior structures, including the abdominal wall, the aorta, and the vena cava, are of insufficient length to allow correction to occur without shortening the spine to remove tension from these structures.[41,81] Many different procedures have been described to shorten the posterior spine to allow the spine to be straightened and put into more normal sagittal alignment.[36,38,51,80,85,113,134] Most of these techniques require fusion of the spine to maintain correction and therefore should be performed only in an adolescent child; otherwise, the lumbar spine will be too short.

A method used to shorten the spine that does not require spinal fusion is to remove the ossific nuclei from the vertebrae above and below the apical vertebra, which is left intact (Fig. 14-8A, B). The pedicle and posterior arch are removed from these two vertebrae. The apical vertebra is pushed forward, correcting the kyphosis[77] (Fig. 14-8C). Approximately 100 degrees of kyphosis can be corrected. Because the vertebral body growth centers are left intact, the growth of the spine continues, often producing a gradual increase in the lordosis. The spine is not fused, thus the procedure can be performed in children of any age, even in

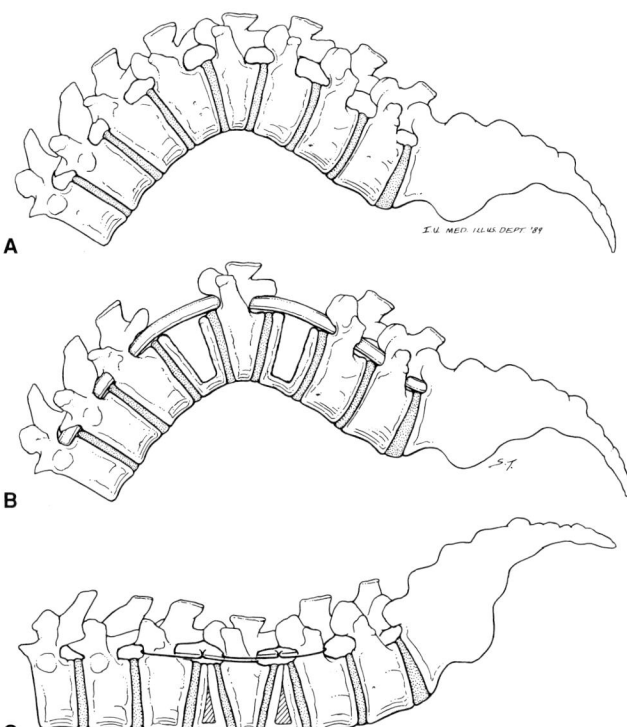

FIGURE 14-8. The C-shaped curve is corrected by removing the ossific nucleus of the vertebrae above and below the apical vertebrae. (**A**) The C-shaped kyphosis before removal of the ossific nucleus from the vertebrae. (**B**) Spinous processes, laminae, pedicles, and ossific nucleus have been removed from the vertebrae above and below the apical vertebra. The growth plate, disc, and anterior cortex are left intact. (**C**) The deformity is reduced by pushing the apical vertebrae forward. Tension band wiring around the pedicles maintains the reduction. (From Lindseth RE: Spine deformity in myelomeningocele. Inst Course Lect. 1991;40:276.)

newborns. It is also possible to perform this surgery without mobilizing the spinal cord or dividing any of the nerve roots. Therefore, it can be performed when nerve function is intact below the level of the kyphosis. If the child is younger than 1 year old, tension band wiring between the pedicles of the apical vertebra and the vertebrae above and below the osteotomy appears to be sufficient. If the child is older than 1 year, Luque instrumentation modified to attach to the sacrum without fusion should be performed[135] (Fig. 14-9). If the child is an adolescent, posterior spinal fusion can be added to the instrumentation.

Skin coverage is often a problem. If the skin is exceedingly scarred or ulcerated over the kyphosis, wound breakdown and infection are likely. The problem with skin coverage should be addressed prior to the spinal correction. A myocutaneous flap should be planned and prepared beforehand.[57]

RIGID S-SHAPED KYPHOSIS. Treatment of the rigid form of upper lumbar kyphosis is difficult and controversial. Conservative nonoperative treatment

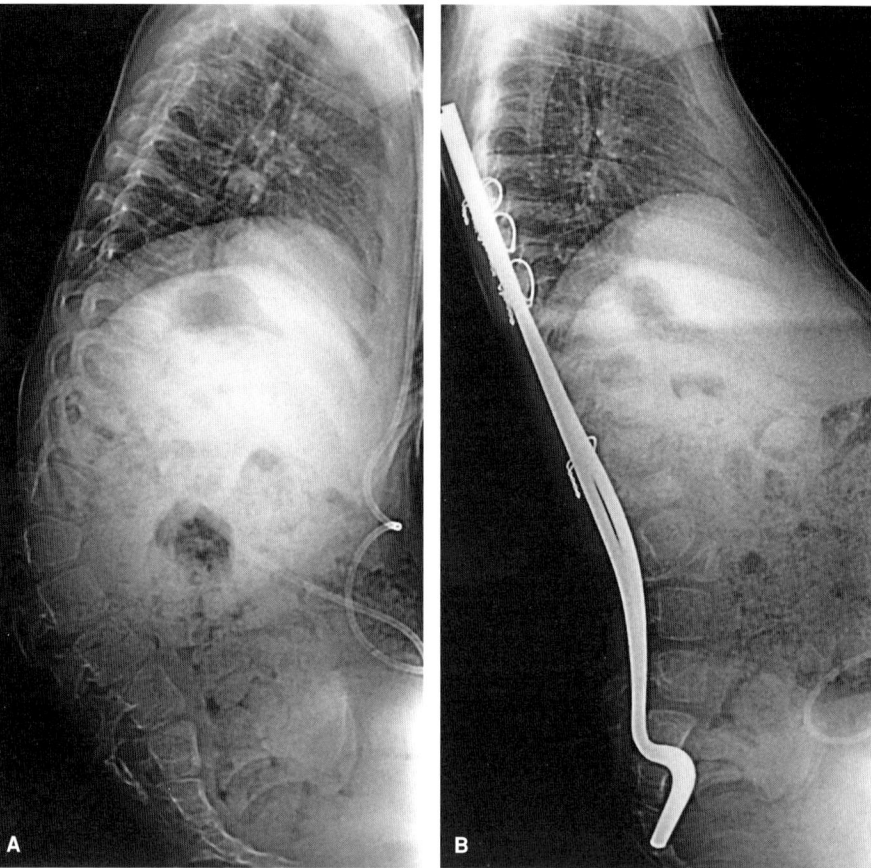

FIGURE 14-9. A 2-year-old child with 65 degrees of progressive kyphosis. (**A**) After excision of the ossific nucleus above and below the apical vertebrae, the correction is held with a specially modified Luque rod, which is inserted into the first sacral formaen.

invariably leads to an increased deformity and difficulty in later correction. In 1968, Sharrard[113] first described resection of the apical vertebral body for the treatment of kyphosis; since then, most authors have recommended vertebral excision as a part of the operative treatment.[57] Most of these reports also showed that excision of the apical vertebra may lead to initial correction of the deformity. However, the deformity has a tendency to recur, often to a worse degree than the initial kyphosis,[80] leading to feelings of futility and frustration.

Treatment of the rigid form of kyphosis requires a different approach. Because both the kyphosis and the proximal lordosis are rigid, it is necessary to correct both deformities at the same time. This can be accomplished by excising the vertebra (usually two) between the kyphosis and lordosis[51,80,81] (Fig. 14-10) and fusing the apical vertebra to the distal end of the thoracic spine at the level of the resection. In a young child, this is the only area fused, and the osteotomy is held in position by tension band wiring around the pedicle above and below the resected vertebrae[80,81] (Fig. 14-11). It is important that the paraspinous muscles be sutured behind the area of the spine in order to add a corrective force, decreasing the likelihood of recurrence of the deformity. The correction can also be held by use of rods anchored in the first sacral foramen distally and sublaminal wires proximally, similar to the fixation used in the collapsing kyphosis. If the child is Risser sign I or above, the spine may be fused along the length of the instrumentation.

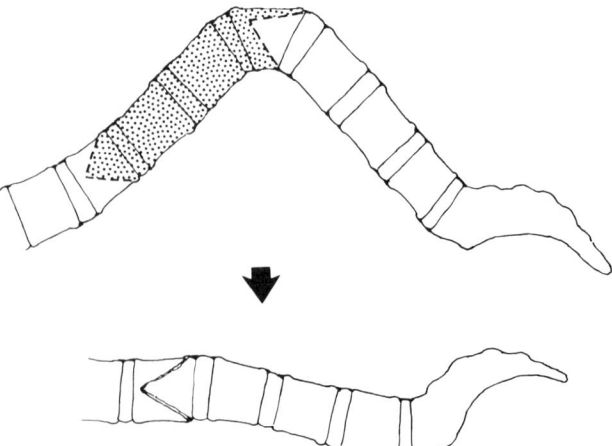

FIGURE 14-10. Bone is removed for correction of a rigid dorsal kyphosis (*shaded area*). The area removed usually includes one or two vertebrae proximal to the apical vertebrae in the area of the fixed lordosis. The vertebrae proximal to the resection and the apical vertebrae are shaped to receive each other in a tongue-and-groove joint to provide stability until bony union is achieved.

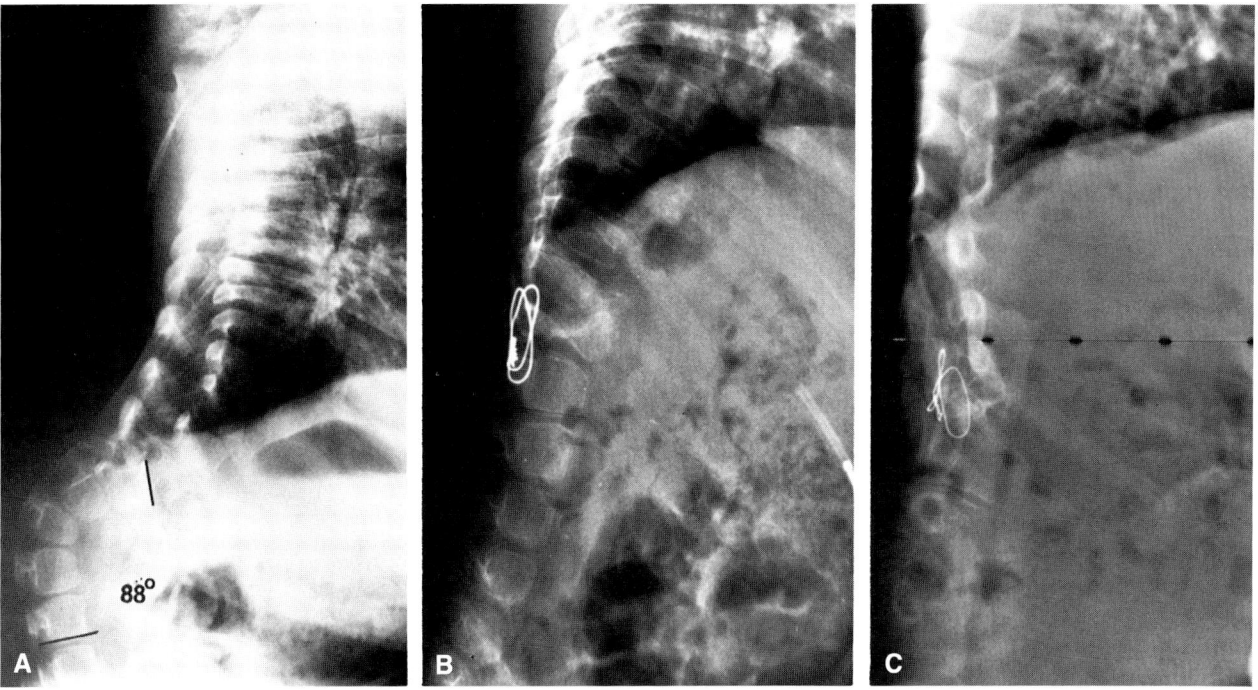

FIGURE 14-11. (A) A 1-year, 10-month-old child with an 88-degree kyphosis. (B) Two years after surgery, the kyphosis is at 13 degrees, and the lumbar spine has increased in height from 6.1 to 9 cm. (C) Twelve years after surgery, the kyphosis is unchanged, and the spine height has increased to 14 cm.

Hip

The function of the hip joint depends on neurologic level. The treatment program therefore is based on the level of sensory and motor paralysis.[5,71,75] In a large proportion of myelomeningocele patients, the hips are reduced at birth with the exception of those children who are breech position (Fig. 14-12). Following birth, normal hips may become dislocated or dysplastic because of the position of the infant following closure of the back. If the infant is laid on his or her side, continued adduction of the superior hip eventually leads to dislocation. However, if the child can be placed in the prone position, with the feet in the "human position" of flexion and 60 degrees of abduction, the hips can be maintained in the reduced position while the spine heals without being soiled by urine or feces (Fig. 14-13). This position also does not preclude placement of a shunt, and the therapist can have access to the feet and knees. If abduction splinting is maintained during nap time and night-time after discharge from the hospital, most children survive the first year of life with their hips reduced. Generally, I do not maintain the splinting after the first 3 months of life; however, in other medical centers splints are maintained throughout the first year.

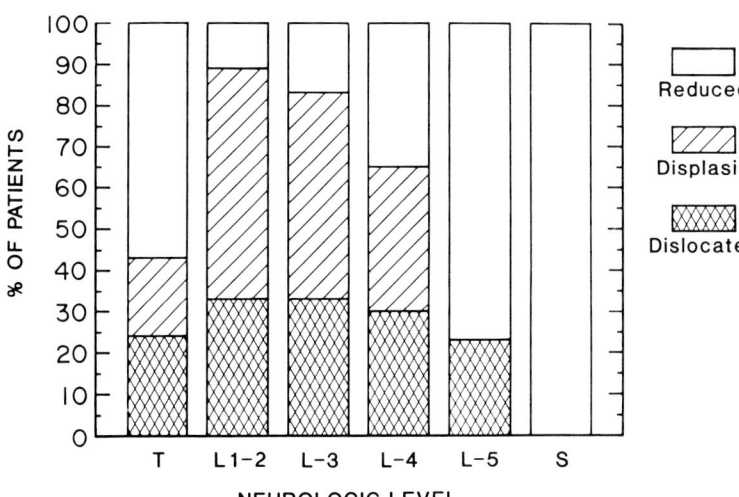

FIGURE 14-12. An evaluation of 100 consecutive infants with myelomeningocele who had not received treatment for their hips.

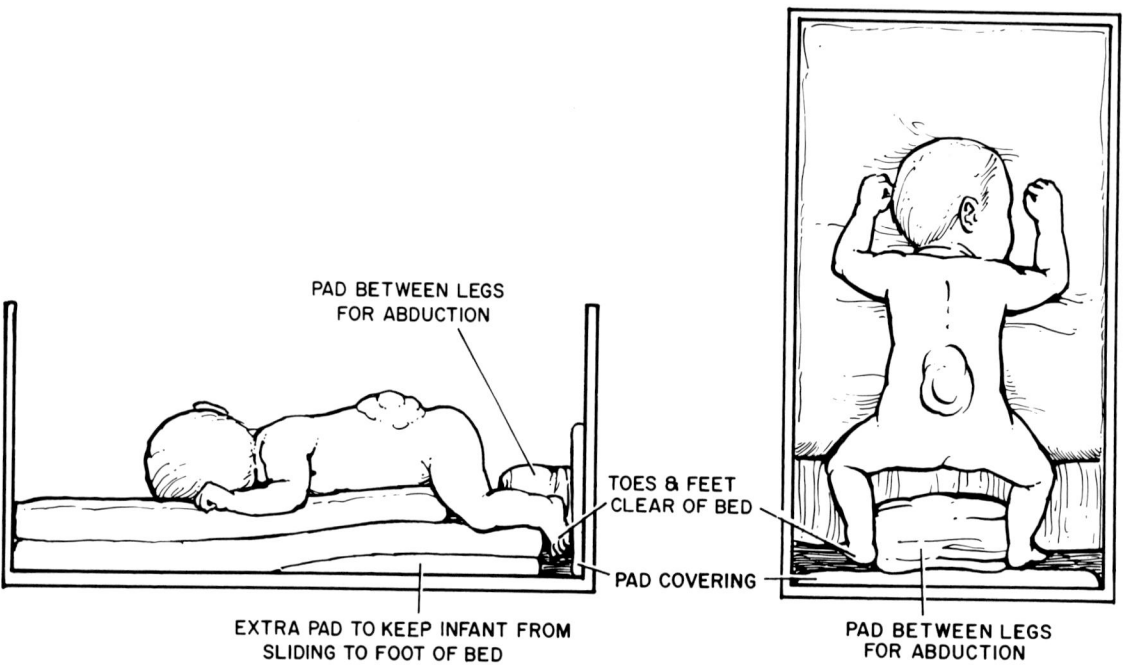

Thoracic Paraplegia

The thoracic level paraplegic child does not have sensation or muscle control over the lower extremities. Surgery cannot provide stability; it must be provided by an orthosis. Without sensation and motor control, reduction of the hip is not necessary for sitting and walking using orthotic aids.[39] However, the child needs a functional range of motion without contracture.[96] Surgical procedures should be used to provide range of motion so that the child can sit satisfactorily in a wheelchair, lie comfortably in bed, and use orthoses for standing and walking, if indicated.

Treating hip contractures in paraplegics is often frustrating because many contractures return promptly, often to a worse degree than before surgical release. A simple sectioning of tight tendons and release of tight ligamentous structures does not appear to be sufficient. The use of a free fat graft to fill the dead space formed by the release of tendon and capsule has helped prevent the recurrence of contracture in a few of my patients. It is important that prolonged bracing and physical therapy be used to maintain whatever motion has been obtained by surgery.

Fortunately, dislocation of the hip is not usually found in the thoracic level paraplegic person because of the lack of muscle function. If a hip is becoming dysplastic or is dislocating, the cause should be found and treated. Increased muscle tone or spasticity should be treated by muscle release or perhaps by neurectomy. Pelvic obliquity caused by developing scoliosis should be treated. Attempts to reduce a dislocated hip are difficult and often unsuccessful. The principal risk of surgically reducing the hip is stiffness. Multiple surgical procedures should be avoided because the risk of stiffness increases with each surgical procedure. It is better to have a supple dislocated hip than a stiff located hip.

The limitation of motion from a dislocated hip usually does not interfere with the overall function of the child. Even in unilateral dislocation, a dislocated hip does not prevent standing in an orthosis, sitting, or lying down unless an associated adduction contracture is present.

The increased incidence of pressure sores because of unilateral or bilateral hip dislocation in the absence of contractures or pelvic obliquity has not been documented. Because of the loss of the greater trochanter as a pressure-accepting area, more pressure is placed on the ischium and sacrum. This would seem to increase the possibility of ulceration. In the presence of hip dislocation, special attention must be made to wheelchair seating.

Orthotic devices are needed to provide stability to the lower extremity, and they must provide pelvic, hip, knee, ankle, and foot stability. The standing frame, the parapodium, the swivel walker, and hip control orthosis and provide stability.[84] At approximately 18 to 24 months of age, if the child has developed head control and sitting balance, a standing brace is prescribed. There are many options for this type of brace; however, I feel that there is little difference between them and all are satisfactory. The child finds these devices to be confining because they are too slow, they require too much energy, and they are too difficult to apply. Consequently, most of these children give up walking by the time they are 8 or 9 years of age and use a wheelchair for their mobility.[75]

Two designs in orthotic devices may change this prognosis for walking. The first is a *reciprocating orthosis* that allows controlled flexion and extension of the hip during walking.[86] This decreases the energy requirement and increases walking speed.[142] However, this orthosis allows for almost no contractures of the hips or knee, and orthotic breakage can be a frequent occurrence. The second development is a *hip guidance orthosis*, which allows for limited hip motion while still providing stability.[108] These braces may be tried after the age of 3 years and the child has developed an interest in walking and standing.

Upper Lumbar Paraplegia

The upper lumbar paraplegic (L4–L2) has sensation in the anterior hip joint and thigh. Motor function includes the iliopsoas and the adductors producing hip flexion and adduction. Flexion adduction contracture of the hip, because of the unrestricted contraction of the hip flexors and adductors, is typical, with a high incidence of hip dislocation. Attempts to reduce the hip without correcting the muscle imbalance are doomed to failure, and severe ankylosis of the hips often results. Although providing hip stability for the child without the use of orthosis is possible, up to the present, surgical attempts have been unsuccessful. Iliopsoas transfer is contraindicated in children with upper lumbar paraplegia and often leads to severe extension contractures and increased disability.[14,59]

The preferred treatment of children with upper lumbar paraplegia is obtaining range of motion by release of the contracture, including the iliopsoas and adductor tendons, and then treating the child in a manner similar to that done for a thoracic level paraplegic. If range of motion can be obtained, the dislocated hip does not cause disability for either walking or sitting.[39,59] Because of the intact sensation across the hip joint, the reciprocating brace and the hip guidance orthosis are useful, and walking may continue to be a major mode of mobility for these children into young adulthood.[108,142]

Middle and Lower Lumbar Paraplegia

The middle to lower lumbar paraplegic (L3–L5) patient has sensation to below the knee. Muscle function includes hip flexion and adduction, knee extension, and weak knee flexion. Foot dorsiflexion and eversion also may be present. These patients have the potential for control of the hip and knee and therefore the potential for independent walking.

Gait studies show almost normal sagittal plane motion of the hip and is responsible for the movement of the child forward. There is an associated increase in hip rotation and abduction and adduction more than normal. This indicates that range of motion and control of the hip are probably the most important factors in walking for these children.

The hip in the middle to lower lumbar level paraplegic is also a major source of deformity and disability. The natural history of the hip is to undergo progressive dysplasia and dislocation associated with hip flexion contracture, which becomes evident when the child begins to walk. Muscle imbalance is caused by strong hip flexors, adductors, and absent or weak hip abductors and extensors. This muscle imbalance is exaggerated by the forces of walking when the hip flexors and adductors are used to stabilize the hip during the stance phase of walking instead of during their typical function in the swing phase. The contraction of the hip flexors and adductors during the stance phase of gait causes the hip to flex and adduct, which produces a shear force across the acetabulum. It is not unusual for these paraplegic children to survive infancy with hips that are not dislocated and then to have them become dislocated at age 3 or 4 years. Attempts to reduce the hip and correct the progressive deformity are unsuccessful unless correction of the forces around the hip can be obtained.

Historically, muscle balance has been obtained at the hip by performing muscle releases. However, taking the muscle control away from the hip does not increase its stability, although the hip stays reduced, but increases its instability because of weakness and requires the use of an orthosis to stabilize the hip for walking.[39] This conclusion is not surprising, considering the severely weakened hip made unstable by surgical procedures.

Sharrard initiated another approach to hip instability by transferring the iliopsoas tendon to the greater trochanter, a modification of procedures suggested by Garceau and Mustard to treat instability of the hip following poliomyelitis.[20,42,101] The purpose of the tendon transfer was to produce an abduction force across the hip joint during the stance phase of walking and thereby eliminate the deforming hip flexion force of the iliopsoas. Long-term studies have shown that this transfer is successful in maintaining hip reduction and decreasing the hip flexion contracture.[14,20,122] However, the iliopsoas is transferred out of phase to normal walking and may decrease the necessary sagittal plane motion necessary for walking, stepping up on a curb, or climbing stairs. The weakness of the hip flexion requires the child to use the rectus femoris and sartorius muscles to flex the hip. This in turn results in extension of the knee, which also makes stair climbing difficult.

Bunch[14] has shown that with careful selection of patients, preservation of the nerve to the sartorius muscle, and intensive physical therapy, stair climbing can be achieved. Because the iliopsoas normally is used as a hip flexor, it continues to contract during the flexion activity of the hip and also may prevent the hip from flexing, leading to an extension contracture. In many instances in the lower lumbar level paraplegic person without pelvic or hip deformity, without spasticity, and with good knee control, gait can be improved to the point that patients may be able to "cruise the mall" using their braces, crutches, or walker rather than a wheelchair.[105]

Transfer of the external oblique muscle from the abdomen to the greater trochanter; posterior transfer of the adductor longus, brevis, and gracilis to the ischium; and transfer of the tensor fascia lata muscle posteriorly on the ilium and to the tendon of the gluteus maximus have been used to control the hip.[103,125,143] Studies have shown a maintenance of hip reduction and improvement in the acetabular index and the center-edge angle after those muscle transfers similar to the results obtained with Sharrard iliopsoas transfer (Fig. 14-14). In addition, after the three muscle transfers, children with L3–L5 paraplegia have shown marked improvement in their walking ability, 70% of whom demonstrated a marked increase in endurance and walking speed. They also have required less bracing. Fifty percent of these children have developed enough stability around their hip to learn to walk independently without crutches or a walker.[103] These muscle transfers are performed after the child has reached 2 years of age and learned to walk.

Although improvement in the hip indices can be produced by muscle transfers around the hip, they are not sufficiently forceful to correct major anatomic deformities. It is therefore necessary to reduce the hip and correct femoral and acetabular deformity at the time of or prior to the muscle transfer. Continued radiographic evaluation must be made following the reconstruction because recurrent dysplasia is possible.

If the hip is dislocated at birth, I prefer to wait until the child is 1 year of age before carrying out hip reduction to avoid interfering with motor development. If the child is between 1 and 6 years of age, an open reduction and capsular plication are carried out to provide stability. If there is deformity of the femoral neck, a varus femoral shortening osteotomy is indi-

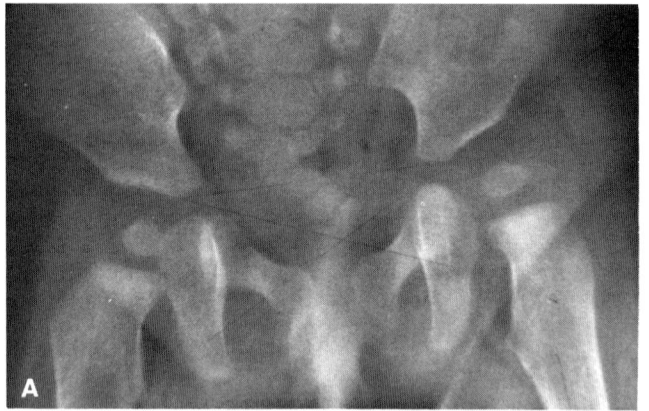
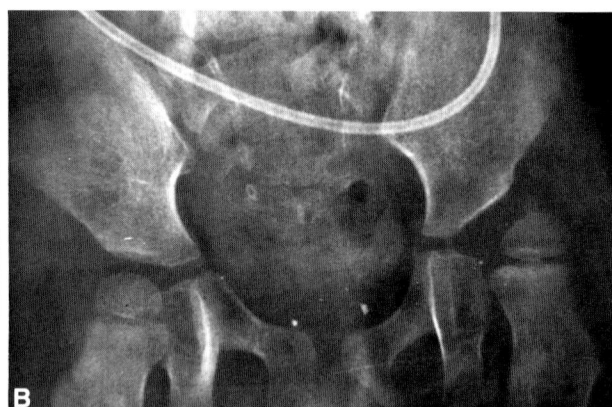
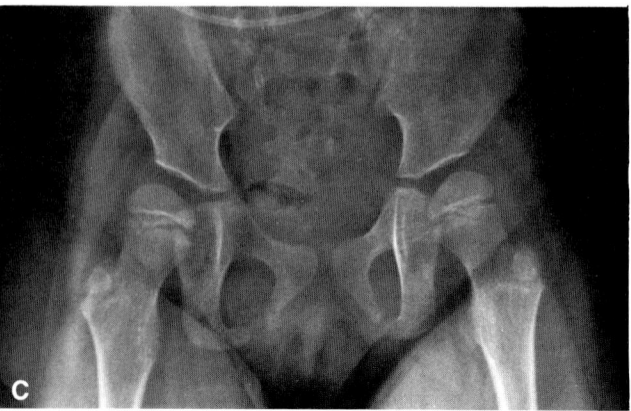

FIGURE 14-14. (A) A 2-year-old child with L4 paraplegia begins to walk with ankle-foot orthoses and a walker. The hips are reduced. (B) One year later, the left hip becomes dysplastic. (C) Two years after bilateral transfer of the external oblique and adductor muscles, the hips are reduced, and the child remains ambulatory.

cated. Pelvic osteotomy is indicated for severe acetabular dysplasia.[18] The type of pelvic osteotomy performed depends on the deformity and the surgeon's preference. An arthrogram and a CT scan may help to establish the area of acetabular insufficiency so that a correct procedure can be selected. The muscle transfers are then performed to help maintain reduction. The muscle transfers work better on a reduced hip than a dislocated one. Therefore, I reduce the hips, even bilateral dislocations, before the age of 4 years. After that age the dysplasia is so great that the success rate is poor, and the hips are left dislocated.

Sacral level paraplegics have intrinsic stability to their hip with sensation and motor control. Dislocation of the hip in these children is rare; however, when it occurs, it should be treated as a developmental dislocation of the hip.

Knee

The function of the knee is important to a child with myelomeningocele. Function of the knee is dependent on both the absence of deformity and the presence of stability. It must be stable during stance to accept the weight of the child without buckling, and flex sufficiently during swing to clear the foot. However, it is possible to walk with a stiff knee, and stability is more important than motion. The three deformities that may seriously diminish the ambulatory ability are extension or hyperextension contractures, flexion contractures, and valgus rotational deformities.

In a study of 16 patients with residual hyperextension contractures of the knee, only three were able to walk.[75] These children also have difficulty sitting. Fortunately, the incidence of extension contractures is relatively low. There are several causes of extension contractures. One of the most common causes is seen in a child born with a breech presentation and with hyperflexed hips, hyperextended knees, and clubfoot. In these infants, the hamstring tendons usually have displaced anterior to the knee axis, perpetuating the hyperextension deformity, although the child may be an L4 or L5 level paraplegic. The next most common cause appears in the middle lumbar level paraplegic person, in which the child has quadriceps function but no perceptible knee flexors. The least common cause is seen in high-level paraplegics people in whom there is spasticity of the quadriceps muscle. Most of these cases can be treated by passive range of motion and splinting during the neonatal period of life. Although normal range of motion is rarely achieved, 60 to 70 degrees of flexion is common.

For those paraplegic children who do not respond to physical therapy, surgical treatment is indicated. If the child has voluntary function of the quadriceps, a

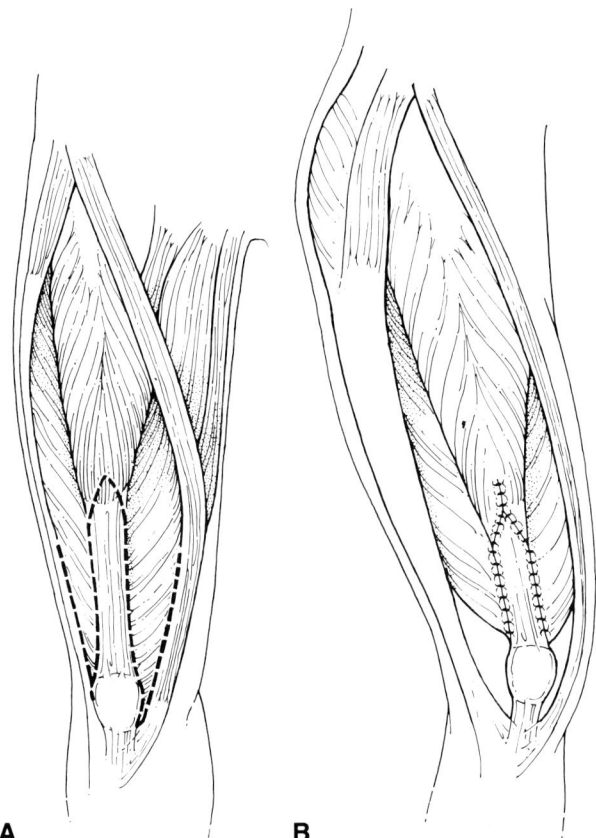

FIGURE 14-15. The V-Y quadricepsplasty for hyperextension contracture of the knee. (**A**) In addition to the detachment of the rectus femoris tendon from the muscle of the rectus femoris, the vastus medialis, and the vastus lateralis muscles, the vastus medialis and lateralis muscles are separated from the iliotibial band, the lateral hamstrings, the medial hamstrings, and the sartorius muscles. (**B**) When the knee is flexed, the hamstring muscles and fascia lata slip posterior to the knee axis, restoring their normal function. The quadriceps muscles are then repaired in the lengthened position. (From Lindseth RE. Extension contracture of the knee. In: McLaurin RL, Oppenheimer S, Dias L, Kaplan WE, eds. Spina bifida: a multidisciplinary approach. New York: Praeger, 1986:40.)

modification of the V-Y plasty of the quadriceps tendons should be performed (Fig. 14-15). This procedure is modified by detaching the vastus medialis and the vastus lateralis from the medial and lateral hamstrings, which slide posterior to the knee axis. This approach often restores the hamstring function, and the child develops both active flexion and extension of the knee. If the quadriceps is not under voluntary control and is spastic, sectioning of the patellar tendon and the retinaculum, as proposed by Kiloyle* is appropriate.

Flexion deformities are common in these children, even in the face of normal quadriceps function.[28]

---

* Kilfoyle RM, personal communication, August 1977.

A small degree of contracture, below 20 degrees, seems to be tolerated well, but contraction greater than 30 degrees decreases the likelihood that the child will continue to walk. Contractures over 20 degrees in the adult have a high incidence of patellofemoral pain.[137]

The cause of the flexion contracture is not always apparent. In some children, spasticity of the hamstrings or gastrocnemius can be implicated. In most middle and low lumbar paraplegic people the cause appears to be a co-contraction of the hamstring and the quadriceps during the entire stance phase of gait. This lack of coordinated activity occurs only during walking and may not be present during manual testing of muscle activity during the neurologic examination. It appears to be related to brain stem abnormalities. The result of the tug of war between the knee flexors and extensors is persistent knee flexion during stance and decreased knee flexion during swing.

In the neonatal period and in infancy, physical therapy may be helpful in decreasing the flexion contracture. In those children who do not respond to physical therapy by 18 months to 2 years of age, surgical correction is indicated.

If the child with flexion contractures has some voluntary function of the medial hamstrings, the hamstrings should be lengthened rather than sectioned. The biceps femoris and the posterior part of the iliotibial band can be sectioned. The gastrocnemius origin should be resected. Almost all children with this deformity need to have a posterior capsulotomy extending from the posterior aspect of the medial collateral ligament to the posterior aspect of the lateral collateral ligament. In most patients, the anterior cruciate ligament also needs to be partially, if not completely, resected to allow the tibia to slide forward on the femur into extension.

Postoperatively, the patient must wear an above-the-knee orthosis for a prolonged period to prevent the development of knee instability. In the child older than 6 or 7 years, sufficient deformity has developed in the femoral condyles to preclude satisfactory soft tissue correction of the contracture, and a distal femoral osteotomy is needed.

Valgus and rotational deformities of the knee primarily are caused by tightness of the iliotibial band and the forces of ambulation. During the Trendelenburg gait pattern, the shift of weight lateral to the hip joint along with contraction of the adductors and fixed position of the foot to the floor produces a valgus thrust to the knee. The young child is best treated by muscle transfers to the hip to stabilize his or her gait pattern, by sectioning of the distal iliotibial band, if it is contracted, and by placing the child in a knee-ankle-foot orthosis to resist the valgus thrust to the knee. If the deformity becomes fixed, a distal femoral osteotomy is required to realign the knee.

Stability for the knee in thoracic and upper lumbar paraplegics is provided by an orthosis. Sufficient sensation and motor control of the knee is not present unless the child has functioning of the L4–L5 nerve roots. Without a good quadriceps, some medial hamstring function, and sensation to the tibial tubercle, the child cannot control the knee adequately. Attempts to stabilize the thoracic upper and middle lumbar level paraplegic patients with a below-the-knee orthosis by means of equinus positioning or with other types of foot positioning should be avoided. Because the child is unable to raise his or her center of gravity to vault over a plantar flexed foot, the knee must hyperextend or externally rotate, producing degenerative changes because of a lack of protective sensation (Fig. 14-16). Functional knee stability can be obtained in the higher level paraplegic person by means of an offset knee

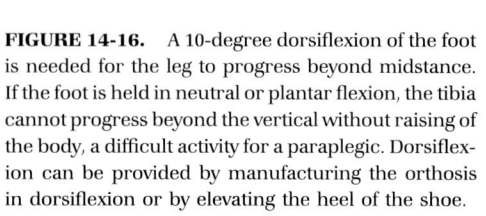
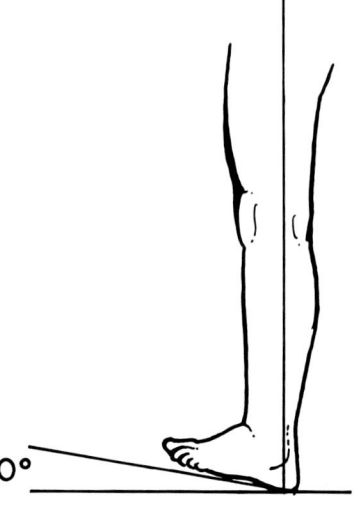
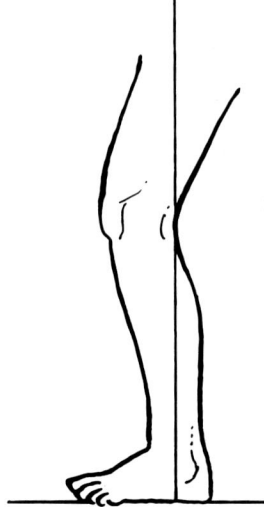

FIGURE 14-16. A 10-degree dorsiflexion of the foot is needed for the leg to progress beyond midstance. If the foot is held in neutral or plantar flexion, the tibia cannot progress beyond the vertical without raising of the body, a difficult activity for a paraplegic. Dorsiflexion can be provided by manufacturing the orthosis in dorsiflexion or by elevating the heel of the shoe.

joint and an elastic knee extension assist. This obviates the need for a knee lock and allows for function at the knee similar to an above-the-knee prosthesis.

Foot

The function of the foot of a child paralyzed by myelomeningocele is significantly impaired.[114] The severe deformity of the leg and foot, limited ankle and subtalar motion, absent weak or spastic muscles, and the lack of sensation make it almost impossible for the foot to function normally by providing shock absorption, control of floor reaction forces, and the transfer of weight that is necessary for gait.[131] Almost all of the myelomeningocele children require treatment of their feet. Even nonambulatory children require adequate positioning of the foot to accept shoe wear, placement on wheel foot rests, and prevent pressure sores. Ambulatory children require an accurate correction of deformity. They are unable to compensate for malposition of the foot because of weakness of the trunk, the hip, and the knee, which causes the weight-bearing line and the floor reaction force to fall outside the zone of stability of the hip, the knee, and the ankle. For example, a foot that has residual inward rotation produces a varus deformity at the knee and inward rotation of the leg during the stance phase of gait. Outward rotation of the foot causes a valgus deformity to the knee and an exaggerated outward rotation of the leg during stance. Residual equinus deformity causes hyperextension of the knee and the inability of the child to move the center of gravity beyond midstance. On the other hand, calcaneus deformity allows the tibia to fall forward during mid stance, producing knee flexion and a crouched gait. The foot must also be able to compensate for deformity of the knee. For example, a knee flexion contracture requires the ability of the ankle to dorsiflex so that the heel will contact the floor.

The correction of the deformity, by itself, is not sufficient. Muscle balance must be achieved in the foot, as well. If this muscle imbalance is left uncorrected when the alignment of the foot is obtained, the deformity will recur. There are only two choices available to correct the muscle imbalance: removing the muscle force by excising the tendon or transferring the force to another location by tendon transfer. The preservation or removal of muscle activity must be considered carefully in relation to the function of the foot during walking. If the child needs an orthosis to walk, then muscle control of the foot is of little importance, and the deforming forces should be eliminated; however, if the child has enough muscular control and sensation to walk without an orthosis the muscle balance must be obtained by performing the appropriate tendon transfer.

The goal of treatment is to align the foot to allow transfer of the floor reaction force through the center of the ankle and to produce stability of the knee and hip during stance phase of gait. The motion of the joints in the foot should be preserved, which allows preservation of the shock absorptive capacity of the foot and lessens the possibility of joint degenerations. A rigid foot also has a high incidence of ulceration, even if the deformity has been corrected by subtalar arthrodesis or triple arthrodesis.[16] It is also important to avoid bony prominences in the weight-bearing area to lessen the likelihood of pressure sores.[110]

Talipes Equinovarus Deformity

Talipes equinovarus, or clubfoot, is the most common deformity in these children and occurs in well over 50%.[114] It is present in all levels of paraplegia, but the treatment differs at each level as a result of the muscle function that may be present. The correction of the equinovarus deformity in myelomeningocele patients is rarely accomplished by nonoperative means. An attempt to manipulate the foot and cast the deformity during the newborn period is worth a try if the foot is reasonably supple and can be manipulated into a satisfactory position prior to the casting.[133] However, most of these feet are rigid and the success rate with manipulation and casting has been poor. The cast cannot be used to obtain correction because pressure sores will develop. Occasionally, after cast treatment, the foot appears to be in satisfactory position; however, evaluation of the foot-thigh axis shows that the foot is still internally rotated approximately 45 degrees. This is the result of the severe deformity of the neck of the talus. As the foot is manipulated into the proper relation to the axis of the leg, the calcaneus is moved laterally from underneath the talus, depriving it of its support and allowing the talar head to drop plantarward, producing a foot that resembles a congenital vertical talus. If this occurs, then further attempts at nonoperative treatment should be abandoned. If satisfactory correction has been achieved, then the child must be placed in splints to prevent recurrence of deformity. The splints must be worn continuously until the age of standing. If the foot has not achieved satisfactory correction by the time the infant is 3 months of age, I abandon conservative treatment and recommend surgical correction when the child is 1 year old. This interim period between nonoperative and surgical treatment allows for normal development of the child without the problem of constant cast change and braces. The advantage of performing surgery at the time the child is ready to stand is that weight bearing can be used to maintain the correction along with the orthosis used for ambulation.

The surgical correction of the clubfoot rarely is

accomplished by limited surgery. A radical complete circumferential subtalar release is necessary in order to allow the calcaneus to rotate sufficiently underneath the talus to align the axis of the foot to the axis of the ankle and knee.[88] Because of the deformity of the neck of the talus, it is then necessary to displace the calcaneus medially beneath the talus so that the posterior facet and the anterior facets are reduced in order to prevent the talar head from sagging or falling into a vertical position. It is important to repair the tibial calcaneal ligaments with nonabsorbable suture to prevent lateral migration of the calcaneus into valgus. A plantar release and capsulotomy of the calcaneal cuboid joint is usually necessary, as well.

Unless the child has a sacral level of paralysis, all of the contracted tendons should be resected rather than lengthened because they are spastic and nonfunctional. A simple cutting of the tendons often results in the tendon being caught in the scar and then acting as a tether as the foot grows. This causes recurrence of the deformity. In the L5 level paraplegic person, the anterior tibialis and peroneal tendons also should be released. Leaving them intact often results in a calcaneal valgus deformity. It is better to have a flaccid braceable foot than a deformed foot with muscle activity that is inappropriate for standing.

A major problem during surgical correction of the deformity is skin coverage for the posteromedial aspect of the foot. Many incisions have been tried, but no one incision is free of complications. For the relatively mild deformity, a Cincinnati incision gives adequate results.[25] It provides excellent exposure to the medial and lateral side of the subtalar joint. The drawback to this incision is exposure of the heelcord; however, in most of these children, the tendon is sectioned rather than lengthened, and lack of exposure is not critical. The medial and lateral calcaneal vessels must be carefully preserved to provide circulation to the heel. Other incisions such as the Turco or the two incisions described by Carroll are equally effective.[19,129]

With severe deformity, the Cincinnati incision does not appear to be sufficient. The axis of the foot often must rotate almost 90 degrees in relation to its ankle at the time of surgery. The skin on the medial aspect of the foot is insufficient to allow this degree of correction. If the skin is closed with excessive tension, it will slough and heal by scar. This scar then contracts as the foot grows and causes recurrent deformity. On the other hand, if the deformity is not completely corrected in order to allow skin closure, then a satisfactory position of the foot is not obtained. I use the modified Cincinnati incision by connecting the medial and lateral ends of the incision over the dorsum of the foot. This allows the redundant lateral skin to be moved medially, where it is needed.[76,135] Experience with this procedure has been gratifying with virtual elimination of skin problems.

In this procedure, the skin incision is started on the medial side of the midfoot, where the anterior tibial tendon crosses the medial cuneiform. The incision curves posteriorly distal to the medial malleolus, upward slightly over the Achilles tendon at the level of the ankle joint, and then continues distally and laterally below the lateral malleolus. The incision is extended anteriorly over the sinus tarsi until the extensor tendons are reached. The incision is not completed over the dorsum of the foot until the conclusion of the surgical procedure, when the foot is in the corrected position. After the foot has been positioned and pinned in the corrected position, an assessment is made about the integrity of the medial skin. If the skin is excessively tight, the incision is extended across the dorsum of the foot approximately 2 cm distal to the anterior ankle joint to connect the two ends of the previous incision. The incision is used to divide the skin and subcutaneous tissue, being careful to preserve cutaneous veins and nerves. The proximal flap is freed by blunt dissection from the fascia for a distance of 2 cm. There is no subcutaneous dissection of the distal skin. The skin is then allowed to find its normal position without tension. This permits the skin of the proximal flap to keep its normal relation with the leg while the foot rotates underneath it. The incision is then closed with interrupted subcutaneous sutures and a running dermal stitch. This incision relieves the tension on the medial side of the incision and decreases the redundant skin on the lateral aspect of the foot. It does not completely relieve the tension on the posterior skin in the area of the Achilles tendon. Should there be insufficient skin in the posterior area, the foot is allowed to assume an equinus position during the immediate postoperative period. The foot is gradually brought up out of equinus after the initial wound healing.

Another approach to obtain skin coverage is to insert a subcutaneous balloon (i.e., tissue expander) well before the planned correction of the foot.[49] The balloon is gradually expanded by the injection of saline, stretching the skin and subcutaneous tissue. At the time of correction of the foot deformity, the balloon is removed and the redundant skin is used to close the incision without tension.

It is rarely possible to correct the metatarsus adductus at the same time as the correction of the hindfoot. I prefer to do this as a separate procedure when the child is 3 or 4 years of age. Although not always necessary, it needs to be done more often than in idiopathic clubfoot. Soft tissue release is rarely effective in achieving a permanent correction of the metatarsus adductus. A closing wedge osteotomy of the cuboid and an opening osteotomy of the first cuneiform with transfer of the wedge of bone from the cuboid to the first cuneiform is preferred.[66,88] The metatarsals II and III are then osteotomized at their base. The correction is held with multiple pins that are removed in 1 month. The child is held in a walking cast for 1 additional month, and then placed in suitable orthoses as needed for ambulation.

Recurrent equinovarus deformity may be treated by talectomy; however, the deformity has a tendency to recur, and its short distance from the medial malleolus in the plantar aspect of the foot makes it difficult to fit with an orthotic device.[98] Another problem with brace wear is that the pressure in the plantar surface of the foot is not distributed evenly, although the foot appears plantigrade. These areas of high pressure may predispose these patients to ulcerations.[30,115,116] Persistent wear of an orthosis is essential despite the difficult fit. In the older child, severe residual deformity may be corrected by a triple arthrodesis.[35] This procedure should be limited to only the extreme cases because of the danger of joint degeneration and skin ulceration caused by the stiffness of the foot. Less severe deformities may be managed by a tarsal metatarsal osteotomy to correct the midfoot deformity and a calcaneal osteotomy to correct the varus deformity of the heel.[128]

Calcaneus Deformity

Calcaneal deformities of the foot in the newborn primarily are due to the unopposed contraction of the anterior tibial muscle, the toe extensor muscles, or the peroneal muscles.[40] There is flaccid paralysis of the triceps surae. The deformity may be calcaneal valgus, calcaneus, or calcaneal varus depending on the predominant muscle activity. The deformity is usually progressive, and the calcaneus eventually becomes positioned vertically underneath the talus (Fig. 14-17). The deformity prevents the forefoot from contacting the floor, interfering with balance, preventing the floor reaction force from stabilizing the knee, and causing the child to walk in a flexed knee or crouched gait. Because of the lack of sensation, this deformity leads to heel ulcerations in the teenage years.

Nonoperative treatment is rarely successful. Manipulations of the foot in the newborn period and bracing as the child becomes older may provide satisfactory position. However, in most cases, the muscles continue to shorten, making brace and shoe wear difficult. In the child younger than 5 years of age with a minor deformity, which includes vertical alignment of the calcaneus, the anterior tibial tendon should be transferred through the interosseous membrane and attached to the calcaneus or released if the deformity is not severe. The remaining tight anterior structures should be released so that the foot can be brought into satisfactory position for bracing.[9,107] The purpose of the anterior tendon transfer is to relieve a deforming force and to counteract the function of the toe extensors. The transfer is insufficient in power to substitute for the gastrocnemius soleus muscles. Although these patients may learn to walk without an orthosis following the tendon transfer, gait studies have shown they walk better with than without the orthosis.[7]

In children older than 5 years of age, soft tissue procedures rarely are sufficient. These patients also require osteotomy of the calcaneus with posterior displacement of the posterior fragment.[24]

If the child has already developed ulceration underneath the calcaneus, the treatment must provide correction of the foot deformity followed by removal of the prominent part of the calcaneus, excision of the ulcer, and primary closure by means of a local flap. To allow the ulcer to heal by secondary intention will

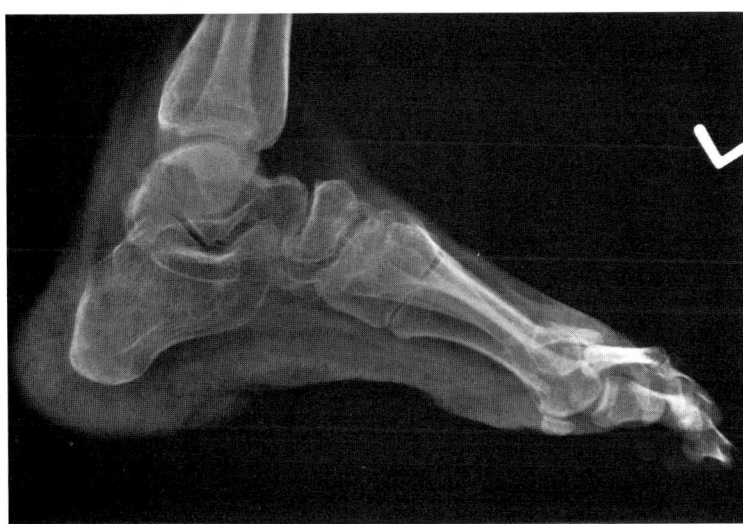

FIGURE 14-17. Lateral radiograph of an L5 paraplegic patient shows the vertical position of the os calcis. Note the hypertrophy of the heel pad.

not provide reconstitution of the normal weight-bearing fat pad. Repeat ulcerations are common. The weight-bearing skin and fat pad must be restored in order to prevent recurrence of the ulceration. Post-healing orthotic wear is essential.

Valgus Deformity in the Newborn

Valgus deformities usually are associated with contracture of the lateral musculature of the foot, equinus deformity of the calcaneus, and a lateral displacement of the calcaneus from beneath the talus.[29,97] The external appearance of the foot resembles that of a congenital vertical talus, but usually it is less rigid. Nonoperative treatment is rarely successful despite the observation that the foot often can be manipulated back into a satisfactory position by plantar flexing the foot and rotating the calcaneus beneath the talus. The lack of active function of the posterior tibial muscle and the spastic activity of the peroneal muscles cause frequent recurrence. Occasionally, a rigid form of congenital vertical talus may be found in myelodysplasia.[31]

If the foot cannot be manipulated passively into the correct deformity and held with an orthosis, then an aggressive surgical approach is needed at about 1 year of age. I prefer an extensive subtalar release to allow reduction of the calcaneus beneath the talus. This may require resection of the Achilles tendon and the peroneal tendons. The posterior ankle capsule is divided along with the fibular calcaneal ligaments. The anterior tibial tendon can be resected or transferred back to the neck of the talus. In most cases, an extraarticular subtalar arthrodesis is needed.[4,27,72]

Valgus Deformity in the Older Child

Valgus deformity is common in the ambulatory child and frequently is associated with outward rotation deformity of the foot and the ankle.[29,93] The cause of the deformity is undetermined but is probably related to the floor reaction force during stance without the appropriate muscle control of the posterior tibial muscle. There usually is a lateral tilt to the ankle mortis with shortening of the fibula. The subtalar joint may be deformed as well. The location of the deformity can be determined by standing anteroposterior radiographs of the ankle mortis and foot. The outward rotation of the ankle axis in relation to the knee should be assessed. It may exceed 60 degrees. Pressure sores caused by shoes and orthotic devices are common.

Nonoperative care, including casts, manipulation, and orthoses, will not correct or prevent the deformity. Most children will require surgical correction. The deformity in the tibia and fibula can be corrected by supramalleolar osteotomy that corrects both the valgus and rotation. If there is minimal outward rotation of the ankle, the valgus deformity of the ankle mortis can be treated by a medial tibial epiphyseodesis.[17] If the child is young, then staples can be used so they can be removed later after the correction has been obtained. If the valgus deformity is mild and associated with a calcaneus deformity and a minimal outward tibial rotation, a calcaneal fibular tendo Achillis tenodesis can prevent progression of the deformity in about 70% of the patients.[17,121] However, stretching of the tenodesis is a major problem, and Dias recommends the addition of an anterior tibial tendon transfer to the calcaneus.[110] If there is subtalar valgus, the foot should be treated similar to the valgus deformity in the newborn.

Cavus Deformity

Cavus deformity of the foot usually is accompanied with claw toe deformity and is seen in the sacral level paraplegic child. These children have normal strength of the anterior tibial and toe extensor muscles, which pull up the midfoot at the base of the first metatarsal and dorsiflex or hyperextend the metatarsal phalangeal joints. The normal functioning peroneus longus plantar flexes the first metatarsal. The paralysis of the gastrocnemius soleus muscles leave the hindfoot in calcaneus position. Active toe flexors flex the interphalangeal joints, and with paralysis, the foot intrinsic muscles cannot flex the metacarpal phalangeal joints or extend the interphalangeal joints. These children have enough sensation and muscle control to walk without an orthosis but frequently develop progressive deformity and ulcerations under their toes and their metatarsal heads. Their gait is also abnormal because of the lack of sufficient power in the gastrocnemius soleus muscles. The cavus deformity is often progressive and may be associated with secondary varus deformity of the foot as the child attempts to use flexor hallucis and digitorum longus muscles to compensate for paralysis of the gastrocnemius soleus muscles.

Conservative treatment by means of an ankle-foot orthosis often provides a temporary solution; however, once the child can walk without the brace, it is difficult to get him or her to wear it again. Therefore, most of these children come to surgical correction.

Surgical treatment must include correction of the bone deformity and soft tissue contracture and restoration of the muscle imbalance. In the young child with mild deformation, a plantar fascia release followed by an ankle-foot orthosis may provide satisfactory correction of the deformity. Rigid cavus due to midfoot deformity can be corrected by a tarsal metatarsal osteotomy associated with plantar release. If the deformity is due to a dorsiflexion deformity of the calcaneus, a calcaneal osteotomy is necessary.[10] The calcaneus is moved backward or laterally, as needed, to correct the cavus or cavovarus deformities. Muscle balancing procedures must consider the phase of the muscle during gait, the power of the muscle available, and the required muscle power necessary for walking.[123,124] The primary goal is to have a plantigrade braceable foot without recurrent deformity or pressure sores. If the residual muscle power in the foot is in the poor to fair range, then the foot cannot be made functional by muscle transfers, and it is best to lengthen a section of the deforming muscle and brace the foot. However, if there is sensation on the sole of the foot and the strength of the toe flexor is good to normal, it may be possible to transfer the muscles to the heel to achieve force balance and a satisfactory brace-free gait.

The anterior tibial muscle is a swing phase muscle and cannot be made into a stance phase muscle to substitute for the gastrocnemius soleus muscle unless electromyogram gait studies show the contrary. In most circumstances, it is better to lengthen the tendon and preserve its necessary function of foot clearance during swing. If the foot is in varus, then transfer of its anterior tibial tendon to the midfoot may be useful. Muscle imbalance of the toes can be helped by transfer of the long extensor tendons to the metatarsal heads with fusion of the interphalangeal joints. This transfer helps elevate the metatarsal heads and prevent recurrent cavus. When the foot is in cavovalgus deformity, the peroneus brevis also can be transferred back to the calcaneus.

Charcot Arthropathy

Charcot, or neurotrophic, arthropathy is a progressive degeneration of a joint caused by a lack of protective sensation. This is a problem that primarily affects ambulatory young adult patients who have decreased sensation of the knee, the ankle, and the foot. Because of the pathologic anatomy of the myelomeningocele, the sensory level is usually higher than the motor level. Consequently, these patients often are able to stand and walk but do not have protective sensation. The patient with paralysis at the L4–L5 level appears to be the most vulnerable (Fig. 14-18). The pathologic process begins following an initial traumatic episode. The initial episode may follow a minor fall that the patient does not consider to be a major injury-producing event. Following this initial traumatic episode, there usually is a considerable amount of swelling and redness around the joint. The appearance of the foot resembles an infection and cellulitis. There may be some minor discomfort but usually no severe pain. Because of the lack of pain, the patient often does not seek medical advice and continues to walk on the joint, causing further microfractures to occur. Even if the patient obtains medical consultation, the initial radiographs often are unremarkable, and the patient is often given antibiotics for the mistaken diagnosis of infection. Once the joint degenera-

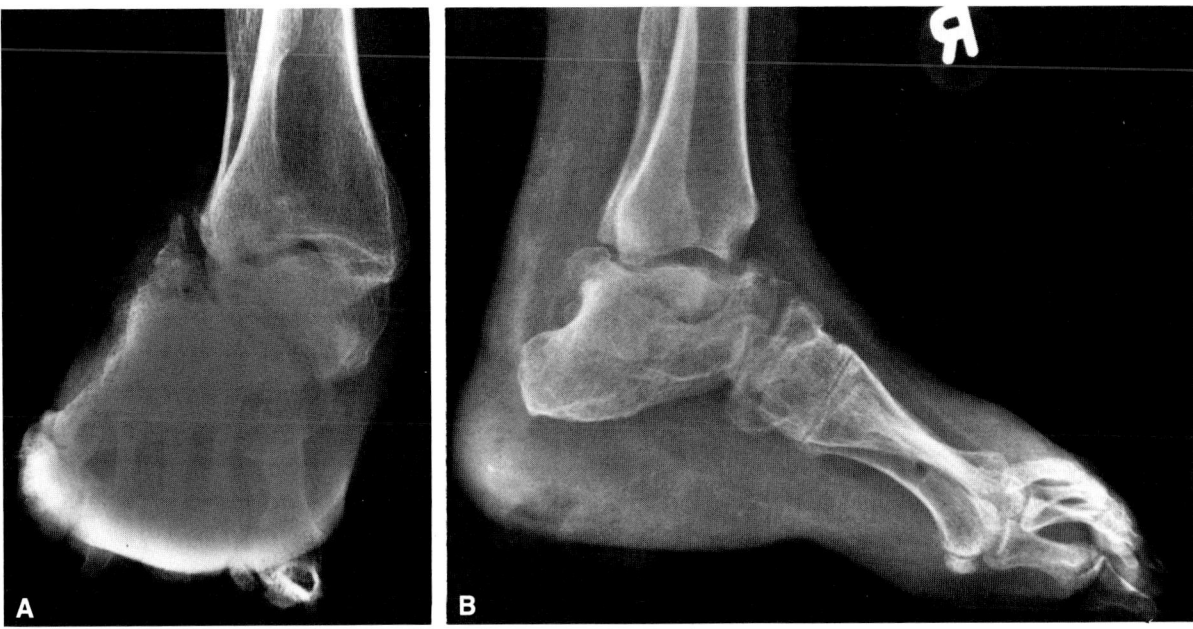

FIGURE 14-18. This Charcot degeneration occurred in a 16-year-old, L5 paraplegic girl who refused to wear her ankle-foot orthosis.

tion has become evident on radiograph, the joint has been destroyed, and satisfactory outcome is difficult to achieve.

Treatment of the Charcot arthropathy must be instituted early and based on suspicion rather than waiting for radiographic confirmation. The best treatment is a vigorous protection of the joint following the initial episode before additional injury occurs. This may be accomplished by a splint or a cast and by non–weight bearing. If the early treatment has been successful, radiographic changes may never be identified. Typically, the swelling and erythema subside after 1 or 2 weeks. If they recur after the beginning of weight bearing, then the protection must be resumed for a longer time. The healing usually takes 6 to 8 weeks. However, if the diagnosis and treatment are delayed until the radiograph becomes positive for joint deformity or degeneration, prolonged immobilization and protection must be provided until the process has run its course. This may take a 6 to 8 months or longer. The joint protection should be maintained until there is radiographic evidence of healing of the avascular segment of the joint and all swelling and erythema has disappeared. Continued orthotic protection of the foot and ankle is essential.

Orthotic Devices

The goal of treatment of the myelomeningocele foot is a braceable plantigrade foot. Only the sacral level paraplegic has sufficient sensation and muscle control to gain stability of the foot and ankle without orthotic support. The orthosis must provide stability to the foot and ankle and, ideally, should be lightweight and cosmetically acceptable. It should limit all unwanted motion of the foot and ankle, and transmit the floor reaction force to the anterior shin, where the child has sensation. The ideal orthosis has not been developed. The closest we can come is a brace made out of polypropylene that controls the ankle but does not allow motion in the ankle.[48] If the ankle is in valgus or if there is instability of the subtalar joint, the brace can be modified with a supramalleolar strap, which uses the principle of the T-strap of the double upright style of orthosis.[73] This helps release the pressure on the medial malleolus and the head of the talus.

I prefer the floor reaction force ankle-foot orthosis that is closed anteriorly over the tibial tubercle so that the floor reaction force can be transmitted directly to the area of intact sensation (Fig. 14-19). It also gives a firm support to the tibia to help extend the knee during midstance.[76] Because the orthosis is in part a cylinder, it is much more resistant to rotation and valgus deformation during walking than the more common posterior polypropylene ankle-foot orthosis. Because the ankle is rigid, the heel of the shoe must act as the

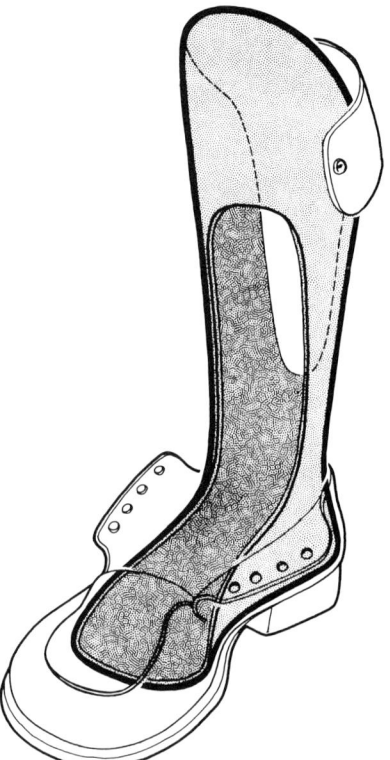

FIGURE 14-19. An ankle-foot orthosis made of a polypropylene shell with a plastazote lining. The orthosis is closed anterior over the tibial tubercle so that the floor reaction force can be transmitted directly to the area of intact sensation. (From Glancy J, Lindseth RE. The polypropylene solid-ankle orthosis. J Orthot Prosthet 1972, 26:16.)

shock absorber at heel strike and should be of a relatively soft, shock-absorbing material. The foot also must be allowed to simulate 10 degrees of dorsiflexion in order to get the tibia beyond midstance to take the next step[63] (see Fig. 14-16). This can be adjusted by the height of the heel or the position of the foot when the mold is made for the brace. The drawback to the floor reaction orthosis is that it is difficult to make and requires a skilled orthotist. There is little margin of error permitted or maximum gait cannot be achieved.

Shoe inserts and modifications are rarely successful in providing correction of alignment and position deformities of the foot. Most of these children do not have the muscle control or the sensation to take advantage of these devices. They may be helpful in protecting the foot of an S1 level paraplegic.

Fractures of the Femur and Tibia

Fractures of the femur and tibia occur commonly in children with myelomeningocele.[64,136] The trauma needed to produce the fracture is often minimal, particularly after cast immobilization. The fractures are usually epiphyseal or metaphyseal.[26,37,67,68] The peak incidence of fracture appears to be between the ages of 3 and 7 years, but fracture may occur at any age. Fracture is related to the level of paralysis and postoperative immobilization. Metabolic abnormalities have been investigated and not found to be present.[106]

Diagnosis of fracture often is missed because of the minimal trauma. If the fracture is not diaphyseal, no instability of the leg may be present, which aids in the diagnosis. The local and systemic response to the fracture also is exaggerated and consists of swelling of the leg, local warmth, erythema, and fever.[33] These signs and symptoms often are misdiagnosed as cellulitis or osteomyelitis. Any unexplained fever in these children in association with a swollen warm leg that appears to be cellulitis should be treated as a fracture until radiographs prove otherwise.

Fracture following postoperative cast immobilization is common, and several studies have reported an incidence of 18% to 45%. Prevention of fractures in the postoperative period include starting the child on weight bearing as soon as possible and keeping the plaster immobilization time to a minimum. After the cast has been removed, extreme caution must be exercised for at least 1 week. Once a fracture has occurred it is best to carry out minimal immobilization and begin weight bearing as soon as possible. If these children are treated with the usual routine of plaster cast and inactivity, the osteopenia increases and repeated fractures are more likely to occur.

In most instances, I prefer a soft cast made of cast padding about 1 inch thick, followed by an elastic bandage and, if necessary, a single lightweight plaster splint. The swelling decreases rapidly, and the soft cast has to be reapplied within 2 or 3 days. The family rewraps the elastic bandage daily. Usually there is sufficient callus to begin weight bearing in 2 or 3 weeks after casting. If a plaster cast is used, weight bearing should be started as soon as possible. If the fracture is close to the hip, internal fixation may be necessary to obtain early mobility.

References

1. Alan LD, Donald I, Gibson AA, et al. Amniotic fluid alpha-fetoprotein in the antenatal diagnosis of spina bifida. Lancet 1973;2:522.
2. Allen BL Jr. The operative treatment of myelomeningocele spinal deformity. Orthop Clin North Am 1979;10:845.
3. American Academy of Allergy and Immunology: Task Force Report on Allergic Reactions to Latex. J Allergy Clin Immunol 1993;92:16.
4. Aronson DD, Middleton DL. Extra-articular subtalar arthrodesis with cancellous bone graft and internal fixation for children with myelomeningocele. Dev Med Child Neurol 1991;33(3):232.
5. Asher M, Olson J. Factors affecting the ambulatory status of patients with spina bifida cystica. J Bone Joint Surg [Am] 1983;65:350.
6. Banta JV, Hamanda JS. Natural history of the kyphotic deformity in myelomeningocele. J Bone Joint Surg [Am] 1976;58:279.
7. Banta JV, Sutherland DH, Wyatt M. Anterior tibial transfer to the os calcis with achilles tenodesis for calcaneal deformity in myelomeningocele. J Pediatr Orthop 1982;1:125.
8. Banta JV. Combined anterior and posterior fusion for spinal deformity in myelomeningocele. Spine 1990;15(9):946.
9. Bliss DG, Menelaus MB. The results of transfer of the tibialis anterior to the heel in patients who have a myelomeningocele. J Bone Joint Surg [Am] 1986;68(8):1258.
10. Bradley GW, Coleman SS. The treatment of the calcaneocavus foot deformity. J Bone Joint Surg [Am] 1981;63:1159.
11. Breningstall GN, Marker SM, Tubman DE. Hydrosyringomyelia and diastematomyelia detected by MRI in myelomeningocele. Pediatr Neurol 1992;8(4):267.
12. Bunch WH. Treatment of the myelomeningocele spine. Instr Course Lect 1976;25:93.
13. Bunch WH. The Milwaukee brace in paralytic scoliosis. Clin Orthop 1975;110:63.
14. Bunch WH, Hakala MW. Iliopsoas transfers in children with myelomeningocele. J Bone Joint Surg [Am] 1984;66:224.
15. Bunch WH, Scarff TB, Dvonch VM. Progressive loss in myelomeningocele patients. Orthop Trans 1983;7:185.
16. Burke SW, Weinse LS, Maynard MJ. Neuropathic foot ulcers in myelodysplasia. Orthop Trans 1991;15:102.
17. Burkus JK, Moore DW, Raycroft JF. Valgus deformity of the ankle in myelodysplastic patients. Correction of stapling of the medial part of the distal tibial physis. J Bone Joint Surg [Am] 1983;65:1157.
18. Canale TS, Hammond NL III, Cotler JM, et al. Pelvic displacement osteotomy for chronic hip dislocation in myelodysplasia. J Bone Joint Surg [Am] 1975;57:177.
19. Carroll NC. Pathoanatomy and surgical treatment of the resistant clubfoot. Instr Course Lect 1988;37:93.
20. Carroll NC, Sharrard WJ. Long term follow up of posterior iliopsoas transplantation for paralytic dislocation of the hip. J Bone Joint Surg [Am] 1972;54:551.
21. Carter CO. Spina bifida and anencephaly—a problem in genetic-environmental interaction. J Biosoc Sci 1969;1:71.
22. Carter CO, Roberts JA. The risk of recurrence after two children with central nervous system malformations. Lancet 1967;1:306.
23. Centers for Disease Control and Prevention. Recommendations for the use of folic acid to reduce the number of cases of spina bifida and other neural tube defects. MMWR 1992;RR-14:41.
24. Coleman SS. Complex foot deformities in children. Philadelphia: Lea & Febiger, 1983:147.
25. Crawford AH, Marxen JL, Osterfield DL. The Cincinnati Incision—a comprehensive approach for surgical procedures of the foot and ankle in childhood. J Bone Joint Surg [Am] 1982;64:1355.
26. Cuxart A, Iborra J, Melendez M, Pages E. Physeal injuries in myelomeningocele patients. Paraplegia 1992;30(11):791.
27. Diamond L. Dowel type subtalar arthrodesis in children. J Bone Joint Surg [Am] 1976;58:725.
28. Dias LS. Surgical management of knee contractures in myelomeningocele. J Pediatr Orthop 1982;2(2):127.
29. Dias LS, Jasty MJ, Collins P. Rotational deformities of the lower limb in myelomeningocele—evaluation and treatment. J Bone Joint Surg [Am] 1984;66(2):215.
30. Dias LS, Stern LS. Talectomy in the treatment of resistant talipes equinovarus deformity in myelomeningocele and arthrogryposis. J Pediatr Orthop 1987;7(1):39.
31. Drennan JC, Sharrard WJW. The pathologic anatomy of convex pes valgus. J Bone Joint Surg [Br] 1971;53:455.

32. Drennan JC. The role of muscles in the development of human lumbar kyphosis. Dev Med Child Neurol 1970;12:33.
33. Drummond DS, Moreau M, Cruess RL. Postoperative neuropathic fractures in patients with myelomeningocele. Dev Med Child Neurol 1981;23:147.
34. Drummond DS, Moreau M, Cruess RL. The results and complicatons of surgery for the paralytic hip and spine in myelomeningocele. J Bone Joint Surg [Br] 1980;62:49.
35. Duncan JW, Lovell WW. Hoke triple arthrodesis. J Bone Joint Surg [Am] 1978;60:795.
36. Dunn HK. Kyphosis of myelodysplasia—operative treatment based on pathophysiology. Orthop Trans 1983;7:19.
37. Edvardsen P. Physeo-epiphyseal injuries of lower extremities in myelomeningocele. Acta Orthop Scand 1972;43:550.
38. Eyring EJ, Wanken JJ, Sayers MP. Spinal osteotomy for kyphosis in myelomeningocele. Clin Orthop 1972;88:24.
39. Feiwell E, Sakar D, Blatt T. The effect of hip reduction on function in patients with myelomeningocele—potential gains and hazards of surgical care. J Bone Joint Surg [Am] 1978;60:169.
40. Fraser RK, Hoffman EB. Calcaneus deformity in the ambulant patient with myelomeningocele. J Bone Joint Surg [Br] 1991;73(6):994.
41. Fromm B, Carstens C, Niethard FU, Lang R. Aortography in children with myelomeningocele and lumbar kyphosis. J Bone Joint Surg [Br] 1992;74(5):691.
42. Garceau GJ, Kinzel JW. Transplantation of the iiacus muscle for loss of hip abduction power. Q Bull Indiana Univ Med Center 1951;13:27.
43. Gardner WJ. Anatomic features common to the Arnold-Chiari and the Dandy-Walker malformations suggest a common origin. Cleve Clin Q 1959;26:206.
44. Gardner WJ. Myelocele—rupture of the neural tube? Clin Neurosurg 1968;15:57.
45. Gardner WJ. Embrylogic origin of spinal malformations. Acta Radiol (Stockh) 1966;5:1012.
46. Gardner WJ. Diastematomyelia and the Klippel-Feil syndrome. Cleve Clin Q 1964;31:19.
47. Gardner WJ. Myelomeningocele—the result of rupture of the embryonic neural tube. Cleve Clin Q 1960;27:88.
48. Glancy JC, Lindseth RE. The polypropylene solid-ankle orthosis. Orthot Prosth 1972;26:16.
49. Grant AD, Silver L, Lehman WB, Altar D. The use of tissue expander in clubfoot surgery. Presented to the Pediatric Orthopaedic Society of North America Meeting, May 7, 1990; San Francisco, CA.
50. Greenberg F, James LM, Oakley GP Jr. Estimate of birth prevalance rates of spina bifida in the United States from computer generated maps. Am J Obstet Gynecol 1983;145:570.
51. Hall JE, Poitra B. The management of kyphosis in patients with myelomeningocele. Clin Orthop 1977;128:33.
52. Hall PV, Campbell RH, Kalsbeck JE. Myelomeningocele and progressive hydromyelia—progressive paresis in myelodysplasia. J Neurosurg 1975;43:457.
53. Hall PV, Lindseth RE, Campbell RL, Kalsbeck JE. Myelodysplasia and developmental scoliosis. Spine 1976;1:48.
54. Hall PV, Lindseth RE, Campbell RH, et al. Scoliosis and hydrocephalus in myelocele patients. The effect of ventricular shunting. J Neurosurg 1979;50:174.
55. Hammar SL. The approach to the adolescent patient. Pediatr Clin North Am 1973;20:799.
56. Heinz ER, Rosenbaum AE, Scarff TB, et al. Tethered spinal cord following myelomeningocele repair. Radiology 1979; 131:153.
57. Heydermann JS, Gillespie R. Management of myelomeningocele kyphosis in the older child by kyphectomy and segmental spinal instrumentation. Spine 1987;12(1):37.
58. Hide DW, Williams HP, Ellis HL. The outlook for the child with a myelomeningocele for whom early surgery was considered inadvisable. Dev Med Child Neurol 1972;14:304.
59. Hoffer MM, Feiwell E, Perry R, et al. Functional ambulation in patients with myelomeningocele. J Bone Joint Surg [Am] 1973;55:137.
60. Hoppenfeld S. Congenital kyphosis in myelomeningocele. J Bone Joint Surg [Br] 1967;49:276.
61. Hostler SL. Development of the infant with myelomeningocele. Instr Course Lect 1975;25:70.
62. Hull WJ, Moe JN, Winter RB. Spinal deformity in myelomeningocele—natural history, evaluation, treatment. J Bone Joint Surg [Am] 1974;56:1767.
63. Hullin MG, Robb JE, Loudon IR. Ankle–foot orthosis function in low level myelomeningocele. J Pediatr Orthop 1992; 12(4):518.
64. James CC. Fractures of the lower limbs in spina bifida cystica—a survey of 44 fractures in 122 children. Dev Med Child Neurol 1970;22(Suppl):88.
65. Johnson WR. Sex education of the mentally retarded. In: Curz F, Levic GD, eds. Human sexuality and the mentally retarded. New York: Brunner Mazel, 1973:57.
66. Kling TF Jr, Schmidt TL, Conklin, MJ. Open wedge osteotomy of the first cuneiform for severe metatarsus adductus. Presented to the Pediatric Orthopaedic Society of North America Meeting, May 7, 1990; San Francisco, CA.
67. Korhonen BJ. Fractures in myelodysplasia. Clin Orthop 1971;79:145.
68. Kumar SJ, Cowell HR, Townsend P. Physeal, metaphyseal, and diaphyseal injuries of the lower extremities in children with myelomeningocele. J Pediatr Orthop 1984;4(1):25.
69. Lawrence KM. Clinical and ethical considerations on alpha-fetoprotein estimated for early prenatal diagnosis of neural tube malformations. Dev Med Child Neurol 1974;16(Suppl 32):117.
70. Lawrence KM. The recurrence risk in spina bifida cystica and anencephaly. Dev Med Child Neurol 1969;(Suppl 20):23.
71. Lee EH, Carroll NC. Hip stability and ambulatory status in myelomeningocele. J Pediatr Orthop 1985;5(5):522.
72. Lee YF, Grogan TJ, Moseley CF. Extra-articular subtalar arthrodesis in myelodysplasia. Orthop Trans 1990;14:590.
73. Lin RS. Application of varus T-strap principle to the polypropylene ankle–foot orthosis. Orthot Prosthet 1982;36:67.
74. Lindseth RE. Posterior iliac osteotomy for fixed pelvic obliquity. J Bone Joint Surg [Am] 1978;60:17.
75. Lindseth RE. Treatment of the lower extremity in children paralyzed by myelomeningocele. Instr Course Lect 1976;25:76.
76. Lindseth RE. Myelomeningocele. In: Drennan JC, ed. The child's foot and ankle. New York: Raven Press, 1992.
77. Lindseth RE. Myelomeningocele spine. In: Weinstein SL, ed. The pediatric spine: principles and practice. New York: Raven Press, 1994.
78. Lindseth RE, Clancy J. Polypropylene lower extremity braces for paraplegia due to myelomeningocele. J Bone Joint Surg [Am] 1975;56(3):566.
79. Lindseth RE, Graziano GP. One-stage anterior transpedicular and unilateral fusion for congenital scoliosis. Orthop Trans 1988;12:184.
80. Lindseth RE, Selzer L. Vertebral excision for kyphosis in children with myelomeningocele. J Bone Joint Surg [Am] 1979;61:699.
81. Lintner SA, Lindseth RE. The long-term follow up after proximal resection in children with myelomeningocele and a kyphos deformity. Orthop Trans 1993;17(1):123.
82. Loder RT, Shapiro P, Towbin R, Aronson DD. Aortic anatomy in children with myelomeningocele and congenital lumbar kyphosis. J Pediatr Orthop 1991;11(1):31.

83. Lorber J. Selective treatment of myelomeningocele—To treat or Not to Treat? Pediatrics 1974;53:307.
84. Lough LK, Nielsen DH. Ambulation of children with myelomeningocele—parapodium versus parapodium with Orlau swivel modification. Dev Med Child Neurol 1986;28(4):489.
85. Lubicky JP, Fredrickson BE. The combined use of kyphectomy, spinal cord resection, luque instrumentation, and myocutaneous flaps for severe kyphosis in the myelomeningocele. Orthop Trans 1985;9:495.
86. McCall RE, Schmidt WT. Clinical experience with the reciprocal gait orthosis in myelodysplasia. J Pediatr Orthop 1986;6(2):157.
87. McDonald CM, Jaffe KM, Shurtleff DB, Menelaus MB. Modifications to the traditional description of neurosegmental innervation in myelomeningocele. Dev Med Child Neurol 1991;33(6):473.
88. McKay DW. New concept of and approach to clubfoot treatment. Section II. Correction of the clubfoot. J Pediatr Orthop 1983;3:10.
89. McLaughlin TP, Banta JV, Gahm NH, Raycroft JF. Intraspinal rhizotomy and distal cordectomy in patients with myelomeningocele. J Bone Joint Surg [Am] 1986;68(1):88.
90. McLone DG, Herman JM, Gabrieli AP, Dias L. Tethered cord as a cause of scoliosis in children with a myelomeningocele. Pediatr Neurosurg 1990;16(1):8.
91. McMaster MJ. Anterior and posterior instrumentation and fusion of thoracolumbar scoliosis due to myelomeningocele. J Bone Joint Surg [Br] 1987;69(1):20.
92. Mackel JL, Lindseth RE. Scoliosis in myelodysplasia. J Bone Joint Surg [Am] 1975;57:1031.
93. Malhotra D, Puri R, Owen R. Valgus deformity of the ankle in children with spina bifida aperta. J Bone Joint Surg [Br] 1984;66(3):381.
94. Maynard MJ, Weiner LS, Burke SW. Neuropathic foot ulceration in patients with myelodysplasia. J Pediatr Orthop 1992;12(6):786.
95. Mazur JM, Menelaus MB, Dicksen DR, Doig WG. Efficacy of surgical management for scoliosis in myelomeningocele—correction of deformity and alteration of functional status. J Pediatr Orthop 1986;6(5):568.
96. Menelaus MB. Progress in the management of the paralytic hip in myelomeningocele. Orthop Clin North Am 1980;11:17.
97. Menelaus MB. Pes plano-valgus. In: McLaurin RL, Oppenheimer S, Dias L, and Kaplan WE, eds. Spina bifida—a multidisciplinary approach. New York: Prager, 1986:431.
98. Menelaus MB. Talectomy for equinovarus deformity in arthrogryposis and spina bifida. J Bone Joint Surg [Br] 1971;53:468.
99. Mintz LJ, Sarwark JF, Dias LS, Schafer MF. The natural history of congenital kyphosis in myelomeningocele. A review of 51 children Spine 1991;16(8 Suppl):S348.
100. Morgagni JB. The Seats and causes of diseases investigated by anatomy. vol. 3. London: A Millar & T Cadell, 1797.
101. Mustard WT. Iliopsoas transfer for weakness of hip abduction. J Bone Joint Surg [Am] 1952;34:647.
102. Osebold WR, Mayfield JK, Winter RB, Moe JH. Surgical treatment of the paralytic scoliosis associated with myelomeningocele. J Bone Joint Surg [Am] 1982;64:841.
103. Phillips DP, Lindseth RE. Ambulation after transfer of adductors, external oblique, and tensor fascia lata in myelomeningocele. J Pediatr Orthop 1992;12(6)712.
104. Raycroft JE, Curtis BH. Spinal curvature in myelomeningocele: natural history and etiology. St Louis: CV Mosby, 1972.
105. Raycroft TF. Posterior iliopsoas transfer—long-term results in patients treated at Newington Children's Hospital. Orthop Trans 1987;11:454.
106. Repasky D, Richard K, Lindseth RE. Ascorbic acid and fractures in children with myelomeningocele. J Am Diet Assoc 1976;69:511.
107. Rodrigues RC, Dias LS. Calcaneus deformity in spina bifida—results of anterolateral release. J Pediatr Orthop 1992;12(4):461.
108. Rose GK, Sankarankutt M, Stallard J. A clinical review of the orthotic treatment of myelomeningocele patients. J Bone Joint Surg [Br] 1983;65(3):242.
109. Scarff TB, Toleikis JR, Bunch WH, Parrish S. Dermatosomal somatosensory evoked potentials in children with myelomeningocele. Z Kinderchir Grenzgeb 1979;28:384.
110. Schafer MF, Dias LS. Myelomeningocele—orthopaedic treatment. Baltimore: Williams & Wilkins, 1983:168.
111. Seller MJ, Nevin NC. Periconceptional vitamin supplementation and the prevention of neural tube defects in southeast England and North Ireland. J Med Genet 1984;21:325.
112. Sharrard WJ. Spinal osteotomy for congenital kyphosis in myelomeningocele. J Bone Joint Surg [Br] 1968;50:466.
113. Sharrard WJ, Drennan JC. Osteotomy-excision of the spine for lumbar kyphosis in older children with myelomeningocele. J Bone Joint Surg [Br] 1972;54:50.
114. Sharrard WJ, Grosfield I. The management of deformity and paralysis of the foot in myelomeningocele. J Bone Joint Surg [Br] 1968;50:456.
115. Sherk HH, Ames MD. Talectomy in the treatment of the myelomeningocele patient. Clin Orthop 1975;75:218.
116. Sherk HH, Marchinski LJ, Clancy M, Melchouni J. Ground reaction forces on the plantar surface of the foot after talectomy in the myelomeningocele. J Pediatr Orthop 1989;9:269.
117. Shurtleff DB, Hayden PW, Chapman WH, Broy AB, Hill ML. Myelodysplasia. West J Med 1975;122:199.
118. Shurtleff DB, Lutly DA, Benedetti TJ, et al. The outcome of pregnancies diagnosed as having a fetus with myelomeningocele. Kinderchir 1987;42(Suppl):50.
119. Sriram K, Bobrtchko WT, Hall JE. Surgical management of spinal deformities in spina bifida. J Bone Joint Surg [Br] 1972;54:666.
120. Stein SC, Feldman JG, Friedlander M, Klein RJ. Is myelomeningocele a disappearing disease? Pediatrics 1982;69:511.
121. Stevens PM, Toomey E. Fibular-achilles tenodesis for paralytic ankle valgus. J Pediatr Orthop 1988;8:169.
122. Stillwell A, Menelaus MB. Walking ability after transplantation of the iliopsoas—a long term follow up. J Bone Joint Surg [Br] 1984;66(5):656.
123. Sutherland DH. Gait disorders in childhood and adolescence. Baltimore: Williams & Wilkins, 1984:631.
124. Sutherland DH. An electromyographic study of the plantar flexors of the ankle in normal walking on the level. J Bone Joint Surg [Am] 1966;48:66.
125. Thomas LI, Thompson TC, Strub LR. Transplantation of the external oblique muscle for adductor paralysis. J Bone Joint Surg [Am] 1950;32:207.
126. Toriello HV, Higgins JV. Occurrence of neural tube defects among first, second, and third degree relatives of proband—results of a USA study. Am J Med Genet 1987;15:601.
127. Tosi LL, Slater JE, Shaer C, Mostello LA. Latex allergy in spina bifida patients—prevalence and surgical implications. J Pediatr Orthop 1993;13:709.
128. Trieshmann H, Millis M, Hall J, Watts H. Sliding calcaneal osteotomy for treatment of hindfoot deformity. Orthop Trans 1980;4:305.
129. Turco VJ. Surgical correction of the resistant clubfoot: one stage posteromedial release with internal fixation: a preliminary report. J Bone Joint Surg [Am] 1971;53:477.
130. Turner A. Hand function in children with myelomeningocele. J Bone Joint Surg [Br] 1985;67(2):266.

131. Tylkowski CM. Assessment of gait in children and adolescents. In: Morrissy RT, ed. Pediatric orthopaedics. Vol. 1. Philadelphia: JB Lippincott, 1990;XX:57.
132. von Recklinghausen F. Untersuchungen uber die spina bifida. Arch Pathol Anat 1886;105:243.
133. Walker G. The early management of varus feet in myelomeningocele. J Bone Joint Surg [Br] 1971;53:462.
134. Warner WC Jr, Fackler CD. Comparison of two instrumentation techniques in treatment of lumbar kyphosis in myelodysplasia. J Pediatr Orthop 1993;13:704.
135. Watts HG. Circumcision as a treatment for clubfeet. Orthop Trans 1984;8:448.
136. Weisl H. Coxa vara in spina bifida. J Bone Joint Surg [Br] 1983;65(2):128.
137. Williams JJ, Graham GP, Dunne KB, Menelaus MB. Late knee problems in myelomeningocele. J Pediatr Orthop 1993;13:701.
138. Winter RB, Moe JN, Eilers VE. Congenital scoliosis. A study of 234 patients treated and untreated. Part I. Natural history. Part II. Treatment. J Bone Joint Surg [Am] 1968;50:1.
139. Wolfe PH. Development and motivational concepts in Piaget's sensory-motor theory of intelligence. J Am Acad Child Adolesc Psychiatry 1963;2:225.
140. Yates JRW, Ferguson-Smith MA, et al. Is disordered folate metabolism the basis for the genetic predisposition to neural tube defects? Clin Genet 1987;31:279.
141. Yen S, MacMahon B. Genetics of anencephaly and spina bifida. Lancet 1968;2:623.
142. Yngve DA, Douglas R, Roberts JM. The reciprocating gait orthosis in myelomeningocele. J Pediatr Orthop 1984;4(3):304.
143. Yngve DA, Lindseth RE. Effectiveness of muscular transfer in myelomeningocele hips measured by radiographic indices. J Pediatr Orthop 1982;2:121.

Chapter 15

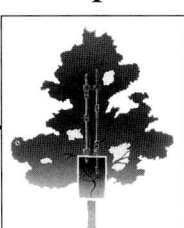

Neuromuscular Disorders

George H. Thompson

Lovell & Winter's Pediatric Orthopaedics, fourth edition, edited by Raymond T. Morrissy and Stuart L. Weinstein. Lippincott–Raven Publishers, Philadelphia © 1996.

History
Physical Examination
Diagnostic Studies
   Hematologic Studies
   Electromyography
   Nerve Conduction Studies
   Muscle Biopsy
   Nerve Biopsy
   Other Studies
   Genetic and Molecular Biology Studies
Muscular Dystrophies
   Sex-Linked Muscular Dystrophies
   Autosomal Recessive Muscular Dystrophies
   Autosomal Dominant Muscular Dystrophies
   Myotonia
   Congenital Myopathies
   Congenital Muscular Dystrophy
Spinal Muscular Atrophy
   Clinical Classification
   Functional Classification
   Genetic Research
   Clinical Features
   Diagnostic Studies
   Radiographic Evaluation
   Treatment
Friedreich Ataxia
   Clinical Features
   Genetic Research
   Treatment
Hereditary Motor Sensory Neuropathies
   Classification
   Diagnostic Studies
   Genetic Research
   Treatment
Poliomyelitis
   Pathology
   Management
   Treatment Guidelines
   Postpoliomyelitis Syndrome

This chapter reviews neuromuscular diseases other than cerebral palsy and myelodysplasia. These disorders are less common than cerebral palsy and myelodysplasia but nevertheless appear in pediatric orthopaedic and neuromuscular clinics. These neuromuscular disorders include the muscular dystrophies, spinal muscular atrophy, Friedreich ataxia, hereditary motor sensory neuropathies (HMSN), and poliomyelitis. It is important that an accurate diagnosis be established, so that an effective treatment program can be planned and initiated. Delaying the diagnosis may lead to inappropriate treatment and perhaps further pregnancies in the presence of genetic diseases.[97] An accurate diagnosis requires a careful history, physical examination, and appropriate diagnostic studies.[40]

HISTORY

The history should include the details of pregnancy, delivery, and growth and development of the involved child. Questions regarding in utero activity, complications of delivery, birth weight, Apgar score, problems during the neonatal period, age at achievement of developmental motor milestones, age at onset of the current symptoms, and information regarding whether the condition is static or progressive should be asked. Systemic symptoms such as fever, weight loss, seizures, or other abnormalities should also be ascertained.

The family history is important in diagnosis because these disorders, with the exception of poliomyelitis, are genetic in origin.[114] Family members of an involved child or adolescent may need to be examined for subtle expressions of the same disorder. These same family members may also require hematologic or other studies to arrive at an accurate diagnosis.

PHYSICAL EXAMINATION

Most children who present for evaluation of suspected neuromuscular disease have either a delay in developmental milestones, abnormal gait, or foot deformity. There usually is a history of progression. Physical examination consists of a thorough musculoskeletal and neurologic evaluation. Observing the child walking and performing simple tasks such as arising from a sitting position on the floor can be beneficial. Observing the gait may reveal decreased arm swing, circumduction of the legs, scissoring, or short cadence. Standing posture may reveal increased lumbar lordosis or wide base position for balance. Also, in the standing position, the appearance of the feet can be observed. Pes cavus or cavovarus deformities are common physical findings in many of these disorders. Having the child walk on the heels and toes gives a gross assessment of motor strength, whereas having the child run may reveal an increase in muscle tone or ataxia.

Inspection of the skin should be performed for evidence of skin rashes or other abnormalities. Typical facies of the patient with spinal muscular atrophy and congenital myotonic dystrophy should become familiar to orthopaedic surgeons. The tongue should be examined to detect evidence of fasciculation suggestive of lower motor neuron diseases. Excessive drooling is common in both cerebral palsy and congenital myotonic dystrophy. In the latter, nasal speech may also be present. A thorough ophthalmologic examination is necessary to elicit external ophthalmoplegia or retinitis pigmentosa. Cataracts may develop during adolescence in myotonic dystrophy.

Muscle testing should be carefully performed. Generally, myopathic disorders selectively affect proximal limb muscles before distal muscles. They also demonstrate proportionally greater weakness than the degree of atrophy early in the disease process. The converse is true in neuropathies.

A careful neurologic evaluation usually completes the musculoskeletal examination. Sensory responses must be checked individually and recorded. Decreased vibratory sensation may be present in HMSN, such as Charcot-Marie-Tooth disease. In spinal muscular atrophy, the deep tendon reflexes may be absent but they are increased in cerebral palsy. A positive Babinski sign confirms upper motor neuron disease. Abnormalities in the Romberg test and rapid alternating movements may indicate cerebellar involvement. Mental function evaluation may be necessary because organic mental deterioration may be part of some neurologic syndromes. In many cases, the assistance of a pediatric neurologist can be invaluable in performing a careful neurologic and mental evaluation because minor subtleties may be a clue to diagnosis.

DIAGNOSTIC STUDIES

Appropriate diagnostic studies are imperative in the accurate diagnosis of the myopathic and neuropathic disorders.[110,114,117,138] These can be divided into hematologic studies, electromyography (EMG), nerve conduction studies, muscle biopsy, and nerve biopsy. Molecular diagnostic studies have become available for several disorders, such as Duchenne and Becker muscular dystrophy.

Hematologic Studies

The measurement of serum creatinine phosphokinase (CPK) is the most sensitive test for demonstrating abnormalities of striated muscle function.[90,136] The level of elevation parallels the rate and amount of muscle necrosis and decreases with time as the muscle is replaced by fat and fibrous tissue. The highest CPK levels are typically seen in the earliest stages of Duchenne or Becker muscular dystrophy, in which increases of 20 to 200 times normal may be found.[114] The level of elevation does not correlate with the severity or rate of progression of the disorder. The highest levels are usually found in Duchenne muscular dystrophy. Umbilical cord blood CPK levels should be obtained in all male infants who are suspected of having this disorder.[149] Birth trauma may elevate the CPK in umbilical cord blood, but in the normal child, this elevation disappears promptly. The enzyme level remains elevated in true muscular dystrophy. Serum CPK may be mildly or moderately elevated in other dystrophic disorders, such as facioscapulohumeral muscle dystrophy, Emery-Dreifuss muscular dystrophy, and spinal muscular atrophy. It is also mildly elevated in female carriers of Duchenne muscular dystrophy, although they are asymptomatic. In congenital myopathies and peripheral neuropathies, the CPK levels are usually normal to only mildly elevated. In other neuromuscular disorders that do not directly affect striated muscle, the CPK levels are normal. Serum enzymes, such as aldolase and serum glutamic oxaloacetic transaminase (SGOT), are also important in the study of striated muscle function. Aldolase levels correlate well with the CPK levels.[138]

Electromyography

EMG can differentiate between a myopathic and neuropathic process but is rarely helpful in establishing a definitive diagnosis. Characteristics of neuropathic disorders include the presence of fibrillation potentials, compared with the normal interference patterns.[114] The fibrillation potential represents individual muscle groups firing spontaneously. These potentials are brief, biphasic, and of low voltage in the early stage of a neuropathic or denervation process but they become prolonged, polyphasic, and high-voltage during the chronic phase.

Myopathic EMG is characterized by low-voltage polyphasic action potentials.[114] Myopathies rarely demonstrate EMG changes characteristic of a neuropathy, but a denervation process may show neuropathic, mixed, or myopathic processes. The use of an experienced electromyographer is imperative in the accurate performance and interpretation of EMG data.

Nerve Conduction Studies

Nerve conduction studies are important in the establishment of the diagnosis of peripheral neuropathy in children. Nerve conduction velocities are normal in children with anterior horn cell diseases, nerve root diseases, and myopathies. The normal value in the child older than 5 years of age is 45 to 65 m/second. In infants and younger children, the velocity is lower because myelinization is incomplete.

Motor conduction velocity may be lowered in HMSN (e.g., Charcot-Marie-Tooth disease) before clinical deficits are present. The nerve conduction studies can help determine whether the neuropathy involves an isolated nerve or is a disseminated process.

Muscle Biopsy

Muscle biopsy is the most important test in determining the diagnosis of a neuromuscular disorder.[33] Muscle biopsy material is usually examined by routine histology, special histochemical stains, and electron microscopy. The criterion for selecting the muscle for biopsy is clinical evidence of muscle weakness. Muscles that are involved but are functioning are selected in chronic diseases such as Duchenne muscular dystrophy because they demonstrate the greatest diagnostic changes. A more severely involved muscle may be chosen in an acute illness because the process has not had sufficient time to progress to extensive destruction. In patients who have proximal lower extremity muscle weakness, biopsy of the vastus lateralis is performed, whereas in those with distal weakness, the gastrocnemius is biopsied. Biopsy of the deltoid, biceps, or triceps is performed for shoulder girdle or proximal upper extremity weakness.

Muscle biopsies can be performed as an open procedure[6,62] or by percutaneous needle.[87] The open technique as described by Banker is preferred.[6] The biopsies are obtained either under general anesthesia, spinal anesthetic, regional nerve block, or with a field block surrounding the area of incision. It is important that local anesthetic not be infiltrated into the muscle because this may alter the morphology of the muscle. The vastus lateralis is the most common muscle chosen. A 4-cm incision is made, and the underlying fascia is incised longitudinally. The muscle is looked at directly to avoid including normal fibrous septae in the specimens. Muscle clamps are used to obtain three specimens. The clamps are oriented in the direction of the muscle fibers. A 2- to 3-mm piece of muscle is grasped in each end of the clamp. The muscle is cut at the outside edge of each clamp and a cylinder of muscle excised. Using a muscle clamp keeps the muscle at its resting length and minimizes artifact. One specimen is quickly frozen in liquid nitrogen ($-160°C$) to prevent loss of soluble enzymes. This specimen is used for light microscopy with a variety of special preparations. The wound is subsequently closed in layers. Electrocautery may be used during the closure. If it is used before the biopsy, it may inadvertently damage the specimens and alter the morphology.

Nerve Biopsy

Occasionally, biopsy of a peripheral nerve is helpful in demyelinating disorders. Usually, the sural nerve is selected for biopsy because of its distal location and lack of autogenous zone of innervation. The patient notices no sensory change or only a mild diminution after excision of the 3- to 4-cm segment of the nerve. Hurley and colleagues reported a single incision for combined muscle and sural nerve biopsy.[62] An incision over the posterolateral aspect of the calf allows access to the nerve and either the soleus or the peroneal muscles. This avoids the necessity for two incisions. This technique was demonstrated to be accurate in diagnosing disorders in which both a muscle and nerve biopsy may be necessary.

Other Studies

Other studies that may be beneficial in establishing the diagnosis of a neuromuscular disorder include electrocardiogram (ECG), pulmonary function studies, magnetic resonance imaging (MRI), ophthalmologic evaluation, amniocentesis, and pediatric neurology evaluation.

Duchenne muscular dystrophy, Friedreich ataxia, and myotonic dystrophy demonstrate ECG abnormalities. Duchenne muscular dystrophy frequently has mitral valve prolapse secondary to papillary muscle involvement.[106,147] Arrhythmias under anesthesia have been reported with both Duchenne and Emery-Dreifuss muscular dystrophy.[36,108]

Pulmonary function studies demonstrate involvement of respiratory muscles but do not establish the diagnosis. If respiratory muscle involvement is present, the rate of deterioration can be followed with periodic studies. This is important if surgery is contemplated in children or adolescents with muscular dystrophy, spinal muscular atrophy, or Friedreich ataxia. The forced vital capacity (FVC) is the most important study after arterial blood gas measurements.[72]

MRI has been demonstrated to distinguish muscles in neuropathic and myopathic disorders.[107] Imaging estimates of the disease severity by degree of muscle involvement correlate well with clinical staging. MRI may also be important in selecting appropriate muscles for biopsy.

Ophthalmologic evaluation may demonstrate subtle or more obvious ocular changes associated with specific disorders.

Genetic and Molecular Biology Studies

Genetic research through molecular biologic techniques has tremendously enhanced our understanding of the genetic aspects of many of these disorders.[123] The exact location of chromosomal and gene defects has led to the possibility of genetic engineering, with correction of these disorders. In each of the various disorders, the current status of genetic and molecular biology research, if any, is discussed.

MUSCULAR DYSTROPHIES

The muscular dystrophies are a group of noninflammatory inherited disorders, with progressive degeneration and weakness of skeletal muscle without apparent cause in the peripheral or central nervous system. These have been divided by clinical distribution, severity of muscle weakness, and pattern of genetic inheritance (Table 15-1). An accurate diagnosis is important, both for prognosis and management of the individual patient and for identification of genetic factors that may be crucial in planning for subsequent children by the involved family.

Sex-Linked Muscular Dystrophies

Duchenne Muscular Dystrophy

Duchenne muscular dystrophy is the most common form of muscular dystrophy. Transmission is by an X-linked recessive trait. A single gene defect is found

TABLE 15-1   ***Classification of Muscular Dystrophies***

Sex-Linked Muscular Dystrophy
Duchenne
Becker
Emery-Dreifuss

Autosomal Recessive Muscular Dystrophy
Limb-Girdle
Infantile fascioscapulohumeral

Autosomal Dominant Muscular Dystrophy
Fascioscapulohumeral
Distal
Ocular
Oculopharyngeal

---

in the short arm of the X chromosome. The disease is characterized by its occurrence in males, except for rare cases associated with Turner syndrome. In this rare event, the XO karyotype who carry the defective gene may demonstrate the phenotype found in involved males.[114] This disorder has a high mutation rate, and a positive family history is present in about 65% of cases. Duchenne muscular dystrophy occurs in about 1 in 3500 live male births, with about one third of involved children having the disease based on a new mutation.[114]

Becker muscular dystrophy is a similar but less common and less severe form of muscular dystrophy. It occurs in about 1 in 30,000 live male births, becomes apparent later in childhood, and has a more protracted and variable course than Duchenne muscular dystrophy. This disorder is discussed later but is introduced here because of the similar inheritance pattern and molecular biology abnormality.

CLINICAL FEATURES. Duchenne muscular dystrophy is generally clinically evident when the child is between 3 and 6 years of age. Earlier onset may also occur. The family may have observed that the child's ability to achieve independent ambulation was delayed or that he has become a toe walker. Children 3 years of age or older may demonstrate frequent episodes of tripping and falling in addition to difficulty in reciprocal motion, such as running or climbing stairs. Inability to hop and jump normally are commonly present.

In Duchenne muscular dystrophy, there is progressive weakness in the proximal muscle groups, which descends symmetrically in both lower extremities—in particular, the gluteus maximus, gluteus medius, quadriceps, and tibialis anterior muscles. The abdominal muscles are involved. Involvement of the shoulder girdle muscles (i.e., trapezius, deltoid, and pectoralis major muscles) and lower facial muscles occurs later. Pseudohypertrophy of the calf muscles caused by the accumulation of fat is common but not invariably present. Most patients have cardiac involvement, most commonly a serious tachycardia and right ventricular hypertrophy. Life-threatening dysrhythmia or heart failure ultimately develops in about 10% of patients. Many also have a static encephalopathy, with mild or moderate mental retardation.[79] Death from pulmonary failure and occasionally from cardiac failure occurs during the second or third decades of life.

During gait, the child's cadence is slow and he develops compensatory changes in gait and stance as weakness progresses. Sutherland and colleagues documented disease progression by measuring the gait variables of cadence, swing phase, ankle dorsiflexion, and anterior pelvic tilt.[131,132] The hip extensors, primarily the gluteus maximus, are the first muscle group to be involved. Initially, the patient compensates by carrying the head and shoulders behind the pelvis, maintaining the weight line posterior to the hip joint and center of gravity (Fig. 15-1). This produces an anterior pelvic tilt and increases lumbar lordosis. Cadence and swing-phase ankle dorsiflexion decrease, and the patient develops a waddling wide-based gait with shoulder sway to compensate for gluteus medius weakness. Muscle weakness requires that the force line remain behind the hip joint and in front of the knee joint throughout single limb support.[60,131,132] Weak hip abductors and quadriceps muscles force the patient to circumduct during the swing phase of gait, while at the same time shifting the weight directly over the hip joint. The generalized pelvic weakness requires considerable forward motion to be generated by the spine for the patient to advance. Ankle plantar flexion becomes fixed, and the stance phase is reduced to the forefoot, resulting in even more difficulty with balance and cadence. Foot inversion develops as peroneal strength diminishes. The tibialis posterior muscle, which is one of the last muscles to be involved, is responsible for the inversion or varus deformity of the foot.

Weakness in the shoulder girdle, which occurs 3 to 5 years later, precludes crutch usage to aid in ambulation. It also makes it difficult to lift the patient from under the arms. This tendency for the child to slip a truncal grasp has been termed Meyeron sign. As the weakness in the upper extremities increases, the child becomes unable to move his arms. Although the hands retain strength longer than the arms, use of the hands is limited because of weakness of the arms.

Clinical diagnosis of Duchenne muscular dystrophy is established by physical examination, including gait and specific muscle weakness, and by the absence

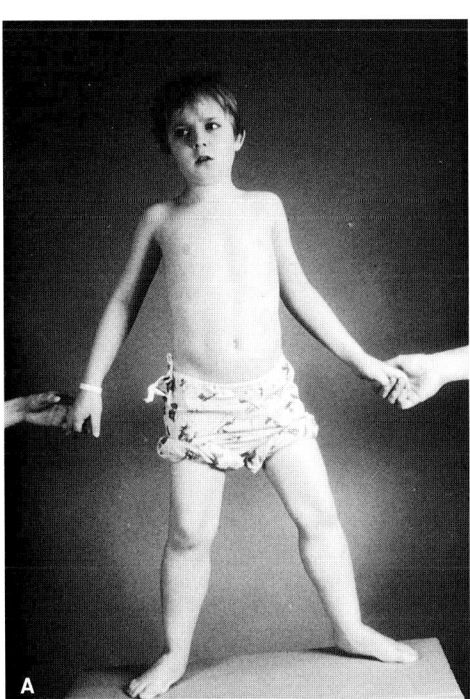
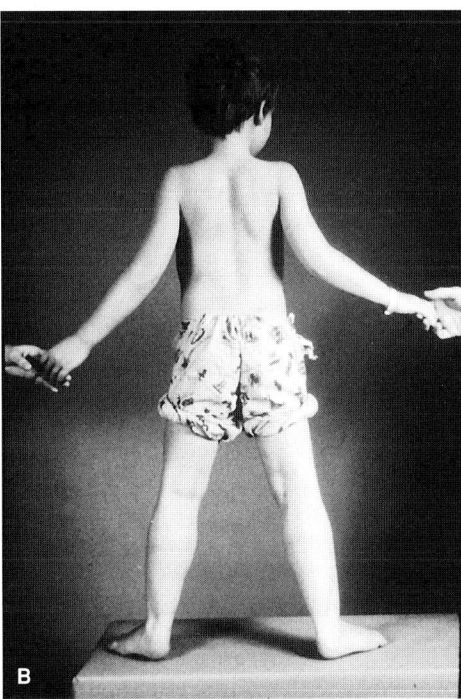
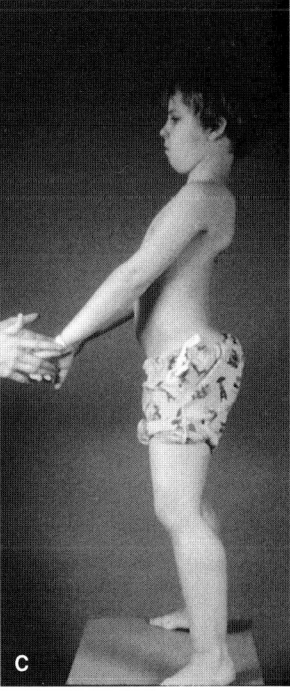

FIGURE 15-1. (**A**) A 7-year-old boy with Duchenne muscular dystrophy demonstrates precarious stance due to mild hip abduction contractures. Observe the pseudohypertrophy of the calves. (**B**) Posterior view demonstrates mild ankle equinus in addition to the calf pseudohypertrophy. (**C**) Side view shows an anterior tilt to the pelvis and increased lumbar lordosis, and the head and the shoulders are aligned posterior to the pelvis. This characteristic posture maintains the weight line posterior to the pelvis and center of gravity, compensates for the muscle weakness, and helps maintain balance.

of sensory deficits. The upper extremity and knee deep tendon reflexes are lost early in the disease, whereas the ankle reflexes remain positive until the terminal phase. A valuable clinical sign is the Gower sign. The patient is placed prone or in the sitting position on the floor and asked to rise. This is usually difficult, and the patient may require the use of a chair for assistance. The patient is then asked to use his or her hands to grasp the lower legs and force the knees into extension. The patient then walks his or her hands up their extremities to compensate for the quadriceps and gluteus maximum weakness. This sign may also be found in congenital myopathies and spinal muscular atrophy. Appreciation of the contracture of the iliotibial band can be measured by the Ober test. To perform this test, the child is placed on his or her side with both hips flexed. The superior leg is then abducted and extended and allowed to fall into adduction. The degree of abduction contracture can be measured by the number of degrees the leg lacks in coming to the neutral position. Tendo Achillis contractures also occur. Contracture of the tendo Achillis and the iliotibial band are the most consistent deformities noted during the physical examination. Macroglossia is also a common finding.

Duchenne muscular dystrophy progresses slowly but continuously. A rapid deterioration may be noted after immobilization in bed, even for short periods after respiratory infections or perhaps extremity fractures. Every effort should be made to maintain a daily ambulatory program. Children are usually unable to ambulate effectively by 10 years of age (range, 8–14 years) in the absence of treatment.[14,37,99,110] With loss of standing ability, the child becomes wheelchair-dependent. This results in a loss of the accentuated lumbar lordosis, which protects the child from kyphoscoliosis.[143] As a consequence, most develop a progressive spinal deformity.

Myocardial deterioration is also a constant finding. ECG changes are present in more than 90% of children with Duchenne muscular dystrophy. The average intelligence quotient of these patients has been shown to be about 80.[79]

HEMATOLOGIC STUDIES. The serum CPK is markedly elevated in the early stages of Duchenne muscular dystrophy. This may be 200 to 300 times normal but decreases as the disease progresses and muscle mass is reduced. CPK levels are also elevated in female carriers, although not as high as in affected boys (two to three times that in normal women and girls). There is an 80% accuracy when the CPK level is repeated at three consecutive monthly intervals.[105] Aldolase and SGOT levels also may be elevated but the elevations are not unique to striated muscle disease.

ELECTROMYOGRAPHY. EMG shows characteristic myopathic changes, with reduced amplitude, short duration, and polyphasic motor action potentials.[114]

MUSCLE BIOPSY. The muscle biopsy specimen reveals degeneration, with subsequent loss of fiber, variation in fiber size, proliferation of connective tissue, and subsequently, adipose tissue.[53] Increased cellularity with occasional internal migration of the sarcolemmal nuclei is present. Histochemical loss of clear-cut subdivisions to fiber types, especially with ATPase reaction and tendency toward type I fiber predominance, are also seen.

GENETIC AND MOLECULAR BIOLOGY RESEARCH. A single gene defect in the short arm of the X chromosome has been identified as being responsible for both Duchenne and Becker muscular dystrophy.[71,118] The status of genetic and molecular biology in Duchenne muscular dystrophy has been summarized by Shapiro and Specht.[114] The gene is located at the Xp21 region and spans 2 million base pairs.[52] It includes 65 exons (i.e., coding regions) and encodes the 400-kd protein dystrophin.[52,54] The large size of the gene correlates with the high rate of spontaneous mutation. Dystrophin is a component of cell membrane cytoskeleton and represents 0.01% of skeletal muscle protein. Its distribution within skeletal, smooth, and cardiac muscle and within the brain correlates well with the clinical features in Duchenne and Becker muscular dystrophy. A structural role for the dystrophin protein is suggested by studies demonstrating concentration of the protein in a lattice organization in the cytoplasmic membrane of skeletal muscle fibers.[27,137] Demonstrable mutations, deletions, or duplications of dystrophin are found in 70% to 80% of involved males.[8,52,54,126] The reading frame hypothesis defines which mutations correlate with the more severe Duchenne muscular dystrophy or with the less severe Becker muscular dystrophy. Mutations that disrupt the translational reading frame or the promoter (i.e., the specific DNA sequence that signals where RNA synthesis should begin) result in a presumably unstable protein, which correlates with Duchenne muscular dystrophy. In contrast, mutations that do not disrupt the translational reading frame or the promoter have a lower molecular weight and semifunctional dystrophin, which correlates with the less severe Becker muscular dystrophy.[52,55]

Dystrophin testing (dystrophin immunoblotting), DNA mutation analysis (polymerase chain reaction or DHA [Southern] blot analysis) or both provide a definitive biochemical diagnosis to differentiate between Duchenne muscular dystrophy, Becker muscular dystrophy, and other initially similar disorders such as dermatomyositis, limb-girdle muscular dystrophy, Emery-Dreifuss muscular dystrophy, and congenital muscular dystrophy.[53,125,126] In the latter disorders, the dystrophin is normal. In patients with Duchenne muscular dystrophy, there is a complete absence of dystrophin, whereas in Becker muscular dystrophy, dystrophin is present but is altered in size, decreased in amount, or both. Nicholson and colleagues[91] reported a positive relation between the amount of dystrophin and the age at loss of independent ambulation in 30 patients with Duchenne muscular dystrophy and 6 patients with Becker muscular dystrophy. They found that even low concentrations of dystrophin in Duchenne muscular dystrophy may have functional significance and may explain the variability of age when ambulation ceases. The presence of partially functional dystrophin protein is sufficient for minimizing the phenotypic expression leading to the milder disorder of Becker muscular dystrophy.[8,52,53] The same tests can be used to improve detection of female carriers.[125,126] Based on smaller than normal dystrophin protein, two atypical forms of Becker muscular dystrophy have been recognized. These include myalgia without weakness in male patients, similar to metabolic myopathy, and cardiomyopathy in male patients, with little or no weakness.[43]

Research involves the possibility of dystrophin replacement in diseased muscles. This involves the implantation of myoblasts, or muscle precursor cells, into the muscles of patients with Duchenne muscular dystrophy.[95] This has been successful in the murine-mdx model of Duchenne muscular dystrophy in producing dystrophin.[94] The results in involved males, however, are unknown.[47,61,74] It is uncertain whether dystrophin replacement will result in recovery of muscle function or whether the myoblasts will be rejected immunologically. Several forms of experimental treatment of Duchenne muscular dystrophy are being investigated. Prednisone has been demonstrated to have some short-term benefits in slowing the progressive weakness.[50] The associated side effects of weight gain, osteoporosis and myopathy limit its usefulness, however.[34,39,81]

TREATMENT. The orthopaedic problems in children with Duchenne muscular dystrophy include decreasing ambulatory ability, soft tissue contractures, and spinal deformity.[40,45,110,114] The goals of treatment should be designed to improve or maintain the functional capacity of the involved child or adolescent.

The treatment modalities in Duchenne muscular dystrophy have been outlined by Drennan and include physical therapy, functional testing, orthoses, fracture management, surgery, wheelchair, cardiopulmonary management, and genetic and psychologic counseling.[29]

PHYSICAL THERAPY. Physical therapy is directed toward prolongation of functional muscle strength, prevention or correction of contractures by passive stretching, gait training with orthoses and transfer techniques, ongoing assessment of muscle strength and functional capacity, and wheelchair and equipment measurements.

After the diagnosis of Duchenne muscular dystrophy has been established and before muscle strength has deteriorated, a program of maximum resistance exercises, performed several times daily, should be instituted.[65,117] This may help prolong strength and delay the onset of soft tissue contractures. Contractures are more effectively delayed or prevented than corrected by physical therapy. Contractures develop in the ambulatory patient as muscle weakness progression results in development of adaptive posturing to maintain lower extremity joint stability. A home exercise program can be effective in minimizing hip and ankle soft tissue contractures. Drennan recommends that exercises be performed twice daily on a firm surface and should include stretching of the tensor fascia lata, hamstrings, knee flexors, and ankle plantar flexors.[29] Occasionally, serial casting may be useful to correct existing deformities before physical therapy. Knee flexion contractures of less than 30 degrees may benefit by serial or wedge casting. This enhances the use of knee-ankle-foot orthoses (KAFOs). Unless orthoses are used after casting and in conjunction with physical therapy, these contractures rapidly recur.

FUNCTIONAL TESTING. Functional testing predominantly involves periodic muscle testing. Muscle strength is tested by measurement of the active range of motion of a joint against gravity. This type of testing allows assessment of the rate of deterioration as well as the functional capacity of the individual.

ORTHOSES. Lightweight molded plastic ankle-foot orthoses (AFOs) or KAFOs are used in independently ambulatory patients when gait becomes precarious, when early soft tissue contractures of the knees and ankle are developing, and after surgical correction of these deformities.[49,127] KAFOs usually are supplemented with a walker because of the excessive weight and the fear of falling. Important prescription components include partial ischial weight-bearing support, posterior thigh cuff, and a spring loaded drop-lock knee joint with an ankle joint set at a right angle. Ambulation may be extended for up to 3 years by the combined use of surgery and orthoses. The maintenance of a straight lower extremity also enables the nonwalking patient to stand with support and thereby assist in transfers.

Spinal orthoses are usually of no value in progressive spinal deformities but wheelchair-bound patients, especially those with severe cardiopulmonary compromise and severe scoliosis, may benefit from the use of a custom wheelchair and a thoracic suspension orthosis. A mobile arm support orthosis attached to the wheelchair may benefit the patient in performing personal hygiene tasks and self-feeding activities.[20,146]

FRACTURE MANAGEMENT. Fractures of the lower extremities occur frequently in children with Duchenne muscular dystrophy. This occurs predominantly after ambulation has ceased and the child is wheelchair-bound. These fractures are best treated by closed reduction and cast immobilization. Occasionally, open reduction and internal fixation may be needed. In children who are still ambulatory, it is important that they be placed on a program of early mobilization to allow weight bearing. This may require the use of an electrically powered circle bed. Once early healing is present, the child can be returned to the KAFO to decrease weight and enhance mobility.

SURGERY. Contractures of the lower extremities and progressive weakness impair ambulation. Surgery is indicated when independent ambulation becomes precarious and when contractures are painful or interfere with essential daily activities. The major contractures amenable to surgical intervention include equinus and equinovarus contractures of the ankle and foot, knee flexion contractures, and hip flexion and abduction contractures. In thin individuals, these contractures may be released by percutaneous techniques.[45,115,121] Orthotic measurements for ambulatory patients should be obtained before surgery. This allows them to be applied shortly after surgery to assist in rapid restoration of ambulation. Correction of contractures and the use of orthoses can prolong effective ambulation by 1 to 3 years.[11,12,32,49,57,60,101,104,110,127,128,144] Hsu and Furumasu reported a mean prolongation of walking of 3.3 years in 24 patients with Duchenne muscular dystrophy, ranging in age from 8 to 12 years at the time of surgery.[60] It is usually not possible to restore functional ambulation once the patient has been unable to walk for more than 3 to 6 months.[11,32,49] Each patient must be individually assessed to determine the functional needs and the best procedures. Common contraindications for correction of lower extremity contractures include obesity, rapidly progressive muscle weakness, or poor motivation in those who prefer to use a wheelchair rather than attempt ambulation.[114]

Equinus contractures occur first, then equinovarus contractures occur. This is due to a combination of tendo Achillis contracture and muscle imbalance induced by the stronger tibialis posterior muscle. This latter muscle retains good function despite the progression of muscle weakness in other areas. These equinovarus deformities can be managed by a combination of tendo Achillis lengthening (percutaneous[12,45,49,57,58,128]; open tenotomy, with or without resection[32]; Vulpius[110,139]; or open Z-lengthening[11,144]) and tibialis posterior lengthening, tenotomy, or transfer through the interosseous membrane to the dorsum of the foot.[11,32,45,46,57,58,84,99,110,127,128] Tibialis posterior transfer prevents recurrence of equinovarus deformities and maintains active dorsiflexion of the foot. Some authors, however, have questioned the necessity of a transfer because it is a more extensive procedure and prefer tenotomy, recession, or lengthening.[12,45,117] Postoperative gait analysis has shown that the transferred tibialis posterior muscle is electrically silent.[80] Greene has reported that tibialis posterior myotendinous junction recession in 6 patients (12 feet) had an increased recurrence rate when compared with transfer in 9 patients (18 feet), which made the former a less desirable procedure.[46] Percutaneous tendo Achillis lengthening under local anesthesia has been reserved for nonambulatory patients who have a typically equinus deformity and cannot wear shoes. The nonambulatory patient with a moderately severe equinovarus deformity may require open tenotomies of the tendo Achillis, the tibialis posterior, and long toe flexors. Severe equinovarus contractures have been managed effectively by talectomy.

Knee flexion contractures coexist with hip flexion contractures and develop rapidly when the patient is wheelchair-bound. These contractures limit proper positioning in bed and may lead to the development of hamstring spasm, causing considerable discomfort when the patient attempts to transfer. A Yount procedure, release of the distal aspect of the tensor fascia lata and iliotibial band, is the most common procedure used in correcting knee flexion contractures.[45,127,128,148] Hamstring tenotomies,[11] recession or Vulpius-type lengthening,[139] and formal Z-lengthening may also be necessary. These procedures enhance quadriceps power and function as well as relieve symptoms. KAFOs are necessary postoperatively to prevent recurrence.

Hip flexion and abduction contractures increase lumbar lordosis and interfere with the ability to stand and to lay comfortably supine. Patients with hip flexion contractures may complain of low back pain. Correction of flexion contractures involves release of the tight anterior muscles, including the sartorius, rectus femoris, and tensor fascia femoris.[45,114] Abduction contractures are improved by release of the tensor fasciae lata proximally with use of the Ober procedure,[92] modified Soutter release,[122] the Yount procedure distally,[148] or by complete resection of the entire iliotibial band.[99,101]

Upper extremity contractures are common in adolescents with Duchenne muscular dystrophy but usually do not require treatment. These contractures include shoulder adduction, elbow flexion, forearm pronation, wrist flexion, metacarpophalangeal and proximal interphalangeal joint flexion, and others. These usually do not preclude the use of wheelchairs. Muscle weakness is the most devastating aspect of upper extremity involvement. Wagner and colleagues[140] demonstrated wrist ulnar deviation and flexion contractures in addition to contractures of the extrinsic and intrinsic muscles of the fingers, producing boutonniere and swan neck deformities and hyperextension of the distal interphalangeal joints in adolescents with Duchenne muscular dystrophy. The treatment of upper extremity contractures involves physical therapy with daily passive range of motion exercises. When passive wrist dorsiflexion is limited to neutral, a nighttime extension orthosis may be beneficial. Surgery for these contractures is rarely indicated.

About 95% of patients with Duchenne muscular dystrophy develop progressive scoliosis.[14,18,41,42,59,89,101,103,116,119,143] This typically begins to occur when ambulation ceases, and it is rapidly progressive. About 25% of older ambulating patients, however, have mild scoliosis.[14,77] Prolongation of ambulation by appropriate soft tissue releases of the lower extremity contractures, which maintains accentuated lumbar lordosis, can delay the onset of scoliosis.[104] The curves are usually thoracolumbar, associated with kyphosis, and lead to pelvic obliquity. Scoliosis cannot be controlled by orthoses or wheelchair seating systems.[18,21,101,109,130,133,141] Orthotic management, although it may slow curve progression, does not slow the systemic manifestations of Duchenne muscular dystrophy (e.g., decreasing pulmonary function and cardiomyopathy). These may complicate spinal surgery at a later time. As the scoliosis progresses, it can result in a loss of sitting balance, produce abnormal pressure, and occasionally cause the patient to become bedridden.[113]

Surgical correction of scoliosis both improves sitting balance and minimizes pelvic obliquity.[9,14,18,41,100,113,130,133,141] It is usually recommended that a posterior spinal fusion be performed once the curve is greater than 20 degrees.[14,18,41,93,100,113,130,133,141] Fusion extends from the upper thoracic spine (T2 or T4) to L5 or the pelvis. It is important to center the patient's head over the pelvis in both the coronal and sagittal planes. This usually allows complete or almost complete correction of the deformity. This maintains sitting balance, improves head control, and allows more independent hand function. Segmental spinal instrumentation techniques using Luque rod instrumentation are most commonly used.[9,15,18,41,45,78,89,100,130,134] Other segmental instrumentation systems such as Cotrel-Dubousset,[24,70] TSRH, or Isola can be used, although there are no published series of long-term results. These allow sufficient fixation, so that postoperative immobilization is not necessary (Fig. 15-2). Fixation to the pelvis with Luque rods, using the Galveston technique or other systems, is debated.[2] Some authors believe that fusion to L5 is sufficient and that there will be no spinopelvic deformity throughout the remainder of the patient's life.[81,88] Others, however, believe that deformity can progress and recommend fusion to the pelvis. Mubarak and colleagues[88,89] recommend fusion to L5 if the curve is greater than 20 degrees, the FVC is greater than 40%, and the patient is using a wheelchair full time, except for occasional standing. If the patient's curve is greater than 40 degrees or if there is pelvic obliquity greater than 10 degrees, then fusion to the sacropelvis is recommended.

Careful preoperative evaluation, including pulmonary function studies and cardiology consultation, is mandatory because of the associated pulmonary and cardiac abnormalities and the risk for malignant hyperthermia.[64,98,102,113,120] Children with Duchenne muscular dystrophy have a decreased FVC, beginning when they are about 10 years of age due to weakness of the intercostal muscles and associated contractures. There is a linear decrease over time.[41,64,72,93,100,113,119] Kurz and colleagues[72] observed a 4% decrease in percentage of FVC for each year of age or each 10 degrees of scoliosis. It stabilizes at about 25% of normal until death. The presence of severe scoliosis may increase the rate of decline in the FVC. Jenkins and colleagues[64] reported that when the FVC is 30% or less, there is an increasing risk for postoperative complication, such as pneumonia and respiratory failure.[64,72,100,113] Smith and colleagues[119] found that most patients with curves of more than 35 degrees had FVC less than 40% of predicted normal values and therefore recommended that spinal arthrodesis be considered for all patients with Duchenne muscular dystrophy when they can no longer walk.

It is debated whether spinal stabilization increases the quantity of life, although it definitely increases the quality of the remaining life. In a study of 55 patients with Duchenne muscular dystrophy, of which 32 underwent spinal fusion and 23 did not, Galasko and colleagues found that FVC remained stable in the operated group for 36 months postoperatively and then fell slightly.[41] In the nonoperated group, it progressively declined. The survival data showed that a significantly

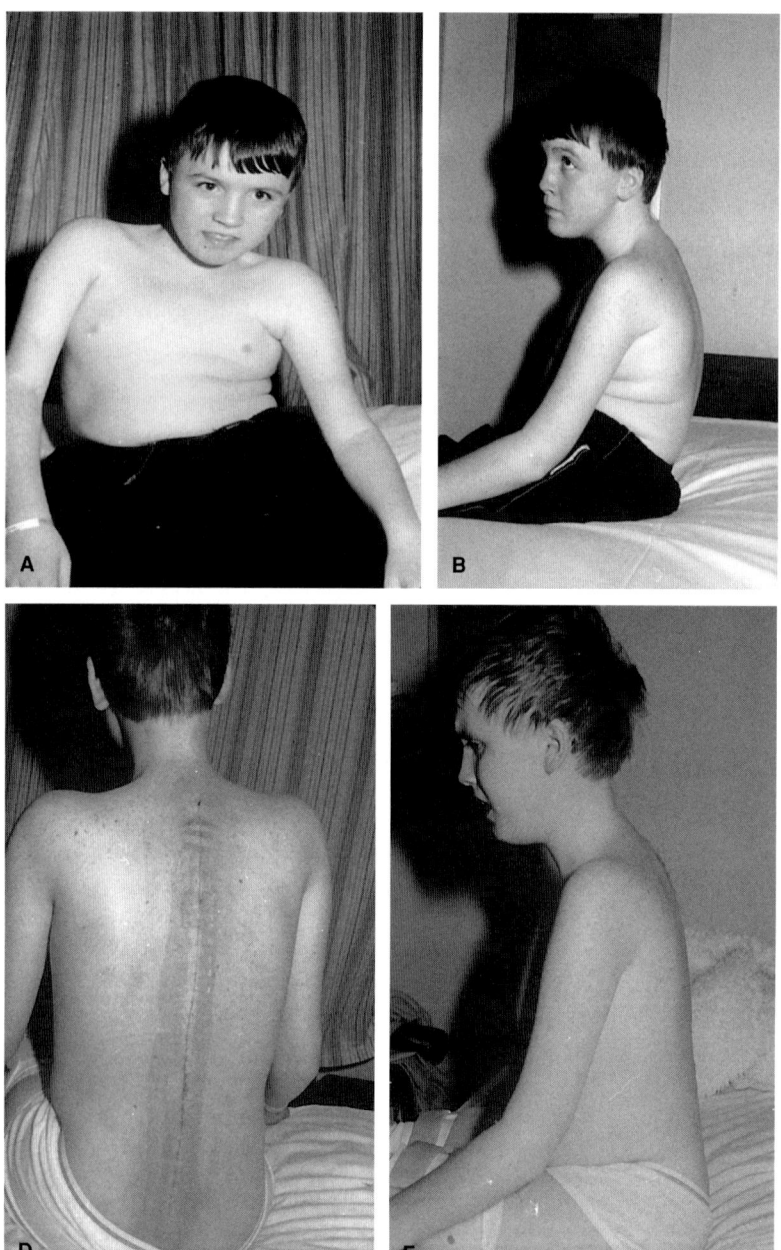
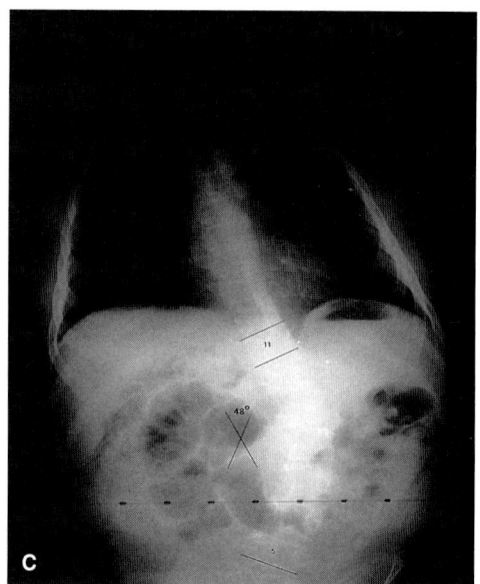

FIGURE 15-2. (A) An 11-year-old boy with Duchenne muscular dystrophy with a rapidly progressive right thoracolumbar scoliosis and decreasing sitting balance. He uses his hands to maintain sitting balance. (B) Side view shows an associated mild kyphotic deformity. (C) Preoperative sitting posteroanterior radiograph demonstrates a long, sweeping, 48-degree thoracolumbar curve between T11 and L5. Six months earlier, no clinical or radiographic deformity was evident. (D) Postoperatively, an immediate improvement in spinal alignment and sitting balance is noted. (E) Side view demonstrates correction of the associated kyphosis. (F) Postoperative sitting radiograph after posterior spinal fusion and Luque rod instrumentation from T4 to the sacrum. The Galveston technique, with insertion of the Luque rod into the wing of the ilium, was used for pelvic fixation. Almost complete correction of his spinal deformity was achieved. (G) Postoperative lateral radiograph shows improved sagittal alignment.

higher mortality rate was seen in the nonoperated group. This study indicated that spinal stabilization can increase survival for several years if it is done early, before significant progression has occurred. Other studies, however, have shown that posterior spinal fusion has no effect on the steady decline in pulmonary function when compared with unoperated patients.[83,86]

Wheelchair. A wheelchair is necessary for patients who are no longer capable of independent ambulation. This is typically a motorized wheelchair to allow the patient to be independent of parents or aides, especially while attending school. The wheelchair may be fitted with a balanced mobile arm orthosis for the purpose of facilitating personal hygiene and feeding.[20,146]

Cardiopulmonary Management. Respiratory failure in Duchenne muscular dystrophy is a constant threat and is the most common cause of death early in the third decade of life. Kurz and colleagues[72] found the vital capacity peaks at the age when standing ceases and then declines rapidly thereafter. The development of scoliosis compounds the problems and leads to further diminution of the vital capacity.[83] The complication rate in spinal surgery increases when the FVC is less than 30% of expected. Programs of vigorous

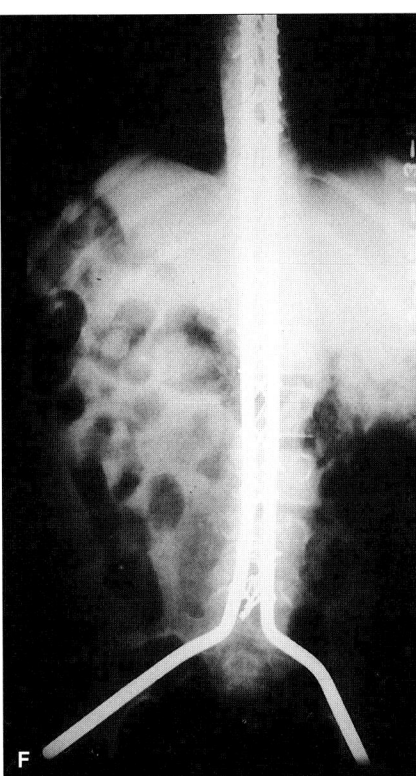
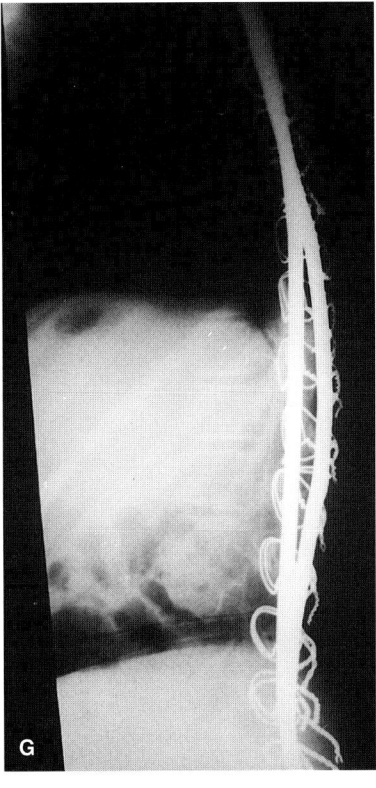

FIGURE 15-2. (Continued)

respiratory therapy and the use of home negative-pressure and positive-pressure ventilators may allow patients with Duchenne muscular dystrophy to survive into the third and fourth decades of life.[1,4,25,51]

Cardiac failure may also occur in the second decade of life. After initially responding to digitalis and diuretics, the involved cardiac muscle becomes flabby and the patient goes into congestive heart failure. Myocardial infarction has been reported in boys as young as 10 years of age. There is no correlation between the severity of pulmonary dysfunction and cardiac function or between age and cardiac function.[129] The cardiomyopathy of Duchenne muscular dystrophy exists clinically as a separate entity.

Genetic and Psychologic Counseling. Proper diagnosis and early genetic counseling may help prevent birth of additional male infants with Duchenne muscular dystrophy. It must be remembered that 20% of families have already conceived and delivered a second involved male infant before the diagnosis is made in the first.[35,73] Genetic counseling with parents and family groups is important in the management of psychologic problems arising when the genetic nature of the diagnosis becomes known.

Becker Muscular Dystrophy

Becker muscular dystrophy is similar to Duchenne muscular dystrophy in clinical appearance and distribution of weakness but it is less severe.[7,13] Onset is generally after the age of 7 years and the rate of progression is slower. The patients usually remain ambulatory until adolescence or early adult years. The Gower maneuver may occur as the weakness progresses (Fig. 15-3). Pseudohypertrophy of the calf is common, and eventually equinus and cavus foot deformities develop (Fig. 15-4). Cardiac involvement is frequent. There may be a family history of atypical muscular dystrophy. Pulmonary problems are less severe and the patient's life expectancy is longer.

TREATMENT. The treatment of the musculoskeletal deformities associated with Becker muscular dystrophy is essentially the same as with Duchenne muscular dystrophy. Ankle and forefoot equinus occur commonly. Shapiro and Specht[114] have reported good success with the Vulpius tendo Achillis lengthening in patients with equinus contractures. A tibialis posterior tendon transfer is performed if necessary. Forefoot equinus may require a plantar release and possibly a midfoot dorsal wedge osteotomy for correction. The use of orthotics is also beneficial because the rate of progression is slower and the remaining muscle strength greater than in Duchenne muscular dystrophy. The incidence of scoliosis is high, especially in those adolescents who have ceased walking. These patients require careful evaluation and periodic spinal radiographs. Posterior spinal fusion and segmental

548 CHAPTER 15 NEUROMUSCULAR DISORDERS

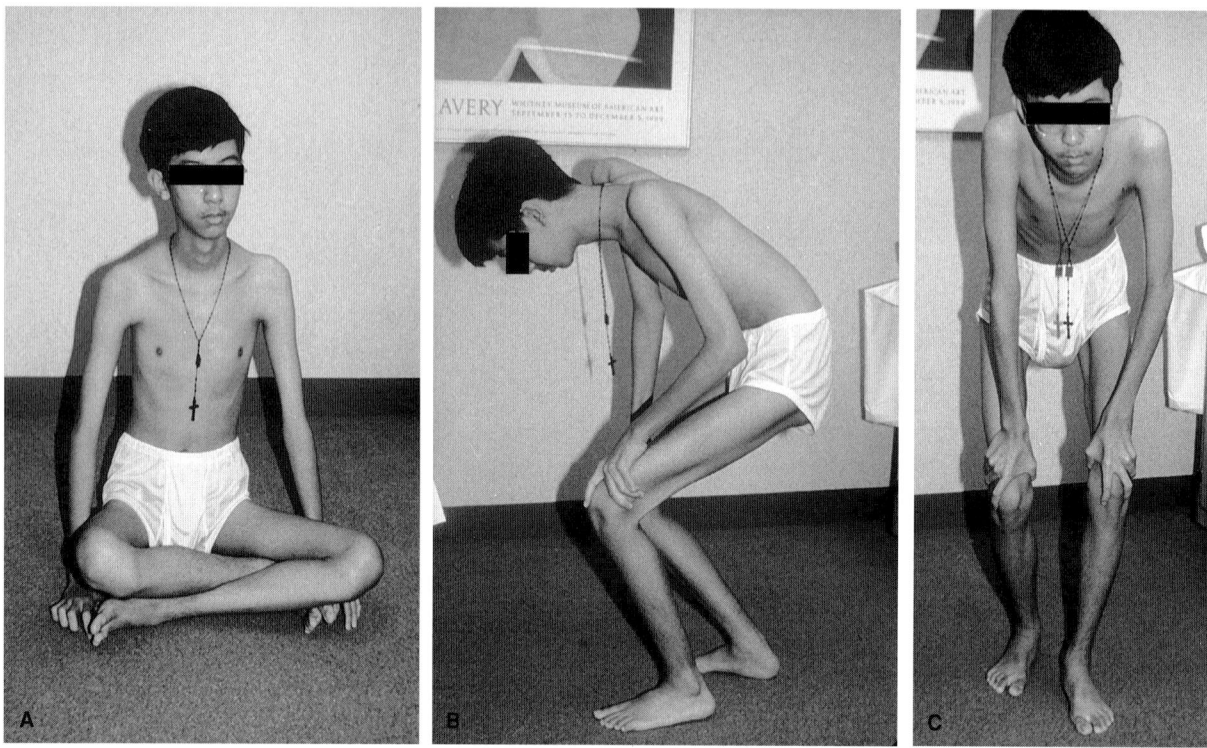

FIGURE 15-3. (A) A 13-year-old boy with suspected Becker muscular dystrophy uses the Gower maneuver to stand from a sitting position. (B) Manually assisted knee extension is necessary to achieve upright stance. (C) Front view.

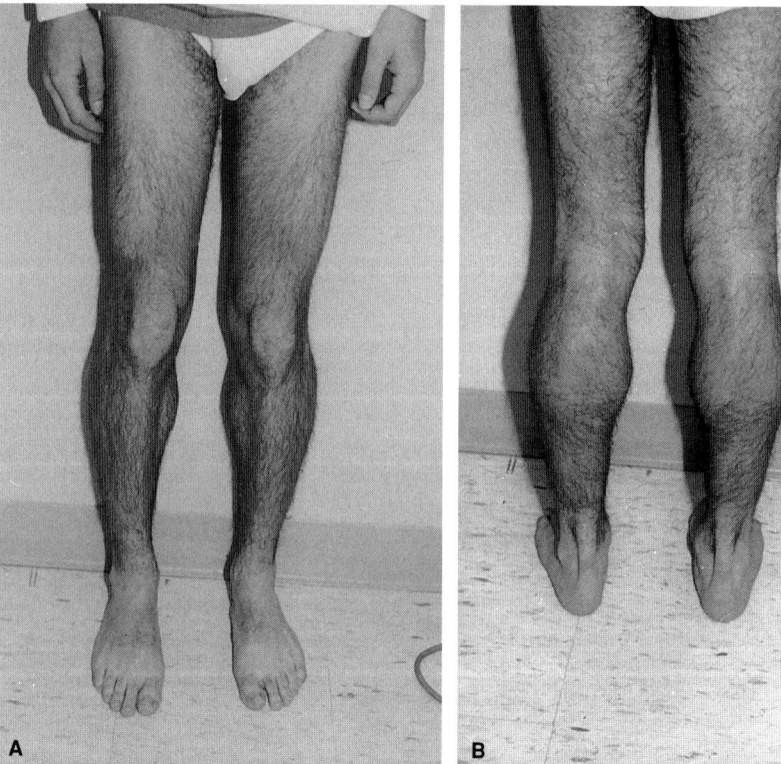

FIGURE 15-4. (A) Pseudohypertrophy of the calves in an 18-year-old man with Becker muscular dystrophy. He is a brace-free ambulator. (B) Posterior view.

instrumentation, usually Luque, are beneficial when progression occurs.[26]

Emery-Dreifuss Muscular Dystrophy

Emery-Dreifuss muscular dystrophy is an uncommon sex-linked recessive disorder characterized by early contractures and cardiomyopathy.[36] The typical phenotype is seen only in males, although milder or partial phenotypes has been reported in female carriers.[28,85,111,124] Involved males show mild muscle weakness in the first 10 years of life and a tendency for toe walking. The Gower maneuver may be present in young children. The distinctive clinical criteria occur in late childhood or early adolescence. These include tendo Achillis contractures, elbow flexion contractures, neck extension contracture, tightness of the lumbar paravertebral muscles, and cardiac abnormalities involving brachycardia, first-degree and eventually a complete heart block.[82,111,124] The muscle weakness is slowly progressive but there may be some stabilization in adulthood. Most patients are able to ambulate into the fifth and sixth decades of life. Obesity and untreated equinus contractures can lead to the loss of ambulatory ability at an earlier age.[114]

The CPK level in patients with Emery-Dreifuss muscular dystrophy is only mildly or moderately elevated. EMG and muscle biopsy are myopathic. The diagnosis of this form of muscular dystrophy should be considered in patients with a myopathic phenotype after Duchenne and Becker muscular dystrophy has been ruled out, usually by dystrophin testing.[114] The condition must also be distinguished from scapuloperoneal muscular dystrophy and the rigid spine syndrome.[44]

GENETIC AND MOLECULAR BIOLOGY STUDIES. The gene locus for Emery-Dreifuss muscular dystrophy has been localized to the long arm of the X chromosome at Xq28 in linkage studies.[22,135]

TREATMENT. The treatment of Emery-Dreifuss muscular dystrophy is similar to that used for other forms of muscular dystrophy. The goals are to prevent or correct deformities and maximize function. Treatment modalities include physical therapy, correction of soft tissue contractures, spinal stabilization, and cardiologic intervention.

PHYSICAL THERAPY. This can be useful in the management of neck extension contractures, elbow flexion contractures and the tightness of the lumbar paravertebral muscles. Decreased neck flexion, which is characteristic of this disorder, can begin as early as the first decade but usually is not present until the second decade. This is due to contracture of the extensor muscles and the ligamentum nuchae. According to Shapiro and Specht,[114] this does not progress past neutral. Lateral bending and rotation of the neck also become limited as the extensor contractures progress. Physical therapy can be beneficial in maintaining limited flexion of the neck.

SOFT TISSUE CONTRACTURES. Tendo Achillis lengthening and posterior ankle capsulotomy combined with anterior transfer of the tibialis posterior tendon can be beneficial in providing long-term stabilization of the foot and ankle.[111,114] Elbow flexion contractures usually do not require treatment. These contractures can be as severe as 90 degrees, although most do not exceed 35 degrees.[111,114] Full flexion from this position and normal forearm pronation and supination are preserved. Physical therapy may be beneficial to slow the progress of the elbow flexion contractures. Surgery has not been shown to be beneficial.

SPINAL STABILIZATION. Scoliosis is common in this form of muscular dystrophy, but it has a lower incidence of progression. This has been attributed to contractures at the lumbar and ultimately the thoracic paravertebral muscles, which seem to prevent progression.[111,114] Those patients with scoliosis need to be followed closely but most do not require treatment. Curves that progress beyond 40 degrees may require surgical stabilization.

CARDIOLOGIC INTERVENTION. Sudden death due to severe brachycardia caused by complete heart block has been a major cause of death in these patients.[82] Most do not have cardiac symptoms preceding death. Merlini and colleagues[82] reported that 30 of 73 patients with Emery-Dreifuss muscular dystrophy died suddenly, and only four were symptomatic. It is recommended that a cardiac pacemaker be inserted shortly after confirmation of the diagnosis.[56,82]

Autosomal Recessive Muscular Dystrophies

Limb-Girdle Muscular Dystrophy

Limb-girdle muscular dystrophy is common and more benign than the other forms of muscular dystrophy. The age of onset and rate of progression of muscle weakness are variable. It usually begins in the second or third decade of life. It is transmitted as an autosomal recessive trait, but an autosomal dominant pattern of inheritance has been reported in some families.[3,17]

The symptoms of limb-girdle muscular dystrophy are similar to fascioscapulohumeral muscular dystrophy, except that the facial muscles are not involved. The initial muscle weakness involves either the pelvic or shoulder girdle. The rate of progression is usually slow, with soft tissue contractures and disability developing 20 years or more after the onset. The patients remain ambulatory for many years.

The distribution of weakness is similar to that seen in Duchenne and Becker muscular dystrophy. The iliopsoas, gluteus maximus, and quadriceps muscles are involved early in the disease process. Usually, shoulder girdle involvement occurs at about the same time. The serratus anterior, trapezius, rhomboid, latissimus dorsi, and sternal portions of pectoralis major muscles are affected most often. The disease later spreads to involve other muscles, such as the biceps brachia and the clavicular portion of the pectoralis major. Deltoid involvement may occur but is usually late. Weakness may involve the distal muscles of the limbs, such as the wrist and finger flexors and extensors, in the more severely involved individuals.

There are two forms of limb-girdle muscular dystrophy. A more common pelvic girdle type, described by Leyden,[76] and a scapulohumeral form, described by Erb.[38] The latter is rare, with symptoms involving primarily the shoulder girdle. Involvement of the pelvic girdle may not occur for many years. In the pelvic girdle type, there is weakness of the hip extensors and abductors, resulting in accentuated lumbar lordosis, gait abnormalities, and hip instability.

The CPK level is moderately elevated in patients with limb girdle muscular dystrophy. The clinical characteristics are indistinguishable from those of sporadic Becker muscular dystrophy, carriers of Duchenne or Becker muscular dystrophy, and those of childhood acid-maltase deficiency.[114] Thus, a dystrophin assay is essential in establishing the diagnosis.

Treatment of limb-girdle muscular dystrophy is similar to that for Duchenne and Becker muscular dystrophy. Significant scoliosis rarely occurs because of the late onset of the disease process. When present, it usually is mild and does not require treatment.[26] Involved individuals usually succumb to their disease process before 40 years of age.

Infantile Fascioscapulohumeral Muscular Dystrophy

Infantile fascioscapulohumeral muscular dystrophy (IFSH MD) has been recognized with increasing frequency. It is a more severe variant of the more common later-onset fascioscapulohumeral muscular dystrophy.[5,19,69,112] It appears to be autosomal recessive, but the affected gene has not been identified. Facial diplegia is noted in infancy, followed by sensorineural hearing loss in childhood (mean age, 5 years). A Mobius type of facial weakness may also be present and progress asymptomatically at a relatively slow pace.[48] Ambulation begins at a normal age, but because of progressive muscle weakness, most patients become wheelchair-bound during the second decade of life. Weakness causes the child to walk with the hands and forearms folded across the upper buttocks to provide support for the weak gluteus maximus muscles.[5,112,114] This marked lumbar lordosis is progressive and is almost pathognomonic for IFSH MD. The lordosis leads to fixed hip flexion contractures after the patient is wheelchair-dependent. Equinus or equinovarus deformities and scoliosis occur less frequently.

TREATMENT. The treatment of patients with IFSH MD is individualized because most patients do not have significant orthopaedic deformities. These patients usually have severely compromised pulmonary functions and succumb in early adolescence. Shapiro and colleagues[112] outlined the possible treatment modalities for children with IFSH MD. Flexible equinus and equinovarus deformities respond well to AFOs. Occasionally, a Vulpius-type tendo Achillis lengthening may be necessary. Hip flexion contractures usually do not require treatment in ambulatory patients and it may decrease function. Spinal orthoses control the lordosis but do not provide correction because the spine remains flexible early in the course of the disorder. Because an orthosis interferes with ambulation, it is usually not employed. When wheelchair use is full-time, a modified wheelchair with an orthosis may be beneficial or perhaps a posterior spinal fusion and segmental instrumentation, depending on the severity of the deformity.[89] Scapulothoracic stabilization is not necessary because the severity of dysfunction is so severe that minimal or no improvement in shoulder function can be achieved.

Autosomal Dominant Muscular Dystrophies

Fascioscapulohumeral Muscular Dystrophy

Fascioscapulohumeral muscular dystrophy is an autosomal dominant disorder having variable expression.[66,73] The disease is manifest by muscular weakness of the face, shoulder girdle, and upper arm. It is caused by a gene defect on chromosome 4q.[142] There is selective sparing of the deltoid, the distal part of the pectoralis major muscle, and the erector spinae muscles. This results in decreased scapulothoracic motion, with scapular winging and a marked decrease in shoulder flexion and abduction. Glenohumeral motion is usually preserved. The onset may occur at any age but is most common in late childhood or early adulthood. It occurs in both genders but is more common in females. Abortive or mild cases are common. Progression is insidious and periods of apparent arrest may occur. Cardiac involvement and central nervous system involvement are absent. Life expectancy is relatively good.

Initially, the face and shoulder girdle muscles are involved but they may be affected only mildly for many years. Facial signs, which can be present at infancy, include lack of mobility, incomplete eye closure, pouting lips with a transverse smile, and absence of eye and forehead wrinkles. It tends to produce a "popeye" appearance. The shoulder girdle weakness leads to scapular winging. The weight of the upper extremities, together with the weakness of the trapezius, permits the clavicles to assume a more horizontal position. It also leads to a forward-sloping appearance of the shoulders. As the disease progresses, pelvic girdle and tibialis anterior muscle involvement may also occur.[66] Scoliosis is rare because of the late onset of the disease process.[116]

The CPK levels in patients with fascioscapulohumeral muscular dystrophy is usually normal. The diagnosis is made by physical examination and muscle biopsy.[10]

TREATMENT. The winging of the scapula, with weakness of shoulder flexion and abduction, is the major orthopaedic problem in fascioscapulohumeral muscular dystrophy. The deltoid, supraspinatus, and intraspinatus muscles are usually normal, however, or minimally involved. Posterior scapulocostal fusion by a variety of techniques can be beneficial in stabilizing the scapula and restoring mechanical advantage of the deltoid and rotator cuff muscles.[16,23,63,67,68,75] This can result in increased active abduction and forward flexion of the shoulder and in improved cosmesis. Jakab and Gledhill[63] reported the results of a simplified technique for scapulocostal fusion. The technique involves wiring of the medial border of the scapula to ribs three through seven. Internal fixation is achieved with 16-gauge wire. The wires ensure firm fixation and eliminate the need for postoperative immobilization and subsequent rehabilitation. The child uses a sling for 3 to 4 days postoperatively and then begins a physical therapy program. They found that shoulder flexion increased 28 degrees (range, 20–40 degrees) and abduction 27 degrees (range, 20–35 degrees) at a mean follow-up of 2.9 years. This allowed all patients to raise their arms and hands above their heads, conferring a greater mechanical advantage. The beneficial effects do not seem to deteriorate with time.[16,23,75]

Distal Muscular Dystrophy

This is a rare form of muscular dystrophy. It is also known as Gower muscular dystrophy. It typically begins after 45 years of age. It is transmitted as an autosomal dominant trait. The initial involvement is in the intrinsic muscles of the hand. The disease process spreads proximally. In the lower extremities, the calves and tibialis anterior are first involved. The absence of sensory, especially vibratory, abnormalities differentiates this from Charcot-Marie-Tooth disease.

Ocular Muscular Dystrophy

Ocular muscular dystrophy, also known as progressive external ophthalmoplegia, is another rare form of muscular dystrophy. It typically begins in the adolescent years. The extract and motor muscles are affected, resulting in diplopia entosis. This is followed by limitation of ocular movement.[145] The upper facial muscles are often affected. The disease is slowly progressive and may involve the proximal upper extremities. The pelvis can be involved late in the disease process.

Oculopharyngeal Muscular Dystrophy

This form of muscular dystrophy begins in the third decade of life and is particularly common in French Canadians.[96] Pharyngeal muscle involvement results in dysarthria and dysphasia, which leads to repetitive regurgitation and weight loss. This condition necessitates cricopharyngeal myotomy, which does not alter pharyngeal function.[30,31] Ptosis develops in middle life.

Myotonia

Myotonia are a group of disorders characterized by the inability of skeletal muscle to relax after a strong contraction from either voluntary movement or mechanical stimulation.[29] This is best demonstrated by a slow relaxation of a clenched fist. The most common myotonias include myotonic dystrophy, congenital myotonic dystrophy, and myotonia congenita. These are all rare disorders that are transmitted by autosomal dominant inheritance.[155,162]

Myotonic Dystrophy

Myotonic dystrophy is a systemic disorder characterized by myotonia, progressive muscle weakness, gonadal atrophy, cataracts, frontal baldness, heart disease, and dementia.[160] The genetic defect is located on chromosome 19q.[161] The distal musculature is affected first and the myotonia begins to disappear as muscle weakness progresses. Onset is usually in late adolescence or early adulthood. In women, the diagnosis is frequently made only after they have given birth to a child who is more severely involved. The disease spreads slowly proximally and involves the quadriceps and hamstrings and eventually the hip extensors. The lower extremities are more involved than the upper extremities. The most common presenting symptoms are weakness of the hands and difficulty in walking. Patients may be unable to relax the fingers after shaking hands and may need to palmar flex the hand to open the fingers. Muscles of the face, mandible, eyes, neck, and distal limbs may also be affected. The level of serum enzymes are normal. Muscle biopsies show type I atrophy of the muscle fibers and the presence of some internal nuclei.[33] These are nonspecific findings. The "dive-bomber" pattern on EMG is diagnostic.[114]

Examination reveals an expressionless face, ptosis, and a fish mouth that is difficult to close. There is marked wasting of the temporal, masseter, and sternocleidomastoid muscles. Deep tendon reflexes are diminished or lost. Slit lamp examination of the eyes reveal that most patients have lenticular opacities, cataracts, and retinopathy. Cardiac involvement is also common and includes mitral valve prolapse and arrhythmias. Organic brain deterioration may also occur. Frontal baldness in men and glaucoma in both genders occurs in midadult life. The course of the disease is one of steady deterioration. Most patients lose the ability to ambulate within 15 to 20 years of onset of symptoms.[154] There are no characteristic orthopaedic deformities, although a slight tendency toward increased hindfoot varus has been observed.[114] Life span is shortened, and death is usually caused by pneumonia or cardiac failure.

Treatment of myotonic dystrophy is primarily orthotic because the onset is usually after skeletal maturity. An AFO may be beneficial in patients with a drop foot due to weakness of the tibialis anterior and peroneal muscles.

Congenital Myotonic Dystrophy

This is a relatively common muscle disorder of variable expression that occurs most frequently with a mother who has either a forme fruste or mild clinical involvement.[150,153,159,165,169] Although it has autosomal dominant transmission, it is predominantly transmitted maternally.[159] This is an exception in autosomal dominant disorders and indicates additional maternal factors. About 40% of patients have severe involvement or die in infancy, whereas 60% will be affected later. The child have may an expressionless long, narrow face; hypotonia; delayed developmental milestones; facial diplegia; difficulty feeding due to pharyngolaryngeal palsy; respiratory failure; and mild mental retardation. Swallowing improves with growth but the hypotonia persists. Examination shows diffuse weakness and absent deep tendon reflexes. It can appear to be similar to spinal muscular atrophy. Ambulation is usually delayed. If the mother is the carrier, there may be other organic disorders later in life.[152] Cataracts usually occur after 14 years of age.

The defective gene has been localized to chromosome 19, and a test for prenatal diagnosis is available.[163] There appears to be an expansion of a highly repeated sequence of three nucleotides; cystosine, thymine, and guanine. The trinucleotide repeat is at the 3' end of a protein kinase gene on chromosome 19, which lengthens as it passed from one generation to another. The length of the sequence correlates with the severity of the disorder.

Orthopaedic problems in congenital myotonia dystrophy include congenital hip dislocation and talipes equinovarus (i.e., clubfeet). There is a tendency to develop soft tissue contractures of other major joints of the lower extremities. Clubfeet may behave like those in arthrogryposis multiplex congenita.[151] Serial casting may be tried, but most require surgery, such as an extensive, complete release. If this fails, a talectomy or Verebelyi-Ogston procedure may be useful.[157] Scoliosis is also common and may require orthotic or surgical intervention.[26] Because life expectancy is at least to the early adult years, aggressive orthopaedic management improves the quality of life.

Myotonia Congenita

Myotonia congenita is usually present at birth but does not become clinically apparent until after 10 years of age. In some cases, it may present as low back pain.[158] The severity of the myotonia varies considerably. The distribution is widespread, although it is more marked in the lower extremities than the upper extremities.[164,166] Myotonia is most evident with initial movement. Repetitive movement decreases the myotonia and facilitates later movements. Usually, within 3 to 4 minutes stiffness disappears, and normal activities including running are possible. Some patients appear herculean because of generalized muscle hypertrophy, particularly in the buttocks, thighs, and calves. Children with myotonia congenita have no associated weakness and no other endocrine or systemic abnormalities. The disease is compatible with a normal life span. A patient's disability is not great when the limits of the disease have been accepted. Procaine amide and dyphenylhydantoin (Dilantin) have been used with some success to decrease the myotonia, but they should be used only in severe cases.[156] There are no characteristic orthopaedic deformities.[114]

Congenital Myopathies

Congenital myopathies and congenital muscular dystrophy is exhibited by a hypotonic or floppy baby at birth or in early infancy. When these conditions occur in an older child, they can present as muscle weakness.[170,176] These disorders are not well understood clinically or at the molecular level. The diagnostic categorization is not uniform or predictive. They are defined histologically from muscle biopsies.[6,114,131] When the biopsy findings are abnormal but not dystrophic, the patient is diagnosed as having a nonspecific myopathy.[114] When considerable fibrosis is present along with necrotic fibers, congenital muscular dystrophy may be diagnosed.[169]

The congenital myopathies include:

- central core disease
- nemaline myopathy (rod-body myopathy)
- myotubular myopathy (central nuclear)
- congenital fiber-type disproportion
- metabolic myopathies.

Differentiation between these types can be accomplished through histochemical analysis and electron microscopy of muscle biopsy specimens.

Central Core Disease

Central core disease is a nonprogressive autosomal dominant congenital myopathy that frequently presents in infancy with hypotonia or in young children with delayed motor developmental milestones.[6,176,180,181,194] Independent ambulation may not be achieved until 4 years of age. The distribution of muscle involvement is similar to that found in Duchenne muscular dystrophy, with the trunk and lower extremities being more involved than upper extremities and the proximal muscles more than the distal muscle groups. The pelvic girdle is more involved than the shoulder. Use of the Gower maneuver is common. No deterioration in strength occurs with time, sensation is normal, and the deep tendon reflexes are either deceased or absent. Muscle wasting is a common finding, but progression of muscle weakness is rare. Muscle biopsies show mostly type I fibers containing central round or oval regions that are devoid of oxidative enzymes, adenosine triphosphate activity, and mitochondria. Serum CPK and nerve conduction studies are normal, whereas EMGs show myopathic abnormalities. Scoliosis, soft tissue contractures, congenital hip subluxation and dislocation, talipes equinovarus, pes planus, and hypermobility of joints, especially the patella, are the most common musculoskeletal problems and can require treatment.[114,168,180,185,192,194] Scoliotic deformities have patterns similar to those of idiopathic scoliosis, progress rapidly, and tend to be rigid. Posterior spinal fusion and segmental instrumentation yields satisfactory results.[114,185] Soft tissue contractures about the hip and knee may need to be released. Clubfeet require extensive soft tissue releases to achieve correction. Congenital dislocation of the hip can be treated by open or closed reduction techniques but the recurrence rate is high and may require osseous procedures such as pelvic or proximal femoral osteotomies.[114,192] Central core disease is one of the disorders in which patients are susceptible to malignant hyperthermia.

Nemaline Myopathy

Nemaline or rod-body myopathy is a variable congenital myopathy that usually begins in infancy or early childhood, with hypotonia affecting all skeletal muscles.[6,114,181,187,193,195,196] There is no involvement of cardiac muscle. Elongated facies, with a high arched palette and a nasal high-pitched voice frequently are noted. Skeletal changes may resemble those seen in arachnodactyly. Martinez and Lake,[187] in a review of the literature regarding 99 patients, recognized these forms: neonatal (severe), congenital (moderate), and adult onset. The neonatal form is characterized by severe hypotonia, with 90% mortality in the first 3 years of life due to respiratory insufficiency. The mean survival after birth was 16 months. The moderate congenital form, which is the most common and prototypic, is diagnosed during or after the neonatal period and has mild or moderate hypotonia, weakness, and delayed developmental milestones. Most patients begin to walk at 2 to 4 years of age, and the weakness is usually nonprogressive or only slowly progressive. The mortality rate is about 5%. Those who die are usually neonates. Death is typically from severe involvement of the pharyngeal and respiratory muscles.[177,186,188] The adult-onset form is characterized by proximal weakness that occasionally progresses acutely. There is no correlation between the number of rods and the phenotype in nemaline myopathy.[193]

Soft tissue contractures are uncommon in nemaline myopathy. The major musculoskeletal problems are scoliosis and lumbar lordosis. Posterior spinal fusion and segmental instrumentation may be indicated in progressive scoliotic deformities.[114] Lower extremity orthoses can be beneficial in providing joint stability and aiding ambulation. Because of diminished pulmonary function and a risk for malignant hyperthermia, patients undergoing surgery require careful administration of anesthesia and monitoring.[174]

Centronuclear Myopathy

Centronuclear (i.e., myotubular) myopathy is a disorder of considerable variability.[6,181] Muscle biopsies demonstrate persistent myotubes of fetal life.[191,197] There is an X-linked recessive and an autosomal recessive form.[175] The defect in the X-linked recessive form is at the locus Xq28. Children have varying degrees of weakness, generally noted in infancy. Patients with X-linked recessive forms are usually severely involved and die in infancy. The autosomal recessive form is hypotonic at birth but is not progressive and may improve with time. Most of these children are able to walk. They may have a myopathic facies, high arched palate, and proximal muscle weakness. There is an increased incidence of cavovarus foot deformities, scoliosis, lumbar lordosis, and scapular winging.[6] By late adolescence or early adult life, some patients lose their ability to ambulate.

Congenital Fiber-Type Disproportion

Congenital fiber-type disproportion is characterized by generalized hypotonia at or shortly after birth. The histologic criteria from muscle biopsies to diagnose this disorder include a predominance in number and a reduction in size of type I fibers and relatively large type II fibers.[6,33] It is recognized as a nonspecific pathologic change that occurs in many patients and has a myopathic, neuropathic, or central nervous system origin.[6,172] The degree of weakness is variable, and sequential examinations determine the prognosis. Most patients become ambulatory. The most serious problem is life-threatening respiratory infections during the first years of life. Proximal muscle weakness is frequently associated with acetabular dysplasia.[171,172]

To prevent postural contractures from developing, an appropriate lower extremity splint should be used until the patient achieves ambulation. Severe, rigid scoliosis can occur. Orthoses are usually ineffective, and early spinal arthrodesis may be necessary.[114]

Metabolic Myopathies

These myopathies represent a broad spectrum of metabolic abnormalities that are generally clinically evident in the first two decades of life.[182] These include disorders of glycogenesis and mitochondrial dysfunction. Myopathies caused by metabolic error in the first step of glycolysis are clinically associated with exercise intolerance, in which there are myophosphorylase and phosphofructokinase deficiencies, or with progressive muscle weakness and wasting, in which there are acid maltase or debrancher enzyme deficiencies.[173] Defects in the second step of glycogenesis are associated with exercise intolerance. Myopathies caused by deficiencies in mitochondrial enzymes are less well defined and may be associated with severe benign exercise intolerance and progressive myopathic syndromes.[173,184,190]

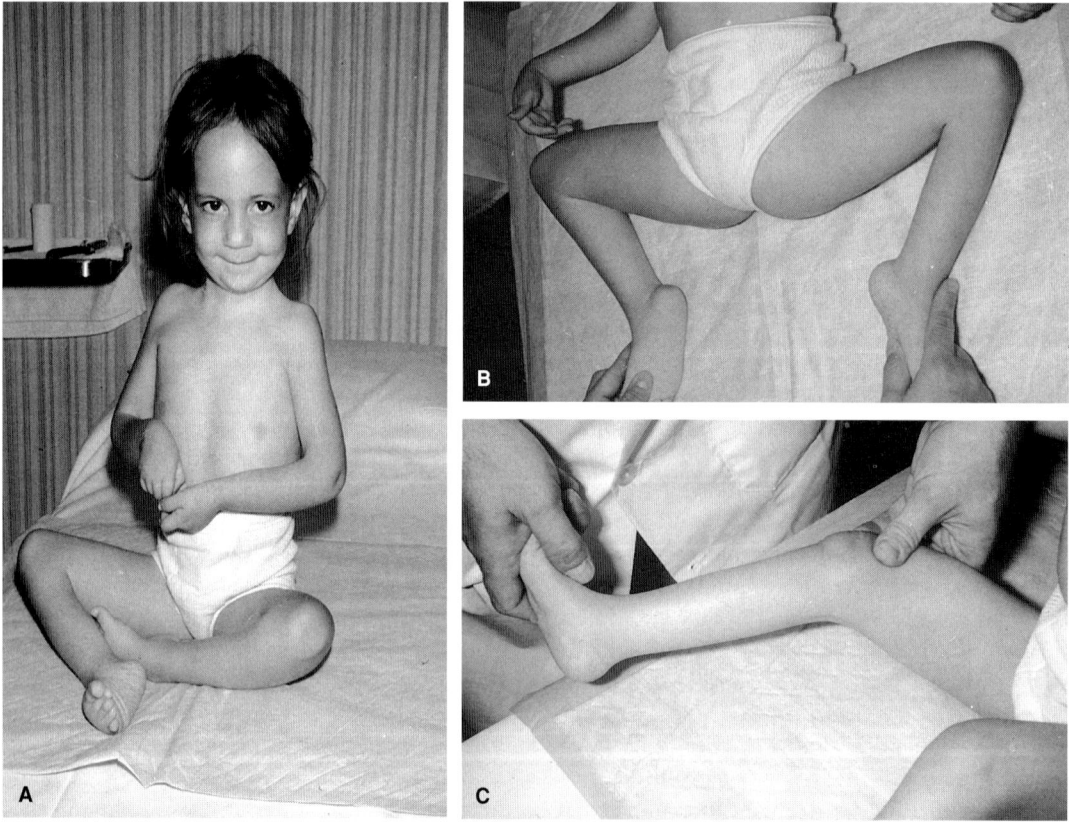

FIGURE 15-5. (A) Clinical photograph of a 3-year-old girl with congenital muscular dystrophy. Observe the position of the upper and lower extremities. (B) The hips are flexed, abducted, and externally rotated. (C) Moderate knee flexion contractures are present.

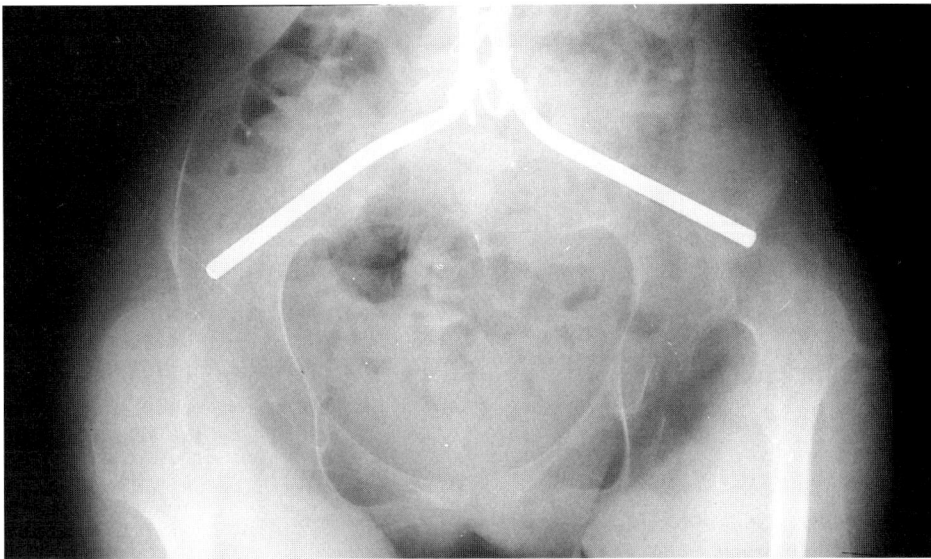

FIGURE 15-6. Pelvic radiograph of an 11-year-old girl with congenital muscular dystrophy, 3 years after posterior spinal fusion and Luque rod instrumentation, including the Galveston technique. She is wheelchair-dependent and has developed bilateral asymptomatic hip dislocations despite extensive soft tissue releases in early childhood.

Congenital Muscular Dystrophy

Congenital muscular dystrophy is a rare disorder that generally presents as a floppy baby during infancy, with generalized muscle weakness with involvement of respiratory and facial muscles. It is a muscle disorder in which the muscle biopsy demonstrates dystrophic features characterized by considerable perimysial and endomysial fibrosis.[169] It is different from Duchenne muscular dystrophy and Becker muscular dystrophy because it affects both males and females, is not associated with massively elevated levels of CPK, does not involve abnormalities of the dystrophin gene or protein, and is associated with a more variable prognosis.[114] There are two forms of congenital muscular dystrophy. In type 1, the infant is weak at birth. Many have severe stiffness of joints, whereas others do not. A few infants have rapid progression and do not survive after the first year of life. Most, however, stabilize and survive into adulthood.[189] Type 2 congenital muscular dystrophy is usually seen in Japanese infants and has been termed Fukuyama congenital muscular dystrophy.[169] It is characterized by a marked developmental defect in the central nervous system.[178,179] There is progressive muscle degeneration and mental retardation. Severe joint contractures develop, and many involved children die in the first decade of life.

Common orthopaedic problems include congenital hip dislocation and subluxation, tendo Achillis contractures, and talipes equinovarus (Fig. 15-5). Because most survive, aggressive orthopaedic management is warranted. This may include physical therapy, orthoses, soft tissue releases, and perhaps osteotomy.[114,183] Early physical therapy may be beneficial in the prevention of soft tissue contractures. Soft tissue releases in the treatment of congenital dislocation of the hip are characterized by a high incidence of recurrent dislocation (Fig. 15-6).[183] Progressive scoliosis may be initially treated by an orthosis, although most require surgical stabilization, similar to other forms of muscular dystrophy.

SPINAL MUSCULAR ATROPHY

Spinal muscular atrophy is a group of disorders characterized by degeneration of the anterior horn cells of the spinal cord and occasionally the neurons of the lower bulbar motor nuclei, resulting in muscle weakness and atrophy. They are autosomal recessive disorders that occur in about 1 in 20,000 live births.[203] The loss of anterior horn cells is considered to be an acute event without progression. The neurologic deterioration may stabilize and remain unchanged for long periods.[174,214,227] The progression of muscle weakness is a reflection of normal growth that exceeds muscle reserve. Respiratory function is compromised, and atelectasis and pneumonia are the usual causes death.

Clinical Classification

The clinical features of spinal muscular atrophy vary widely and are based on the age at onset and the functional capacity of the child at the time of diagnosis. This has led to the disorder being classified into three types. These include type I (severe), or acute Werdnig-Hoffman disease; type II (intermediate), or chronic Werdnig-Hoffman disease; and type III (mild), or Kugelberg-Welander disease.[174,200] All three are a spectrum of the same disorder, but each has specific diagnostic criteria and prognosis. There is a considerable overlap between these three disorders, however, and most authors consider them to be a single disorder—spinal muscular atrophy.[226] Generally, the earlier the onset, the worse the prognosis.

Functional Classification

Evans and colleagues[206] have developed a four-group functional classification that may be useful prognostically.

- Group I: children who never sit independently, have poor head control, and develop early progressive scoliosis
- Group II: children who have head control and the ability to sit if placed in a sitting position but are unable to stand or walk, even with orthotics
- Group III: children with the ability to pull to stand and to walk with external support, such as orthoses
- Group IV: children with the ability to walk and run independently

Other studies have supported the use of this classification.[218,220,225,227]

Genetic Research

Linkage studies have established that the genetic homogeneity for the three types of spinal muscular atrophy occur at the same locus on chromosome 5q.[203,209,210,216,217] The gene product has not been identified, however. The three forms of spinal muscular atrophy appear to result from different mutations at the same single locus. Prenatal diagnosis is available with the use of restriction fragment length polymorphisms. No specific gene therapy is available.

Clinical Features

The clinical features of spinal muscular atrophy vary according to the clinical classification. The clinical characteristics common to all groups are relatively symmetric limb and trunk weakness and muscle atrophy that affects the lower extremities more than the upper extremities and the proximal muscles more than the distal muscles. Hypotonia and areflexia are present. Sensation and intelligence are normal. In infants, gross fasiculations of the tongue and fine tremors of the fingers are commonly present.[214,219] The only muscles not involved are the diaphragm, sternothyroid, sternohyoid, and the involuntary muscles of the intestine, bladder, heart, and sphincters.[220]

Diagnostic Studies

The studies used in the initial diagnosis of spinal muscular atrophy include laboratory studies, EMG, nerve conduction studies, and muscle biopsies. Hematologic studies in spinal muscular atrophy are not particularly useful.[229] The CPK and aldolase levels are normal to only slightly elevated. Electrophysiologic studies, such as EMG, in patients with spinal muscular atrophy show typical neuropathic changes, such as increased amplitude and duration of response.[229] Nerve conduction studies in spinal muscular atrophy are typically normal. Muscle biopsies are usually diagnostic, demonstrating muscle fiber degeneration and atrophy of fiber groups.[229]

Radiographic Evaluation

There are no specific radiographic characteristics that are useful in making the diagnosis of spinal muscular atrophy. The most common radiographic abnormalities are nonspecific and include hip subluxation or dislocation and progressive spinal deformity.[229] Bowen and Forlin[199] recommended that spinal radiographs, posteroanterior and lateral, be obtained in the sitting position to avoid the compensations seen in the standing and supine positions.

Type I, Acute Werdnig-Hoffman Disease

Type I spinal muscular atrophy is characterized by clinical onset between birth and 6 months of age. These children typically have severe involvement, with marked weakness and hypotonia. They usually die from respiratory failure between 1 and 24 months of age. Because of their young age and severe involvement, they usually do not require orthopaedic intervention. Pathologic multiple fractures may occur due to in utero osteoporosis secondary to decreased movement at birth and suggest osteogenesis imperfecta.[204] These fractures heal rapidly with immobilization.

Type II, Chronic Werdnig-Hoffman Disease

The clinical onset of type II spinal muscular atrophy varies between 6 and 24 months of age. These children are less involved than those with type I spinal muscular atrophy but are never able to walk. They may, however, live into the fourth and fifth decades.

Type III, Kugelberg-Welander Disease

The clinical onset of type III spinal muscular atrophy occurs after 2 years of age and usually before age 10 years. Walking is usually possible until late childhood or early adolescence. These patients usually are not able to run. Their motor capacity decreases with time, however, and they have difficulty rising from the floor because of weakness of the pelvic girdle muscles; this is known as the Gower sign. There is atrophy of the lower limbs, with pseudohypertrophy of the calves. Cranial nerve muscles are usually not affected. They have normal intelligence and may function effectively in society. Both the quality and quantity of life may be extended in type II and type III spinal muscular atrophy by the use of nighttime or full-time assisted ventilation.[208]

Treatment

The major orthopaedic abnormalities associated with spinal muscular atrophy include the presence of soft tissue contractures of the lower extremities, hip subluxation and dislocation, and spinal deformity.[229]

Lower Extremity Soft Tissue Contractures

Soft tissue contractures of the lower extremities are the result of progressive muscle degeneration and replacement with fibrous tissue. Ambulation may be promoted and soft tissue contractures delayed by the use of orthoses, such as KAFOs.[211] Contractures tend to occur most frequently after the child becomes wheelchair-bound. The prolonged sitting posture enhances hip and knee flexion contractures. Hip soft tissue contractures may also result in abnormal growth of the proximal femur and predisposes the patient to coxa valga and progressive hip subluxation. Soft tissue contractures without an associated osseous deformity usually do not require treatment. Even when they are released, the sitting posture of the child enhances their recurrence.

Hip Subluxation and Dislocation

Progressive hip subluxation leading to dislocation occurs predominantly in spinal muscular atrophy types II and III. It is important that this be prevented to provide comfort, sitting balance, and maintain pelvic alignment. A comfortable sitting posture is important if the adolescent or young adult is to function in society. Periodic anteroposterior radiographs of the pelvis, beginning in midchildhood to late childhood, are important to allow early recognition of coxa valga and subluxation. Once diagnosed, it is usually progressive because of the continued muscle weakness and soft tissue contractures. Procedures that have been used with some success in the past include soft tissue releases, such as adductor tenotomy, iliopsoas recession, and medial hamstring lengthening. This restores some balance to the proximal musculature. Most children also require varus derotation osteotomy if the hip is severely subluxated.[229] If the hip is dislocated, an open reduction with capsulorrhaphy and pelvic osteotomy of the Chiari type may be beneficial. The usual rotation osteotomies (e.g., Salter, Sutherland, Steel) sacrifice posterior coverage to gain lateral (superior) and anterior coverage. In the child who will be predominantly in a sitting position, this lack of posterior coverage may predispose the patient to a posterior subluxation. Therefore, the pelvic osteotomy method chosen must allow improved posterior coverage. This is usually accomplished with the Chiari osteotomy or perhaps a shelf procedure. Even after satisfactory alignment of the hip, resubluxation and dislocation can occur due to the progressive degeneration of the proximal muscles.[230] These children require annual clinical and radiographic evaluation to assess the hips postoperatively. Thompson and Larsen[230] reported four cases of recurrent hip dislocation after corrective surgery. Two patients had second operations followed by recurrent dislocation. They questioned the advisability of treatment of hip dislocations in patients with spinal muscular atrophy; this approach remains controversial.

Spinal Deformity

Most children who survive into adolescence develop a progressive spinal deformity. This occurs in 100% of the spinal muscular atrophy children and adolescents with type II and most of those with type III, especially when they lose their ability to walk.[199,202,206,212,221,224,227] As in other neuromuscular disorders, as the curve progresses, there is an adverse effect on pulmonary functions.[199,224]

The deformity typically begins in the first decade due to severe truncal weakness. Once the deformity begins, it is steadily progressive and can reach severe magnitude unless appropriately managed. The thoracolumbar paralytic C-shaped and single thoracic patterns, usually curved to the right, are most common. About 30% of children also have an associated kyphosis, which is also progressive.[212,223] In type II spinal muscular atrophy, the mean expected increase in scoliosis is 8.3 degrees per year, whereas in type III it is 2.9 degrees per year.

Orthotic Management

Bracing is ineffective in preventing or halting the progression of scoliosis or kyphosis in children with spinal muscular atrophy.[198,206,212,213,218,221,222,223,227,228] It can be effective in slowing the rate of progression in young ambulatory children, however. This has the advantage of allowing them to reach an older, more suitable age to undergo surgical intervention. Bowen and Forlin[199] recommended orthotic treatment to help maintain posture or slow curve progression in a child 9 years of age or younger with a deformity between 20 and 40 degrees. The thoracolumbar spinal orthosis (TLSO) is the most common orthosis used in children with spinal muscular atrophy. This orthosis must be carefully molded to distribute the forces over a large surface area to prevent skin irritation and breakdown, a major problem for children with neuromuscular diseases. Furumasu and colleagues[207] found that orthoses decreased function because of less spinal flexibility.

Occasionally, wheelchair modifications can also be effective in controlling truncal alignment and improving sitting posture.[229] This also may be beneficial in slowing the rate of curve progression.

Surgery

The criteria for surgical spinal stabilization in spinal muscular atrophy include curve magnitude greater than 40 degrees, satisfactory flexibility on supine lateral bending radiographs, and an FVC greater than 40% of normal.[229] When these criteria are met, a posterior spinal fusion using segmental spinal instrumentation techniques, such as Luque rod instrumentation and sublaminar wires, are used (Fig. 15-7).[9,78,134,198,199,201,202,205-207,212,213,215,218,221,222,227,228] Other systems, such as Cotrel-Dubousset, Texas Scottish Rite Hospital, and Isola can also be considered. These, however, do not usually distribute the forces of instrumentation throughout the spine as well as the Luque rods with sublaminar wiring. The spine is usually osteopenic, and there is a risk for bone failure unless the forces of instrumentation are minimized through extensive distribution. Fixation to the pelvis using the Galveston technique[1,3] or other techniques is controversial. In most children who are nonambulatory and have pelvic obliquity, fusion to the pelvis provides improved spinopelvic stability and alignment. Anterior spinal fusion and instrumentation is rarely indicated because of the compromised pulmonary status of these children. This may predispose the patient to pulmonary complications postoperatively.[198,218] Anterior fusions alone are also too short and do not adequately stabilize the entire spine. When performed, it is combined with a simultaneous or staged posterior spinal fusion, usually with Luque rod instrumentation.[9,199] Whatever posterior instrumentation system is used, it is important that no postoperative immobilization be necessary; this enhances sitting balance and pulmonary status and makes transfers easier.

Decreased function has been observed after spine fusion.[202,207] Although spinal alignment and sitting balance are improved the loss of spinal mobility decreases the function of the upper extremities and activities of daily living such as performing transfers and personal hygiene.

Operative complications are similar to other neuromuscular disorders. These include excessive blood loss, pulmonary complications, wound infection, loss of fixation due to osteopenia, pseudarthrosis, and death.[9,134,198,202,205,221,222,223] The use of segmental spinal instrumentation techniques and aggressive preoperative and postoperative respiratory therapy can result in decreased complications.

FRIEDREICH ATAXIA

Spinocerebellar degenerative diseases are a group of relatively uncommon disorders that are hereditary and progressive. Friedreich ataxia is the most common form and has orthopaedic implications because of its high incidence of scoliosis. Friedreich ataxia is characterized by slow, progressive spinocerebellar degeneration. It occurs in about 1 in 50,000 live births.[235] It is autosomal recessive and occurs most commonly in North America in people of French Canadian heritage. Males and females are affected equally.

Clinical Features

Friedreich ataxia is characterized by a clinical triad consisting of ataxia, which is usually the presenting symptom, areflexia of the knees and ankles, and a positive plantar response, or the Babinski sign.[229] Geoffroy and colleagues[236] established strict criteria for the clinical diagnosis of typical Friedreich ataxia. This has been modified by Harding.[237] The primary symptoms and signs that occur in all involved patients include onset before the age of 25 years; progressive ataxia of limbs and gait; absent knee and ankle deep tendon reflexes; positive plantar response; decreased nerve conduction velocities in the upper extremities, with small or absent sensory action potentials; and dysarthria. The secondary symptoms and signs that are present in more than 90% of cases include scoliosis, pyramidal weakness in the lower extremities, absent reflexes in the upper extremities, loss of position and vibratory sense in the lower extremities, and an abnormal ECG. Accessory symptoms and signs present in fewer than 50% of cases include optic atrophy, nystag-

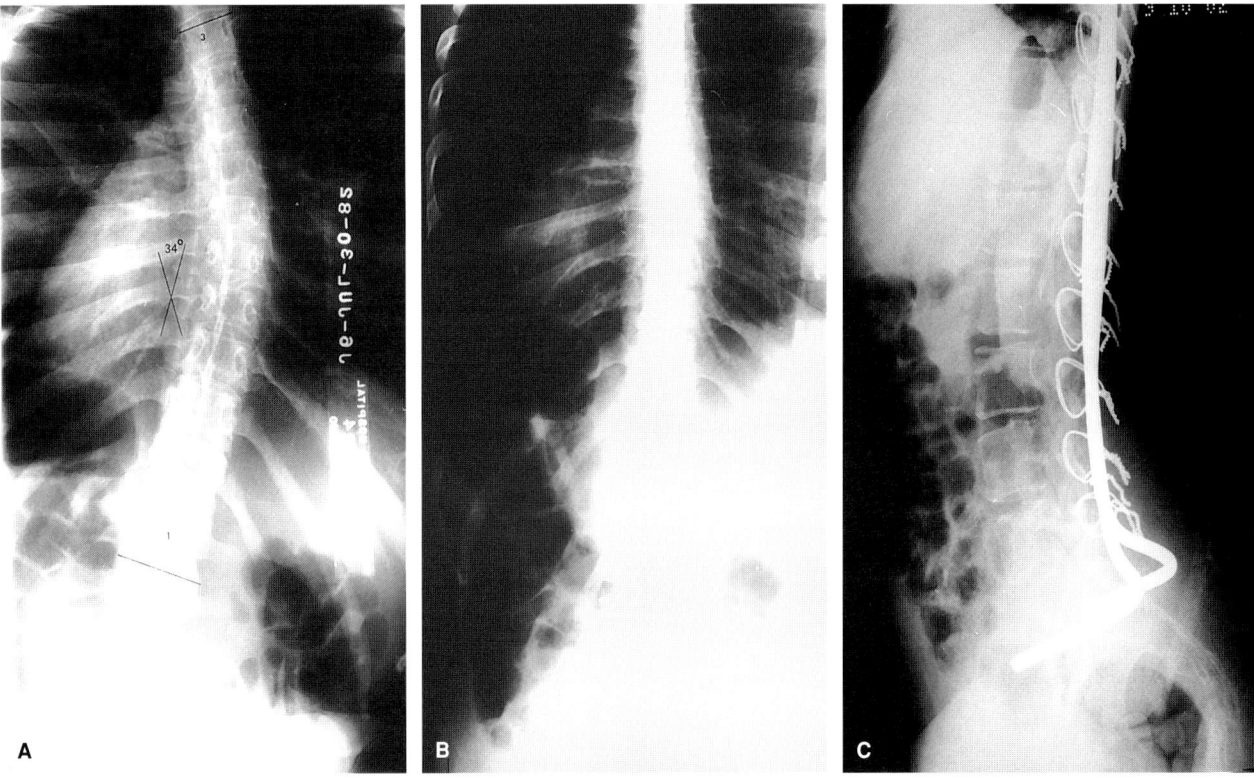

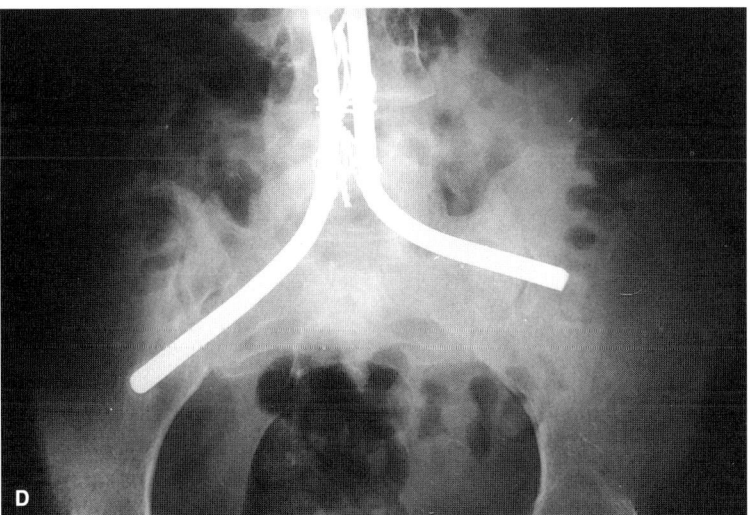

FIGURE 15-7. (A) Sitting posteroanterior spinal radiograph of an 18-year-old woman with spinal muscular atrophy. A slowly progressive scoliosis has affected her wheelchair sitting balance. (B) Postoperative radiograph after posterior spinal fusion and Luque rod instrumentation using the Galveston technique, provided almost complete correction of the spinal deformity. Thirteen years postoperatively, she functions independently despite the subsequent need for a tracheostomy and ventilator support. (C) Lateral view demonstrates preservation of lumbar lordosis, which is important for proper sitting balance. (D) Anteroposterior view of the pelvis shows proper positioning of the Luque rods in the ilium. They should penetrate as far into the ilium as possible for maximum strength.

mus, distal weakness and wasting, partial deafness, pes cavus, and diabetes mellitus.

The mean age at onset is between 7 and 15 years, although the range is wide, from 4 years to as late as 25 years of age.[231,233,234,236,237,243] Most involved individuals lose their ability to walk and are wheelchair-bound by the second or third decade. Labelle and colleagues[241] demonstrated that the muscle weakness is always symmetric, initially proximal rather than distal, more severe in the lower extremities, and rapidly progressive when the patients become nonambulatory. The first muscle to be involved is the hip extensor, (gluteus maximus). They also demonstrated that muscle weakness is not the primary cause of loss of ambulatory function. Ataxia and other factors also play a role. Death usually occurs in the fourth or fifth decade due to progressive hypertrophic cardiomyopathy, pneumonia, or aspiration.[237,239]

Nerve conduction studies show decreased or absent sensory action potentials in the digital and sural nerves. Conduction velocity in the motor and sensory fibers of the median and tibial nerves are moderately slowed. An EMG shows a loss of motor limits and an increase in polyphasic potentials. The ECG in adults typically shows a progressive hypertrophic cardiomyopathy. Hematologic tests such as CPK are normal but there is increased incidence of clinical and chemical diabetes mellitus.

Genetic Research

Chamberlain and colleagues,[232] in genetic research, have demonstrated that individuals with Friedreich ataxia have a defect on chromosome 9. Additional studies have identified two loci on chromosome 9 (D9S5 and D9S15) that are linked to Friedreich ataxia.[235] The biochemical disorder produced by this defect is unknown, however. The condition appears to be a single gene defect, with variations in characteristics such as age at onset and the rate of progression due to different mutations at one of the loci.

Treatment

The major orthopaedic problems in Friedreich ataxia are pes cavovarus, scoliosis, and painful muscle spasms.[229]

Pes Cavovarus

Pes cavovarus is common in patients with Friedreich ataxia. It is slowly progressive and tends to become rigid. When combined with ataxia, it can result in decreased ability to stand and walk. Orthotic management is usually ineffective in preventing the deformity, but an AFO can be used after surgery to stabilize the foot and ankle and to prevent recurrent deformity. Surgical procedures can be used in ambulatory patients to improve balance and walking ability. Procedures that have been shown to be effective include tendo Achillis lengthening and tibialis posterior tenotomy, lengthening, or anterior transfer to the dorsum of the foot.[229] The tibialis anterior muscle may also be involved and may require either tenotomy, lengthening, or centralization to the dorsum of the foot to prevent recurrence. In fixed, rigid deformities, a triple arthrodesis may be necessary to achieve a plantigrade foot.

Scoliosis

Scoliosis occurs in essentially all patients with Friedreich ataxia.[231,234,237,240,242] The age at onset is variable and usually begins while the patient is still ambulatory. The incidence of curve progression has been shown to correlate to the age at clinical onset of the disease process. Labelle and colleagues[240] demonstrated that when disease onset is before 10 years of age and scoliosis occurs before 15 years of age, most patient curves progress to greater than 60 degrees and require surgical intervention. When the disease onset is after 10 years of age and the scoliosis occurs after 15 years of age, curve progression is not as severe; most do not reach 40 degrees by skeletal maturity or progress thereafter. There was no correlation between curve progression, degree of muscle weakness, level of ambulatory function, and duration of the disease process. The patterns of scoliosis in patients with Friedreich ataxia are similar to those of idiopathic adolescent scoliosis rather than to those of neuromuscular scoliosis. The pathogenesis of scoliosis in Friedreich ataxia appears to be not muscle weakness but the ataxia that causes a disturbance of equilibrium and postural reflexes. Double major (i.e., thoracic and lumbar) and single thoracic or thoracolumbar curves are the most common curve patterns.[231,233,240,242] Only a few patients have lumbar or long C-shaped thoracolumbar curves. About two thirds of patients with Friedreich ataxia develop an associated kyphosis greater than 40 degrees.[233,240] The treatment of scoliosis in Friedreich ataxia can be either by orthotic or surgical methods.

Orthoses

A thoracolumbar spinal orthosis may be tried in ambulatory patients having 25 to 40 degree curves. It is usually not well tolerated but it may slow the rate of progression, although rarely does it stabilize the curve.[231,233,242] In ambulatory patients, an orthosis may interfere with walking because it prevents compensatory truncal movement necessary for balance and movement.

Surgery

In progressive curves greater than 60 degrees, especially in older adolescents confined to a wheelchair, a single-stage posterior spinal fusion stabilizes the curve and yields moderate correction. Curves between 40 and 60 degrees can be either observed or treated surgically, depending on the patient's age at clinical onset, the age when scoliosis was first recognized, and evidence of curve progression. Posterior segmental instrumentation using Harrington rods and sublaminar wires or Luque rod instrumentation has been demonstrated to be effective in achieving correction and a solid arthrodesis.[9,134,231,233,238,242] Other segmental systems (e.g., Cotrel-Dubousset, Isola, TSRH) should also be effective. Fusions are typically from the upper thoracic (T2 or T3) to lower lumbar regions. Fusion to the sacrum is usually unnecessary, except in C-shaped thoracolumbar curves with associated pelvic obliquity.[233,242] Autogenous bone supplemented with banked bone, when necessary, usually produces a solid fusion. Anterior surgery, with or without instrumentation, usually followed by a posterior spinal fusion and instrumentation is limited to rigid curves greater than 60 degrees associated with poor sitting balance.[242] Surgery is performed only after a thorough cardiopulmonary evaluation and under careful intraoperative and postoperative monitoring. Postoperative immobilization should be avoided. Vertebral osteopenia and spinal stenosis is not a problem with this disorder.

Painful Muscle Spasms

Painful muscle spasms occur in some patients with Friedreich ataxia.[229] They usually begin in the late adolescent or early adult years and worsen with time. The spasms are characterized by a sudden onset and short duration. The hip adductors and the knee extensors are commonly involved. Initial treatment is usually by massage, heat, and perhaps muscle relaxants, such as diazepam and baclofen. In adults, if the adductor or quadriceps spasms are interfering with perineal care or sitting balance, the patient may benefit by tenotomies. This is rarely necessary.

HEREDITARY MOTOR SENSORY NEUROPATHIES

HMSNs are a large group of variously inherited neuropathic disorders.[174] Charcot-Marie-Tooth disease is the prototype, but there are other disorders with similar but different manifestations.

Classification

The classification system for HMSN is presented in Table 15-2. HMSNs types I, II, and III are encountered predominantly in pediatric orthopaedic and neuromuscular clinics, whereas HMSN types IV, V, VI, and VII tend to be late-onset and occur in adults.[229]

HMSN type I is an autosomal dominant disorder and includes disorders referred to the peroneal atrophy, Charcot-Marie-Tooth disease (hypertrophic form), or Roussy-Lévy syndrome. It is a demyelinating disorder that is characterized by peroneal muscle weakness, absent deep tendon reflexes, and slow nerve conduction velocities. HMSN type II is the neuronal form of Charcot-Marie-Tooth disease. It is characterized by persistently normal reflexes, sensory and motor nerve conduction times that are only mildly abnormal, and variable inheritance patterns.[229] These two types are clinically similar, although HMSN type II often causes less severe weakness and has a later onset than HMSN type I. HMSN type III is the autosomal recessive disorder, Déjérine-Sottas disease. This disorder begins in infancy and is characterized by more severe alterations in nerve conduction and by

TABLE 15-2 Classification of Motor Sensory Neuropathies

TYPE	TERMINOLOGY	INHERITANCE
I	Charcot-Marie-Tooth syndrome (hypertrophic form) or Roussy-Lévy syndrome (areflexic dystaxia)	Autosomal dominant
II	Charcot-Marie-Tooth (neuronal form)	Variable
III	Déjérine-Sotta disease	Autosomal recessive
IV	Refsum disease	
V	Neuropathy with spastic paraplegia	
VI	Optic atrophy with peroneal muscle atrophy	
VII	Retinitis pigmentosa with distal muscle weakness and atrophy	

sensory disturbances that are more extensive than in HMSN types I and II. HMSN types I and III are due to demyelinization of peripheral nerves. These are characterized by muscle weakness in the feet and hands, absent deep tendon reflexes, and diminution of distal sensory capabilities—in particular, light touch position and vibratory sensation.[229]

The four additional types are late onset and rarely seen by pediatric orthopaedists or in pediatric neuromuscular clinics. HMSN type IV, Refsum disease, is characterized by excessive phytanic acid. HMSN type V is an inherited spastic paraplegia, with distal weakness in the limbs presenting in the second decade of life with an awkward gait and equinus foot deformities. HMSN type VI is characterized by optic atrophy in association with peroneal muscle atrophy. HMSN type VII has retinitis pigmentosa, with distal weakness in the limbs and muscle atrophy.

Diagnostic Studies

Diagnosis of HMSN is made by physical examination in combination with EMG, nerve conduction studies, muscle biopsy, and perhaps peripheral nerve biopsy. The EMG findings in HMSN show typical neuropathic changes, with increased amplitude and duration of response. Nerve conduction studies show marked slowing of the rate of impulse conduction in the involved muscles. A biopsy specimen of muscles such as the gastrocnemius demonstrates typical neuropathic findings, including atrophy of the fiber group, with all of the fibers in an abnormal group having uniformly small diameter. A biopsy specimen of a peripheral nerve, usually the sural nerve, shows typical demyelinization, confirming the diagnosis of peripheral neuropathy.

Genetic Research

Many individuals with the HMSN type I appear to have a DNA duplication of a portion of the short arm of chromosome 17 in the region of p 11.2 to p 12.[256,270,271] Additional studies have shown a human peripheral myelin protein-22 gene to be contained within the duplication.[262,268,269] It is thought that the abnormality in the peripheral myelin protein-22 gene that encodes the myelin protein has a causative role in Charcot-Marie-Tooth disease. Either a point mutation in peripheral myelin protein-22 or duplication of the region that contains the peripheral myelin protein-22 gene can result in the disorder.[265,271]

Treatment

Children with HMSN typically present with gait disturbance or foot deformities. The severity of involvement is variable. In severe involvement, there may be proximal muscle weakness. The major orthopaedic problems include pes cavovarus, hip dysplasia, scoliosis, and hand and upper extremity dysfunction.

Pes Cavovarus

The pathogenesis of cavovarus deformities in children with HMSN and other neuromuscular disorders is becoming better understood.[244,258,259,263,267] The components of the pes cavovarus deformity include claw toes; plantar flexed first metatarsal, with adduction and inversion of the remaining metatarsals; midfoot malposition of the navicular, cuboid and cuneiforms, leading to a high arch (cavus) and hindfoot varus malposition between the talus and calcaneus (Fig. 15-8). HMSNs affect the more distal muscles initially. The mildest cases affect the toes and forefoot, whereas the midfoot and hindfoot are progressively affected with progression of the disease process. Price and colleagues,[264] in a computed tomography study of 26 patients with HMSN I, II, or III, found that the interossei and lumbrical muscles of the feet demonstrated earlier and more severe involvement, compared with the extrinsic muscles. These intrinsic muscles have the most distal innervation. Even with minimal weakness, the invertor muscles, such as the tibialis anterior and tibialis posterior muscles, are stronger than the evertors such as the peroneus longus; this relation favors the development of adduction and varus deformities.

Pes cavovarus deformities are progressive, but the rate is variable, even among involved family members. Initially, the deformity is flexible but later becomes rigid. Shapiro and Specht point to the plantar flexed first metatarsal as the key finding.[229] As the first metatarsal becomes increasingly plantar flexed, this is followed by increasing hindfoot varus and forefoot and midfoot supination and cavus. The block test is useful

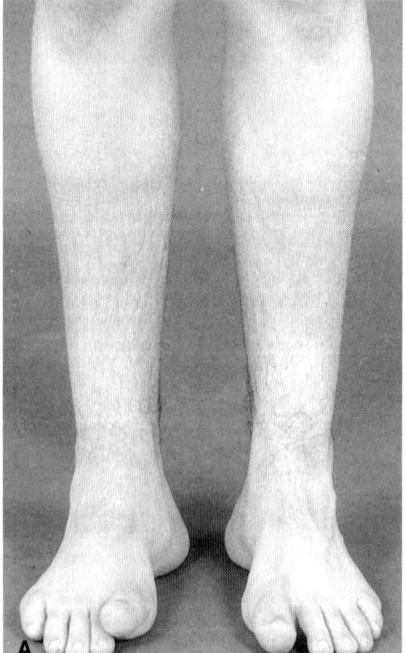 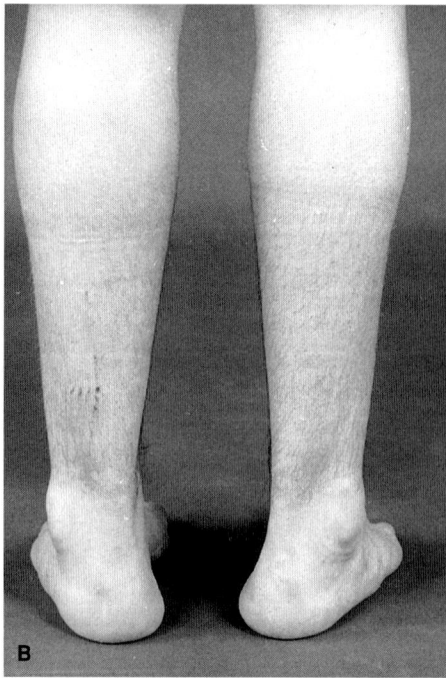 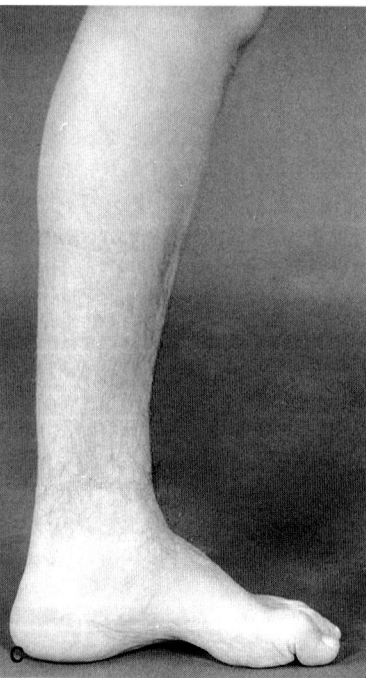

FIGURE 15-8. (A) Front view of the lower legs and feet of a 16-year-old boy with hereditary motosensory neuropathy type I (i.e., Charcot-Marie-Tooth disease). His calves are thin, and he has mildly symptomatic cavus feet. Clawing of the toes is minimal. (B) Posterior view demonstrates moderate heel varus. (C) The cavus foot deformity is most apparent when viewed from the medial side. A mild flexion deformity of the great toe interphalangeal joint is present.

in defining the mobility of the remainder of the foot in children with a rigid plantar flexed first metatarsal.[263]

The goals in the treatment of foot deformities in children with HMSN include maintenance of a straight plantigrade and relatively flexible foot during growth. This maximizes function and minimizes the development of osseous deformities that may require more extensive surgery in adolescence and early adult years, such as triple arthrodesis.

The treatment options for the management of foot deformities include:

- plantar release
- plantar-medial release
- tendon transfers
- calcaneal osteotomy
- midtarsal osteotomy
- triple arthrodesis
- correction of toe deformities.

Plantar Release

In children younger than 10 years of age who have a mild cavovarus deformity, a plantar release may be beneficial in correcting the plantar flexed first metatarsal and providing correction of the associated flexible hindfoot and midfoot deformities.[263]

Plantar-Medial Release

If the hindfoot deformity in the child younger than 10 years of age is rigid, leading to fixed varus deformity, the plantar release may be combined with a medial release. The medial structures to be released include the tendon sheaths of the muscles posterior to the medial malleolus, which include the tibialis posterior, flexor digitorum longus, and flexor hallucis longus; the capsule of the talonavicular joint; and the superficial tibiotalar or deltoid ligament. Once the incision has healed, a weight-bearing cast or series of corrective casts are applied. Excellent correction of the entire foot has been reported after this technique.[263]

Tendon Transfers

In children and adolescents who have a flexible cavovarus deformity in which active inversion is associated with relative weakness of the evertor muscles, a transfer of the tibialis anterior tendon to the dorsum of the midtarsal region in line with the third metatarsal may be helpful.[266] The transfer is designed to balance strength, but the foot must be aligned initially by a plantar release and perhaps the plantar-medial release.

Other tendinous procedures that may be used depend on the individual needs of the patient. These may include tendo Achillis lengthening, anterior transfer at the tibialis posterior tendon, a plantar release, and when needed, flexor-to-extensor tendon transfers for claw toes.[266] Tendo Achillis lengthening is rarely necessary, however, because the calcaneus position of the hindfoot is due to an equinus deformity distal to the talonavicular and calcaneocuboid joints.

Calcaneal Osteotomy

In children who are younger than 10 years of age and who have mild but fixed deformity, a calcaneal osteotomy may be beneficial in correcting the varus deformity of the hindfoot.[229] This osteotomy does not interfere with growth because it is not made through a cartilaginous growth area. To allow lateral translation, the osteotomy is cut slightly obliquely, passing from a superior position on the lateral surface to a more inferior position on the medial surface. It is possible to translate the distal fragment as much as one third of its transverse diameter, thus allowing conversion of weight bearing from varus to slight valgus. In patients who are older than 10 years of age or who are more severely affected, a lateral closing-wedge calcaneal osteotomy, with lateral translation of the distal and posterior fragments, is performed.[229] In both procedures, the osteotomy is stabilized with staples or Steinmann pins.

Midtarsal Osteotomy

The midtarsal osteotomy provides correction by removal of a dorsal and slightly laterally based wedge, with the proximal osteotomy cut through the navicular and cuboid bones and the distal cut through the cuboid and three cuneiforms.[248] Mild or moderate deformities can be corrected satisfactorily with this procedure, especially if it is augmented with a plantar release, calcaneal osteotomy, and perhaps an anterior transfer of the tibialis anterior tendon. Equinus deformities of the midfoot and varus deformities of the forefoot can be corrected with appropriate wedge resections. Growth retardation and limitation of mobility are minimal, compared with those after a triple arthrodesis.

Triple Arthrodesis

In adolescents who have reached skeletal maturity and have a severe deformity, walk with difficulty, and cannot run, a triple arthrodesis can be performed. Every attempt should be made to avoid this procedure because of the associated complications of undercorrection, overcorrection, pseudoarthrosis of the talonavicular joint, and degenerative changes in the ankle and midfoot joints.[245,250,257,274,275] The Ryerson triple arthrodesis is preferred as the joint surfaces of the talocalcaneal, talonavicular, and calcaneal cuboid joints are removed, along with appropriate sized wedges to correct the various components of the hindfoot and midfoot deformities.[253] In patients who have marked equinus of the midfoot and forefoot in relation to a relatively well-positioned hindfoot, the Lambrinudi triple arthrodesis may be performed.[251] Once an arthrodesis has been performed to straighten the foot, tendon transfers to balance muscle power are of great importance.

Toe deformities in adolescents or after a triple arthrodesis may be corrected by proximal and distal interphalangeal fusion or flexor-to-extensor tendon transfer. The great toe may require an interphalangeal joint fusion and transfer of the extensor hallucis longus from the proximal phalanx to the neck of the first metatarsal (Jones procedure). The latter then serves as a foot dorsiflexor.

Hip Dysplasia

Hip dysplasia in HMSN occurs in about 6% to 8% of involved children.[261,272] Occasionally, hips may be dislocatable at birth, although the neuropathy does not become apparent for several years. It is more likely to occur in HMSN type I than HMSN type II because of the more severe neurologic involvement in the former. Walker and colleagues[272] thought that the slight muscle weakness about the hip in growing children with HMSN may be sufficient to distort growth and development, leading to dysplasia. Usually, hip dysplasia is diagnosed between 5 and 15 years of age because of mild discomfort.[255,261,272] Dysplasia may be present in asymptomatic patients, however (Fig. 15-9). Annual anteroposterior radiographs of the pelvis have been recommended to allow early diagnosis and treatment. Typical radiographic findings include acetabular dysplasia, coxa valga, and subluxation. The treatment of HMSN hip dysplasia includes soft tissue releases to correct contractures and restore muscle balance and pelvic or proximal femoral varus derotation osteotomies or both to stabilize and adequately realign the hip.[255,261]

Scoliosis

A spinal deformity was initially thought to occur in about 10% of children with HMSN.[249,252] These children were usually ambulatory, with age of onset of spinal deformity of about 10 years. A study by Walker and colleagues[273] found a 37% incidence of scoliosis or kyphoscoliosis in involved children. The incidence increases to 50% in those who were skeletally mature. Spinal deformity is more common in girls and HMSN type I. Curve progression requiring orthoses or surgery is uncommon. The curve patterns and management are similar to those for idiopathic adolescent scoliosis, except for an increased incidence of kyphosis. As a consequence, orthotic management can be effective in arresting progression of the deformity. If progression reaches 45 to 50 degrees, a posterior spinal fusion and segmental spinal instrumentation can effectively stabilize and partially correct the deformity.[246,249,252] Intraoperative spinal cord monitoring with somatosensory cortical evoked potentials may show no signal transmission. This is due to the demyelination of the peripheral nerves and perhaps to degeneration of the dorsal root ganglion and dorsal column of the spinal cord.[254] A wake-up test may need to be performed.

Hand and Upper Extremity Dysfunction

The upper extremities are involved in about two thirds of individuals with HMSN.[247,260] The involvement

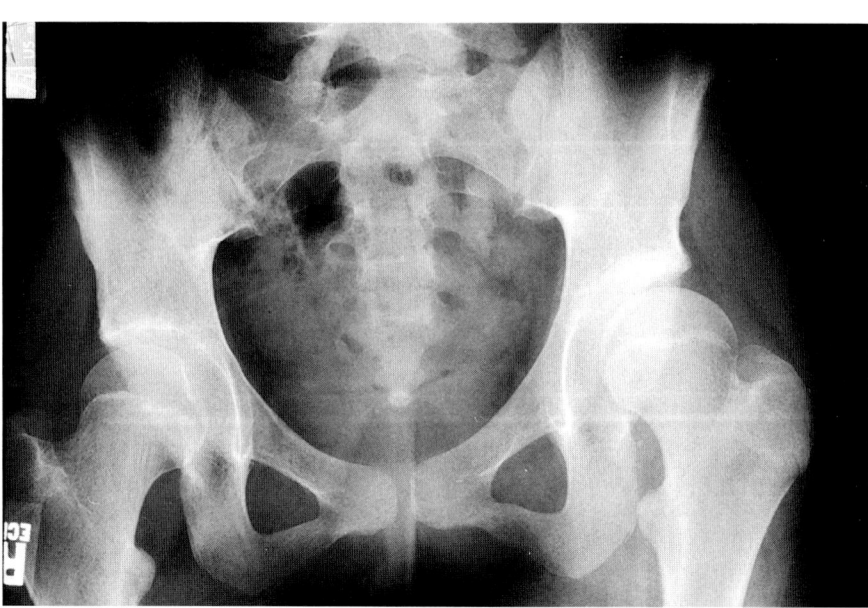

FIGURE 15-9. Anteroposterior pelvic radiograph of a 15-year-old girl with Charcot-Marie-Tooth disease. Asymptomatic acetabular dysplasia of the left hip is visible. The medial joint is slightly widened. The Shenton line is disrupted, and the center-edge angle is 16 degrees. This condition was first observed 6 years previously and did not progress.

tends to be milder, however, and does not appear until a later age. Intrinsic muscle weakness with decreased stability is a relatively common finding. In a study of 68 patients with Charcot-Marie-Tooth disease, the mean age at onset of symptoms in the hands and upper extremities was 19 years. Intrinsic muscle function was initially impaired, and patients became aware of motor weakness and a lack of dexterity. Sensory changes such as numbness are usually present concomitantly. Physical and occupational therapy may be helpful. In some patients, operative intervention, such as transfer of the flexor digitorum sublimis to restore opposition, nerve compression releases, soft tissue contracture releases, and joint arthrodeses, may be effective in improving function.

POLIOMYELITIS

Acute poliomyelitis results from an acute viral infection, with localization in the anterior horn cells of the spinal cord and certain brain stem motor nuclei. It is caused by one of three polioviruses known as Brunhilde (type 1), Lansing (type 2), and Leon (type 3). Humans are the natural host for poliovirus, transmitting the disease by the oropharyngeal route. Each one of the polioviruses has varying virulence. Most poliovirus infections have an abortive course, with only mild gastrointestinal symptoms. Fewer than 1% of infections develop the paralytic form of the disease. Development of prophylactic vaccines has greatly reduced the incidence of polio, although the disease remains a major health problem in developing countries. Fewer than 10 cases occur in the United States annually, and these most commonly result from the use of the active oral polio vaccine.[285,305]

Pathology

The poliovirus invades the body through the oropharyngeal route and multiplies in the gastrointestinal tract lymph nodes before spreading to the central nervous system by the hematogenous route. The incubation period ranges from 6 to 20 days. Motoneuron cells of the anterior horn cells of the spinal cord and brain stem are acutely attacked. In the spinal cord, the lumbar and cervical regions are particularly involved. The medulla, cerebellum, and midbrain may be also involved. Except for the motor areas, the white matter of the spinal cord and the cerebral cortex are uninvolved.

Damage to the anterior horn cells may be due directly to viral multiplication, toxic by-products of the virus, or indirectly from ischemia, edema, and hemorrhage in the glial tissues surrounding the anterior horn cells. In addition to acute inflammatory cellular reaction, edema with perivascular mononuclear cuffing occurs.

The inflammatory response gradually subsides, and the necrotic ganglion cells are surrounded and partially dissolved by macrophages and neutrophils. After 4 months, the spinal cord is left with residual areas of gliosis and lymphocytic cell collections occupying the area of the destroyed motor cells. Evidence exists of continuous disease activity in spinal cord segments examined two decades after the onset of the disease. Histopathologic sections demonstrate a loss or atrophy of motor neurons, severe reaction gliosis, and mild to moderate perivascular interparenchymal inflammation, with sparing of corticospinal tracts. Skeletal muscle demonstrates gross atrophy and replacement by fat and connective tissue histologically. The percentage of motor units destroyed in an individual muscle varies markedly, and the resultant clinical weakness is proportionate to the number of lost motor units. Sharrard has stated that clinically detectable weakness is present only when more than 60% of the motor nerve cells supplying the muscle have been destroyed.[302] Involved muscles can range from those of one extremity to those of all four extremities, the trunk, and the bulbar musculature.

Muscles innervated by the cervical and lumbar segments are most frequently involved. This process occurs twice as frequently in the lower extremity than in the upper extremity muscles. Sharrard[303,304] combined clinical and histologic studies, which demonstrated that muscles with short motor nerve cell columns often are severely paralyzed, whereas those with long motor cell columns are more frequently left paretic or weak. The quadriceps, tibialis anterior, medial hamstrings, and hip flexors are the lumbar innervated muscles most frequently involved. The deltoid, triceps, and pectoralis major are most frequently affected in the upper extremities. The sacral nerve roots are usually spared, resulting in the characteristic preservation of the intrinsic muscles of the foot.[289]

Recovery of muscle function depends on return to function of those anterior horn cells damaged but not destroyed. Clinical recovery begins during the first month after the acute illness and is nearly complete by the sixth month, although there is limited potential for additional recovery through the second year. Sharrard has stated that the mean final grade of a muscle is two grades above its assessment at 1 month and one grade above it at 6 months.

Management

Management of poliomyelitis varies according to the stage of the disease process. These are designated acute, convalescent, and chronic stages. Because the acute and convalescent stages are rarely encountered, in this country, orthopaedic management is usually confined to the chronic stage. Most pediatric orthopaedic programs see several children or more per year with poliomyelitis in the chronic stage. These children are usually adopted from nonindustrialized nations or from parents who have immigrated from such countries.

Acute Stage

Acute poliomyelitis may cause symptoms ranging from mild malaise to generalized encephalomyelitis with widespread paralysis. Diagnosis is based on clinical findings because there are no diagnostic laboratory tests. This phase generally lasts 7 to 10 days. The return to normal temperature for 48 hours and the absence of progressive muscle involvement indicates the end of the acute phase. This phase is usually managed by pediatricians because there may be medical problems, especially respiratory, that may be life-threatening.

The orthopaedist should be familiar with the clinical signs of acute poliomyelitis. Meningismus is reflected in the characteristic flexor posturing of the upper and lower extremities. Involved muscles are tender, even to gentle palpation. Clinical examination can be difficult because of pain during the acute stage.

Orthopaedic treatment during this phase emphasizes prevention of deformity and comfort. This approach consists of physical therapy with gentle, passive range of motion exercises and splinting. Muscle spasms, which can lead to shortening and contractures, may respond to the application of warm moist heat. This can relieve muscle sensitivity and discomfort. Sharrard[302] emphasized that rapid loss of elasticity coupled with shortening of tendons, fascia, and ligaments leads to contractures.

Convalescent Stage

The convalescent phase of poliomyelitis begins 2 days after the temperature returns to normal and progression of the paralytic disease ceases. The phase continues for 2 years, during which spontaneous improvement of muscle power occurs. The assessment of the rate of recovery in poliomyelitis is made by serial examination of the muscle strength. Muscle assessment should be performed monthly for 6 months and then at 3-month intervals during the remainder of the convalescent stage.

Johnson[288] demonstrated that an individual muscle demonstrating less than 30% of normal strength at 3 months should be considered to be permanently paralyzed. Muscles showing evidence of more than 80% return of strength require no specific therapy. He emphasized that muscles that fall between these two parameters retain the potential for useful function and that therapy should be directed toward recreating hypertrophy of the remaining muscle fibers.

The treatment goals during this phase include efforts to prevent contractures and deformity, restoration and maintenance of normal joint range of motion, and assisting individual muscles in achieving maximum recovery.[281] Physical therapy and orthotics are the main treatment modalities. Physical therapy is directed toward having individual muscles assume maximum capability within their pattern of normal motor activity and not permitting adaptive or substitute patterns of associated muscles to persist. Hydrotherapy can also be helpful in achieving these goals. Orthoses, both ambulatory and nighttime, are necessary to support the extremity during this phase.

Chronic Stage

The chronic stage of poliomyelitis begins after 2 years, and it is during this stage that the orthopaedist assumes responsibility for the long-term management resulting from muscle imbalance.

The management goal during the chronic stage is to achieve maximal functional capacity. This is accomplished by restoring muscle balance, preventing or correcting soft tissue contractures, correcting osseous deformities, and directing allied personnel such as physical therapists, occupational therapists, and orthotists.

Soft Tissue Contractures

Flaccid paralysis, muscle imbalance, and growth all contribute to soft tissue contractures and fixed deformities in poliomyelitis. Contractures occur from increased mechanical advantage of the stronger muscles and continue the attenuation of their weaker antagonists. The greater the disparity in muscle balance, the sooner a contracture may develop.

Joint instability does not result in fixed deformity, except in cases in which it is allowed to occur over a period of years in a growing child. Static instability can be controlled readily and indefinitely by orthoses. Dynamic joint instability readily produces a fixed deformity, and orthotic control is difficult. Deformities are initially confined to soft tissues but later, bone growth and joint alignment may be affected.

The age at onset of poliomyelitis is important. The osseous growth potential of young children makes them more vulnerable to secondary osseous deformities. The worst deformities occur in young children and those with severe muscle imbalance. Release of soft tissue contractures and appropriate tendon transfers performed in a young child are important in preventing structural changes.

Tendon Transfers

Achievement of muscle balance in patients with dynamic instability effectively halts progression of paralytic deformity.[301] Tendon transfers are performed when dynamic muscle imbalance is sufficient to produce deformity and when orthotic protection is required. Transfers should be delayed until the paralyzed muscle has been given adequate postural treatment to ensure that it has regained maximum strength and that the proposed tendon transfer is required. The objectives of tendon transfer are to provide active motor power to replace function of a paralyzed muscle or muscles, to eliminate the deformity caused by a muscle when its antagonist is paralyzed, and to produce stability through better muscle balance. The principles of tendon transfer have been well established.[287,294]

- The muscle to be transferred should rate good or fair before transfer and must have adequate strength to actively perform the desired function. On the average, one grade of motor power is lost after muscle transfer.
- The length and range of motion of the transferred muscle and that of the muscle being replaced must be similar.
- Loss of original function resulting from tendon transfers must be balanced against potential gains.
- Free passive range of motion is essential in the absence of deformity at the joint to be moved by the tendon transfer.
- A transfer as an adjunct to bony stabilization cannot be expected to overcome a fixed deformity.[290]
- The smooth gliding channel for the tendon transfer is essential.
- Atraumatic handling of the muscle tissue can prevent injury to its neurovascular supply and prevent adhesions.
- The tendon should be rooted in a straight line between its origin and new insertion.
- Attachment of the tendon transfer should be under sufficient tension to correspond to normal physiologic conditions and should allow the transferred muscle to achieve a maximum range of contraction.

Osteotomies

Osseous deformities may produce joint deformities that impair extremity alignment and limit function. This most commonly occurs in the lower extremity. Osteotomies can be beneficial in restoring extremity alignment and improving function. Because of possible recurrence during subsequent growth, these procedures are usually postponed if possible until late childhood or early adolescence.

Arthrodeses

Arthrodeses are usually performed for salvage except in the foot, where a subtalar, triple, or pantalar arthrodesis may be useful in stabilizing and realigning the foot.

Treatment Guidelines

The basic treatment guidelines for chronic or postpoliomyelitis in children have been outlined by Watts.[307] These guidelines include restoring ambulation, correcting factors that cause deformities with growth, correcting factors that obviate or reduce dependency on orthoses, correcting upper extremity problems, and treating spinal deformities. Understandably, these guidelines allow the child or adolescent to achieve maximum functional level. The specific methods to achieve each guideline are multiple, sometimes complex, and based on careful evaluation of the patient. Because children with previous poliomyelitis are infrequently encountered, specific details on the various procedures are not presented. Such information can be obtained from the references in the various sections.

The orthopaedist must establish a comprehensive plan for each child, based on a thorough musculoskeletal examination, in particular joint range of motion, existing deformities, and manual testing of the individual muscles of the extremities and trunk. The latter should be individually recorded on a worksheet, so that it can be used for future reference. It is important to remember that a muscle normally loses one grade of power when transferred. To be functionally useful, a muscle grade of at least 4 is necessary, although a grade 3 muscle, when transferred, may be an effective tenodesis in preventing deformity by balancing an opposing muscle.

Upper Extremity

In polio, upper extremity involvement tends to be less severe than in the lower extremity. A stable upper extremity, especially the shoulder, is necessary for support of the body weight with a walker or crutches. It is also necessary for transfers or shifting the trunk if wheelchair-bound. A functional elbow, wrist, and hand is necessary for maximum independent function.

SHOULDER. Shoulder stability is essential for all upper extremity activities. Satisfactory level of function of the hand, forearm, and elbow is a prerequisite for any shoulder reconstructive surgery. The major problems affecting the shoulder are predominantly muscle paralysis of the deltoid, pectoralis major, subscapularis, supraspinatus, and infraspinatus muscles. Rarely are all muscles involved because of the multiple levels of innervation. Tendon transfers can occasionally be effective in restoring shoulder stability. When there is extensive weakness, shoulder arthrodesis may be helpful. It can also be indicated whether there is a painful subluxation or dislocation. A strong trapezius serratus anterior muscle is necessary to allow increased function after fusion.

ELBOW. The major problem affecting the elbow is loss of flexion. When the biceps and brachialis are paralyzed, a tendon transfer may be helpful in restoring useful elbow flexion. Possible procedures include a Steindler flexorplasty, which transfers the origin of the wrist flexors to the anterior aspect of the distal humerus.[293] The best functional results occur in patients whose elbow flexors are only partially paralyzed and whose fingers and wrist flexors are normal. Transfer of the sternal head of the pectoralis major also may be considered. Other possible procedures include transfer of the sternocleidomastoid, latissimus dorsi, and anterior transfer of the triceps brachii. Paralysis of the triceps brachii muscle may occur in poliomyelitis but seldom interferes with elbow function because gravity passively extends the elbow. Triceps brachii function is necessary, however, in activities in which the body weight is shifted to the hands, such as in transferring from bed to wheelchair or in crutch walking.

FOREARM. Fixed deformities of the forearm seldom create major functional disabilities in children and adolescents with poliomyelitis. Pronation contractures are the most common disability. Function can be improved with release of the pronator teres and transfer of the flexor carpi ulnaris muscle.

HAND. Tendon transfers and fusions to improve hand function can be considered in selected cases. The number of possible transfers is extensive, and each patient requires a careful evaluation to ensure maximum functional improvement. Carpal tunnel syndrome has also been reported as a long-term sequela of poliomyelitis.[306] This is associated with prolonged use of crutches or cane.

Lower Extremity

Lower extremity problems are most common in poliomyelitis. They can have a significant impact on function, especially ambulation.

HIP. Hip problems in poliomyelitis include muscle paralysis, soft tissue contractures, internal or medial femoral torsion, coxa valga, and hip subluxation and dislocation. Periodic anteroposterior radiographs of the pelvis are necessary to assess growth and the relation between the femoral head and acetabulum. Function can be improved and subluxation-dislocation prevented with appropriate soft tissue releases, tendon transfers, proximal femoral varus derotation osteotomy, and pelvic osteotomy (Fig. 15-10).[291,304] It is important that the procedures be coordinated to provide as balanced musculature as possible, so that hip stability can be maintained. Lau and colleagues[291] reported good or satisfactory results in 70% of patients with paralytic hip instability due to poliomyelitis. The key factors for success were muscle balance, the femoral neck shaft and anteversion angles, and the acetabular geometry.

KNEE. Flexion contractures, extension contractures, genu valgum, and external rotation of the tibia are common knee deformities in poliomyelitis that can have an adverse effect on functional ambulation. Hamstring release, distal femoral extension osteotomy, proximal femoral extension osteotomy, and rotational tibial osteotomies are common procedures.[276,277,296,297] One of the most common soft tissue procedures is that described by Yount, in which the distal iliotibial band, including the intermuscular septum, is released.[148] This may be combined with an Ober release proximally if hip flexion contractures are also present.[92]

FOOT AND ANKLE. Deformities of the foot and ankle are among the most common in adolescents with poliomyelitis. Drennan[281] has discussed possible procedures to correct the deformities and improve muscle balance. This is again achieved with a combination of correction of soft tissue contractures, tendon transfers, and bone stabilizing procedures such as calcaneal osteotomy, subtalar arthrodesis, triple arthrodesis, and pantalar arthrodesis.[278,284,299,308] The patient requires a careful evaluation to determine the appropriate procedures.

Scoliosis

Scoliosis occurs in about one third of patients with poliomyelitis.[279] The type and severity of the curvature depends on the extent of paralysis and residual muscle power of the involved trunk muscles and pelvic obliquity. The most common curve patterns are the double major thoracic and lumbar curves, followed by the long paralytic C-shaped thoracolumbar curve.[295] Pelvic obliquity occurs in about 50% of cases of spinal deformity. Because of severe rotation, kyphosis in the lum-

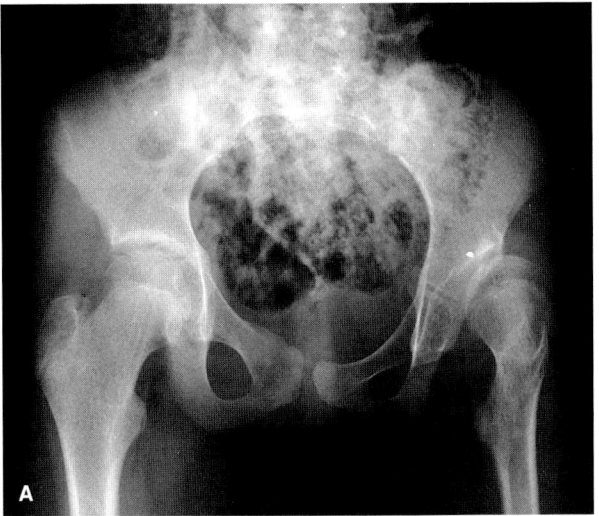
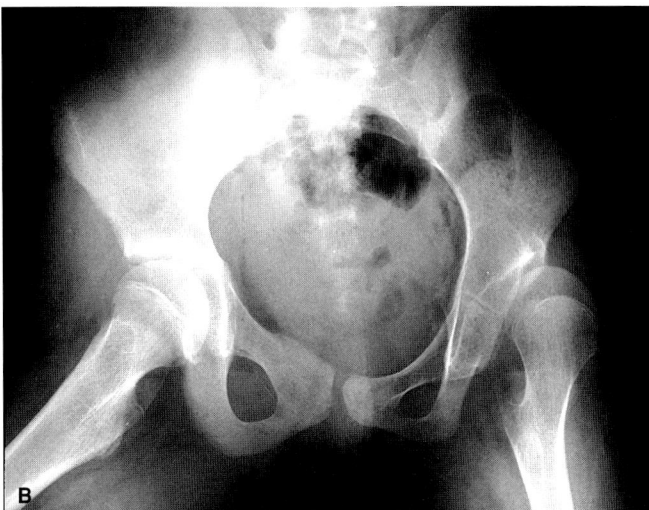
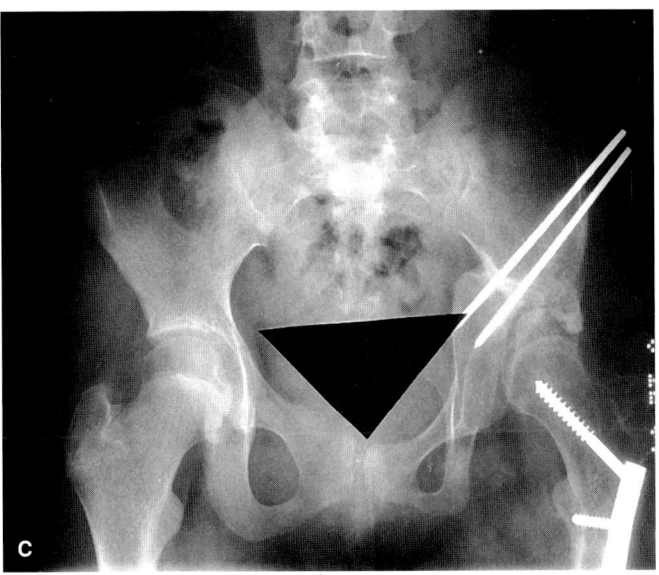

FIGURE 15-10. (A) Anteroposterior radiograph of the pelvis of a 13-year-old Korean girl who had poliomyelitis. She has a painful subluxation of her left hip. The acetabulum is dysplastic, the center-edge angle is −6 degrees, and a coxa valga deformity of the proximal femur is present. (B) Frog-leg or Lauenstein lateral. (C) Two years after a proximal femoral varus derotation osteotomy and Chiari pelvic osteotomy, there is markedly improved alignment of the left hip, and she is asymptomatic.

bar spine and lordosis in the thoracic spine are also common.

The goals of treatment are to obtain a balanced vertical torso over a level pelvis. This permits stable sitting and hands-free activities. It also helps prevent decubiti and paralytic hip dislocation. In young children with curves between 20 and 40 degrees, orthotic management with a TLSO can be tried. It rarely provides complete stability but can be effective in slowing the rate of progression and allowing the child to reach a more suitable age for surgery. In severe cases in young children, segmental spinal instrumentation without fusion may be considered. Eberle,[283] however, reported failure of segmental spinal instrumentation in 15 of 16 children with poliomyelitis between 5 and 12 years of age. Thus, children who undergo instrumentation without fusion should be treated with TLSO and undergo fusion as soon as possible to prevent late complications. For adolescents with a supple spine and a curve of less than 60 degrees, a posterior spinal fusion with segmental instrumentation, usually Luque rod instrumentation, provides stability and a low pseudoarthrosis rate.[9,78,279,280,295] Other segmental systems (e.g., TSRH, Cotrel-Dubousset,[24] Isola) should also be effective. In severe curves of 60 to 100 degrees, a combined anterior and posterior spinal fusion is usually necessary. Anterior spinal instrumentation with a Dwyer or Zielke system may be used in thoracolumbar and lumbar curves. Anterior discectomy and fusion is preferred for thoracic curves. The posterior spinal fusion and instrumentation is performed 1 or 2 weeks later. Leong and colleagues[292] and others[298] have demonstrated that combined anterior and posterior spinal fusions provide excellent correction for postpoliomyelitis spinal deformity, including the associated pelvic obliquity (Fig. 15-11). Rarely is preoperative traction or traction between staged anterior and posterior procedures necessary for additional correction. Fusion

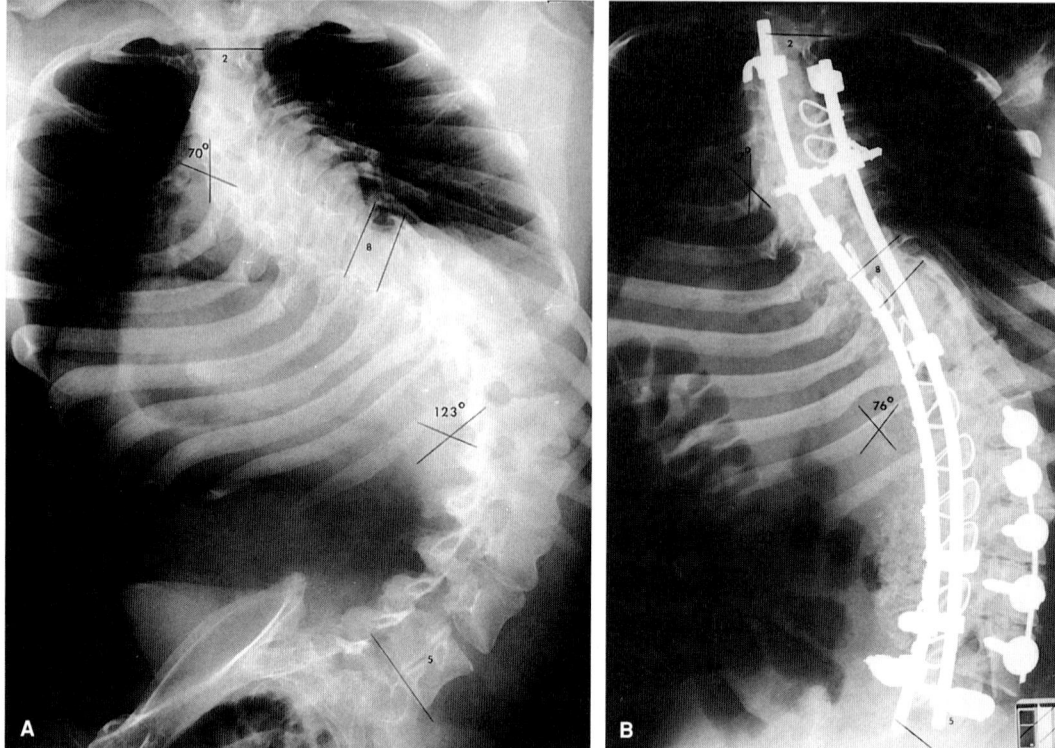

FIGURE 15-11. (A) Anteroposterior sitting spinal radiograph of a 17-year-old girl from the Middle East who has a severe paralytic scoliosis. There is a 123-degree left thoracolumbar scoliosis and a 70-degree right thoracic scoliosis. She contracted poliomyelitis at the age of 2 years, which left her with flail lower extremities and essentially normal upper extremities. She is wheelchair-dependent and has pain from rib-pelvis impingement. (B) Postoperative radiograph after staged anterior spinal fusion and Zielke instrumentation and posterior spinal fusion using Isola instrumentation from T3 to the sacrum. Pain relief was complete, and sitting balance improved. The left thoracolumbar curve has been reduced to 70 degrees and the right thoracic curve to 47 degrees.

to the pelvic or sacrum is usually necessary in patients with severe pelvic obliquity.[279,282,286]

Postpoliomyelitis Syndrome

Postpoliomyelitis syndrome is a true entity, occurring in adults, and a sequela to previous poliomyelitis. Reactivation of the poliovirus has been confused with amyotrophic lateral sclerosis. Postpoliomyelitis syndrome is thought to be an overuse syndrome.[300] Diagnosis is based on five criteria and is essentially a diagnosis of exclusion. The criteria include:

1. A confirmed history of previous poliomyelitis
2. Partial to fairly complete neurologic and functional recovery
3. A period of neurologic and functional stability of at least 15 years duration
4. Onset of two or more of the following health problems since achieving a period of stability: unaccustomed fatigue, muscle and joint pain or both, new weakness in muscles previously affected or unaffected, functional loss, cold intolerance, and new atrophy
5. No other medical diagnosis to explain the aforementioned health problems.[29]

Postpoliomyelitis syndrome is more likely to develop in those with onset later than 10 years of age because older children are more likely to have severe poliomyelitis. Management of these patients is conservative and consists of muscle strengthening, decreasing the duration of effort, and orthotics.[300] Reconstructive surgery is rarely indicated or necessary.

References

Muscular Dystrophies

1. Alexander MA, Johnson EW, Petty J, Stauch D. Mechanical ventilation of patients with late stage Duchenne muscular dystrophy. Management in the home. Arch Phys Med Rehabil 1979;60:289.
2. Allen BL Jr, Ferguson AL. The Galveston technique for L-rod instrumentation of the scoliotic spine. Spine 1982;7:119.
3. Arikawa E, Hoffman EP, Kaido M, et al. The frequency of patients with dystrophin abnormalities in a limb-girdle patient population. Neurology 1991;41:1491.
4. Bach JR, O'Brien J, Krolenberg R, Alba AS. Muscular dystrophy. Management of end stage respiratory failure in Duchenne muscular dystrophy. Muscle Nerve 1987;10:177.

5. Bailey RO, Marzulo DC, Hans MB. Muscular dystrophy. Infantile facioscapulohumeral muscular dystrophy. New observations. Acta Neurol Scand 1986;74:51.
6. Banker BQ. Myology. Basic and clinical. vol. 2. New York: McGraw-Hill, 1986:1527.
7. Becker PE. Two new families of benign sex-linked recessive muscular dystrophy. Rev Can Biol 1962;21:551.
8. Beggs AH, Hoffman EP, Snyder JR, et al. Exploring the molecular basis for variability among patients with Becker muscular dystrophy. Dystrophin gene and protein studies. Am J Hum Genet 1991;49:54.
9. Boachie-Adjei O, Lonstein JE, Winter RB, et al Management of neuromuscular spinal deformities with Luque segmental instrumentation. J Bone Joint Surg [Am] 1989;71:548.
10. Bodensteiner JB, Schochet SS. Facioscapulohumeral muscular dystrophy. The choice of a biopsy site. Muscle Nerve 1986;9:544.
11. Bonnet I, Burgot D, Bonnard C, Glorion B. Surgery of the lower limbs in Duchenne muscular dystrophy. Fr J Orthop Surg 1991;5:160.
12. Bowker JH, Halpin PJ. Factors determining success in reambulation of the child with progressive muscular dystrophy. Orthop Clin North Am 1978;9:431.
13. Bradley WG, Jones MZ, Mussini JM, Fawcett PRW. Becker-type muscular dystrophy. Muscle Nerve 1978;1:111.
14. Brooke MH, Fenichel GM, Griggs RC, et al. Duchenne muscular dystrophy. Patterns of clinical progression and effects of supportive therapy. Neurology 1989;39:475.
15. Broom MJ, Banta JV, Renshaw TS. Spinal fusion augmented by Luque rod segmental instrumentation for neuromuscular scoliosis. J Bone Joint Surg [Am] 1989;71:32.
16. Bunch WH, Siegal IM. Scapulothoracic arthrodesis in fascioscapulohumeral muscular dystrophy. Review of seventeen procedures with three to twenty-one year follow-up. J Bone Joint Surg [Am] 1993;75:372.
17. Bushby K. Report on the 12th ENMC sponsored international workshop—the "limb-girdle" muscular dystrophies. Neuromuscul Disord 1992;2:3
18. Cambridge W, Drennan JC. Scoliosis associated with Duchenne muscular dystrophy. J Pediatr Orthop 1987;7:436.
19. Carroll JE, Brooke MH. Infantile facioscapulohumeral dystrophy. In: Serratrice G, Roux H, eds. Peroneal atrophies and related disorders. New York: Masson, 1978:305.
20. Chyatte SB, Long C, Vignos PJ. The balanced forearm orthosis in muscular dystrophy. Arch Phys Med Rehabil 1965;46:633.
21. Colbert AP, Craig C. Scoliosis management in Duchenne muscular dystrophy. Prospective study of modified Jewett hyperextension brace. Arch Phys Med Rehabil 1987;68:302.
22. Consalez GG, Thomas NST, Stayton CL, et al. Assignment of Emery-Dreifuss muscular dystrophy to the distal region of Xq28. The results of a collaborative study. Am J Hum Genet 1991;48:468.
23. Copeland SA, Howard RC. Thoracoscapular fusion for facioscapulohumeral dystrophy. J Bone Joint Surg [Br] 1978;60:547.
24. Cotrel Y, Dubousset J, Guillaumat M. New universal instrumentation in spinal surgery. Clin Orthop 1988;227:10.
25. Curran FJ. Night ventilation by body respirators for patients in chronic respiratory failure due to late stage Duchenne muscular dystrophy. Arch Phys Med Rehabil 1981;62:270.
26. Daher YH, Lonstein JE, Winter RB, Bradford DS. Spinal deformities in patients with muscular dystrophy other than Duchenne. A review of 11 patients having surgical treatment. Spine 1985;10:614.
27. Darras BT. Molecular genetics of Duchenne and Becker muscular dystrophy. J Pediatr 1990;117:1.
28. Dickey RP, Ziter FA, Smith RA. Emery-Dreifuss muscular dystrophy. J Pediatr 1984;104:555.
29. Drennan JC. Neuromuscular disorders. In: Morrissy RT, ed. Lovell and Winter's pediatric orthopaedics. Philadelphia: JB Lippincott, 1990:381.
30. Dobrowski JM, Zajtchuck JT, LaPiana FG, Hensley SJ Jr. Oculopharyngeal muscular dystrophy. Clinical and histopathologic correlations. Otolaryngol Head Neck Surg 1986;95:131.
31. Duranceau A, Forand MD, Fautaux JP. Surgery in oculopharyngeal muscular dystrophy. Am J Surg 1980;139:33.
32. Dubousset J, Queneau P. Place et indication de la chirurgie dans la dystrophie musculaire de Duchenne de boulogne a evolution rapide. Rev Chir Orthop 1983;69:207.
33. Dubowitz V. Muscle biopsy. 2nd ed. London: Bailliere Tindall, 1985.
34. Dubowitz V. Prednisone in Duchenne dystrophy (editorial). Neuromuscul Disord 1991;1:161.
35. Emery AEH, Watt MS, Clack ER. The effects of genetic counseling in Duchenne muscular dystrophy. Clin Genet 1972;3:147.
36. Emery AEH. X-linked muscular dystrophy with early contractures and cardiomyopathy [Emery-Dreifuss type]. Clin Genet 1987;32:360.
37. Emery AEH. Duchenne muscular dystrophy. 2nd ed. New York: Oxford University Press, 1988.
38. Erb W. Uber die 'juvenile form' der progressiven muskelatrophie ihre beziehunger zur sogennanten pseudohypertrophie der muskeln. Deutsch Arch Klin Med 1884;34:467.
39. Fenichel GM, Florence JM, Pestronk A, et al. Long-term benefit from prednisone therapy in Duchenne muscular dystrophy. Neurology 1991;41:1874.
40. Florence JM, Brocke MH, Carroll JE. Evaluation of the child with muscular weakness. Orthop Clin North Am 1978;9:409.
41. Galasko CSB, Delaney C, Morris P. Spinal stabilisation in Duchenne muscular dystrophy. J Bone Joint Surg [Br] 1992;74:210.
42. Gibson DA, Wilkins KE. The management of spinal deformities in Duchenne muscular dystrophy. A new concept in spinal bracing. Clin Orthop 1975;108:41.
43. Gospe SM Jr, Lazaro RP, Lava NS, et al. Familial X-linked myalgia and cramps. A nonprogressive myopathy associated with a deletion in the dystrophin gene. Neurology 1989;39:1277.
44. Goto I, Ishimoto S, Yamada T, et al. The rigid spine syndrome and Emery-Dreifuss muscular dystrophy. Clin Neurol Neurosurg 1986;88:293.
45. Green NE. The orthopaedic care of children with muscular dystrophy. Instr Course Lect 1987;36:267.
46. Greene WB. Transfer versus lengthening of the posterior tibial tendon in Duchenne's muscular dystrophy. Foot Ankle 1992;13:526.
47. Gussoni E, Pavlath GK, Lanctot AM, et al. Normal dystrophin transcripts detected in Duchenne muscular dystrophy patients after myoblast transplantation. Nature 1992;356:435.
48. Hanson PA, Rowland LP. Mobius syndrome and facioscapulohumeral muscular dystrophy. Arch Neurol 1971;24:31.
49. Heckmatt JZ, Dubowitz V, Hyde SA, et al. Prolongation of walking in Duchenne muscular dystrophy with lightweight orthoses; review of 57 cases. Dev Med Child Neurol 1985;27:149.
50. Heckmatt J, Rodillo E, Dubowitz V. Management of children. Pharmacological and physical. Br Med Bull 1989;45:788.
51. Hilton T, Orr RD, Perkin RM, Ashwal S. End of life care in Duchenne muscular dystrophy. Pediatr Neurol 1993;9:165.
52. Hoffman EP, Brown RH Jr, Kunkel LM. Dystrophin. The protein product of the Duchenne muscular dystrophy locus. Cell 1987;51:919.
53. Hoffman EP, Fischbeck KH, Brown RH, et al. Characterization of dystrophin in muscle-biopsy specimens from patients with

Duchenne's or Becker's muscular dystrophy. N Engl J Med 1988;318:1363.
54. Hoffman EP, Kunkel LM. Dystrophin abnormalities in Duchenne/Becker muscular dystrophy. Neuron 1989;2:1019.
55. Hoffman EP, Kunkel LM, Angelini C, et al. Improved diagnosis of Becker muscular dystrophy by dystrophin testing. Neurology 1989;39:1011.
56. Hopkins LC, Jackson JA, Elsas LJ. Emery-Dreifuss humeroperoneal muscular dystrophy. An X-linked myopathy with unusual contractures and bradycardia. Ann Neurol 1981; 10:230.
57. Hsu JD. The management of foot deformity in pseudohypertrophic muscular dystrophy (DMD). Orthop Clin North Am 1976;7:979.
58. Hsu JD, Hoffer MM. Posterior tibial tendon transfer through the interosseous membrane. A modification of the technique. Clin Orthop 1978;131:202.
59. Hsu JD. The natural history of spine curvature progression in the nonambulatory Duchenne muscular dystrophy patient. Spine 1983;8:771.
60. Hsu JD, Furumasu J. Gait and posture changes in the Duchenne muscular dystrophy child. Clin Orthop 1993;288:122.
61. Huard J, Bouchard JP, Roy R, et al. Human myoblast transplantation; preliminary results of 4 cases. Muscle Nerve 1992;15:550.
62. Hurley ME, Davids JR, Mubarak SJ. Single-incision combination biopsy (muscle and nerve) in the diagnosis of neuromuscular disease in children. J Pediatr Orthop 1994;14:740.
63. Jakab E, Gledhill RB. Simplified technique for scapulocostal fusion in facioscapulohumeral dystrophy. J Pediatr Orthop 1993;13:749.
64. Jenkins JG, Bohn D, Edmonds JF, et al. Evaluation of pulmonary function in muscular dystrophy patients requiring spinal surgery. Crit Care Med 1982;10:645.
65. Johnson EW, Kennedy JH. Comprehensive management of Duchenne muscular dystrophy. Arch Phys Med Rehabil 1971;52:110.
66. Kazakov VM, Bogorodinsky DK, Znoyko ZV, Skorometz AA. The facioscapulo-limb (or the facioscapulohumeral) type of muscular dystrophy. Clinical and genetic study. European Neurol 1974;11:236.
67. Ketenjian AY. Scapulocostal stabilization for scapular winging in facioscapulohumeral muscular dystrophy. J Bone Joint Surg [Am] 1978;60:476.
68. Kocialkowski A, Frostick SP, Wallace WA. One-stage bilateral thoracoscapular fusion using allografts. A case report. Clin Orthop 1991;273:264.
69. Korf BR, Bresnan MJ, Shapiro F, et al. Facioscapulohumeral dystrophy presenting in infancy with facial diplegia and sensorineutral deafness. Ann Neurol 1985;17:513.
70. Kostuik JP. Current concepts review. Operative treatment of idiopathic scoliosis. J Bone Joint Surg [Am] 1990;72:1108.
71. Kunkel LM, Monaco AP, Hoffman E, et al. Molecular studies of progressive muscular dystrophy (Duchenne). Enzyme 1987;38:72.
72. Kurz LT, Mubarak SJ, Schultz P, et al. Correlation of scoliosis and pulmonary function in Duchenne muscular dystrophy. J Pediatr Orthop 1983;3:347.
73. Landouzy L, Dejerine J. De la myopathie atrophique progressive (myopathie hereditaire), dubutant, dans l'enfance, par le face, sans alteration du system nerveux. CR Acad Sci Paris 1884;98:53.
74. Law PK, Goodwin TG, Fang Q, et al. Feasibility, safety and efficacy of myoblast transfer therapy on Duchenne muscular dystrophy boys. Cell Transplant 1992;1:235.
75. Letournel E, Fardeau M, Lytle JO, et al. Scapulothoracic arthrodesis for patients who have fascioscapulohumeral muscular dystrophy. J Bone Joint Surg [Am] 1990;72:78.
76. Leyden E. Klinik der ruckenmarks-krankheiten, vol 2. Berlin: Hirschwalk, 1876.
77. Lord J, Behrman B, Varzos N, et al. Scoliosis associated with Duchenne muscular dystrophy. Arch Phys Med Rehabil 1990;71:13.
78. Luque ER. Segmental spinal instrumentation for correction of scoliosis. Clin Orthop 1982;163:192.
79. Marsh GG, Munsat TL. Evidence for early impairment of verbal intelligence in Duchenne muscular dystrophy. Arch Dis Child 1974;49:118.
80. Melkonian GJ, Cristafaro RL, Perry J, Hsu JD. Dynamic gait electromyography study in Duchenne muscular dystrophy (DMD) patients. Foot Ankle 1983;1:78.
81. Mendell JR, Moxley RT, Griggs RC, et al. Randomized double-blind six-month trial of prednisone in Duchenne's muscular dystrophy. N Engl J Med 1989;320:1592.
82. Merlini L, Granata C, Dominici P, Bonfiglioli S. Emery-Dreifuss muscular dystrophy. Report of five cases in a family and review of the literature. Muscle Nerve 1986;9:481.
83. Miller F, Moseley CF, Koreska J, Levison H. Pulmonary function and scoliosis in Duchenne dystrophy. J Pediatr Orthop 1988;8:133.
84. Miller GM, Hsu JD, Hoffer MM, Rentfro R. Posterior tibial tendon transfer. A review of the literature and analysis of 74 procedures. J Pediatr Orthop 1982;2:363.
85. Miller RG, Layzer RB, Mellenthin MA, et al. Emery-Dreifuss muscular dystrophy with autosomal dominant transmission. Neurology 1985;35:1230.
86. Miller RG, Chalmers AC, Dao H, et al. The effects of spine fusion on respiratory function in Duchenne muscular dystrophy. Neurology 1991;41:38.
87. Mubarak SJ, Chambers HG, Wenger DR. Percutaneous muscle biopsy in the diagnosis of neuromuscular disease. J Pediatr Orthop 1992;12:191.
88. Mubarak SJ, Morin WD, Leach J. Spinal fusion in Duchenne muscular dystrophy-fixation and fusion to the sacropelvis? J Pediatr Orthop 1993;13:752.
89. Mubarak SJ, Miller LS. Muscular dystrophy. In: Weinstein SL, ed. The pediatric spine. Principles and practice. New York: Raven Press, 1994:1101.
90. Munsat TL, Baloh R, Pearson CM, Fowler W Jr. Serum enzyme alterations in neuromuscular disorders. JAMA 1973;226:1536.
91. Nicholson LVB, Johnson MA, Bushby KMD, Gardiner-Modwin D. Functional significance of dystrophin positive fibres in Duchenne muscular dystrophy. Arch Dis Child 1993;68:632.
92. Ober FR. The role of the iliotibial band and fascia lata as a factor in the causation of low back disabilities and sciatica. J Bone Joint Surg 1936;18:105.
93. Oda T, Shimizu N, Yonenobu K, et al. Longitudinal study of spinal deformity in Duchenne muscular deformity. J Pediatr Orthop 1993;13:478.
94. Partridge TA, Morgan JE, Coulton GR, et al. Conversion of mdx myofibres from dystrophin-negative to-positive by injection of normal myoblasts. Nature 1989;337:176.
95. Partridge TA. Invited review. Myoblast transfer. A possible therapy for inherited myopathies? Muscle Nerve 1991;14:197.
96. Pratt MF, Meyers PK. Oculopharyngeal muscular dystrophy. Recent ultrastructural evidence for mitochondrial abnormalities. Laryngoscope 1986;96:368.
97. Read L, Galasko CS. Delay in diagnosing Duchenne muscular dystrophy in orthopaedic clinics. J Bone Joint Surg [Br] 1986;68:481.
98. Rideau Y, Jankowski LW, Grellet J. Respiratory function in the muscular dystrophies. Muscle Nerve 1981;4:155.

99. Rideau Y, Glorion B, Duport G. Prolongation of ambulation in the muscular dystrophies. Acta Neurol 1983;38:390.
100. Rideau Y, Glorion B, Delaubier A, et al. the treatment of scoliosis in Duchenne muscular dystrophy. Muscle Nerve 1984;7:281.
101. Rideau Y, Duport G, Delaubier A. Premieres remissions reproductibles dans l'evolution de la dystrophie musculaire de Duchenne. Bull Acad Natl Med 1986;170:605.
102. Rideau Y, Delaubier A. Neuromuscular respiratory deficit. Setting back mortality. Semin Orthop 1987;2:203.
103. Robin GC, Brief LP. Scoliosis in childhood muscular dystrophy. J Bone Joint Surg [Am] 1971;53:4666.
104. Rodillo EB, Fernandez-Bermejo E, Heckmatt JZ, Dubowitz V. Prevention of rapidly progressive scoliosis in Duchenne muscular dystrophy by prolongation of walking with orthoses. J Child Neurol 1988;3:269.
105. Roses AD, Roses MJ, Miller SE, et al. Carrier detection in Duchenne muscular dystrophy. N Engl J Med 1976;294:193.
106. Sanjal SK, Leung RK, Tierney RC, et al. Mitral valve prolapse syndrome in children with Duchenne's progressive muscular dystrophy. Pediatrics 1979;63:116.
107. Schreiber A, Smith WL, Ionasescu V, et al. Magnetic resonance imaging of children with Duchenne muscular dystrophy. Pediatr Radiol 1987;17:495.
108. Seay AR, Ziter FA, Thompson JA. Cardiac arrest during induction of anesthesia in Duchenne muscular dystrophy. J Pediatr 1978;93:88.
109. Seeger BR, Sutherland AD'A, Clark MS. Orthotic management of scoliosis in Duchenne muscular dystrophy. Arch Phys Med Rehabil 1984;65:83.
110. Shapiro F, Bresnan MJ. Current concepts review. Orthopaedic management of childhood neuromuscular disease. Part III: diseases of muscle. J Bone Joint Surg [Am] 1982;64:1102.
111. Shapiro F, Specht L. Orthopedic deformities in Emery-Dreifuss muscular dystrophy. J Pediatr Orthop 1991;11:336.
112. Shapiro F, Specht L, Korf BR. Locomotor problems in infantile fascioscapulohumeral muscular dystrophy. Retrospective study of 9 patients. Acta Orthop Scand 1991;62:367.
113. Shapiro F, Sethna N, Colan S, et al. Spinal fusion in Duchenne muscular dystrophy: a multidisciplinary approach. Muscle Nerve 1992;15:604.
114. Shapiro F, Specht L. Current concepts review. The diagnosis and orthopaedic treatment of inherited muscular diseases of childhood. J Bone Joint Surg [Am] 1993;75:439.
115. Siegel IM, Miller JE, Ray RD. Subcutaneous lower limb tenotomies in treatment of pseudohypertrophic muscular dystrophy. J Bone Joint Surg [Am] 1968;50:1437.
116. Siegel IM. Scoliosis in muscular dystrophy: some comments about diagnosis, observations on prognosis, suggestions for therapy Clin Orthop 1973;93:235.
117. Siegel IM. Diagnosis, management and orthopaedic treatment of muscular dystrophy. Instr Course Lect 1981;30:3.
118. Slater GR. The missing link in Duchenne muscular dystrophy. Nature 1987;330:693.
119. Smith AD, Koreska J, Moseley CF. Progression of scoliosis in Duchenne muscular dystrophy. J Bone Joint Surg [Am] 1989;71:1066.
120. Smith PEM, Calverley PMA, Edwards RHT, et al. Practical problems in the respiratory care of patients with muscular dystrophy. N Engl J Med 1987;316:1197.
121. Smith SE, Green NE, Cole RJ, et al. Prolongation of ambulation in children with Duchenne muscular dystrophy by subcutaneous lower limb tenotomy. J Pediatr Orthop 1993;13:331.
122. Soutter R. A new operation for hip contractures in poliomyelitis. Boston Med Surg J 1914;170:380.
123. Specht LA. Molecular basis and clinical applications of neuromuscular disease in children. Curr Opin Pediatr 1991;3:966.
124. Specht LA. Case records of the Massachusetts General Hospital. Case 34-1992. N Engl J Med 1992;327:548.
125. Specht LA, Beggs AH, Korf B, et al. Prediction of dystrophin phenotype by DNA analysis in Duchenne/Becker muscular dystrophy. Pediatr Neurol 1992;8:432.
126. Specht LA, Kunkel LM. Duchenne and Becker muscular dystrophies. In: Rosenberg RN, Prusiner SB, DiMauro S, Barchi RL, Kunkel LM, eds. The molecular and genetic basis of neurological disease. Boston: Butterworth-Heinemann, 1993:613.
127. Spencer GE Jr, Vignos PJ Jr. Bracing for ambulation in childhood progressive muscular dystrophy. J Bone Joint Surg [Am] 1962;44:234.
128. Spencer GE Jr. Orthopaedic care of progressive muscular dystrophy. J Bone Joint Surg [Am] 1967;49:1201.
129. Stewart CA, Gilgoff Baydur A, Prentice W, Applebaum D. Gated radionuclide ventriculography in the evolution of cardiac function in Duchenne's muscular dystrophy. Chest 1988;94:1245.
130. Sussman MD. Advantage of early spinal stabilization and fusion in patients with Duchenne muscular dystrophy. J Pediatr Orthop 1984;4:532.
131. Sutherland DH, Olshen R, Cooper L, et al. The pathomechanics of gait in Duchenne muscular dystrophy. Dev Med Child Neurol 1981;23:3.
132. Sutherland DH. Gait analysis in neuromuscular diseases. Instr Course Lect 1990;39:333.
133. Swank SM, Brown JC, Perry RE. Spinal fusion in Duchenne's muscular dystrophy. Spine 1982;7:484.
134. Taddonio RF. Segmental spinal instrumentation in the management of neuromuscular spinal deformity. Spine 1982;7:305.
135. Thomas NS, Williams H, Elsas LJ, et al. Localization of the gene for Emery-Dreifuss muscular dystrophy to the distal long arm of the X-chromosome. J Med Genet 1986;23:596.
136. Thomson WH, Leyburn P, Walton JN. Serum enzyme activity in muscular dystrophy. Br Med J 1960;2(5208):1276.
137. Uchino M, Araki S, Miike T, et al. Localization and characterization of dystrophin in muscle biopsy specimens for Duchenne muscular dystrophy and various neuromuscular disorders. Muscle Nerve 1989;12:1009.
138. Vignos PJ Jr. Diagnosis of progressive muscular dystrophy. J Bone Joint Surg [Am] 1967;49:1212.
139. Vulpius O, Stoffel A. Orthopaedische operationsiehre. 2nd ed. Stuttgart: Ferdinand Enke, 1920.
140. Wagner MB, Vignos PJ Jr, Carlozzi C. Duchenne muscular dystrophy: a study of wrist and hand function. Muscle Nerve 1989;12:236.
141. Weimann RL, Gibson DA, Moseley CF, Jones DC. Surgical stabilization of the spine in Duchenne muscular dystrophy. Spine 1983;8:776.
142. Wijmenga C, Frants RR, Brouwer OF, et al. Location of facioscapulohumeral muscular dystrophy gene on chromosome 4. Lancet 1990;336:651.
143. Wilkins KE, Gibson DA. The patterns of spinal deformity in Duchenne muscular dystrophy. J Bone Joint Surg [Am] 1976;58:24.
144. Williams EA, Read L, Ellis A, et al. The management of equinus deformity in Duchenne muscular dystrophy. J Bone Joint Surg [Br] 1984;66:546.
145. Wosick WF, Alker G. CT manifestation of ocular muscular dystrophy. Comput Radiol 1984;8:391.
146. Yasuda YL, Bowman K, Hsu JD. Mobile arm supports: criteria

146. for successful use in muscle disease patients. Arch Phys Med Rehabil 1986;67:253.
147. Yazawa Y. Mitral valve prolapse related to geometrical changes of the heart in cases of progressive muscular dystrophy. Clin Cardiol 1984;7:198.
148. Yount CC. The role of the tensor fasciae femoris in certain deformities of the lower extremities. J Bone Joint Surg [Am] 1926;8:171.
149. Zellweger H, McCormick WF, Mergner W. Severe congenital muscular dystrophy. Am J Dis Child 1967;114:591.

Myotonia

150. Bell DB, Smith DW. Myotonic dystrophy in the neonate. J Pediatr 1972;81:83.
151. Bowen RS Jr, Marks HG. Foot deformities in myotonic dystrophy. Foot Ankle 1984;5:125.
152. Calderon R. Myotonic dystrophy. A neglected cause of mental retardation. J Pediatr 1966;68:423.
153. Carroll JE, Brooke MH, Kaiser K. Diagnosis of infantile myotonic dystrophy. Lancet 1975;2:608.
154. Cook AW, Bird TD, Spence AM, et al. Myotonic dystrophy, mitral-valve prolapse and stroke. Lancet 1978;1:335.
155. Cruz-Martinez A, Arpa J, Perez-Conde MC, Ferrer MT. Bilateral carpal tunnel in childhood associated with Schwartz-Jampel syndrome. Muscle Nerve 1984;7:66.
156. Geschwind N, Simpson JA. Procaine amide in the treatment of myotonia. Brain 1955;78:81.
157. Gross RH. The role of the Verebelyi-Ogston procedure: the management of the arthrogrypotic foot. Clin Orthop 1985;194:99.
158. Haig AJ. The complex interactions of myotonic dystrophy in low back pain. Spine 1991;16:580.
159. Hanson PA. Myotonic dystrophy in infancy and childhood. Pediatr Ann 1984;13:123.
160. O'Brien TA, Harper PS. Course, prognosis and complications of childhood-onset myotonic dystrophy. Dev Med Child Neurol 1984;26:62.
161. Schonk D, Coerwinkel-Driessen M, van Dalen I, et al. Definition of subchromosomal intervals around the myotonic dystrophy gene region at 19q. Genomics 1989;4:384.
162. Schwartz O, Jampel RS. Congenital blepharophimosis associated with a unique generalized myopathy. Arch Ophthalmol 1962;68:52.
163. Speer MC, Pericak-Vance MA, Yamaoka L, et al. Presymptomatic and prenatal diagnosis in myotonic dystrophy by genetic linkage studies. Neurology 1990;40:671.
164. Thomsen J. Tonisch krampfe in willkurlich beweglichen muskeln in folge von erebter psychischer disposition. Arch Psychiatr Nerv 1876;6:706.
165. Vanier TM. Dystrophia myotonia in childhood. Br Med J 1960;2(5208):1284.
166. Winters JL, McLaughlin LA. Myotonia congenita. J Bone Joint Surg [Am] 1970;52:1345.
167. Zellweger H, Ionasescu V. Early onset of myotonic dystrophy in infants. Am J Dis Child 1973;125:601.

Congenital Myopathies

168. Armstrong RM, Koenigsberg R, Mellinger J, Lovelace RE. Central core disease with congenital hip dislocation: study of two families. Neurology 1971;21:369.
169. Banker BQ. Myology. Basic and clinical. vol. 2. New York: McGraw-Hill, 1986:1367.
170. Brooke MH. A clinician's view of neuromuscular diseases. Baltimore: Williams & Wilkins, 1977.
171. Brooke MH. A neuromuscular disease characterized by fiber types disproportion. In: Kakulas BA, ed. Proceedings of the Second International Congress on Muscle Diseases, Perth, Australia, November 1971. Amsterdam: Excerpta Medica, 1973.
172. Cavanagh NPC, Lake BD, McMeniman P. Congenital fibre type disproportion myopathy. A histological diagnosis with an uncertain clinical outlook. Arch Dis Child 1979;54:735.
173. Cornelio F, DiDonato S. Myopathies due to enzyme deficiencies. J Neurol 1985;232:329.
174. Cunliffe M, Burrows FA. Anesthetic implications of nemaline rod myopathy. Can Anaesth Soc J 1985;32:543.
175. Darnsfors Catarina, Larsson HEB, Oldfors A, et al. X-linked myotubular myopathy: a linkage study. Clin Genet 1990;37:335.
176. Dubowitz V. Muscle disorders in childhood. Philadelphia: WB Saunders, 1978.
177. Eeg-Olofsson O, Henriksson KG, Thornell LE, Wesstroom G. Early infant death in nemaline (rod) myopathy. Brain Dev 1983;5:53.
178. Fukuyama Y, Osawa M, Suzuki H. Congenital progressive muscular dystrophy of the Fukuyama type—clinical, genetic and pathological considerations. Brain Dev 1981;3:1.
179. Fukuyama Y, Osawa M. A genetic study of the Fukuyama type congenital muscular dystrophy. Brain Dev 1983;6:373.
180. Gamble JG, Rinsky LA, Lee JH. Orthopaedic aspects of central care disease. J Bone Joint Surg [Am] 1988;70:1061.
181. Goebel HH. Congenital myopathies. In: Adachi M, Ser JH, eds. Neuromuscular discoid. New York: Igaku-Schoin, 1990:197.
182. Gullotta F. Metabolic myopathies. Pathol Res Pract 1985;180:10.
183. Jones R, Kahn R, Hughes S, Dubowitz V. Congenital muscular dystrophy. The importance of early diagnosis and orthopaedic management in the long-term prognosis. J Bone Joint Surg [Br] 1979;61:13.
184. Kearns TP, Sayre GP. Retinitis pigmentosa, external ophthalmoplegia and complete heart block. Arch Ophthalmol 1958;60:280.
185. Kumano K. Congenital non-progressive myopathy, associated with scoliosis—clinical, histological, histochemical and electron microscopic studies of seven cases. Nippon Seikeigeka Gakkai Zasshi 1980;54:381.
186. Maayan C, Springer C, Armon T, et al. Nemaline myopathy as a cause of sleep hypoventilation. Pediatrics 1986;77:390.
187. Martinez BA, Lake BD. Childhood nemaline myopathy: a review of clinical presentation in relation to prognosis. Dev Med Child Neurol 1987;29:815.
188. McComb RD, Markesbery WR, O'Connor WN. Fatal neonatal nemaline myopathy with multiple congenital anomalies. J Pediatr 1979;95:47.
189. McManamin JB, Becker LE, Murphy EG. Congenital muscular dystrophy: a clinicopathologic report of 24 cases. J Pediatr 1982;100:692.
190. Mechler F, Mastaglia FL, Serena M, et al. Mitochondrial myopathies. A clinico-pathological study of cases with and without extra-ocular muscle involvement. Aust NZ J Med 1986;16:185.
191. Munsat TL, Thompson LR, Coleman RF. Centronuclear ("myotubular") myopathy. Arch Neurol 1969;20:120.
192. Ramsey PL, Hensinger RN. Congenital dislocation of the hip associated with central core disease. J Bone Joint Surg [Am] 1975;57:648.
193. Shimomura C, Nonaka I. Nemaline myopathy: comparative muscle histochemistry in the severe neonatal, moderate congenital and adult-onset forms. Pediatr Neurol 1989;5:25.
194. Shuaib A, Paasuke RT, Brownell KW. Central core disease. Clinical features in 13 patients. Medicine 1987;66:389.
195. Shy GM, Magee KR. A new congenital nonprogressive myopathy. Brain 1956;79:610.

196. Shy GM, Engel WK, Somers JE, Wanko T. Nemaline myopathy. A new congenital myopathy. Brain 1963;86:793.
197. Spiro AJ, Shy GM, Gonatas NK. Myotubular myopathy. Persistence of fetal muscle in an adolescent boy. Arch Neurol 1966;14:1.

Spinal Muscular Atrophy

198. Aprin H, Bowen JR, MacEwen GD, Hall JE. Spine arthrodesis in patients with spinal muscular atrophy. J Bone Joint Surg [Am] 1982;64:1179.
199. Bowen JR, Forlin E. Spinal muscular atrophy. In: Weinstein SL, ed. The pediatric spine. Principles and practice. New York: Raven Press, 1994:1025.
200. Brooke MH. A clinician's view of neuromuscular diseases. 2nd ed. Baltimore: Williams and Wilkins, 1986:36.
201. Broom MJ, Banta JV, Renshaw TS. Spinal fusion augmented by Luque-rod segmental instrumentation for neuromuscular scoliosis. J Bone Joint Surg [Am] 1989;71:32.
202. Brown CJ, Zeller JL, Swank SM, et al. Surgical and functional results of spine fusion in spinal muscular atrophy. Spine 1989;14:763.
203. Brzustowicz LM, Lehner T, Castilla LH, et al. Genetic mapping of chronic childhood-onset spinal muscular atrophy to chromosome 5q 11.2–13.3 Nature 1990;334:540.
204. Burke SW, Jameson VP, Roberts JM, et al. Birth fractures in spinal muscular atrophy. J Pediatr Orthop 1986;6:34.
205. Daher YH, Lonstein JE, Winter RB, Bradford DS. Spinal surgery in spinal muscular atrophy. J Pediatr Orthop 1985;5:391.
206. Evans GA, Drennan JC, Russman BS. Functional classification and orthopaedic management of spinal muscular atrophy. J Bone Joint Surg [Br] 1981;63:516.
207. Furumasu J, Swank SM, Brown JC, et al. Functional activities in spinal muscular atrophy patients after spinal fusion. Spine 1989;14:771.
208. Gilgoff IS, Kahlstrom E, McLaughlin E, Keens TG. Long-term ventilitory support in spinal muscular atrophy. J Pediatr 1989;115:904.
209. Gilliam TC, Brzustowicz LM, Castilla LH, et al. Genetic homogeneity between acute and chronic forms of spinal muscular atrophy. Nature 1990;345:823.
210. Gordon N. The spinal muscular atrophies. Dev Med Child Neurol 1991;33:930.
211. Granata C, Cornelio F, Bonfiglioli S, et al. Promotion of ambulation of patients with spinal muscular atrophy by early fitting of knee-ankle-foot orthoses. Dev Med Child Neurol 1987;29:221.
212. Granata C, Merlini L, Magni E, et al. Spinal muscular atrophy. Natural history and orthopaedic treatment of scoliosis. Spine 1989;14:760.
213. Hensinger RN, MacEwen GD. Spinal deformity associated with heritable neurological conditions. Spinal muscular atrophy. Friedreich's ataxia, familial dysautonomia, and Charcot-Marie-Tooth disease. J Bone Joint Surg [Am] 1976;58:13.
214. Iannaccone ST, Browne RH, Samaha FJ, Buncher CR. Prospective study of spinal muscular atrophy before age 6 years. Pediatr Neurol 1993;9:187.
215. Liu GT, Specht LA. Progressive juvenile segmental spinal muscular atrophy. Pediatr Neurol 1992;9:54.
216. Melki J, Sheth P, Abdelhak S, et al. The French spinal muscular atrophy investigators. Mapping of acute (type 1) spinal muscular atrophy to chromosome 5q12–q14. Lancet 1990;336:271.
217. Melki J, Abdelhak S, Sheth P, et al. Gene for chronic proximal spinal muscular atrophies maps to chromosome 5q. Nature 1990;344:767.
218. Merlini L, Granata C, Bonfiglioli S, et al Scoliosis in spinal muscular atrophy. Natural history and management. Dev Med Child Neurol 1989;31:301.
219. Miles JM. Diagnosis and discussion. Type I spinal muscular atrophy (Werdnig-Hoffman disease). Am J Dis Child 1993;147:908.
220. Pearn J. Classifications of spinal muscular atrophies. Lancet 1980;1:919.
221. Phillips DP, Roye DP Jr, Farcy J-P, et al. Surgical treatment of scoliosis in a spinal muscular atrophy population. Spine 1990;15:942.
222. Piasecki JO, Mahinpour S, Lovine DB. Long-term follow-up of spinal fusion in spinal muscular atrophy. Clin Orthop 1986;207:44.
223. Riddick MF, Winter RB, Lutter LD. Spinal deformities in patients with spinal muscle atrophy. A review of 36 patients. Spine 1982;7:476.
224. Rodillo E, Marini ML, Heckmaht JZ, Dubowitz V. Scoliosis in spinal muscular atrophy. Review of 63 cases. J Child Neurol 1989;4:118.
225. Russman BS, Melchreit R, Drennan, JC. Spinal muscular atrophy. The natural course of the disease. Muscle Nerve 1983;6:179.
226. Russman BS, Iannascone ST, Buncher CR, et al. Spinal muscular atrophy. New thoughts on the pathogenesis and classification schema. J Child Neurol 1992;7:347.
227. Schwentker EP, Gibson DA. The orthopaedic aspects of spinal muscular atrophy. J Bone Joint Surg [Am] 1976;58:32.
228. Shapiro F, Bresnan MJ. Current concepts review. Orthopaedic management of childhood neuromuscular disease. Part I. Spinal muscular atrophy. J Bone Joint Surg [Am] 1982;64:785.
229. Shapiro F, Specht L. Current concepts review. The diagnosis and orthopaedic treatment of childhood spinal muscular atrophy, peripheral neuropathy, Friedreich ataxia and arthrogryposis. J Bone and Joint Surg [Am] 1993;75:1699.
230. Thompson CE, Larsen LJ. Recurrent hip dislocation in immediate spinal atrophy. J Pediatr Orthop 1990;10:638.

Friedreich Ataxia

231. Cady RB, Bobechko WP. Incidence, Natural history and treatment of scoliosis in Friedreich's ataxia. J Pediatr Orthop 1984;4:673.
232. Chamberlain S, Shaw J, Rowland A, et al. Mapping of mutation causing Friedreich's ataxia to human chromosome 9. Nature 1988;334:248.
233. Daher YH, Lonstein JE, Winter RB, Bradford DS. Spinal deformities in patients with Friedreich ataxia. A review of 19 patients. J Pediatr Orthop 1985;5:553.
234. Filla A, DeMichele G, Caruso G, et al. Genetic data and natural history of Friedreich's disease. A study of 80 Italian patients. J Neurol 1990;237:345.
235. Fujita R, Hanauer A, Vincent A, et al. Physical mapping of two loci (D9S5 and D9S15) tightly linked to Friedreich ataxia locus (FRDA) and identification of nearby CpG Islands by pulse-field gel electrophoresis. Genomics 1991;10:915.
236. Geoffroy G, Barbeau A, Breton G, et al. Clinical description and roentgenologic evaluation of patients with Friedreich's ataxia. Canadian J Neurol Sci 1976;3:279.
237. Harding AE. Friedreich's ataxia. A clinical and genetic study of 90 families with an analysis of early diagnostic criteria and intrafamilial clustering of clinical features. Brain 1981;104:589.
238. Hensinger RN, MacEwen GD. Spinal deformity associated with heritable neurological conditions. Spinal muscular atrophy, Friedreich's ataxia, familial dysautonomia, and Charcot-Marie-Tooth disease. J Bone Joint Surg [Am] 1976;58:13.
239. Hewer RL. Study of fatal cases of Friedreich's ataxia. Br Med J 1968;3:649.

240. Labelle H, Tohme S, Duhaime M, Allard P. Natural history of scoliosis in Friedreich's ataxia. J Bone Joint Surg [Am] 1986;68:564.
241. Labelle H, Beauchomp M, LaPierre Duhaime M, Allard P. Pattern of muscle weakness and its relation to loss of ambulatory function in Friedreich's ataxia. J Pediatr Orthop 1987;7:496.
242. Labelle H, Duhaime M, Allard P. Spinal deformities in Friedrieich's ataxia. In: Weinstein SL, ed. The pediatric spine: principles of practice. New York: Raven Press, 1994:999.
243. Shapiro F, Bresnan MJ. Current concepts review. Orthopaedic management of childhood neuromuscular disease. Part II: peripheral neuropathies, Friedreich's ataxia and arthrogryposis multiplex congenita. J Bone Joint Surg [Am] 1982;64:949.

Hereditary Motor Sensory Neuropathy

244. Alexander TJ, Johnson KA. Assessment and management of pes cavus in Charcot-Marie-Tooth disease. Clin Orthop 1989;246:273.
245. Angus PD, Cowell HR. Triple arthrodesis. A critical long-term review. J Bone Joint Surg [Br] 1986;68:260.
246. Brown JC, Zeller JL, Swank SM, et al. Surgical and functional results of spine fusion in spinal muscular atrophy. Spine 1989;14:763.
247. Brown RE, Zamboni WA, Zook EG, Russell RC. Evaluation and management of upper extremity neuropathies in Charcot-Marie-Tooth disease. J Hand Surg 1992;17-A:523.
248. Cole WH. The treatment of claw-foot. J Bone Joint Surg 1940;22:895.
249. Daher YH, Lonstein JE, Winter RB, Bradford DS. Spinal deformities in patients with Charcot-Marie-Tooth disease. A review of 12 patients. Clin Orthop 1986;202:219.
250. Gould N. Surgery in advanced Charcot-Marie-Tooth disease. Foot Ankle 1984;4:267.
251. Hall JE, Calvert PT. Lambrinudi triple arthrodesis. A review with particular reference to the technique of operation. J Pediatr Orthop 1987;7:19.
252. Hensinger RN, MacEwen GD. Spinal deformity associated with heritable neurological conditions. Spinal muscular atrophy, Friedreich's ataxia, familial dysautonomia, and Charcot-Marie-Tooth disease. J Bone Joint Surg [Am] 1976;58:13.
253. Ingram AJ. Paralytic disorders. In: Crenshaw AH, ed. Campbell's operative orthopaedics. 7th ed. vol. 4. St Louis: CV Mosby, 1987:2925.
254. Krishna M, Taylor JF, Brown MC, et al. Failure of somatosensory-evoked-potential monitoring in sensorimotor neuropathy. Spine 1991;16:479.
255. Kumar SJ, Marks HG, Bowen JR, MacEwen GD. Hip dysplasia associated with Charcot-Marie-Tooth disease in the older child and adolescent. J Pediatr Orthop 1985;5:511.
256. Lupski JR, de Oca-Luna RM, Slaugenhaupt S, et al. DNA duplication associated with Charcot-Marie-Tooth disease type 1A. Cell 1991;66:219.
257. Mann DC, Hsu JD. Triple arthrodesis in the treatment of fixed cavovarus deformity in adolescent patients with Charcot-Marie-Tooth disease. Foot Ankle 1992;13:1.
258. Mann RA, Missirian J. Pathophysiology of Charcot-Marie-Tooth disease. Clin Orthop 1988;234:221.
259. McCluskey WP, Lovell WW, Cummings RJ. The cavovarus foot deformity. Etiology and management. Clin Orthop 1989;247:27.
260. Miller MJ, Williams LL, Slack SL, Nappi JF. The hand in Charcot-Marie-Tooth disease. J Hand Surg [Br] 1991;16:191.
261. Pailthorpe CA, Benson MKD'A. Hip dysplasia in hereditary motor and sensory neuropathies. J Bone Joint Surg [Br] 1992;74:538.
262. Patel PI, Roa BB, Welcher AA, et al. The gene for the peripheral myelin protein pmp-22 is a candidate for Charcot-Marie-Tooth disease type 1A. Nat Genet 1992;1:159.
263. Paulos L, Coleman SS, Samuelson KM. Pes cavovarus. Review of a surgical approach using selective soft-tissue procedures. J Bone Joint Surg [Am] 1980;62:942.
264. Price AE, Maisel R, Drennan JC. Computed tomographic analysis of the pes cavus. J Pediatr Orthop 1993;13:646.
265. Roa BB, Garcia CA, Suter U, et al. Charcot-Marie-Tooth disease type 1A. Association with a spontaneous point mutation in the PMP22 Gene. N Engl J Med 1993;329:96.
266. Roper BA, Tibrewal SB. Soft tissue surgery in Charcot-Marie-Tooth disease. J Bone Joint Surg [Br] 1989;71:17.
267. Sabir M, Lyttle D. Pathogenesis of Charcot-Marie-Tooth disease. Gait analysis and electrophysiologic, genetic, histopathologic, and enzyme studies in a kinship. Clin Orthop 1984;184:223.
268. Timmerman V, Nelis E, Van Hul W, et al. The peripheral myelin protein gene pmp-22 is contained within the Charcot-Marie-Tooth disease type 1A duplication. Nat Genet 1992;1:171.
269. Valentijn LJ, Bolhuis PA, Zorn I, et al. The peripheral myelin gene PMP-22/GAS-3 is duplicated in Charcot-Marie-Tooth disease type IA. Nat Genet 1992;1:166.
270. Vance JM, Nicholson GA, Yamaoka LH, et al. Linkage of Charcot-Marie-Tooth neuropathy type 1A to chromosome 17. Exp Neurol 1989;104:186.
271. Vance JM. Hereditary motor and sensory neuropathies. J Med Genet 1991;28:1.
272. Walker JL, Nelson KR, Heavilon JA, et al. Hip abnormalities in children with Charcot-Marie-Tooth disease. J Pediatr Orthop 1994;14:54.
273. Walker JL, Nelson KR, Stevens DB, et al. Spinal deformity in Charcot-Marie-Tooth disease. Spine 1994;19:1044.
274. Wetmore RS, Drennan JC. Long-term results of triple arthrodesis in Charcot-Marie-Tooth Disease. J Bone Joint Surg [Am] 1989;71:417.
275. Wukich DK, Bowen JR. A long-term study of triple arthrodesis for correction of pes cavovarus in Charcot-Marie-Tooth disease. J Pediatr Orthop 1989;9:433.

Poliomyelitis

276. Asirvatham R, Watts HG, Rooney RJ. Rotation osteotomy of the tibia after poliomyelitis. J Bone Joint Surg [Br] 1990;72:409.
277. Asirvatham R, Rooney RJ, Watts HG. Proximal tibial extension medial rotation osteotomy to correct knee flexion contracture. J Pediatr Orthop 1991;11:646.
278. Asirvatham R, Watts HG, Rooney RJ. Tendoachilles tenodesis to the fibula. A retrospective study. J Pediatr Orthop 1991;11:652.
279. Chen P-Q, Shen Y-S. Poliomyelitis scoliosis. In: Weinstein SL, ed. The pediatric spine. Principles and practice. New York: Raven Press, 1994:1069.
280. DeWald RL, Faut M. Anterior and posterior spinal surgery for paralytic scoliosis. Spine 1979;4:401.
281. Drennan JC. Poliomyelitis. In: Drennan JC, ed. The child's foot and ankle. New York: Rowen Press, 1992:305.
282. Eberle CF. Pelvic obliquity and the unstable hip after poliomyelitis. J Bone Joint Surg [Br] 1982;64:300.
283. Eberle CF. Failure of fixation after segmental spinal instrumentation without arthrodesis in the management of paralytic scoliosis. J Bone Joint Surg [Am] 1988;70:696.

284. El-Batonty MM, Aly El-S, El-Lakkany MR, Abdellatif FY. Triple arthrodesis for paralytic valgus—a modified technique: brief report. J Bone Joint Surg [Br] 1988;70:493.
285. Gaebler JW, Kleiman MB, French ML, et al. Neurologic complications in oral polio vaccine recipients. J Pediatr 1986; 108:878.
286. Gau YL, Lonstein JE, Winter RB, et al Luque-Galveston procedure for correction and stabilization of neuromuscular scoliosis and pelvic obliquity. A review of 68 patients. J Spinal Disord 1991;4:399.
287. Herndon CH. Tendon transplantation of the knee and foot. Instr Course Lect 1961;18:145.
288. Johnson EW Jr. Results of modern methods of treatment of poliomyelitis. J Bone Joint Surg 1945;27:223.
289. Kojima H, Furuta Y, Fujita M, et al. Onuf's motorneuron is resistant to poliovirus. J Neurol Sci 1989;93:85.
290. Kuhlmann RF, Bell JF. A clinical evaluation of tendon transplantations for poliomyelitis affecting the lower extremities. J Bone Joint Surg [Am] 1952;34:915.
291. Lau JHK, Parker JC, Hsu LCS, Leong JCY. Paralytic hip instability in poliomyelitis. J Bone Joint Surg [Br] 1986;68:528.
292. Leong JCY, Wilding K, Mok CD, et al. Surgical treatment of scoliosis following poliomyelitis: a review of 110 cases. J Bone Joint Surg [Am] 1981;63:726.
293. Liu T-K, Yang R-S, Sun J-S. Long-term results of the steindler flexorplasty. Clin Orthop 1993;276:104.
294. Mayer L. The physiologic method of tendon transplants. review after forty years. Instr Course Lect 1956;13:116.
295. Mayer PJ, Edwards JW, Dove J, et al. Post-poliomyelitis paralytic scoliosis. A review of curve patterns and results of surgical treatment in 118 consecutive patients. Spine 1981;6:573.
296. Mehta SN, Mukherjee AK. Flexion osteotomy of the femur for genu recurvatum after poliomyelitis. J Bone Joint Surg [Br] 1991;73:200.
297. Men H-X, Bian C-H, Yang C-D, et al. Surgical treatment of the flail knee after poliomyelitis. J Bone Joint Surg [Br] 1991; 73:195.
298. O'Brien JP, Yau ACMC, Gertzbien S, Hodgson AR. Combined staged anterior and posterior correction of the spine in scoliosis following postmyelitis. Clin Orthop 1975;110:81.
299. Pandy AK, Pandy S, Prasnd V. Calcaneal osteotomy and tendon sling for the management of calcaneus deformity. J Bone Joint Surg [Am] 1989;71:1192.
300. Perry J, Barnes G, Gronley JK. The postpolio syndrome. An overuse phenomenon. Clin Orthop 1988;233:145.
301. Schottsdaedt ER, Larsen LJ, Bost FC. Complete muscle transportation. J Bone Joint Surg [Am] 1955;37:897.
302. Sharrard WJW. Muscle recovery in poliomyelitis. J Bone Joint Surg [Br] 1955;37:63.
303. Sharrard WJW. The segmental innervation of the lower limb musculature in man. Ann R Coll Surg Engl 1964;35:106.
304. Sharrard WJW. Posterior iliopsoas transplantation in the treatment of paralytic dislocation of the hip. J Bone Joint Surg [Br] 1964;46:426.
305. Strebel PM, Sutter RW, Cochi SL, et al. Epidemiology of poliomyelitis in the United States one decade after the last reported case of indigenous wild virus-associated disease. Clin Infect Dis 1992;14:568.
306. Waring WP, Werner RA. Clinical management of carpal tunnel syndrome in patients with long-term sequelae of poliomyelitis. J Hand Surg [Am] 1989;14:865.
307. Watts HG. Management of common third world orthopaedic problems. Paralytic poliomyelitis, tuberculosis of bones and joints, hansen's disease (leprosy), and chronic osteomyelitis. Instr Course Lect 1992;41:471.
308. Westin GW, Dingeman RD, Gausewitz SH. The results of tenodesis of the teondo achilles to the fibula for paralytic pes calcaneus. J Bone Joint Surg [Am] 1988;70:320.

Chapter 16

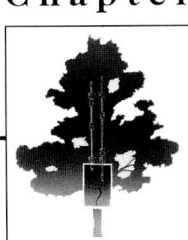

Bone and Joint Sepsis

Raymond T. Morrissy

Bone and Joint Infection
  Definition
  Epidemiology
  Etiology
  Pathophysiology of Osteomyelitis
  Pathophysiology of Septic Arthritis
Diagnosis
  History
  Examination
  Laboratory
  Organisms
  Imaging
  Aspiration
Differential Diagnosis
  Osteomyelitis
  Septic Arthritis
Treatment
  Organism Identification
  Antibiotic Selection
  Antibiotic Delivery
  Surgery
Results
Special Conditions
  The Spine
  Pelvis and SI Joint
  The Neonate
  Sickle Cell Disease
  Chronic Recurrent Multifocal
    Osteomyelitis
  Subacute Osteomyelitis
  Puncture Wounds of the Foot
  Lyme Arthritis
  Gonococcal Arthritis
  Tuberculosis

BONE AND JOINT INFECTION

Bone and joint sepsis is a relatively common disorder in the pediatric population. This makes it likely that all orthopaedic surgeons will be faced with the problems inherent in the diagnosis and treatment of these disorders. If diagnosis was always easy, this would be of little concern, but bone and joint sepsis in childhood is characterized by protean manifestations. The infant may only appear to be septic. The cause of the limp may not be obvious. The bone changes may resemble a tumor. The joint swelling may be due to an acute onset of juvenile rheumatoid arthritis (JRA).

After diagnosis, other problems remain. What antibiotic is correct for use before culture results are known? What should be done if the cultures are negative? What is the best way to administer the antibiotic and for how long? When is surgery indicated? The diversity of organisms, the variety of locations where infection is possible, and the numerous conditions associated with bone and joint sepsis increase the difficulty.

Definition

Osteomyelitis is an inflammation of the bone, and arthritis is an inflammation of the joint. Although it is assumed that osteomyelitis and septic arthritis are caused by bacteria, in certain cases, the bacteria cannot be isolated, making it necessary to develop criteria that establish the diagnosis in the absence of a bacteria. A useful definition is proposed by Petola and Vahvanen.[165] They consider the diagnosis to be firm when two of the following four criteria are present: pus aspirated from bone; positive bone or blood culture; classic symptoms of localized pain, swelling, warmth, and limited range of motion (ROM) of the adjacent joint; and radiographic changes typical of osteomyelitis. Another useful classification is that proposed by Morey and Peterson,[149] in which the diagnosis is considered to be definite when an organism is isolated from the bone or adjacent soft tissue or there is histologic evidence of osteomyelitis; probable when there is a positive blood culture in addition to clinical and roentgenographic features of osteomyelitis; or likely when there are typical clinical findings in addition to definite roentgenographic evidence of osteomyelitis and a response to antibiotics.

Because so many patients with septic arthritis have negative cultures, it is important to use criteria that include those patients. Morey included those patients with negative cultures when five of the following six criteria are present: temperature greater than 38.3°C, pain in the suspected joint that is made worse with motion, swelling of the suspected joint, systemic symptoms, absence of other pathologic processes, and a satisfactory response to antibiotics.[148]

Epidemiology

Knowledge of the epidemiology of osteomyelitis and septic arthritis is derived from institutional studies and governmental morbidity data.[41,60,76]

Osteomyelitis shows a clearly increased incidence in childhood, with a slight increase after 50 years of age. In contrast, the incidence of septic arthritis, although greatest in childhood, is markedly increased in the older age groups.[75] In childhood, septic arthritis occurs about twice as often as osteomyelitis and tends to have its peak incidence in the early years of the first decade, whereas osteomyelitis has a peak incidence in the later years of the first decade. The disease is more common in males and actually tends to increase with age through adolescence, according to hospital morbidity data.[77]

There is an impression among clinicians and in some institutional reports of a seasonal variation in the incidence of acute hematogenous osteomyelitis (AHO). Gillespie[75] confirmed this, showing an increase in the early autumn and late summer in both the Northern and Southern hemispheres.

Gillespie[75] has shown that incidence of AHO varies among races, with a higher incidence in New Zealand Maoris and Australian aboriginals than in children of European descent in these countries. At the same time, groups of similar ethnic background show differences in the incidence of AHO for which social or environmental factors may be responsible.

The idea that osteomyelitis is a changing disease is not new and perhaps indicates that it is a disease that is capable of continuous change, depending on various circumstances. In the city of Glasgow, Scotland, the incidence of AHO in children younger than 13 years of age has dropped by more than 50%, due mainly to a decrease in long bone infections. At the same time, the incidence of subacute infections increased from 12% to 42% during the period of study.[41]

Jones and colleagues[109] also suggest that the incidence of subacute osteomyelitis is increasing while the incidence of acute AHO is decreasing. In a review of 60 patients having AHO between 1980 and 1985, 35% had subacute infection.

A study from Denmark that reviewed 30 years' experience with bone and joint infection due to *Staphylococcus aureus* found that although *S aureus* bacteremia had increased over the last decade of the study (coinciding with an increase in hospital admissions), the prevalence of AHO in patients 1 to 20 years of age decreased. There was a significant increase in joint infections among patients between 1 and 20 years of age during a 4-year period in this decade. The investigators thought this likely to be due to a change in the type of *S aureus* that was predominant during this period, illustrating the complex bacterial-host interaction.[60]

In the 1970s, a change in the causative organism in septic arthritis was noted, with *Haemophilus influenzae* type B becoming the most common cause in children 1 and 4 years of age.[5] The reason for this is not clear. In the mid-1990s, *H influenzae* is becoming less common as a cause of joint sepsis, which is attributable to a vaccine against *H influenzae* that numerous children in the United States have received.

Etiology

Koch's postulates are the basis of the germ theory of infections:

- the organism must be identified at the site of the disease
- the organism must not be found in other diseases
- the organism must be able to produce the disease in other animals
- the organism must be identified in the disease that is produced.[119]

Pasteur[160a] failed to satisfy Koch's postulates when he injected staphylococci intravenously into guinea pigs, as did many others after him. Rodet[175] was reportedly successful but details in his report are sketchy. Others have reported variable success.[229]

The reproducible creation of a bone or joint infection requires some other intervention, usually something that has the potential to change the local environment. The standard model for the study of antibiotics for treatment of osteomyelitis involves the injection of sodium morrhuate directly into the bone to produce necrosis, followed by the injection of bacteria directly into the area.[156]

Some of the earliest attempts to produce osteomyelitis in animals involved trauma to the bone, and many of these were reportedly successful. Trauma to the growth plate, followed by the intravenous injection of *S aureus*, has produced an AHO that resembles the human form of the disease.[152,234] These studies allow observations on the pathology of AHO.

How bacteria lodge in a bone or joint and then establish a clinical infection cannot be completely explained. There are numerous bacteria in and on our body, and bacteremia is a daily event in childhood, giving ample opportunity for bacteria to gain access to the bones and joints.[62] The answer lies in a better understanding of the factors that influence host resistance, of bacteria pathogenicity, and of factors that relate both, an exploration of which is beyond the scope of this chapter.

Among the factors that have been observed to be associated with infection, none is so common as trauma. The idea of trauma as a predisposing factor to infection is not new. As mentioned, it was one of the earliest methods in experimental efforts to produce AHO. The entire subject was summarized by Burrows[28] in 1932, when he popularized the term *locus minoris resistentiae* to describe the effect injury had on decreasing resistance to infection. Clinically, trauma to the affected part is noted in 30% to 50% of those who have clinical AHO.[49,78,133,188,238] Although there are no similar clinical data for septic arthritis, experimental models demonstrate the role of trauma in the production of the disease.[158,186]

The conclusion that may be drawn from the clinical and laboratory data is that trauma is not always essential for an infection to be established but that it makes it easier in some circumstances.

Just as trauma is a factor, so is the function of the immune system. This is easily illustrated by the increased susceptibility to infections of all types in those patients with diseases characterized by deficient or altered immune function and in the neonate with immature immune function.

More mysterious are those factors that may cause temporary and transient depression of immune function (e.g., intercurrent viral illness, anesthesia, surgery, trauma, and malnutrition); all are known to impair certain aspects of immune function and have been related to an increased incidence of clinical infection.

Despite our partial understanding of the interrelated factors between host and bacteria, many aspects of AHO and septic arthritis in children remain unexplained; for example, the predilection for males, increased incidence of infection in the lower extremities, and peak age incidence.

Pathophysiology of Osteomyelitis

Bone is unique as a tissue and as an organ, not only for its rigid and variable structure but also for its ability to heal and replace itself with entirely normal tissue without scar.

There are two types of cortical bone that are especially evident in childhood. That which is found in the metaphyseal region is little more than a compact version of cancellous bone. Its maze-like structure allows easy communication between the subperiosteal space and the medullary space. The cortical bone of the diaphysis is dense lamellar bone, which is relatively acellular. Consequently, it is impenetrable and renews itself more slowly. This structure is more obvious in the larger bones (Fig. 16-1A).

The cancellous bone that makes up the central part is also differentiated both by structure and function. The central cellular part, known as the medullary cavity, has little bone but contains a rich reticuloendothelial system. The metaphyseal region has more bone structure but is relatively acellular, containing few cells of the reticuloendothelial system. These differences are more pronounced in the long bones, particularly at the rapidly growing ends (see Fig. 16-1A and B).

The periosteum of a child's bone is thick. Although it is easily separated from the bone, it is not easily penetrated by infection. Because its blood supply is from the outside, elevation from the bone does not impair function and it continues to produce osteoid and bone. In children, this response of an elevated periosteum is often dramatic, producing a layer of bone around the original bone.

In a classic article, Hobo[97] described his experiments on the localization of both India ink particles and bacteria in bone after intravenous injection. He noted that although most bacteria lodged in the medullary cavity, they were rapidly phagocytized and no infection resulted. In the area beneath the epiphyseal plate, few bacteria lodged. These bacteria were not phagocytized, however, due to the absence of phagocytic cells in this region of the bone and infection subsequently developed. Hobo thought that the vessels beneath the physeal plate were small arterial loops that emptied into venous sinusoids and that the resulting turbulence was the cause of localization. Electron microscopic studies have shown these to be small terminal branches, however,[185] whereas the endothelial wall of new metaphyseal capillaries have gaps that allow the passage of blood cells and presumably bacteria.[200]

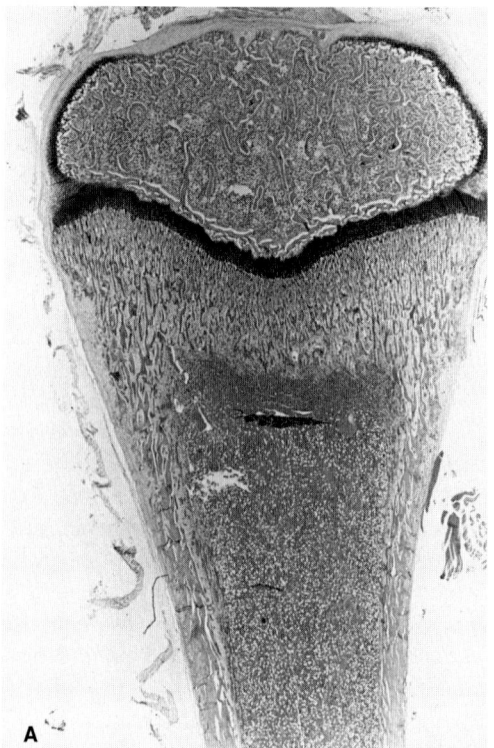
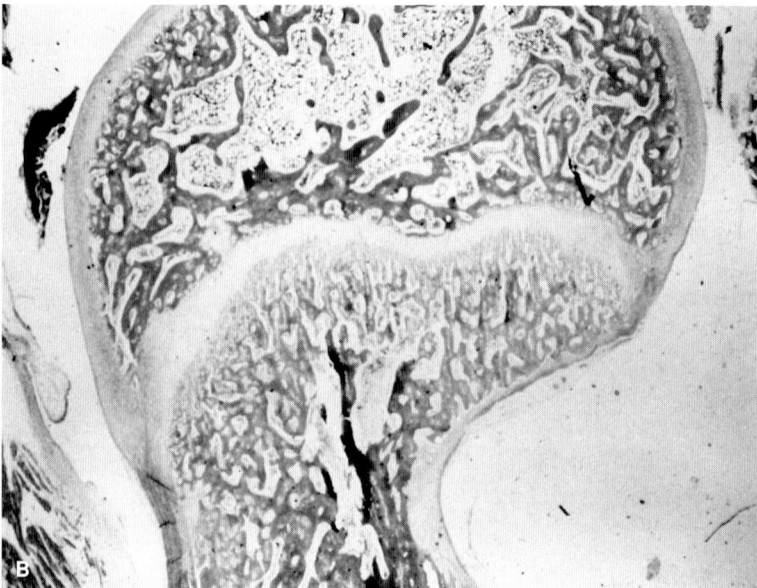

FIGURE 16-1. (A) Proximal tibia and (B) proximal radius of a 6-week-old rabbit, demonstrating the difference in the cortical bone between the metaphysis and the diaphysis. The diaphyseal cortex is composed of thick, relatively acellular bone, whereas the metaphyseal cortex is a condensation of the spongy metaphyseal bone. Also note the difference in the cellularity between the metaphyseal and the diaphyseal area. The size of this metaphyseal area separating the cellular marrow from the area beneath the epiphyseal plate is different in the rapidly growing bones, such as the proximal tibia (A), than in the slow-growing bones, such as the proximal radius (B).

How and why bacteria lodge in the area beneath the epiphyseal plate and establish an infection in this region is poorly understood. In closed experiments with trauma as a model, infection did not develop in fractures of the diaphysis of the fibula or in the uninjured metaphysis of the tibia but developed in the injured metaphysis.[152,234] Thus, bacterial seeding of a hematoma cannot be the explanation. It is possible that specific bacteria-substrate interactions play a role (e.g., those that occur for the localization of certain bacteria in the nasopharynx or on damaged heart valves). Possibly, the injury to the unique physeal plate cartilage produces a new substrate that is attractive to certain bacteria—specifically, those that cause AHO. There are numerous other possibilities.[152,234]

Trueta[222] was the first to note the importance of the changing anatomy of the interosseous blood supply with age. In the infant, before the ossific nucleus is formed, the vessels from the metaphysis penetrate directly into the cartilaginous anlage of the epiphysis (Fig. 16-2A). As the ossific nucleus develops, a separate blood supply to this epiphysis develops and the metaphyseal vessels crossing the developing physeal plate disappear (see Fig. 16-2B). The change is signaled by the development of the ossification of the epiphysis and is generally complete with the distinct formation of a physeal plate (see Fig. 16-2C and D).

Because of this blood supply pattern in the infant, the initial bacterial localization is in the cartilaginous precursor of the epiphysis. Infection results in its early destruction, with the consequent alteration of future growth. When the physeal plate is formed, it provides a temporary barrier to the spread of infection into the epiphysis because the vessels end beneath the plate.

A unique characteristic of hematogenous osteomyelitis is its predilection for the most rapidly growing end of the large long bones, especially those of the lower extremity. This may be explained by the observation that in rapidly growing bones, the phagocytic cells are further from where the bacteria localize because of the structure of these bones (see Fig. 16-1A and B). Thus, the inflammatory response takes longer to reach the bacteria, allowing a clinical infection to become established.

Bone formation and resorption are integrally linked. Diseases that result in net bone loss may be viewed as being processes that alter this linkage. The earliest change observed in osteomyelitis is the death

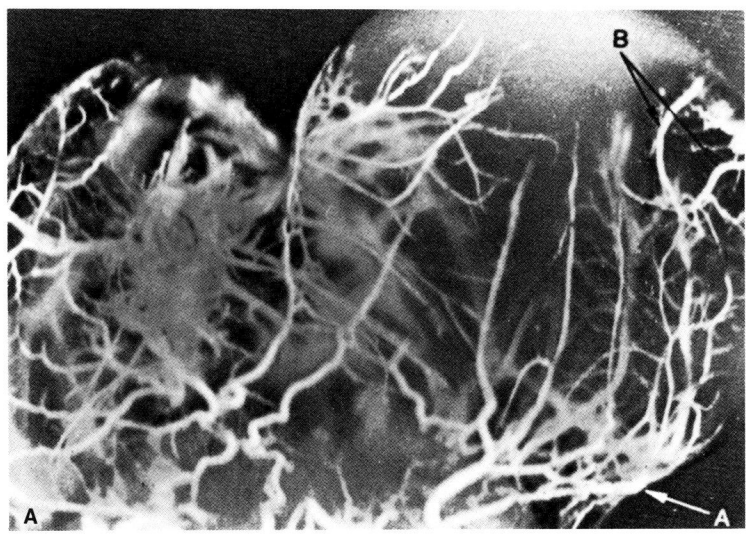
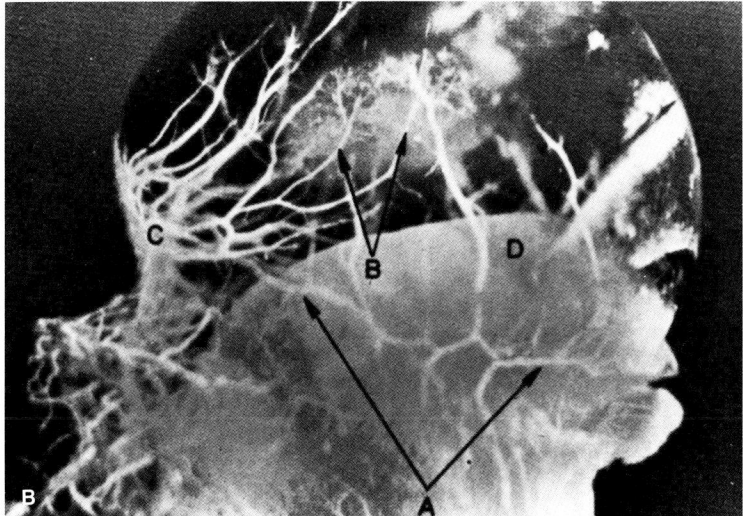
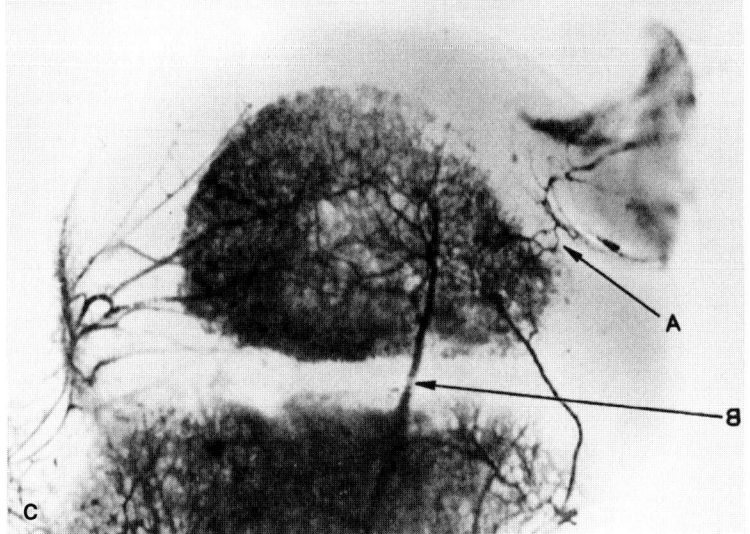

FIGURE 16-2. Human specimens of the proximal femur that are injected with barium sulfate demonstrate the changing blood supply to the developing femoral head with growth. (**A**) In the 3-day-old infant, the vessels proceed directly from the metaphysis into the cartilaginous precursor of the femoral head. (**B**) By 9 months of age, separate vessels (**C**) have developed to supply the ossifying nucleus of the femoral head. (**C**) At 3 years, 4 months of age, the vessels crossing from the metaphysis have disappeared. Only peripheral vessels remain to supply the epiphysis. (From Chung SMK. The arterial supply of the developing proximal end of the human femur. J Bone Joint Surg [Am] 1976;58:961.)

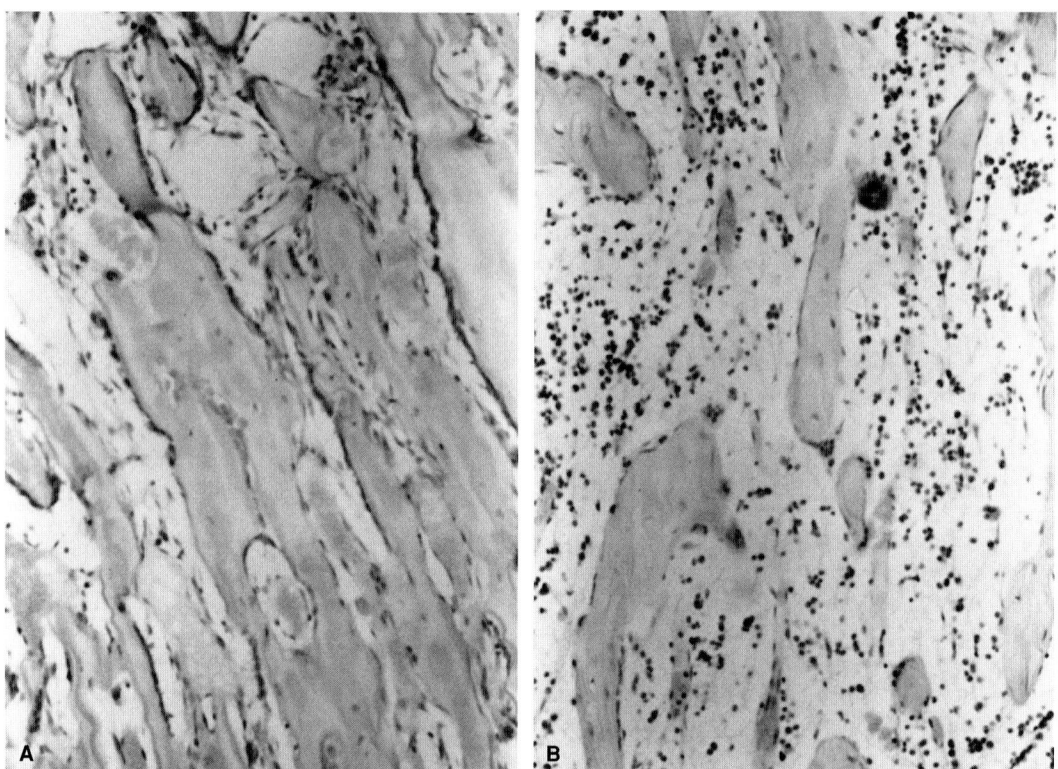

FIGURE 16-3. (A) A photomicrograph of the proximal tibial metaphysis of a 6-week-old rabbit demonstrates trabecular bone lined with osteoblasts. (B) Twenty-four hours after induction of experimental hematogenous osteomyelitis by injury to the physis and intravenous injection of *Staphylococcus aureus*, the osteoblasts have disappeared, and the trabeculae are being resorbed by osteoclasts.

of the osteoblasts, followed by resorption of the bony trabeculae by numerous osteoclasts (Fig. 16-3A and B). This occurs over a wide area of the metaphysis surrounding the infection, beginning within 12 to 18 hours. In experimental situations, it has also been shown that lymphocytes may release an osteoclastic activating factor, whereas macrophages, monocytes, and vascular endothelial cells may all directly resorb both the crystalline and matrix components of bone.

Although the complete mechanism of this finding is yet to be elucidated, it is known that in response to toxins and bacterial antigens, interleukin-1 is produced by macrophages and polymorphonuclear leukocytes.[218] Interleukin-1 is known to cause most of the events known as inflammation and to stimulate the production of prostaglandin E_2, which stimulates osteoclast bone resorption.[50] In response to these stimuli, inflammatory cells accumulate and migrate to the area of bacterial localization beneath the physis. As these inflammatory cells migrate to the accumulating bacteria, the bone in the path of the migration is resorbed (Fig. 16-4A and B).

In response to products liberated by the increasing number of bacteria as well as host factors, inflammatory cells begin to accumulate.[131] Because there are few such cells in the area of bacterial localization beneath the physeal plate, this response begins in a region closer to the medullary cavity. Over the next few days this inflammatory response migrates to the area of the bacteria, and the bone in its path is resorbed (Fig. 16-5A). As the accumulation of pus continues, it finds egress through the maze-like cortex of the metaphysis (see Fig. 16-5A). If the infection continues, a subperiosteal abscess forms, the periosteum is elevated, and new osteoid is formed under the elevated periosteum (see Fig. 16-5B).

If the metaphysis lies within the joint, septic arthritis results early in the process because the periosteum within the joint is thin and the pus quickly ruptures through it. This occurs in four locations in the older child: proximal femur, proximal humerus, distal lateral tibia, and proximal radius. As the periosteum is elevated, the cortical bone is deprived of its blood supply and may become necrotic, forming a sequestrum. Because the blood supply to the periosteum comes from the muscle side, it remains healthy and begins to lay down new bone, known as the involucrum.

It is important to note that the pus does not usually spread down the medullary cavity because it is successfully walled off by the inflammatory response (see Fig. 16-5B). Contrary to how it may first appear, the

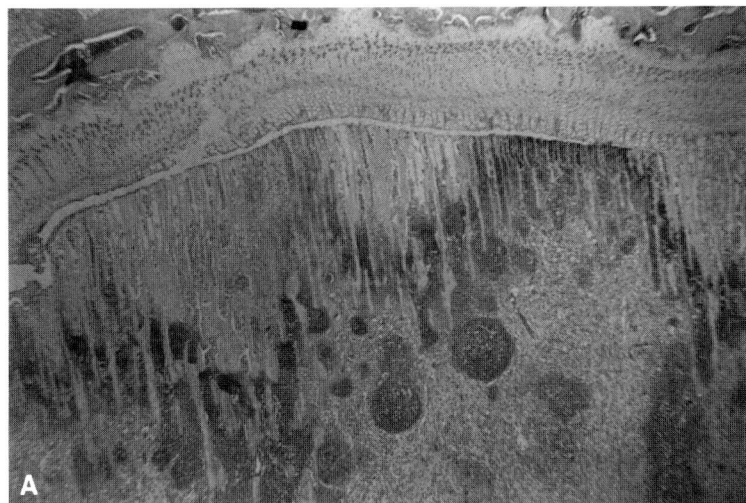
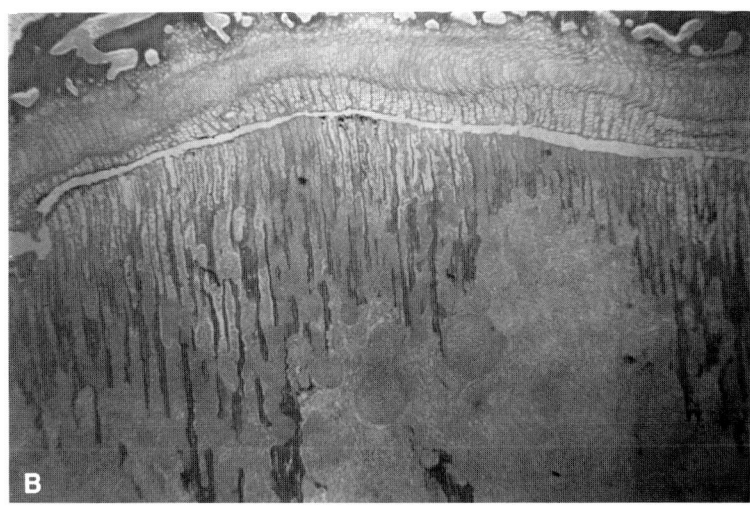

FIGURE 16-4. (A) In a hematoxolin and eosin–stained specimen of a 3-day-old hematogenous infection in the proximal tibia of a rabbit, the accumulation of inflammatory cells and microabscesses can be seen. (B) In an adjacent Gram-stained section, the remaining bony and cartilaginous columns and microabscesses can be seen. In addition, small clumps of organisms can be seen beneath the physis.

path of least resistance in the presence of a healthy inflammatory response is through the metaphyseal cortex. The spread of pus into the medullary cavity is seen either in a neglected case or in a patient whose immunity is impaired.

Pathophysiology of Septic Arthritis

As in bone, the unique anatomic features of a joint should be considered in relation to infection. The synovial lining of the joint is a unique and vascular tissue that does not have a basement membrane. It secretes a fluid that is essentially a transudate of serum. The remainder of the joint surface is avascular cartilage. The interior of the joint provides a unique environment for bacterial proliferation, similar to a culture tube.

It is probable that the transient bacteremia experienced by children results in bacteria entering the joint. It has been demonstrated that the joint has the ability to clear bacteria from the joint, thus avoiding clinical infection.[108] There are two important limitations to this ability: the mechanism is not so effective with pathogenic bacteria (e.g., S aureus) and there is a limit to the amount of bacteria that can be cleared.

Localization of bacteria in a joint is not so well understood as it is in bone. Although trauma has been implicated as being a factor,[186] it may not completely explain the propensity for large joints and those of the lower extremity to be involved. What is apparent, however, is that bacteria are present not only in the synovium but also gain access to the joint cavity early in the process. Within a matter of hours, this is associated with a synovitis and fibrinous exudate, followed shortly by areas of synovial necrosis.

The mechanisms of cartilage destruction have been extensively studied in both bacterial and nonbacterial arthritis. Although the specific mechanisms of cartilage destruction may differ, depending on the infecting organism, it is important that the clinician understand the biology of the process that he is attempting to alter.

A large variety of enzymes (e.g., proteases, peptidases, collagenases) are released from the leukocytes,

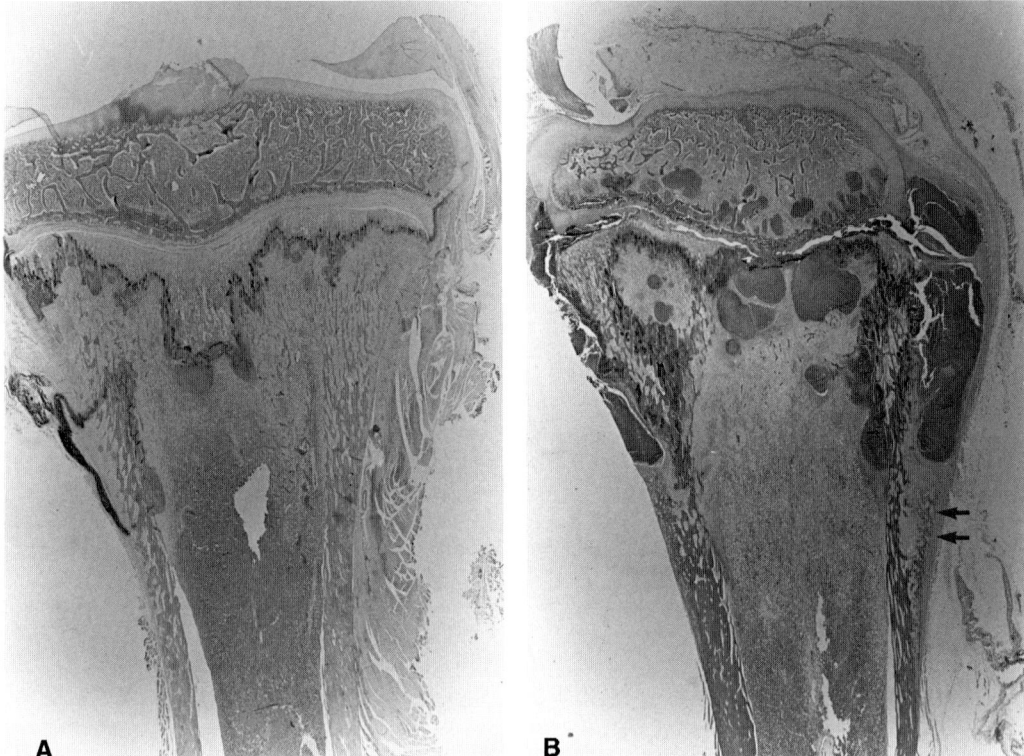

FIGURE 16-5. (**A**) Rabbit's tibia with 3-day-old hematogenous osteomyelitis. A small amount of pus has found its way through the metaphyseal cortex into the subperiosteal space. (**B**) Rabbit's tibia with 7-day-old infection. Note the well-developed intraosseous abscesses in addition to the large subperiosteal abscess. New bone formation is occurring beneath the elevated periosteum (*arrow*). (From Morrissy RT, Haynes DH. Acute hematogenous osteomyelitis: a model with trauma as an etiology. J Pediatr Orthop 1989;9:447.)

the synovial cells, and the cartilage. These enzymes are capable of degrading the matrix and the collagen of articular cartilage. In addition, organisms (e.g., *S aureus*, several gram-negative bacteria) liberate extracellular proteolytic enzymes.[7,51,90,159,209]

These enzymes initiate the first measurable change in the articular cartilage, the loss of glycosaminoglycan. This can occur as early as 8 hours in experimental models and is not detectable by visual inspection.[195] It renders the cartilage less stiff and perhaps subject to increased wear.[91] Collagen destruction occurs later in the process and is responsible for the visual changes that may be seen.[44–46] It is important to understand that these destructive mechanisms do not require the continued presence of live organisms to be sustained.

DIAGNOSIS

History

Among the expected symptoms in any case of bone or joint sepsis, pain leads the list.[63,187] This common symptom is not always verbalized by children. Thus, it is important for the physician to realize that it may be expressed in many different ways: refusal to walk, refusal to bear weight, limping, or simple disuse of a part.

A careful history should do more than lead to a suspicion of infection. It should lead to the consideration of the possible organism, the reason the particular organism established a clinical infection, the stage of the infection, and the possible extent of damage.

Although it is difficult to relate the stage of infection seen in experimental animals to the onset of clinical symptoms of a child, there seems to be a relatively close correlation, which suggests that symptoms begin shortly after the establishment of the inflammatory reaction in the bone or joint. The ease of access to expert medical care in some parts of the United States demonstrates this. It is no longer unusual to see children within 12 hours of the onset of limp who have only normal or mildly elevated laboratory values and a positive bacterial aspirate from the bone or joint.

A good clinical correlation is that pus is seldom found on aspiration of bone with fewer than 3 days of symptoms. The same is not true for joints, wherein elevated leukocyte counts are found in the joint fluid within 24 hours of symptoms.

This response is frequently blunted by the unintentional or ill-advised use of antibiotics before establishing the diagnosis of bone or joint infection. Thus, when recent antibiotic administration is a part of the history, care must be taken in interpreting each clinical symptom, sign, and laboratory value.

In the history, a careful search should be made for concomitant infections, recent infection, or reasons for lowered resistance to infection. A history of recent upper respiratory infection or other seemingly unrelated illness is frequent and may explain an organism's access to the circulation. Recent rash or swollen nodes are important for their association with diseases such as rheumatoid arthritis, Lyme arthritis, or leukemia.

Chickenpox is probably the most common childhood illness that produces a temporary suppression of immunity, leading to an increased incidence of skin infections, usually due to *S aureus* and group A *Streptococcus*. This in turn leads to an increased opportunity for bone or joint infections with these organisms.[87]

Trauma has been mentioned as a possible etiologic factor in both osteomyelitis and septic arthritis. Its importance in the history is twofold. First, it should be recognized that symptoms after trauma may not be due to trauma, particularly when they are more severe day by day or fail to improve as expected. Secondly, the history of trauma may successfully direct the search for the location in children too young to communicate.

Examination

The entire purpose of the examination is to search for signs of infection and to localize the process.

The typical child who is seen in the first 3 to 4 days of osteomyelitis or septic arthritis may appear unhappy and out of sorts but rarely appears to be ill or moribund, as has often been described. Fever is not a consistent accompaniment of what would seem to be such a serious infection.[63,187]

Because most cases of AHO and septic arthritis involve the lower extremities, a common finding is limp. This usually is an antalgic limp, defined by a shortened stance phase on the affected leg. Failure to use an upper extremity in the usual manner or discomfort noted by the mother in dressing the child are common symptoms in the upper extremity.

Swelling and erythema, cardinal signs of infection, are of value early in the process only in bones that are not covered by muscles and in joints that are easily palpated. Loss of normal concavities and loss of normal skin wrinkles may be the only subtle clues. Visual comparison of the normal and affected limb symmetrically positioned should always be done.

After the affected part is identified by limp or disuse, palpation of the bones and joints is used to identify the specific location of the inflammation. In the case of small children who cry at the mere presence of a stranger and panic at being touched, it is often beneficial to instruct the parent how to elicit the tender area. After showing the parent how to palpate the area, the physician should leave the room and allow the parent to first examine the unaffected and then the affected part and report the results.

Joints are more effectively examined by ROM than tenderness, although palpation of those joints that are not covered by muscle may reveal both the presence of an effusion and tenderness. Involvement of large joints covered by large amounts of tissue is detected by a decreased ROM. In the axial skeleton, such as the spine and the sacroiliac (SI) region, percussion and compression, respectively, are more effective in eliciting symptoms than palpation.

An infected joint usually has neither full flexion nor extension and may be painful through anything but a small ROM. In the case of the hip, internal rotation, which tightens the hip capsule, is painful and limited.

Laboratory

The leukocytes count is not a reliable indication of inflammation in its early stages and when normal often leads the physician away from the correct diagnosis of sepsis. In a series from the Mayo clinic, only 25% of infants and children with osteomyelitis had a leukocyte count above normal for their age and only in 65% was the differential count abnormal.[149] The results were similar for a series of patients from the same institution with septic arthritis.[148] This has been confirmed in other series.[49,63,187]

The erythrocyte sedimentation rate (ESR) is one of the nonspecific acute-phase reactants found in the serum in response to inflammation. Although nonspecific and poorly understood, it reflects the concentration of fibrinogen and immunoglobulins. The ESR is almost always elevated within 48 to 72 hours of the onset of infection and returns over a period of 2 to 4 weeks to normal after elimination of the infection. In the Mayo clinic series, the ESR was below 20 mm in only 5 of 76 patients with septic arthritis.[148] It appears that an elevated ESR can be anticipated in about 90% of cases that subsequently prove to be AHO.[63,187] Although noted to be elevated just as often in patients with osteomyelitis, the ESR was significantly higher in those with septic arthritis.[148] These authors did not find the value of the ESR diminished by previous antibiotic therapy.

The ESR is unreliable in the neonate, in the presence of significant anemia, in patients with sickle cell disease, or when the patient is taking steroids. It is less reliable when symptoms have been present for less than 48 to 72 hours. Although the ESR continues to rise for 3 to 5 days after institution of successful therapy, a continuing rise beyond the fourth to fifth day of treatment is an indication of failure to eradicate the infection. For this reason, the ESR is not a good means of assessing the resolution of sepsis during the first week of treatment because its fall lags behind resolution of the infection.[166]

The C-reactive protein (CRP) is a substance found in the serum in response to inflammation and trauma. The CRP may begin to rise within 6 hours of the triggering stimulus and then increases several hundredfold, reaching a peak within 50 hours. In contrast to the ESR, it may be of greater value, not only for earlier diagnosis of infection but also for determining resolution of the inflammation.[164]

One report comparing serial determinations of ESR and CRP in 44 children with proved bacteriologic osteomyelitis demonstrated the ESR to be elevated initially in 92% of the patients and the CRP to be elevated in 98%.[223] The peak ESR was measured on days 3 through 5, whereas the peak CRP was measured on day 2. Thereafter, it took the ESR about 3 weeks to return to normal, whereas the CRP returned to normal within 1 week. Thus, the CRP is more likely to be helpful in diagnosing the early case of infection and is more useful after its resolution.

Blood cultures are indispensable because they frequently demonstrate the organism. In most series, the yield from blood culture ranges between 30% and 50% in both septic arthritis and osteomyelitis. The yield from both blood culture and aspirated material decreases with previous antibiotic therapy.[148] Even with previous antibiotic treatment, however, the chances of obtaining positive cultures when all sources (blood, bone, and joint fluid) are cultured remain high.[187]

The importance of needle aspiration of the bone or direct biopsy at the time of surgery before antibiotic administration is emphasized by the frequency with which positive cultures are obtained. In 91 aspirations of bone for osteomyelitis, pus was obtained in 58% and positive cultures were obtained in 70% of these aspirates, yielding 40 positive cultures from all aspirates.[187] In other series, the yield of positive cultures from bone has been even higher, ranging from 51% to 73%.[63,165]

Aspiration of joint fluid provides the opportunity to gather more information than does bone aspiration. The question, however, is which tests in addition to the culture and Gram stain are worthwhile. The answer appears to be that only the leukocyte count and the percentage of polymorphonuclear cells are of value.[66,191] Because fluid from an infected joint frequently clots, it may be helpful to rinse the syringe with heparin before aspirating the joint. Because only a small amount of fluid may be obtained, care must be taken to not leave any significant volume of heparin in the syringe, which may alter the cell count.

TABLE 16-1   Synovial Fluid Analysis

DISEASE	LEUKOCYTES*	POLYMORPHS* (%)
Normal	<200	<25
Traumatic	<5000 with many erythrocytes	<25
Toxic synovitis	5000–15,000	<25
Acute rheumatic fever	10,000–15,000	50
Juvenile rheumatoid arthritis	15,000–80,000	75
Septic arthritis	>80,000	>75

* The leukocyte count and percentage of polymorphs can vary in most diseases, depending on the severity and duration of the process. Overlap greater than shown in these averages is possible.
Morrissy RT. Septic arthritis. In: Gustilo RB, Genninger RP, Tsukayama DT, eds. Orthopaedic infection: diagnosis and treatment. Philadelphia: WB Saunders, 1989.

Although it is generally assumed that septic joints have a leukocyte count from 80,000/mL to more than 100,000/mL and other inflammatory disorders in the differential diagnosis have counts of 50,000/mL and less, there is considerable overlap (Table 16-1). In a series of 126 bacteriologically proved cases of septic arthritis, Fink and Nelson[66] found leukocyte counts of 50,000 mL or less in 55%, with 34% having counts less than 25,000/mL. Only 44% of the patients had counts of 100,000/mL. At the same time, inflammatory diseases (e.g., rheumatoid arthritis) may have counts in excess of 80,000/mL.[9]

As in osteomyelitis, the frequency of positive cultures seems to be slightly higher with open biopsy than with needle biopsy but the difference is not great. In addition, the positive yields are generally not as high as in osteomyelitis, ranging in various reports from 36% to 80%.[63,165,237]

The importance of obtaining material from blood and bone or joint aspiration is emphasized in a report by Vaughan and colleagues,[224] in which many children with osteomyelitis had only positive blood cultures, whereas others had only positive bone cultures.

Gram staining is the only opportunity for presumptive identification of the organism within a few hours of initial patient contact and is thus a valuable test that should not be ignored. It appears from reports of both septic arthritis and osteomyelitis that the Gram stain demonstrates an organism in about one third of the bone or joint aspirates.[63,66,187]

Certain bacteria growing in the body release their type-specific polysaccharide capsule into the circulation. Detection of this antigen by either counterimmunoelectrophoresis or cold agglutination tests can provide presumptive evidence for the organism.[120,143] The release of this antigen does not depend on the presence of live organisms. Therefore, this test has the potential of rapid identification of the organism and may be especially useful in patients who have received previous antibiotics.

Initially performed by counterimmunoelectrophoresis, the test can also be performed by more simple and rapid agglutination tests. It can be used to detect the presence of those bacteria with a type-specific capsular antigen: *H influenzae* type B, *Streptococcus pneumoniae*, group B streptococcus, and *Neisseria meningitidis*. Although the test can theoretically be performed on any fluid, it is best done on urine or synovial fluid. False-positive results can occur from surface bacteria that are inadvertently gathered with the specimen (e.g., a urine bag).

The test is positive in about 20% of patients and depends on the incidence of organisms that are detectable by this method. There are few data on how often the test is positive in the presence of negative blood and joint cultures.[48] Personal experience using this test has not proved rewarding.

Organisms

The value of knowing the relative incidence of causative organisms is threefold:

1. to aid in selecting a likely effective antibiotic before the organism is positively identified by culture
2. to understand the unique characteristics of the organism, if any, so that treatment may be modified accordingly
3. to appreciate that it is impossible to accurately predict which organism is responsible without a positive culture.

When only hematogenous osteomyelitis and septic arthritis are considered, age is the most important factor in the incidence of a particular organism. The most useful age division is the neonate, the infant younger than 2 years of age, and the child. The neonate is considered separately. In reviewing different series, there are often wide variations in the percentage of cases caused by a particular organism. This may be because of the years over which the data were gathered, the population being evaluated, and the diligence in identifying the organisms. Despite these variations, some useful generalizations can be made.

S aureus is the most common causative organism in AHO after infancy, with the incidence ranging between 25% and 64%, depending largely on the age mix of the patients in the study.[49,63,166,187] Streptococcal organisms, including group A *Streptococcus* and *S pneumoniae*, are also common, ranging from 4% to 21%. Infections with streptococcal organisms tend to occur in the younger age groups.[49,163]

H influenzae type B has been reported as becoming a more common organism in hematogenous osteomyelitis. In one report, it was the second most common organism identified in 21% of the positive cultures.[63] All of the children were younger than 3 years of age and as in other reports, there seems to be a tendency for such cases to occur in the upper extremity.

In septic arthritis, *H influenzae* has been the most common organism in patients younger than 5 years of age, whereas *S aureus* is the most common organism in children older than 5 years of age.[10,66,190] It is important to recognize that as many as 30% of children with *H influenzae* septic arthritis may also have meningitis.[179,190] This is especially likely to occur in children younger than 2 years of age. With the use of the vaccine, *H influenzae* as a cause of septic arthritis (the incidence of which has increased during the past three decades) should no longer be seen. As does *H influenzae*, several other organisms (e.g., group B streptococci and *Escherichia coli*) found in septic arthritis show a predilection for the younger age groups.

An organism that is increasingly identified in osteoarticular infections, particularly in the younger child, is *Kingella kingae*. This organism was initially identified and characterized in the late 1960s. It has been isolated in slightly more than 1% of pharyngeal cultures but may be more prevalent. In one series of infections due to *K kingae*, 56% of the patients had a respiratory infection.[242] It is described as an opportunistic pathogen and is thought to colonize the nasopharynx and then invade the bloodstream. Favored sites are bone, joints, disk space, and heart.

The increased incidence of *K kingae* infection may be due to better methods of isolation. It has been demonstrated that inoculation of the material into a BACTEC culture bottle (Johnston Laboratories, Towson, MD) can dramatically increase the rate of recovery of *K kingae*.[243]

Like *H influenzae*, *K kingae* infections most often occur in children younger than 5 years of age. Most children are healthy before the onset of the infection. The organism affects joints most frequently. The clinical course and laboratory findings do not differ significantly from septic arthritis caused by other organisms. The bone infections are often insidious and frequently occur in the epiphysis. Treatment failures are unusual. The organism is sensitive to penicillin and to many of the semisynthetic penicillins and cephalosporins that are used to treat bone and joint infections.[72,123]

Imaging

Plain Radiographs

Deep soft tissue swelling is the earliest radiographic evidence of osteomyelitis.[31] The role of radiography in the diagnosis of early bone and joint sepsis is often undervalued. This is because it is often considered only to seek changes in the bone, which in osteomyelitis may not occur for 5 to 7 days after the onset of symptoms. Radiographs are a two-dimensional representation of density difference and as such can detect changes in the soft tissues as well as in the bone. Because the inflammation in the bone or joint produces edema in the soft tissues adjacent to the area of inflammation, there is swelling in this region, with enlargement of this muscle layer detectable on the radiograph. In addition, the edema obliterates the normal fat planes that can be seen between the muscle layers. All of this can be detected with routine radiographs if they are properly obtained.

Detection of deep soft tissue swelling and loss of normal fat planes depends on comparison of one limb with the other. Therefore, radiographs should be ordered of symmetrically positioned views of both limbs, using a technique to demonstrate the soft tissues (Fig. 16-6).

Radiographs to detect deep soft tissue swelling are of most value in suspected sepsis of the long bones. The technique becomes less useful in the axial skeleton because of the large overlapping muscles. An additional problem in interpretation occurs around the hip. In this location, the normal external rotation and abduction position assumed by the irritable hip (regardless of the cause) causes the appearance of capsular bulging.[24] Another sign that is often sought in suspected sepsis of the hip joint is joint space widening. Although this may be seen frequently in the neonate, it is often lacking in older children. It is a late sign and its absence is not to be interpreted as lack of sepsis.[226]

The more classic radiographic signs of osteomyelitis—resorption of bone and periosteal new bone formation—are easily recognized. The forms that the bone destruction can take are myriad, however, and particularly in children can be confused with bone neoplasms.[29,129] This is another point that illustrates the importance of a definitive tissue or bacteriologic diagnosis before treatment can be confidently pursued (Fig. 16-7).

Bone Scan

Radionuclide scanning of the skeleton is done with three different radiopharmaceuticals: technetium 99m (^{99m}Tc) diphosphonate, gallium 67 citrate, and indium 111. Because of the high diagnostic accuracy of the scan; easy availability; relatively low cost; high resolution, compared with other methods; and rapidity, ^{99m}Tc diphosphonate is the clear choice for detecting physiologic alterations in the skeletal tissues of children.

An understanding of the uptake and mechanism of ^{99m}Tc diphosphonate in bone is useful in the interpretation of scans.[70] Although isotope uptake depends on a combination of vascularity and calcium phosphate deposition, there is not a proportional relation between isotope uptake and vascularity, as is seen in the epiphyseal plate, bone tumors, and healing fractures. This is because the material deposited during earliest stages of calcium phosphate deposition differs from more mature calcium phosphate deposition in terms of calcium to phosphorus ratio, hydration, and density. Diphosphonate adsorption to this new calcium phosphate material has been shown to be considerably greater than to more mature calcium phosphate.

Bone scans are often referred to as three-phase bone scans. This relates to the time after injection of the radiopharmaceutical that the scan is made and

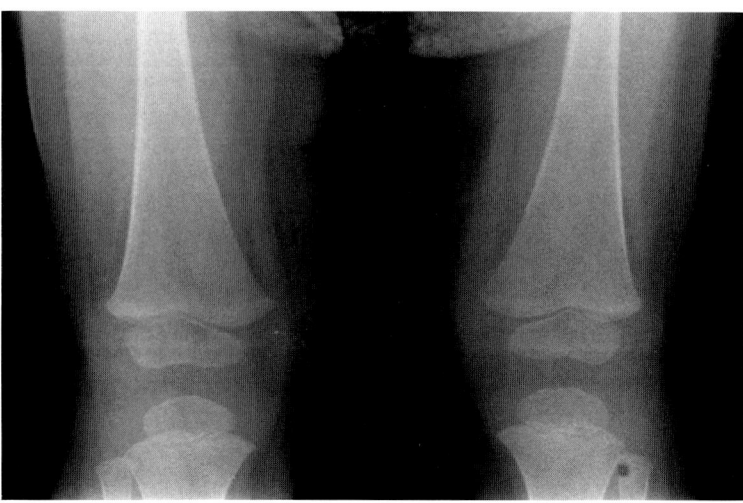

FIGURE 16-6. Plain radiograph of a 16-month-old toddler with a 36-hour history of increasing difficulty bearing weight and pain in the region of the left knee. Note the deep soft tissue swelling about the medial side of the distal left femur. Deep soft tissue swelling is the earliest finding in osteomyelitis.

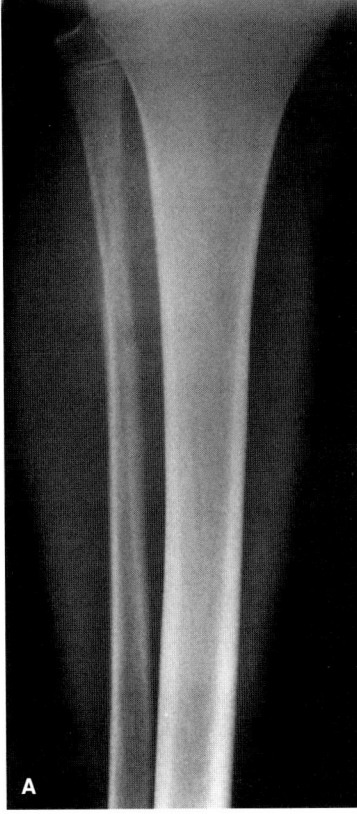
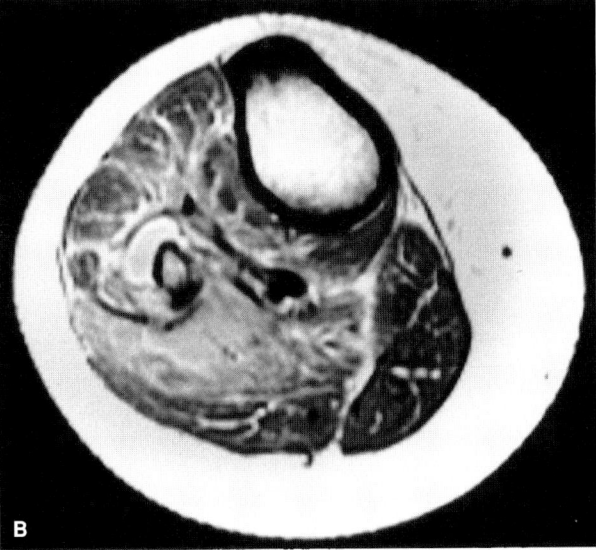

FIGURE 16-7. (A) Radiograph of the leg of a 14-year-old boy who presented with swelling and pain for the past 6 weeks. He related the onset to twisting his leg when he fell into a hole. Is this osteomyelitis or tumor? Note the deep soft tissue swelling, the bone destruction, and the periosteal new bone around the fibula. (B) The magnetic resonance imaging scan demonstrated bone destruction, fluid in one area around the fibula, and extensive edema in the surrounding muscles, all of which suggest that osteomyelitis is more likely. The fibula was biopsied as though the lesion were malignant. Pus and gram-positive staphylococci were identified.

what is being imaged. The first phase is actually an angiogram, performed immediately after injection. This is immediately followed by the second or "blood pool" phase, during which the vascular pooling is examined. These stages reflect soft tissue flow and are helpful in distinguishing cellulitis from osteomyelitis.[100,136] The third phase occurs 2 to 4 hours after injection. This allows clearing of the background material and uptake in the skeletal tissues.

It is during the third phase that the most important images are obtained. The bladder should be empty, so that accumulated isotope does not obstruct the sacrum. It is important that symmetrically positioned views of both sides be obtained. In children, it is important that pinhole or converging-collimator images be obtained of suspected areas of infection. Because most AHO occurs in the metaphysis adjacent to the physeal plate, such views are necessary to separate early metaphyseal changes from the large amount of uptake found in the physeal plate (Fig. 16-8A and B). Because these images are time-consuming to obtain, it is important that the physician communicate the desired areas of interest to the radiologist.

The value of radionuclide scans in children with suspected bone or joint sepsis differs, depending on the diagnosis. In a large series of 280 patients referred with a clinical diagnosis of osteomyelitis, the scan correctly identified osteomyelitis at 55 of 62 sites of proved osteomyelitis in the appendicular skeleton.[100] This report demonstrated a sensitivity of 89% and a specificity of 94%, with an overall accuracy of 92% for this method. Considering differences in populations and methodologies, these results are not too different from other reports in the literature.

The accepted criterion for diagnosis of septic arthritis on radionuclide scan is equally increased uptake on both sides of the joint. The interpretation is not so simple in practice. As compared with osteomyelitis, the diagnosis of septic arthritis presents a different problem: although the scan may correctly identify the site of joint sepsis in about 90% of infected joints, it does not accurately separate bone from joint sepsis

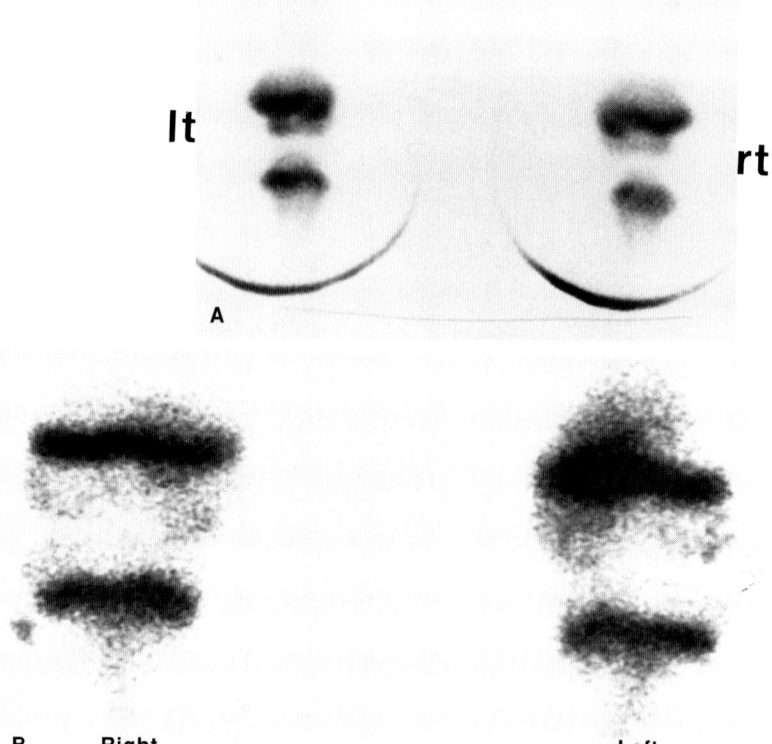

FIGURE 16-8. (A) Bone scan of lower extremities of the same patient in Figure 16-6. Note the activity around the physis. Differences in isotope uptake between the two sides are equivocal. (B) Pinhole views of the distal femurs clearly demonstrate a difference between the left and right. In addition, the pattern of "peaking" in the metaphysis is typical of early osteomyelitis and corresponds to the expected pathologic process.

nor differentiate infectious from noninfectious arthritis.[100,213] This is a particular problem in the hip, in which the differential diagnoses may include transient synovitis, septic arthritis, or osteomyelitis of the femoral neck.

Not all "positive" scans indicate infection, and because skeletal scintigraphy is "interpreted," it suggests that many factors need to be included if the scan is to be helpful.[211,212] Foremost among these factors is that the scan should be interpreted in the context of the clinical facts. This was illustrated by McCoy and colleagues, who demonstrated improved specificity and sensitivity when the scan was interpreted with knowledge of the clinical findings and initial laboratory studies than when the interpretation was a blind reading of the scan.[138] The importance of this has been emphasized by others.[100,213]

The interpretation of the scan is important. There is a tendency to call a bone scan "positive" or "negative," depending on areas of increased, normal, or decreased uptake. Linking knowledge of the pathophysiology of the disease process to the scan, which actually reflects localized physiologic changes in the bone, is more useful and more accurate.

Although localized increased isotope uptake may be due to osteomyelitis, it may also be due to any other process that increases the vascularity or deposition of calcium phosphate. Among the most common disorders seen in children are tumors and bone resorption due to disuse. Therefore, the bone scan can localize the area of the skeleton where there is altered physiology but it cannot determine the cause (Fig. 16-9A and B).

The importance of a "cold scan," in which there is an area of decreased isotope uptake, has been recognized as a serious problem, indicating acute devascularization of the bone caused by subperiosteal abscess.[15,100,213,220]

The diagnosis and treatment of an acute bone or joint infection should not be delayed by the bone scan. As important as bone scans may be in some cases, they should be available at all reasonable hours and all days of the week. In requesting or waiting for a bone scan, the question often arises regarding whether aspiration of the bone or joint alters the results of the scan. McCoy and colleagues[138] demonstrated in the clinical situation that the aspiration did not alter the scan, whereas Canale and colleagues[30] showed the same results in an experimental situation. This suggests that when the site of pathology is known and aspiration is indicated, it need not and in many cases probably should not be delayed while waiting for a bone scan.

Computed Tomography

CT is valuable in the detection of focal areas of bone destruction and detection and delineation of soft tissue abscess associated with bone and joint infection. Positive bone scans of the spine and pelvis often fail

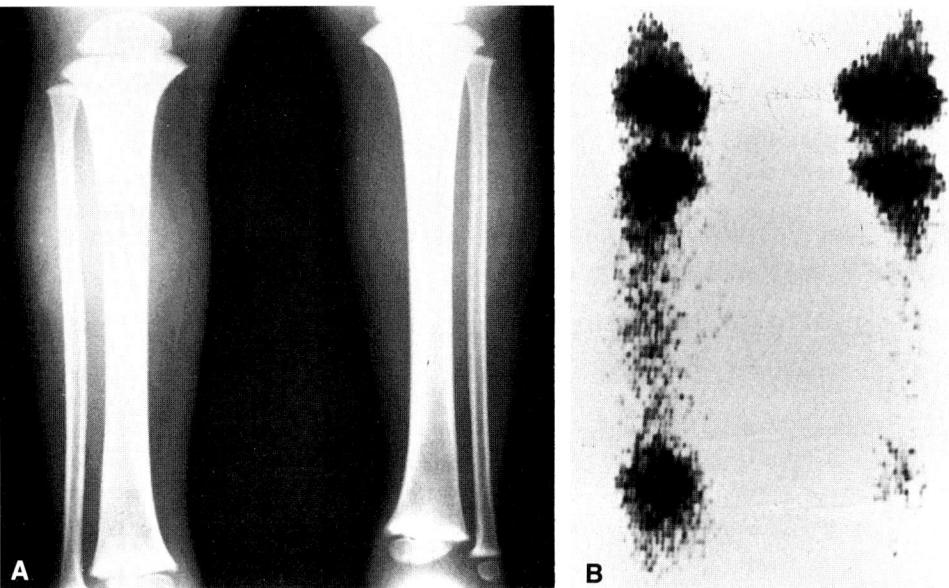

FIGURE 16-9. (A) Seven-year-old girl complained of pain in her leg for about 24 hours. Examination revealed diffused swelling in the leg and a rapidly spreading erythema. Radiographs show superficial soft tissue swelling on the right leg but the deep soft tissue layers are not swollen. This appearance indicates cellulitis. (B) Bone scan was obtained on this patient and mistakenly interpreted as showing osteomyelitis. The diffused pattern of uptake is not typical of osteomyelitis but represents the effects of increased circulation throughout the bone secondary to inflammation and acute disuse.

to provide the surgeon with the exact location of the lesion, which would permit either aspiration or planning of a surgical approach. In such circumstances, CT examination of the area localized by the bone scan can prove useful (see Fig. 16-12).[96]

Magnetic Resonance Imaging

MRI is a useful technique in the evaluation of both acute and chronic osteomyelitis because of its ability to provide good anatomic detail in many planes and to detect pathologic changes within the marrow and soft tissues. Its actual use, however, is mitigated by its cost and the frequent necessity for sedation or general anesthesia in small children coupled with it simply not being necessary for the diagnosis and treatment of the usual case of osteomyelitis or septic arthritis.

MRI for the evaluation of sepsis should include both T1- and T2-weighted sequences because the difference between the two is important. In acute osteomyelitis, the low-intensity signal seen on the T1-weighted image becomes a high-intensity signal on the T2-weighted image. These changes reflect the increased water in the marrow produced by the edema, hyperemia, and purulent exudate that characterize the pathologic process.[216]

MRI is most often needed in the unusual case that has been previously treated, especially those infections in the spinal column and the pelvis and those that cannot be clearly differentiated from neoplasm (see Fig. 16-7).

Ultrasound

Following its use in evaluation of developmental dislocation of the hip, ultrasound examination has been suggested as a tool for diagnosis of septic arthritis of the hip. Several reports leave no doubt that ultrasound can detect the presence of fluid within the hip as well as the presence of a bulging capsule.[4,245,246]

Ultrasound examination can be useful when the physician is unable to elicit the clinical signs of an irritable hip (limited and painful internal rotation) that accompany a joint effusion. The degree to which the ultrasonographer is able to detect synovial and capsular thickening and the reliability of these findings in distinguishing toxic synovitis from septic arthritis probably need further evaluation.[53,180]

Ultrasound also has been applied to the diagnosis of osteomyelitis, based on the ultrasound detection of the soft tissue changes in the periosteum and surrounding soft tissues, including subperiosteal abscess.[99] If further evaluations confirm the accuracy of this technique, it may replace the bone scan in many cases of suspected osteomyelitis in the appendicular skeleton.

Aspiration

The history, physical examination, and all of the radiographic procedures have been used to locate the area of abnormality. None of these examinations has the ability to confirm whether this abnormal area is caused by infection or some other process, such as neoplasia. In addition, none of these modalities allow identification of the organism—an essential step in confirming the diagnosis, selecting the correct antibiotic, and determining the need for surgical debridement.

Aspiration is the step most often omitted in the workup of a suspected osteomyelitis and to lesser extent, septic arthritis. The reasons are many: the physician is reluctant to introduce a needle into the bone or joint for fear of causing an infection; the physician is afraid of hurting the patient; the physician does not believe that it is necessary. None of these are valid reasons. There is little risk of introducing new organisms when sterile technique is used; with intravenous sedation and local anesthetic the aspiration of bone or joint can be performed with little discomfort; and aspiration of the bone or joint often yields organisms that are not found by culture of blood and other materials.

Aspiration of joints is a relatively simple matter, causing no more discomfort than placing an intravenous needle. Aspiration of the bone may be more difficult. Depending on the age and cooperation of the patient, various amounts of sedation may be necessary. Oral or intravenous midazolam (Versed) has proved to be quick and effective. After the area is prepared with a skin disinfectant, sterile towels are used to drape the area. A large-bore, shallow, tapered needle is used. The needle is first inserted into the most likely area until it contacts bone. Aspiration at this point may withdraw pus, indicating a subperiosteal abscess. If no pus is obtained, the needle is twisted like a drill until it is felt to penetrate the bone. Aspiration is again performed. The needle easily penetrates the thin metaphyseal bone.

Any material obtained should be sent for both culture and Gram staining, even if it does not appear to be purulent, because it may contain organisms. It is an unfortunate mistake to think that it is only blood and discard it. The next most common error is to be too far from the metaphysis. Fear of being in the physis or epiphysis coupled with difficulty in discerning the landmarks in a small, fat, and swollen extremity leads to this error. The physician knows this is the case when it is difficult to penetrate the bone with the needle because the metaphyseal bone is easy to penetrate, whereas the cortical bone of the diaphysis is impenetrable with the usual needle (see Fig. 16-1A).

DIFFERENTIAL DIAGNOSIS

Osteomyelitis

Although most cases of osteomyelitis in infants and children are relatively easy to diagnose there are always cases having an atypical presentation and appearance and osteomyelitis can be a great imitator. It is therefore helpful for the physician to always keep in mind those conditions that may present with the characteristics of bone infection and thus be mistaken for infection.

Trauma is perhaps the most common. It is easily confused with osteomyelitis because the latter often presents with a history of injury to the part and is characterized by the same features: pain, swelling, tenderness, and soft tissue swelling on radiographs. Trauma may be associated with an elevation of the CRP but not of the ESR, whereas both are usually elevated in osteomyelitis. The pain of trauma usually improves within 36 to 48 hours, whereas that of osteomyelitis worsens.

Most troublesome are those cases that are difficult to distinguish from neoplasia. The most common malignancy in childhood is leukemia and about 30% of these children present with bone pain.[88] To complicate matters even more, 39% of these children present with constitutional symptoms such as lethargy, 18% with fever, and 60% have an elevated leukocyte count and elevated ESR.[176] Although lucent metaphyseal bands are said to be characteristic of leukemia, other bone changes are also seen. One study found lytic lesions in 19%, sclerotic lesions in 4%, and periosteal new bone in 2%.[176]

The treating physician should be suspicious when other signs associated with leukemia are noted (e.g., bleeding, easy bruising, bone pain in multiple sites). A low leukocyte count, seen in 35% of patients presenting with leukemia, should also raise suspicion, although it may also indicate serious systemic sepsis. An anemia that is not explained by acute symptoms of osteomyelitis and abnormally low platelets should also arouse suspicion. An additional clue is when the bone scan does not demonstrate the findings that would be expected in the presence of osteomyelitis. The typical finding in leukemia is a lytic lesion without increased uptake because the lesion is purely lytic, without new bone formation or reaction.[35]

Other less common neoplasms may mimic osteomyelitis.[29,129] Whenever the characteristic appearance of one of these neoplasms is recognized, the physician should immediately run through the differential diagnosis in his or her mind, remembering that the differential diagnosis is the possibilities arranged in order of probability. In the younger child, an irregular lytic lesion and or the presence of periosteal new bone, with or without a lytic lesion, should always suggest osteomyelitis, metastatic neuroblastoma, and eosinophilic granuloma, along with leukemia. In the older child and adolescent, the various forms of subacute osteomyelitis discussed below most often mimic tumors. The most difficult to differentiate from osteomyelitis when periosteal new bone characterizes the lesion is Ewing sarcoma.[137] In all such cases, the diagnosis must be established before treatment is begun. The lesion should be approached as a malignancy, with complete radiographic staging and a biopsy approach that would not jeopardize limb salvage surgery if the lesion is malignant.

Bone infarction can mimic AHO. (The differential diagnosis of bone infarct and osteomyelitis in sickle cell disease is discussed later.) Gaucher disease is another less common disorder in which acute bone infarction occurs. Similar to those with sickle cell disease, these patients can also have AHO, although it is less common than bone infarction. In one series of 49 patients with Gaucher disease, 11 were admitted to the hospital with acute lower extremity pain, constitutional symptoms, fever, an elevated leukocyte count, and an elevated ESR.[12] Of these, 5 were diagnosed as AHO, whereas the others had a bone infarction. There was no difference between the clinical signs and laboratory data for the two groups. Because bone destruction was rapid in those with osteomyelitis, the authors recommended early biopsy for culture. Because these patients seem to be unusually susceptible to infection after bone surgery, it is best to perform this biopsy by aspiration and in the sterile environment of the operating room.

Septic Arthritis

The differential diagnoses of septic arthritis, which is that of an acutely swollen and painful joint, include many more possibilities than that for osteomyelitis. The culture results are even more important because many disorders mimicking septic arthritis are not diagnosed by biopsy but by many complex laboratory tests and often by the passage of time. In considering the differential diagnoses of septic arthritis, the urgency of making the correct diagnosis is important. The physician should always consider what must be diagnosed today, what can be diagnosed tomorrow, and what can be diagnosed next week. For example, septic arthritis, particularly of the hip should be diagnosed as soon as possible, whereas there is little harm to the patient if JRA is diagnosed next week.

One of the most difficult and yet important differentials is between septic arthritis of the hip and toxic synovitis because of the importance of immediate drainage of the hip in the presence of sepsis. Both may present with a history of a few to several days of hip pain, with limp progressing to the inability to walk. A longer history of improvement and worsening suggests toxic synovitis. The physical signs are similar in both, with limited and painful internal rotation, abduction, and extension. The pain is usually worse and the motion more restricted in septic arthritis.

One study comparing 94 patients with toxic synovitis and 38 with septic arthritis found that there was significant overlap of the temperature, leukocyte count, and ESR between the two groups.[47] That the ESR is often elevated in toxic synovitis is not always appreciated. These authors found that of those with toxic synovitis, 28% had an ESR greater than 20 mm/hour; in 14%, it was greater than 30 mm/hour. The percentage of patients with septic arthritis whose ESR was greater than 20 mm/hour and 30 mm/hour was 79% and 71%, respectively. The use of ultrasound in the diagnosis has been discussed. Although the ability to differentiate these two conditions becomes better with experience, whenever the physician is in doubt, aspiration of the joint is indicated.

JRA is frequently a consideration, especially when it presents as a single acutely swollen joint. Clinically different from septic arthritis, the history is often a more gradual onset, particularly regarding pain. The patient usually remains ambulatory. The examination is characterized by motion that is good, with surprisingly little pain, compared with the large amount of swelling that is usually present. The joint is only mildly tender and the synovium may be thickened. Immediate laboratory tests are not helpful in the differential diagnosis. The synovial fluid leukocyte count usually contains fewer than 100,000 leukocytes/mL, whereas in sepsis, the count is typically more than 100,000 leukocytes/mL. This is not always true, however, and the leukocyte count can be more than 100,000 leukocytes/mL in JRA.[9] In many cases, the aspirate from the joint has the appearance of pus from a septic joint; in such cases, the physician has little choice but to begin treatment for septic arthritis while searching for other clues.

Rheumatic fever, a sequela of group A streptococcal infection, is another childhood illness that often is associated with swollen and painful joints. For reasons that are not clear, there was a resurgence of rheumatic fever beginning in the late 1980s after years of decline.[16] The problem for the orthopaedic surgeon is to think of this disorder in the initial evaluation because those additional findings that lead to the diagnosis must be sought. The joint pain is typically in the large joints (knees, ankles, elbows, and wrists) and is evanescent and migratory. Also characteristic is that the pain, which is severe, is out of proportion to the amount of swelling, which is usually mild. The history should seek evidence of an untreated pharyngitis or febrile illness, a rash, or some other infection due to group A *Streptococcus* about 2 weeks before the onset of joint swelling. Inquiry should also be made about any joint symptoms preceding the presenting complaint, especially the involvement of multiple joints.

The diagnosis of rheumatic fever is based on the Jones criteria. The major criteria are carditis, arthritis, chorea, subcutaneous nodules, and erythema marginatum. The minor criteria are fever; arthralgia; elevated ESR or CRP; heart block, as evidenced on an electrocardiogram; and a previous history of rheumatic fever. The diagnosis is made when there are two major or one major and two minor criteria. A heart murmur usually is not present this early in the course of the disease. Rheumatic fever is one diagnosis that must be considered in the differential diagnosis of any patient with septic arthritis.

Another disorder that causes either arthralgia or arthritis is Henoch-Schönlein purpura. This disorder is a vasculitis of unknown origin (possibly allergic) that affects mainly children between the ages of 2 and 11 years of age. In the full-blown case having all of the clinical manifestations (nonthrombocytopenic purpuric rash, abdominal pain, arthritis, and nephritis), the diagnosis is not difficult. The joint manifestations, which occur in up to 75% of the patients, precede the other symptoms in about 25% of those affected. For this reason, the orthopaedist should be familiar with the features of the joint findings. The joints most commonly involved are the knees and ankles. The swelling and tenderness are more periarticular than that in septic arthritis and if an effusion is present, it is usually mild. Joint fluid will not contain blood. The earliest signs of purpura must be sought, which may be fine pinpoint hemorrhagic lesions, usually seen below the waist. The joint symptoms do not require treatment and usually disappear within days. These patients require medical management for the other, sometimes more serious manifestations of the disease.

There are many other causes of joint swelling that merit consideration. Enteroarthritis secondary to *Salmonella* or *Yersinia* infection may be suspected when abdominal symptoms coincide. The arthritis may precede the abdominal symptoms, however. These patients can be confused with those having septic arthritis because as with septic arthritis, the ESR and CRP are often elevated to high levels. Kawasaki disease, a vasculitis of unknown etiology, may present with joint symptoms in its early stage. It is characterized by a rash, with red eyes and lips, erythema of the palms and soles with edema, and lethargy. The child does not like to be moved and may seem to be more ill than the visible signs suggest. Serum sickness, which is often manifest by joint swelling and an urticarial rash, usually affects more than one joint and most commonly follows treatment with penicillin or a cephalosporin antibiotic, especially Ceclor. Other considerations are discussed later in this chapter.

TREATMENT

There are four principles that the physician must always keep in mind when treating an infection:
1. Identify the organism.
2. Select the correct antibiotic.
3. Deliver the antibiotic to the organisms.
4. Stop the tissue destruction.

Organism Identification

The first principle, to identify the organism, is part of the diagnosis. The diagnosis of septic arthritis is difficult to establish with certainty unless an organism is identified, and it is even more difficult to treat until the specific organism is identified.

Antibiotic Selection

If the organism is not identified on the Gram stain of aspirated material, the initial antibiotic must be selected by an educated guess. Difficult as this may seem, there should be several clues, such as the usual organisms causing osteomyelitis and septic arthritis in various age groups and the presence or absence of any predisposing reasons for the infection. All of these factors have been discussed and some of the special circumstances are discussed below.

The most likely organism in the typical patient older than 1 year of age, without any other special circumstances, is *S aureus*.

Recommendations for the initial antibiotic management in such a patient are either a semisynthetic penicillin (oxacillin or methicillin) or a first- or second-generation cephalosporin (cefazolin or cefuroxime, respectively). If the patient is allergic to the penicillins, the cephalosporins may be used. In the rare patient who is allergic to both, clindamycin is a good choice. Selection of the oral antibiotic for continuing treatment should be based on the culture results. If *S aureus* is identified, cephalexin suspension is a good choice for the child younger than 6 or 7 years of age because it is more palatable than a semisynthetic penicillin and thus compliance will be greater. If the child is older and can swallow capsules, a semisynthetic penicillin (e.g., dicloxacillin) can be used (Table 16-2).

For the patient with septic arthritis, the choice may depend somewhat on age. In infants and children between the ages of 4 weeks and 4 years, the most likely organism is *S aureus* if the patient has been immunized against *H influenzae*. If they have not been immunized, *H influenzae* is the most likely. Group A and B streptococci are likely organisms in children younger than the age of 1 year. Therefore, a good choice in these patients is cefuroxime. In the older patient, in whom *H influenzae* is not a likely consideration, a semisynthetic penicillin or first-generation cephalosporin, as recommended for osteomyelitis, remains a good choice. The selection of an oral antibiotic should be based on Gram stain and culture results. For the child younger than the age of 5 years, cefprozil is a good choice. For the older child, cephalexin suspension or dicloxacillin capsules are a good choice (see Table 16-2).

These initial antibiotic choices can be modified, depending on the results of cultures. If Gram stains

TABLE 16-2 Antibiotics Commonly Used in the Treatment of Bone and Joint Sepsis

DRUG*	ROUTE	DOSAGE†‡	COMMENTS
Amoxicillin	Oral	80 mg/kg/d, q 8 h	
Ampicillin	IV	100–150 mg/kg/d, q 6 h	
Dicloxacillin	Oral	100 mg/kg/d, q 6 h	
Methicillin	IV	150 mg/kg/d, q 6 h	
Nafcillin	IV	150 mg/kg/d, q 6 h	
Penicillin G	IV	150,000 U/kg/d, q 4–6 h	
Penicillin V	Oral	100 mg/kg/d, q 6 h	
Oxacillin	IV	150 mg/kg/d, q 6 h	
Cefaclor (Ceclor)	Oral	80 mg/kg/d, q 8 h	
Cefazolin (Ancef, Kefazol)	IV	100 mg/kg/d, q 8 h	
Cephalexin (Keflex)	Oral	100 mg/kg/d, q 6 h	
Cefotaxime (Claforan)	IV	100–150 mg/kg/d, q 6–8 h	
Cefprozil (Cefzil)	Oral	60 mg/kg/d, q 12 h	
Ceftazidime (Fortaz)		100–150 mg/kg/d, q 8 h	
Ceftriaxone (Rocephin)	IV/IM	50 mg/kg/d, q 12–24 h	Maximum dose, 2 g/d
Cefuroxime (Zinacef)	IV	100–150 mg/kg/d, q 8 h	
Clindamycin	IV/oral	25–40 mg/kg/d, q 6 h	
Gentamicin	IV	7.5 mg/kg/d, q 8 h	Monitor peak and trough blood levels
Vancomycin	IV	40 mg/kg/d, q 6 h	Administer over 1 h and monitor peak and trough blood levels

* Complete blood count should be monitored weekly for neutropenia or anemia in any patient on high-dose penicillin or cephalosporin therapy.
† Doses recommended are for normal children with normal renal function for the treatment of bone and joint infections; recommended doses for the treatment of other conditions may be lower.
‡ For doses in the neonatal period, see Nelson JD. Pocket book of pediatric antimicrobial therapy, 10th ed. Baltimore: Williams & Wilkins, 1993.

and cultures fail to identify an organism, selection is based on the most likely organism in the particular circumstance of that case (e.g., age, other illness, predisposing factors) and the response to the antibiotic that was selected. Recommendations for initial antibiotic choice in the neonate and other special circumstances are discussed below.

Antibiotic Delivery

Giving an antibiotic to a patient who has an infection is not sufficient. The physician must ensure that the antibiotic both reaches all of the organisms and effectively kills them. This involves several issues. Does it matter whether the antibiotic is given intravenously or orally? How long should the antibiotic be given and why? Where can the antibiotic be expected to penetrate? Can it kill the organism when it gets there?

Route of Administration

Initial antibiotic therapy for bone or joint infections should always begin with intravenous administration. Intravenous administration is more expensive than oral administration, however, and certainly less convenient for the patient.[58] An advantage to intravenous administration is that high concentrations of antibiotic can be achieved quickly with certainty. These levels exceed those usually necessary, whereas the levels achieved with oral administration are usually adequate. The difficulty with oral administration is in ensuring that absorption from the gut is adequate and that the patient is compliant. Despite these potential pitfalls, the efficacy of oral antibiotics in the treatment of bone and joint sepsis has been well documented.[27,121,153]

It is imperative to recognize that the success of oral therapy depends on certain conditions being fulfilled. The criteria for oral therapy of bone and joint sepsis are listed in Table 16-3. The single most important criterion is the assurance that there is an adequate blood level of the antibiotic from the oral therapy. This is determined by measuring the serum bactericidal titers from blood drawn about 1 hour after oral administration of the drug. A titer of 1 : 8 or greater should be achieved. This may require larger oral doses than those usually given. In one series, about 10% of the patients failed to achieve adequate serum concentrations of the antibiotic after oral administration.[153] Despite this standard of measuring the

TABLE 16-3 *Criteria for Oral Therapy of Bone and Joint Sepsis*

1. Course of disease is resolving
2. Surgical debridement is adequate
3. Oral antibiotic is well tolerated
4. Parents are reliable
5. Organism is identified
6. Adequate serum levels of antibiotic have been demonstrated

peak level of antibiotic, there is some evidence that it may actually be the trough level that is more significant.[231,240]

Because the direct measurement in the blood of the level of commonly used antibiotics (e.g., semisynthetic penicillins, cephalosporins) is not feasible, it is measured indirectly by the serum bactericidal test. This test uses serial dilutions of patient serum to test against the bacteria, which is isolated to determine the minimal dilution that is bactericidal for the organism.[130,210]

Blood is drawn after the administration of the oral antibiotic to determine the peak level. For antibiotic given in suspension, the blood is drawn 1 hour after administration; for antibiotic administered in capsule or tablet, blood is drawn about 1.5 to 2 hours after administration. If the trough level is to be measured, blood is drawn just before the next dose. Dilutions of the serum are prepared and tested against the isolated organism. If an organism is not isolated, a laboratory strain of the presumed organism is used. Although it is controversial regarding how much the peak serum level should exceed the bactericidal concentration, a 1 : 8 dilution is generally accepted as being effective. This usually requires larger oral doses (usually two times larger) than commonly recommended. When adequate levels are not present, the dose may be increased: probenecid (Benemid) to inhibit renal excretion may be added; or intravenous therapy may be reinstituted.

Other antibiotics (e.g., gentamicin, vancomycin) can be measured directly in the blood. In addition, the blood level of these intravenous antibiotics varies significantly between individuals, and their toxic side effects are significant. Both the peak and trough levels need to be measured and monitored. For gentamicin, blood is drawn about 30 minutes after administration and just before the next dose. The peak level should be between 5 to 10 μg/mL, and the trough should be 1.9 μg/mL or less. For vancomycin, blood is drawn 1 hour after administration and just before the next dose. The peak level should be between 20 to 40 μg/mL and the trough between 5 to 10 μg/mL.

Generally, blood levels of gentamicin or vancomycin should be measured every 3 to 4 days in addition to those of blood urea nitrogen and creatinine. For prolonged (longer than 3 weeks) or recurrent therapy with these drugs, it is wise to monitor the patient for ototoxicity also. Vancomycin should be infused over no less than 1 hour to avoid the release of histamine by the drug (red man syndrome). If a rash occurs, it usually can be circumvented by administering the drug over 90 to 120 minutes or by the use of intravenous diphenhydramine (Benadryl) 1 mg/kg (total dose not to exceed 50 mg) just before the infusion.

Compliance of the parents and child in administration of the antibiotic is an important consideration. For that reason, most patients are given an oral cephalosporin (e.g., Claforan) rather than an oral semisynthetic penicillin (e.g., dicloxacillin) because the latter has a bitter taste, a factor in noncompliance. If the causative organism is not identified, it is only a relative contraindication for oral therapy if the other criteria are met. An oral antibiotic with the same coverage as that given intravenously is selected and tested against a laboratory strain of the presumed organism, usually *S aureus*. This should provide reasonable assurance that adequate serum levels are achieved.

Penetration

After an adequate serum level of the antibiotic is achieved, it must reach all of the areas harboring bacteria. In evaluating data on antibiotic penetration, it is necessary to consider the antibiotic in addition to the methods used to measure its concentration.[194] Methicillin, dicloxacillin, cephaloridine, and cefazolin all penetrate into pus and bone in children with osteomyelitis in concentrations several times greater than the mean inhibitory and mean bactericidal concentrations for *S aureus*.[217] The same is true for orally administered ampicillin, cephalexin, cloxacillin, dicloxacillin, and penicillin G in the synovial fluid of children with septic arthritis.[154] There is no evidence that antibiotics penetrate into dead bone.

Efficacy of Antibiotic

It seems that all that is necessary for a cure is to administer the correct antibiotic in the correct dosage. There are, however, several factors that may interfere with the antibiotic action and that also explain why more than the administration of antibiotic is required in many cases. One factor that is poorly studied is the effect the local environment has on the ability of the antibiotic to kill bacteria. It is known that the interaction of purulent material from some gram-negative organisms can interfere with the action of certain antibiotics.[25,26]

With a large inoculum and the production of large amounts of β-lactamase, β-lactam antibiotics such as semisynthetic penicillins and cephalosporins are susceptible to breakdown, rendering them ineffective.[52,65,181] In addition, the low pH at the site of infection is known to interfere with the action of some antibiotics. These factors suggest that the local environment is important to the effective action of the antibiotic and that the site of infection may not be the ideal environment.

Duration of Administration

There are no good data that indicate how long antibiotics should be administered in any particular case. The old recommendation of 6 weeks of intravenous administration is often based on difficult and complicated referral cases from large tertiary medical centers, which do not represent the "usual" case.[227] Conversely, there is no evidence other than clinical experience that a shorter duration can be effective. More important than rigid rules is an understanding of the pathophysiology of each case, so that the treatment can be based on the particulars of that case. The correct answer is that the antibiotic should be continued until all of the organisms have been killed.

To illustrate, consider two different cases. A 5-year-old boy presents with a history of increasing pain in the distal thigh for 3 days and inability to walk on the day of presentation. His radiographs are normal, except for deep soft tissue swelling. Aspiration demonstrates pus and he undergoes surgical debridement the same day. He is started on the correct antibiotic. Over the next 5 days, the pain, swelling, and fever subside, the CRP is falling, and he begins to walk. He can be safely treated with 5 to 7 days of intravenous antibiotics followed by oral antibiotics for an additional 3 or 4 weeks.

Another 5-year-old boy is seen 2 weeks after the onset of pain in the distal thigh. His physician had placed him on oral antibiotics after 3 days but the pain and limp continued to worsen. His radiographs show extensive involvement of the distal femoral metaphysis, with radiolucent areas and periosteal new bone. He undergoes surgical debridement but it is not deemed possible to debride all of the bone that is involved. At the end of 7 days, his fever is decreasing, the CRP has not fallen, and although his signs and symptoms are improving, he still has some swelling and tenderness. This patient should remain on intravenous antibiotics.

These two cases illustrate the factors to consider when deciding the duration of antibiotic therapy. How long has the infection been present and how much bone is involved? Is there abscess formation? Has the patient had adequate surgical debridement to remove the pus and other materials that interfere with effective antibiotic action? Has all of the dead bone been removed to expose organisms to antibiotic? Is the patient getting better? These clinical observations can be aided to a limited extent by radiographic and laboratory studies, remembering that radiographic changes lag the actual bone changes and that the ESR and to a lesser degree the CRP also lag resolving infection during the first week.[166]

Current practice is a sequential course of intravenous antibiotic followed by an oral course. Clinical parameters determine when oral antibiotics begin. In the typical case, which resolves quickly with treatment, oral therapy starts after 5 days of intravenous antibiotic administration; in the case of osteomyelitis, it continues for 4 to 6 weeks and in septic arthritis, for an additional 2 to 3 weeks.

Surgery

Destruction of tissue is the final result of infection. Although bone has the ability to repair itself, articular and epiphyseal cartilage do not. Therefore, one of the main goals of treatment is to stop tissue destruction. Killing the bacteria is the first part of the treatment but not the only part. Tissue destruction is mainly the result of the complex process known as the "inflammatory reaction." Although this reaction is initiated by bacteria, the presence of live bacteria is not necessary for its continuation. It is well recognized that the products liberated by bacteria, cell wall fragments of dead bacteria, products liberated from leukocytes, and products of tissue destruction are all capable of causing an inflammatory reaction, which results in tissue destruction.[21,51,79,80,159]

With an understanding of the mechanisms of tissue destruction and the delivery of antibiotic to the bacteria in an environment where it can be effective, the basis for surgery becomes more meaningful. Surgery is for debridement. It removes the inflammatory products more rapidly than the host defense mechanisms. In so doing, it provides a more effective environment in which antibiotics can work. It reduces the size of the inoculum, ensuring more effective antibiotic action of many commonly used antibiotics. Lastly, it removes all of the dead and avascular bone or the thick fibrinous exudate from joints, thus exposing all of the organisms to antibiotic. This provides a more rapid end to tissue destruction and requires a shorter course of antibiotic therapy.

The indications for surgical debridement of AHO remain controversial and in flux. Difficulty in evaluating published reports recommending various points of view arise because of failure to identify the important characteristics of those who were treated with surgery and those who were not (e.g., duration and severity of infection, type of organism, appropriateness of antibiotic use). In addition, the necessity for longer hospitalization and intravenous antibiotic administration is difficult to justify.

I have used the aspiration of pus or failure of signs and symptoms to resolve within 36 to 48 hours as an indication for surgical debridement. This practice is based on the same principles used to treat infection in other parts of the body. Especially important is the age-old wisdom of draining an abscess, regardless of location. With these criteria, many cases avoid surgery, few require prolonged intravenous therapy, and recurrence is unusual. This is a mainstream opinion that is supported by others.[85,124]

Surgical debridement of a focus of hematogenous osteomyelitis requires an incision only large enough to expose the area of bone involved. Incision and circumferential stripping of the periosteum in the involved area is performed first, to drain the subperiosteal abscess. Next, using a drill, an entry hole is made into the bone. This can be enlarged with a rongeur to allow access with a curet but should not be any larger than necessary to curet the involved bone. The diseased area is easily distinguished from more normal bone by "feel" with the curet and the appearance of the material removed.

Specimens should be sent for both culture and routine histology. The importance of routine histologic examination of material from the bone is twofold. Some tumors have a tendency to become necrotic and when surgically explored may look similar to pus; the most common is metastatic neuroblastoma, followed by Ewing sarcoma. In addition, if positive identification of the organism is not obtained, it is reassuring to have a histologic diagnosis of osteomyelitis.

The indications for arthrotomy in the treatment of septic arthritis are perhaps even more controversial (except for the hip), although more sharply divided between the orthopaedic and pediatric literature. Experimental evidence supports lavage of the joint but interpretation of individual experiences constitutes the evidence that drives clinical decisions.

In experimental staphylococcal septic arthritis in rabbits who were treated with antibiotic, the beneficial effect of surgical lavage was demonstrated.[46] During the first arthrotomy at 4 days, all of the material in the knee could be washed out; at 7 days, it had to be removed manually. All cultures were negative at 7 days. Both the surgically treated and nonsurgically treated animals showed loss of glycosaminoglycan. There was no collagen degradation in those treated by surgical lavage, however. A similar study has shown that arthrotomy and irrigation may be more effective than repeated aspirations, as the above data suggest.[82]

In my experience, there is little question that some joint infections can be cured with antibiotics alone. This seems to be especially true in the smaller joints, such as the wrist, and in younger children. Attempts to treat joints such as the knee without drainage have never been as prompt to resolve as those treated with a small arthrotomy and irrigation followed by a brief period of splinting.

Effective drainage of most joints can be performed through a small incision. The incision should be large enough to permit a small retractor to be inserted into the joint. On the knee, this can be accomplished with an incision of no more than 2.5 cm. After suctioning the purulent material from the joint, a swab of the synovium for culture is obtained. A small biopsy of the synovium may also be sent for culture. Irrigation is then performed with saline through a small rubber catheter directed into all of the recesses of the joint. A drain (or irrigation system, if preferred) is inserted into the joint and the wound is closed.[126,161]

Repeated aspiration has been recommended but suffers from two drawbacks: it is ineffective in draining the joint (Fig. 16-10), and it becomes a difficult trial for both the patient and the physician because it must

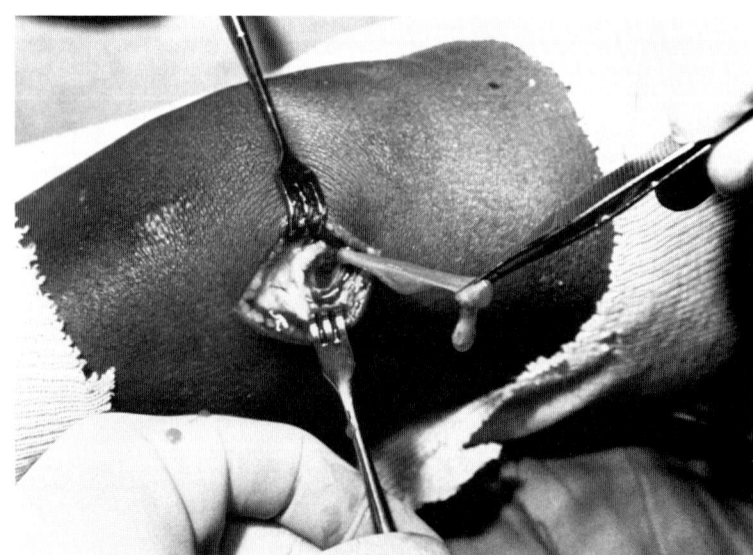

FIGURE 16-10. This patient with 3 days of symptoms was diagnosed as having septic arthritis after aspiration of the joint. Within 2 hours of aspiration, the knee joint was opened through a small arthrotomy with the patient under general anesthesia. Before and after irrigation, large amounts of thick fibrinous pus were removed with a forceps, illustrating the inadequacy of aspiration as a method to debride the joint.

be repeated. Arthroscopy has also been recommended.[192,203] The claimed advantages of decreased morbidity do not seem to be any different than for open arthrotomy, whereas the operative time and resources are more costly for arthroscopy.

RESULTS

Most children who are seen for AHO or septic arthritis can expect to recover without sequelae. These disorders are curable. Untoward consequences are usually due to advanced disease at the time of presentation or problems in the initial management.[227] Other than these two factors, the literature sheds little light on other reasons for failure, because the reports cover decades during which organisms, antibiotics, and principles of management changed.[18,36,49,124,146,224,227]

Most complications from musculoskeletal sepsis occur in the hip for reasons documented elsewhere in this chapter. Other than the hip, joint destruction is expected only in the late-presenting and neglected case. Chronic osteomyelitis remains distinctly unusual, probably because of the rapid bone turnover in children. Epiphyseal destruction with growth arrest is occasionally seen but usually in cases in which appropriate treatment is delayed.

SPECIAL CONDITIONS

Spine

For decades, physicians have recognized hematogenous infections of both the disk space and the vertebral body. Descriptions of the disorder as "a benign form of osteomyelitis of the spine" provide a clue to its natural history,[193] whereas the various descriptions in the literature of vertebral osteomyelitis and diskitis over the past several decades reflect the uncertainty that these are indeed two separate conditions.[22,73] Modern imaging modalities such as scintigraphy, CT scanning, and MRI have resolved the confusion by demonstrating evidence of bone involvement in children with the clinical presentation of diskitis. It thus appears that both vertebral osteomyelitis and diskitis are the result of a hematogenous infection beginning in the bone adjacent to the cartilaginous vertebral end plate.

The vascular anatomy of the vertebral body and disk has been well studied.[39,43,93,236] These studies demonstrate that the blood supply to the disk comes from the contiguous bone of the vertebral bodies. In the young child, vessels can be identified traversing the cartilaginous vertebral end plate and entering the annulus. By the age of 8 years these vessels have largely disappeared but a rich anastomotic network of vessels remains along the periphery of the disk that can persist until 30 years of age.

The etiology of the syndrome of diskitis is most likely infectious. Occasionally, the question of traumatic injury to the vertebral end plate similar to a Salter-Harris I fracture is raised; however, substantial proof is lacking. The different presentations, the characteristic age range (average age, 7 years), and the isolation of bacteria from many cases also militates against this being a traumatic disorder. It is recognized, however, that this is an infection that behaves differently than most musculoskeletal infections.

The presentation of patients with diskitis is variable and insidious, with fewer than half presenting with the characteristic symptoms of refusal to walk or back pain.[174] In addition, signs of infection such as fever are usually minimal or absent. Despite this, three different patterns of clinical presentation have been described.[201,233] The first presentation is in the younger child, usually younger than 3 years of age, who has difficulty walking. In the very young child, this may begin with a reluctance and then refusal to walk and may be confused with more common causes, such as a septic hip. In the child who is attempting to walk, there is often a characteristic gait, with the child bending forward and hands on the thighs for support.

The second presentation, usually occurring in children 7 to 15 years of age, is abdominal pain. This can be vague and associated with a poor appetite and listlessness. Sometimes the pain radiates anteriorly and can be confused with an intraabdominal condition, although localized physical signs in the abdomen are lacking.

The final presentation is back pain. In the classic presentation, the patient complains of back pain, has loss of the normal lumbar lordosis, and is painful to percussion. In some children, this onset may be gradual, whereas in others, who often have radiographic evidence of vertebral osteomyelitis, the onset may be rapid and may suggest infection. In most cases, fever is absent or low. It is also important to remember that these presentations may overlap greatly in age, symptoms, and findings.

The laboratory evaluation, as with most cases of skeletal sepsis, is not helpful unless the underlying disease is suspected and all of the correct tests are obtained. The leukocyte count may or may not be elevated or show a leftward shift. The ESR and CRP are usually elevated and blood cultures may be positive but not so reliably as in the usual infection involving a major bone or joint.

Radiographs at the initial presentation are often normal and usually show no changes in the first 1 to 3 weeks of symptoms. One of the earliest findings, often seen only in retrospect, is an irregularity of the vertebral end plate. This is followed by narrowing of the disk space and then erosion of the vertebral end plate as evidence of involvement of more than just the disk space (Fig. 16-11).

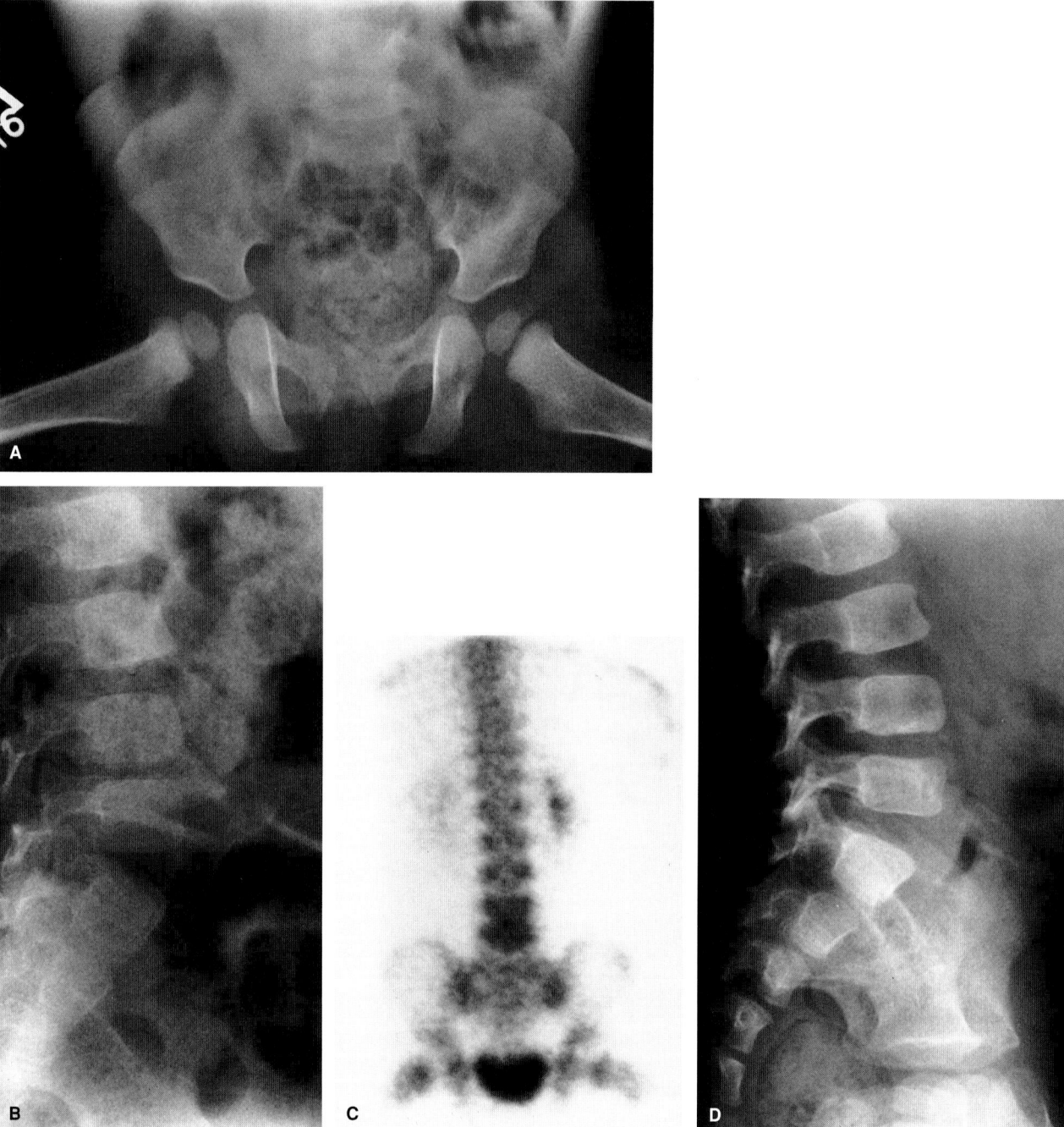

FIGURE 16-11. (A) Anteroposterior view of the pelvis of a 14-month-old child who stopped walking after several days of limping, falling, and irritability. This radiograph was ordered by the initial treating physician because of the suspicion of hip infection. Note the narrowing of the L4–5 disc space. (B) The lateral view was subsequently taken when examination by the orthopaedic surgeon demonstrated pain on percussion of the lower spine. Again, note the narrowing of the L4–5 disc space. (C) Increased isotope uptake in the vertebral bodies of L4 and L5 is typical of discitis. (D) At 10-month follow-up, disc space has almost recovered its normal height.

Bone scintigraphy is useful in suspected cases, demonstrating increased isotope uptake at the affected disk space. This usually occurs sooner than the radiographic changes but I have seen negative bone scans after 2 weeks of symptoms in patients with proved diskitis. CT scanning is a useful technique to delineate the anatomic changes in the vertebral bodies. When performed on patients having classic disk space narrowing, it usually shows unsuspected areas of vertebral involvement. MRI is rarely indicated because of the expense and lack of need, except in the most difficult cases. It also shows the vertebral body involvement earlier than the plain radiograph. Differential diagnosis of the causes of disk space narrowing and vertebral body involvement is usually not difficult.

Collapse of the vertebral body, with preservation of the disk space, is seen in eosinophilic granuloma (vertebra plana) and to a lesser extent in leukemia. Neither of these conditions demonstrates increased isotope uptake on bone scan early in their course. Destruction of bone with subsequent involvement of one or two disk spaces suggests infection. A large amount of bone destruction, especially in adjacent vertebrae, suggests tuberculosis. Primary bone tumors of the spine are unusual in childhood but must also be considered when bone destruction is present.

In almost all other cases of musculoskeletal infection, aspiration or biopsy for culture is considered to be mandatory. With infections of the vertebrae and disk, however, difficulty, potential complications, morbidity, and cost are factors that usually lead to treatment without biopsy. This course is supported by the usually benign natural history of this condition and the excellent results that are achieved with empiric treatment in the absence of positive cultures. In those series in which biopsy has been performed, the yield of positive cultures is slightly less than 50%. Open biopsy is more likely to yield positive cultures than needle biopsy and there is a trend toward better identification of organisms in more recent series. The results of the positive biopsies show a preponderance of S aureus as the causative organism.[20,174,201,233]

The treatment of disk space infections reflects both past observations and contemporary knowledge. Past observations of this disease demonstrated that it was largely self-limited, with occasional morbidity that was successfully treated with rest, despite recognition of a likely infectious etiology.[22,142] Despite these observations, current treatment consists of antistaphylococcic antibiotics (e.g., a semisynthetic penicillin or first-generation cephalosporin, as used in the initial treatment of AHO).[233] This has resulted in less morbidity. Antibiotic therapy is usually started intravenously, with hospitalization and bed rest. Careful observation for the onset of neurologic signs that would indicate epidural abscess formation is advisable until the patient shows resolution of symptoms. Immobilization may also be used but the trend is to avoid it. If the patient's symptoms resolve, intravenous antibiotics are switched to oral antibiotics after 5 to 7 days, with verification of adequate serum bactericidal levels. Oral antibiotics are continued for 3 to 5 weeks.

Resolution of symptoms usually occurs within the first 72 hours. If this is not the case, the physician should begin to question the diagnosis or the specific bacterial etiology. Further imaging studies such as CT scan or MRI may be justified in such circumstances to search for tumor or abscess formation. Biopsy is indicated in a patient who fails to respond to antibiotics and bed rest or has findings on imaging studies that suggest a diagnosis other than typical diskitis.

Pelvis and Sacroiliac Joint

Infections of the pelvis and SI joint share two features with each other and diskitis: they present with a wide variety of symptoms and are thus difficult to diagnose, and they can usually be treated successfully without surgery. The debate over whether the process in the SI joint is an osteomyelitis or true septic arthritis is largely irrelevant to the clinician. Both are possible and probably occur.

The presentation is not always acute, as in most forms of septic arthritis and osteomyelitis. In one series, only one third of the cases were acute and the average time from onset to diagnosis was 3.9 weeks.[184] Morgan and Yates[150] described four different presentations of osteomyelitis of the pelvis, depending on the initial area of pain: hip joint, abdominal, buttocks, and sciatic. In addition, they described a systemic presentation with malaise and fever. Beaupre and Carroll[11] described three presentations of SI joint osteomyelitis, which they termed gluteal, abdominal, and lumbar disk. The lumbar disk syndrome presents with pain in the lower back, hip, and thigh; the gluteal syndrome presents with pain and possibly a mass in the buttocks; and the abdominal syndrome can mimic acute appendicitis.

The most important step in the diagnosis of pelvic osteomyelitis is to consider it as a possibility. Failure to perform an adequate examination for symptoms in the SI joint and careful palpation of the other pelvic bones is a common cause of delay in diagnosis and confusion with other sites of infection. At the same time, it is important to remember that the pelvis and the SI joint are the site for many different pathologic processes, of which infection is only one.[171]

Perhaps the most common diagnosis that is confused with SI joint sepsis is septic hip. SI joint infection is generally seen in older children, with the mean age being 10 years, whereas septic hip is more common in the younger child.[184] Despite the complaint of pain around the hip, children with SI joint infection often remain ambulatory and have relatively free internal rotation of the hip, in contrast to those with a septic hip. Conversely, patients with SI joint infection frequently experience pain on external rotation of the hip. If the fabere test (*f*lexion, *ab*duction, *e*xternal *ro*tation) is performed, it usually elicits pain in the presence of SI joint sepsis, as does compression of the pelvis (Gaenslen test). Tenderness almost always is found over the SI joint if sought. Other areas (e.g., the ischium, pubis, ilium) should always be palpated for tenderness in children with gait disturbance or hip pain.

It is important to remember that osteomyelitis can occur in any location in any pelvic bone, and failure to elicit symptoms in the SI joint does not rule out pelvic osteomyelitis.[34,55] Bony tenderness is usually present at the site of involvement, emphasizing the importance of suspicion followed by a careful examination.[55]

Osteomyelitis of the ischiopubic synchondrosis presents a confusing picture despite tenderness being present. This synchondrosis, which fuses between 5 and 12 years of age and occasionally later, shows a radiographic picture of expansion and uneven mineralization before fusion. In addition, it is often asymmetric to the opposite side, which may have fused earlier, and radioisotope uptake is increased in many cases.[105] Kloiber and colleagues report that if the radioisotope activity at the ischiopubic synchondrosis is equal to or greater than that adjacent to the triradiate cartilage or if the activity extends into the adjacent pubic ramus or ischium, it is indicative of a pathologic process.[117]

Oblique radiographic views demonstrating the SI joint should be obtained. In most cases of pelvic osteomyelitis, the initial radiographs are normal. This is especially true when symptoms have been present for fewer than 1 or 2 weeks. The earliest sign of infection on the radiograph is disappearance of the subchondral margins and erosion; however, this should be considered to be a late finding. If radiographic changes are present with less than 1 week of symptoms, careful consideration should be given to other disorders, such as tumor or chronic inflammatory SI disease. It has been well recognized that ^{99m}Tc bone scanning is the most effective test in localizing a focus of pathology within the pelvic bones, making this the radiographic procedure of choice when pelvic osteomyelitis is suspected and the radiographs are normal (Fig. 16-12).[3,64,144,171]

CT scans can be helpful in several respects but are not necessary in all cases.[64,151,171] CT can better delineate the extent of bone involvement than can the radionuclide scan. This may be important in the atypical location or presentation when tumor or some other pathology is suspected. If pelvic osteomyelitis is strongly suspected but the bone scan is normal, CT scanning may demonstrate the lesion. Perhaps most important is the ability of the CT scan to delineate soft tissue abscess. This may be important if surgical drainage is contemplated because the abscess may be either anterior, posterior, or both (see Fig. 16-11C).

Schaad and colleagues reported that the bacterial etiology was established in 57% of the cases they studied from their own patients and a literature review.[184] In most cases, *S aureus* is the organism that is cultured from blood, direct aspiration, or biopsy.[11,40,64,171,184] *Staphylococcus epidermidis* and *Streptococcus* species are also reported but in many cases may be contaminants.[64] An occasional *Salmonella* species may be isolated in patients who are not otherwise predisposed.[171,184]

Laboratory findings in SI joint sepsis and pelvic osteomyelitis parallel other bone and joint infections, with the leukocytes often being normal and the ESR and CRP levels usually elevated. Blood cultures are positive in about 50% of cases; therefore, considering the difficulty in obtaining cultures from the SI joint and pelvis, they should always be obtained. *Salmonella* are always a possibility, even in those not predisposed to this organism, and thus stool cultures should be obtained. Joint aspirates are positive for the organism less often than in other cases of bone and joint sepsis.[40,171,184] Although this is partly due to the difficulty in entering the joint, even biopsy specimens and pus seem to yield positive culture results less often than would be expected.

In the report by Reilly and colleagues,[171] six of ten cultures from aspiration or biopsy of the SI joint were positive—the same yield as obtained from blood cultures. I prefer to aspirate only those cases that do not respond promptly to antibiotics or exhibit atypical features for the following reasons:

Morbidity and expense associated with this procedure, which usually requires general anesthesia, are high.
Blood or stool culture can identify at least 60% of the organisms.
Most organisms are *S aureus*.
The literature indicates that most of these patients respond to antistaphylococcic antibiotics.

The technique for aspirating the SI joint has been described.[95,145]

Reports in the literature demonstrate that surgical debridement of pelvic osteomyelitis is usually not necessary.[11,40,171] This contradicts reports in the older literature.[184] The ability of this process to resolve with antibiotic therapy alone is probably due to a variety of factors: the large and diffuse blood supply to the bones, which makes sequestrum formation unlikely; the rigid ligament structure around the SI joint, which contains the spread of infection; and negligible long-term morbidity, even when the joint becomes ankylosed.[40] Indications for surgery are those for biopsy in the case of suspected tumor, an unusual presentation, or failure to achieve resolution of the symptoms in a reasonable amount of time. Drainage of a large abscess may be necessary, especially in the presence of systemic symptoms.

Initial antibiotic therapy should be with an intravenous semisynthetic penicillin or first-generation cephalosporin, as used in the treatment of AHO (see Table

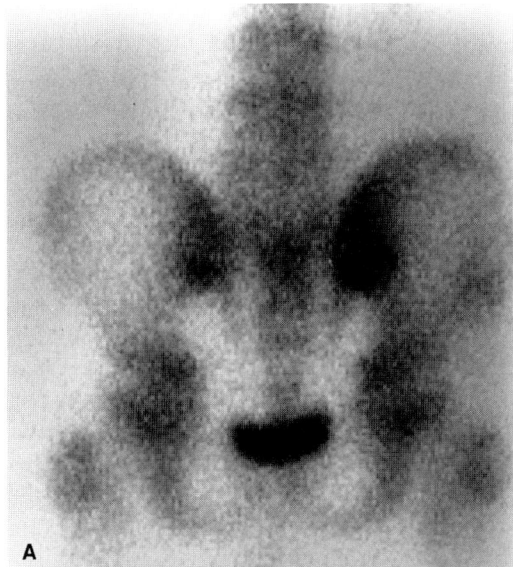
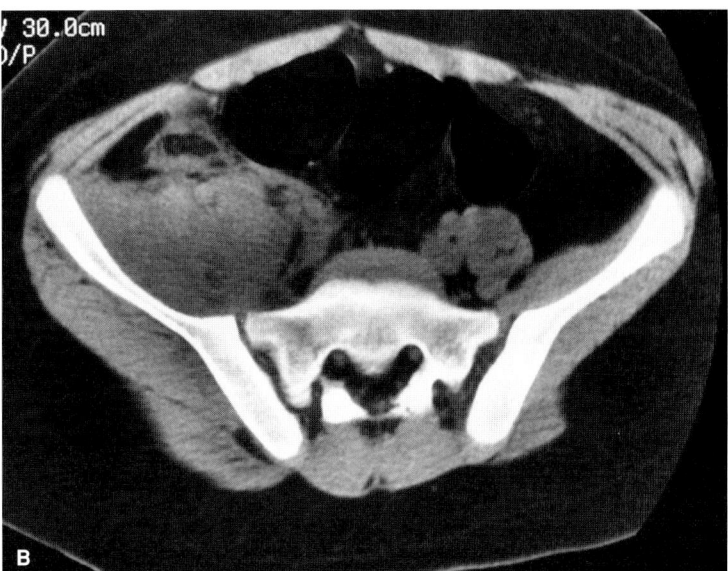
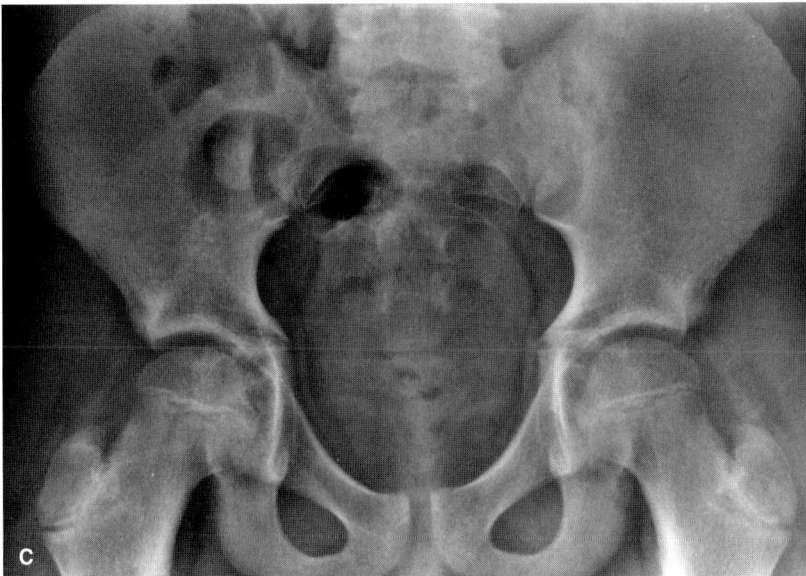

FIGURE 16-12. (A) Anteroposterior radiograph of the pelvis of a 13-year-old boy who had several days of vague hip pain. The day before this radiograph was made, he was unable to walk and became ill with fever, chills, and lethargy. Clinical findings pointed toward the right sacroiliac (SI) joint as the source of the infection. The oblique views of the SI joints were normal. (B) The technetium bone scan demonstrates increased uptake in the region of the SI joint. (C) Because surgical drainage was considered to be necessary, a computed tomography scan was performed to search for an abscess. The large collection of pus anterior demonstrated that the correct approach was anterior. (Courtesy of Douglas K. Kehl, M.D., Atlanta, Georgia.)

16-2). If symptoms resolve and the CRP begins to fall, the patient may be switched to oral antibiotics in 5 to 7 days if adequate blood levels are obtained with oral administration. Initial and subsequent antibiotics should be adjusted to reflect information from blood and stool cultures, in addition to biopsy material if that has been obtained. Failure of a response suggests that the antibiotic is not effective against the causative organism, a large abscess persists, or the etiology is not infectious.

The Neonate

Both AHO and septic arthritis can occur in the neonatal period. The classic definition of the neonatal period is the first 28 days of life. For the purposes of antibiotic selection in community-acquired infection, however, the physician is well advised to consider this period to extend to the first 8 weeks of life. The pathogenesis, diagnosis, and treatment of bone and joint sepsis differ significantly in the neonate.

The immune system in the neonate is immature. The factors are multiple, with some being specific and others nonspecific and many of them incompletely understood.[83,122] There are two important effects of this lack of well-developed immunity. First, neonates are susceptible to a wide range of organisms that are less virulent under normal circumstances. Second, because they lack a well-developed immune system, neonates do not have the usual inflammatory response that creates the signs and symptoms so important to early diagnosis.

In most circumstances, the organisms reach the bone or joint by the hematogenous route. In addition to their unusual susceptibility to many organisms that may be considered normal flora, neonates may be subjected to a wider range of organisms and to opportunities for these organisms to gain access to the circulation. This is particularly true of the neonate (especially the premature infant) who is sick and remains in the intensive care unit in the presence of nosocomial pathogens coupled with invasive monitoring, intravenous feeding, drug administration, and blood sampling. Indwelling vascular catheters, particularly those in the umbilical vessels, have long been recognized as being one of the main sources of infection.[128]

There appears to be two types of infection in the neonate: that recognized in the hospital in premature infants, and that which becomes apparent after discharge from the nursery in otherwise healthy neonates. The type manifest in the hospital usually occurs in premature infants undergoing invasive monitoring. These infants are more likely to have infection caused by S aureus or gram-negative organisms, to have multiple sites of involvement, and to be systemically ill. More than 40% of affected infants have more than one site of involvement.[14,69] The other type is usually manifest between 2 to 4 weeks of life (sometimes as late as 8 weeks) in infants who are not systemically ill and are developing and feeding normally. These infections are more likely to be due to group B *Streptococcus* and involve a single site.

Most cases of bone and joint sepsis in the neonate are caused by S aureus, with group B *Streptococcus* being the next most common. Gram-negative organisms probably comprise 10% to 15% of the infections.[14,56,69,101,118,141,147,232] *Candida albicans* is not uncommon but usually occurs along with or after other infection, often in patients on prolonged antibiotic therapy or hyperalimentation.[244] It is characterized by an even greater lack of the usual symptoms (e.g., increased warmth, tenderness).

A unique feature of neonatal bone and joint sepsis is the frequent association of contiguous bone and joint involvement and high morbidity due to the subsequent destruction of the growth plate or joint. This association, which has been reported to be as high as 76%,[14,69] leads to another important difference between the neonate and the older child regarding the changing anatomy with growth and maturation. Trueta[221,222] described the changing vascular anatomy of the physis and in particular the femoral head during growth. Ogden[157] extensively studied the role that this unique vascular anatomy plays in neonatal osteomyelitis, and Chung[33] beautifully demonstrated this changing anatomy with injected human specimens.

The changing anatomy of the blood supply within the physis has been addressed previously in this chapter. Its importance in neonatal osteomyelitis is that the vascular channels penetrating the physis and the chondroepiphysis (cartilaginous anlage of the epiphysis) permit an early destruction of both, with consequent disturbance of growth and joint congruity. This probably occurs by both lysis of the cartilage through the direct action of the organisms and destruction of the blood vessels (and the consequent avascular changes) by the inflammatory process.[114,157]

Ogden's studies led him to conclude that the frequent association of bone and joint involvement was the result of primary bone infection and was mainly due to the vascular canals traversing the physeal plate and the chondroepiphysis, allowing early abscess formation in the chondroepiphysis, which could rupture into the joint. An additional factor is that the metaphysis in neonates may lie within the capsule of the joint, thus creating septic arthritis when the pus penetrates the metaphysis and elevates the periosteum.[114,157] The lesson for the physician is that when a septic joint is diagnosed in the neonate, a thorough search for osteomyelitis in an adjacent metaphysis or epiphysis is mandatory.

The diagnosis of bone and joint sepsis in the neonate is not easy, largely because of the absence of signs and symptoms secondary to the immature immune system. The most common presenting findings are swelling, followed by pseudoparalysis and tenderness. The large amount of fat surrounding the limbs of the neonate often makes detection of swelling difficult, whereas the lack of apparent illness often leads the unsuspecting physician to ascribe the lack of motion or apparent pain to some other cause. The diagnosis in the septic premature neonate is often delayed while other causes such as meningitis or pneumonia are sought.

Because early diagnosis is so important, the evaluation of the septic infant for osteomyelitis or septic arthritis should be serial and not sequential. Any neonate with sepsis should be suspected of musculoskeletal sepsis. Any infant who exhibits disuse, discomfort of a joint with motion, or tenderness of a limb should be suspected of having bone or joint sepsis.

Other than possible soft tissue swelling, radiographic changes do not accompany an early diagnosis. The ^{99m}Tc bone scan is useful because it can survey the entire skeleton and detect changes before they are radiographically apparent. Ash and Gilday,[7a] however, found that only 32% of proved sites of osteomyelitis in 10 neonates were positive on the bone scan. This lack of ability to detect osteomyelitis may be partly due to the lack of inflammatory response to the infection or because the infectious focus lies adjacent to the active growth plate and is thus obscured by the uptake of the isotope in the growth plate. Subsequently, Bressler and colleagues[23] reported a more favorable experience, detecting all 25 sites of proved osteomyelitis in 15 affected infants. The improved results appear to be due to higher-resolution equipment and magnification views of all suspected areas.

Routine laboratory evaluation is of little value. The leukocyte count and differential leukocyte count are not reliably elevated. The sedimentation rate is usually elevated but is a nonspecific finding. The blood cultures are positive in about 50% of patients with proved infection.

Once the area of involvement is identified, aspiration is mandatory. This permits confirmation, either through obtaining pus, positive Gram-staining, or positive culture. I strongly believe that in any infant with known osteomyelitis or septic arthritis, both hip joints should be aspirated because:

- multiple sites of involvement are common
- the proximal femur and hip joint are frequently involved
- symptoms and signs are often subtle or lacking
- the hip is the most difficult joint to examine
- the window of opportunity for effective treatment is small
- the hip joint is the most frequent site of permanent sequelae.

The antibiotic management of the neonate is difficult and should be undertaken in conjunction with a physician having such experience. The selection of the antibiotic is guided by the probable causative organisms and modified by positive Gram staining and culture. The dosage varies, depending on the degree of prematurity and the status of hepatic or renal function. Because penicillinase-resistant forms of *S aureus* in addition to gram-negative enteric organisms are possible, initial antibiotic selection should cover these organisms as well as group B *Streptococcus*. Choices may include oxacillin or nafcillin along with gentamicin. A third-generation cephalosporin such as cefotaxime or ceftazidime may also be used. If methicillin-resistant *S aureus* is suspected, vancomycin should be considered in the initial therapy.

Although some authors have implied that surgical drainage may worsen the result[69] and others have implied success without surgical drainage,[101] such studies suffer from treatment of only the most severe case with surgery, acceptance of a high incidence of complications, and inadequate follow-up to detect the magnitude of growth alteration. It would seem to be even more imperative to treat the neonate with surgical debridement because adequate immune mechanisms are lacking. Therefore, when pus is found, its removal is advised. This cannot be adequately accomplished with repeated aspiration and therefore this form of therapy is not recommended.

Sickle Cell Disease

Sickle cell disease is the result of an autosomal recessive gene that produces abnormal hemoglobin, with numerous effects. Marrow hyperplasia as a mechanism to compensate for the reduced oxygen-carrying capacity of the erythrocytes resorbs both trabeculae and cortex, whereas reactive bone formation thickens the existing trabeculae. Susceptibility to infections other than osteomyelitis (e.g., sepsis, pneumonia) is increased, growth and sexual development are retarded, and infarction of bone and other organs is common. This section discusses only with those factors relating to bone and joint infection.

The gene responsible for production of the abnormal hemoglobin (hemoglobin S gene) occurs predominantly in those of African descent but is also present in Caucasians in Greece, Turkey, Italy, and India. It is estimated that between 8% to 30% of African Americans carry the hemoglobin S gene.[13,208] About 2.5% of African Americans are estimated to be homozygous for the gene that produces the clinical picture of sickle cell anemia. Although patients who are homozygous for the sickle cell gene are those most likely to be affected with bone infarction and infection, those who have hemoglobin SC disease or hemoglobin S thalassemia are also predisposed. The pathophysiologic effects of the abnormal hemoglobin molecule are discussed in Chapter 10.

Although the orthopaedist is most familiar with the bone manifestations of this disease, it is important to remember that the most serious, common, and important infections result from the pneumococcus organism. This is because those children who are homozygous for the sickle gene have defects in the alternate complement pathway, defects in opsonic activity, and impaired splenic function, which renders them susceptible to infection from pneumococci.[125] In addition, these children may have an increased susceptibility to *H influenzae*. Neither of these organisms play a large role in the bone and joint sepsis seen by the orthopaedist.

The incidence of osteomyelitis in patients with sickle cell anemia is low (particularly in the United States), despite the attention it receives in the literature. In 1971, Specht[199] found only 82 cases in the literature, whereas the few cases reported over several years in other large centers attest to the infrequent occurrence.[59,113] This low incidence is even more important to the orthopaedist when considered relative to the number of admissions for sickle cell crisis, a clinically similar presentation.[113]

The presentation of osteomyelitis or sickle cell crisis in patients with sickle cell disease does not differ significantly. Because infection is thought to follow bone infarction, both conditions may coexist. The patient with known sickle cell disease in crisis presents as an uncomfortable child with pain in one or more joints or bones. Mild swelling is often present, joint effusions are not uncommon, and bone tenderness is usual. A late but differentiating feature is that with proper management, the pain of infarction is usually markedly diminished by 3 to 5 days, whereas that of infection is not unless antibiotics are also administered.

The leukocyte count and differential are not helpful in distinguishing infection from infarction. The ESR must be interpreted with caution because it is elevated in both infarction and infection. In addition, the ESR tends to be falsely low in patients with sickle cell disease. The ESR is more likely be above 20 mm/hour in those with infection[132,215] and significant elevations should raise the suspicion of sepsis.

The initial radiologic manifestations of osteomyelitis in sickle cell disease are indistinguishable from those of bone infarction and consist of periosteal new bone along the diaphysis. As the infection proceeds, however, a diffuse moth-eaten appearance of the bone occurs, with longitudinal fissuring and increasing periosteal bone formation. This results in the typical radiographic findings of a chronic diaphyseal bone infection with involucrum and sequestrum. Frequently, the other changes of sickle cell disease are seen also—the result of marrow hyperplasia and previous bone infarction (Fig. 16-13).

The role of bone scintigraphy to differentiate marrow infarction from infection has been controversial.[113,115,169] An understanding of the local pathophysiology in both conditions explains the problem and the potential usefulness of this modality. Bone infarction initially produces an area of decreased vascularity and thus decreased isotope uptake. Once the inflammatory reaction to the infarction is established, however, the vascularity around the infarction results in increased isotope uptake. This probably occurs between 3 and 7 days after the infarction. Once it occurs, the scintigraphic appearance is the same as that of infection, which also produces increased vascularity and increased isotope uptake.

Therefore, if bone scintigraphy is to be useful, it must be performed early, preferably within 72 hours of the onset of symptoms. Two different scans must be used: a ^{99m}Tc bone scan followed by a bone marrow scan with a different isotope. Increased uptake on the ^{99m}Tc scan with decreased uptake on the marrow scan suggests infection.[113,115] Although gallium 67 citrate scanning after ^{99m}Tc scanning has been recommended,[6] it has not been found useful by others[113] and its high radiation dose to the child is an additional factor to consider.

A unique manifestation of this disorder is a condition known as sickle cell dactylitis or hand-foot syndrome.[228,241] The condition occurs in infants and young children, usually those younger than 4 years of age. No case of a child older than 7 years of age has been reported. It may precede the diagnosis of sickle cell disease. The actual incidence is probably between 10% and 20% of children with sickle cell disease, and it seems to be more common in Africa. Although it is logical to assume that it is due to infarction, there is also evidence that it may be secondary to acute marrow hyperplasia because is is not seen once the hands and feet are no longer the site of active hematopoietic production.

Patients present with acute symmetric or asymmetric painful swelling of the hands and feet. Although considered to be a benign condition, obviating further evaluation,[241] *Salmonella* osteomyelitis has been associated with this condition.[86,155] Laboratory tests do not help in the differential diagnosis. Radiographic findings in the hand-foot syndrome at first demonstrate only soft tissue swelling, followed in 7 to 14 days by the formation of subperiosteal new bone. This is followed by medullary resorption and the appearance of irregular densities in addition to cortical thinning. The changes revert to normal in weeks to months. Thus, radiographs do not help in the differential diagnosis.

With so few objective findings and tests to help in the differential diagnosis of bone infarction and osteomyelitis, how should the orthopaedist approach the patient in a clinical situation wherein the diagnosis could be either? Awareness, repeated examination, and blood cultures are basic and important. High fever, an elevated ESR, and a sequential bone scan early in the course of the disease may raise the suspicion of osteomyelitis. Aspiration of the suspected bone, with Gram staining and culturing of all material, should not be postponed when the orthopaedist or other caring for the child suspect infection. This is the only test

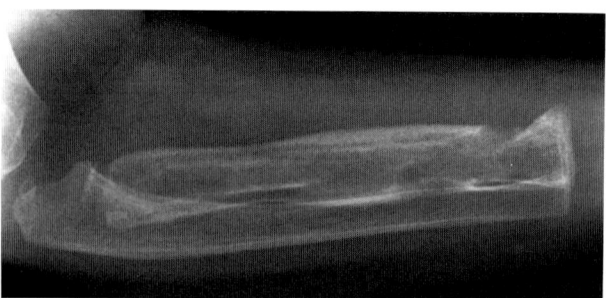

FIGURE 16-13. Lateral radiographs of the forearm in this infant demonstrate the typical changes of sickle cell osteomyelitis: longitudinal fissuring, diaphyseal location of the infection, and developing involucrum. These changes would be expected in any chronic infection of bone and are not unique to sickle cell osteomyeltits.

that confirms the diagnosis and allows appropriate early treatment.

In the literature, recommendations for or against surgical debridement are variable: some believe it to be the best treatment,[183] some believe that patients do well without surgery,[1,132,215] and others report surgery without specific indications.[132,215] A close look at the outcomes and complications of this disease lead the modern orthopaedist to question the treatment of osteomyelitis without surgical drainage in the 1990s. Although in children the diaphyseal infections eventually heal, the contemporary standard of care seeks to avoid the diaphyseal destruction commonly seen and the morbidity of prolonged hospitalization, intravenous antibiotic administration, and late sequelae. In other words, early diagnosis (not common in reports in the literature) and prompt drainage of an abscess, especially in an area of infarction, may result in outcomes comparable with normal children having the usual course of pyogenic osteomyelitis.

The question of using a tourniquet in patients with sickle cell disease who are undergoing extremity surgery is frequently raised because of the possibility that the ischemia may provoke thrombosis. This does not seem to be a problem; when the patient is properly prepared for surgery, no complications from the use of a tourniquet should result.[2,208]

Which organism is the most common cause of osteomyelitis in sickle cell disease—S aureus or Salmonella? This is a frequent test question, although it has little relevance in practice because both are so common that antibiotic agents must be given against both organisms until cultures establish the etiology. In addition, the literature is contradictory on which organism is the most common.[1,132,182] Initial antibiotic choices include ampicillin or chloramphenicol to cover Salmonella species and a semisynthetic penicillin to cover those of Staphylococcus. An alternative choice would be cefotaxime or ceftriaxone, each of which covers both S aureus and Salmonella species, including those Salmonella resistant to ampicillin, chloramphenicol, or trimethoprim-sulfamethoxazole (Bactrim; see Table 16-2).

Arthritis may be seen in various forms in patients with sickle cell disease.[94] The most common is an aseptic arthritis, most likely due to the sickle cell disease. It may be seen during crisis but is more often a transient synovitis, usually involving the knee, which resolves within 5 days.[61,160] A second form of aseptic arthritis is that associated with a remote Salmonella infection.[214] This may be seen with other organisms and the exact mechanism is not clear. Finally, the patient with sickle cell disease may have a septic arthritis. When this is the case, Salmonella is not the most likely organism. Salmonella is a rare organism in septic arthritis[102]; when it occurs, it is most often in patients without sickle cell disease. When Salmonella septic arthritis occurs in sickle cell patients, it is most often from contiguous spread of osteomyelitis. More likely organisms in septic arthritis are Staphylococcus species.[54,183] As with osteomyelitis, there is a difference of opinion on the advisability of arthrotomy for drainage.[54,183]

Chronic Recurrent Multifocal Osteomyelitis

In 1972, a condition described as "subacute and chronic symmetrical osteomyelitis" was reported in the radiology literature.[74] Since then, more than 50 cases of this disorder, which has come to be known as chronic recurrent multifocal osteomyelitis, have been described. Females are affected in about 70% of the cases.[110] This entity is distinct from pyogenic osteomyelitis and is associated with a variety of other curious disorders of bone and skin. These associations include chronic sclerosing osteomyelitis of Garré, condensing osteitis of the clavicle, sternocostoclavicular hyperostosis, and palmarplantar pustulosis.

The clinical picture is characterized by the insidious onset of pain, often with swelling and occasionally erythema, suggesting infection of the bone. Patients usually remain ambulatory. Although more often multifocal, the initial presentation may be unifocal, progressing to multifocal. Although arthritis is more common in adults, it may be seen in adolescents.[32] This and subsequent attacks are usually associated with symptoms of malaise and occasionally low-grade fever.

A curious associated condition is palmarplantar pustulosis, a descriptive term for vesicles that may appear on the hands or feet. The association of these lesions with a variety of bone lesions is common, and all of these various conditions previously described as being associated with palmarplantar pustulosis are probably the same disease.[112] These lesions do not occur in all cases but seem to recur with recurrence of the bone symptoms. The bone lesions and the clinical course do not seem to differ between patients with and those without these skin manifestations.

The subsequent course of resolution and then recurrence months later is characteristic of this disease. Subsequent flare-ups are associated with the same findings and symptoms of the initial attack. The same or different bones may be involved. Generally, the symptoms recur over a period of 2 years; however, symptoms may recur as many as 5 years later. Growth arrest has both been absent[32] and present[134] in different series.

Laboratory findings are distinct from the usual findings in pyogenic osteomyelitis because the leukocyte count remains normal. The sedimentation rate is elevated and cultures of bone and blood are nega-

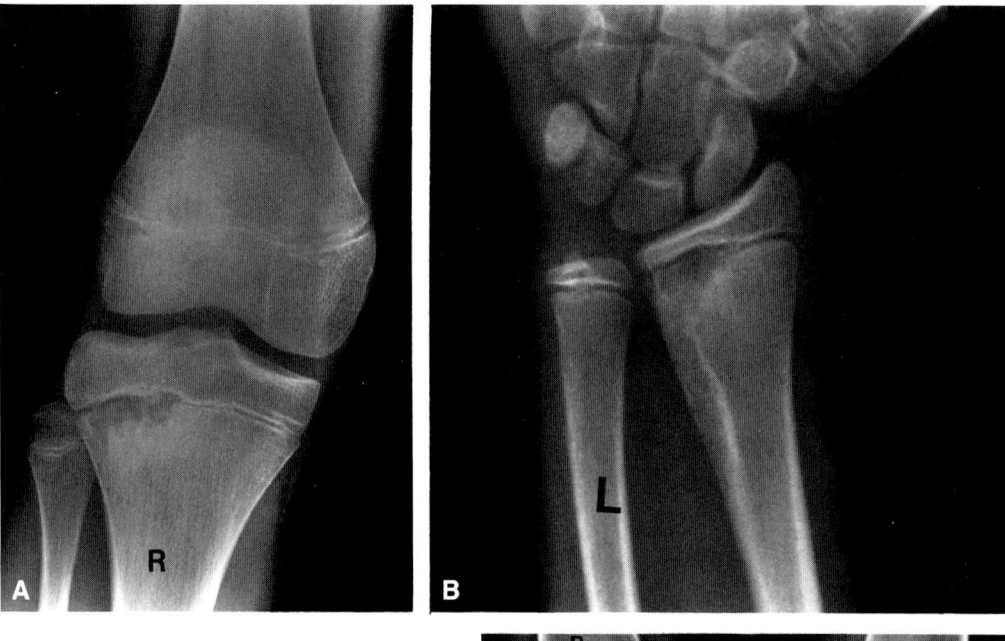
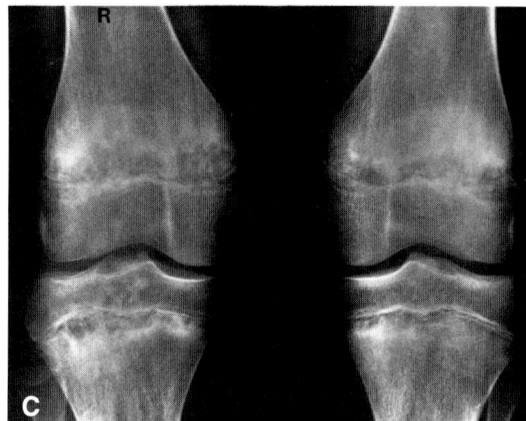

FIGURE 16-14. (A) A 12-year-old girl presented with recurrent limp over a period of 18 months. She complained of pain in the right knee. Examination demonstrated tenderness about the right knee but no other signs of inflammation. Radiographs of the right knee showed metaphyseal irregularity of the proximal tibia. (B) Skeletal survey demonstrated additional similar lesions in the opposite knee, distal tibia, and radius. These lesions were asymptomatic. (C) Radiographs 1 year later show diffuse metaphyseal changes of the distal femur and proximal tibia of both legs. No antibiotics were administered, and the symptoms resolved over the next several months.

tive. It has been noted that the chemotactic activity of the polymorphonuclear cells is increased, whereas in the presence of bacterial infection, this activity is decreased.[110]

The descriptions of the pathology in the bony lesions vary in the literature.[17,32,111] This variation probably results from sampling differences and the stage of the lesion at the time of the biopsy. It seems that early lesions consist of infiltration with predominantly neutrophils. This is followed by infiltration with fibrovascular tissue and inflammatory cells, predominantly lymphocytes and plasma cells. Osteoblasts and trabecular thickening follow.

At the time of presentation, the characteristic metaphyseal lesions are usually well developed. These lesions consist of poorly delimited eccentric metaphyseal lucencies along the physeal border. These lesions have been shown to cross into the epiphysis.[32,134] The most common sites for these lesions are the distal and proximal metaphyses of the tibia and femur. Other affected sites are the distal radius and ulna, the distal fibula, and the metatarsals (Fig. 16-14). From a review of the literature, it seems that almost every bone has been reported as being involved, including the pelvis.

As healing occurs, sclerosis surrounds the lesion. When the lesion extends into the cortex, periosteal reaction may occur. This is more likely to be seen early in the course in the small tubular and flat bones. This picture can be confused with bony neoplasm, such as leukemia, Ewing sarcoma, or eosinophilic granuloma.

The clavicle is frequently involved, presenting as a chronic sclerosing osteomyelitis.[111] When present, this starts in the medial end of the clavicle and may present with both lucencies and an onionskin periosteal reaction.

Bone scintigraphy shows increased uptake in radiographically apparent lesions and also helps to identify lesions that are inapparent on plain radiographs.

It is doubtful that every case needs to undergo biopsy. If the picture is characteristic, little is to be gained. There may well be circumstances wherein the diagnosis is in doubt, in which case biopsy is necessary to rule out a malignancy or obtain culture from a lesion suspected of being pyogenic or tuberculous.

The most likely confusion is between subacute osteomyelitis and chronic recurrent multifocal osteomyelitis. Gamble and Rinsky[71] compared groups of patients with each other. From their data, the only helpful initial finding is the the presence of multiple bone lesions in patients with chronic recurrent multifocal osteomyelitis. The age, symptoms, and laboratory findings were similar in both groups. Occasionally, the periosteal reaction can indicate a more serious bone lesion such as Ewing sarcoma when it is the only lesion.

There is no specific treatment for this disorder, and the symptoms resolve without treatment. In most cases, nonsteroidal antiinflammatory medications ameliorate the pain. Antibiotics have not been demonstrated to have any effect on the course of the disorder and are not indicated.

Subacute Osteomyelitis

In 1965, Harris and Kirkaldy-Willis[92] called attention to a subacute form of pyogenic osteomyelitis in which there had been no acute symptoms and the patient had received no antibiotics. Four years later, King and Mayo[116] reported a similar group of patients. The characteristic presenting features were no previous acute attack to suggest evolution of an acute osteomyelitis to a chronic form, insidious onset of pain, absence of systemic signs, and radiographic presence of a bone lesion at the time of presentation. They found these lesions in both the epiphysis and diaphysis and described the various radiographic presentations.

Regardless of the location within the bone, the presentation is usually the same: weeks to months of worsening pain that started insidiously and limp and tenderness with swelling visible, depending on the location. In addition, the laboratory findings are similar in most cases and are distinct from AHO. The leukocyte count is usually normal or only slightly elevated. The ESR is usually elevated, although usually not as high as in AHO. Blood cultures are usually negative, although curettings from the lesions are frequently culture-positive, usually for *S aureus*. Histology is compatible with acute and chronic inflammation.

Radiographic lesions are usually seen at the time of presentation. Far from being uniform, these lesions can present in many different locations and with a plethora of radiographic features. This highlights the main problem that faces the treating physician: the differential diagnosis of the lesion. Gledhill's classification[81] was further expanded by Roberts and colleagues[173] (Fig. 16-15).

The most common type of subacute osteomyelitis in the pediatric age group is the metaphyseal lesion (types IA and IB).[19] This represents a true Brodie abscess, a localized abscess of bone without previous acute illness. The lesion is located eccentrically in the metaphysis, frequently with visible extension into the epiphysis (Fig. 16-16). The lesion may have a sclerotic border or may be irregular and ill-defined. The second most common type is the epiphyseal lesion (type V).[8,84,197] The radiographic appearance is similar to the lesion in the metaphysis; it also may extend across the plate into the metaphysis. The other lesions—erosion of the metaphyseal cortex (type II); localized conical and periosteal reaction (type III); onionskin cortical reaction in the diaphysis (type IV); and those involving the vertebral body (type VI)—are seen less commonly.

As mentioned, the differential diagnosis of these lesions is the most important step in correct treatment and is often the most difficult. In a series of 71 children with subacute osteomyelitis, Ross and Cole[178] divided the lesions into two categories: aggressive lesions (26) and cavities in the region of the metaphysis and epiphysis (45). All of the lesions in the "aggressive" group that were in the diaphysis or metaphysis demonstrated onionskin periosteal new bone. Two lesions were in the spine. The other lesions were all in the metaphysis or epiphysis and had the typical radiologic features of type I and V lesions described above. The differential diagnoses of a type V lesion in the epiphysis include chondroblastoma and osteoid osteoma (and osteoblastoma), with eosinophilic granuloma, enchondroma, and chondromyxoid fibroma being less common. Of these, only chondroblastoma produces a periosteal response. The differential diagnoses of the typical type I lesion include eosinophilic granuloma and perhaps giant cell tumor. Computerized tomography can be useful in the questionable case. The type III metaphyseal lesion with erosion of the cortex can be confused with osteosarcoma.

The appearance of the typical lesion of a bone abscess in the epiphysis or metaphysis is so characteristic that Ross and Cole believed that it was diagnostic and could be treated without biopsy or curettage. For these patients, they recommended 48 hours of intravenous semisynthetic penicillin or first-generation cephalosporin, followed by 6 weeks of oral antibiotic. Eighty-seven percent of 37 children were healed with one course of antibiotics. Failure increased with the age of the child and led to curettage and a further course of antibiotic. The authors do not mention the dosage of oral antibiotic nor whether adequate serum levels of antibiotic were verified in these patients. This 13% failure rate may be improved with a longer course

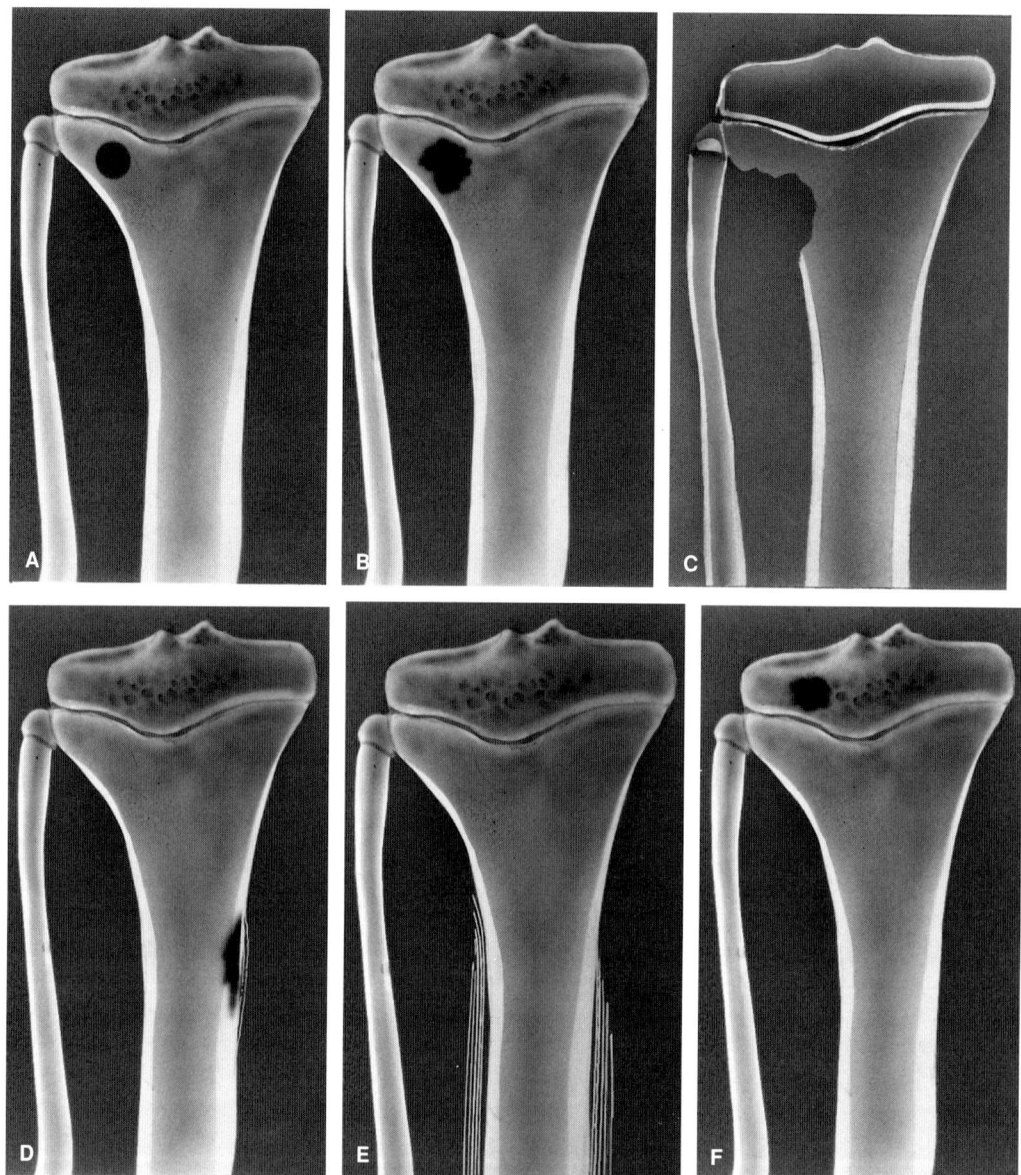

FIGURE 16-15. The variety of presentations of subacute hematogenous osteomyelitis in the classification of Roberts and colleagues.[173] (**A**) Type 1A is a punched-out metaphyseal lesion resembling an eosinophilic granuloma. (**B**) Type 1B is similar to type 1A but has a sclerotic cortex. (**C**) Type 2 lesions erode the metaphyseal bone, often including the cortex, and appear as aggressive lesions. (**D**) Type 3 lesions are localized cortical and periosteal reactions, simulating osteoid osteoma. (**E**) Type 4 lesions produce onion-skin–like periosteal reactions in the diaphysis and resemble Ewing sarcoma. (**F**) Type 5 lesions are epiphyseal erosions. (**G**) Type 6 lesions involve the vertebral bodies.

of intravenous antibiotic without resort to surgical treatment. All of the cases of "aggressive" lesions underwent biopsy and curettage.

Puncture Wounds of the Foot

Since Johanson's 1968 report,[107] orthopaedic surgeons have become increasingly aware of the association between puncture wounds of the foot and *Pseudomonas aeruginosa* as the causative organism of deep infections that follow. It was subsequently demonstrated that *Pseudomonas* can be recovered from the inner spongy sole of well-worn tennis shoes.[67] *P aeruginosa* is a gram-negative aerobic organism with anaerobic tolerance that is found widely in soil, water, and on the skin. As a human pathogen seen in orthopaedic conditions, it seems to have an affinity for cartilage.

Fitzgerald and Cowan[68] identified puncture wounds of the foot as the reason for an emergency room visit in 0.8% of children younger than the age of 15 years. Of the total number with puncture wounds, 8.4% who were seen within the first 24 hours

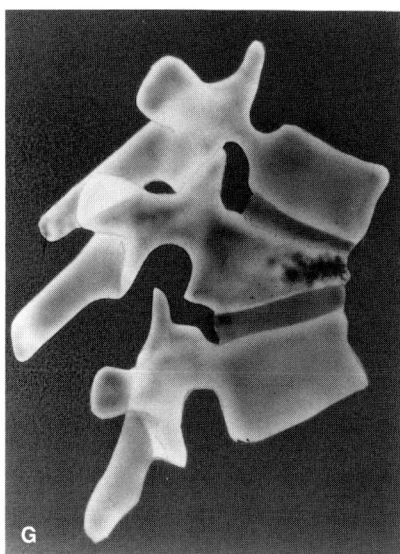

FIGURE 16-15 (Continued)

after the injury either had cellulitis at the time of presentation or returned within the first 4 days with cellulitis. Of those presenting 1 to 7 days after the injury, cellulitis was present in 57%. Only 0.6% of those who were not referred to the emergency room for an established infection subsequently developed osteomyelitis. Of 132 patients seen with soft tissue infection after puncture wound of the foot, 112 had a prompt response to soaks, rest, elevation, and antibiotics. The importance of these data is that most infections after puncture wounds of the foot do not develop osteomyelitis or septic arthritis. The cases of cellulitis that do not develop osteomyelitis or septic arthritis are mostly infections after puncture wounds of the foot and represent the denominator usually not seen by the orthopaedist. Most of these infections respond to nonoperative therapy such as rest, elevation, and oral antibiotics.

A major dilemma is the initial management of the puncture wound. Suggestions for "debridement and irrigation with loose closure over small irrigation tubes" are impractical, given the number of puncture wounds occurring annually in the United States and the infrequency of serious infection.[107] Similarly, the recommendation that "any deep wounds should be surgically debrided" seems impractical because the treating physician would not know how deep the puncture wound is without anesthesia and surgical exploration.[170]

Given the data on the development of cellulitis and osteomyelitis after puncture wounds, it appears that subsequent development of osteomyelitis and septic arthritis is largely determined by whether the nail punctures the bone or joint. It is usually impossible for the initial treating physician to know this, although there should be a high degree of suspicion if the wound is over the metatarsal heads, the lateral border of the foot, or the heel—areas where the bone is in close approximation to the skin of the sole of the foot.

A reasonable approach to the initial management of a puncture wound of the foot includes superficial debridement of the skin and inspection for a foreign body because a foreign body is found in almost 3% of cases.[68] Tetanus prophylaxis is important. Because of the possibility of cellulitis developing in the first several days, patients should be advised to return at the first sign of infection. There does not seem to be any solid evidence either for or against the routine use of antibiotics in the initial management. They can be used effectively in the management of cellulitis and there is no effective oral antibiotic for *Pseudomonas* osteomyelitis or septic arthritis in the pediatric age group.

The typical course of osteomyelitis or septic arthritis is the onset of pain and swelling 2 to 5 days after

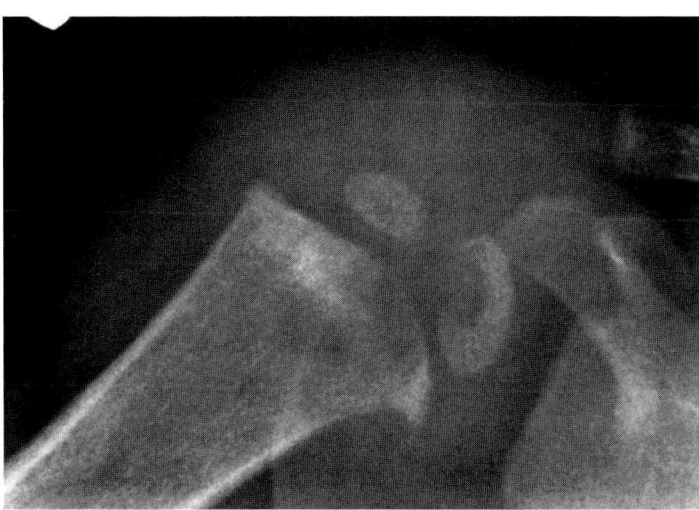

FIGURE 16-16. A 13-month-old girl presented for examination when her mother noted the child experienced discomfort when lifting her arms while her mother changed the child's clothes. *Haemophilus influenzae* was cultured from the lesion. The epiphyseal lesion communicates with the metaphyseal lesion.

the puncture, when the initial symptoms should be gone. At this time, soaks, elevation, and an oral antistaphylococcic antibiotic are prescribed. If the patient has cellulitis, this regimen usually results in a cure. When osteomyelitis or septic arthritis is present, the symptoms may improve but do not disappear. This is probably due to the mixed flora in these infections. Finally, either continued pain and swelling or radiographic changes prompt the correct diagnosis. Good treatment includes close follow-up of those puncture wounds having signs of infection and appropriate treatment if signs and symptoms of cellulitis do not resolve promptly on oral antibiotic treatment.

Initially, the signs and symptoms of cellulitis and osteomyelitis or septic arthritis can be difficult to differentiate. Pain on motion of a specific metatarsophalangeal joint is usually indicative of a septic arthritis in that joint. Dorsal swelling on the forefoot or swelling laterally and medially around the heel is often an additional sign of a serious deep infection (Fig. 16-17). Aspiration is helpful, not only in locating pus but in obtaining material for culture. If no pus is obtained, bone scintigraphy may help in the early differentiation of cellulitis from osteomyelitis or septic arthritis.

Pseudomonas infection of a bone or joint is a surgical disease; the failure of antibiotics alone to resolve these infections has been adequately demonstrated.[103] The surgical approach may be either dorsal or volar but must give adequate access to both the bones and joints in the region of the puncture because *P aeruginosa* is a "cartilage-seeking" organism. Some surgeons believe that the volar approach leaves a potentially painful scar. When properly placed, however, this should not be the case. This approach has the advantage of directly exposing the puncture track, which is an essential part of the surgery because of the high incidence of foreign material found at surgical debridement.[68,104] The dorsal approach allows direct access to the joints and bones through a more anatomic and easier to extend approach that is not limited by the considerations of placement on the sole of the foot. This can be combined with a limited debridement of the volar puncture wound. Except in the most extensive cases of destruction of the calcaneus, in which the "cloven hoof" incision can be used, this bone should be approached from a medial or lateral incision or from both.

Infections due to puncture wounds have two characteristics: they are caused by multiple organisms, and *P aeruginosa* is usually one of them. For this reason, it makes sense to begin antibiotic therapy with a combination of antibiotics effective against both gram-positive organisms and gram-negative organisms, including *P aeruginosa*. An initial choice may be ceftazidime and gentamicin or oxacillin and gentamicin (see Table 16-2). Jacobs and coworkers[103,104] suggest that 7 days

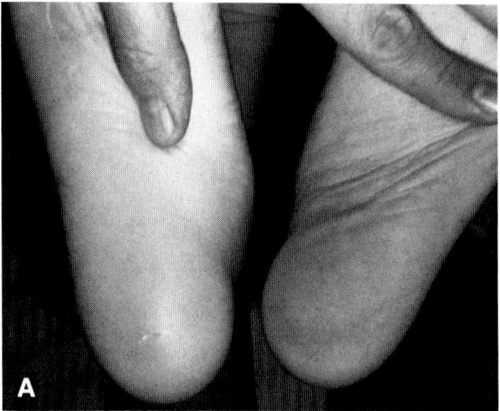
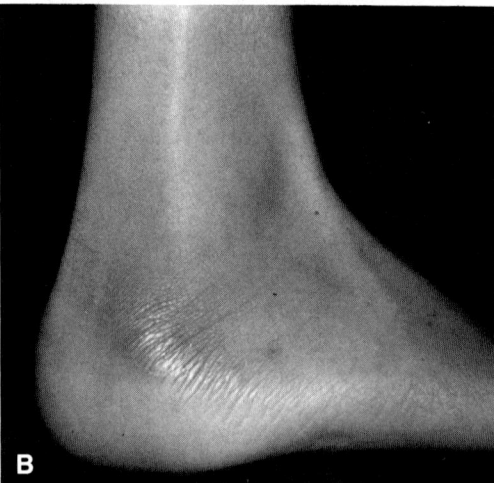
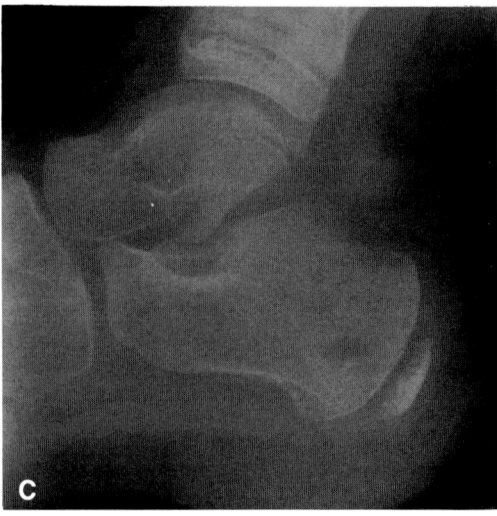

FIGURE 16-17. This patient was seen with pain 2 weeks after a puncture wound of the heel. He returned to the emergency department 3 days after the puncture wound because of increasing pain and swelling. Therapy was begun with a first-generation cephalosporin antibiotic. He experienced temporary improvement, but later the pain became worse. (**A**) Note the swelling of the affected heel when compared with the opposite contralateral heel side. (**B**) Because of the dense septated tissue in the heel, osteomyelitis of the calcaneus usually is seen laterally. The swelling and erythema on the lateral side of the heel indicates deep infection. (**C**) A radiograph demonstrates a lytic lesion of the heel in addition to the soft tissue swelling. *Pseudomonas aeruginosa* was cultured from the infected site.

of intravenous antibiotic after adequate surgical debridement are adequate, although others recommend longer treatment (e.g., 10 days to 2 weeks).

In cases that fail to respond to the above treatment, the fast-growing mycobacteria (e.g., *Mycobacterium chelonei* and *Mycobacterium fortuitum*) should be considered as possible pathogens.

Lyme Arthritis

Lyme disease was first described as a disorder transmitted by a tick in the mid-1970s after the investigation of an epidemic of arthritis in both children and adults in the region of Old Lyme, Connecticut.[205,206] The infectious agent is a spirochete, *Borrelia burgdorferi*, and it is transmitted by *Ixodes* ticks, the common 'deer tick'. Most infections occur during the months of May through August because that is when both outdoor activity by children and the activity of the tick are greatest. It is important for the orthopaedist to recognize that this disease in children has several characteristics that differ from the usual descriptions of adults who are affected.

The pathogenesis of the disease in all of its various stages is not completely understood. The identification of *B burgdorferi* in the synovial tissue and its isolation from synovial fluid suggest a direct infectious mechanism as with any other bacteria. Because the chronic form of the arthritis (occurring in 10% of adults) is unresponsive and tends to develop in patients with the haplotype HLA-DR4, additional immunologic factors are suggested.

The disease is usually heralded by the onset of a characteristic spreading skin lesion called erythema migrans. It begins between 3 and 30 days after the bite by the tick and is caused by the spirochete's spread in the skin. Although it is present in 60% to 80% of adults, its occurrence in children seems to be less.[42,57]

The other early signs are fever, headache, malaise, and myalgia—all nonspecific symptoms. In addition to the joint manifestations, children may also present with neurologic or cardiac findings. The most common neurologic finding is seventh cranial nerve palsy, although a fluctuating meningoencephalitis and peripheral neuropathy may also be seen. The most common cardiac manifestation is an atrioventricular block seen on electrocardiography. Myocarditis is also seen.

In children, the most common early symptom that brings the child to medical attention is the arthritis.[57,177] This may present as an acute arthritis and be difficult to distinguish from other bacterial arthritis; more commonly, the arthritis is less debilitating and less painful. The second difficult differential diagnosis is JRA. As with JRA, several joints (usually fewer than four and most commonly the large joints such as the knee) may be involved and the swelling is usually greater than the symptoms experienced by the child. Both acute septic arthritis and acute Lyme arthritis are treated by antibiotics, with those used for common bacterial causes usually being adequate for Lyme arthritis. In suspected cases, blood may be drawn for serologic testing. The difficulty with false-positive and false-negative results makes clinical diagnosis most important in an endemic area, however. A diagnosis of JRA requires 6 or more weeks of unremitting arthritis (which can occur in Lyme disease) that does not respond to antibiotics, which Lyme arthritis does. It is important to note that the antinuclear antibody titers can be elevated in Lyme arthritis.

The only consistent laboratory finding is an elevated ESR. The most common test to detect infection with *B burgdorferi* is an enzyme-linked immunosorbent assay. Although this test is reported to be highly sensitive and specific in some laboratories, it is not standardized and results vary considerably among different laboratories, making a laboratory diagnosis suspect.[198,207] Bacterial isolation is most specific but is difficult and not widely available. This makes the clinical findings even more important in the diagnosis.

The treatment of choice is penicillin or amoxicillin. In the early localized stages of the disease, these can be given orally but in later stages, most prefer intravenous penicillin.[42,57,198] Tetracycline can be used in children older than 8 years of age who are allergic to penicillin (see Table 16-2). More than 4 weeks of therapy is probably not indicated.[204] Children do not develop the chronic disease, unlike adults, and the arthritis is usually cured with antibiotics.

Gonococcal Arthritis

Gonococcal arthritis is usually a sexually transmitted disease caused by the gram-negative diplococcus *Neisseria gonorrhoeae*. In the newborn, the disease is contracted from the mother during passage through the birth canal and results most commonly in conjunctivitis and scalp abscesses. When the disease is noted after the newborn period, before puberty, and in sexually inactive adolescents, sexual abuse should be suspected. Gonococcal infection is most common in women in the second and third decade and therefore is seen frequently in the adolescent age group. Although gonococcal infection can take many forms, the orthopaedist is most likely to encounter this infection as septic arthritis in the disseminated form of the disease.

In the adolescent, the infection most often results from dissemination of a genitourinary infection, which is frequently asymptomatic. The delay between the genitourinary infection and the arthritis is variable, ranging from a few days to several weeks. In adolescence, the disseminated form of the disease is associated with pregnancy and menstruation, periods of low progesterone activity.[98]

The orthopaedist needs to be especially aware of the possibility of sexual abuse in patients with gonococcal arthritis. Sexual abuse may occur in as many as 10% of all abuse cases, and it is estimated that between 5% and 20% of sexually abused children have a sexually transmitted disease, most commonly gonococcal infection.[172,235] Children who are identified with or suspected of having a gonococcal infection should have cultures of all mucous membranes, including pharynx, vagina, and rectum, before the administration of antibiotics. These cultures should be handled in a manner that permits them to be used as evidence in court. In addition, reporting of suspected cases is mandated by the Child Abuse Reporting Law. For all of these reasons, the orthopaedist should involve a knowledgeable pediatrician in the evaluation of these patients.

The classic presentation is rash, tenosynovitis, and migratory polyarthralgia. Only about one third of the cases develop a distinctive but not pathognomonic rash, which is a result of gonococcal septicemia. The initial lesion is a small erythematous macule. This may disappear or develop a small vesicle, followed by a necrotic center that may form a pustule. The tenosynovitis, when seen, often affects the dorsal surface of the wrist and hand. This finding, like the skin rash, is nonspecific and can be caused by other organisms.

The clinical presentation of the disseminated disease with septic arthritis begins with chills and fever in about three fourths of the patients. Joint involvement is polyarticular in 80% of cases. The knee is most often affected but it is important to remember that any joint, large or small, can be involved. The size of the effusion may vary widely and may even be absent. The involved joints are usually painful. The nature of the arthritis does not appear to have changed over the past several decades, although treatment with antibiotics has resulted in the virtual elimination of joint destruction.[37,38,202,230,239] Osteomyelitis still may be seen as an occasional complication.[219]

The leukocyte count is elevated in two thirds of the patients. Culture is the only way to confirm the diagnosis. Culture and Gram-staining of joint fluid and of the cervix of postpubertal girls and the vagina of prepubertal girls should be performed. Any urethral or prostatic discharge in the male should also be cultured and examined by Gram staining. Blood cultures should be routine. The organism may occasionally be isolated from skin lesions but Gram staining gives a higher yield.

N gonorhoeae is a difficult organism to grow and special care is needed in the handling of the material for culture. Because the organism is sensitive to cold, material for culture should be plated directly onto a warm medium whenever possible. Special culture tubes for transport of gonococcal cultures are available and should be used in addition to prompt delivery of specimens to the bacteriology laboratory when direct-plating is not feasible. Cultures from sterile sites (e.g., blood, synovial fluid) are plated on chocolate blood agar. Cultures from nonsterile sites (e.g., the vagina, skin lesions) should be plated on selective media (e.g., Thayer-Martin agar) that contains antibiotics to inhibit the growth of other organisms. Cultures are grown in a 5% to 10% CO_2 atmosphere.

The increasing resistance of *N gonorrhoeae* to penicillin and tetracycline makes parenteral administration of a third-generation cephalosporin (e.g., ceftriaxone, 50 mg/kg/day, intramuscularly or intravenously, once daily) the initial drug of choice (see Table 16-2). If the organism is demonstrated to be sensitive to penicillin, it can be used. Recommendation for drainage of the joints remains variable. In the hip joint, there is no controversy; surgical drainage as for pyogenic septic arthritis caused by any organism is required. In other large joints with large amounts of purulent fluid, surgical drainage may be preferable to repeated needle aspiration. If surgical drainage is used, it is wise to leave a closed suction drain in the joint because the tendency to reaccumulate fluid is greater than with other forms of septic arthritis.

Tuberculosis

1985 is the year in which fewer cases of tuberculosis were reported in the United States since reporting began in 1953. Between 1985 and 1991, the incidence rose sharply, only to slightly decrease in both 1992 and 1993 for all age groups except those younger than 15 years of age. During this period, the largest increase was reported for patients born outside of the United States and its territories. In 1993, these patients comprised almost 30% of the reported cases. California, New York, and Texas saw the largest increases. The increased incidence has been accompanied by human immunodeficiency virus infection and multi-drug–resistant organisms.

Because extrapulmonary tuberculosis is more common among children, particularly those younger than 5 years of age, the orthopaedic surgeon must again become aware of this possibility when evaluating chronic joint inflammation or chronic bone lesions.

Patients who are exposed to tuberculosis may or may not become infected, and those who are infected may or may not become diseased. There is a time lag between infection and diagnosis of the extrapulmonary disease of about 1 year.

Most patients are infected by human contact because bovine tuberculosis has been eliminated in this country by the pasteurization of milk. The lungs are the most common site of initial infection in children; the kidneys are not. The tubercle bacilli may disseminate to bones or joint during the lymphatic and hematogenous spread of the initial infection. If the initial lung infection remains untreated, involvement of the bones and or joints occurs in 5% to 10% of children.[195a] The development of the lesions in bone is time- and location-related. Dactylitis may occur within a few months in younger children. Long bone involvement may occur in 1 to 3 years.

The initial focus in the bone is usually the epiphysis or metaphysis, rarely the diaphysis. As the osteomyelitis develops, it enlarges the area of bone destruction in a centrifugal fashion, producing a characteristic round cystic lesion with ill-defined margins. These lesions are filled with an inflammatory granulation tissue, creating a reactive hyperemia, which produces a wide area of osteopenia surrounding the lesion. This process is almost purely destructive or lytic, with little or no bone reaction (Fig. 16-18); thus, the lack of sclerotic margins and a periosteal response. Because of the chronicity and hyperemia, widening and accelerated growth of the epiphysis may be seen. The physeal plate offers little resistance to the spread of the infection, as it does in other pyogenic infections. Before extraosseous abscess formation, the bone lesions may mimic pyogenic infection or tumors such as eosinophilic granuloma.

Most skeletal tuberculosis affects the spine. The infection almost always begins in the vertebral body, usually the anterior one third. The most frequent site of involvement in the spine is the lower thoracic and upper lumbar spine. Paravertebral abscess formation is characteristic, and calcification developing within the abscess is almost diagnostic of a tuberculous abscess. The disks become involved when two adjacent vertebral bodies are affected. The bone lesions in the vertebral bodies are mainly destructive (Fig. 16-18).

Skeletal tuberculosis outside of the axial skeleton usually affects the major joints, particularly the hip and knee. Isolated joint infections, unusual in childhood, are initially characterized by effusion in addition to synovial proliferation and thickening. In the early stages, there are no radiographic characteristics that separate tuberculous arthritis from any chronic inflammation of the joint. As with the bone lesions, the hyperemia causes widespread osteopenia and may cause overgrowth of the epiphyses. The infection proceeds by both pannus formation over the articular cartilage and erosion of the subchondral bone, beginning at the synovial margins.[167] The result is joint space narrowing and subchondral cystic erosion. Early in the process, the clinical and radiologic findings may closely resemble those of JRA or pigmented villonodular synovitis. Laboratory studies, however, should easily separate these entities.

As the infection continues untreated, large amounts of caseous material and pus accumulate and dissect along normal tissue planes. Eventually, a sinus track to the surface is formed—a hallmark of a long-standing neglected case. The abscess formed by tuber-

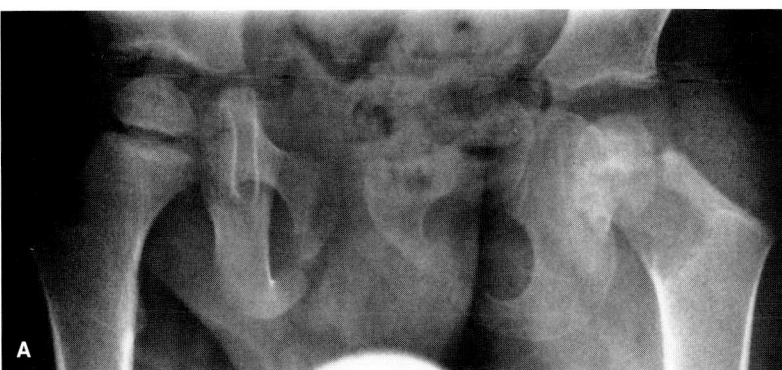
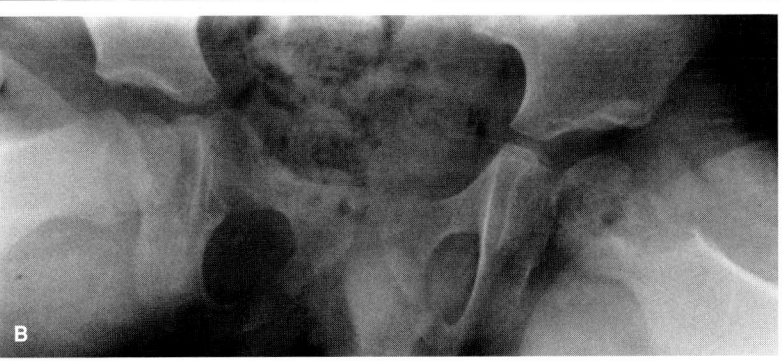

FIGURE 16-18. (A and B) Radiographs of a 3-year-old boy who recently moved to the United States from Mexico. The child had complaints of increasing limp on the left, pain that worsened at night, and no significant limitation of activity. Examination demonstrated limited motion with irritability. Laboratory studies showed a normal complete blood count, erythrocyte sedimentation rate of 25 mm/hour, and a positive purified protein derivative test. Open biopsy confirmed the diagnosis of tuberculosis by histology and culture. (Courtesy of Hugh Watts, M.D., Los Angeles.)

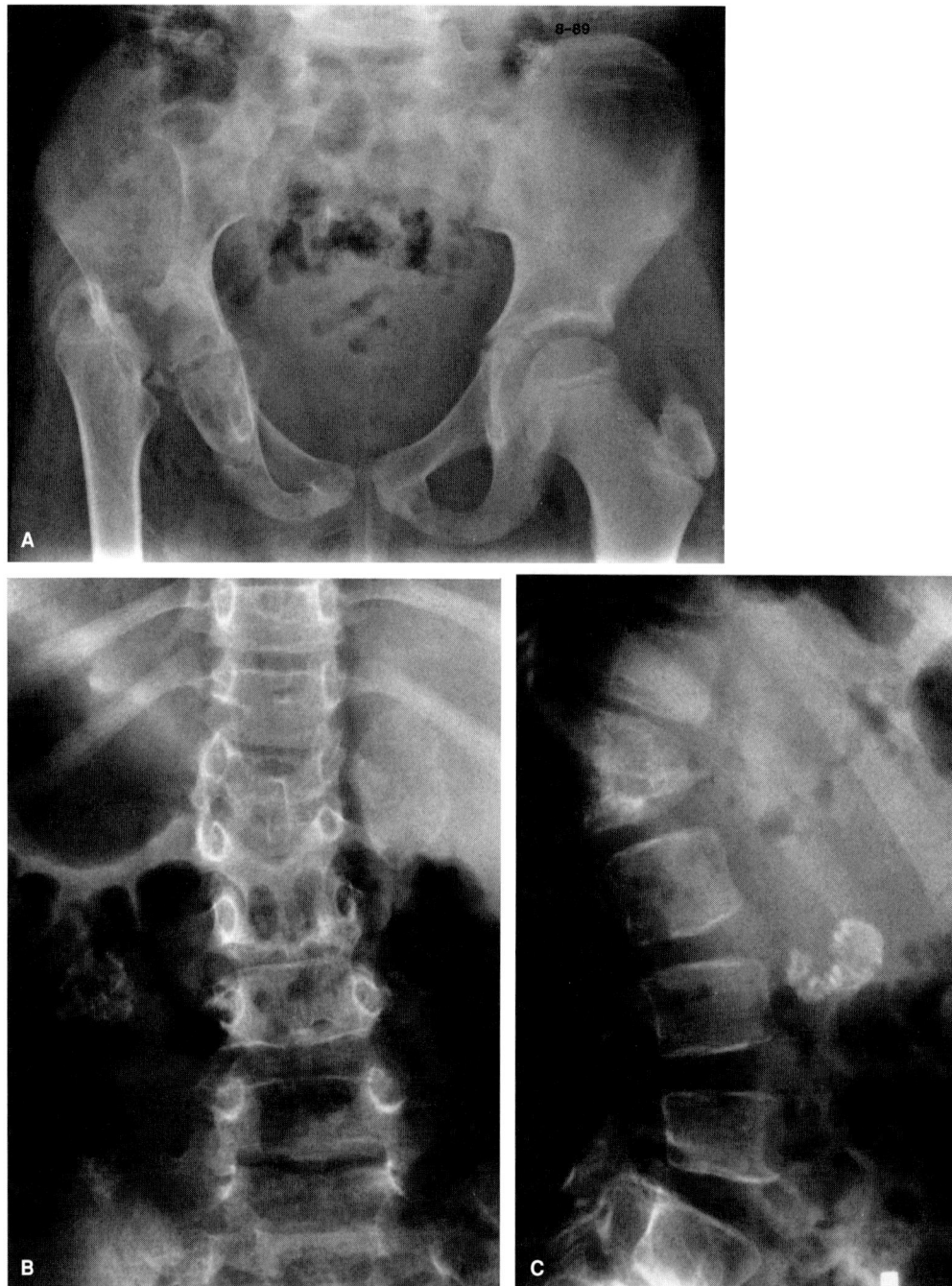

FIGURE 16-19. (A) Anteroposterior (AP) radiograph of a 10-year-old girl from Mexico who had a past history of several operations on the right hip for tuberculosis presented with increasing back pain and kyphosis. (B and C) AP and lateral views of the spine show bony destruction of the vertebral body with relative preservation of the intervertebral disc and the calcified node; both are features of tuberculosis. Open biopsy confirmed the diagnosis of tuberculosis. (Courtesy of Hugh Watts, M.D., Los Angeles.)

culous infection is called a "cold abscess" because of the lack of any signs of acute inflammation.

Two other presentations occur in childhood. The first, tuberculous dactylitis, may resemble sickle cell dactylitis, with swelling of the phalanges, metacarpals, and metatarsals. Tuberculous dactylitis is usually not very painful, however, and onset is usually consecutive rather than simultaneous. Before the availability of radiographs, this was called spina (Latin for "a short bone") ventosa (meaning "inflated with air"). The radiographs show a cyst-like expansion of the tubular bones, with thinning of the cortex.[89] A second presentation is with multifocal cystic involvement of the bone. This is characterized by areas of simultaneous destruction in the shafts of long bones and in flat bones, with a strong tendency to symmetry.[189]

The first and most important step in the diagnosis of tuberculous infection of the bone or joint is to consider it as a possibility. Tuberculosis should be considered whenever a chronic-appearing bone lesion is encountered. Early diagnosis is important to prevent spread to a contiguous joint. The clinical picture is variable, depending on the location and the stage of the disease. It is characterized by its insidious onset; lack of characteristic inflammatory features, such as erythema; and bone destruction or joint involvement greater than the symptoms would suggest.

Laboratory studies usually show a normal leukocyte count and an elevated ESR. The purified protein derivative skin test usually is positive. Radiographic changes are usually present at the time of presentation. The diagnosis depends on the identification of the organism, *Mycobacterium tuberculosis*. Positive cultures are obtained in 85.5% of patients who have both pulmonary and extrapulmonary disease, in 83.5% of those with only pulmonary disease, and in 76.5% of those who have only extrapulmonary disease.[106]

Tuberculosis produces a widespread inflammatory response, which may mislead the surgeon in obtaining biopsy material, especially if the synovium is to undergo biopsy. In cases with bone lesions, the granulation tissue filling the cystic bone lesion is the best material for biopsy. In tuberculosis arthritis without bone involvement, the biopsy should be taken from the peripheral junction of the synovium with the bone or preferably from the junction of the synovium with a cyst.[225]

The treatment of skeletal tuberculosis is medical. Surgical debridement of the bone lesions is not necessary for a cure, although drainage of large abscesses often improves the patient's overall constitutional symptoms.[135,189,225] In addition, open surgical biopsy is often necessary. Because of the effectiveness of drug therapy, there is little chance that surgical biopsy will lead to sinus formation. It is important to always be aware that superinfection with pyogenic organisms can occur, and this may be a reason for apparent treatment failure with antitubercular drugs. This is particularly true when a sinus has formed.[135]

Several studies on tuberculous spondylitis demonstrate that surgery is necessary primarily to treat the kyphosis and not the tuberculosis; many cases do well with only medical management.[127,139,140,168] Indications for surgery remain relative and include neurologic involvement, spinal instability, and failure of medical treatment. Although patients with neurologic involvement can recover with medical management, they seem to do so faster with surgical management.[127] Surgical treatment of the kyphosis produces a higher rate of union and less deformity than regimens without surgical stabilization.[139,140] Thus, it appears that with contemporary surgical and anesthetic techniques, tuberculous kyphosis is best treated early with anterior surgery for debridement and strut grafting. The treatment of spinal instability, especially that spanning more than two disk spaces, is difficult and probably requires both anterior arthrodesis with strut-grafting and posterior arthrodesis with instrumentation.[168]

Although the effectiveness of ambulatory drug treatment has been demonstrated,[139,140] there is evidence of an increasing incidence of resistant strains due most likely to inadequate treatment of the initial infection.[106] This emphasizes both the need for constant surveillance for drug resistance and the importance of careful supervision of outpatient oral therapy to be certain that compliance is optimal.

Initial antimicrobial agent selection depends on the likelihood of drug-resistant organisms, whereas long-term selection should be guided by susceptibility testing. In those who are not at high risk for drug-resistant organisms, various regimens of isoniazid, rifampin, and pyrazinamide are recommended.[162] In children who come from areas where antibiotics are sold "over the counter" and incomplete treatment may have resulted in multi-drug–resistant strains, ethambutol or streptomycin should be added to the standard three-drug regimen. Treatment of bone and joint tuberculosis in children should be continued for 1 year.

References

1. Adeyokunnu AA, Hendrickse RG. *Salmonella* osteomyelitis in childhood. Arch Dis Child 1980;55:175.
2. Adu-Gyamfi Y, Sankarankutty M, Marwa S. Use of a tourniquet in patients with sickle-cell disease. Can J Anaesth 1993;40:24.
3. Ailsby RL, Staheli LT. Pyogenic infections of the sacroiliac joint in children. Radioisotope bone scanning as a diagnostic tool. Clin Orthop 1974;100:96.
4. Alexander JE, Seibert JJ, Glasier CM, et al. High-resolution hip ultrasound in the limping child. J Clin Ultrasound 1989;17:19.
5. Almquist EE. The changing epidemiology of septic arthritis in children. Clin Orthop 1970;68:96.
6. Amundsen TR, Siegel MJ, Siegel BA. Osteomyelitis and infarction in sickle cell hemoglobinopathies: differentiation by combined technetium and gallium scintigraphy. Radiology 1984;153:807.
7. Arvidson S, Holme T, Lindholm B. The formation of extracellular proteolytic enzymes by *Staphylococcus aureus*. Acta Pathol Microbiol Scand 1972;80:835.
7a. Ash JM, Gilday DL. The futility of bone scanning in neonatal osteomyelitis: concise communication. J Nucl Med 1980;21:417.
8. Azouz EM, Greenspan A, Marton D. CT evaluation of primary epiphyseal bone abscesses. Skeletal Radiol 1993;22:17.
9. Baldassare AR, Chang F, Zuckner J. Markedly raised synovial fluid leucocyte counts not associated with infectious arthritis in children. Ann Rheum Dis 1978;37:404.

10. Barton LL, Dunkle LM, Habib FH. Septic arthritis in childhood. A 13-year review. Am J Dis Child 1987;141:898.
11. Beaupre A, Carroll N. The three syndromes of iliac osteomyelitis in children. J Bone Joint Surg [Am] 1979;61:1087.
12. Bell RS, Mankin HJ, Doppelt SH. Osteomyelitis in Gaucher disease. J Bone Joint Surg [Am] 1986;68:1380.
13. Bennett OM, Namnyak SS. Bone and joint manifestations of sickle cell anaemia. J Bone Joint Surg [Br] 1990;72:494.
14. Bergdahl S, Ekengren K, Eriksson M. Neonatal hematogenous osteomyelitis: risk factors for long-term sequelae. J Pediatr Orthop 1985;5:564.
15. Berkowitz ID, Wenzel W. 'Normal' technetium bone scans in patients with acute osteomyelitis. Am J Dis Child 1980;134:828.
16. Bisno AL. Group A streptococcal infections and acute rheumatic fever. N Engl J Med 1991;325:783.
17. Bjorksten B, Boquist L. Histopathological aspects of chronic recurrent multifocal osteomyelitis. J Bone Joint Surg [Br] 1980;62:376.
18. Blockey NJ, Watson JT. Acute osteomyelitis in children. J Bone Joint Surg [Br] 1970;52:77.
19. Bogoch E, Thompson G, Salter RB. Foci of chronic circumscribed osteomyelitis (Brodie's abcess) that traverse the epiphyseal plate. J Pediatr Orthop 1984;4:162.
20. Boston HC, Bianco AJJ, Rhodes KH. Disk space infections in children. Orthop Clin North Am 1975;6:953.
21. Braude AI, Jones JL, Douglas HI. The behavior of *Escherichia coli* endotoxin (somatic antigen) during infectious arthritis. J Immunol 1963;90:297.
22. Bremner AE, Neligan GA. Benign form of acute osteitis of the spine in young children. Br Med J 1953;1:856.
23. Bressler EL, Conway JJ, Weiss SC. Neonatal osteomyelitis examined by bone scintigraphy. Radiology 1984;152:685.
24. Brown I. A study of the "capsular" shadow in disorders of the hip in children. J Bone Joint Surg [Br] 1975;57:175.
25. Bryan LE, Van den Elzen HM. Streptomycin accumulation in susceptible and resistant strains of *Escherichia coli* and *Pseudomonas aeruginosa*. Antimicrob Agents Chemother 1976;9:928.
26. Bryan RE, Hammond D. Interaction of purulent material with antibiotics used to treat *Pseudomonas* infection. Antimicrob Agents Chemother 1974;6:700.
27. Bryson YJ, Connor JD, Leuers M, et al. High dose dicloxacillin treatment of acute staphyloccal osteomyelitis in children. J Pediatr 1979;94:673.
28. Burrows H. Some factors in the localization of disease in the body. New York: William Wood, 1932:.
29. Cabanela ME, Sim FH, Beabout JW, et al. Osteomyelitis appearing as neoplasms: a diagnostic problem. Arch Surg 1974;109:68.
30. Canale ST, Harkness RM, Thomas PA, et al. Does aspiration of bones and joints affect results of later bone scanning? J Pediatr Orthop 1985;5:23.
31. Capitanio MA, Kirkpatrick JA. Early roentgen observations in acute osteomyelitis. AJR 1970;108:488.
32. Carr AJ, Cole WG, Roberton DM, et al. Chronic multifocal osteomyelitis. J Bone Joint Surg [Br] 1993;75:582.
33. Chung SMK. The arterial supply of the developing proximal end of the human femur. J Bone Joint Surg [Am] 1976;58:961.
34. Chung SMK, Borns P. Acute osteomyelitis adjacent to the sacro-iliac joint in children. J Bone Joint Surg [Am] 1973;55:630.
35. Clausen N, Gotze H, Pedersen A, et al. Skeletal scintigraphy and radiography at onset of acute lymphocytic leukemia in children. Med Pediatr Oncol 1983;11:291.
36. Cole WG, Dalziel RE, Leitl S. Treatment of acute osteomyelitis in childhood. J Bone Joint Surg [Br] 1982;64:218.
37. Cooperman MB. Gonococcus arthritis in infancy. A clinical study of forty-four cases. Am J Dis Child 1927;33:932.
38. Cooperman MB. End results of gonorrheal arthritis. A review of seventy cases. Am J Surg 1928;5:241.
39. Coventry MB, Ghormley RK, Kernohan JW. The intervertebral disc: its microscopic anatomy and pathology. Part I. Anatomy, development and physiology. J Bone Joint Surg 1945;27:105.
40. Coy JTI, Wolf CR, Brower TD, et al. Pyogenic arthritis of the sacro-iliac joint: long-term follow-up. J Bone Joint Surg [Am] 1976;58:845.
41. Craigen MA, Watters J, Hackett JS. The changing epidemiology of osteomyelitis in children. J Bone Joint Surg [Br] 1992;74:541.
42. Cristofaro RL, Appet MH, Gelb RI, et al. Musculoskeletal manifestations of Lyme disease in children. J Pediatr Orthop 1987;7:527.
43. Crock HV, Yoshizawa H. The blood supply of the vertebral column and spinal cord in man. New York: Springer-Verlag, 1977.
44. Curtiss PHJ, Klein L. Destruction of articular cartilage in septic arthritis. I. In vitro studies. J Bone Joint Surg [Am] 1963;45:797.
45. Curtiss PHJ, Klein L. Destruction of articular cartilage in septic arthritis. II. In vivo studies. J Bone Joint Surg [Am] 1965;47:1595.
46. Daniel D, Akeson W, Amiel D, et al. Lavage of septic joints in rabbits: effects of chondrolysis. J Bone Joint Surg [Am] 1976;58:393.
47. Del BMA, Champoux AN, Bockers T, et al. Septic arthritis versus transient synovitis of the hip: the value of screening laboratory tests. Ann Emerg Med 1992;21:1418.
48. DeLuca PA, Gutman LT, Ruderman, RJ. Counterimmunoelectrophoresis of synovial fluid in the diagnosis of septic arthritis. Pediatr Orthop 1985;5:167.
49. Dich VQ, Nelson JD, Haltalin KC. Osteomyelitis in infants and children. Am J Dis Child 1975;129:1273.
50. Dinarello CA, Cannon JG, Mier JW, et al. Multiple biological activities of human recombinant interleukin-1. J Clin Invest 1986;77:1734.
51. Dingle JT. The role of lysosomal enzymes in skeletal tissue. J Bone Joint Surg [Br] 1973;55:87.
52. Donowitz GR, Mandell GL. Beta-lactam antibiotics. N Engl J Med 1988;318:419.
53. Dorr U, Zieger M, Hauke H. Ultrasonography of the painful hip. Prospective studies in 204 patients. Pediatr Radiol 1988;19:36.
54. Ebong WW. Septic arthritis in patients with sickle-cell disease. Br J Rheumatol 1987;26:99.
55. Edwards MS, Baker CJ, Granberry WM, et al. Pelvic osteomyelitis in children. Pediatrics 1978;61:62.
56. Edwards MS, Baker CJ, Wagner ML, et al. An etiologic shift in infantile osteomyelitis: the emergence of the group B *Streptococcus*. J Pediatr 1978;93:578.
57. Eichenfield AH, Goldsmith DP, Benach JL, et al. Childhood Lyme arthritis: experience in an endemic area. J Pediatr 1986;109:753.
58. Eisenberg JM, Kitz DS. Savings from outpatient antibiotic therapy for osteomyelitis. Economic analysis of a theraputic strategy. JAMA 1986;255:1584.
59. Engh CA, Hughes JL, Abrams RC, et al. Osteomyelitis in the patient with sickle-cell disease. J Bone Joint Surg [Am] 1971;53:1.
60. Espersen F, Frimodt MN, Thamdrup RV, et al. Changing pattern of bone and joint infections due to *Staphylococcus aureus*: study of cases of bacteremia in Denmark, 1959–1988. Rev Infect Dis 1991;13:347.
61. Espinoza LR, Spilberg I, Osterland CK. Joint manifestations of sickle-cell disease. Medicine 1974;53:295.

62. Everett ED, Hirschmann JV. Transient bacteremia and endocarditis prophylaxis: a review. Medicine 1977;56:61.
63. Faden H, Grossi M. Acute osteomyelitis in children. Reassessment of etiologic agents and their clinical characteristics. Am J Dis Child 1991;145:65.
64. Farley T, Conway J, Shulman ST. Haematogenous pelvic osteomyelitis in children. Am J Dis Child 1985;139.
65. Farrar WE, O'Dell NM. Comparative β-lactamase resistance and antistaphylococcal activities of parenterally and orally administered cephalosporins. J Infect Dis 1978;137:490.
66. Fink CW, Nelson JD. Septic arthritis and osteomyelitis in children. Clin Rheum Dis 1986;12:423.
67. Fisher MC, Goldsmith JF, Gilligan PH. Sneakers as a source of *Pseudomonas aeruginosa* in children with osteomyelitis following puncture wounds. Pediatrics 1985;106:607.
68. Fitzgerald RH, Cowan JDE. Puncture wounds of the foot. Orthop Clin North Am 1975;6:965.
69. Fox L, Sprunt K. Neonatal osteomyelitis. Pediatrics 1978;62:535.
70. Francis MD, Fogelman I. 99m Tc diphosphonate uptake mechanism on bone. In: Fogelman I, ed. Bone scanning in clinical practice. London: Springer-Verlag, 1987:7.
71. Gamble JG, Rinsky LA. Chronic recurrent multifocal osteomyelitis: a distinct clinical entity. J Pediatr Orthop 1986;6:579.
72. Gamble JG, Rinsky LA. *Kingella kingae* infection in healthy children. J Pediatr Orthop 1988;8:445.
73. Ghormley RK, Bickel WH, Dickson DD. A study of acute infectious lesions of the intervertebral disks. South Med J 1940;33:347.
74. Giedion A, Holthusen W, Masel LF, et al. Subacute and chronic "symmetrical" osteomyelitis. Ann Radiol 1972;15:329.
75. Gillespie WJ. The epidemiology of acute haematogenous osteomyelitis of childhood. Int J Epidemiol 1985;14:600.
76. Gillespie WJ. Epidemiology in bone and joint infection. Infect Dis Clin North Am 1990;4:361.
77. Gillespie WJ, Nade SML. Musculoskeletal infections. Melbourne: Blackwell Scientific Publications, 1987:35.
78. Gilmour WN. Acute hematogenous osteomyelitis. J Bone Joint Surg [Br] 1962;44:842.
79. Ginsburg I, Sela MN. The role of leukocytes and their hydrolases in the persistence, degradation, and transport of bacterial constituents in tissues: relation to chronic inflammatory processes in staphylococcal, streptococcal, and mycobacterial infections and in chronic peridontal disease. Crit Rev Microbiol 1976;249.
80. Ginsburg J, Goultchin A, Stabholtz N, et al. Streptococcal and staphylococcal arthritis. Agents Actions 1980;7:260.
81. Gledhill RB. Subacute osteomyelitis in children. Clin Orthop 1973;96:57.
82. Goldstein WM, Gleason TF, Barmada R. A comparison between arthrotomy and irrigation and multiple aspirations in the treatment of pyogenic arthritis. Orthopedics 1983;6:1309.
83. Gotoff SP. Neonatal immunity. J Pediatrics 1974;85:149.
84. Green NE, Beauchamp RD, Griffin PP. Primary subacute epiphyseal osteomyelitis. J Bone Joint Surg [Am] 1981;63:107.
85. Green NE, Edwards K. Bone and joint infections in children. Orthop Clin North Am 1987;18:555.
86. Greene WB, McMillan CW. *Salmonella* osteomyelitis and hand-foot syndrome in a child with sickle cell anemia. J Pediatr Orthop 1987;7:716.
87. Griebel M, Nahlen B, Jacobs RF, et al. Group A streptococcal postvaricella osteomyelitis. J Pediat Orthop 1985;5:101.
88. Hann IM, Gupta S, Palmer MK, et al. The prognostic significance of radiological and symptomatic bone involvement in childhood acute lymphoblastic leukaemia. Med Pediatr Oncol 1979;6:51.
89. Hardy JB, Hartmenn JR. Tuberculous dactylitis in childhood. J Pediatr 1947;30:146.
90. Harris ED, McCroskery PA. The influence of temperature and fibril stability on degradation of cartilage collagen by rheumatoid synovial collagenase. N Engl J Med 1974;290:1.
91. Harris EDJ, Parker HG, Radin EL, et al. Effects of proteolytic enzymes on structural and mechanical properties of cartilage. Arthritis Rheum 1972;15:497.
92. Harris NG, Kirkaldy-Willis WH. Primary subacute pyogenic osteomyelitis. J Bone Joint Surg [Br] 1965;47:526.
93. Hassler O. The human intervertebral disc: a microangiographical study on its vascular supply at various ages. Acta Orthop Scand 1969;40:765.
94. Henderson RC, Rosenstein BD. *Salmonella* septic and aseptic arthritis in sickle-cell disease. A case report. Clin Orthop 1989.
95. Hendrix RW, Lin P-J, Kane WJ. Simplified aspiration or injection technique for the sacro-iliac joint. J Bone Joint Surg [Am] 1982;64:1249.
96. Hernandez RJ, Conway JJ, Poznanski AK, et al. The role of computed tomography and radionuclide scintigraphy in the localizaion of osteomyelitis in flat bones. J Pediatr Orthop 1985;5:151.
97. Hobo T. Zur pathogenese de akuten haematogenen osteomyelitis, mit berucksichtigungder vitalfarbungs leher. Acta Scolar Med Kioto 1921;4:1.
98. Holmes K, Counts G, Beaty H. Disseminated gonococcal infection. Ann Intern Med 1971;74:979.
99. Howard CB, Einhorn M, Dagan R, et al. Ultrasound in diagnosis and management of acute haematogenous osteomyelitis in children. J Bone Joint Surg [Br] 1993;75:79.
100. Howie DW, Savage JP, Wilson TG, et al. The technetium phosphate bone scan in the diagnosis of osteomyelitis in childhood. J Bone Joint Surg [Am] 1983;65:431.
101. Ish-Horowicz MR, McIntyre P, Nade S. Bone and joint infections caused by multiply resistant *Staphylococcus aureus* in a neonatal intensive care unit. Pediatr Infect Dis J 1992;11:82.
102. Jackson MA, Nelson JD. Etiology and medical management of acute suppurative bone and joint infections in pediatric patients. J Pediatr Orthop 1982;2:313.
103. Jacobs RF, Adelman L, Sack CM, et al. Management of *Pseudomonas* osteochondritis complicating puncture wounds of the foot. Pediatrics 1982;69:432.
104. Jacobs RF, McCarthy RE, Elser JM. *Pseudomonas* osteochondritis complicating puncture wounds of the foot in children: a 10-year evaluation. J Infect Dis 1989;160:657.
105. Jarvis J, McIntyre W, Udjus K, et al. Osteomyelitis of the ischiopubic synchondrosis. J Pediatr Orthop 1985;5:163.
106. Jereb JA, Cauthen GM, Kelly GD, et al. The epidemiology of tuberculosis. In: Friedman LN, ed. Tuberculosis: current concepts and treatment. Boca Raton: CRC Press, 1994:17.
107. Johanson PH. *Pseudomonas* infections of the foot following puncture wounds. JAMA 1968;204:170.
108. Johnson AH, Campbell WG, Callahan BC. Infection of rabbit knee joints after intra-articular injection of *Staphylococcus aureus*. Am J Pathol 1970;60:165.
109. Jones NS, Anderson DJ, Stiles PJ. Osteomyelitis in a general hospital. A five-year study showing an increase in subacute osteomyelitis. J Bone Joint Surg [Br] 1987;69:779.
110. Jurik AG, Helmig O, Ternowitz T, et al. Chronic recurrent multifocal osteomyelitis: a follow-up study. J Pediatr Orthop 1988;8:49.
111. Jurik AG, Moller BN. Chronic sclerosing osteomyelitis of the clavicle: a manifestation of chronic recurrent multifocal osteomyelitis. Arch Orthop Trauma Surg 1987;106:144.
112. Kawai K, Doita M, Tateishi H, et al. Bone and joint lesions associated with pustulosis palmaris et plantaris: a clinical and histological study. J Bone Joint Surg [Br] 1988;70:117.

113. Keely K, Buchanan GR. Acute infarction of long bones in children with sickle cell anemia. J Pediatr 1982;101:170.
114. Kemp HBS, Lloyd-Roberts GC. Avascular necrosis of the capital epiphysis following osteomyelitis of the proximal femoral metaphysis. J Bone Joint Surg [Br] 1974;56:688.
115. Kim HC, Alavi A, Russell MO, et al. Differentiation of bone and bone marrow infarcts from osteomyelitis in sickle cell disorders. Clin Nucl Med 1989;14:249.
116. King DM, Mayo KM. Subacute haematogenous osteomyelitis. J Bone Joint Surg [Br] 1969;51:458.
117. Kloiber R, Udjus K, McIntyre W, et al. The scintigraphic and radiographic appearance of the ischiopubic synchondroses in normal children and in osteomyelitis. Pediatr Radiol 1988;18:57.
118. Knudsen CJM, Hoffman EB. Neonatal osteomyelitis. J Bone Joint Surg [Br] 1990;72:846.
119. Koch R. Die aetiologie der tuberkulose. Berl Klin Wochenschr 1882;19:779.
120. Kohler RB, Wheat LJ. Rapid diagnosis by the detection of microbial antigens. Med Microbiol 1982;1:327.
121. Kolyvas E, Shronheim G, Marks MI, et al. Oral antibiotic therapy of skeletal infections in children. Pediatrics 1980;65:867.
122. Kuo KN, LLoyd-Rogerts GC, Orme IM, et al. Immunodeficiency and infantile bone and joint infection. Arch Dis Child 1975;50:51.
123. Lacour M, Duarte M, Beutler A, et al. Osteoarticular infections due to Kingella kingae in children. Eur J Pediatr 1991;150:612.
124. LaMont RL, Anderson PA, Dajani AS, et al. Acute hematogenous osteomyelitis in children. J Pediatr Orthop 1987;7:579.
125. Landesman SH, Rao SP, Ahonkhai VI. Infections in children with sickle cell anemia. Am J Pediatr Hematol Oncol 1982;4:407.
126. Letts RM, Wong E. Treatment of acute osteomyelitis in children by closed-tube irrigation: a reassessment. Can J Surg 1975;18:60.
127. Lifeso RM, Weaver P, Harder EH. Tuberculous spondylitis in adults. J Bone Joint Surg [Am] 1985;67:1405.
128. Lim MO, Gresham EL, Franken EAJ, et al. Osteomyelitis as a complication of umbilical artery catheterization. Am J Dis Child 1977;131:142.
129. Lindenbaum S, Alexander H. Infections simulating bone tumors. Clin Orthop 1984;184:193.
130. MacLowry JD. Perspective: The serum dilution test. J Infect Dis 1989;160:624.
131. Malech HL, Gallin JI. Neutrophils in human disease. N Engl J Med 1987;317:687.
132. Mallouh A, Talab Y. Bone and joint infection in patients with sickle cell disease. J Pediatr Orthoop 1985;5:158.
133. Manche E, Rombouts GV, Rombouts JJ. Acute hematogenous osteomyelitis due to ordinary germs in children with closed injuries. Study of a series of 44 cases. Acta Orthop Belg 1991;57:91.
134. Manson D, Wilmot DM, King S, et al. Physeal involvement in chronic recurrent multifocal osteomyelitis. Pediatr Radiol 1989;20:76.
135. Martini M, Adjrad A, Boudjemaa A. Tuberculous osteomyelitis. A review of 125 cases. Int Orthop 1986;10:201.
136. Maurer AH, Chen DCP, Camargo EE, et al. Utility of three-phase skeletal scintigraphy in suspected osteomyelitis: concise communication. J Nucl Med 1981;22:941.
137. McCormack LJ, Dockerty MB, Ghormley RK. Ewing's sarcoma. Cancer 1952;5.
138. McCoy JR, Morrissy RT, Seibert J. Clinical experience with the technetium-99 scan in children. Clin Orthop 1981;154:175.
139. Medical Reaearch Council Working Party on Tuberculosis of the Spine. Five-year assessment of controlled trials of ambulatory treatment, debridement and anterior spinal fusion in the management of tuberculosis of the spine; studies in Bulawayo (Rhodesia) and in Hong Kong. J Bone Joint Surg [Br] 1978;60:163.
140. Medical Reaearch Council Working Party on Tuberculosis of the Spine. Five-year assessment of controlled trials of inpatient and outpatient treatment and of plaster-of-paris jackets for tuberculosis of the spine in children on standard chemotherapy. Studies in Masan and Pusan, Korea. J Bone Joint Surg [Br] 1976;58:399.
141. Memon IA, Norman MB, Jacobs NM, et al. Group B streptococcal osteomyelitis and septic arthritis. Am J Dis Child 1979;133:921.
142. Menelaus MB. Discitis: An inflammation affecting the intervertebral disc in children. J Bone Joint Surg [Br] 1964;46:16.
143. Merritt K, Boyle WE, Dye SK, et al. Counter immunoelectrophoresis in the diagnosis of septic arthritis caused by Haemophilus influenzae. J Bone Joint Surg [Am] 1976;58:414.
144. Miller JH, Gates GF. Scintigraphy of sacroiliac pyarthrosis in children. JAMA 1977;238:2701.
145. Miskew DB, Block RA, Witt PF. Aspiration of infected sacroiliac joints. J Bone Joint Surg [Am] 1979;61:1071.
146. Molan RAB, Piggot J. Acute osteomyelitis in children. J Bone Joint Surg [Br] 1977;59.
147. Monk PM, Reilly BJ, Ash JM. Osteomyelitis in the neonate. Radiology 1982;145:677.
148. Morey BF, Bianco AJ Jr, Rhodes KH. Septic arthritis in children. Orthop Clin North Am 1975;6:923.
149. Morey BF, Peterson HA. Hematogenous pyogenic osteomyelitis in children. Orthop Clin North Am 1975;6:935.
150. Morgan A, Yates A. The diagnosis of acute osteomyelitis of the pelvis. Postgrad Med J 1966;42:74.
151. Morgan JG, Schlegelmilch JG, Spiegel PK. Early diagnosis of septic arthritis of the sacroiliac joint by use of computed tomography. J Rheumatol 1981;8:879.
152. Morrissy RT, Haynes DW. Acute hematogenous osteomyelitis: a model with trauma as an etiology. J Pediatr Orthop 1989;9:447.
153. Nelson JD, Bucholz RW, Kusmiesz H, et al. Benefits and risks of sequential parenteral-oral cephalosporin therapy for suppurative bone and joint infections. J Pediatr Orthop 1982;2:255.
154. Nelson JD, Howard JB, Shelton S. Oral antibiotic therapy for skeletal infection of children: I. Antibiotic concentration in suppurative synovial joint. J Pediatr 1978;92:131.
155. Noonan WJ. Salmonella osteomyelitis presenting as "hand-foot syndrome" in sickle-cell disease. Br Med J 1982;284:1464.
156. Norden CW. Experimental osteomyelitis. I. A description of the model. J Infect Dis 1970;122:410.
157. Ogden JA. Pediatric osteomyelitis and septic arthritis: the pathology of neonatal disease. Yale J Biol Med 1979;52:423.
158. Olney BW, Papasian CJ, Jacobs RR. Risk of iatrogenic septic arthritis in the presence of bacteremia: a rabbit study. J Pediatr Orthop 1987;7:524.
159. Oronsky A, Ignarro L, Perrer R. Release of cartilage mucopolysaccharide-degrading neutral protease from human leukocytes. J Exp Med 1973;138:461.
160. Orozoco-Alcala J, Baum J. Arthritis during sickle cell crisis. N Engl J Med 1973;288:420.
160a. Pasteur L. De l'extension de la theorie des germes a l'etiologie de quelques maladies communes. Bull Acad Med 1880;9:435.
161. Patterson DC. Acute suppurative arthritis in infancy and childhood. J Bone Joint Surg [Br] 1970;52:474.
162. Pediatrics AAo. Tuberculosis. In: Peter G, ed. 1994 Red book: Report of the Committee on Infectious Diseases, 23rd ed. Elk Grove Village, IL: American Academy of Pediatrics, 1994:488.

163. Peltola H, Vahvanen V. A comparative study of osteomyelitis and purulent arthritis with special reference to aetiology and recovery. Infection 1984;12:75.
164. Pepys MB. C-reactive protein fifty years on. Lancet 1981;1:653.
165. Petola H, Vahvanen V. 1. A comparative study of osteomyelitis and purulent arthritis with special reference to aetiology and recovery. Infection 1984;12:75.
166. Petola H, Vahvanen V, Aalto K. Fever, C-reactive protein, and erythrocyte sedimentation rate in monitoring recovery from septic arthritis: a preliminary study. J Pediatr Orthop 1984;4:170.
167. Phemister DB, Hatcher CH. Correlation of pathological and roentgenological findings in the diagnosis of tuberculous arthritis. AJR 1933;29:736.
168. Rajasekaran S, Soundarapandian S. Progression of kyphosis in tuberculosis of the spine treated by anterior arthrodesis. J Bone Joint Surg [Am] 1989;71:1314.
169. Rao S, Solomon N, Miller S, et al. Scintigraphic differentiation of bone infarction from osteomyelitis in children with sickle cell disease. Pediatrics 1985;107:685.
170. Reichl M. Septic arthritis following puncture wound of the foot. Arch Emerg Med 1989;6:277.
171. Reilly JP, Gross RH, Emans JB, et al. Disorders of the sacroiliac joint in children. J Bone Joint Surg [Am] 1988;70:31.
172. Rimsza M, Niggemann E. Medical evaluation of sexually abused children: a review of 311 cases. Pediatrics 1982;69:8.
173. Roberts JM, Drummond DS, Breed AL, et al. Subacute hematogenous osteomyelitis in children: a retrospective study. J Pediatr Orthop 1982;2:249.
174. Rocco HD, Erying EJ. Intervertebral disk infections in children. Am J Dis Child 1972;123:448.
175. Rodet A. Etude experimental aur l'osteomyelite infectieuse. In: Bick EM, ed. Classics of orthopaedics. Philadelphia: JB Lippincott, 1976:461.
176. Rogalsky RJ, Black GB, Reed MH. Orthopaedic manifestations of leukemia in children. J Bone Joint Surg [Am] 1986;68:494.
177. Rose CD, Fawcett PT, Eppes SC, et al. Pediatric Lyme arthritis: clinical spectrum and outcome. J Pediatr Orthop 1994;14:238.
178. Ross ERS, Cole WG. Treatment of subacute osteomyelitis in childhood. J Bone Joint Surg [Br] 1985;67:443.
179. Rotbart HA, Glode MP. *Haemophilus influenzae* type B septic arthritis in children: report of 23 cases. Pediatrics 1985;75:254.
180. Royle SG. Investigation of the irritable hip. J Pediatr Orthop 1992;12:396.
181. Sabath LD, Garner C, Wilcox C, et al. Effect of inoculum and of beta-lactamase on the anti-staphylococcal activity of thirteen penicillins and cephalosporins. Antimicrob Agents Chemother 1975;8:344.
182. Sadat-Ali Sankaran-Kutty K. Recent observations on osteomyelitis in sickle-cell disease. Int Orthop 1985;9:97.
183. Sankaran KM, Sadat AM, Kutty MK. Septic arthritis in sickle cell disease. Int Orthop 1988;12:255.
184. Schaad UB, McCracken GH, Nelson JD. Pyogenic arthritis of the sacroiliac joint in pediatric patients. Pediatrics 1980;66:375.
185. Schenk RK, Wiener J, Spiro D. Fine structural aspects of vascular invasion of the tibial epiphyseal plate of growing rats. Acta Anat 1968;69.
186. Schurman DJ, Mirra J, Ding A, et al. Experimental *E. coli* arthritis in the rabbit: a model of infectious and post-infectious inflammatory synovitis. J Rheumatol 1977;4:118.
187. Scott RJ, Christofersen MR, Robertson WWJ, et al. Acute osteomyelitis in children: a review of 116 cases. J Pediatr Orthop 1990;10:649.
188. Shandling B. Acute hematogenous osteomyelitis: a review of 300 cases treated during 1953–1959. South Afr Med 1960;34:520.
189. Shannon BF, Moore M, Houkom JA, et al. Multifocal cystic tuberculosis of bone. J Bone Joint Surg [Am] 1990;72:1089.
190. Shaw BA, Kasser JR. Acute septic arthritis in infancy and childhood. Clin Orthop 1990;257:212.
191. Shmerling RH, Delbanco TL, Tosteson AN, et al. Synovial fluid tests. What should be ordered? JAMA 1990;264:1009.
192. Skyhar MJ, Mubarak SJ. Arthroscopic treatment of septic knees in children. J Pediatr Orthop 1987;7:647.
193. Smith AIDF. A benign form of osteomyelitis of the spine. JAMA 1933;101:335.
194. Smith BR, Rolston KV, LeFrock JL, et al. Bone penetration of antibiotics. Orthopedics 1983;6:187.
195. Smith L, Schurman dJ, Kajiyama G, et al. The effect of antibiotics on the destruction of cartilage in experimental infectious arthritis. J Bone Joint Surg [Am] 1987;69:1063.
195a. Smith MHD, Stack JR, Marquis JR. Tuberculosis and opportunistic mycobacterial infections. In: Fegin RO, Cherry JD. Pediatric infectious diseases, 3rd ed. Philadelphia: WB Saunders, 1992:1327.
196. Society AT. Treatment of tuberculosis infection in adults and children. Am J Respir Crit Care Med 1994;149:1359.
197. Sorensen TS, Hedeboe J, Christensen ER. Primary epiphyseal osteomyelitis in children. Report of three cases and review of the literature. J Bone Joint Surg [Br] 1988;70:818.
198. Spach DH, Liles WC, Campbell GL, et al. Tick-born disease in the United States. N Engl J Med 1993;329:936.
199. Specht EE. Hemoglobinopathic *Salmonella* osteomyelitis. Clin Orthop 1971;79:110.
200. Speers DJ, Nade SML. Ultrastructural studies of *Staphylococcus aureus* in experimental acute haematogenous osteomyelitis. Infect Immun 1985;49:443.
201. Spiegel PG, Kengla KW, Isaacson AS, et al. Intervertebral discspace inflammation in children. J Bone Joint Surg [Am] 1972;54:284.
202. Spink WW, Keefer CS. Gonococcic arthritis: pathogenesis, mechanism of recovery and treatment. JAMA 1938;109:1448.
203. Stanitski CL, Harvell JC, Fu FH. Arthroscopy in acute septic knees. Management in pediatric patients. Clin Orthop 1989.
204. Steere AC. Lyme disease. N Engl J Med 1989;321:586.
205. Steere AC, Broderick TF, Malawista SE. Erythema chronicum migrans and Lyme arthritis: epidemiologic evidence for a tick vector. Am J Epidemiol 1978;108:312.
206. Steere AC, Malawista SE, Snydman DR. Lyme arthritis: an epidemic of oligoarticular arthritis in children and adults in three Connecticut communities. Arthritis Rheum 1977;20:7.
207. Steere AC, Taylor E, McHugh GL, et al. The overdiagnosis of Lyme disease. JAMA 1993;269:1812.
208. Stein RE, Urbaniak J. Use of the tourniquet during surgery in patients with sickle cell hemoglobinopathies. Clin Orthop 1980;151:231.
209. Steinberg JJ, Sledge CB. Co-cultivation models of joint destruction. In: Dingle JT, Gordon JL, ed. Cellular interactions. Amsterdam: Elsevier/North-Holland Biomedical Press, 1981:263.
210. Straton CW. Serum bactericidal test. Clin Microbiol Rev 1988;1:19.
211. Sullivan DC, Rosenfield NS, Ogden J, et al. Problems in the scintigraphic detection of osteomyelitis in children. Radiology 1980;135:731.
212. Sullivan JA, Vasileff T, Leonard JC. An evaluation of nuclear scanning in orthopaedic infections. J Pediatr Orthop 1980;1:73.
213. Sundberg SB, Savage JP, Foster BK. Technetium phosphate bone scan in the diagnosis of septic arthritis of childhood. J Pediatr Orthop 1989;9:579.
214. Swaak AJG, Van Soesbergen RM, Van Der Korst JK. Arthritis

215. Syrogiannopoulos GA, McCracken GHJ, Nelson JD. Osteoarticular infections in children with sickle cell disease. Pediatrics 1986;78:1090.
216. Tang JS, Gold RH, Bassett LW, et al. Musculoskeletal infection of the extremities: evaluation with MR imaging. Radiology 1988.
217. Tetzlaff TR, Howard JB, McCracken GH, et al. Antibiotic concentrations in pus and bone of children with osteomyelitis. J Pediatr 1978;92:135.
218. Tiku K, Tiku ML, Skosey JL. Interleukin-1 production by human polymorphonuclear neutrophils. J Immunol 1986;136:3677.
219. Tindall EA, Regan-Smith MG. Gonococcal osteomyelitis complicating septic arthritis. JAMA 1983;250:2671.
220. Trackler RT, Miller KE, Sutherland DH, et al. Childhood pelvic osteomyelitis presenting as a "cold" lesion on bone scan: case report. J Nucl Med 1976;17:620.
221. Trueta J. The normal vascular anatomy of the human femoral head during growth. J Bone Joint Surg [Br] 1957;39:358.
222. Trueta J. The three types of acute haematogenous osteomyelitis. A clinical and vascular study. J Bone Joint Surg [Br] 1959;41:671.
223. Unkila-Kallio L, Kallio MJT, Eskola J, et al. Serum C-reactive protein, erythrocyte sedimentation rate, and white blood cell count in acute hematogenous osteomyelitis of children. Pediatrics 1994;93:59.
224. Vaughan PA, Newman NM, Rosman MA. Acute hematogenous osteomyelitis in children. J Pediatr Orthop 1987;7:652.
225. Versfeld GA, Solomon A. A diagnostic approach to tuberculosis of bones and joints. J Bone Joint Surg [Br] 1982;64:446.
226. Volberg FM, Summer TE, Abramson JS, et al. Unreliability of radiographic diagnosis of septic hip in children. Pediatrics 1984;74:118.
227. Waldvogle FA, Medoff G, Swartz MN. Osteomyelitis: a review of clinical features, therapeutic considerations and unusual aspects. N Engl J Med 1970;282:198.
228. Watson RJ, Burko H, Megas H, et al. The hand-foot syndrome in sickle cell disease in young children. Pediatrics 1963;31:975.
229. Weaver JB, Tyler MW. Experimental staphylococcaemia and hematogenous osteomyelitis. J Bone Joint Surg 1943;25:791.
230. Wehrbein HL. Gonococcus arthritis—a study of six hundred cases. Surg Gynecol Obstet 1929;49:105 associated with *Salmonella* infection. Clin Rheumatol 1982;4:275.
231. Weinstein MP, Stratton CW, Hawley HB, et al. Multicenter collaborative evaluation of a standardized serum bactericidal test as a predictor of therapeutic efficacy in acute and chronic osteomyelitis. Am J Med 1987;83:218.
232. Weissberg ED, Smith AL, Smith DH. Clinical features of neonatal osteomyelitis. Pediatrics 1974;53:505.
233. Wenger DR, Bobechko WP, Gilday DL. The spectrum of intervertebral disc-space infection in children. J Bone Joint Surg [Am] 1978;60:100.
234. Whalen JL, Fitzgerald RHJ, Morrissy RT. A histological study of acute hematogenous osteomyelitis following physeal injuries in rabbits. J Bone Joint Surg [Am] 1988;70:1383.
235. White ST, Loda FA, Ingram DL. Sexually transmitted diseases in sexually abused children. Pediatrics 1983;72:16.
236. Wiley AM, Trueta J. The vascular anatomy of the spine and its relationship to pyogenic vertebral osteomyelitis. J Bone Joint Surg [Br] 1959;41:796.
237. Wilson NIL, DiPaola M. Acute septic arthritis in infancy and childhood. J Bone Joint Surg [Br] 1986;68:584.
238. Winters JL, Cahen I. Acute hematogenous osteomyelitis. J Bone Joint Surg [Am] 1960;42:691.
239. Wise CM, Morris CR, Wasilauskas BI, et al. Gonococcal arthritis in an era of increasing penicillin resistance. Presentations and outcomes in 41 recent cases (1985–1991). Arch Intern Med 1994;154:2690.
240. Wolfson JS, Swartz MN. Serum bactericidal activity as a monitor of antibiotic therapy. N Engl J Med 1985;312:968.
241. Worrel VT, Burera V. Sickle-cell dactylitis. J Bone Joint Surg [Am] 1976;58:1161.
242. Yagupsky P, Dagan R, Howard CB, et al. Clinical features and epidemiology of invasive *Kingella kingae* infections in southern Israel. Pediatrics 1993;92:800.
243. Yagupsky P, Dagan R, Howard CW, et al. High prevalence of *Kingella kingae* in joint fluid from children with septic arthritis revealed by the BACTEC blood culture system. J Clin Microbiol 1992;30:1278.
244. Yousefzadeh DK, Jackson JH. Neonatal and infantile candidal arthritis with or without osteomyelitis: a clinical and radiographical review of 21 cases. Skeletal Radiol 1980;5:77.
245. Zawin JK, Hoffer FA, Rand FF, et al. Joint effusion in children with an irritable hip: US diagnosis and aspiration. Radiology 1993;187:459.
246. Zieger MM, Dorr U, Schulz RD. Ultrasonography of hip joint effusions. Skeletal Radiol 1987;16:607.

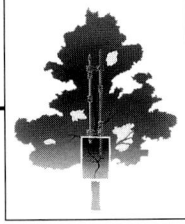

Index

Page numbers followed by f indicate illustrations; those followed by t indicate tabular materials.

A

Abduction, 1078t
Abduction contracture
  assessment of, 77f
  of hip, spastic quadriplegia and, 482
Abduction orthosis, Legg-Calve-Perthes syndrome and, 980f
Absent tibial syndromes, 123
Accessory navicular, 1099–1101, 1100f
Acetabular cartilage, hypertrophied, 907, 908f
Acetabular cartilage complex, 904–905, 905f
Acetabulum, 906f
  coronal section through, 905f
  determinants of shape and depth, 906–907
  dysplasia of
    treatment of, 931
    treatment of hip dysplasia and, 931–937, 933–937f
  fracture of, 1270–1271, 1272f
  growth and development of, 904–905
  hypertrophic labrum in, 914f
Acheiria, 1137
Achilles tendinitis, 1191–1192
Achondroplasia, 122, 205–213, 206–209f, 211f
  autosomal dominance and, 125–126
  bowlegs and, 1059, 1059t
  clinical features of, 205–206
  growth and development and, 206
  kyphotic deformity and, 705, 707f
  medical considerations in, 207–209
  orthopaedic implications in, 209–213
  point mutations and, 119
  radiographic features of, 206–207
Acidosis, renal tubular, vitamin D-resistant rickets and, 152–153
Acquired amputation, 1158–1164
Acquired coxa vara, 1024, 1025f
Acquired immunodeficiency syndrome (AIDS), 132, 357–358
Acrocephalosyndactyly, 123, 806f
Acromioclavicular separation, 1237–1238
Actin, 4
Actinomycin D, musculoskeletal tumors and, 463
Acute hematogenous osteomyelitis (AHO), 580
Adactylia, 1137
Adamintonoma, osteofibrous dysplasia and, 447–448
Adduction, 1078t
Adduction contracture, of hip, spastic diplegia and, 492
Adenoidectomy, Grisel syndrome and, 751

ADI. *See* Atlantodens interval
Adolescent bunion, 1116–1119, 1117–1118f
Adolescent idiopathic scoliosis, 638–639, 644–667
  progression of, 644–645, 644t
    curve magnitude/Risser sign and, 646t
  spondylolysis/spondylolisthesis and, 720
Adolescent tibia vara, 1055
Adriamycin. *See also* Doxorubicin
  Langerhans cell histiocytosis and, 368
AER. *See* Apical ectodermal ridge
Agammaglobulinemia, X-linked, 356–357
Aglucerase, Gaucher disease and, 362
AHO. *See* Acute hematogenous osteomyelitis
AIDS. *See* Acquired immunodeficiency syndrome
Ainhum, 317
Albers-Schonberg disease, 172
Albright syndrome, 190, 446
Alcohol, teratogenicity and, 132, 275
Allergy, transient synovitis of hip and, 1033
Aluminum, phosphate absorption and, 145
Alveolar rhabdomyosarcoma, 458
Amelia, 1137
Amino acids, DNA triplets encoding for, 3f
Amniocentesis, prenatal diagnosis and, 134
Amniotic bands, prenatal amputations and, 1138–1139, 1139f
Amniotic band syndrome, 1139f
Amoxicillin, bone and joint infection and, 597t
Ampicillin, bone and joint infection and, 597t
Amputation
  above-knee, 1162
    prosthesis for, 1168–1170
  acquired, 1158–1164
  below-knee, 1162–1164, 1163f
    prosthesis for, 1172–1173
  complete tibial hemimelia and, 1156–1157
  congenital, 784–785, 785f
    multiple, 1164–1166, 1165f
  fibular deficiency and, 1154f
  Klippel-Trenaunay syndrome and, 307
  macrodactyly and, 315
  osteosarcoma and, 438
  phantom pain and, 1161
  prostheses for, 1160f

  proximal focal femoral deficiency and, 1146–1147, 1146f, 1171
  purpura fulminans and, 1159–1160, 1161f
  upper extremity, 1164
Ancef. *See* Cefazolin
Anderson lengthening device, 881f
Androgens, bone formation and, 140
Anemia
  Diamond-Blackfan, 346–347
  Fanconi, 347
    radial deficiencies and, 789
  iron deficiency, 345–346
  sickle cell, 347–353, 348f, 350f, 352f
    osteomyelitis and, 349–350, 349f
  thalassemia and, 353
Aneurysmal bone cysts, 450–451, 450–451f
  cervical spine and, 773
Angelman syndrome, 285
  genomic imprinting in, 130
Angiography, 31
  bone and soft tissue tumors and, 428
Angular deformity, 891–896
  Blount disease and, 895f
  hypophosphatemic rickets and, 894f, 896f
Ankle
  anterolateral impingement on, 1201
  epiphyseal injuries and, 1301–1302
  excessive dorsiflexion of, gait and, 108
  excessive plantar flexion of, gait and, 108
  fractures of, 1300–1303
    pronation and external rotation, 1300–1301, 1302f
    supination-inversion, 1300, 1301f
    transitional, 1302–1303, 1304f
  juvenile rheumatoid arthritis and, 417
  normal motion, moments, and powers of, 102f
  pediatric orthopaedic examination and, 84–89
  plantar-flexion injuries and, 1301
  poliomyelitis and, 568
  sprains of, 1199–1201
  stance phase of gait and, 100–103
  swing phase of gait and, 103
Ankle drawer test, 1200f
Ankle equinovalgus, spastic diplegia and, 490–491
Ankle equinovarus, spastic diplegia and, 489–490
Ankle equinus, spastic diplegia and, 488–489
Ankle reflex, testing, 57
Ankle synovectomy, hemophilia and, 377
Ankylosing spondylitis, 397–398

1

Anlage, ulnar deficiency and, 799
Anterior cruciate ligament injuries, 1203–1204
Anterior fusion, spondylolisthesis and, 730
Anterior talofibular ligament, evaluating stability of, 1200f
Antibiotics
  bone and joint infection and, 596–599, 597t
  chronic granulomatous disease and, 356
Anticipation, 122
Anticonvulsant medication, rickets and, 153–154
Antiinflammatory drugs, sports medicine and, 1184–1185
Antinuclear antibody (ANA) test, juvenile rheumatoid arthritis and, 394
Anus, imperforate, 7
Apert hand, 806f
Apert syndrome, cervical spine anomalies and, 761
Apical ectodermal ridge (AER), 14–15
Apodia, 1137
Apophyseal conditions, young athlete and, 1188–1191
Apophysitis, young athlete and, 1191
Apoptosis, 15
Arachnodactyly, 180f
  Marfan syndrome and, 179
Arnold-Chiari malformation, 505, 505f, 746f
  cervical spine and, 754
  gait assessment analysis in, 506f
  myelomeningocele and, 508
Arthralgia, childhood, differential diagnosis of, 401–404, 402t
Arthritis
  childhood, management of, 407–409
  Down syndrome and, 274
  gonococcal, 615–616
  idiopathic chondrolysis of hip and, 1038
  inflammatory, chronic in childhood, 395t
  juvenile, periosteal reaction and, 174t
  Lyme, 615
  psoriatic, 398
  Reiter syndrome and, 398
  rheumatoid. See Juvenile rheumatoid arthritis
  septic
    definition of, 579–580
    diagnosis of, 586–594
    differential diagnosis of, 402, 595–596
    epidemiology of, 580
    etiology of, 580–581
    imaging of, 37f
    pathophysiology of, 586
    synovial fluid analysis in, 588t
    treatment of, 596–601
  sickle cell disease and, 350–351
  X-linked agammaglobulinemia and, 356–357
Arthrocentesis, juvenile rheumatoid arthritis and, 406–407
Arthrochalasis multiplex congenita, 181
Arthrodesis
  hereditary motor sensory neuropathies and, 563–564
  juvenile rheumatoid arthritis and, 412–413
  poliomyelitis and, 567
  proximal focal femoral deficiency and, 1146–1147, 1146f
  slipped capital femoral epiphysis and, 1015–1016, 1016f
  spondylolisthesis and, 726
  spondylolysis and, 724–725, 726f
  subtalar, 490, 490f
Arthrography, 31–32
  idiopathic chondrolysis of hip and, 1039, 1040
Arthrogryposis, 19, 262–271, 808–810, 809–810f
  clubfoot and, 1103
  distal, 267–268, 268f
  hip dislocations in newborns and, 911
Arthrogryposis multiplex congenita, 262–265, 263f, 808
  at birth, 264f
  manifestations and diagnosis of, 262–264
  treatment of, 264–265
Arthroophthalmopathy, progressive, hereditary, 287
Arthropathy
  Charcot, 531f
    myelomeningocele and, 531–532
  hemophilic, 372–376
    of knee, 375f
    radiographic grading of, 375t
Arthroplasty
  Legg-Calve-Perthes syndrome and, 982
  slipped capital femoral epiphysis and, 1016–1017
  total joint, juvenile rheumatoid arthritis and, 67f
Arthrotomography, 32f
Articular cartilage, 138–139, 905
  osteochondritis dissecans and, 1065–1067, 1066f
Aspiration, bone and joint infection and, 593–594
Aspirin
  juvenile rheumatoid arthritis and, 408t
  transient synovitis of hip and, 1037
  young athlete and, 1185
Ataxia, Friedreich, 558–561
Ataxia-telangiectasia, 308
Ataxic cerebral palsy, 471
Athetoid cerebral palsy, 470–471
  management of, 494
Athletic trainers, sports trauma and, 1199
Atlantoaxial instability, Down syndrome and, 756–757
Atlantoaxial ligament, transverse, ruptures of, 765
Atlantoaxial rotary displacement, 748–751, 749–751f
Atlantodens interval (ADI), 741–742
Atlantooccipital anomalies, 745–747
Atlantooccipital dislocation, 764
  BC/OA ration and DB distance and, 765f
Atlantooccipital hypermobility, Down syndrome and, 757
Atlantooccipital instability, measuring, 743f
Atlantooccipital motion, 741–742
Atlas, 740
  formation of, 10
  fractures of, 764–765
Auranofin, juvenile rheumatoid arthritis and, 408
Aurothioglucose, juvenile rheumatoid arthritis and, 408
Autosomal chromosomes, abnormalities of, 121–122
Avascular necrosis, growth of leg and, 861
Axis, 740
  formation of, 10

B

Back pain
  Gaucher disease and, 361–362
  spinal infection and, 601
Baclofen, spastic diplegia and, 483
Barlow maneuver, 911
Basilar impression, 744–745, 745f
Bayne classification system, 788
Becker muscular dystrophy. See Muscular dystrophy, Becker
Beckwith-Wiedemann syndrome, 286–287, 287f, 313
  differential diagnosis of, 311t
  genomic imprinting in, 130
  Klippel-Trenaunay syndrome and, 306
Bed rest, spondylolisthesis and, 730
Behcet syndrome, differential diagnosis of, 404
Benign familial hypermobility, 181
Beryllium, phosphate absorption and, 145
Biceps reflex, testing, 57
Bicortical fracture, 1262f
Bilaminar disc, inner cell mass of, 8f
Biopsy
  bone and soft tissue tumors and, 431–433
  developmental coxa vara and, 1026–1027, 1026f
  Duchenne muscular dystrophy and, 542
  idiopathic chondrolysis of hip and, 1040, 1041f
  juvenile rheumatoid arthritis and, 406–407
  neuromuscular disorders and, 539
Bipartite patella, 1065
Birth injury, cervical spine and, 769
Birth palsy, 828–828, 827f
Blanch sign of Steel, 999
Bleomycin, musculoskeletal tumors and, 462–462
Block test, 87f
Blood donation, acquired immunodeficiency syndrome and, 357
Blount disease, 1055–1057, 1056–1057f
  angular deformity in, 895f
  unilateral, 1058f
Blue rubber bleb nevus syndrome, 307
Body segments, relation of center of gravity to, 61f
Bone
  blood supply to, 22f
  cortical, 582f
  cysts of
    aneurysmal, 450–451, 450–451f, 773
    unicameral, 448–450, 449f
  disorders of, localized, 305–341
  eosinophilic granuloma of, 363–369, 365–369f, 448, 448f
  formation of, 18–24
    growth plate development and, 20–24
    intramembranous, 18
    mechanical loading and, 19–20, 20f
    periosteal, 1231f
    regulation of, 140–141
  growing-remodeling process of, 23f
  growth arrest patterns in, 1234f
  infection of, 579–586
    criteria for oral therapy of, 598t
    diagnosis of, 586–594
    newborn and, 605–607

sickle cell disease and, 607–609
  treatment of, 596–601
 physiology of, 163–164
 trabecular, 584f
  rickets and, 148f
 tuberculosis of, 616–619, 617–618f
 tumors of. See Tumors, bone
Bone densitometry, 30–31
Bone disease, metabolic, 137
Bone-forming tumors, 433–439
Bone graft
 congenital pseudoarthrosis of tibia and, 325f, 325t, 326–328
 fibrous dysplasia and, 190
 giant cell tumor of bone and, 452
Bone infarction, osteomyelitis and, 595
Bone marrow transplantation, sickle cell disease and, 352
Bone peg epiphyseodesis, slipped capital femoral epiphysis and, 1008–1009, 1010f
Bone scan
 bone and joint infection and, 590–592, 592f
 osteochondritis dissecans and, 1066–1067
 spondylolysis/spondylolisthesis and, 722
Boston bracing system, 651
Botryoid rhabdomyosarcoma, 458
Botulinum-A toxin, spastic diplegia and, 485
Bowlegs, 1054–1061
 causes and treatment of, 1055–1060
 genetic disorders and, 1059, 1059f
 physiologic, 1055
 rickets and, 1057–1059
Brachial plexus, obstetric injury to, 826–828
Brachydactyly, 60
Brain, development of, cerebral palsy and, 469–470
Brain stem, Arnold-Chiari type II malformation of, 505, 505f
Breaststroker's knee, 1195
Brown procedure, 1159f
Brown-Sequard syndrome, instrumentation in Down syndrome and, 757
Bunion, 88, 88f
 adolescent, 1116–1119, 1117–1118f
 cerebral palsy and, 488
Burns, periosteal reaction and, 175t
Buschke-Ollendorff syndrome, 320

C
Cafe-au-lait spots, neurofibromatosis and, 256–257, 256f
Caffey disease, 176, 319
 mandible in, 176f
 periosteal reaction and, 175t
 ulna in, 177f
Calcaneal apophysitis, young athlete and, 1191
Calcaneal osteotomy
 hereditary motor sensory neuropathies and, 563
 tarsal coalition and, 1098–1099
Calcaneocavus, 1123–1124, 1124f
Calcaneonavicular osteocartilaginous coalition, 1097f
Calcaneous gait, 108
Calcaneous osteotomy, cavus and, 1122–1123
Calcaneovalgus foot, congenital, 1083–1085, 1084f

Calcaneus
 facets of, 1097f
 deformity of, 529f
  myelomeningocele and, 529–530
 fracture of, 1307, 1308f
Calcification
 ectopic, renal osteodystrophy and, 154
 soft tissue, 178–179
Calcinosis, tumoral, 178
Calcitonin
 hypercalcemia and, 146
 physiology of, 140
Calcitriol, calcium transport and, 142
Calcium
 absorption of, 144–145
 kinetics in hypercalcemic state, 146f
 kinetics in hypocalcemic state, 146f
 kinetics in normocalcemic state, 145f
 transport by gut cell, 142
  parathyroid hormone and, 142f
  vitamin D and, 143f
Calcium deficiency, rickets and, 150
Calcium homeostasis, 141–146
Calorimetry, gait analysis and, 114
Camptodactyly, 811–813, 812f
Capillary hemangioma, 307, 455
Capillary lymphangioma, 309
Capitellum
 osteochondral lesions of, 1195–1197, 1196f
 Panner disease of, 338f
CAPP terminal device, 1175f
Carbohydrate loading, young athlete and, 1182
Carpal deformity, 795
Carpal injury, 839f, 840
Carpal synostosis, 802f
Car seat injury, cervical spine and, 769, 769f
Cartilage, 138–139
 articular, 138–139, 905
  osteochondritis dissecans and, 1065–1067, 1066f
 elastic, 138–139
 humoral factors and, 140
 hyaline, 138–139, 904–905
 triradiate, 904–905, 906f
Cartilage-hair hypoplasia, 357
Cartilaginous tumors, 439–444
Casting
 congenital clubfoot and, 1107
 spastic diplegia and, 485
Castle procedure, 481f
Cauda equina syndrome, postoperative, 735
Cavernous hemangioma, 307, 455
Cavernous lymphangioma, 309
Cavus, 87, 1120–1123, 1121–1123f
 myelomeningocele and, 530–531
Ceclor. See Cefaclor
Cefaclor, bone and joint infection and, 597t
Cefazolin, bone and joint infection and, 596, 597t
Cefotaxime, bone and joint infection and, 597t
Cefprozil, bone and joint infection and, 597t
Ceftazidime, bone and joint infection and, 597t
Ceftriaxone, bone and joint infection and, 597t
Cefuroxime, bone and joint infection and, 596, 597t
Cefzil. See Cefprozil

Cells
 differentiation of, gene-directed protein synthesis and, 2
 pleuripotential, 2
 programmed death of, 15
Center-edge angle, leg-length discrepancy and, 851f
Center of gravity
 normal gait and, 95, 96f
 relation to body segments, 61f
Central core disease, 553
Central deficiency, 797–798, 797f
Central hypoplasia, 797
Centralization, 794f
 congenital radial deficiency and, 792–793
 inadequate, 793f
Central nervous system, cerebral palsy and, 472
Central polydactyly, 819, 819f
Centronuclear myopathy, 553–554
Cephalexin, bone and joint infection and, 596, 597t
Cephalosporin, bone and joint infection and, 596
Cerebral infarction, sickle cell disease and, 352
Cerebral palsy, 469–497
 anatomic patterns in, 471
 ataxic, 471
 athetoid, 470–471
  management of, 494
 brain development and, 469–470
 cervical spine and, 759–760, 759f
 classification of, 470–471
 developmental milestones and, 473t
 diagnosis of, 472–473
 etiology of, 470
 hip management in, 479–482
 hip problems in, 477–479
 hyperkyphosis and, 475–476
 hyperlordosis and, 475
 hypotonic, 471
 instrumented motion analysis and, 94
 in-toeing and, 1049
 management of, 473–494
 mixed, 471
 other systems and, 472
 prevalence of, 470
 Sandifer syndrome and, 754
 scoliosis and, 476–477
 spastic, 470
 stiff knee gait in, 109
 upper extremity involvement in, 494–497
 walking prognosis criteria in, 483t
Ceredase. See Aglucerase
Cervical spine, 739–774
 atlantodens interval in, 741–742
 atlantooccipital anomalies and, 745–747
 atlantooccipital instability in, measuring, 743f
 atlantooccipital motion in, 741–742
 basilar impression and, 744–745, 745f
 battered children and, 769
 birth injury and, 769
 car seat injury and, 769, 769f
 cerebral palsy and, 759–760, 759f
 congenital and developmental problems in, 744–763
  neurogenic types, 754
  nonosseus types, 751–754
  osseus types, 744–751
 congenital muscular torticollis and, 751–754

Cervical spine (continued)
  craniofacial syndromes and, 760–761
  craniosynostosis syndromes and, 761–762
  deformity of, postlaminectomy, 760
  Down syndrome and, 742f, 756–758, 758f
  dysplasia of, familial, 748, 748f
  embryology of, 739–740
  fetal alcohol syndrome and, 760
  fibrodysplasia ossificans progressive and, 763
  growth and development of, 740–741
  gunshot wounds and, 769–770
  inflammation and infection of, 770–773
  intervertebral disc calcification and, 771–772, 771f
  juvenile rheumatoid arthritis and, 770–771, 770f
  Klippel-Feil syndrome and, 755
  lower, normal motion of, 743–744
  neurofibromatosis and, 761f, 762–763
  occipitoatlantal instability in, 758–759
  os odontoideum and, 755–756
  posterior line of Swischuk in, 743f
  pseudosubluxation in, 742–743
  pyogenic osteomyelitis and discitis and, 772
  radiography and, 741–744
  Sandifer syndrome and, 754–755
  transient quadriparesis and, 767–769
  trauma to, 763–770, 768f
    positioning with backboard in, 764f
  tuberculosis and, 772–773
  tumors of, 773–774
    benign, 773–774
    malignant, 774
  unilateral absence of C1 in, 747–748, 747f
  variations in curvature and growth of, 744
Charcot arthropathy, 531f
  myelomeningocele and, 531–532
Charcot-Marie-Tooth disease, 123, 561, 562f
  pelvis and, 564f
Charleston brace, 651
Cheilectomy, Legg-Calve-Perthes syndrome and, 982
Chemotherapy
  acquired amputation and, 1159
  Ewing sarcoma and, 453
  Langerhans cell histiocytosis and, 367–368
  musculoskeletal tumors and, 462–463
  spinal tuberculosis and, 709
Chiari osteotomy, Legg-Calve-Perthes syndrome and, 982
Chickenpox, bone and joint infection and, 587
Child abuse, 1315–1332
  cervical spine and, 769
  clinical manifestations of, 1317–1319
  dating fractures in, 1325–1326, 1327f
  decision making in, 1323–1326
  definition of, 1316
  diagnosis of, 1316–1317
  law and, 1331–1332
  management of, 1327–1331
  orthopaedic manifestations of, 1319–1323
  preparation for court testimony in, 1331–1332
  prevalence of, 1316
  radiologic findings in, 1327t

  suspected, skeletal imaging strategy in, 38–39, 38f
Childhood, early, normal development in, 57–61
Children, hip dislocation in, treatment of, 925–932
Choline magnesium trisalicylate, juvenile rheumatoid arthritis and, 408t
Chondral shaving, patellofemoral pain syndrome and, 1214
Chondroblastoma, 443–444, 443–444f
Chondrocytes, 139
Chondrodysplasia, 123
  missense mutation in, 119
Chondrodysplasia punctata, 235–237, 236f
Chondroectodermal dysplasia, 216–218, 216–217f
Chondroitin sulfate, repeating disaccharide units of, 5t
Chondrolysis
  idiopathic of hip, 1037–1043, 1039–1042f
  slipped capital femoral epiphysis and, 1018–1019
Chondromalacia, 1215
Chondromatosis, synovial, 461, 461f
Chondromyxofibroma, 442–443, 442f
Chordoma, 11
  cervical spine and, 774
Chorionic villus sampling, prenatal diagnosis and, 134
Christmas disease, 371
Chromosome 11p15, Beckwith-Wiedemann syndrome and, 287
Chromosome 15
  Angelman syndrome and, 285
  Prader-Willi syndrome and, 285
Chromosome 21, Down syndrome and, 271
Chromosome disorders, 121–122
Chromosomes, 117–118
  autosomal, abnormalities of, 121–122
  sex, abnormalities of, 122
Chronic granulomatous disease, 355–356, 356f
Cisplatin, musculoskeletal tumors and, 462
Claforan. See Cefotaxime
Clavicle
  congenital pseudoarthrosis of, 330–331, 330f
  fractures of, 1236–1237, 1237f
Clawing, 89
Claw toes, 1122
  juvenile rheumatoid arthritis and, 417
Cleavage, 5–7, 6t
Cleft foot, 1127–1128, 1128f
  cleft hand and, 798
Cleft hand, 797–798, 797f
Cleft lip
  cervical spine anomalies and, 760
  cleft hand and, 798
Cleft palate
  cervical spine anomalies and, 760
  cleft hand and, 798
  congenital constriction band syndrome and, 316
  Diamond-Blackfan anemia and, 346
Cleidocranial dysostosis, 331
Cleidocranial dysplasia, 240–242, 241–242f
Clindamycin, bone and joint infection and, 596, 597t
Clinodactyly, 60, 813–814, 813f
Closing wedge osteotomy, tibia vara and, 1057

Clubfoot
  arthrogryposis multiplex congenita and, 265
  congenital, 1103–1116, 1105–1106f
    resistant, 1111–1112f
  congenital constriction band syndrome and, 316, 316f
  evaluating, prone position for, 86f
  fetal alcohol syndrome and, 276
  functional rating system for, 1109t
  Larsen syndrome and, 266
  myelomeningocele and, 527–529
  posteromedial tibiotalar release and, 1115f
  untreated, 1106f
Clubhand, 785–795, 786f
  ulnar, 798–801, 799–800f
Codman tumor, 443
Coleman block test, 1121f
Collagen, 4–5, 138, 164
  types of, 4t, 139t
Compartment syndrome, 1298–1299
  chronic, 1193–1194
Complex syndactyly, 802
Compression plates and screws
  femoral shaft fractures and, 1284–1285, 1286f
  tibial fracture and, 1299–1300
Computed tomography (CT), 25, 32–34
  bone and joint infection and, 592–593
  bone and soft tissue tumors and, 428–429
  femoral rotation and, 1050
  idiopathic chondrolysis of hip and, 1040, 1040f
  pelvis and, 33f
  scoliosis and, 632
  single-photon emission, 36
    spine and, 36f
  slipped capital femoral epiphysis and, 999–1000
  spondylolysis/spondylolisthesis and, 722
  tarsal coalition and, 1096, 1097f
  tibial osteosarcoma and, 35f
Condyle fracture, 1251–1252
  lateral, 1247–1251, 1249–1251f
    classification of, 1249f
Confusion test, 62f
Congenital amputation, 784–785, 785f
  multiple, 1164–1166, 1165f
Congenital calcaneovalgus foot, 1083–1085, 1084f
Congenital cleft foot, 1127–1128, 1128f
Congenital clubfoot, 1103–1116, 1105–1106f
  resistant, 1111–1112f
Congenital constriction band syndrome, 315–317, 316f, 822–825, 823–824f
Congenital coxa vara, 1024, 1024f
Congenital fiber-type disproportion, 554
Congenital hallux varus, 1124–1125, 1124f
Congenital hip dysplasia, 29
Congenital kyphosis
  effect of traction on, 694f
  type I, 690f, 692f, 693
  type II, 690f, 693–694
Congenital muscular dystrophy, 554–555f, 555
Congenital muscular torticollis, 751–754
Congenital myopathy, 552–554
Congenital myotonic dystrophy, 552
Congenital quadriceps fibrosis, 338–339
Congenital radial deficiency, 785–795, 786f
Congenital scoliosis, 518

Congenital vertical talus, 1089–1093, 1090–1091f
Congenital wry neck, 751
Conjunctivitis, Reiter syndrome and, 398
Connective tissue syndromes, 179–182
Constriction band syndrome
 congenital, 315–317, 316f, 822–825, 823–824f
 congenital pseudoarthrosis of tibia and, 323
Contracture
 abduction, assessment of, 77f
 adduction of hip, spastic diplegia and, 492
 Duchenne muscular dystrophy and, 545–546
 Emery-Dreifuss muscular dystrophy and, 549
 extension and abduction of hip, spastic quadriplegia and, 482
 flexion of hip, spastic diplegia and, 492
 hemophilia and, 378–379, 379f
 hip flexion, examination for, 76–77
 iliotibial band, detecting, 78
 pediatric orthopaedic examination and, 61–62
 poliomyelitis and, 566
 quadriceps, 338–339
 radial, 795f
 soft tissue, spinal muscular atrophy and, 557
Contrast media, biologic effect of, 27
Cornelia de Lange syndrome, 279–280, 279–280f
Corset Lyonaisse, 651
Cortical bone, 582f
Cortical desmoid, 29f
Corticosteroids
 Diamond-Blackfan anemia and, 347
 unicameral bone cysts and, 449
 young athlete and, 1185
Corticotomy, leg-length discrepancy and, 886, 886f
Coxa plana, 951
Coxa vara
 acquired, 1024, 1025f
 congenital, 1024, 1024f
 developmental, 1023–1033, 1025f
  clinical presentation of, 1027
  etiology of, 1026–1027, 1026f
  historical review of, 1025–1026
  incidence of, 1026
  natural history of, 1027–1028
  preoperative/postoperative, 1030–1032f
  radiographic findings in, 1027, 1028f
  recurrent, 1032f
  treatment of, 1028–1032
Cranial-caudal resegmentation, 13f
Craniofacial syndromes, cervical spine anomalies and, 760–761
Craniosynostosis syndromes, cervical spine anomalies and, 761–762
Cretinism, hypothyroidism and, 186
Crouch gait, 109
Crouzon syndrome, cervical spine anomalies and, 761
Cruciate ligament injury
 anterior, 1203–1204
 posterior, 1205
Cryosurgery, giant cell tumor of bone and, 453
CT. See Computed tomography
Cuneiform osteotomy, slipped capital femoral epiphysis and, 1012, 1013f

Curly toes, 1125–1126, 1125f
Cushing syndrome, steroid-induced osteoporosis in, 189f
Cyclophosphamide, musculoskeletal tumors and, 462
Cylinderization, 23, 23f
Cystathionine synthetase, homocystinuria and, 182
Cystic fibrosis
 autosomal recessiveness and, 126
 cystic fibrosis transmembrane conductance regulator and, 127
Cystic lymphangioma, 309
Cysts
 bone
  aneurysmal, 450–451, 450–451f, 773
  unicameral, 448–450, 449f
 dural, Scheuermann disease and, 696
 popliteal, 1065
Cytoxan. See Cyclophosphamide

D
Dactinomycin. See Actinomycin D
Dactylitis
 sickle cell disease and, 348–349
 tuberculous, 618
DDH. See Developmental dislocation of hip
Decompression, spondylolisthesis and, 727–728
Degenerative spondylolisthesis, 717
7-Dehydrocholesterol
 calcium transport system and, 142–143
 conversion to vitamin D3, 143f
Dejerine-Sottas disease, 561
de Lange syndrome, 279–280, 279–280f
Delta phalanx, 814–815, 814f
Dentinogenesis imperfecta, 165
Depo-Medrol. See Methylprednisolone acetate
Dermatan sulfate, repeating disaccharide units of, 5t
Dermatome, 8–9, 11f
Derotation osteotomy, rotational abnormalities and, 1051–1052
Development
 achondroplasia and, 206
 average achievement by age, 58t
 brain, cerebral palsy and, 469–470
 cervical spine, 740–741
 myelomeningocele and, 509–510
 normal, 54–61
  in early childhood, 57–61
  of hip joint, 904–907
  in newborn, 55–57
 skeletal, factors influencing, 137–141
 stages of, 92
Developmental coxa vara. See Coxa vara, developmental
Developmental dislocation of hip (DDH), 40
Diabetes insipidus, Langerhans cell histiocytosis and, 365
Diabetes mellitus
 fibrous dysplasia and, 446
 teratogenicity and, 132
Diamond-Blackfan anemia, 346–347
Diaphyseal dysplasia, progressive, 317–319, 318f
Diaphyseal fracture, 1323f
 child abuse and, 1321–1322
Diastematomyelia, 671f
Diastrophic dwarfism, kyphotic deformity and, 708

Diastrophic dysplasia, 218–222, 218f, 220–221f
Dicloxacillin, bone and joint infection and, 596, 597t
Digital radiography, 25, 30
1,25-Dihydroxyvitamin D
 hypercalcemia and, 162
 vitamin D-resistant rickets and, 152–153
1,25-Dihydroxyvitamin D3, osteopetrosis and, 173–174
Dilantin. See Diphenylhydantoin
Diphenylhydantoin, myotonia congenita and, 552
Diplegia
 cerebral palsy and, 471
 spastic, management of, 482–493
Directional tomography, 30
Disappearing bone disease, 309
Discitis, 601–603, 602f
 cervical spine and, 772
Discoid lateral meniscus, 1067–1069, 1068f
Dislocation. See specific type
Disomy, uniparental, 130
Distal arthrogryposis, 267–268, 268f
Distal femoral physeal fracture, 1285–1287, 1286–1288f
Distal humeral physeal fracture-separation, 1252–1253, 1254f
Distal humerus
 ossification of secondary centers of, 1242f
 radiographic lines of, 1243f
Distal muscular dystrophy, 551
Distal osteotomy, rotational abnormalities and, 1052
Distal phalanx fracture, 830, 831f
Distal radial physis fracture, 1264, 1266f
Distal radius
 epiphysiolysis of, 1188, 1188–1189f
 short, 787, 787f
Distal tibia, growth arrest in, 1234f
Distal tibial physeal injury, 1303f
Distal tibiofibular sprains, 1201–1202
Distraction epiphysiolysis, leg-length discrepancy and, 883
Disuse osteoporosis, 163
DNA, 2
 encoding for amino acids, 3f
 translation of, 118–119
Dolichostenomelia, Marfan syndrome and, 179
Dome osteotomy, tibia vara and, 1057
Down syndrome, 271–274, 272f
 cervical spine in, 273–274f, 742f, 756–758, 758f
 chromosome abnormality in, 121
 hip dysplasia in, 275f
 polyarthritis in, 276f
Doxorubicin, musculoskeletal tumors and, 462
Drug abuse, young athlete and, 1184
Duchenne muscular dystrophy. See Muscular dystrophy, Duchenne
Duplicate thumbs, 815–817, 816–817f
Dural cysts, Scheuermann disease and, 696
Dwarfism
 diastrophic, kyphotic deformity and, 708
 Russell-Silver, 284, 284f
 short-limb, 125, 205–213
Dynamic electromyography, gait analysis and, 112–113
Dysautonomia, familial, 280–281, 281f

Dyschondrosteosis, 239–240, 240f
Dysplasia. *See specific type*
Dysplasia epiphysealis hemimelia, 331–332, 332f
Dysplastic spondylolisthesis, 717, 718f
　isthmic spondylolisthesis compared, 719t
Dystonia, cerebral palsy and, 471
Dystrophin, Duchenne muscular dystrophy and, 542–543
Dystrophin gene, muscular dystrophy and, 255

E

Ear, Goldenhar syndrome and, 288–289, 289f
Ectopic calcification, renal osteodystrophy and, 154
Ectrodactyly, 797
EDS. *See* Ehlers-Danlos syndrome
Ehlers-Danlos syndrome (EDS), 2, 123, 180–181
　congenital pseudoarthrosis of tibia and, 323
　instrumentation in Down syndrome and, 757
　type I, 181f
Elastic cartilage, 138–139
Elbow
　carrying angle of, 72f
　cerebral palsy and, 495
　dislocation of, 804f, 1255–1257
　fractures of, 1241–1257
　juvenile rheumatoid arthritis and, 419
　pediatric orthopaedic examination and, 72–73
　poliomyelitis and, 568
　valgus overload injuries of, 1195–1197
Elbow synovectomy, hemophilia and, 377
Electrical stimulation, congenital pseudoarthrosis of tibia and, 324–325, 325f, 325t
Electromyography (EMG)
　Duchenne muscular dystrophy and, 542
　gait analysis and, 112–113
　neuromuscular disorders and, 539
Ellis-van Creveld syndrome, 216
Elmslie-Trillat technique, 1220, 1220f
Ely test, 80, 80f
Embryo, dermatome, myotome, sclerotome in, 11f
Embryogenesis, 5–9
　stages of, 6t
Embryology, molecular, 2–5
Embryonal rhabdomyosarcoma, 458
Emery-Dreifuss muscular dystrophy, 549
EMG. *See* Electromyography
Enchondroma, 440–441, 440f
Endochondral ossification, 18–19
Endocrine abnormalities, 137–190
　slipped capital femoral epiphysis and, 995–996
Endocrinopathies, with indefinite pathophysiology, 182–190
Energetics, gait analysis and, 114
Engelmann-Camurati disease, periosteal reaction and, 174t
Enthesopathy, 398
Enzyme replacement therapy, Gaucher disease and, 362–363
Eosinophilic granuloma
　of bone, 363–369, 365–369f, 448, 448f
　cervical spine and, 773

Epicondyle fracture, 1247–1251
　medial, 1251–1252, 1252f
Epiphyseal cartilage, blood vessels in, 23f
Epiphyseal fracture, Salter-Harris classification of, 859f
Epiphyseal plate, rickets and, 148f, 149f
Epiphyseodesis
　juvenile rheumatoid arthritis and, 413–414
　leg-length discrepancy and, 877–879, 878f
　posteromedial bowing of tibia and, 1071
　slipped capital femoral epiphysis and, 1008–1009, 1010f
Epiphysiolysis
　distal radius and, 1188, 1188–1189f
　proximal humerus and, 1187–1188, 1187f
Equinovalgus, foot and ankle, spastic diplegia and, 490–491
Equinovarus
　foot and ankle, spastic diplegia and, 489–490
　talipes
　　congenital, 1103–1116, 1105–1106f
　　congenital scoliosis and, 672f
　　myelomeningocele and, 527–529
Equinus, ankle, spastic diplegia and, 488–489
Equinus contracture, hemophilia and, 378, 379f
Equinus gait, 108
Erb palsy, 827f
Ergosterol
　calcium transport system and, 142–143
　conversion to vitamin D2, 143f
Erlenmeyer-flask deformity, 360f
Erythrocytes, disorders of, 345–354
Escobar syndrome, 269
Estrogens
　bone formation and, 140
　slipped capital femoral epiphysis and, 996
　Turner syndrome and, 285
Ethambutol, extrapulmonary tuberculosis and, 619
Etoposide, Langerhans cell histiocytosis and, 367
Eversion, 1078t
Ewing sarcoma, 453–454, 454f
　cervical spine and, 774
　osteomyelitis and, 594
Exercise, patellofemoral rehabilitation and, 1212
Exostosis, 441–442, 441f
　subungual, 1131
Expert witness, guidelines for, 1333–1334
Extension contracture, of hip, spastic quadriplegia and, 482
Extensor thrust, 59, 60f
　of hip, spastic quadriplegia and, 482
External compression-distraction, congenital pseudoarthrosis of tibia and, 325f, 325t, 328–329
External fixation
　femoral shaft fracture and, 1281–1282, 1283f
　tibial fracture and, 1299
External tibial torsion, spastic diplegia and, 491
Extracellular matrix, formation of, 4–5
Eye, Goldenhar syndrome and, 288–289, 289f

F

Factor VIII deficiency, 371–372
　knee and, 374f
　pseudotumor of ilium and, 380f
Factor IX deficiency, 371–372
Familial cervical dysplasia, 748, 748f
Familial dysautonomia, 280–281, 281f
Familial hypercholesterolemia, 2
Familial Mediterranean fever, differential diagnosis of, 404
Fanconi anemia, 347
　radial deficiencies and, 789
Fascioscapulohumeral muscular dystrophy, 550–551
　infantile, 550
Fat pad impingement, 1216
Femoral anteversion, 29
　measuring, 1049
　natural history of, 1050–1051
Femoral condyle, hypoplasia of, 859f
Femoral deficiency, proximal focal, 857f
Femoral derotation osteotomy, rotational abnormalities and, 1052
Femoral epiphysis
　blood supply to, 1008f
　slipped capital. *See* Slipped capital femoral epiphysis
Femoral head
　cartilage of, 957f
　classification of, 940t
　idiopathic chondrolysis and, 1041f
　osteonecrosis of, sickle cell disease and, 351, 351t
Femoral intramedullary nailing, rotational abnormalities and, 1052
Femoral neck
　blood supply to, 1008f
　cartilage in, 958f
　fracture of, 1275–1276f
Femoral neck osteotomy, slipped capital femoral epiphysis and, 1012, 1014f
Femoral shaft fractures, 1277–1285
　bilateral, 1282f
　compression plates and screws and, 1284–1285, 1286f
　external fixation of, 1281–1282, 1283f
　intramedullary fixation and, 1282–1283, 1284–1285f
　spiral, 1280f
Femoral shortening, leg-length discrepancy and, 879–880
Femur
　aneurysmal cyst of, 450f
　developing, blood supply to, 583f
　dysplasia of, treatment of hip dysplasia and, 931–937, 933–937f
　dysplasia epiphysealis hemimelia of, 332f
　enchondroma of, 440f
　fracture of, myelomeningocele and, 532–533
　giant cell tumor of, 452f
　juvenile osteoporosis and, 171f
　nonossifying fibroma of, 445f
　pedunculated exostosis of, 441f
　progressive diaphyseal dysplasia and, 318f
　proximal. *See* Proximal femur
　scurvy and, 178f
　short, congenital, 1024f
　unicameral cyst of, 449f
Fenoprofen calcium, juvenile rheumatoid arthritis and, 408t
Fertilization, 5–7, 6t, 7f
Fetal alcohol effects, 275

Fetal alcohol syndrome, 274–277, 277f
  cervical spine and, 760
alpha-Fetoprotein screening, prenatal diagnosis and, 133–134
Fibrillin gene, Marfan syndrome and, 122, 179
Fibrocartilage, 138
Fibrocartilaginous dysplasia
  focal, 323, 324f
  proximal tibial, 1059–1060
Fibrodysplasia ossificans progressiva, 178, 332–334, 334–335f
  cervical spine and, 763
Fibroma
  nonossifying, 444–446, 445f
  ossifying, 447–448, 447f
Fibromatosis, 456–457, 457f
Fibrous ankylosis, slipped capital femoral epiphysis and, 1019
Fibrous dysplasia, 189–190, 446–447, 446f
  congenital pseudoarthrosis of tibia and, 323
  deformity of left hip and, 190f
  rickets and, 153
Fibrous histiocytoma, malignant, 457–459, 458f
Fibula
  centralization of, 1159f
  congenital pseudoarthrosis of, 329–330, 330f
  Ewing sarcoma involving, 454f
Fibular deficiency, 1149–1154, 1149–1154f
  prosthetics for, 1172
  Syme amputation and, 1154f
Fibular hemimelia, 1149
  bilateral, 1155f
  classification of, 1151f
  complete, 1153f
  left, 1152f
  partial, 1152f, 1153f
Fifth metatarsal, apophysitis of, young athlete and, 1191
Finger, mallet, 829–830, 830f
Flatfoot, flexible, 1085–1089, 1086–1087f
Flexible flatfoot, 1085–1089, 1086–1087f
Flexion contracture, of hip, spastic diplegia and, 492
Flexor digitorum profundus avulsion, 830–831, 832f
Flexor muscles, congenital radial deficiency and, 786f
Flexor tone, pediatric orthopaedic examination and, 55–56
Floating knee, 1299
Fluids, heat illness and, 1182–1183
Fluoroscopy, 28–30, 29f
Focal fibrocartilaginous dysplasia, 323, 324f
Focused examination, 51–54
Foot. See also Pediatric foot
  cavus, 87
  congenital absence of, 1160f
  deformity of, diastrophic dysplasia and, 221
  fractures of, 1303–1310
  juvenile rheumatoid arthritis and, 417, 417f
  macrodactyly of, 314f
  myelomeningocele and, 527–532
  pediatric orthopaedic examination and, 84–89
  poliomyelitis and, 568
  prostheses for, 1170
    partial, 1173
  puncture wounds of, 612–615, 614f

supination and pronation of, 85f
  effect on ankle motion, 88f
  terminology of, 1078t
Foot deficiency, 1157–1158, 1160f
Foot equinovalgus, spastic diplegia and, 490–491
Foot equinovarus, spastic diplegia and, 489–490
Foot placement reaction, 59, 60f
Foot-progression angle, 1048, 1048f
Force platform, gait analysis and, 113
Forearm
  disuse atrophy of, 172f
  fracture-dislocation of, 1264–1268, 1267–1268f
  fractures of, 1257–1268
    both-bone, 1261f
    distal-third, 1262–1264, 1262–1265f
    midshaft, 1259–1262, 1259f, 1261f
  greenstick fracture of, 73f, 1259–1260
  malunion of, 1261f
  pediatric orthopaedic examination and, 72–73
  poliomyelitis and, 568
Foreign body synovitis, differential diagnosis of, 403
Fortaz. See Ceftazidime
Fracture
  acetabular, 1270–1271, 1272f
  ankle, 1300–1303
    pronation and external rotation, 1300–1301, 1302f
    supination-inversion, 1300, 1301f
    transitional, 1302–1303, 1304f
  arthrogryposis multiplex congenita and, 264
  atlas, 764–765
  avulsion of pelvis, 1207–1208, 1207f
  C1-C2 complex, 764–765
  C3-C7, 765–767
  calcaneous, 1307, 1308f
  in children, 1230–1231
  clavicle, 1236–1237, 1237f
  condyle, 1251–1252
  congenital pseudoarthrosis of tibia and, 324–329
  diaphyseal, 1323f
    child abuse and, 1321–1322
  distal femoral physeal, 1285–1287, 1286–1288f
  distal phalanx, 830, 831f
  distal physis, 1264, 1266f
  Duchenne muscular dystrophy and, 544
  elbow, 1241–1257
  epicondyle, 1247–1251
    medial, 1251–1252, 1252f
  epiphyseal, Salter-Harris classification of, 859f
  familial dysautonomia and, 281
  femoral neck, 1275–1276f
  femoral shaft, 1277–1285
    bilateral, 1282f
    compression plates and screws and, 1284–1285, 1286f
    external fixation of, 1281–1282, 1283f
    intramedullary fixation and, 1282–1283, 1284–1285f
    spiral, 1280f
  foot, 1303–1310
  forearm
    both-bone, 1261f
    distal-third, 1262–1264, 1262–1265f
    midshaft, 1259–1262, 1259f, 1261f
  forearm and wrist, 1257–1268

Gaucher disease and, 361
greenstick, 73f, 1259–1260
growth of leg and, 862
growth plate, location of, 860f
Hangman, 765
hemophilia and, 380
humeral, 1238–1241, 1239–1241f
  child abuse and, 1324f
intraarticular, 834, 834f
Jefferson, 764
knee, 1285–1293
lateral condylar, 1247–1251, 1249–1251f
leg-length discrepancy and, 856–858
management of, 1229–1310
metacarpal, 836–837, 837f
metaphyseal, 1320–1321f
  child abuse and, 1319–1321
metatarsal, 1307–1310, 1309f
middle phalanx, 832, 833f
myelomeningocele and, 532–533
neurofibromatosis and, 259
occipital complex, 764–765
odontoid, 765, 766f
olecranon, 1254–1255, 1256–1257f
open, 1298
  classification of, 1298t
osteogenesis imperfecta and, 169
osteopetrosis and, 174
pelvic, 1268–1271, 1271f
phalangeal neck, 831–832, 833f
physeal, 1232–1233, 1232f, 1320f
  child abuse and, 1319
proximal femoral, 1271–1277
  classification for, 1274f
proximal phalanx shaft, 834–836, 835f
radial, proximal, 1253–1257
radial neck, 1254, 1255f
radiographic changes in, timetable of, 1328t
renal osteodystrophy and, 159
reverse mallet finger, 830–831, 832f
rib, 1325f
  child abuse and, 1322
rickets and, 155, 158
scapular, 1238
shoulder region, 1236–1242
sickle cell disease and, 350
stress, 1185–1187
  of tibia, 1069–1070
supracondylar, 831–832, 833f, 1242–1247
  fracture line in, 1244f
  type II, 1245f
  type III, 1246–1247f
talus, 1303–1307, 1306f
T-condylar, 1247, 1248f
thalassemia and, 353
tibial, 1293–1300
  child abuse and, 1326f, 1327f
  diaphyseal, 1295
  high-energy, 1297f
  mid-diaphyseal, 1300f
  proximal epiphyseal, 1293–1294, 1294f
  proximal metaphyseal, 1294–1295, 1295f
tibial tubercle, 1292–1293, 1293f
  classification of, 1292f
Tillaux, 1303, 1304f
toddler's, 1069, 1069f, 1296–1298
triplane, 1303, 1304–1305f
ulnar, 1253–1257
unicameral bone cysts and, 448–449
Fragile X syndrome, 128–129
Fragilitas ossium, 165

Freeman-Sheldon syndrome, 268–269, 268–269f
Freiberg infarction, 1101–1103, 1103f
Friedreich ataxia, 558–561
Fulkerson modification, 1220, 1220f
Functional testing, Duchenne muscular dystrophy and, 543
Funnelization, 23, 23f

G
Gait
  calcaneous, 108
  cerebral palsy and, 94
  crouch, 109
  deviations of, 107–110
  Duchenne muscular dystrophy and, 541
  equinus, 108
  initial contact in, 99f
  initial swing in, 101f
  jump, 109
  Legg-Calve-Perthes syndrome and, 983
  leg-length discrepancy and, 850
  loading response in, 99f
  maturation of, 107
  midstance in, 99f
  midswing in, 101f
  myelodysplasia and, 95
  normal, 95–97
  pediatric orthopaedic examination and, 53
  pelvis motion during, 850f
  preswing in, 100f
  stance phase of, 98t
    ankle and, 100–103
    hip and, 103–104
    knee and, 103
  stiff knee, 109
  swing phase of, 100t
    ankle and, 103
    hip and, 104
    knee and, 103
  terminal stance in, 100f
  terminal swing in, 101f
Gait analysis, 110–114
  cerebral palsy and, 473
  idiopathic toe walking and, 1071
  instrumented, 112–114
  lower limb prostheses and, 1171–1174
  observational, 110–112, 11f
  spastic diplegia and, 487–488
Gait cycle, 97–105, 97f
  running, 106–107
  walking and running compared, 106f
Galeazzi procedure, 1219f, 1220
Galeazzi sign, 76
Gallium 67 imaging, bone and soft tissue tumors and, 428
Gangrene, amputation and, 1159–1160, 1161f
Gastroesophageal reflux, Sandifer syndrome and, 754–755
Gastrointestinal rickets, 150–152
Gastrointestinal system, cerebral palsy and, 472
Gastrulation, 6t, 7–8
Gaucher crisis, 360–361
Gaucher disease, 127, 359–363, 360–362f
  osteomyelitis and, 595
Genes, 2
  deletions and insertions and, 120
  homeotic, morphogenesis and, 3–4
  structure of, 118, 118f

Gene therapy, 135
Genetic counseling, 131, 132–134
  Duchenne muscular dystrophy and, 547
Genetic disease
  burden of, 133
  treatment of, 134–135, 134t
Genitourinary system, cerebral palsy and, 472
Genomic imprinting, 130
  Prader-Willi syndrome and, 285
Gentamicin, bone and joint infection and, 597t
Genu valgum, 1054–1061
  Down syndrome and, 272
  expected change with age, 1054f
  juvenile rheumatoid arthritis and, 416f
  Proteus syndrome and, 261
Genu varum, 1054–1061
  achondroplasia and, 212
  expected change with age, 1054f
  metaphyseal chondrodysplasia and, 239
  thrombocytopenia with absent radius syndrome and, 371
German measles. See Rubella
Germ layers, 7–8
Germline mosaicism, 129–130
Giant cell tumor of bone, 451–453, 452f
Glenohumeral dislocation, 1238
Glucocerebrosidase gene, 359
Glucocorticoids
  bone formation and, 140
  growth and, 188–189
Glycosaminoglycans
  attaching to core proteins, 6f
  repeating disaccharide units of, 5t
Goldenhar syndrome, 288–290, 289f
  cervical spine anomalies and, 761
  surgery for, cervical spine and, 752f
Gold sodium thiomalate, juvenile rheumatoid arthritis and, 408
Gonadal abnormalities, growth and, 187–188
Gonococcal arthritis, 615–616
Gorham disease, 309, 310f
Gower muscular dystrophy, 551
Granulocytes, disorders of, 354–356
Granuloma, eosinophilic
  bone and, 363–369, 365–369f, 448, 448f
  cervical spine and, 773
Granulomatous disease, chronic, 355–356, 356f
Grasp reflex, 56
  testing, 56f
Gravity, center of
  normal gait and, 95, 96f
  relation to body segments, 61f
Greenstick fracture, 73f, 1259–1260
Grisel syndrome, 750–751, 751f
Growth
  achondroplasia and, 206
  cervical spine and, 740–741
  fetal alcohol syndrome and, 275–276
  glucocorticoid-related abnormalities and, 188–189
  gonadal abnormalities and, 187–188
  growth hormone deficiency and, 185–186
  hypopituitarism and, 185–186
  hypothyroidism and, 186–187
  idiopathic scoliosis and, 638
  leg-length discrepancy and, 853–856, 854–856f
  normal charts for boys, 183f

normal charts for girls, 184f
normal of hip joint, 904–907
patterns of disturbance in, 185f
sex steroids and, 187–188
spondylolysis and, 720
velocity curves for, 185f
Growth factors, 138t
Growth hormone
  achondroplasia and, 209
  growth plate and, 140
  hypochondroplasia and, 213
  postnatal skeletal development and, 952
  scoliosis and, 639
  slipped capital femoral epiphysis and, 996
  Turner syndrome and, 285
Growth hormone deficiency, linear growth and maturation and, 185–186
Growth plate
  bone tracers and, 39f
  damage in knee, imaging of, 46f
  humoral factors and, 140
  location of fractures in, 860f
  zones of, 139
Growth plate development
  bone formation and, 20–24
  primary spongiosa in, 19f
Growth retardation
  de Lange syndrome and, 279
  human immunodeficiency virus infection and, 358
  Turner syndrome and, 284
Growth spurt, scoliosis and, 638
Gunshot wounds, cervical spine and, 769–770

H
Hallux valgus
  adolescent, 1116–1119, 1117–1118f
  cerebral palsy and, 488
  juvenile rheumatoid arthritis and, 417
Hallux varus, congenital, 1124–1125, 1124f
Hand. See also Pediatric hand
  central deficiency of, 797–798, 797f
  cerebral palsy and, 496–497, 496f
  cleft, 797–798, 797f
  cleidocranial dysplasia and, 242
  distal arthrogryposis and, 267–268, 268f
  hereditary motor sensory neuropathies and, 564–565
  juvenile rheumatoid arthritis and, 418–419
  landmarks in, 868f
  pediatric orthopaedic examination and, 73–74
  poliomyelitis and, 568
  pseudohypoparathyroidism and, 162f
  sensory distribution of, 74f
Handedness, 58
Hand-foot syndrome, 348
Hand-Schuller-Christian disease, 363, 448
Hangman fracture, 765
Happy puppet syndrome, 285
Harris growth arrest line, 1234f
Head injuries, child abuse and, 1318–1319
Heat illness
  fluids and, 1182–1183
  guidelines for preventing, 1183t
Heat stroke, 1183
Heavy metal poisoning, 163
Heel bisector, 1080f

Heel pain, 1119–1120
 differential diagnosis of, 1120t
Helfet test, 83, 83f
Hemangioma, 455–456, 455–456f
 conditions associated with, 307–308, 308t
 Klippel-Trenaunay syndrome and, 305–307, 306f
Hemarthrosis
 acute of knee, 1292
 hemophilia and, 375
Hematology
 Duchenne muscular dystrophy and, 542
 neuromuscular disorders and, 538
Hematopoietic system, diseases related to, 345–383
 skeletal changes in children and, 346t
Hemi-3 syndrome
 differential diagnosis of, 311t
 hemihypertrophy and, 313
Hemihypertrophy, 310–313
 differential diagnosis of, 310, 311t
 idiopathic, 312f
Hemihypotrophy, 310–313
 differential diagnosis of, 310, 311t
Hemimelia, 1137
 fibular, 1149
  bilateral, 1155f
  classification of, 1151f
  complete, 1153f
  left, 1152f
  partial, 1152f, 1153f
  Syme amputation and, 1154f
 radial, bilateral, 371f
 tibial
  bilateral complete, 1156f
  classification of, 1156f
  complete, 1158f
  right, 1158f
  type II partial, 1157f
Hemiplegia
 cerebral palsy and, 471
 spastic, management of, 493–494
Hemispherization, 23, 23f
Hemivertebra, congenital scoliosis and, 668–669, 678f
Hemivertebra excision, congenital scoliosis and, 679
Hemoglobin C, 347
Hemoglobin S, sickle cell disease and, 347
Hemophilia, 371–380
 acquired immunodeficiency syndrome and, 357
 factor VIII infusion in, fall-off curve after, 373f
 patellar erosions in, 374f
 synovium in, 373f
Hemophilic arthropathy, 372–376
 of knee, 375f
 radiographic grading of, 375t
Hemorrhage, hemophilia and, 377–378, 378f
Hemostasis, disorders of, 369–380
Henoch-Schonlein purpura
 differential diagnosis of, 403
 septic arthritis and, 596
Heparan sulfate, repeating disaccharide units of, 5t
Hepatomegaly, Gaucher disease and, 359–360
Hereditary motor sensory neuropathies, 561–565, 562f

Hereditary progressive arthroophthalmopathy, 287
Hereditary telangiectasia, 308
Hernia
 inguinal, arthrogryposis multiplex congenita and, 263
 Legg-Calve-Perthes syndrome and, 953
Heuter-Volkmann principle, 695, 700
Hip. See also Legg-Calve-Perthes syndrome
 adduction contracture of, spastic diplegia and, 492
 cerebral palsy and, 477–482
 chondrolysis of, idiopathic, 1037–1043, 1039–1042f
 congenital dysplasia of, 29
 course in adults, 916–917
 deformity of
  diastrophic dysplasia and, 221–222
  spondyloepiphyseal dysplasia congenita and, 227
 dislocation of, 903–942, 1277
  bilateral, 917–918f
  closed reduction of, 927f
  complete, 917f
  developmental of, 40
  Fanconi anemia and, 347
  high-riding, 857f
  infants and, 912–913f
  Larsen syndrome and, 243
  newborn and, 907–908
  open reduction of, 930f
  spinal muscular atrophy and, 557
  traction and, 926f
  traumatic, 1278f
  treatment of, 922–931, 922–931f
  untreated, 907f
 dysplasia of, 903–942
  acetabular development in, 908, 909f
  causes of, 908–910
  closed reduction of, 927f
  course in newborns, 916
  diagnosis of, 911–916
  Down syndrome and, 275f
  hereditary motor sensory neuropathies and, 564
  risk factors and incidence of, 910–911, 911t
  sequelae and complications of, 931–942
  subluxation and, 917–922, 919–921f
 embryonic, 904f
 excessive abduction of, gait and, 110
 excessive adduction of, gait and, 109–110
 fibrous dysplasia and, 190f
 flexion contracture of, 76–77
  spastic diplegia and, 492
 fractures of, 1271–1277
 growth and development of, normal, 904–907
 inadequate extension and excessive flexion of, gait and, 109
 juvenile rheumatoid arthritis and, 414, 414f
 leg-length discrepancy and, 851, 851f
 Morquio syndrome and, 293–294, 293f
 multiple epiphyseal dysplasia and, 232–233
 myelomeningocele and, 521, 521f
 normal motion, moments, and powers of, 105f
 pediatric orthopaedic examination and, 74–79

 poliomyelitis and, 568
 stance phase of gait and, 103–104
 toxic synovitis of, differential diagnosis of, 403
 transient synovitis of, 1033–1037, 1035f
 ultrasonography of, 41f, 42f
  protocol for infants, 42f
 unstable, displacing in infant, 75f
Hip arthrography, 31
Hip disarticulation, 1170, 1171f
Hip disarticulation prosthesis, bilateral, 1168f
Hip subluxation
 cerebral palsy and, 479–481
 developmental dysplasia and, 917–922, 919–921f
 spinal muscular atrophy and, 557
Histiocytoma, fibrous, malignant, 457–459, 458f
Histiocytosis, Langerhans cell, 363–369, 448
 criteria of organ dysfunction in, 364t
Histiocytosis X, 364, 448
HIV. See Human immunodeficiency virus
HLA-B27 antigen, juvenile rheumatoid arthritis and, 406
Holt-Oram syndrome, radial deficiencies and, 789
Homeostasis
 calcium, 141–146
 phosphorus, 141–146
Homeotic genes, morphogenesis and, 3–4
Homocystinuria, 127, 181–182
Hounsfield unit (HU), 32
HOX genes, 3–4
Hueter-Volkmann principle, 140–141, 158
Human genome, 2–3
Human immunodeficiency virus (HIV), 357–358
 teratogenicity and, 132
Humeral head, osteonecrosis of, sickle cell disease and, 351–352, 352t
Humeral shaft, fracture of, 1240–1241
Humerus
 chondroblastoma in, 443f
 congenital deficiency of, 796–797
 distal
  ossification of secondary centers of, 1242f
  radiographic lines of, 1243f
 fractures of, 1238–1241, 1239–1241f
  child abuse and, 1324f
 proximal, epiphysiolysis of, 1187–1188, 1187f
 rachitic changes in, 149f
Huntington disease, 2
 genomic imprinting in, 130
 transmission of, parental sex bias in, 129
Hurler syndrome, 127
 kyphotic deformity and, 708
Hutchinson-Gilford syndrome, 283
Hyaline cartilage, 138–139, 904–905
Hyaluronic acid, 139
 repeating disaccharide units of, 5t
Hydrocephaly, myelomeningocele and, 505, 507–508
Hydromyelia, scoliosis and, 513
Hydrosyringomyelia, scoliosis and, 513
Hydroxyapatite, 141, 164
Hydroxychloroquine, juvenile rheumatoid arthritis and, 408
1-Hydroxyvitamin D, hypercalcemia and, 162

Hypercalcemia, 146, 162–163
Hypercholesterolemia, familial, 2
Hyperhomocysteinemia, 182
Hyperkyphosis, cerebral palsy and, 475–476
Hyperlordosis
  cerebral palsy and, 475
  spastic diplegia and, 492
Hypermobility syndrome, differential diagnosis of, 403–404
Hyperostosis, prostaglandin-induced, periosteal reaction and, 175t
Hyperparathyroidism, 141, 161
  renal osteodystrophy and, 157f
  rickets and, 155
Hyperphosphatemia, periosteal reaction and, 175t
Hypersensitivity, latex, myelomeningocele and, 509
Hypertelorism, 60
Hyperthyroidism, fibrous dysplasia and, 446
Hypertrophic osteoarthropathy, periosteal reaction and, 175t
Hypervitaminosis A, 176–177
  periosteal reaction and, 175t
Hypervitaminosis D, hypercalcemia and, 162
Hypocalcemia, 146
Hypochondroplasia, 126, 213–214, 214f
Hypoparathyroidism, 161
Hypophosphatasia, 159–161
  ossification defects in, 160f
Hypophosphatemic rickets, 128
  angular deformity in, 894f, 896f
Hypopituitarism, growth retardation and, 185–186
Hypoplastic radius, 787, 788f
Hypothyroidism, 186–187
  congenital, 187f
  femoral epiphyses in, 187f, 188f
Hypotonic cerebral palsy, 471
Hypovitaminosis, Scheuermann disease and, 696
Hysterical scoliosis, 636, 637f

I

Ibuprofen
  juvenile rheumatoid arthritis and, 408t
  young athlete and, 1185
Idiopathic hypertrophic subaortic stenosis, sudden death in young athletes and, 1198
Idiopathic juvenile osteoporosis, 170–172, 171f
Idiopathic scoliosis. See Scoliosis, idiopathic
Ifosfamide, musculoskeletal tumors and, 462
Iliac apophysitis, young athlete and, 1191
Iliotibial band, contracture of, detecting, 78
Iliotibial band friction syndrome, young athlete and, 1194–1195, 1195f
Ilium, pseudotumor of, factor VIII deficiency and, 380f
Ilizarov technique
  leg-length discrepancy and, 883, 885f
  relapsed clubfeet and, 1114
Imaging
  bone and joint infection and, 590–594
  bowlegs and, 1055
  in-toeing/out-toeing and, 1049–1050
  Legg-Calve-Perthes syndrome and, 974

Immobilization
  hypercalcemia and, 162–163
  spondylolisthesis and, 730
Immune system, disorders of, 356–358
Imperforate anus, 7
Inborn errors of metabolism, autosomal recessive disease and, 127
Indomethacin, juvenile rheumatoid arthritis and, 408t
Infant, hip dislocation in, treatment of, 922–925
Infantile coxa vara, 1024
Infantile fascioscapulohumeral muscular dystrophy, 550
Infantile idiopathic scoliosis, 637–638, 640–642, 641f
Infantile poliomyelitis, 19
Infantile tibia vara, 1055
Infection
  bone and joint, 579–586
    criteria for oral therapy of, 598t
    diagnosis of, 586–594
    neonatal, 605–607
    sickle cell disease and, 607–609, 608f
    treatment of, 596–601
  cervical spine, 770–773
  chronic granulomatous disease and, 355–356
  growth of leg and, 860
  pelvic, 603–605, 605f
  postenteric Reiter syndrome and, 398
  sacroiliac joint, 603–605
  sickle cell disease and, 349–350
  spinal, 601–603
  teratogenicity and, 132
  X-linked agammaglobulinemia and, 356
Inflammation
  cervical spine and, 770–773
  growth of leg and, 862
  slipped capital femoral epiphysis and, 995
Ingrown toenails, 1129–1131
Inguinal hernia, arthrogryposis multiplex congenita and, 263
Inheritance
  autosomal dominant, 123
  autosomal recessive, 126–127
  camptodactyly and, 812
  central polydactyly and, 819
  cleft hand and, 798
  clinodactyly and, 813
  congenital constriction band syndrome and, 823
  delta phalanx and, 814–815
  macrodactyly and, 821
  Madelung deformity and, 825
  molecular basis of, 117–119
  multifactorial, 131, 506
  postaxial polydactyly, 820
  radial head dislocation and, 804
  single-gene, 129–130
  syndactyly and, 806
  thumb polydactyly and, 815
  triphalangeal thumb and, 817
  upper extremity malformation and, 783
  X-linked, 127–129, 127f
Inhibition casting, spastic diplegia and, 485
Innominate bone, 907f
Innominate osteotomy, Legg-Calve-Perthes syndrome and, 981–982
Instrumentation
  adolescent idiopathic scoliosis and, 661–663
  Down syndrome patient and, 757
  spondylolisthesis and, 730

Instrumented gait analysis, 112–114
Instrumented motion analysis, 94–95
Insulin
  bone formation and, 140
  growth plate function and, 140
Integrins, 141
Interferon, chronic granulomatous disease and, 356
Internal injuries, child abuse and, 1319
Intersegmental deficiency, 796–797
Intertrochanteric osteotomy, slipped capital femoral epiphysis and, 1012–1015, 1015f
Intervertebral disc calcification, cervical spine and, 771–772, 771f
In-toeing, 85, 1047–1054
  clinical features of, 1048–1049, 1049
  complications of, 1052–1054
  etiology of, 1048
  imaging and, 1049–1050
  natural history of, 1050–1051
  spastic diplegia and, 492–493
  treatment of, 1051–1052
    nonsurgical, 1051
    surgical, 1051–1052
Intraarticular avulsion, 1289–1290, 1290f
Intraarticular fracture, 834, 834f
Intramedullary fixation, femoral shaft fracture and, 1282–1283, 1284–1285f
Intramedullary nail fixation, tibial fracture and, 1299, 1300f
Intramedullary rod
  congenital pseudoarthrosis of tibia and, 325f, 325t, 326
  leg lengthening over, 883–886
Intramuscular injection, spastic diplegia and, 485
Intravenous pyelography (IVP), scoliosis and, 632
Inversion, 1078t
Iridocyclitis, chronic, juvenile rheumatoid arthritis and, 395–396
Iritis, juvenile rheumatoid arthritis and, 396f
Iritis surveillance, routine schedule of, 395t
Iron deficiency anemia, 345–346
Irradiation, biologic effect of, 26
Isokinetic exercise, patellofemoral rehabilitation and, 1212
Isoniazid
  extrapulmonary tuberculosis and, 619
  spinal tuberculosis and, 709
Isthmic spondylolisthesis, 717, 718f
  dysplastic spondylolisthesis compared, 719t
IVP. See Intravenous pyelography

J

Jefferson fracture, 764
Joint
  deformity of, multiple epiphyseal dysplasia and, 232
  infection of, 579–586
    criteria for oral therapy of, 598t
    diagnosis of, 586–594
    newborn and, 605–607
    sickle cell disease and, 607–609
    treatment of, 596–601
  motion and function of, examining and recording, 61–63
  synovial, development of, 16–17
Jones criteria, diagnosis of rheumatic fever and, 403t

JRA. *See* Juvenile rheumatoid arthritis
Jumper's knee, 1190
Jump gait, 109
Juvenile arthritis, periosteal reaction and, 174t
Juvenile idiopathic scoliosis, 642–644, 643f
Juvenile osteoporosis
　idiopathic, 170–172, 171f
　kyphotic deformity and, 709–710, 710f
　Scheuermann kyphosis and, 695–696
Juvenile rheumatoid arthritis (JRA), 394–397
　arthrocentesis and synovial biopsy in, 406–407
　arthrodesis in, 412–413
　cervical spine and, 770–771, 770f
　differential diagnosis of, 401–404, 402t
　epiphyseodesis in, 413–414
　etiology of, 398–399
　history in, 404–405
　idiopathic chondrolysis of hip and, 1038
　intraarticular steroid injections in, 409
　iritis surveillance in, 395t
　joint-specific treatment in, 414–419
　laboratory tests in, 406
　management of, 407–409
　medical therapy for, 407–409, 408t
　orthopaedic surgical treatment in, 410–414
　osteotomy in, 412
　pathology of, 399–401
　pauciarticular-onset, 394–396
　　iritis in, 396f
　physical examination and, 405–406
　physical and occupational therapy in, 409
　polyarticular-onset, 396, 412f
　　apple-core odontoid in, 400f
　radiology of, 399–401, 400–401f, 406
　septic arthritis and, 595
　soft tissue release in, 411–412
　synovectomy in, 410–411
　synovial fluid analysis in, 588t
　systemic-onset, 396–397, 401f
　　cervical spine in, 401f
　　maculopapular rash of, 397f
　total joint arthroplasty in, 413
Juvenile tibia vara, 1055

K
Karyotype, 117
Kasabach-Merritt syndrome, 306
Kefazol. *See* Cefazolin
Keflex. *See* Cephalexin
Keratin sulfate, repeating disaccharide units of, 5t
Kidney, vitamin D conversion in, 143, 144f
Kidney failure, nail-patella syndrome and, 277
King-Denborough syndrome, 285
Klein line, 999, 999f
Klinefelter syndrome, 122
Klippel-Feil syndrome, 65, 269, 276, 284, 745, 760
　cervical spine and, 755
　congenital kyphosis and, 691
　Diamond-Blackfan anemia and, 346
　Fanconi anemia and, 347
Klippel-Trenaunay syndrome, 260, 305–307, 306f
　differential diagnosis of, 311t
　limb-length inequality and, 313

Knee
　breaststroker's, 1195
　collateral ligaments of, 1202f
　　injuries of, 1202–1203
　constant-friction, 1169
　deformity of, recurvatum, 1061–1063, 1063f
　discoid lateral meniscus in, 1067–1069, 1068f
　dislocation of, 1287–1289
　　congenital, 1061–1062, 1062f
　　Larsen syndrome and, 243
　disorders of, 1061–1069
　excessive flexion and inadequate extension of, gait and, 109
　factor VIII deficiency and, 374f
　floating, 1299
　fluid-controlled, 1169–1170
　fractures of, 1285–1293
　giant cell tumor in, 425f
　growth plate damage in, imaging of, 46f
　hemarthrosis of, acute, 1292
　hemophilic arthropathy of, 375f
　inadequate flexion and excessive extension of, gait and, 108–109
　intraarticular avulsions and, 1289–1290, 1290f
　jumper's, 1190
　juvenile rheumatoid arthritis and, 405, 414–417, 415f
　Larsen-Johansson disease and, 1064–1065
　Larsen syndrome and, 266
　lead poisoning and, 163f
　leg-length discrepancy and, 851
　manual-locking, 1169
　myelomeningocele and, 525–527, 525–526f
　normal motion, moments, and powers of, 104f
　Osgood-Schlatter disease and, 1063–1064
　osteochondritis dissecans and, 1065–1067, 1066f
　pediatric orthopaedic examination and, 79–84
　plicas of, 1216f
　poliomyelitis and, 568
　polycentric/four-bar, 1169
　popliteal cyst in, 1065
　pterygium syndromes and, 271
　stance-control/weight-activated friction, 1169
　stance phase of gait and, 103
　stress fractures about, 1186
　swing phase of gait and, 103
　thrombocytopenia with absent radius syndrome and, 371
Knee arthrodesis, proximal focal femoral deficiency and, 1146–1147, 1146f
Knee disarticulation, 1162, 1162f, 1170
　complete tibial hemimelia and, 1156–1157
Knee flexion contracture, hemophilia and, 378–379
Knee flexion deformity, spastic diplegia and, 491–492
Knee pain, anterior, 1209–1215
Knee reflex, testing, 57
Knee synovectomy, hemophilia and, 376
Kniest dysplasia, 222–224, 223f
Knock-knees, 1054–1061
　causes and treatment of, 1060–1061
　genetic disorders and, 1061

　physiologic, 1060
　rickets and, 1060
Koehler disease, 1101, 1102f
Kugelberg-Welander disease, type III, 557
Kyphoscoliosis
　achondroplasia and, 212
　diastrophic dysplasia and, 219–221
　Kniest dysplasia and, 222
　neurofibromatosis and, 709
　spondyloepiphyseal dysplasia congenita and, 226
Kyphosis, 687–710
　achondroplasia and, 705, 707f
　cerebral palsy and, 475–476
　cervical, neurofibromatosis and, 761f
　chondrodysplasia punctata and, 237
　collapsing, 519
　congenital, 690–694
　　effect of traction on, 694f
　　type I, 690f, 692f, 693
　　type II, 690f, 693–694
　C-shaped, 519f
　diastrophic dwarfism and, 708
　diastrophic dysplasia and, 219–221
　familial dysautonomia and, 280
　juvenile osteoporosis and, 709–710, 710f
　lumbar, types of, 518f
　Marfan syndrome and, 708–709, 708f
　metatropic dysplasia and, 215
　mucopolysaccharidosis and, 708
　myelomeningocele and, 518–520
　neurofibromatosis and, 709
　postlaminectomy, 699–703, 702–703f, 760, 762f
　posttraumatic, 709
　postural, 689–690
　pseudoachondroplasia and, 705–708
　radiation, 704–705, 706f
　Scheuermann, 694–699, 695f
　　lower thoracic, 701f
　spinal disorders resulting in, 689t
　spondyloepiphyseal dysplasia congenita and, 708
　spondylolisthesis and, 728–729
　S-shaped, 519–520
　structural, thoracic hump of, 68f
　thoracic, 694–699, 695f
　　secondary to Scheuermann disease, 700f
　thoracolumbar, achondroplasia and, 210–211
　treatment of, 519–521f
　tuberculosis and, 709

L
Lachman test, 82
Laminectomy
　cervical spine deformity and, 760, 762f
　kyphosis and, 699–703, 702–703f
Laminography, scoliosis and, 632
Laminoplasty, postlaminectomy kyphosis and, 703
Langer-Giedion syndrome, 122, 290
Langerhans cell histiocytosis, 363–369, 448
　criteria of organ dysfunction in, 364t
Larsen-Johansson disease, 1064–1065
　young athlete and, 1190–1191, 1190f
Larsen syndrome, 242–244, 243–244f, 265–267, 265–267f
Lateral clavicle, fracture of, 1237, 1237f
Lateral condylar fracture, 1247–1251, 1249–1251f
　classification of, 1249f

Lateral condyle, nonunion of, 1251f
Lateral meniscus, discoid, 1067–1069, 1068f
Lateral pillar classification, 971f
Lateral retinacular release, patellofemoral pain syndrome and, 1214
Latex hypersensitivity, myelomeningocele and, 509
Law, child abuse and, 1331–1332
Lead poisoning, 163
 radiograph of knee in, 163f
Leg. *See also* Leg-length discrepancy; Lower extremity
 growth of
  inhibition of, 858–861
  patterns of, 862
  stimulation of, 861–862
Legg-Calve-Perthes syndrome, 951–983
 abduction orthosis in, 980f
 Catterall group 1 disease, 959f
 Catterall group 2 disease, 969f
 Catterall group 3 disease, 961f, 965f, 975f
 Catterall group 4 disease, 960f, 962–964f, 973f, 976–977f, 983f
 clinical presentation in, 973
 deformity in
  pathogenesis of, 958–961
  patterns of, 961–963
 differential diagnosis in, 974–977, 974t
 epidemiology and etiology of, 952–954
 imaging in, 974
 lateral pillar classification in 970t, 971f
 left hip, 955f
 long-term follow-up results in, 965–968, 966–967f
 Mose sphericity scale and, 967f
 natural history of, 963–973
 ossific nucleus in, 960f
 pathogenesis of, 954–963
 patient management in, 978–979
 physical examination in, 973–974
 prognostic factors in, 968–973, 968t
 radiographic stages in, 956–958
 results of untreated, 963t
 Stulberg classification of, 968t
 total head involvement in, 964f
 transient synovitis of hip and, 1036
 treatment of, 977–983, 978t
  late-presenting case and, 982–983
  nonoperative, 979–980
  surgical, 980–982
Legg-Perthes disease, 234
Leg length
 as function of skeletal age, 852t, 853–854f
 measurement of, 863–864, 863f
 radiologic assessment of, 864–867, 865–866f
Leg-length discrepancy, 849–891
 arithmetic method in, 869f, 871–872
 center-edge angle and, 851f
 classification of causes of, 857t
 corticotomy in, 886, 886f
 data analysis in, 868–875
 distraction epiphysiolysis in, 883
 effects of, 850–853
 epiphyseodesis in, 877–879, 878f
 etiology of, 856–862
 femoral shortening in, 879–880
 growth and, 853–856, 854–856f
 growth remaining method in, 870f, 872
 hamartomatous disorders and, 313
 Ilizarov technique in, 883, 885f
 intramedullary rod in, 883–886

 leg lengthening in, 880–891
 lengthening hardware in, 888–891
 lumbar scoliosis and, 67f
 measuring, 64f
 metaphyseal lengthening in, 887f
 Orthofix technique in, 883, 885f
 patient assessment in, 862–868
 pediatric orthopaedic examination and, 63–65
 posteromedial bowing of tibia and, 1070–1071
 prosthetic fitting in, 876–877
 scoliosis and, 636–636, 636f
 shoe lift in, 876
 straight-line graph method in, 871f, 872–874, 873f
 treatment in, 875–891
 Wagner technique in, 882, 882–884f
Leg lengthening, leg-length discrepancy and, 880–891
Letterer-Siwe disease, 363, 448
Leukemia, 380–383, 381–382f
 acute lymphoblastic, diagnosis of, 381t
 acute lymphocytic, 382f
 acute myelogenous, 382f
 cervical spine and, 774
 differential diagnosis of, 402
 osteomyelitis and, 594
 periosteal reaction and, 175t
Ligamentous instability, evaluation of, 81–82
Limb. *See also* Lower extremity; Upper extremity
 development of, timeline of, 17f
 developmental sequence of, 15f
 formation of, 14–15
 lengths of, assessing, 63–65
 movement of, biomechanical analysis of, 112
 precursors of, 13–14
 rotation of, 15–16
Limb anomalies, congenital, 1137–1142
 chance of recurrence in, 1139–1140
 classification of, 1138f
 etiology of, 1138–1139
 timing of, 1139
Limb bud, 14
Limb deficiency, 1137–1177
 prosthetics for, 1166–1177
Limb-girdle muscular dystrophy, 549–550
Limb lengthening, proximal focal femoral deficiency and, 1149
Limb-salvage surgery, osteosarcoma and, 438
Linear tomography, bone and soft tissue tumors and, 428
Lipomeningocele, 504
Little disease, 94f
Little-finger polydactyly, 819–821, 820f
Liver, vitamin D conversion in, 144f
Loading response, 99f
Lobstein disease, 164
Lobster claw, 797
Locus minoris resistentiae, 581
Longitudinal deficiency, 785f, 796–801
Lordosis
 cerebral palsy and, 475
 Larsen syndrome and, 243
 lumbar, 687–689
 myelomeningocele and, 512–518
 thoracic, 67f
Lower extremity, 1047–1072
 acquired amputations and, 1158–1164
 angular configuration of, assessment from behind, 80f

 bone scan of, 592f
 bowlegs. *See* Bowlegs
 deficiencies of, 1142–1158
 deformity of, angular, 891–896, 894–896f
 idiopathic toe walking, 1071–1072
 in-toeing. *See* In-toeing
 knee disorders, 1061–1069
 knock-knees. *See* Knock-knees
 normal angular relations in, 892f
 normal muscle-firing patterns for, 487f
 out-toeing. *See* Out-toeing
 pediatric orthopaedic examination and, 79–84
 poliomyelitis and, 568
 prosthetics for, 1167–1174, 1167–1168f, 1171f
 soft tissue contractures of, spinal muscular atrophy and, 557
 thrombocytopenia with absent radius syndrome and, 371
 tibial disorders, 1069–1071
Lumbar kyphosis
 myelomeningocele and, 518
 types of, 518f
Lumbar level paraplegia, 511
Lumbar lordosis, 687–689
Lumbar paraplegia, 523–525
Lumbar scoliosis
 leg-length discrepancy and, 67f
 progressive, 515–517f
Lumbar spine
 kyphotic posture of, 69f
 spondylolisthesis and, 68f
Lyme arthritis, 615
Lyme disease, differential diagnosis of, 403
Lymphangiohemangioma, 309
Lymphangioma, 308–310, 309f
 differential diagnosis of, 311t
 limb length inequality and, 313
Lymphocytes, disorders of, 356–358
Lyon hypothesis, 127
Lysosomal storage disease, 127

M
Macrodactyly, 313–315, 314f, 821–822, 822f, 1128, 1129f
 pathology of, 314–315
 Proteus syndrome and, 260–261
Madelung deformity, 239–240, 240f, 825–826, 825f
Maffucci syndrome, 260, 308
 Klippel-Trenaunay syndrome and, 306
 malignany and, 440–441
Magnesium, parathyroid hormone and, 143
Magnetic resonance imaging (MRI), 25, 43–46
 biologic effect of, 27
 bone and joint infection and, 593
 bone and soft tissue tumors and, 429–430
 congenital kyphosis and, 691–692, 692f
 developmental dysplasia of hip and, 916
 growth plate damage in knee and, 46f
 osteochondritis dissecans and, 1067
 scoliosis and, 632
 slipped capital femoral epiphysis and, 1000
 spondylolysis/spondylolisthesis and, 722
 tarsal coalition and, 1096
 tethered cord and, 44f
 tibial osteosarcoma and, 45f

Malignancy
  neurofibromatosis and, 259–260
  osteomyelitis and, 594–595
  somatic mosaicism and, 129
Malignant fibrous histiocytoma, 457–459, 458f
Mallet finger, 829–830, 830f
Mandible, Caffey disease and, 176f
Manipulation, spastic diplegia and, 485
Maquet procedure, 1220f, 1221
Marble bone disease, 172
Marfan syndrome, 122, 123, 129, 179–180, 180f
  kyphotic deformity and, 708–709, 708f
Maroteaux-Lamy syndrome, 127
  kyphotic deformity and, 708
McCune-Albright syndrome, 129
McMurray sign, 81
Measles, German. See Rubella
Meclofenemate sodium, juvenile rheumatoid arthritis and, 408t
MED. See Multiple epiphyseal dysplasia
Medial clavicle, fracture of, 1237
Medial epicondyle fracture, 1251–1252, 1252f
Medial epicondyle injury, 1197
Medial tibial stress syndrome, 1193
Medical neglect, child abuse and, 1331
Medrol. See Methylprednisolone
Megaspondylodysplasia, 261
Melorheostosis, 319–320, 320f
Meningocele, 504
Meniscal tears, 1205–1206
Meniscus
  lateral, discoid, 1067–1069, 1068f
  vascularity of, 1206f
Menkes kinky hair syndrome, periosteal reaction and, 174t
Mental retardation, cerebral palsy and, 472
6-Mercaptopurine, Langerhans cell histiocytosis and, 368
Metabolic abnormalities, 137–190
Metabolic bone disease, 137
Metabolic myopathies, 554
Metabolism, inborn errors of, autosomal recessive disease and, 127
Metacarpal fracture, 836–837, 837f
Metacarpophalangeal deformity, 795–796
Metacarpophalangeal joint injury, 837–840, 838f
Metaphyseal chondrodysplasia, 237–239, 238f
Metaphyseal fracture, 1320–1321f
  child abuse and, 1319–1321
Metatarsal fracture, 1307–1310, 1309f
Metatarsalgia, juvenile rheumatoid arthritis and, 417
Metatarsus adductus, 1078–1081, 1079–1080f, 1082f
Metatropic dysplasia, 214–216, 215f
Methicillin, bone and joint infection and, 596, 597t
Methotrexate
  juvenile rheumatoid arthritis and, 409
  Langerhans cell histiocytosis and, 368
  musculoskeletal tumors and, 462
Methylprednisolone
  postoperative radiculopathy and, 733
  sickle cell disease and, 349
  unicameral bone cysts and, 449
Meyerding grading system, spondylolisthesis and, 722
Micrognathia, thrombocytopenia with absent radius syndrome and, 371

Middle phalanx fracture, 832, 833f
Midtarsal osteotomy, hereditary motor sensory neuropathies and, 563
Milk alkali syndrome, 141
Milwaukee brace, 641, 643f, 648–652, 648f, 672–673, 698, 699f, 705
Mineralization, defects in, 164
Missense mutation, 119
Mitchell osteotomy, adolescent bunion and, 1118
Mitosis, 117–118
Mixed cerebral palsy, 471
Molecular embryology, 2–5
Monocyte-macrophage system, disorders of, 358–369
Monteggia-equivalent lesion, 1269f
Monteggia lesion, 1264–1268, 1267–1268f
Moro response, 56, 58
  testing, 56f
Morphogenesis, 1–2
  errors in, schema illustrating, 55f
  homeotic genes in, 3–4
Morquio syndrome, 127, 224, 292–294, 293f
  genu valgum and, 1061
  kyphotic deformity and, 708
Mosaicism, 129–130
  germline, 129–130
  somatic, 129
  Turner syndrome and, 284
Mose sphericity scale, 967f
Motion analysis, instrumented, 94–95
Motor sensory neuropathies
  classification of, 561t
  hereditary, 561–565, 562f
MRI. See Magnetic resonance imaging
mRNA splicing, mutations of, 120
Mucopolysaccharidosis, 291–294, 291t, 292f
  kyphotic deformity and, 708
Multifactorial disorders, 131
Multifactorial inheritance, 506
Multiple congenital amputation, 1164–1166, 1165f
Multiple congenital contracture syndromes, 262
Multiple epiphyseal dysplasia (MED), 232–235, 233–234f
Multiple pterygia syndrome, 269–271, 270–271f
Muscle biopsy
  Duchenne muscular dystrophy and, 542
  neuromuscular disorders and, 539
Muscle hemorrhage, hemophilia and, 377–378, 378f
Muscle herniation, young athlete and, 1194
Muscle spasm, Friedreich ataxia and, 561
Muscular atrophy, spinal, 555–558, 559f
Muscular dystrophy, 540–555
  autosomal dominant, 550–551
  autosomal recessive, 549–550
  Becker, 547–549, 548f
    DMD gene in, 120
    kyphotic deformity and, 708
  classification of, 540t
  congenital, 554–555f, 555
  distal, 551
  Duchenne, 2, 58, 128, 540–547, 541f, 546–547f
    dystrophin gene in, 255
  Emery-Dreifuss, 549
  fascioscapulohumeral, 550–551
  infantile, 550

  Gower, 551
  limb-girdle, 549–550
  ocular, 551
  oculopharyngeal, 551
  sex-linked, 540–549
Muscular torticollis, congenital, 751–754
Musculoskeletal tumors, chemotherapy for, 462–463
Mutation
  detection of, 120–121
  missense, 119
  molecular basis of, 119–121
  mRNA splicing, 120
  nonsense, 119
  point, 119
  promoter, 119
Myelodysplasia, 503
  hip dislocations in newborns and, 911
  instrumented motion analysis and, 95
Myelography, 32
  scoliosis and, 632
Myelomeningocele, 11f, 19, 503–533
  Arnold-Chiari deformity and, 508
  calcaneus deformity and, 529–530
  cavus deformity and, 530–531
  Charcot arthropathy and, 531–532
  classification and pathology of, 503–505
  clubfoot and, 1104
  congenital scoliosis and, 518
  cross section of, 504f
  developmental sequence and, 509–510
  foot and, 527–532
  genetics, etiology, prenatal diagnosis of, 506–507
  hip and, 521, 521f
  hydrocephaly and, 507–508
  knee and, 525–527, 525–526f
  kyphosis and, 518–520
  latex hypersensitivity and, 509
  natural history of, 507–509
  neurologic abnormality in, 505–506
  orthotic devices and, 532–533
  position of infant after closure of spine, 522f
  scoliosis and lordosis and, 512–518
  spine deformity in, 511–520
  talipes equinovarus and, 527–529
  tethered cord syndrome and, 508–509
  treatment of, 510–533
  valgus deformity and, 530
Myopathy
  centronuclear, 553–554
  congenital, 552–554
  metabolic, 554
  nemaline, 553
  rod-body, 553
Myosin, 4
Myositis, pseudomalignant, 179
Myositis ossificans, 334–337, 336f
Myositis ossificans circumscripta, 178–179
Myositis ossificans traumatica, 179
Myotome, 8–9, 11f
Myotonia, 551–552
Myotonia congenita, 552
Myotonic dystrophy, 551–552
  congenital, 552
  genomic imprinting in, 130
  transmission of, parental sex bias in, 129

N
Nafcillin, bone and joint infection and, 597t
Nail bed, injury to, 830, 831f

Nail-patella syndrome, 277–279, 278f
Naproxen
  juvenile rheumatoid arthritis and, 408t
  young athlete and, 1185
Navicular, dorsal subluxation of, 1116f
Neck pain, intervertebral disc calcification and, 771
Neck-righting reflex, 58, 59f
Nemaline myopathy, 553
Neonatal diagnosis, 133–134
Neonate. See Newborn
Neoplasm, osteomyelitis and, 594–595
Nerve biopsy, neuromuscular disorders and, 539
Nerve conduction, neuromuscular disorders and, 539
Neural tube, 9–10, 10f
Neural tube defects, 503
  inheritance of, 506–507
Neurilemoma, 457–458, 457f
Neuroblastoma
  metastatic
    cervical spine and, 774
  periosteal reaction and, 175t
Neurofibroma, 457–458
  in neurofibromatosis, 257, 257f
Neurofibromatosis (NF), 256–260
  cervical kyphosis and, 761f
  cervical spine and, 762–763
  congenital pseudoarthrosis of fibula and, 329
  congenital pseudoarthrosis of tibia and, 323
  cutaneous markings in, 256–257, 256f
  differential diagnosis of, 311t
  Klippel-Trenaunay syndrome and, 306
  kyphotic deformity and, 709
  limb length inequality and, 313
  neurofibroma in, 257, 257f
  orthopaedic manifestations in, 258–260, 258–261f
  rickets and, 153
Neurofibromatosis 1, 123
  autosomal dominance and, 126
  genomic imprinting in, 130
Neurogenesis, 8
Neurologic maturation, in early childhood, 57–59
Neuromuscular development, 15
Neuromuscular disorders, 537–570
  diagnostic studies and, 538–540
  history and, 537–538
  physical examination and, 538
Neuromuscular integration, 9–17
Neuropathy, motor sensory
  classification of, 561t
  hereditary, 561–565
Neurulation, 6t, 8
Newborn
  bone and joint infection in, 605–607
  hip dislocation in, 907–908
    treatment of, 922–925
  normal development of, 55–57
  physiologic periosteal reaction of, characteristics of, 174t
NF. See Neurofibromatosis
Niemann-Pick disease, 363
Night splints, tibial torsion and, 1051
NOF. See Nonossifying fibroma
Nonossifying fibroma (NOF), 444–446, 445f
Nonsense mutation, 119
Nonsteroidal antiinflammatory drugs (NSAIDs)
  juvenile rheumatoid arthritis and, 408, 408t
  progressive diaphyseal dysplasia and, 319
  sports medicine and, 1184–1185
  transient synovitis of hip and, 1037
Noonan syndrome, 285
Normal variant short statute (NVSS), 184–185
Notochord, 9–10
NSAIDS. See Nonsteroidal antiinflammatory drugs
Nutrition
  growth plate function and, 140
  young athlete and, 1182
NVSS. See Normal variant short stature

O
Ober test, 78, 78f, 1194, 1195f
Obesity
  infantile tibia vara and, 1055–1056
  slipped capital femoral epiphysis and, 993–995
Oblique osteotomy, tibia vara and, 1057
Observational gait analysis, 110–112
  spastic diplegia and, 487
  standardized form for, 111f
Obstetric brachial plexus injury, 826–828
Occipital complex, fractures and ligamentous injuries of, 764–765
Occipitoatlantal instability, nontraumatic, 758–759
Occipitoaxioatlas complex, 739–740
Occupational therapy, juvenile rheumatoid arthritis and, 409
Ocular-auricular-vertebral dysplasia, 288
Ocular dysfunction, torticollis and, 754
Ocular muscular dystrophy, 551
Oculopharyngeal muscular distrophy, 551
Odontoid, fractures of, 765, 766f
Odontoid hypoplasia, spondyloepiphyseal dysplasia congenita and, 226
Olecranon apophysitis, young athlete and, 1191
Olecranon fractures, 1254–1255, 1256–1257f
Ollier disease, secondary chondrosarcoma and, 440
Open fracture, 1298
  classification of, 1298t
Ophthalmoplegia, external, progressive, 551
Organogenesis, 6t, 8–9
Orofaciodigital syndrome, congenital pseudoarthrosis of tibia and, 323
Orthofix technique, leg-length discrepancy and, 883, 885f
Orthopaedic examination, pediatric, 51–89
  patient profile chart in, 91
Orthopaedic surgeon
  child abuse and, 1315–1332
  preparation for court testimony in child abuse, 1331–1332
Orthopaedic syndromes, 255–294. See also specific syndrome
Orthoradiography, 865f, 866
Orthosis, Friedreich ataxia and, 560
Orthotic devices
  adolescent idiopathic scoliosis and, 648–651, 648–649f
  congenital scoliosis and, 672–673
  Duchenne muscular dystrophy and, 543–544
  Legg-Calve-Perthes syndrome and, 979–980, 980f
  myelomeningocele and, 532–533
  spastic diplegia and, 485–486
  spinal muscular atrophy and, 557–558
Ortolani maneuver, 76
Ortolani sign, 903, 910
Os acetabuli, 907f
Osgood-Schlatter disease, 1063–1064
  young athlete and, 1188–1190, 1189f
Osler-Weber-Rendu, 308
Os odontoideum
  cervical spine and, 755–756
  spondyloepiphyseal dysplasia congenita and, 226
Ossification
  ectopic, renal osteodystrophy and, 154
  endochondral, 18–19
  primary centers of, 19f, 137
  soft tissue, 178–179
Ossifying fibroma, 447–448, 447f
Osteitis fibrosa, renal osteodystrophy and, 154
Osteitis fibrosa cystica disseminata, 189
Osteoarthritis
  cerebral palsy and, 481–482
  Kniest dysplasia and, 224
  slipped capital femoral epiphysis and, 1017
Osteoarthropathy, hypertrophic, periosteal reaction and, 175t
Osteoblast, 138
Osteoblastoma, 435
  cervical spine and, 773
Osteochondritis dissecans, 1065–1067, 1066f
  Legg-Calve-Perthes syndrome and, 982
Osteochondrodysplasias, 203–244
  achondroplasia, 119, 122, 125–126, 205–213, 206–209f, 211f
  chondrodysplasia punctata, 235–237, 236f
  chondroectodermal dysplasia, 216–218, 216–217f
  classification of, 250–254
  cleidocranial dysplasia, 240–242, 241–242f
  diastrophic dysplasia, 218–222, 218f, 220–221f
  dyschondrosteosis, 239–240, 240f
  hypochondroplasia, 126, 213–214, 214f
  Kniest dysplasia, 222–224, 223f
  Larsen syndrome, 242–244, 243–244f
  metaphyseal chondrodysplasia, 237–239, 238f
  metatropic dysplasia, 214–216, 215f
  multiple epiphyseal dysplasia, 232–235, 233–234f
  pseudoachondroplastic dysplasia, 229–232, 229–231f
  spondyloepiphyseal dysplasia congenita, 224–227, 225–227f
  spondyloepiphyseal dysplasia tarda, 227–229, 228f
Osteochondroma, cervical spine and, 773
Osteochondroses, 337–338, 338f, 1101–1103, 1102–1103f
  examples by regions, 337t
Osteoclast, 138
Osteocyte, 138
Osteofibrous dysplasia, 447–448, 447f

Osteogenesis imperfecta, 164–170
    autosomal dominance and, 123–125
    classification of, 166–169, 166t
    clinical manifestations of, 165–166
    management of, 169–170
    missense mutation in, 119
    mRNA splicing mutation in, 120
    nonsense mutation in, 119
    type I 166, 166t, 167f
    type I collagen chains in, 124f
    type II 166, 166t, 167f
    type III 166, 166t, 168f
    type IV 166, 166t, 168f
Osteoid osteoma, 433–435, 434f
    cervical spine and, 773–774
    stress fracture and, 1186
Osteomalacia, 146–154
    causes of, 151t
Osteomalacia congenita, 165
Osteomyelitis
    definition of, 579–580
    diagnosis of, 586–594
        differential, 594–595
    epidemiology of, 580
    etiology of, 580–581
    Gaucher disease and, 361
    growth of leg and, 860
    hematogenous, 586f
        acute, 580
    imaging of, 37f
    infective, periosteal reaction and, 174t
    multifocal, chronic recurrent, 609–611, 610f
    pathophysiology of, 581–585
    pyogenic, cervical spine and, 772
    sickle cell disease and, 349–350, 349f, 607–609, 608f
    subacute, 611–612, 612f
        imaging of, 34f
    treatment of, 596–601
    vertebral, 601–603
Osteonecrosis
    femoral head, sickle cell disease and, 351, 351t
    Gaucher disease and, 362, 362f
    humeral head, sickle cell disease and, 351–352, 352t
    slipped capital femoral epiphysis and, 1017–1018, 1018f
Osteopathia striata, 321–322, 322f
Osteopenia, Gaucher disease and, 360
Osteopetrosis, 172–174, 173f
Osteopithia condensans disseminata, 320
Osteoplasty, slipped capital femoral epiphysis and, 1017
Osteopoikilosis, 320–321, 321f
Osteoporosis
    disuse, 163
    juvenile
        idiopathic, 170–172, 171f
            kyphotic deformity and, 709–710, 710f
            Scheuermann kyphosis and, 695–696
        steroid-induced, 189f
        Turner syndrome and, 285
Osteoporosis fetalis, 165
Osteosarcoma, 435–439
    classic high-grade, 436–438, 436–437f
    juxtacortical, 438–439, 439f
    tibial, imaging of, 35f, 45f
Osteosclerosis, renal osteodystrophy and, 154
Osteosclerosis fragilis generalisata, 172
Osteotomy
    adolescent bunion and, 1118

cavus and, 1122–1123
developmental coxa vara and, 1029–1030
hereditary motor sensory neuropathies and, 563
juvenile rheumatoid arthritis and, 412
Legg-Calve-Perthes syndrome and, 981–982
poliomyelitis and, 567
proximal femoral, methods of, 1029f
rotational, radioulnar synostosis and, 804f
rotational abnormalities and, 1051–1052
slipped capital femoral epiphysis and, 1011–1015, 1013–1015f
tarsal coalition and, 1098–1099
tibia vara and, 1057
Otitis media, achondroplastic children and, 208
Out-toeing, 85, 1047–1054
    clinical features of, 1048–1049, 1049
    complications of, 1052–1054
    etiology of, 1048
    imaging and, 1049–1050
    natural history of, 1050–1051
    treatment of, 1051–1052
        nonsurgical, 1051
        surgical, 1051–1052
Overriding fifth toe, 1126–1127, 1126f
Overuse syndromes, 1185–1197
Oxacillin, bone and joint infection and, 596, 597t

P
Pain
    back
        Gaucher disease and, 361–362
        spinal infection and, 601
    chronic recurrent multifocal osteomyelitis and, 609
    heel, 1119–1120
        differential diagnosis of, 1120t
    idiopathic chondrolysis of hip and, 1038
    juvenile osteoporosis and, 710
    juvenile rheumatoid arthritis and, 404–405
    knee, anterior, 1209–1215
    musculoskeletal tumors and, 425
    neck, intervertebral disc calcification and, 771
    osteoid osteoma and, 434
    pediatric orthopaedic examination and, 52–53
    phantom, amputation and, 1161
    Scheuermann disease and, 696
    shin, young athlete and, 1192–1194
    spondylolisthesis and, 719
    spondylolysis and, 719
    tethered cord syndrome and, 509
Palmarplantar pustulosis, 609
Palsy
    birth, 828–828, 827f
    Erb, 827f
Pancytopenia, Fanconi anemia and, 347
Panhypopituitarism, 186f
Panner disease, 338f, 1195–1196
Parachute reflex, 59, 59f
Paralysis, growth of leg and, 860–861
Paraplegia
    level of, scoliosis and, 512f
    lumbar, 523–525
    lumbar level, 511

sacral level, 511
spondyloepiphyseal dysplasia congenita and, 226
thoracic level, 511, 522–523
    scoliosis and, 512
Paraspinal muscles, idiopathic scoliosis and, 639
Parathyroid disorders, 161–162
Parathyroid hormone (PTH)
    calcium transport in gut cell and, 142f
    physiology of, 140
Parkes-Webber syndrome, Klippel-Trenaunay syndrome and, 306
Paroxysmal torticollis of infancy, 754
Patella
    bipartite, 1065
    dislocation of, 1290–1292
        acute, 1217–1218
        congenital, 1062–1063
        Galeazzi procedure and, 1219f
        recurrent, 1218–1221, 1219t
        Roux-Goldthwait procedure and, 1219f
    dorsal defects of, 1215–1216, 1215f
    fracture of, 1290, 1291f
    mobility of, testing, 82–83
Patellofemoral disorders, young athlete and, 1208–1221
Patellofemoral joint
    anatomy and biomechanics of, 1208–1209, 1210f
    evaluating, 1211f
    quadriceps strengthening technique and, 1213f
    rehabilitating, 1212f
    testing, 83
Patellofemoral pain syndrome, 1209–1215
Pathologic spondylolisthesis, 717
Pavlik harness, 922f, 923–925
Pectus deformities, Marfan syndrome and, 179
Pediatric foot, 1077–1131
    accessory navicular, 1099–1101, 1100f
    adolescent bunion, 1116–1119, 1117–1118f
    calcaneocavus, 1123–1124, 1124f
    cavus, 1120–1123, 1121–1123f
    cleft foot, 1127–1128, 1128f
    congenital calcaneovalgus foot, 1083–1085, 1084f
    congenital clubfoot, 1103–1116, 1105–1106f
    congenital hallux varus, 1124–1125, 1124f
    congenital vertical talus, 1089–1093, 1090–1091f
    curly toes, 1125–1126, 1125f
    flexible flatfoot, 1085–1089, 1086–1087f
    heel pain, 1119–1120
    idiopathic toe walking, 1127
    ingrown toenails, 1129–1131
    macrodactyly, 1128, 1129f
    metatarsus adductus, 1078–1081, 1079–1080f, 1082f
    normal alignment in, 1078
    osteochondroses, 1101–1103, 1102–1103f
    overriding fifth toe, 1126–1127, 1126f
    polydactyly, 1128–1129, 1130f
    radiography and, 1078
    skewfoot, 1081–1083, 1083f, 1084f
    subungual exostosis, 1131
    tailor bunionette, 1119
    tarsal coalition, 1093–1099, 1095f

Pediatric hand
  carpal injury, 840
  distal phalanx fracture, 830, 831f
  flexor digitorum profundus avulsion, 830–831, 832f
  intraarticular fractures, 834, 834f
  mallet finger, 829–830, 830f
  metacarpal fractures, 836–837, 837f
  metacarpophalangeal joint injury, 837–840, 838f
  middle phalanx fractures, 832, 833f
  nail bed injury, 830, 831f
  nail beds in, 829f
  phalangeal neck fractures, 831–832, 833f
  proximal interphalangeal joint injury, 837–840, 838f
  proximal phalanx shaft fractures, 834–836, 835f
  reverse mallet finger fracture, 830–831, 832f
  supracondylar fractures, 831–832, 833f
  trauma to, 828–840
  zone of hypertrophy and, 828f
Pediatric orthopaedic examination, 51–89
  patient profile chart in, 91
Pelvis
  Charcot-Marie-Tooth disease and, 564f
  cleidocranial dysplasia and, 241–242
  computed tomography and, 33f
  Down syndrome and, 272
  Ewing sarcoma of, 454
  fracture of, 1268–1271, 1271f
    avulsion, 1207–1208, 1207f
  infection of, 603–605, 605f
  juvenile osteoporosis and, 171f
  motion during gait, 850f
  oblique, scoliosis and, 852f
  osteogenesis imperfecta and, 165
  poliomyelitis and, 569f
  renal osteodystrophic changes in, 156f, 157f
Penetrance, 122
Penicillin, bone and joint infection and, 596
Penicillin G, bone and joint infection and, 597t
Penicillin V, bone and joint infection and, 597t
Periosteal chondroma, 444, 444f
Periosteal reaction, 174–176
  causes of, 174–175t
Periosteum, fracture healing and, 1230
Periostitis, young athlete and, 1193
Peroneal nerve compression, superficial, young athlete and, 1194
Peroneal spastic flatfoot, 1094–1095
Pes cavovarus, Friedreich ataxia and, 560
Pes planovalgus, 88
Pes planus, 1087
  calcaneal lengthening and, 1088–1089
Pes valgus, 1087
Pfeiffer syndrome, cervical spine anomalies and, 761
PFFD. See Proximal focal femoral deficiency
Phalangeal neck fracture, 831–832, 833f
Phantom pain, amputation and, 1161
Phemister technique, 787f
Phenylketonuria, 127
Phocomelia
  bilateral, 797f
  thalidomide and, 9, 783, 796

Phosphate
  calcium transport system and, 142
  kinetics of, 145f
Phosphate deficiency, rickets and, 150
Phosphate diabetes, vitamin D-resistant rickets and, 152–153
Phosphorus, absorption of, 145
Phosphorus homeostasis, 141–146
Physeal arrest, 1233–1235, 1234f
Physeal bar resection, 1235f
Physeal fracture, 1232–1233, 1232f, 1320f
  child abuse and, 1319
Physeal injuries, 1231–1235
  repetitive, 1187–1188
Physeal morphology, variations in, 21f
Physical development, in early childhood, 59–61
Physical therapy
  Duchenne muscular dystrophy and, 543
  Emery-Dreifuss muscular dystrophy and, 549
  juvenile rheumatoid arthritis and, 409
  spastic diplegia and, 483–485
Physiologic bowing, 1055
Physiologic knock-knees, 1060
Pigmented villonodular synovitis (PVNS), 461–462
  differential diagnosis of, 403
  idiopathic chondrolysis of hip and, 1038
Piroxicam, juvenile rheumatoid arthritis and, 408t
Plain film, 28–30, 29f
  bone and joint infection and, 590, 590–591f, 593f
  bone and soft tissue tumors and, 426–427
Plantar-medial release, hereditary motor sensory neuropathies and, 563
Plantar release, hereditary motor sensory neuropathies and, 563
Pleomorphic rhabdomyosarcoma, 458
Plica syndrome, 1216–1217, 1216f
PMMA. See Polymethyl methacrylate
Point mutation, 119
Poisoning, lead, 163
  radiograph of knee in, 163f
Poland syndrome, 54
Poliomyelitis, 565–570
  calcaenocavus and, 1123
  infantile, 19
Politeus tendinitis, 1192, 1192f
Polyarteritis nodosa, differential diagnosis of, 404
Polyarticular arthropathy, Down syndrome and, 274
Polydactyly, 54, 1128–1129, 1130f
  central, 819, 819f
  postaxial, 819–821, 820f
  preaxial, 815–817, 816–817f
Polymethyl methacrylate (PMMA), giant cell tumor of bone and, 453
Polyostotic fibrous dysplasia, 319
Polysyndactyly, 819, 819f
Popliteal angle, 69f
Popliteal cyst, 1065
Popliteal pterygium syndrome, 270, 271f
Port wine stain, 307
Postaxial polydactyly, 819–821, 820f
Posterior cruciate ligament injuries, 1205
Postlaminectomy kyphosis, 699–703, 702–703f
Postpoliomyelitis syndrome, 570

Postural kyphosis, 689–690
Postural scoliosis, 635
Posture, spondylolysis and, 720
Prader-Willi syndrome, 188, 285–286, 286f
  genomic imprinting in, 130
Preaxial polydactyly, 815–817, 816–817f
Prednisolone, Langerhans cell histiocytosis and, 367
Prednisone, progressive diaphyseal dysplasia and, 319
Prenatal counseling, 134
Prenatal diagnosis, 133–134
  neural tube defects and, 506–507
Primary ossification center, 19f
Procaine amide, myotonia congenita and, 552
Progeria, 283–284, 283f
Programmed cell death, 15
Progressive diaphyseal dysplasia, 317–319, 318f
Progressive external ophthalmoplegia, 551
Promoter mutation, 119
Pronation, 1078t
  evaluation of, 72f
  of foot, 85f
    effect on ankle motion, 88f
Prostaglandin E2, bone formation and, 140
Prosthetic fitting, leg-length discrepancy and, 876–877
Prosthetics
  acquired amputation and, 1160f
  below-knee, 1172–1173
  fibular deficiency and, 1172
  foot, 1170
    partial, 1173
  limb deficiency and, 1166–1177
  lower extremity, 1167–1174, 1167–1168f, 1171f
    bilateral, 1173
  proximal femoral deficiency and, 1151f
  proximal focal femoral deficiency and, 1145–1149, 1146–1147f
  tibial deficiency and, 1172
  upper extremity, 1174–1177, 1175–1177f
Proteins, posttranslational modification of, 119
Proteoglycan, 139
Proteus syndrome, 260–261, 262f
  differential diagnosis of, 311t
  Klippel-Trenaunay syndrome and, 306
  limb length inequality and, 313
Proximal femoral osteotomy, methods of, 1029f
Proximal femur, 906f
  arterial supply of, 1273f
  blood supply to, 954f
  in child, 956f
  focal deficiency of, 1142–1149
  fractures of, 1271–1277
    classification for, 1274f
  growth of, 905–906
  growth disturbance of
    classification of, 941f
    treatment of hip dysplasia and, 937–942, 939f
  stress fracture of, 1186
  variation of neck-shaft angle with age, 1024f
Proximal focal femoral deficiency (PFFD), 54, 1142–1149
  Aitken classification of, 1142, 1142f
  Aitken type A, 1143f
  Aitken type B, 1143f

Aitken type C, 1144f
Aitken type D, 1144f
  bilateral, 1149f
  femoral segment fusion in, 1148f
  Hamanishi classification of, 1144f
  knee arthrodesis for, 1146f
  knee walking and, 1145f
  prosthetics for, 1170–1172
  rotationplasty for, 1147, 1147f
  untreated, 1145f
Proximal humerus
  epiphysiolysis of, 1187–1188, 1187f
  fracture of, 1238–1240, 1239–1241f
Proximal interphalangeal joint
  injury to, 837–840, 838f
  intraarticular fracture of, 834, 834f
Proximal intertrochanteric osteotomy, rotational abnormalities and, 1052
Proximal phalanx shaft fracture, 834–836, 835f
Proximal radius fracture, 1253–1257
Proximal tibia
  fibrocartilaginous dysplasia of, 1059–1060
  fracture of, child abuse and, 1327f
  stress fracture of, 1069–1070
Proximal tibial metaphyseal fracture, 1294–1295, 1295f
Pseudarthrosis
  spinal fusion and, 702
  spondylolisthesis and, 733
Pseudoachondroplasia, kyphotic deformity and, 705–708
Pseudoachondroplastic dysplasia, 229–232, 229–231f
Pseudoarthrosis
  congenital of clavicle, 330–331, 330f
  congenital of fibula, 329–330, 330f
  congenital of tibia, 322–329, 323f, 329f
    classification of treatment of, 323t
    options for treatment of, 325f, 325t
  neurofibromatosis and, 259, 259–260f
Pseudohypoparathyroidism, 161–162
  radiograph of hand in, 162f
Pseudomalignant myositis, 179
Pseudoosteomyelitis, Niemann-Pick disease and, 363
Pseudosubluxation, cervical spine and, 742–743
Pseudotumor, hemophilia and, 379–380, 380f
Psoriatic arthritis, 398
Psychosocial development, in early childhood, 61
Pterygia syndromes, 269–271, 270–271f
PTH. See Parathyroid hormone
Puberty
  Scheuermann disease and, 696
  slipped capital femoral epiphysis and, 993
Pulmonary function testing, scoliosis and, 632–633
Pump bump, 1120
Puncture wounds, of foot, 612–615, 614f
Purpura fulminans, amputation and, 1159–1160, 1161f
PVNS. See Pigmented villonodular synovitis
Pyelography, scoliosis and, 632
Pyogenic osteomyelitis, cervical spine and, 772
Pyrazinamide, extrapulmonary tuberculosis and, 619

Q

Q angle, 82, 82f
Quadriceps contusion, 1206–1207
Quadriceps fibrosis, 1063
Quadriceps strengthening technique, 1213f
Quadriparesis, transient, cervical spine and, 767–769
Quadriplegia
  cerebral palsy and, 471
  instrumentation in Down syndrome and, 757
  metatropic dysplasia and, 215
  spastic
    hip dislocation in, 480f, 481
    management of, 473–482
Quengel cast antisubluxation hinge, 380f

R

Rachischisis, 8
Rachitic disease. See Rickets
Radial artery, anomalies of, 787f
Radial head
  dislocation of, 1256–1257, 1258f
    congenital, 804–805, 805f
  osteochondral lesions of, 1197
Radialization, Buck-Gramcko's method of, 792, 792f
Radial neck, fracture of, 1254, 1255f
Radial physis, distal, fracture of, 1264, 1266f
Radial ray, congenital deficiency of, differential diagnosis of, 790t
Radiation, teratogenicity and, 132
Radiation kyphosis, 704–705, 706f
Radiation therapy, Ewing sarcoma and, 453
Radiculopathy
  instrumentation in Down syndrome and, 757
  spondylolisthesis and, 733–735
Radioactive synovectomy, hemophilia and, 377
Radiography
  accessory navicular and, 1100, 1100f
  bone and joint infection and, 590, 590–591f, 593f
  bone and soft tissue tumors and, 426–427
  cavus and, 1121, 1122f
  cervical spine and, 741–744
  congenital vertical talus and, 1090–1091, 1091f
  with contrast, 31–32
  without contrast, 28–31
  developmental coxa vara and, 1027, 1028f
  developmental dysplasia of hip and, 913–916, 913–916f
  digital, 25, 30
  flexible flatfoot and, 1086
  Freiberg infarction and, 1102, 1103f
  idiopathic chondrolysis of hip and, 1038–1040, 1039f
  Koehler disease and, 1101, 1102f
  Legg-Calve-Perthes syndrome and, 956–958
  leg-length assessment and, 864–867, 865–866f
  pediatric foot and, 1078
  Scheuermann disease and, 697–698, 698f
  scoliosis and, 627–629, 628–629f
  skewfoot and, 1083, 1083f
  slipped capital femoral epiphysis and, 998–1000, 999–1001f
  spinal muscular atrophy and, 556
  spondylolysis/spondylolisthesis and, 721–722, 722f
  subacute osteomyelitis and, 34f
  tarsal coalition and, 1095–1096, 1095f
  tibia vara and, 1056, 1056f
  transient synovitis of hip and, 1034–1035
Radiohumeral fusion, 800f
Radionuclide scan, bone and soft tissue tumors and, 427–428
Radioulnar synostosis, 803f
Radius
  congenital deficiency of, 785–795, 786f, 785–795f
    bilateral, 790f
    centralization and, 791f
    differential diagnosis of, 790t
    incidence by type, 788t
    recurrent, 796f
    thumb deficiencies and, 789t
    unilateral, 791f
  contracture of, 795f
  cortical bone in, 582f
  distal
    epiphysiolysis of, 1188, 1188–1189f
    short, 787, 787f
  hypoplastic, 787, 788f
  partial absence of, 787–788, 788f
  proximal, fractures of, 1253–1257
  total absence of, 788, 789f
Range of motion, spasticity and, 62
Reduction, spondylolisthesis and, 728–730, 728–729f
Reflex neurovascular dystrophy, differential diagnosis of, 403
Reflex sympathetic dystrophy, 339–341
  algorithm for treatment of, 340f
  criteria for diagnosis and stages, 339t
Refsum disease, 561
Reiter syndrome, cardinal manifestations of, 398
Renal osteodystrophy, 141, 154–159
  chemical and bony changes in, mechanism of development of, 155f
  clinical manifestations of, 155–157, 156f
  management of, 157–159
  pathophysiology of, 154–155
Renal tubular acidosis, vitamin D-resistant rickets and, 152–153
Retinitis pigmentosa, 561
Retinoblastoma
  genomic imprinting in, 130
  periosteal reaction and, 175t
  somatic mosaicism and, 129
Retinoic acid, teratogenicity and, 132
Reverse mallet finger fracture, 830–831, 832f
Rhabdomyosarcoma, 458
  staging system for, 459t
Rheumatic fever
  diagnosis of
    differential, 402
    modified Jones criteria for, 403t
  septic arthritis and, 595–596
  synovial fluid analysis in, 588t
  synovitis and, 1034
Rheumatoid arthritis, juvenile. See Juvenile rheumatoid arthritis
Rheumatoid factor, juvenile rheumatoid arthritis and, 396

Rhizotomy, selective posterior, spastic diplegia and, 486–487
Rib, rickets and, 150f
Rib fracture, 1325f
 child abuse and, 1322
Rib-vertebral angle difference (RVAD), 627, 640
Rickets, 141, 146–154. See also Renal osteodystrophy
 anticonvulsant medication and, 153–154
 bowlegs and, 1057–1059
 causes of, 150, 151t
 chemical findings in, 151t
 clinical manifestations of, 147
 gastrointestinal, 150–152
 healing phase of, periosteal reaction and, 175t
 histologic changes in, 147–149, 148f
 hypophosphatasia and, 159–161
 hypophosphatemic, 128
  angular deformity in, 894f, 896f
 knock-knees and, 1060
 management of, 157–159
 radiographic changes in, 149–150, 149f
 unusual forms of, 153–154
 vitamin D-resistant, mechanism of development of, 152f
Ridge phenomenon, 911
Rifampicin, spinal tuberculosis and, 709
Rifampin, extrapulmonary tuberculosis and, 619
Riley-Day syndrome, 280
Risser sign, untreated adolescent idiopathic scoliosis and, 646t
RNA, transcription and, 118
Rocephin. See Ceftriaxone
Rod-body myopathy, 553
Rotational osteotomy, radioulnar synostosis and, 804f
Rotationplasty, proximal focal femoral deficiency and, 1147, 1147f
Roux-Goldthwait procedure, 1219f, 1220
Rubella
 organogenesis and, 9
 teratogenicity and, 132
Rubinstein-Taybi syndrome, 281–283, 281–282f
Running cycle, 106–107
Russell-Silver dwarfism, 284, 284f
 differential diagnosis of, 311t
 idiopathic hemihypotrophy and, 313
RVAD. See Rib-vertebral angle difference

S
Sacral agenesis, 7
Sacral level paraplegia, 511
Sacroiliac joint, infection of, 603–605
Sagittal rotation, measurement of, 722–723, 723f
Salter-Harris classification, 1232f, 1233
Sandifer syndrome, 754–755
Sanfilippo syndromes, 127
Saphenous nerve entrapment, 1215
Sarcoidosis, differential diagnosis of, 403
Sarcoma
 Ewing, 453–454, 454f
  cervical spine and, 774
  osteomyelitis and, 594
 soft tissue, revised AJC staging system for, 430t
 synovial cell, 460–461, 460f
SARDs. See Slow-acting remittive drugs
Scanography, 866, 866f

Scapula, fracture of, 1238
Scapular winging, 71, 71f
SCFE. See Slipped capital femoral epiphysis
Scheie syndrome, 127
Scheuermann disease, 140, 694–699, 695f
 kyphotic deformity in, 698f
 lower thoracic, 701f
 thoracic kyphosis secondary to, 700f
Schwachman-Diamond syndrome, 355
Schwannoma, 457–458, 457f
Scintigraphy, 25, 34–39
 idiopathic chondrolysis of hip and, 1039–1040, 1040f
 osteomyelitis and, 37f
 septic arthritis and, 37f
 subacute osteomyelitis and, 34f
SCIWORA. See Spinal cord injury without radiographic abnormality
Sclerotome, 8–9, 11f
Scoliometer, 67f
Scoliosis, 29, 625–679
 adult sequelae of untreated, 633–635, 634–635f
 anomalies causing, 667f
 arthrogryposis multiplex congenita and, 263
 Becker muscular dystrophy and, 547
 Beckwith-Wiedemann syndrome and, 287
 cerebral palsy and, 476–477
 chondrodysplasia punctata and, 237
 congenital, 518, 667–679
  bilateral talipes equinovarus and, 672f
  hemivertebra in, 668–669, 678f
  left lumbar, 670f
  left thoracic, 676f
  progressive, 674f
  progressive thoracolumbar, 677f
  right, 669f
  right thoracic, 671f, 675f
  right upper thoracic, 668f
 curve evaluation in, 629–631, 630–631f
 curve patterns of thoracic curves in, 653t
 curve rotation in, 630–631
 diastrophic dysplasia and, 219–221
 Down syndrome and, 272
 Duchenne muscular dystrophy and, 545
 familial dysautonomia and, 280–281
 Freeman-Sheldon syndrome and, 268
 Friedreich ataxia and, 560
 Goldenhar syndrome and, 289–290
 hereditary motor sensory neuropathies and, 564
 hysterical, 636, 637f
 idiopathic, 636–667
  adolescent, 638–639, 644–667
  double, 656–657f
  double thoracic, 662f
  infantile, 637–638, 640–642, 641f
  juvenile, 642–644, 643f
  left lumbar, 664f
  left thoracic, 647–648
  presentation in, 639–640
  progressive left lumbar, 660–661f
  progressive thoracolumbar, 659f
  right rib hump of, 67f
  right thoracic, 645–646f, 650f, 655f, 658f, 664f
  right thoracolumbar, 651f
 Larsen syndrome and, 242–243, 266
 leg-length discrepancy in, 636–636, 636f

level of paraplegia and, 512f
lumbar
 leg-length discrepancy and, 67f
 progressive, 515–517f
Marfan syndrome and, 179
maturity of child and, 631–632
metatropic dysplasia and, 215
myelomeningocele and, 512–518
neurofibromatosis and, 258, 258–259f
nonstructural, 635–636, 636f
oblique pelvis with, 852f
osteogenesis imperfecta and, 170
patient evaluation in, 625–633
patient positioning for radiography in, 627–629, 628–629f
poliomyelitis and, 568–570, 570f
postural, 635
Prader-Willi syndrome and, 286
right thoracic prominence in, 626f
Scheuermann disease and, 696
spasm, 732–733f, 733
spondyloepiphyseal dysplasia congenita and, 226
spondylolisthesis and, 730–733, 732–733f
spondylolysis/spondylolisthesis and, 720
structural, 636–679
treatment by posterior spinal fusion, 478f
Scurvy, 177–178, 178f
 periosteal reaction and, 175t
SED. See Spondyloepiphyseal dysplasia
Selective posterior rhizotomy, spastic diplegia and, 486–487
SEMD. See Spondylepimetaphyseal dysplasia
Septic arthritis. See Arthritis, septic
Seronegative spondyloarthropathies. See Spondyloarthropathies, seronegative
Serpentine foot, 1081
Sever disease, 1120
Sex chromosomes, abnormalities of, 122
Sex-linked muscular dystrophy, 540–549
Sex steroids, growth and, 187–188
Shelf arthroplasty, Legg-Calve-Perthes syndrome and, 982
Shelf augmentation, multiple epiphyseal dysplasia and, 234
Shin pain, young athlete and, 1192–1194
Shoe lift, leg-length discrepancy and, 876
Short-limb dwarfism, 125, 205–213
Shoulder
 cerebral palsy and, 495
 dislocation of, 1238
 fractures of, 1236–1242
 juvenile rheumatoid arthritis and, 419
 motion of, assessment of, 70f
 pediatric orthopaedic examination and, 68–72
 poliomyelitis and, 567–568
 renal osteodystrophic changes in, 156f
Shoulder arthrography, 31–32
Shoulder disarticulation prosthesis, 1175f, 1177f
Sickle cell crisis, 349
Sickle cell disease, 347–353, 348f, 350f, 352f
 bone and joint infection and, 607–609
 femoral head osteonecrosis in, 351, 351t
 humeral head osteonecrosis in, 351–352, 352t
 osteomyelitis and, 349–350, 349f
Sickle cell osteomyelitis, 607–609, 608f

Sillence classification, 166
Single-gene disorders, 122–130
    autosomal dominant, 123–126
    autosomal recessive, 126–127
    genomic imprinting in, 130
    X-linked, 127–129
Single-photon emission computed tomography (SPECT), 36
    spine and, 36f
Sirenomelia, 7
Skeletal age
    estimating, 867–868, 868f
    length of leg as function of, 852t, 853–854f
Skeletal dysplasia. See Osteochondrodysplasias
Skeletal imaging, suspected child abuse and, 38–39, 38f
Skeletal traction, femoral shaft fracture and, 1281
Skeletogenesis, 9–17
Skeleton, development of, factors influencing, 137–141
Skewfoot, 1081–1083, 1083f, 1084f
    calcaneal lengthening and, 1089
Skin, pediatric orthopaedic examination and, 65
Skin lesions, child abuse and, 1317–1318, 1318f
Slip angle, spondylolisthesis and, 722–723, 723f
Slipped capital femoral epiphysis (SCFE), 993–1019
    clinical presentation of, 996–998, 997–998f
    complications of, 1017–1019, 1018f
    early displacement of, 994f
    epidemiology of, 993–994
    etiology of, 994–996
    in situ fixation in, 1004–1007f
    multiple pin fixation in, 1008f
    natural history of, 1000–1002
    pathoanatomy of, 994, 994–995f
    pinning of contralateral hip in, 1017
    preventing further slippage in, 1002–1009
    radiographic features in, 998–1000, 999–1001f
    reducing degree of slippage in, 1009–1015
    salvage procedures in, 1015–1017, 1016f
    treatment of, 1002–1017
Slip percentage, spondylolisthesis and, 722
Slow-acting remittive drugs (SARDs), juvenile rheumatoid arthritis and, 408
Sly syndrome, 127
SMED. See Spondylometepiphyseal dysplasia
Soft tissue
    disorders of, localized, 305–341
    tumors of. See Tumors, soft tissue
Soft tissue calcification, 178–179
Soft tissue contracture
    Emery-Dreifuss muscular dystrophy and, 549
    poliomyelitis and, 566
    spinal muscular atrophy and, 557
Soft tissue hemorrhage, hemophilia and, 377–378, 378f
Soft tissue release, juvenile rheumatoid arthritis and, 411–412
Somatic mosaicism, 129
Somatomedin C, postnatal skeletal bone maturation and, 952

Somatomedins, growth plate and, 140
Somites, differentiation of, 8–9
Spasm scoliosis, 732–733f, 733
Spastic cerebral palsy, 470
Spastic diplegia, management of, 482–493
Spastic hemiplegia, management of, 493–494
Spastic hemiplegic hand, 496f
Spasticity, joint motion and, 62
Spastic quadriplegia
    hip dislocation in, 480f, 481
    management of, 473–482
SPECT. See Single-photon emission computed tomography
Spica cast
    developmental coxa vara and, 1028–1029
    femoral shaft fracture and, 1279–1281
    slipped capital femoral epiphysis and, 1002–1003
Spike osteotomy, tibia vara and, 1057
Spina bifida, 744
    craniofacial syndromes and, 760
Spina bifida aperta, 503
Spina bifida occulta, 11f, 504
Spinal cord, caudal end of, 13f
Spinal cord injury without radiographic abnormality (SCIWORA), 767
Spinal deformity, spinal muscular atrophy and, 557
Spinal dysraphia, 503
Spinal injury
    child abuse and, 1322–1323, 1326f
    young athlete and, 1208
Spinal instrumentation
    adolescent idiopathic scoliosis and, 661–663
    Down syndrome patient and, 757
    Drummond system of, 663f
Spinal muscular atrophy, 555–558, 559f
Spinal stabilization, Emery-Dreifuss muscular dystrophy and, 549
Spinal stenosis, achondroplasia and, 209–210
Spine
    aneurysmal bone cyst of, 451
    cervical. See Cervical spine
    chondrodysplasia punctata and, 236–237
    congenital defects of, Larsen syndrome and, 243
    curvatures of, 688f
    deformity of. See also specific deformity
        adult sequelae of untreated, 633–635, 634–635f
        myelomeningocele and, 511–520
    development of, 9–13
    disorders resulting in kyphosis, 689t
    Goldenhar syndrome and, 289
    imaging of, 36f
    infection of, 601–603
    juvenile osteoporosis and, 171f
    kyphosis. See Kyphosis
    leg-length discrepancy and, 851–853, 852f, 852t
    lumbar. See Lumbar spine
    neurofibromatosis and, 258–259, 258–259f
    pediatric orthopaedic examination and, 65–68
    physical examination of, 626–627
    scoliosis. See Scoliosis
    thoracic, kyphotic deformity of, 688f
    tuberculosis of, 617
Splenomegaly, Gaucher disease and, 359

Split hand, 797
Spondylepimetaphyseal dysplasia (SEMD), 224
Spondyloarthropathies, seronegative, 397–398
    differential diagnosis of, 401–404, 402t
    etiology of, 398–399
    idiopathic chondrolysis of hip and, 1038
    management of, 407–409
    orthopaedic surgery in, 419–420
    pathology of, 399–401
    radiology of, 399–401, 400–401f
Spondyloepiphyseal dysplasia (SED), 1061f
    autosomal dominance and, 125
    mRNA splicing mutation in, 120
Spondyloepiphyseal dysplasia congenita, 224–227, 225–227f
    kyphotic deformity and, 708
Spondyloepiphyseal dysplasia tarda (SED tarda), 227–229, 228f
Spondylolisthesis, 717–735
    of C2, 765
    cerebral palsy and, 477
    classification of, 717
    degenerative, 717
    Down syndrome and, 272
    dysplastic, 717, 718f
    dysplastic and isthmic compared, 719t
    etiology of, 719–720
    isthmic, 717, 718f
    lumbar spine and, 68f
    measurement of, 723f
    natural history of, 719
    pathologic, 717
    patient evaluation in, 720–723
    scoliosis and, 730–733, 732–733f
    traumatic, 717
    treatment of, 725–735, 728–729f, 731–734f
    typical findings of, 721f
Spondylolysis, 717–735, 724–725f
    cerebral palsy and, 477
    etiology of, 719–720
    natural history of, 719
    patient evaluation in, 720–723
    Scheuermann disease and, 696
    treatment of, 723–725, 726–727f
Spondylometepiphyseal dysplasia (SMED), 224
Sports medicine, 1181–1221
    atlantoaxial instability and, 757
    care of young athlete in, 1181–1185
    instrumented motion analysis and, 95
    overuse syndromes and, 1185–1197
    patellofemoral disorders and, 1208–1221
Sports trauma, 1197–1208
Sprains
    ankle, 1199–1201
    tibiofibular, distal, 1201–1202
Sprengel deformity, 71
    Diamond-Blackfan anemia and, 346
    Fanconi anemia and, 347
S-shaped foot, 1081
Stance phase, of gait, 98t
    ankle and, 100–103
    hip and, 103–104
    knee and, 103
Stature
    cartilage-hair hypoplasia and, 357
    Down syndrome and, 274
    normal variant short, 184–185
    Prader-Willi syndrome and, 286
    Scheuermann disease and, 695

Sternoclavicular separation, 1236f
Sternocleidomastoid muscle, congenital muscular torticollis and, 752–753
Steroids
　juvenile rheumatoid arthritis and, 409
　progressive diaphyseal dysplasia and, 319
Sterols, calcium transport system and, 142–143
Stickler syndrome, 125, 287–288
Storage diseases, 127
Strawberry hemangioma, 307
Street syndrome, 1138
Strength training, young athlete and, 1184
Streptomycin
　extrapulmonary tuberculosis and, 619
　spinal tuberculosis and, 709
Stress fracture, 1185–1187
　proximal and middle tibia and, 1069–1070
Stride, analysis of, 113–114
Stroke, sickle cell disease and, 352
Stulberg classification, 968–969, 968t
Sturge-Weber syndrome, 307–308
Subluxation, atlantoaxial rotary, 748–751, 749–751f
Subtalar arthrodesis, 490, 490f
Subungual exostosis, 1131
Sulfasalizine, juvenile rheumatoid arthritis and, 408
Sulindac, juvenile rheumatoid arthritis and, 408t
Supination, 1078t
　evaluation of, 72f
　of foot, 85f
　　effect on ankle motion, 88f
Supination-inversion ankle fracture, 1300, 1301f
Supracondylar fracture, 831–832, 833f, 1242–1247
　fracture line in, 1244f
　type II, 1245f
　type III, 1246–1247f
Surgery
　adolescent idiopathic scoliosis and, 652–666
　bone and joint infection and, 599–601, 600f
　cavus and, 1122–1123
　congenital clubfoot and, 1108–1116
　congenital scoliosis and, 673–679
　developmental coxa vara and, 1029–1030
　Duchenne muscular dystrophy and, 544–546
　flexible flatfoot and, 1088–1089
　Friedreich ataxia and, 560–561
　hallux valgus and, 1118–1119
　idiopathic chondrolysis of hip and, 1043
　idiopathic toe walking and, 1127
　Legg-Calve-Perthes syndrome and, 980–982
　metatarsus adductus and, 1081
　rotational abnormalities and, 1051–1052
　Scheuermann disease and, 699
　spinal muscular atrophy and, 558
　spondylolisthesis and, 725–730
　spondylolysis and, 724–725, 727f
　tarsal coalition and, 1098–1099
　tibial fractures and, 1296
Sutalar motion, evaluating, 86, 86f
Swing phase, of gait, 99, 100t
　ankle and, 103
　　hip and, 104
　　knee and, 103
Symbrachydactyly, 797–798
Syme amputation
　complete tibial hemimelia and, 1156–1157
　fibular deficiency and, 1154f
　proximal focal femoral deficiency and, 1146–1147, 1146f, 1171
Symphalangism, 802
　diastrophic dysplasia and, 219
Syndactyly, 15, 805–808, 805–808f
　cleft hand and, 798
　complex, 802
　Fanconi anemia and, 347
Synostosis
　carpal, 802f
　radioulnar, 803f
　type 1, 802f
　upper extremity, 801–804, 802–804f
Synovectomy
　hemophilia and, 376–377
　juvenile rheumatoid arthritis and, 410–411
Synovial biopsy, juvenile rheumatoid arthritis and, 406–407
Synovial cell sarcoma, 460–461, 460f
Synovial chondromatosis, 461, 461f
Synovial fluid analysis, 588t
Synovial joints, development of, 16–17
Synovial tumors, 461–462
Synovitis
　foreign body, differential diagnosis of, 403
　hemophilia and, 375–377
　pigmented villonodular, 461–462
　　differential diagnosis of, 403
　　idiopathic chondrolysis of hip and, 1038
　　slipped capital femoral epiphysis and, 995
　toxic
　　septic arthritis and, 595
　　synovial fluid analysis in, 588t
　toxic of hip, differential diagnosis of, 403
　transient
　　of hip, 1033–1037, 1035f
　　Legg-Calve-Perthes syndrome and, 953
Syphilis
　congenital, periosteal reaction and, 174t
　teratogenicity and, 132
Systemic lupus erythematosus, differential diagnosis of, 402

T

Tache cerebrale, reflex sympathetic dystrophy and, 339
Tailor bunionette, 1119
Talipes equinovarus
　bilateral, congenital scoliosis and, 672f
　congenital, 1103–1116, 1105–1106f
　myelomeningocele and, 527–529
Talocalcaneal coalition, 1095–1096, 1095f
Talus fractures, 1303–1307, 1306f
TAR. See Total absence of radius
Tarsal coalition, 1093–1099, 1095f
Tarsal-metatarsal displacement, 1309f
Tarsal-metatarsal joint injury, 1309f
Tarsoepiphyseal aclasia, 331
T-condylar fracture, 1247, 1248f
Technetium scan, bone and soft tissue tumors and, 427–428

Telangiectasia, hereditary, 308
Teleoradiography, 865, 865f
Tendelenburg gait, Legg-Calve-Perthes syndrome and, 983
Tendinitis
　Achilles, 1191–1192
　popliteus, 1192, 1192f
Tendinoses, young athlete and, 1191–1192
Tendon transfer
　hereditary motor sensory neuropathies and, 563
　poliomyelitis and, 567
Teratogenic agents, 131–132
Teratologic disorders, 131–132
Terminal deficit, 1137
Testosterone
　bone formation and, 140
　slipped capital femoral epiphysis and, 996
Tethered cord syndrome
　myelomeningocele and, 508–509
　scoliosis and, 513
Tetraplegia, 471
Thalassemia, 353–354, 354f
Thalidomide
　limb anomalies and, 1138
　phocomelia and, 9, 783, 796
　proximal focal femoral deficiency and, 1142
　teratogenicity and, 132
Thigh-foot angle, measurement of, 1049, 1049f
Thomas test, 76–77, 77f
Thoracic curves, curve patterns of, 653t
Thoracic kyphosis, 694–699, 695f
　secondary to Scheuermann disease, 700f
Thoracic level paraplegia, 511, 522–523
　scoliosis and, 512
Thoracic lordosis, 67f
Thoracic spine, kyphotic deformity of, 688f
Thoracolumbar kyphosis, achondroplasia and, 210–211
Thoracolumbarsacral orthosis (TLSO), 648–652, 649f, 664f, 724
Thoracoplasty, adolescent idiopathic scoliosis and, 666–667
Thrombin, formation of, 370f
Thrombocytopenia with absent radius (TAR) syndrome, 370–371
　skeletal deficiency in, 370t
Thumb
　congenital deficiency of, radial deficiencies and, 789t
　duplicate, 815–817, 816–817f
　triphalangeal, 817–819, 818f
Thumb-in-palm deformity, repertoire of operations for, 496f
Thyroid hormones
　bone formation and, 140
　slipped capital femoral epiphysis and, 996
Tibia
　body deformity of, 84f
　chondromyxofibroma of, 442f
　classic high-grade osteosarcoma of, 436f
　congenital pseudoarthrosis of, 322–329, 323f, 329f
　　classification of treatment of, 323t
　　options for treatment of, 325f, 325t
　cortical bone in, 582f

disorders of, 1069–1071
distal, growth arrest in, 1234f
fracture of, 1293–1300
  child abuse and, 1326f, 1327f
  high-energy, 1297f
  mid-diaphyseal, 1300f
  myelomeningocele and, 532–533
hematogenous osteomyelitis in, 586f
infection in, 585f
osteosarcoma of, imaging of, 35f, 45f
posteromedial bowing of, 1070–1071, 1070f
progressive diaphyseal dysplasia and, 318f
proximal, fibrocartilaginous dysplasia of, 1059–1060
stress fracture of, 1069–1070
toddler's fracture of, 1069, 1069f
trabecular bone in, 584f
Tibial deficiency, 1154–1157
  prosthetics for, 1172
Tibial derotation osteotomy, rotational abnormalities and, 1052
Tibial diaphyseal fracture, 1295
Tibial eminence avulsion, 1289–1290, 1290f
Tibial epiphysis, proximal, fracture of, 1293–1294, 1294f
Tibial hemimelia
  bilateral complete, 1156f
  classification of, 1156f
  complete, 1158f
  right, 1158f
  type II partial, 1157f
Tibial metaphysis, proximal, fracture of, 1294–1295, 1295f
Tibial physeal injury, distal, 1303f
Tibial rotation osteotomy, rotational abnormalities and, 1052
Tibial torsion
  external, spastic diplegia and, 491
  measuring, 1049, 1049f
  unilateral external, 1053f
Tibial tubercle avulsion, 1292–1293, 1293f
  classification of, 1292f
Tibial valgus, posttraumatic, 1060–1061, 1060f
Tibial valgus deformity, traumatic, 1295f
Tibia vara, 1055–1057, 1056f–1057f
Tibiofibular sprains, distal, 1201–1202
Tillaux fracture, 1303, 1304f
Tissue fatigue, cyclic loading of tissues and, 1186f
TJA. See Total joint arthroplasty
TLSO. See Thoracolumbarsacral orthosis
Toddler's fracture, 1296–1298
Toenails, ingrown, 1129–1131
Toe walking, idiopathic, 1071–1072, 1127
Tolmetin sodium
  juvenile rheumatoid arthritis and, 408t
  young athlete and, 1185
Tomography
  computed. See Computed tomography
  directional, 30
  linear, bone and soft tissue tumors and, 428
Tonic neck reflex, 56–57
  asymmetrical, 57f, 58
  symmetrical, 58, 59f
Tonsillectomy, Grisel syndrome and, 751
Torsional profile, 77, 78f
Torticollis, 744, 746f, 747f
  cervical cord tumors and, 754
  muscular, congenital, 751–754

ocular dysfunction and, 754
paroxysmal of infancy, 754
posterior fossa tumors and, 754
presenting position of, 66f
rotary displacement of, 749
Sandifer syndrome and, 754–755
Z-plasty procedure for, 753f
Total absence of radius (TAR), 788, 789f
Total joint arthroplasty (TJA), juvenile rheumatoid arthritis and, 413
Toxic synovitis
  of hip, differential diagnosis of, 403
  septic arthritis and, 595
  synovial fluid analysis in, 588t
Trabecular bone, 584f
  rickets and, 148f
Traction
  bilateral hip dislocation and, 926f
  femoral shaft fracture and, 1281
Transcription, RNA processing and, 118
Transient quadriparesis, cervical spine and, 767–769
Transient synovitis
  of hip, 1033–1037, 1035f
  Legg-Calve-Perthes syndrome and, 953
Transitional fracture, 1302–1303, 1304f
Transmalleolar-axis, measurement of, 1049
Transtrochanteric rotational osteotomy, slipped capital femoral epiphysis and, 1012
Transverse arrest, 784–796, 785f
Transverse atlantoaxial ligament, ruptures of, 765
Transverse defect, 1137
Trauma
  cervical spine and, 763–770, 768f
    positioning with backboard and, 764f
  growth of leg and, 858–860
  kyphotic deformity and, 709
  Legg-Calve-Perthes syndrome and, 953
  osteomyelitis and, 587, 594
  pediatric hand and, 828–840
  quadriceps contracture and, 339
  septic arthritis and, 587
  slipped capital femoral epiphysis and, 995
  spondylolisthesis and, 720
  spondylolysis and, 720
  sports, 1197–1208
  tibial valgus and, 1060–1061, 1060f
Traumatic spondylolisthesis, 717
Trendelenburg lurch, 1174
Trendelenburg test, 79, 79f
Trevor disease, 331
Trichorhinophalangeal syndrome, 290–291, 290f
Trigger digit, 810–811, 811f
Trilaminar disc, 7–8
  formation of, 8f
Triphalangeal thumb, 817–819, 818f
Triplane fracture, 1303, 1304f–1305f
Triple arthrodesis, hereditary motor sensory neuropathies and, 563–564
Triradiate cartilage, 904–905, 906f
Trisomy, 121
Trisomy 13, trigger digit and, 811
Trisomy 17, radial deficiencies and, 789
Trisomy 21, Down syndrome and, 271
Trisomy X, 122
Tuberculosis
  cervical spine and, 772–773
  extrapulmonary, 616–619, 617–618f
  kyphotic deformity and, 709

Tuberculous arthritis, idiopathic chondrolysis of hip and, 1038
Tuberculous dactylitis, 618
Tuberculous spondylitis, 619
Tumoral calcinosis, 178
Tumors
  bone, 423–463
    biopsy of, 431–433
    chemotherapy for, 462–463
    classification of, 424
    evaluation of, 424–433
    giant cell, 451–453, 452f
    surgical sites/surgical stages, 431t
  bone-forming, 433–439
  cartilaginous, 439–444
  cervical spine, 773–774
    benign, 773–774
    malignant, 774
  growth of leg and, 861–862
  malignant, somatic mosaicism and, 129
  musculoskeletal, chemotherapy for, 462–463
  origins of, 423–424
  soft tissue, 454–463
    benign of nerve origin, 457–458, 457f
    biopsy of, 431–433
    chemotherapy for, 462–463
    classification of, 424
    evaluation of, 424–433
    staging for, 430–431, 430t
    surgical sites/surgical stages, 431t
  synovial, 461–462
Turco procedure, congenital clubfoot and, 1109–1110
Turner syndrome, 122, 186, 188, 284–285
  differential diagnosis of, 311t
  hemihypotrophy and, 313

U

Ulna
  Caffey disease and, 177f
  complete absence of, 800f
  fractures of, 1253–1257
  hypoplasia of, 799f
  partial absence of, 799f
Ulnar clubhand, 798–801, 799–800f
Ulnar deficiency, 798–801, 799–800f
Ultrasonography, 25, 39–43
  biologic effect of, 27
  bone and joint infection and, 593
  developmental dysplasia of hip and, 913–914
  femoral/tibial rotation and, 1050
  prenatal diagnosis and, 134
  slipped capital femoral epiphysis and, 999
Unicameral bone cysts, 448–450, 449f
Uniparental disomy, 130
Upper extremity, 781–840
  amputation, 1164
  arthrogryposis, 808–810, 809–810f
  camptodactyly, 811–813, 812f
  central polydactyly, 819, 819f
  cerebral palsy and, 494–497
  clinodactyly, 813–814, 813f
  congenital constriction band syndrome, 822–825, 823–824f
  delta phalanx, 814–815, 814f
  duplicate thumbs, 815–817, 816–817f
  duplication of, 815–821
  failure of differentiation of parts, 801–815
  failure of formation of parts, 783–801

Upper extremity (continued)
  hereditary motor sensory neuropathies and, 564–565
  longitudinal deficiencies in, 785f, 796–801
  macrodactyly, 821–822, 822f
  Madelung deformity, 825–826, 825f
  malformations of
    classification of, 783, 784t
    incidence of, 782–783
    inheritance of, 783
  multiple epiphyseal dysplasia and, 232
  neurofibromatosis and, 258f
  obstetric brachial plexus injury, 826–828
  pediatric orthopaedic examination and, 68–72
  poliomyelitis and, 567–568
  postaxial polydactyly, 819–821, 820f
  prosthetics for, 1174–1177, 1175–1177f
  syndactyly, 805–808, 805–808f
  synostosis, 801–804, 802–804f
  transverse arrest in, 784–796, 785f
  trigger digit, 810–811, 811f
  triphalangeal thumb, 817–819, 818f
Urethritis, Reiter syndrome and, 398

V

VACTER association, 13
VACTERLS, 288
Valgus deformity, myelomeningocele and, 530
Valgus hindfoot, calcaneal lengthening and, 1089
Vancomycin, bone and joint infection and, 597t
van der Hoeve disease, 165
Varus osteotomy, Legg-Calve-Perthes syndrome and, 981–982
VATER syndrome, radial deficiencies and, 789
Verrucous hemangioma, 307
Vertebra
  C1, unilateral absence of, 747–748, 747f
  C1-C2, fractures and ligamentous injuries of, 764–765
  C2, spondylolisthesis of, 765
  C3-C7, fractures and ligamentous injuries of, 765–767
  cervical
    embryology of, 740
    growth and development of, 740–741
  hypoplasia and aplasia of, common patterns of, 691f
  morphogenesis of, 12f
  osteopetrosis and, 173f
Vertebral arch, formation of, 11f
Vertebral body
  formation of, 11f
  hemangioma of, 456f
Vertical talus, congenital, 1089–1093, 1090–1091f
Vinblastine, Langerhans cell histiocytosis and, 367–368
Vincristine, musculoskeletal tumors and, 462
Vitamin C deficiency. See Scurvy
Vitamin D
  calcium transport and, 142
  calcium transport by gut cell and, 143f
  conversion in kidney, 143, 144f
  conversion in liver, 144f
  hypercalcemia and, 162
  metaphyseal chondrodysplasia and, 239
  physiology of, 140
  rickets and, 150
Vitamin D deficiency. See Rickets
Vitamin D-resistant rickets, 152–153
  mechanism of development of, 152f
Voluntary-opening hook terminal device, 1176f
Von Hippel-Lindau disease, 308
von Recklinghausen disease, 256
  neurofibroma and, 457
Vrolik disease, 164–165

W

Wagner lengthening device, 882, 882–884f
Warfarin, teratogenicity and, 132
Weight control, achondroplastic dwarfs and, 207
Weight lifting, young athlete and, 1184
Werdnig-Hoffman disease
  type I, acute, 556
  type II, chronic, 556
Wheelchair
  Duchenne muscular dystrophy and, 546
  spastic diplegia management and, 474–475, 475f
Whip, prostheses and, 1173
Wilmington brace, 651
Wilms tumor, hemihypertrophy and, 312–313
Wilson test, 82
Wolff's law, 140–141, 164, 695
Wounds
  gunshot, cervical spine and, 769–770
  puncture, of foot, 612–615, 614f
Wrist
  cerebral palsy and, 495–496
  disuse atrophy of, 172f
  fractures of, 1257–1268
  juvenile rheumatoid arthritis and, 418–419, 418–419f
  landmarks in, 868f
  pediatric orthopaedic examination and, 72–73
Wry neck, congenital, 751

X

X chromosome
  single-gene defects and, 122
  uniparental disomy and, 130
X-linked agammaglobulinemia, 356–357
X-linked disorders, 127–129
  atypical, 128–129
  dominant, 128
  recessive, 128
X-linked recessive pedigree, 127f

Y

Y chromosome, uniparental disomy and, 130

Z

Z-foot deformity, 1081
Zinacef. See Cefuroxime
Zone of Ranvier, 21f
Zygote, 1